Reproductive Endocrinology and Infertility

Douglas T. Carrell · C. Matthew Peterson
Editors

Reproductive Endocrinology and Infertility

Integrating Modern Clinical and Laboratory Practice

Springer

Editors
Douglas T. Carrell, PhD, H.C.L.D.
Professor of Surgery (Urology),
Obstetrics and Gynecology and Physiology
University of Utah School of Medicine
Director of IVF and Andrology Laboratories
Salt Lake City, Utah 84132, US
douglas.carrell@hsc.utah.edu

C. Matthew Peterson, MD
John A. Dixon Presidential Professor and Chair
Department of Obstetrics and Gynecology
University of Utah School of Medicine
Practice Director
Utah Center for Reproductive Medicine
Salt Lake City, UT
c.matthew.peterson@hsc.utah.edu

ISBN 978-1-4419-1435-4 ISBN 978-1-4419-1436-1 (eBook)
DOI 10.1007/978-1-4419-1436-1

Springer New York Dordrecht Heidelberg London

Library of Congress Control Number: 2010922889

Printed on acid-free paper

Springer is part of Springer Science+Business Media (www.springer.com)

We dedicate this book to our mentors, students, residents, and fellows who have continually refreshed our excitement for reproductive medicine as we learn with them, and to our families who have sacrificed much to assist us in our professions.

Preface

More than 30 years after the birth of Louise Brown, the first child born as a result of in vitro fertilization, the practice of reproductive medicine has grown and evolved in a dramatic and profound fashion. Classical reproductive endocrinology and surgery remain important components of clinical practice, but they are joined with major developments in the laboratory and clinic that have opened the doors of therapy to millions. Furthermore, the outlook for the future is stunning, including novel technologies that may facilitate quantum advances in the clinic and laboratory.

The advances made in the treatment of infertility have made the care of infertile patients more successful, rewarding, and exciting. However, management of the modern reproductive endocrinology and infertility clinic has become very complex. In addition to the medical and scientific knowledge necessary to manage a clinic and laboratory, the modern director must have an understanding of such disparate fields as marketing, accounting, management, and regulatory issues. It is impractical to obtain such a broad range of experience during a doctoral or fellowship program and difficult to follow the advances of each field through traditional methods. This book was developed to assist the practicing reproductive endocrinologist and/or laboratory director by providing an overview of relevant scientific, medical, and management issues in a single volume. While no book can cover everything associated with managing a reproductive endocrinology clinic and laboratory, we have enlisted experts from all relevant areas to provide concise, practical, and evidence based summaries of relevant topics. It is our hope that this resource will be of assistance to physicians and scientists engaged in this exciting field of medicine.

Salt Lake City, UT Douglas T. Carrell, Ph.D., H.C.L.D
Salt Lake City, UT C. Matthew Peterson, M.D

Preface

Contents

Contributors

Jose R. Alagretti, BS
Huntington Center for Reproductive medicine of Brazil, Sao Paulo, Brazil

Joseph P. Alukal, MD
Scott Department of Urology, Baylor College of Medicine, Houston, TX, USA

Vincent W. Aoki, PhD
Eastside Fertility Laboratory, Bellevue, WA, USA

Kenneth I. Aston, PhD
Department of Urology, University of Utah School of Medicine, Salt Lake City, UT, USA

Barry Behr, PhD
Department of Obstetrics & Gynecology, Stanford University, Palo Alto, CA, USA

Lars Bjorndahl, MD, PhD
Center for Andrology and Sexual Medicine, Endocrinology Clinic Karolinska University Hospital, Huddinge and Department of Medicine, Huddinge, Karol inska Institutet, Stockholm, Sweden

Attila Bokor, MD
Leuven University Fertility Center, UZ Gasthuisberg, K.U.Leuven, Belgium

Carolyn A. Bondy, MD
Developmental Endocrinology Branch, National Institute of Child Health and Human Development, National Institutes of Health, Bethesda, MD, USA

Charles L. Bormann, PhD
Departments of Obstetrics and Gynecology and Urology, University of Michigan, Ann Arbor, MI, USA

D. Ware Branch, MD
Division of Maternal Fetal Medicine, Department of Obstetrics and Gynecology, University of Utah School of Medicine, Salt Lake City, UT, USA

Mats Brännström, MD, PhD
Department of Obstetrics and Gynecology, Sahlgrenska Academy at Göteborg University, Göteborg, Sweden

Douglas T. Carrell, PhD
Departments of Surgery (Urology), Obstetrics and Gynecology, and Physiology, University of Utah School of Medicine, Salt Lake City, Utah 84132, US

Grace M. Centola, PhD
LifeCell DX, Inc., Buffalo, NY, USA
New England Cryogenic Center, Newton, MA, USA

Ri-Cheng Chain, PhD
Department of Obstetrics and Gynecology, Royal Victoria Hospital Women's Pavilion, McGill University, Montreal, QC, Canada

Greg L. Christensen, PhD
The Fertility Center at University Women's Healthcare, University of Louisville, Louisville, KY, USA

Mary Croughan, PhD
Departments of Obstetrics, Gynecology, Reproductive Sciences, and Epidemiology and Biostatistics, University of California, San Francisco, CA, USA

Pernilla Dahm-Kähler, MD, PhD
Department of Obstetrics and Gynecology, Sahlgrenska Academy at Göteborg University, Göteborg, Sweden

Eduardo L.A. da Motta, MD
Huntington Center for Reproductive Medicine of Brazil, Sao Paulo, Brazil

Joy Delhanty, PhD
UCL Center for Obstetrics & Gynecology, University College London, Gower Street, London, England

Ezgi Demirtas, MD
Department of Obstetrics and Gynecology, Royal Victoria Hospital Women's Pavilion, McGill University, Montreal, QC, Canadá

Thomas M. D'Hooghe, MD, PhD
Leuven University Fertility Center, UZ Gasthuisberg, K.U. Leuven, Belgium

Jessie Dorais, MD
Department of Obstetrics and Gynecology, University of Utah School of Medicine, Salt Lake City, UT, USA

Kenneth C. Drury, PhD
Department of Obstetrics and Gynecology, University of Florida College of Medicine, Gainesville, FL, USA

Tonya Edvalson
Department of Obstetrics and Gynecology, University of Utah School of Medicine, Salt Lake City, UT, USA

Hasan M. El-Fakahanya, MD
Department of Obstetrics, Gynecology and Reproductive Sciences, Yale University School of Medicine, New Haven, CT, USA

Benjamin R. Emery, MPhil
Department of Urology, Andrology & IVF Laboratories, University of Utah School of Medicine, Salt Lake City, UT, USA

Enrico Ferrazzi, MD
Department of Obstetrics and Gynecology, Sacco Clinical Sciences Institute, University of Milan Medical School, Milan, Italy

Mark Gibson, MD
Department of Obstetrics & Gynecology, University Center for Reproductive Medicine, University of Utah School of Medicine, Salt Lake City, UT, USA

Antonia V. Gilligan
Alpha Environmental, Inc. Emerson, NJ, USA

Shawn Gurtcheff, MD
Department of Obstetrics & Gynecology, Utah Center for Reproductive Medicine, University of Utah School of Medicine, Salt Lake City, UT, USA

Ahmad O. Hammoud, MD
Department of Obstetrics & Gynecology, Utah Center for Reproductive Medicine, University of Utah School of Medicine, Salt Lake City, UT, USA

Harry H. Hatasaka, MD
Department of Obstetrics & Gynecology, Utah Center for Reproductive Medicine, University of Utah School of Medicine, Salt Lake City, UT, USA

Louis Hermo, PhD
Departments of Anatomy & Cell Biology, McGill University, Montreal, QC, Canada

Cara Heuser, MD
Division of Maternal Fetal Medicine, Department of Obstetrics and Gynecology, University of Utah School of Medicine, Salt Lake City, UT, USA

Emily Hixson, MBA
Department of Obstetrics and Gynecology, University of Utah School of Medicine, Salt Lake City, UT, USA

Hananel Holzer, MD, BSc
Department of Obstetrics and Gynecology, Royal Victoria Hospital Women's Pavilion, McGill University, Montreal, QC, Canada

Maj Hultén, MD, PhD
Warwick Medical School, University of Warwick, Coventry, England

Katharine V. Jackson, BS, ELD
Department of Obstetrics, Gynecology and Reproductive Biology, Brigham and Women's Hospital, Harvard Medical School, Boston, MA, USA

Kirtly Parker Jones, MD
Department of Obstetrics & Gynecology, Utah Center for Reproductive Medicine, University of Utah School of Medicine, Salt Lake City, UT, USA

Brooks A. Keel, PhD
Departments of Biological Sciences and Research and Economic Development, Louisiana State University, Baton Rouge, LA, USA

Anne Kennedy, MD
Department of Radiology, Health Sciences Center, University of Utah, Salt Lake City, UT, USA

William R. Keye, MD
Department of Obstetrics and Gynecology, Utah Center for Reproductive Medicine, University of Utah School of Medicine, Salt Lake City, UT, USA

Lisa Kolp, MD
Department of Obstetrics and Gynecology, Johns Hopkins Medicine, Johns Hopkins at Green Spring Station, Lutherville, MD, USA

Csilla Krausz, MD, PhD
Andrology Unit, Department of Clinical Physipathology, University of Florence, Florence, Italy

Maria Lalioti, MD
Department of Obstetrics, Gynecology and Reproductive Sciences, Yale University School of Medicine, New Haven, CT, USA

Dolores J. Lamb, PhD
Scott Department of Urology, Baylor College of Medicine, Houston, TX, USA

Wendy D. Latash, PhD
Jade Tree Solutions, LLC, Northbrook, IL, USA

Richard S. Legro, MD
Department of Obstetrics and Gynecology, Penn State College of Medicine, M.S. Hershey Medical Center, Hershey, PA, USA

Anna Karin Lind, MD, PhD
Department of Obstetrics and Gynecology, Sahlgrenska Academy at Göteborg University, Göteborg, Sweden

Erika Lindley, MBA
Department of Obstetrics & Gynecology, University of Utah School of Medicine, Salt Lake City, UT, USA

Germaine Buck Louis, PhD, MS
Epidemiology Branch, Division of Epidemiology, Statistics, and Prevention Research, Eunice Kennedy Shriver National Institute of Child Health and Human Development, Bethesda, MD, USA

Lindsay Mains, MD
Department of Obstetrics and Gynecology, University of Iowa, Iowa City, IA, USA

Renée Halo Martin, PhD
Department of Medical Genetics, University of Calgary, Calgary, AB, Canada

Christel Meuleman, MD
Department of Obstetrics and Gynecology, Leuven University Fertility Center, UZ Gasthuisberg, K.U. Leuven, Belgium

Ben W.J. Mol, MD, PhD
Center for Reproductive Medicine, Academic Medical Center, Amsterdam, The Netherlands

Donald G. Morrison, PhD
Anderson Graduate School of Management, University of California at Los Angeles, Los Angeles, CA, USA

Sergey I. Moskovtsev, MD, PhD
Andrology Laboratory, Department of Pathology and Laboratory Medicine, Mount Sinai Hospital, Toronto, ON, Canada

Brendan M. Mullen, MD
Andrology Laboratory, Department of Pathology and Laboratory Medicine, Mount Sinai Hospital, Toronto, ON, Canada

Mark A. Munger, PharmD
Department of Pharmacology, University of Utah College of Pharmacy, Salt Lake City, UT, USA

Kutluk Oktay, MD
Department of Obstetrics & Gynecology, New York Medical College-Westchester Medical Center, Valhalla, NY, USA
The Institute for Fertility Preservation, Center for Human Reproduction, New York, NY, USA

Ozgur Oktem, MD
Department of Obstetrics & Gynecology, New York Medical College-Westchester Medical Center, Valhalla, NY, USA
The Institute for Fertility Preservation, Center for Human Reproduction, New York, NY, USA

C. Matthew Peterson, MD
Department of Obstetrics & Gynecology, Utah Center for Reproductive Medicine,
University of Utah School of Medicine, Salt Lake City, UT, USA

Michael A. Poch, MD
Department of Urology, Brown University, Providence, RI, USA

Catherine Racowsky, PhD
Department of Obstetrics, Gynecology and Reproductive Biology, Brigham and Women's Hospital and Harvard Medical School Boston, MA, USA

Uma M. Reddy, MD, MPH
Pregnancy and Perinatology Branch, Department of Health and Human Services,
Eunice Kennedy Shriver National Institute of Child Health and Human Development,
NIH, Bethesda, MD, USA

Bernard Robaire, PhD
Department of Pharmacology & Therapeutics and Obstetrics & Gynecology,
McGill University, Montreal, QC, Canada

Denny Sakkas, PhD
Department of Obstetrics, Gynecology and Reproductive Sciences,
Yale University School of Medicine, New Haven, CT, USA

Valeria Savasi, MD, PhD
Department of Obstetrics and Gynecology, Sacco Clinical Sciences Institute,
University of Milan Medical School, Milan, Italy

Tammie K. Schalue, PhD
Birenbaum and Associates, St. Louis, MO, USA

Peter N. Schlegel, MD
Departments of Urology and Reproductive Medicine, Weill Medical College of Cornell University, New York, NY, USA

Lone Schmidt, MD, DMSci, PhD
Institute of Public Health, University of Copenhagen, Copenhagen, Denmark

David C. Schmittlein, PhD, MPH
Massachusetts Institute of Technology Sloan School of Management, Cambridge, MA, USA

Lynette Scott, PhD
Fertility Centers of New England, Reading, MA, USA

Emre Seli, MD
Department of Obstetrics, Gynecology and Reproductive Sciences,
Yale University School of Medicine, New Haven, CT, USA

Paulo Serafini, MD
Huntington Center for Reproductive Medicine of Brazil, Sao Paulo, Brazil

Mark Sigman, MD
Department of Urology, Brown University, Providence, RI, USA

Caroline Signore, MD, MPH
Pregnancy and Perinatology Branch, Department of Health and Human Services,
National Institute of Child Health and Human Development, NIH,
Bethesda, MD, USA

Howard T. Sharp, MD
Division of General Gynecology, Department of Obstetrics & Gynecology,
University of Utah School of Medicine, Salt Lake City, UT, USA

Yimin Shu, MD, PhD
Stanford Fertility and Reproductive Medicine Center, Palo Alto, CA, USA

Edward Smith, PhD
Department of Biological Sciences, University of Warwick, Coventry, England

Gary D. Smith, PhD
Departments of Obstetrics and Gynecology, Molecular and Integrative Physiology, Urology, and Reproductive Sciences Program, University of Michigan, Ann Arbor, MI, USA

Weon-Young Son, PhD
Department of Obstetrics and Gynecology, Royal Victoria Hospital Women's Pavilion, McGill University, Montreal, QC, Canadá

Joseph Stanford, MD, MPH
Department of Family and Preventive Medicine, University of Utah Health Sciences Center, Salt Lake City, UT, USA

Pieternel Steures, MD
Center for Reproductive Medicine, Academic Medical Center, Amsterdam, The Netherlands

Ashley J. Stevens, DPhil
Institute for Technology Entrepreneurship and Commercialization School of Management and Technology Transfer, Boston University, Boston, MA, USA

Peter Sutovsky, PhD
Animal Science and Clinical Obstetrics & Gynecology, Section Editor for Reproductive Biology, Cell & Tissue Research, University of Missouri-Columbia, Columbia, MO, USA

Seang Lin Tan, MD, MBBS, FRCOG, FRCSC, MMed (O&G), MBA
Department of Obstetrics and Gynecology, Royal Victoria Hospital Women's Pavilion, McGill University, Montreal, QC, Canada

Cigdem Tanrikut, MD
Massachusetts General Hospital Fertility Center, Massachusetts General Hospital, Boston, MA, USA

Helen Ghislaine Tempest, PhD
Department of Medical Genetics, University of Calgary, Calgary, AB, Canada

Paul J. Turek, MD
Department of Urology, University of California San Francisco, San Francisco, CA, USA

Laurence C. Udoff, MD
Department of Obstetrics, Gynecology and Reproductive Sciences, University of Maryland School of Medicine, Baltimore, MD, USA

Fulco van der Veen, MD, PhD
Center for Reproductive Medicine, Academic Medical Center, Amsterdam, The Netherlands

Bradley J. Van Voorhis, MD
Department of Obstetrics and Gynecology, University of Iowa, Iowa City, IA, USA

Michael Varner, MD
Department of Obstetrics and Gynecology, University of Utah school of Medicine, Salt Lake City, UT, USA

Catherine J. Wheeler, MD
Department of Obstetrics and Gynecology, University of Utah School of Medicine, Salt Lake City, UT, USA

Klaus E. Wiemer, PhD
Northwest Center for Reproductive Sciences, Kirkland, WA, USA

Karen Wilson, MA
University Medical Billing and University Health Care Compliance,
University of Utah School of Medicine, Salt Lake City, UT

Kenneth H.H. Wong, MD, MBA
Loma Linda University Medical Center, Southern California Permanente Medical Group,
Loma Linda, CA, USA

Melissa Yates, MD
Department of Obstetrics and Gynecology, Johns Hopkins Medicine,
Johns Hopkins at Green Spring Station, Lutherville, MD, USA

Johnny Yi, MD
Division of General Gynecology, Department of Obstetrics & Gynecology,
University of Utah School of Medicine, Salt Lake City, UT, USA

Howard Zacur, MD, PhD
Department of Obstetrics and Gynecology, Johns Hopkins Medicine,
Johns Hopkins at Green Spring Station, Lutherville, MD, USA

Grant Zhang, PhD
Center for Integrative Medicine, University of Maryland School of Medicine,
Baltimore, MD, USA

Yulian Zhao, PhD, MD, MBA
Department of Obstetrics and Gynecology, Johns Hopkins Medicine,
Johns Hopkins at Green Spring Station, Lutherville, MD, USA

Part I
Management of the R.E.I. Clinic and Laboratories

Chapter 1
Characteristics of a Successful R.E.I. Clinic and Laboratory

Douglas T. Carrell and C. Matthew Peterson

Abstract This chapter explores a few hallmarks of successful REI clinics and laboratories. While all clinics should fulfill minimal guidelines set for in government oversight and regulations, the successful laboratory will go beyond such guidelines to actively improve the quality of service provided to patients. Pursuit of a high level of success necessitates ongoing employee education, monitoring and evaluation of patient outcomes, and a focus on the objectives set for the institution.

Keywords Leadership • Management • Quality assurance • Continuing education • Focus

1.1 Introduction

> The definition of success – To laugh much; to win respect of intelligent persons and the affections of children; to earn the approbation of honest critics and endure the betrayal of false friends; to appreciate beauty; to find the best in others; to give one's self; to leave the world a little better, whether by a healthy child, a garden patch, or a redeemed social condition; to have played and laughed with enthusiasm, and sung with exultation; to know even one life has breathed easier because you have lived – this is to have succeeded.
>
> Ralph Waldo Emerson

The other chapters of this book are aimed at assisting an infertility clinic or laboratory director in understanding the clinical, scientific, business, and management principles necessary to establish and maintain a successful organization. But, what is meant by a "successful organization"? Judging success, in our life or the lives of others, is commonly performed, but nebulous, difficult, and potentially dangerous. The task of defining a successful clinic and laboratory is no easier, and also fraught with danger. However, the definition of "success" quoted above should on one level reassure all infertility clinics that they are to a certain degree "successful" since every healthy baby born as a result of the clinic's service has indeed caused "one life to breathe easier." However, most would agree that truly successful infertility clinics and laboratories have important characteristics beyond pregnancies.

Each medical and laboratory director of an REI clinic has a distinct set of values that define his perception of a successful clinic or laboratory, and the director's values and perceptions likely differ from other directors. So, this chapter is not meant to be a blueprint, rather as a starting point for consideration and discussion.

Perhaps, one of the major difficulties in defining a successful laboratory and clinic is the misconception that success is defined by checking off a list of activities or achievements, analogous to a graduate receiving a diploma after completing a required list of coursework. However, there is no "certificate of success" for clinics and laboratories, nor is success bestowed as an honorary degree. Arthur Ashe, the respected tennis player and civil rights leader, has said, "Success is a journey, not a destination. The doing is often more important than the outcome." In our opinion, establishing a successful clinic and laboratory is similar; destinations are defined, some common to all labs, and the journey is undertaken. However, as situations, regulations, personnel, technologies, and other factors change, new destinations are charted. Therefore, the success in the clinic and laboratory may be looked at as dependent on setting a good course and in the methods employed and the interactions of all during "the journey."

The journey of becoming a successful clinical operation and laboratory contains distinct and necessary guideposts necessary to mark the journey. Such guideposts include compliance with legal and regulatory mandates, accreditation, and employing good management principles, and other items. Below are a few brief characteristics that, in our opinion, are evident in all successful laboratories. The characteristics

D.T. Carrell
Departments of Surgery (Urology), Obstetrics and Gynecology, and Physiology, University of Utah School of Medicine, Salt Lake City, UT, USA

C.M. Peterson (✉)
Utah Center for Reproductive Medicine, Department of Obstetrics and Gynecology, University of Utah School of Medicine, Salt Lake City, UT, USA
e-mail: c.matthew.peterson@hsc.utah.edu

D.T. Carrell and C.M. Peterson (eds.), *Reproductive Endocrinology and Infertility: Integrating Modern Clinical and Laboratory Practice*,
DOI 10.1007/978-1-4419-1436-1_1, © Springer Science+Business Media, LLC 2010

are provided as guideposts, with the inherent understanding that each clinic or lab's priorities and circumstances affect the implementation of the characteristics. The list is not complete, but rather a formulation of some essential characteristics, and simple ideas to assist in the implementation of a successful clinic or laboratory. If there is one firm hallmark of successful people and organizations, it is the attempt to go beyond expectations. The successful team will be constantly looking for ways to improve and set new standards in these, and other, characteristics.

1.2 Successful Leadership Principles

There is a fundamental difference between leadership and management. Leadership has been defined as "…the art of persuading people to work toward a common goal [1]." However, a clinic or laboratory director relies on leadership in setting the expectations and goals of the institution. Leadership shapes the opinions and attitudes of a team of people dedicated to achieving common goals [2]. In short, a director sets a culture of success, mediocrity, or failure through his leadership.

Four approaches have commonly been used to describe and teach effective leadership. The first approach, the *trait approach*, is the most commonly considered method and involves defining characteristics of a successful leader [3]. Such characteristics would undoubtedly include integrity, character, communication skills, patience, passion, energy, vision, credibility, and maturity. According to this approach, the clinical and laboratory directors should continually assess and refine his skills to become more effective. This approach is useful and should be implemented, but it is apparent that other approaches to leadership are also required.

The *behavior approach* to leadership focuses on the manner in which a person acts, particularly in times of stress or in situations relevant to the rest of the group [3]. The approach focuses more on the actions than on a defined set of characteristics. This approach accentuates the "example" set by a director both in routine clinical and lab work, and in striving to move the norms of the operation to higher levels. IVF laboratory directors are often inundated with office work, but this approach highlights the need for a continual, positive presence in the lab itself. Clinical directors are most successful when they grasp the day-to-day operational activities with patients, nursing, laboratory and management staff. The behavioral approach to defining leadership has resulted in the description of various leadership styles, such as authoritative, democratic, and laissez-faire, and others.

The *situational approach* to leadership maintains that each of these styles may be necessary in different situations [4]. This theory implies that a leader should be flexible and perceptive to the specific styles and techniques needed for different individuals or situations. In a sense, most effective leaders have learned this approach. A successful director will be authoritative on issues of critical importance, and will do so with the traits described earlier, but will learn that effective mentoring of staff also requires flexibility and patience.

It is important to note that leadership in the ART clinic and laboratory does not just come from the director, but also from supervisors, technicians, nurses, staff, referring physicians, and possibly others. In fact, both positive and negative leadership may, and often is, exerted from a nonmanagerial staff member. This effect highlights the *reciprocal approach* to leadership and the need to consider the effect and feedback of others on the team and take actions to implement useful input and eliminate negative influences [5, 6]. For some, this is the most difficult part of leadership.

In summary, leadership consists in doing what needs to be done in the way it needs to be done. The styles and actions will vary dependent on the situation and personalities involved. Laboratory directors should never attempt to bluff or imitate other leaders, but instead cultivate positive characteristics skills, with sensitive application to specific situations. Lastly, the leader sets the goals and expectations and is the example in working toward their achievement.

1.3 Effective Management

Management can be defined as the implementation of processes necessary to keep an organization functioning properly. In the laboratory, this includes such diverse functions as budgeting, accounting, employment policies, organizational issues, and technical and scientific policies [7]. The management needs of ART clinics and laboratories vary depending on the size of the clinic, ownership arrangements, and the scope of services provided, but in any situation, successful laboratories contain systems that effectively manage the resources of the lab. An excellent review of many of these processes is found in this book in the chapter by Peterson and Hammoud.

Two keys to successful management of the both the clinic and the laboratory are organization and accountability. In most laboratories, it is imperative to have an organized, consistent manager available to assist the lab director. While the director should set policies that assist in the mission of the laboratory, the manager is usually responsible for the day to day implementation of the policies [8]. The laboratory director assures that the policies are correctly implemented by oversight of the manager and supervisors, and by daily "hands on" involvement, but usually does not have the time to manage all situations personally. Likewise, clinical directors will make the most effective use of their time and expertise with a seasoned clinic manager.

Leadership without management usually results in failure to achieve goals, and may also result in an increased propensity of errors and problems. This highlights the importance of hiring a good manager/supervisor. Perhaps, no other personnel decision made will be as important as selecting a supervisor or manager to assist you in managing the laboratory. The traits that are most beneficial include organization, consistency, and dedication.

One tool that is of great help in managing the many complex tasks and processes involved in managing the clinical enterprise and laboratory is accountability. Successful operations typically delegate responsibilities to all staff, and then demand accountability. This is done by an organized record keeping of projects and responsibilities coupled with group and private follow-up. The annual review of employees is invaluable in this regard, but more frequent follow-ups are also needed. Staff meetings and quality assurance meetings are also invaluable, but often simple "hallway reminders" are necessary. The good manager will be organized and consistent in following-up on projects, while the good leader will recognize that different techniques and motivations are necessary for each situation.

1.4 Skill

While difficult to define, successful laboratories and clinical operations exhibit a high skill level. The purpose of the ART office is to assist couples in achieving a healthy pregnancy. While the pregnancy rate alone is not very helpful in determining success, good clinics and laboratories do have a good pregnancy rate based on the situations and regulations specific for their clinic. High skill levels are also demonstrated by low error levels.

The factors that contribute to good skills include proper management and application of the quality assurance program [9, 10]. An effective quality assurance program should lead to improvement on all levels of performance. Additionally, proper design and monitoring of facilities and equipment is essential. High expectations by the directors, combined with good training, monitoring, and continuing education, are also necessary [3].

Skill implies accuracy. Several programs are essential in assuring that the results produced by the laboratory are accurate. Internal programs include continual monitoring of key indicators as part of the quality assurance program. One useful tool is internal proficiency testing for semen analysis and other assays in which aliquots of a specimen are independently analyzed by all technicians (Discussed extensively in chapter by Keel). Additionally, periodic "recertification" of employee competence should be performed by testing accuracy in specific skills. As a whole, the laboratory should be monitored by monthly and quarterly indicators of skill and accuracy.

External proficiency testing programs are also available, and obligatory under CLIA regulations to monitor and improve accuracy and skill. All laboratories are mandated to participate in proficiency testing programs, but the successful laboratory uses the process to identify problems and improve performance. The quality laboratory looks at such programs as beneficial tools rather than regulatory requirements.

1.5 A Focus on Patients

As strange as it may seem, clinics and laboratories sometimes lose sight of the fact that their reason for existing is to serve the patient. Reference laboratories assist the patient indirectly without any direct contact with the patient, but ART laboratories are usually in close and direct contact. The truly successful clinic and laboratory goes beyond providing skillful analysis and therapies to educate the patient and provide a private, comfortable environment.

Patient education can be facilitated through several means, including the production and distribution of literature such as handouts and pamphlets. While pharmaceutical companies often provide useful patient literature, the clinical and laboratory programs can improve the quality by customizing the literature to clinic specific protocols. Websites can be invaluable in providing information, and pamphlets can easily be posted online. Lastly, patients seminars are also useful in educating patients about the specific processes the clinic and lab undergo to assure quality and safety during therapy.

Within the clinic, privacy is imperative. While HIPPA assures minimal levels of privacy, the successful clinic goes further. For example, patients should not be exposed to crowded waiting rooms through accurate scheduling and overflow areas. Registration should be performed in private offices rather than in the common waiting area. CAP accreditation inspections include inspection of the collection rooms for privacy, but laboratories can improve further by providing soundproofing, comfortable facilities, and private exits.

One useful method of improving patient service is to provide useful feedback mechanisms for patients. Patient surveys can help identify areas in need of improvement and should be carefully developed to encourage useful feedback. Another useful technique is to periodically invite a patient to give feedback at a staff or laboratory meeting regarding their experiences and concerns. This technique is useful in increasing empathy to the needs of the patients. In summary, the successful laboratory strives to understand protocols and procedures through the patients' eyes, then improve the process for the patient.

1.6 A Focus on the Staff

The greatest asset of a clinic and laboratory is the staff. Facilities and equipment are important in providing high quality service, but nearly useless without trained nurses, technicians, and office staff. Therefore, a major focus of any clinic and laboratory director should be on training, assessing, educating, and motivating staff. The investment in developing high quality staff must be protected by providing an environment where employees are respected and treated in a manner that it is their desire to remain as a member of the team for a long time [11, 12].

The most basic factors in developing a high quality team are common sense actions, such as treating staff with respect and honesty. But, a director can go beyond that to develop highly committed and loyal staff. Efforts should be made to continue the growth and education of staff, such as by sending staff to symposia, courses, and meetings. Another technique is to involve staff in the education process within the clinic or laboratory. Annual retreats focused on education, planning, and building teamwork are effective team-building activities. To increase ownership of the staff members, many of the talks and activities should be assigned to them.

An internal continuing education program can be developed to help in the education and development of staff. For example, continuing education program for laboratory technicians requires that they obtain a certain number of continuing education units (CEUs) in three different areas: (1) attendance at journal clubs, symposia, courses, etc., (2) talks and presentations, and (3) personal study of journals, or other topics beneficial to the lab. Completion of the required number of CEUs, along with other factors, is necessary for annual recertification as an andrology or embryology technician.

Directors are prudent to solve employee issues while they are minor. This can be done by periodic one on one discussions, either formally or informally. Additionally, periodic lunches with one or a few employees, or as a whole group, can inspire an employee's confidence and a feeling of worth. Periodic group social activities may help resolve petty issues from festering between staff members.

1.7 Conclusions

This chapter has briefly highlighted a few characteristics of clinics and laboratories that are essential to providing a high level of service and a quality workplace for staff. Each clinic and laboratory can build further upon this foundation to build a truly "successful" organization that serves patients with the highest level of skill and caring.

References

1. Goleman D (1997) Emotional intelligence. Bantam Books, New York, NY
2. Zalesnick A (1977) Managers and leaders: are they different? Harv Bus Rev 55(3):67–78
3. Kearns E, Sun F (2007) Principles of leadership: past, present, and future. In: Harmening D (ed) Laboratory management: principles and processes. D.H. Publishing & Consulting, Inc, St. Petersburg, FL, pp 23–41
4. Fiedler F (1967) A theory of leadership effectiveness. McGraw-Hill, New York, NY
5. Burns J (1977) Leadership. Harper and Row, New York
6. Trishy N, Devanna M (1986) The transformational leader. Wiley, New York
7. Hudson J (ed) (2004) Principles of clinical laboratory management: a study guide and workbook. Pearson Prentice Hall, Upper Saddle River, NJ
8. Freeman V (2007) Managerial problem solving and decision making. In: Harmening D (ed) Laboratory management: principles and processes. D.H. Publishing & Consulting, Inc., St. Petersburg, FL
9. Holmboe ES, Wang Y, Meehan TP et al (2008) Association between maintenance of certification examination scores and quality of care for medicare beneficiaries. Arch Intern Med 168(13):1396–1403
10. Henning SE, Cohen EL (2008) The competency continuum: expanding the case manager's skill sets and capabilities. Prof Case Manag 13(3):127–148
11. Holland P (2004) Team building. In: Hudson J (ed) Principles of clinical laboratory management: a study guide and workbook. Pearson Prentice Hall, Upper Saddle River, NJ
12. Burdick I (1995) Implementing the work teams in the clinical laboratory. MLO Med Lab Obs 27(1):44–47

Chapter 2
Assisted Reproductive Technology Practice Management

C. Matthew Peterson, Ahmad O. Hammoud, Erika Lindley, Douglas T. Carrell, and Karen Wilson

Abstract A basic knowledge of management issues is required in the operation of any medical practice. This chapter highlights the critical practice management principles necessary for effective interaction with other professionals in business management, human resources, payer organizations, legal counsel, accounting, and risk management who interface with the practice.

Keywords Management • Regulations • Legal rulings • Quality assurance • Accounting • Root cause analysis

2.1 AIM

The successful practice of reproductive endocrinology and infertility demands strict attention to service and educational missions, and in the academic setting, research. Whether operating under a profit or not-for-profit, hospital-based or free-standing setting, these missions cannot be adequately addressed without policies and procedures as well as active management strategies that direct the practice's business operations. While many physicians and scientists prefer to avoid this aspect of their career, a basic knowledge of these management issues is required. This chapter highlights the critical practice management principles necessary for effective interaction with other professionals in business management, human resources, payer organizations, legal counsel, accounting, and risk management who interface with the practice. The aim of this chapter is to serve as a resource and provide references to more detailed information available in specialty publications. The American Society for Reproductive Medicine (ASRM) has a number of management resources on it's web site: www.asrm.org.

2.2 Revenue Cycle

The revenue cycle begins with patient registration (Fig. 2.1). Critical information that must be collected and verified before each visit includes demographics, primary and secondary insurance information, policy holder/responsible party, eligibility for benefits and coverage, and updating patient account balances for the collection of copays/ balances at the point of service. Studies estimate that 42% of practice-generated denials are attributable to a failure to set up the patient's insurance correctly and that 88% of patient-generated errors are due to inaccurate personal information. Thus, insurance verification and updated information from the patient at each encounter are critical steps in the revenue cycle [1]. Industry experts estimate that it costs $25 or more to rework a single claim [2]. Registration can be accomplished over the telephone, on-line, or using written forms. Key strategies to successful registration include appropriate staffing, training, and monitoring of performance indicators. Time studies can be performed to determine new and follow-up patient registration requirements, and staffing should respond appropriately to the findings. The dollar amount of claims denied for registration/ insurance related reasons as a percentage of total denied dollars may be used to assess registration function. Furthermore, registration edit reports track locations and individuals on the team who would benefit by additional training.

Healthcare providers in best practices submit the encounter form, commonly called a superbill, within 24 h of the encounter. Monitoring strategies include nightly reconciliation of missing encounter forms with schedules documenting

C.M. Peterson (✉) and A.O. Hammoud
Utah Center for Reproductive Medicine, Department of Obstetrics and Gynecology, University of Utah School of Medicine, Salt Lake City, UT, USA
e-mail: c.matthew.peterson@hsc.utah.edu

E. Lindley
Departments of Obstetrics and Gynecology, University of Utah School of Medicine, Salt Lake City, UT, USA

D.T. Carrell
Departments of Surgery (Urology), Obstetrics and Gynecology, and Physiology, University of Utah School of Medicine, Salt Lake City, UT, USA

K. Wilson
University Medical Billing and University Health Care Compliance, University of Utah School of Medicine, Salt Lake City, UT, USA

D.T. Carrell and C.M. Peterson (eds.), *Reproductive Endocrinology and Infertility: Integrating Modern Clinical and Laboratory Practice*,
DOI 10.1007/978-1-4419-1436-1_2,

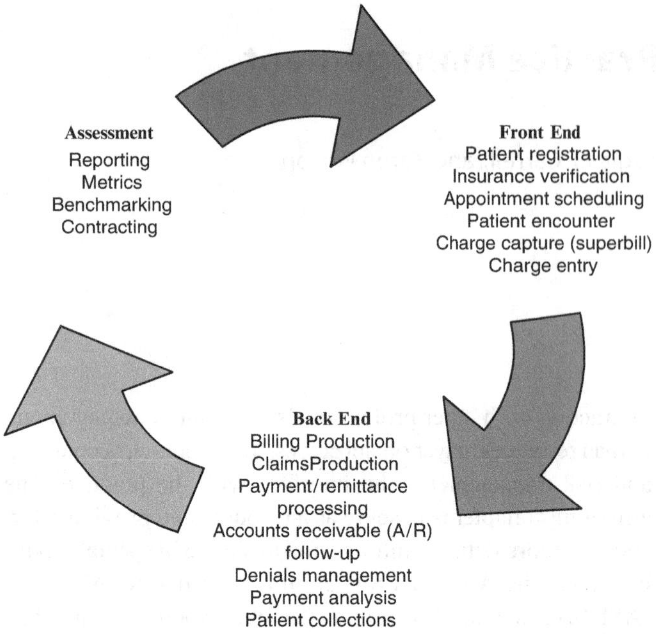

Fig. 2.1 The revenue cycle. The revenue cycle consists of a number of interrelated processes that are categorized as front end, backend and analysis/planning activities. Each process within an activity has numerous subparts which must be analyzed and optimized, for example, the patient encounter component of the front end activities includes check-in, point-of-service collections, provider encounter, checkout, scheduling/referrals and financial counseling

"arrived" patients. Superbills should be designed to facilitate coding the ICD-9 diagnostic codes and CPT procedural codes common to the practice. The superbill should be reviewed annually and reviewed with professional coders. Chart audits insure appropriate documentation of the encounter and its codes. New providers should be audited the first few months in the practice to insure appropriate and maximum coding and completion rates.

Charge entry after a patient encounter should be completed within 48 h. Within 24 h after the encounter, the superbills are collected and batched. In the next 24 h period, the charges should be entered. Best practices reconcile missing charges daily to weekly.

Submission of claims and subsequent payments are improved by the use of a clearinghouse that filters the claim for errors or through the use of a claim scrubber. Claim scrubbers allow the provider to utilize the same software that payers use to deny claims and hold reimbursements longer. Furthermore, practices can identify undercoding in services. Larger volume practices may find the cost/ benefit ratio favors automated claim scrubbing. Payment posting should be reconciled to the maximal contracted amount. Payer policy changes are techniques designed to reduce payments and must be monitored carefully. Larger organizations can consider software that will monitor charges, and contracted payments to actual payments to insure payers adhere to contracted rates.

Analysis/assessment tools include practice metrics and reports that will flag difficulties with the revenue cycle. Useful metrics include accounts receivable (AR), claim denials, write-offs, collection rates, patient complaints, volume of unanswered payer and patient correspondence, claim edits, timely submission of charges, lag days, missing charges, and turnover in revenue cycle employees. An example of a functioning revenue cycle metrics report is found in Fig. 2.2 and in the Appendix. Periodically, supervising individuals should call for a reevaluation of the revenue cycle and the metrics being utilized. Strategic management of the revenue cycle will result in greater margin for the missions undertaken by the practice. Of all improvements that can be recommended for revenue cycle processes, standardization is proven to benefit not only revenue, but also quality and patient satisfaction [3]. Continuous training and cross training in job specific policies and procedures, technology and systems, and practice-specific revenue-cycle-activities will also result in improved financial and patient, provider and employee satisfaction scores. Open discussions of revenue cycle activities will reveal bottlenecks, dropped handoffs, and duplication of work. Figures 2.3 and 2.4 are examples of ambulatory services dashboards, which can facilitate discussions regarding critical practice parameters that affect the revenue cycle. Instituting controls on cash handling/ deposits for point-of-service collections, reconciliation of missing charges, batching/ hashing for charge entry, productivity measures for A/R follow-up and job specific information system access will protect the assets of the practice.

Useful resources regarding the revenue cycle include The Physician Billing Process: Avoiding Potholes in the Road to Getting Paid by Deborah L. Walker, MBA, FACMPE; Sara M. Larch, MSHA, FACMPE; Elizabeth W. Woodcock, MBA, FACMPE, CPC (ISBN 1-56829-230-9) and Financial Management for Medical Groups by Ernest J. Pavlock, PhD, CPA (ISBN 1568290217). The Medical Group Management Association (MGMA) is a professional association providing many resources (http://www.mgma.com) (Figs. 2.5 and 2.6, respectively).

2.3 Employment Cycle

Staffing issues are a time consuming aspect of REI practice management. Concerns related to hospital-based settings include staff unionization and difficulty in providing performance incentives. Furthermore, in hospital-based settings, a clinic staffing model is often applied inappropriately. An optimal staffing ratio for an ART program can be higher than the standard clinic staffing model and ranges from 4 to 12 full-time equivalents per physician with efficiencies gained in multiple provider models. This relatively high fixed cost

13 months provides trending

Previous allows for seasonality- such as: annual conference attendance, etc.

Current Month variance compared to average for fast assessment of status

Year to Year Variance

Measures	2007/Apr	2008/Mar	2008/Apr	12 Mo Total	Prev 12 Mo Tot	12 Mo Tot Var	12 Mo Avg	CM Var	PFYTD	FYTD	FY Var
Charges	$ 516,065	$ 587,332	$ 445,066	$ 4,805,934	$ 1,450,842	$3,355,092	$ 400,494	$44,571	$ 1,173,455	$ 4,274,286	$3,100,830
Payments	$ 241,785	$ 280,658	$ 274,525	$ 2,317,468	$ 873,820	$1,443,647	$ 193,122	$81,403	$ 682,573	$ 2,099,792	$1,417,219
Net Payments	$ 239,779	$ 278,667	$ 270,568	$ 2,296,101	$ 851,197	$1,444,905	$ 191,342	$79,226	$ 663,281	$ 2,079,504	$1,416,224
Contract Adj	$ 182,506	$ 243,076	$ 258,305	$ 1,665,848	$ 517,881	$1,147,966	$ 138,821	$119,484	$ 404,273	$ 1,546,604	$1,142,332
Refunds	$ 2,006	$ 1,991	$ 3,958	$ 21,367	$ 22,624	($1,257)	$ 1,781	$2,177	$ 19,293	$ 20,288	$995
Work RVU	3,730.18	4,371.16	3,367.12	41,471.43	12,545.59	28,925.84	3,455.95	(88.83)	10,118.74	36,277.79	26,159.05
Total Discounts	$ 24,348	$ 20,170	$ 9,204	$177,087	$19,456	$157,632	$14,757	($5,553)	$16,740	$167,563	$150,824

COLLECTION AGENCY ACTIVITY											
TO COLLECTIONS	$ 11,979	$ 6,289	$ 12,784	$ 119,879	$ 63,243	$ 56,636	$ 9,990	$ 2,794	$ 48,262	$ 107,667	$ 59,404

ORIGINAL INSURANCE INFO CAPTURED				12 Mo Totals	12 Mo Avg	Mix 12 Mo	Prev 12 Mo Tot	Prev 12 Mo Mix	Mix CM	Mix PYTD	Mix FYTD
BLUE SHIELD	$ 93,326	$ 122,022	$ 134,471	$ 1,097,872	$ 91,489	22.84%	$ 372,628	25.68%	30.21%	26.57%	22.83%
COMMERCIAL INS	$ 3,253	$ 5,761	$ 1,759	$ 46,191	$ 3,849	0.96%	$ 19,659	1.36%	0.40%	0.87%	0.93%
CONTRACTS	$ 143,248	$ 161,619	$ 109,720	$ 1,410,186	$ 117,516	29.34%	$ 548,134	37.78%	24.65%	38.65%	27.80%
MEDICAID	$ 156,184	$ 166,431	$ 111,425	$ 1,309,426	$ 109,119	27.25%	$ 351,728	24.24%	25.04%	22.66%	27.76%
MEDICARE	$ 542	$ 3,912	$ 358	$ 17,699	$ 1,475	0.37%	$ 4,764	0.33%	0.08%	0.41%	0.33%
MISC GOVT	$ 18,941	$ 18,580	$ 14,582	$ 131,397	$ 10,950	2.73%	$ 35,577	2.45%	3.28%	2.39%	2.94%
OOS MEDICAID	$ 24,582	$ 10,037	$ 8,688	$ 103,897	$ 8,658	2.16%	$ 30,351	2.09%	1.95%	2.25%	2.16%
SELF PAY	$ 75,989	$ 98,971	$ 64,063	$ 689,266	$ 57,439	14.34%	$ 88,001	6.07%	14.39%	6.21%	15.25%

These categories are based on system set-up. Allows for visual of payer charge mix vs. payer payment mix.

PAYER				12 Mo Totals	12 Mo Avg	Mix 12 Mo	Prev 12 Mo Tot	Prev 12 Mo Mix	Mix CM	Mix PYTD	Mix FYTD
BLUE SHIELD	$ 66,414	$ 68,320	$ 57,137	$ 571,665	$ 47,639	24.83%	$ 220,753	25.32%	21.00%	26.08%	24.16%
COMMERCIAL INS	$ 1,321	$ 3,046	$ 1,463	$ 20,431	$ 1,703	0.89%	$ 5,110	0.59%	0.54%	0.66%	0.96%
CONTRACTS	$ 77,682	$ 91,017	$ 69,635	$ 803,750	$ 66,979	34.91%	$ 373,552	42.85%	25.59%	43.37%	34.23%
MEDICAID	$ 67,049	$ 79,316	$ 83,450	$ 608,071	$ 50,673	26.41%	$ 151,933	17.43%	30.67%	16.61%	27.33%
MEDICARE	$ 619	$ 230	$ 2,110	$ 8,490	$ 707	0.37%	$ 1,110	0.13%	0.78%	0.15%	0.35%
MISC GOVT	$ 6,850	$ 4,654	$ 9,208	$ 57,580	$ 4,798	2.50%	$ 16,205	1.86%	3.38%	2.06%	2.57%
OOS MEDICAID	$ 6,740	$ 9,115	$ 14,846	$ 47,825	$ 3,985	2.08%	$ 17,546	2.01%	5.46%	1.30%	2.23%
SELF PAY	$ 13,827	$ 22,023	$ 34,270	$ 184,216	$ 15,351	8.00%	$ 85,509	9.81%	12.59%	9.77%	8.17%

OUTSTANDING ACCOUNTS RECEIVABLE

CURRENT INSURANCE	FEB	MAR	APR	FPSC BENCHMARKS		
A/R 31-60 Days	$ 182,719	$ 159,963	$ 141,606			
% A/R 31-60 Days	21.30%	17.83%	17.96%	15.29%	6.70%	34.00%
A/R 61-90 Days	$ 76,879	$ 127,462	$ 103,444			
% A/R 61-90 Days	8.96%	14.20%	13.12%	8.80%	4.90%	14.40%
A/R 91-120 Days	$ 78,029	$ 62,194	$ 82,893			
% A/R 91-120 Days	9.09%	6.93%	10.51%	6.34%	3.80%	12.50%
A/R >120 Days	$ 121,490	$ 172,324	$ 163,937			
% of AR > 120	14.16%	19.20%	20.79%	18.76%	3.30%	52.30%
A/R Balance	$ 857,944	$ 897,405	$ 788,640			

Use a benchmark that pertains to your size and structure. MGMA or FPSC are some examples

CURRENT FSC	91-120 DAYS	121-150 DAYS	151-180 DAYS	> 180 DAYS	TOTAL AR
BLUE SHIELD	$ 2,284	$ 2,330	$ 496	$ 272	$ 123,507
% OF BLUE SHIELD	1.85%	1.89%	0.40%	0.22%	100.00%
COMMERCIAL INSURANCE	$ 405	$ 509	$ 118	$ 1,461	$ 13,167
% OF COMMERCIAL INS	3.08%	3.87%	0.90%	11.09%	100.00%
CONTRACTS	$ 10,971	$ 4,261	$ 4,698	$ 9,799	$ 160,320
% OF CONTRACTS	6.84%	2.66%	2.93%	6.11%	100.00%
MEDICAID	$ 11,165	$ 8,693	$ 4,685	$ 12,632	$ 108,126
% OF MEDICAID	10.33%	8.04%	4.33%	11.68%	100.00%
MEDICARE	$ 151	$ 99	$ 164	$ 2,724	$ 4,068
% OF MEDICARE	3.71%	2.44%	4.03%	66.97%	100.00%
MISC GOVERNMENT	$ 2,039	$ 236	$ 2,571	$ 694	$ 25,643
% OF MISC GOVERNMENT	7.95%	0.92%	10.03%	2.71%	100.00%
OOS MEDICAID	$ 4,980	$ 901	$ 5,244	$ 19,798	$ 45,819
% OF OOS MEDICAID	10.87%	1.97%	11.44%	43.21%	100.00%
RESPONSIBLE PARTY	$ 50,897	$ 22,908	$ 32,102	$ 26,625	$ 308,072
% OF RESPONSIBLE PARTY	16.52%	7.44%	10.42%	8.64%	100.00%
TOTAL AR	$ 82,893	$ 39,936	$ 50,078	$ 73,923	$ 788,640
% OF TOTAL	10.51%	5.06%	6.35%	9.37%	100.00%

Please see Appendix for step-by-step, detailed information on revenue cycle report.

TOP 5 REJECTIONS - OP CODING	Chg	2007/Apr	2008/Jan	2008/Feb	2008/Mar	2008/Apr	FYTD
97-SERVICE NOT PAID SEPARATELY	Chg Amt	$ 262	$ 1,049	$ 1,455	$ 387	$ 799	$ 6,134
	Rej Count	5	9	8	2	9	63
11-DIAGNOSIS SUBMITTED INCONSISTENT WITH PROCEDURE	Chg Amt	$ 16	$ 82	$ 82	$ 92	$ 164	$ 1,791
	Rej Count	2	1	3	7	2	28
7-INVALID PROC CODE INCONSISTENT WITH PT GENDER	Chg Amt	$ -	$ -	$ -	$ -	$ 151	$ 151
	Rej Count	-	-	-	-	1	1
50-NOT MEDICALLY NECESSARY	Chg Amt	$ -	$ 151	$ -	$ 359	$ 547	$ 1,057
	Rej Count	-	1	-	2	1	4
112-SVC NOT DOCUMENTED	Chg Amt	$ -	$ -	$ -	$ -	$ (85)	$ -
	Rej Count	-	-	-	-	1	2

REGISTRATION	Chg	2007/Apr	2008/Jan	2008/Feb	2008/Mar	2008/Apr	FYTD
28-CLIENT NOT ELIGIBLE ON DATE OF SERVICE	Chg Amt	$ 1,889	$ 1,650	$ 2,395	$ 568	$ 2,824	$ 13,521
	Rej Count	13	15	11	6	21	97
49-NON COVERED SERVICE IN CONJUNCTION WITH ROUTINE	Chg Amt	$ 1,205	$ 328	$ 1,064	$ 257	$ 857	$ 5,424
	Rej Count	10	4	8	2	5	46
L10-PROVIDE DATE OF LMP/ONSET OF ILLNESS	Chg Amt	$ 1,642	$ 113	$ 2,114	$ 1,805	$ 1,599	$ 13,297
	Rej Count	11	1	7	7	5	67
31-INVALID ID NUMBER-UNABLE TO IDENTIFY INSURED	Chg Amt	$ -	$ -	$ 151	$ -	$ 509	$ 874
	Rej Count	-	-	1	-	4	7
27-COVERAGE TERMINATED BEFORE DOS	Chg Amt	$ 660	$ 233	$ 233	$ 793	$ 747	$ 4,432
	Rej Count	5	2	2	6	3	29

FOLLOW UP	Chg	Apr	2008/Jan	2008/Feb	2008/Mar	2008/Apr	FYTD
96-NON-COVERED CHARGES	Chg Amt	$ 692	$ 1,199	$ 6,216	$ 1,823	$ 2,854	$ 15,574
	Rej Count	6	10	27	12	17	104
D6-INS REQUESTS COPY OF REPORT	Chg Amt	$ -	$ -	$ -	$ 372	$ 2,896	$ 5,281
	Rej Count	-	-	-	2	15	30
18-DUPLICATE CLAIM	Chg Amt	$ 2,844	$ 878	$ 1,613	$ 883	$ 1,453	$ 14,963
	Rej Count	10	2	11	9	10	100
16-ADDITIONAL INFO NEEDED	Chg Amt	$ 2,188	$ 164	$ 360	$ 269	$ 151	$ 4,545
	Rej Count	5	1	1	2	5	26
17-ADDITIONAL INFO NEEDED-REQ INFO INSUFFICIENT OR INCOMPLETE	Chg Amt	$ 82	$ -	$ 943	$ 442	$ 1,071	$ 2,538
	Rej Count	1	-	2	2	4	9

% of change between fiscal years.

	2008/Feb	2008/Mar	2008/Apr	12 Mo Total	12 Mo Avg	CM Var	PFYTD	FYTD	% Change
Charges	$ 516,065	$ 587,332	$ 445,066	$ 4,805,934	$ 400,494	$44,571	$ 1,173,455	$ 4,274,286	264.25%
Coding Rejections	$ 7,279	$ 10,239	$ 8,301	$ 54,883	$ 4,574	$3,728	$ 14,483	$ 48,111	232.19%
Coding Rej %	1.41%	1.74%	1.87%	1.14%	1.14%	0.72%	1.23%	1.13%	−0.11%
Follow up Rej	$ 41,437	$ 21,390	$ 41,300	$ 267,783	$ 22,315	$18,985	$ 82,567	$ 251,896	205.08%
Follow up Rej %	8.03%	3.64%	9.28%	5.57%	5.57%	3.71%	7.04%	5.89%	−1.14%
Registration Rej	$ 13,504	$ 7,386	$ 14,368	$ 95,382	$ 7,949	$6,420	$ 40,455	$ 84,663	109.28%
Registration Rej %	2.62%	1.26%	3.23%	1.98%	1.98%	1.24%	3.45%	1.98%	−1.47%
Total Rejections	$ 62,220	$ 39,015	$ 63,970	$ 418,049	$ 34,837	$29,132	$ 137,505	$ 384,671	179.75%
Total Rej ections %	12.06%	6.64%	14.37%	8.70%	9.06%	5.32%	11.72%	9.00%	−2.72%

Fig. 2.2 ART practice management divisional revenue cycle report (for illustrative purposes only and does not represent actual operational data)

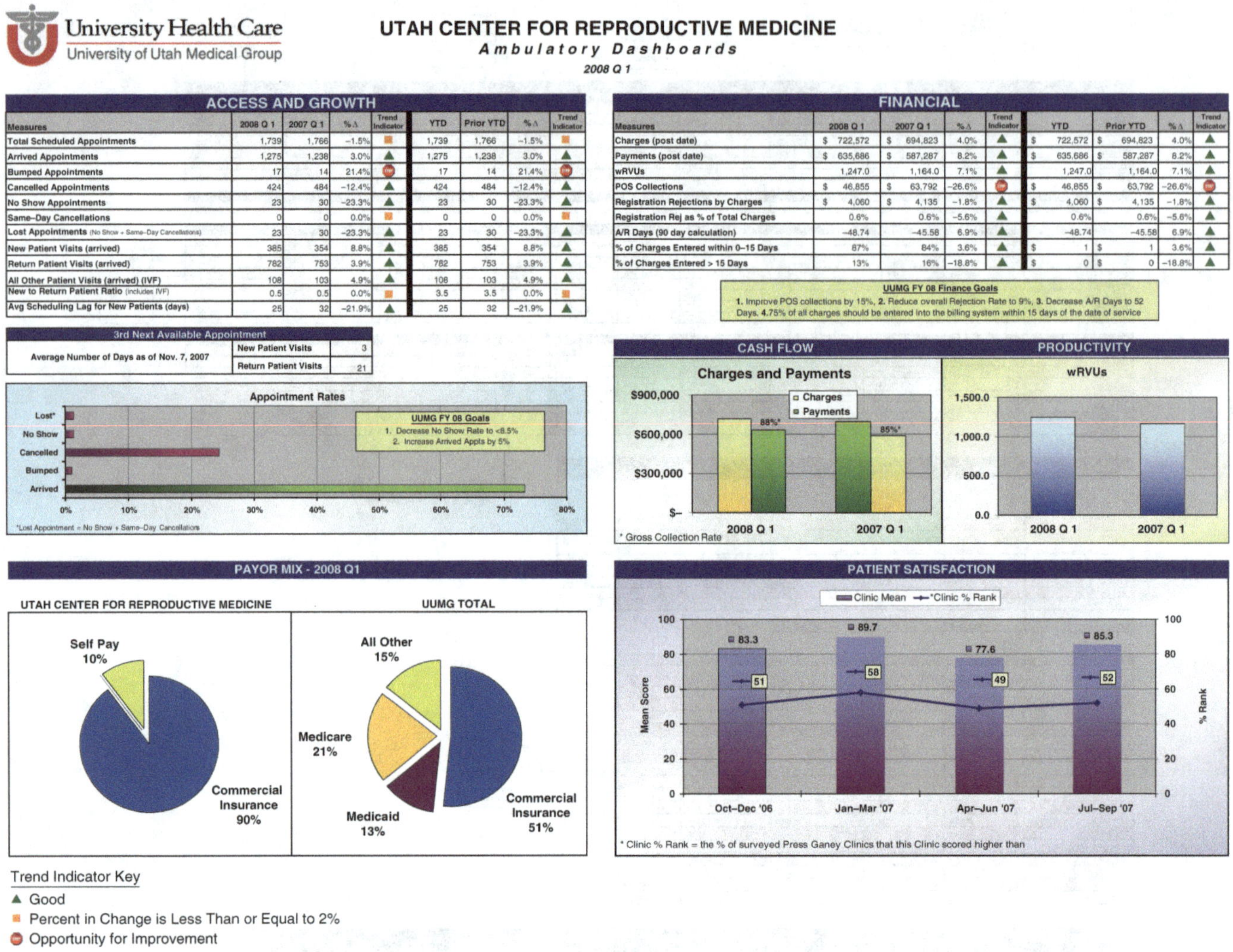

Fig. 2.3 UCRM ambulatory dashboard (for illustrative purposes only and does not represent actual operational data)

requires a significant volume of ART cycles to be economically viable. For these reasons, sound employment principles are mandatory.

Employment advertising should include only the requirements of the position, Equal Opportunity Employer (EEO) statement and avoidance of problematic language which could be construed as discriminatory. Key components of the employment application are found in Table 2.1.

In the offer letter or contract an Employment-At-Will statement is helpful, if applicable in the clinic's governance situation: "You should understand that you will be employed at-will, which means that either you or the company can terminate your employment at any time."

Interviewing questions are governed by federal and state laws. The Department of Labor for each state often has websites that detail laws concerning employment. There are a number of illegal questions to avoid, which can be worked around through proper questioning noted in Table 2.2. Experienced human resource managers suggest a question, which is often quite revealing: Assume you could have anyone to write a letter of reference for you, who would it be and what would they say? Human resource managers should regularly check the federal and state employment laws.

In those positions where an offer letter is appropriate, the letter should include a start date, rate of pay, wage payment schedule, hours of employment, position, remaining steps to be accomplished before hire, employment at-will disclosure, statement that nothing in the offer letter should be interpreted as a contract, signature and date-line. To reduce staff management difficulties, all clinics should have an employee handbook (Table 2.3).

Wage and Hour Laws define "Exempt" employees as those who are exempt from overtime pay such as physicians, embryologists, registered nurses, and managers. "Nonexempt" employees must be paid at least the mini-

University Health Care
University of Utah Medical Group

REPRODUCTIVE ENDOCRINOLOGY

Ambulatory Dashboard

2008 Q 1

ARRIVED APPOINTMENT TOTALS BY PROCEDURE CATEGORY

Measures	2008 Q 1	2007 Q 1	% Δ	Trend Indicator	YTD	Prior YTD	% Δ	Trend Indicator
Egg Retrieval	80	77	3.9%	▲	80	77	3.9%	▲
ET Totals	97	95	2.1%	▲	97	95	2.1%	▲
IVF ET	73	70	4.3%	▲	73	70	4.3%	▲
Cryo ET	25	22	13.6%	▲	25	22	13.6%	▲
Ovum Donar	5	5	0.0%	■	5	5	0.0%	■
Surrogacy	0	0	0.0%	■	0	0	0.0%	■
Insemination	291	300	-3.0%	STOP	291	300	-3.0%	STOP
Ultrasound	762	747	2.0%	■	762	747	2.0%	■
Viability	67	68	-1.5%	■	67	68	-1.5%	■
Super Ovulation Start	109	116	-6.0%	STOP	109	116	-6.0%	STOP

PROVIDER PRODUCTIVITY

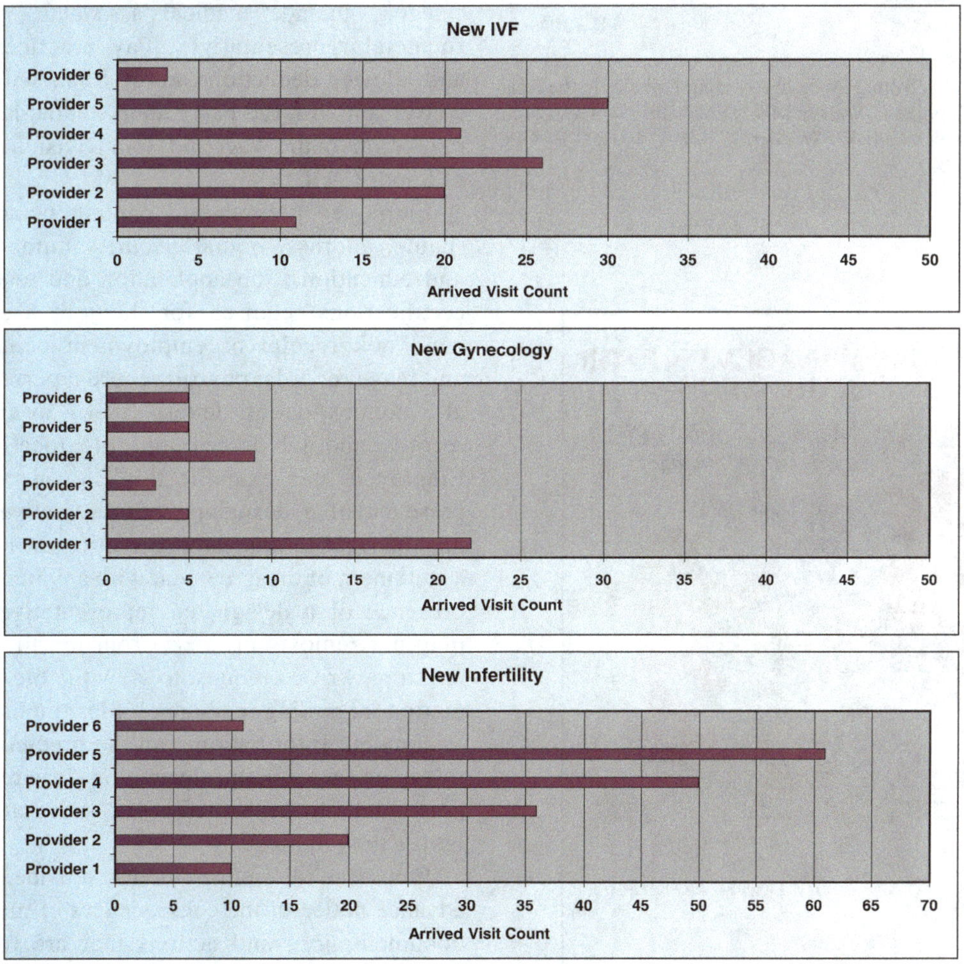

Fig. 2.4 Reproductive endocrinology ambulatory dashboard (for illustrative purposes only and does not represent actual operational data)

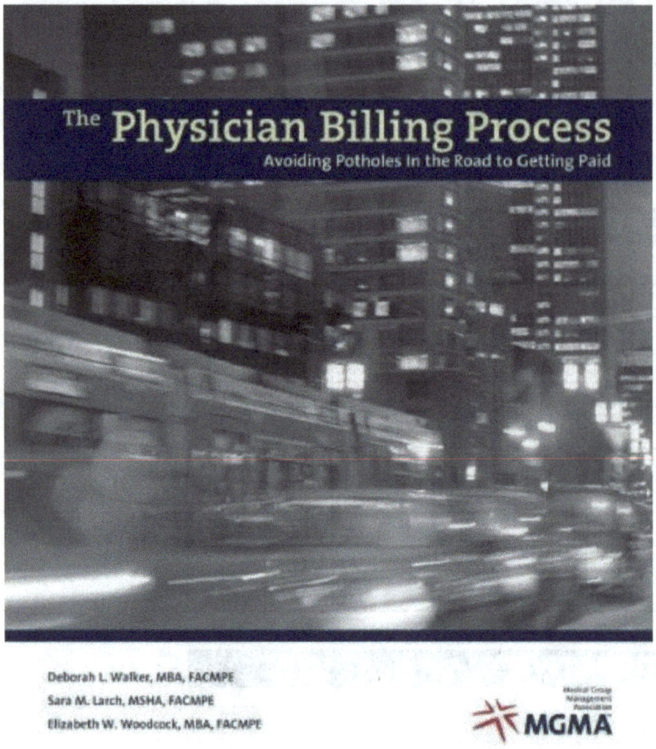

Fig. 2.5 The Physician Billing Process: Avoiding Potholes in the Road to Getting Paid by Deborah L. Walker, MBA, FACMPE; Sara M. Larch, MSHA, FACMPE; Elizabeth W. Woodcock, MBA, FACMPE, CPC (ISBN 1-56829-230-9)

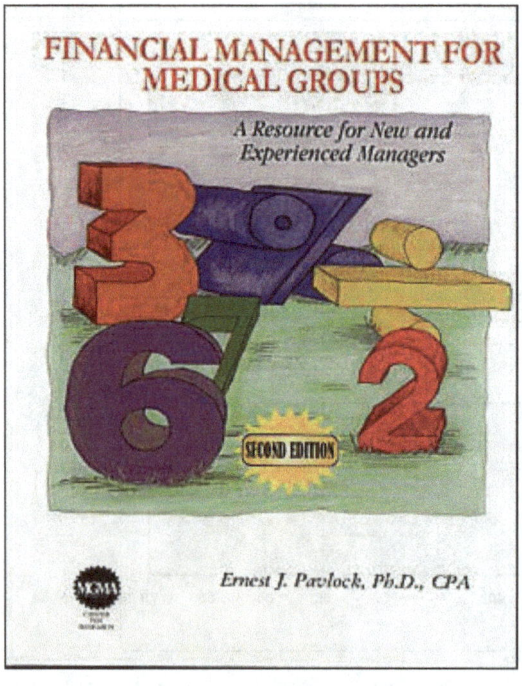

Fig. 2.6 Financial Management for Medical Groups by Ernest J. Pavlock, PhD,CPA. (ISBN 1568290217)

Table 2.1 Key components of the employment application

An employment application has a signed and dated certification that:
The applicant was truthful in completing the application
No information that would affect the application was withheld
The employer may terminate the applicant (if hired) if the employer later discovers that the applicant was not truthful or withheld material information
The applicant agrees to abide by all of the rules and policies of the employer, or be subject to termination
The applicant agrees to the employer's ability to check references and/or verify information
Acknowledges the employer may change the applicant's hours at will
Contains an Employment-At-Will statement (if applicable): "You should understand that you will be employed at-will, if hired, which means that either you or the company can terminate your employment at any time"

mum wage for all hours worked and one-and-one-half times their regular rate of pay for all hours worked over 40 h in a single work week (state laws may differ). Employees in this category include medical assistants, receptionists and financial representatives. Pay practices, withholdings, and allowed deductions are best handled by professionals conversant with the Fair Labor Standards Act (FLSA) and regulations of the Wage and Hour Division of the Department of Labor (DOL).

Employee files should contain personal information (name, address, Social Security number, date of birth and education); job application and resume; licenses or certifications required for the job; a signed employee handbook receipt or employment contract; attendance and leave records; payroll records; performance appraisals, commendation letters, merit awards; disciplinary records; and, job description, title, location and schedule. Employees can examine this file once per year in the presence of a designated representative. The employee has the right to request a correction or a deletion or write a statement of disagreement with any item in the file in the presence of a designated representative. The employee may not remove any item from the file. Employers can require a written request to view the file. Exempted information regarding personnel files include potential job assignment information, and the prediction of any future salary or career path information. It is recommended that personnel file be kept for 4–7 years after an employee leaves the practice.

Employee discipline should provide, where possible, advance notice of the consequences of misconduct; written documentation; and actions that are timely, consistent and impartial. In the articulation of a disciplinary policy, reserve the right to choose the level of discipline, up to and including termination without resorting to less severe

Table 2.2 Illegal employment que.stions and their legal workarounds

Category	Illegal questions	Legal questions
National origin/ citizenship	Are you a U.S. citizen? Where were you/your parents born? What is your native tongue?	Are you authorized to work in the United States? What languages do you read, speak, or write fluently? (This question is okay, as long as this ability is relevant to the performance of the job)
Age	How old are you? When is your birth date? When did you graduate from high school?	Are you over the age of 18?
Marital/family status	What's your marital status? With whom do you live? Do you plan to have a family? When? How many kids do you have? What are your child care arrangements?	Would you be willing to relocate if necessary? Travel is an important part of the job. Would you be able and willing to travel as needed by the job? (This question is okay, as long as all applicants for the job are asked it) This job requires overtime occasionally. Would you be willing and able to work overtime as necessary? (Again, as long as all applicants for the job are asked it)
Affiliations	What clubs or social organizations do you belong to?	List any professional or trade groups or other organizations that you belong to that you consider relevant to your ability to perform this job
Personal	How tall are you? How much do you weigh?	Are you able to lift a 50-pound weight and carry it 100 yards, as this is part of the job? (Questions about height and weight are not acceptable unless minimum standards are essential to the safe performance of the job)
Disabilities	Do you have any disabilities? Please complete the following medical history Have you had any recent or past illnesses or operations? If yes, list and give dates What was the date of your last physical exam? How's your family health? When did you lose your eyesight? How? Do you need an accommodation to perform the job? (Can be asked only after a job offer is made)	Based on the job description, are you able to perform the essential functions of this job? Can you demonstrate how you would perform the following job-related functions? Are you willing to complete a medical exam after we've made you a job offer? (The results of the exam must be kept strictly confidential, except medical/safety personnel may be informed if emergency medical treatment is required, and supervisors/managers may be informed about necessary accommodations to the job, based on the results of the exam) Do you understand that any offer of employment is conditional based on the results of a medical exam?
Arrest record	Have you ever been arrested?	Have you ever been convicted of _______? (The crime named should be reasonably related to the performance of the job in question)
Military	If you've been in the military, were you honorably discharged?	In what branch of the armed forces did you serve? What type of training or education did you receive in the military?

Illegal questions are problematic and information gained in such questions may be used to discriminate against members of protected classes. In order to avoid illegal questions ask objective questions that determine if an applicant can fulfill the legitimate job requirements. Human Resource personnel should frequently assess federal and state employment laws regarding legal and illegal questions

Table 2.3 Critical components of the employee handbook

Employment At-Will Disclaimer Statement (if applicable)
Handbook Acknowledgement Statement
Employee Confidentiality Agreement
Equal Employment Opportunity (EEO) Statement
Sexual Harassment and Other Harassment Guidelines
Summary of Benefits
COBRA
Family Medical Leave Act (FMLA), if applicable
Patient Confidentiality/Substance Abuse Statement
Electronic Communications and Internet Use Policy

measures. There should be a nonexhaustive list of the types of infractions that will result in immediate termination. If your policy includes progressive discipline, it is mandatory that it is followed to avoid a breach of contract or discrimination action. Disciplinary actions including warnings and counseling should be documented in the personnel file. Future expectations should be written and state clearly, "we expect that you will…".

Federal employment laws have compliance thresholds based on the number of employees outlined in Table 2.4, and these laws are briefly described in Table 2.5. Successful ART Programs create a level of professionalism that is expected in the practice by conducting the employment cycle and employee relations with the same level of attention required in the practice of ART. HIPAA is a standard all employees must clearly understand as the standard of patient confidentiality required in the practice. A brief summary of its core elements are outlined in Table 2.6.

Table 2.4 US Federal Employment Law Compliance thresholds by number of employees

Discrimination laws and application of the statute The respective state Department of Labor and attorney should be consulted regarding application	
Federal statutes	Minimum employees
Americans with Disabilities Act of 1990	15
Age Discrimination in Employment Act of 1967	20
Civil Rights Act of 1964 Title VII-Equal Employment Opportunities	15
Consolidated Omnibus Benefits Reconciliation Act (COBRA)	20
Fair Labor Standards Act of 1938 (FLSA)	1
Family and Medical Leave Act of 1993 (FMLA)	50
Health Insurance Portability and Accountability Act of 1996 (HIPAA)	1
Immigration Reform and Control Act of 1986 (IRCA)	1
Occupational Safety and Health Act of 1970 (OSHA)	1
Pregnancy Discrimination Act (PDA)	2

Table 2.5 US Federal Employment Laws Summary

US Federal Employment Laws Summary Please check with your state DOL, and / or attorney.
Americans with Disabilities Act
Prohibition of discrimination based on disabilities
Requires "Reasonable Accommodations" for disabled individuals
Provide equal opportunity in application process
Enable performance of "Essential functions" of position
Enable equal benefits and privileges
Avoid undue hardship in the workplace
Age Discrimination Act of 1967
Prohibits discrimination with respect to any term, condition, or privilege of employment, including hiring, firing, promotion, layoff, compensation, benefits, job assignments, and training
Protects employees and job applicants 40 years of age or older from employment discrimination
Prohibits retaliation against an individual for opposing employment practices that discriminate based on age or for filing an age discrimination charge, testifying, or participating in any way in an investigation, proceeding, or litigation under the ADEA
Title VII of the Civil Rights Act of 1964
Prohibits race, color, gender, national origin, and religious discrimination
Applies to hiring, discharge, compensation, promotion and other terms and conditions of employment
Gender discrimination includes pregnancy discrimination and sexual harassment
Comprehensive Omnibus Budget Reconciliation Act of 1985 (COBRA)
If an employer provides health coverage, it is required to comply with COBRA unless it falls within the following exceptions:
Small businesses that employ fewer than 20 employees on at least 50% of its working days during the preceding calendar year
Note: Employers must provide COBRA-type converge to employees on uniformed service leave, pursuant to the Uniformed Services Employment and Reemployment Rights Act of 1994 (USERRA), regardless of the number of employees they have
Fair Labor Standards Act (FLSA)
The Fair labor Standards Act (FLSA) prescribes standards for wages and overtime pay
The act is administered by the Wage and Hour Division of the Employment Standards Administration
Requires employers to pay covered employees who are not otherwise exempt at least the federal minimum wage ($5.15/h) and overtime pay of one-and-one-half-times the regular rate of pay
The Family and Medical Leave Act (FMLA)
Federal Eligibility Requirements
To be eligible for Federal FMLA leave, an employee must be employed by a covered employer:
For at least 12 months
For a minimum of 1,250 h in the 12 months immediately preceding the commencement of the leave
At a worksite employing 50 or more employees within a 75-mile radius of the worksite
FMLA (1993) gives eligible employees the right to take up to 12 weeks of unpaid leave, or paid leave if it has been earned, in any 12-month period:
For the birth of a child or the placement of a child with the employee by adoption or foster care
If the employee is needed to assist in care for a family member with a serious health condition
If the employee's own serious health condition renders the employee unable to do his/her job
FMLA entitles employees to be restored to the same or an equivalent position with equivalent pay, benefits, and working conditions upon their return from FMLA leave
In determining whether a company's workforce falls under the FMLA, are part-time employees included in the 50-employee count? Yes, every employee on the payroll must be counted. Employers also must also include workers on paid or unpaid leave and who are reasonably expected to return to active employment
When calculating the 1,250 h, should time spent on vacation, suspensions, etc., be included? No. Time spent on vacations or holidays, disciplinary suspension, medical leaves, etc., are not considered time worked in calculating the 1,250 h
Health Insurance Portability and Accountability Act of 1996 (HIPAA)
Ensures that all medical records, medical billing, and patient accounts meet certain consistent standards with regard to documentation, handling and privacy
Requires that all patients be able to access their own medical records, correct errors or omissions, and be informed how their personal information will be shared and used
Immigration Reform Control Act (IRCA)

(continued)

Table 2.5 (continued)

US Federal Employment Laws Summary
Please check with your state DOL, and / or attorney.
IRCA prohibits employers from knowingly hiring, recruiting, referring, or continuing the employment of aliens who are not authorized to work in the United States due to entering the country illegally or because of their immigration status
All public-and private-sector employers, regardless of size or number of employees, must verify the citizenship or employment status of new hires
Employers with more than three but fewer than 15 employees may not discriminate according to citizenship status or national origin
Verification requirements
When an applicant is hired, the employer must sign a Form I-9 attesting that it has examined appropriate documents, provided by the applicant, which verify the applicant's identity and authorization to work in the United States
The applicant must also attest on the form that he/she qualifies for employment
Verification must be done within 3 days of hire, but it could be extended to 90 days if the employee presents a receipt proving that an application for replacement of the authorization document has been filed
If employees are hired for fewer than 3 days, the I-9 form must be completed at the time of hire
Occupational Safety and Health Act (OSHA)
Employers have a duty under the OSHA to provide their employees with work and a workplace free from recognized, serious hazards
OSHA enforcement occurs through workplace inspections and investigations which can be prompted by employee complaints
Pregnancy Discrimination Act
An amendment to Title VII of the Civil Rights Act of 1964
Discrimination on the basis of pregnancy, childbirth or related medical conditions constitutes unlawful sex discrimination under Title VII
Women affected by pregnancy or related conditions must be treated in the same manner as other applicants or employees with similar abilities or limitations

Table 2.6 Health Information Privacy Act Requirements and Authorizations (HIPAA) for Release of Information

Requirements of the Privacy Rule
1. Notifying patients of the office privacy policy
2. Making a good faith effort to receive acknowledgement that the patient has received the office privacy policy
3. Training employees in the privacy procedures adopted by the office
4. Designating a privacy officer to oversee the implementation and progress of the privacy procedures
5. Securing patient information so that they are not readily available to unauthorized persons
Elements required in Authorization for Release of Information under HIPAA
1. A description of the information to be used or disclosed
2. Identification of the person (or class of persons) authorized to use or disclose the personal health information
3. Identification of the person (or class of persons) authorized to whom the covered entity may make the authorized disclosure of the personal health information
4. A description of each purpose of the use or disclosure
5. An expiration date or event
6. The patient's signature and date
Additional notifications required in the authorization
1. A statement that the patient may revoke the authorization in writing and instructions on how to exercise that right
2. A statement regarding the conditioning of the treatment on first obtaining authorization, and the consequence of not providing authorization
3. A statement regarding the potential for the personal health information to be re-disclosed by the recipient
An authorization is not valid if it contains any of the following defects
1. The expiration date has passed, or the expiration event has occurred, and the health care provider is aware of that fact
2. Any of the core elements or required notification statements are not present in the authorization
3. The authorization violates specifications in the Privacy Rule regarding authorizations or
4. The health care provider knows that the information in the authorization is not true

2.4 Site of Service Designation

Site of service considerations in the practice of reproductive endocrinology and infertility are multilayered. A recent study suggests that IVF is underutilized in the United States (<250 cycles /100,000 women) and this is primarily due to the lack of insurance coverage [4]. Comparing states with mandated insurance coverage to nonmandated states shows a significant increase in available providers, and higher utilization rates. The same study shows a positive correlation between the number of physicians in a fertility center and the number of cycles performed by each physician, encouraging a group model for physicians desiring a robust REI practice.

Over the last 30 years, there has been a shift from academic REI practices to private practice. Soules pointed out that the resources of an academic medical center should provide a competitive advantage to an academic ART program. However, a number of impediments found in the academic model must be addressed in order to create a successful marriage between academics and REI [5]. One of the first issues is to determine the site of service designation and hence management model. In order to complete effectively, many would argue that the academic ART program must designate the practice as a free-standing clinic also known as a site of service 11 designation, or function as such within a provider/hospital-based, site of service 22 clinical designation.

Recent developments in federal reimbursements for provider-based ambulatory services within academic medical centers (AMC) have prompted a reevaluation of outpatient reimbursements on the basis of site of service designation. Although Medicare is not a supplier of fertility services, many of the codes that apply to procedure and evaluation and management codes are based indirectly on Medicare reimbursement levels. Furthermore, most ART Centers began within the confines of the academic umbrella, but increasingly have found this financial and governance arrangement to be suboptimal in achieving maximal efficiency, growth and competitive footing. Thus, the ART centers associated with academic institutions must be aware of the history, advantages and disadvantages of various site of service designations and their resultant flow of funds and governance models.

In the early 1980s, Medicare implemented cost control mechanisms including an inpatient prospective payment system (PPS). Hospital payments were based on the cost-basis, but the Tax Equity and Fiscal Responsibility Act of 1982 (TEFRA) included a 40% discount on professional fees for Medicare services in provider-based facilities. Accordingly, many outpatient practices were designated as freestanding to avoid these professional fee discounts. In 1989, Medicare regulations relating to indirect medical education (IME) costs were changed so that IME was to be paid only for costs incurred in provider-based settings. Additionally, the resource-based relative value scale (RBRV) was deployed. The TEFRA discount was replaced with a site-of-service discount to be applied only to only certain services. In order to adjust to these Medicare reimbursement course changes, many AMCs countered by converting many outpatient freestanding clinics to hospital-based clinics in order to enhance Medicare reimbursements.

In 1997, the Balanced Budget Act (BBA) changed the reimbursement structures again and later implemented an outpatient PPS (2000). This system replaced a host of hospital outpatient payment mechanisms (e.g., lower of costs or charges, fee schedules, blended payment amounts) with 350+ ambulatory payment classifications (APCs). These changes caused significant concern that the APC implementation would remove the advantages of provider/hospital-based clinics. However, simultaneously the BBA established specific detailed guidelines defining provider/hospital-based clinics, causing AMCs serious reservations about converting these clinics to free-standing clinics because of the costly and labor intensive governance and operational changes that would be required, which were not familiar to many of these AMCs.

At present, designation as a freestanding or provider-based clinic affects the dollar value of the professional fee received and whether a facility fee is to be paid. Specifically, in free standing clinics, the physicians receive a full Medicare RBRV payment rate but no separate facility fee since the full RBRV payment includes a practice expense payment component. In the provider/hospital-based clinic, the physicians receive a reduced Medicare professional fee (meant to cover work and malpractice expenses and a reduced practice expense component). The hospital in a provider/hospital-based clinic model receives a separate facility fee from Medicare (i.e., practice expense reimbursement). The provider/hospital-based clinic receives a significantly higher amount when both the professional and facility fee are combined compared with the free-standing clinic model. Despite this fact, many services, including ART practices find that a detailed analysis of reimbursement flow of funds, and governance shows a distinct advantage to the free-standing clinic model.

Many academic medical centers have found it useful to evaluate the potential advantages/disadvantages of site of service designation, in a clinic-by-clinic fashion, using a detailed analysis of patient billing information that includes CPT codes, CPT code volumes, and location of service for all Medicare and third party payer charges. The patient level data must be categorized based on APCs, and relative values units calculated under both the freestanding and provider-based scenarios and adjusted by the various third party payer contracted rates.

Potential benefits of provider/hospital-based clinics include a significantly higher combined Medicare reimbursement, which likely does not affect an REI clinic; higher reimbursement from selected payers; opportunity for joint hospital-physician management; and, potentially greater flexibility to finance/grow physician practices through increased hospital revenue sharing. The potential disadvantages of provider/hospital-based clinics include: higher practices costs related to the hospital's employment wage and benefit rates, costly facilities and less efficient cost control; greater governance complexities and regulatory burdens and their associated inefficient bureaucracies; compliance issues related to hospital-based clinic standing, and the negative impact of split billings.

Advantages found in free-standing clinics include a practice expense payment component, which in the case of many REI practices outweighs the Medicare-based reimbursement model; a higher reimbursement from selected payers determined through an analysis of codes and reimbursements; the opportunity to solely manage the operation without restrictions imposed on the provider-based model; and greater flexibility and freedom in directing profit margins solely to the practice missions. Disadvantages include capitalization of the practice including clinic, equipment (ultrasounds, laboratory, furnishings, supplies), and staff; assuming responsibility for employment and discipline and other human resource management issues; assuming responsibility for all regulatory burdens associated with the practice including the College of American Pathologists (CAP); Certified Laboratory Improvement Amendments (CLIA), Society for Assisted Reproductive Technology (SART); and Food and Drug Administration regulations.

ART facilities in the United States have a complex mixture of self pay, and third party payers who base their reimbursement levels indirectly on Medicare rates. Many academic ART centers have, over the years, found the loss of or inadequate sharing of facility fee payments made to the hospital gradually drains the incentive of hardworking practitioners. In these cases, either an unfortunate complete separation of the ART center from academia, or a less drastic separation of the ART clinic from the hospital have been the outcome. Alternatively, well governed and transparent hospital systems accounting for the differences between the site of service designations have been successful despite the designation. Regardless of the site of service designation utilized, transparency and clear communication regarding the facts surrounding the individual practice must be visible and understood by departmental, hospital and school of medicine leadership in order to perpetuate the successful union of academia and ART.

2.5 Optimizing Practice Outcomes Through Quality Improvement

Because REI practices combine both medical and laboratory medicine, understanding of a number of quality improvement management tools is required. Fertility practices function under a number of federal regulations [HCFA (CMS)-88; FDA-21CFR 606 and 21CFR211; FDA GTPs-21CFR 1271; CMS-CLIA 42 CFR] and accrediting organizations (Joint Commission on Accreditation of Healthcare Organization (JACAHO), the College of American Pathologists (CAP); and, the Society for Assisted Reproductive Technology (SART)). Recent establishment of the Food and Drug Administration's Good Tissue Practices regulations (Section 361 Public Health Services Act 21 CFR 1271.160) regarding egg and sperm donors and surrogacy arrangements mandate that each center establish and maintain a quality program which is designed to prevent, detect, and correct deficiencies that could lead to the risk of introduction, transmission, or spread of communicable diseases.

The major requirements of these regulations are to develop standard operating procedures (SOPs) for the following: the organization's quality improvement program; training and education; resource management; equipment management and upkeep; supplier and client issues; process control; documents and record management; deviation, nonconformance, and adverse (error) event management; internal and external assessment (audits); process improvement through corrective and preventative actions; and facilities management and safety programs. Furthermore, any software that is part of the center must be validated (installation, operational, and product qualification). In the past, the majority of these regulations could be managed through the andrology/embryology component of the fertility center. However, the broad reach of the regulations now applicable require the full participation and adherence of both REI and andrology/embryology supervisors and staff. Supervisors of academic, free-standing or hospital-based clinics must assume these responsibilities and insure that an effective and functional program is operational.

The optimization of practice outcomes also suggests a reworking of the SART CORS IVF data collection system, which is considered by many to be inadequate for the appropriate biostatistical analysis of outcomes from IVF. Hopefully, future leaders will accept this challenge and make the necessary changes.

The American Society for Reproductive Medicine (ASRM) recommends that all ART practices participate in the Centers for Disease Control (CDC)-SART registry data collection. From this data, each practice releases identifiable, clinic-specific success rates. The embryology laboratory is required to maintain a policies and procedures manual and personnel employment, training, evaluations, and continuing education. Details of employees who handle gametes and embryos during a cycle must be documented. All of the laboratory records and documentation must be maintained for time periods specified in federal, state and local laws or for a minimum of 10 years beyond the final disposition of embryos or gametes. The records must be maintained on site for 2 years. In the event that the laboratory ceases operation, provisions must be made for these records to be maintained according to the time frame required.

Practices must adhere to ASRM, SART, and Federal Trade Commission guidelines relating to advertising and the use of SART statistics [6]. These guidelines, presently under revision, state that all claims be supported by reliable data and avoid misleading the public into believing that the chances for success are greater than they actually are. Furthermore, practice statistics should include all initiated cycles, including research cycles, and that the method used to calculate success. The numerator and denominator must be specified (such as live births per cycle initiated, retrieved, and transferred). The number of cycles that comprise both the numerator and denominator must also be reported. If advertised procedures or protocols are investigational or experimental, authorization by a properly constituted institutional review board (IRB) must be documented. Whenever rates are quoted the following statement must be included, "A comparison of clinic success rates may not be meaningful because patient medical characteristics and treatment approaches may vary from clinic to clinic." This statement clarifies for patients that comparing success rates between practices is invalid. Using SART Clinic specific data for advertising/marketing that ranks or compares clinics or practices is unacceptable and is not permitted.

2.6 Uniform Laws, Regulations, and Case Law Pertaining to Art

In light of the complex situations that can evolve in ART, many now recommend separate legal counsel for couples undergoing nontraditional parenting arrangements, such as sperm donation, egg donation, surrogacy, disposition of frozen genetic materials, and same-sex parenting. Laws regarding these issues vary by state. A nonexhaustive review of case law and Uniform Laws regarding ART and its variations is included below to highlight potential conflicts that may arise. The ART practice requires competent legal counsel in developing appropriate informed consent and disposition documents.

2.6.1 Case Law Regarding Sperm Donation

(laws vary by state)

2.6.1.1 Re Marriage of Witbeck-Wildhagen (IL 1996)

Consents required for sperm donation from both intended parents. Married couple utilized sperm donation, but husband had not consented to sperm donation, therefore husband could not be held responsible to assume parentage.

2.6.1.2 Laura G. v. Peter G. (NY 2007)

Intended fathers allowing donor sperm give implied consent. State law required written consent for sperm donation, however, husband's actions implied consent and child support was required from the intended father. Intended fathers should sign consent in writing for sperm donation.

2.6.1.3 Thomas S. v. Robin Y. (NY 1994)

Sperm donor authorization document determines donor status. Same-sex female couple were using a friend as a known donor without consent document. The court awarded the donor the right to pursue visitation privileges, which likely would not have occurred if a sperm donation consent had been signed.

2.6.1.4 Stevens v. Deborah D. (CA 2005)

Single women using donor sperm should obtain "donor" consent. A single woman with a known partner provided sperm without consent or agreement. The court held that the sperm donor was not the legal father despite the lack documentation of "donor" status. A sperm donor has no rights and the fertility center should verify that the sperm donor is actually a "donor" and that there is no other alternative understanding.

2.6.1.5 Ferguson v. McKierman (PA 2004)

Sperm donor authorization required to avoid responsibility. A verbal agreement between a single woman and male friend, whereby male would act as a sperm donor and have no obligations to the child, was challenged. Court held that sperm donor was liable for child support and oral agreement was not enforceable.

2.6.1.6 Jackson v. Jackson (OH 2000)

Contemporaneous consent with end dates advised. Husband had initially consented to sperm donation and wife then used donor sperm 2 years after original consent and husband had the burden of proof to document a withdrawal of consent. Consents should have end dates.

2.6.2 Egg Donors

ART practices should be cautious to consider the rights of both the intended parents and the egg donor. Both indeed are patients, and in consideration of the potential complications associated with egg donation, many ethicists and legal scholars suggest that a supplemental insurance policy should be purchased by the intended parents for the donor. Furthermore, some would recommend that the donor be treated by a physician other than the physician monitoring the egg recipient cycle to avoid conflicts of interest. A study by Mastroianni revealed that potential donors were given inadequate information regarding potential risks of the donation stimulation regimen, retrieval and post procedure risks [7].

2.6.2.1 Case Law Regarding Egg Donation

(laws vary by state)

McDonald v. McDonald (NY 1994)

Intent governs parentage when questions arise regarding parentage after egg donation. Husband argued for the custody of child born through donor egg IVF based on ex-wife's lack of a genetic relationship to the child. Court ruled that the gestational intended mother is considered the mother.

2.6.3 *Traditional Surrogacy*

(laws vary by state)

2.6.3.1 Baby M (NJ 1988)

Risk of traditional surrogacy includes potential for parental rights to the surrogate. Traditional surrogate asserted and was granted parental rights and visitation. Baby M has since terminated the rights of her intended parents and was adopted by the surrogate.

2.6.3.2. C of on behalf of T. v. G. (NY 2001)

In traditional surrogacy, parental rights could be granted to the surrogate. Same-sex male couple who executed a traditional surrogacy arrangement, but after birth, the surrogate sought and was granted custody if she would return the fee paid by the intended parents and pay child support.

2.6.3.3. T. v. G. (NY 2001)

Risk of traditional surrogacy includes potential for parental rights to the surrogate. Same-sex male couple entered into traditional surrogacy and surrogate later sought custody of the children. Despite unenforceable contract, there was evidence of intent and visitation, only privileges given to surrogate if she relinquished the fee to intended parents and to paying child support.

2.6.4 *Gestational Surrogacy*

(laws vary by state)

2.6.4.1 Belsito v. Clark (OH 1994)

Gestational surrogacy upheld by court that deemed genetics over birth in assigning motherhood. Court in this case held that birth test is secondary to genetics in determining "motherhood."

2.6.4.2 J.F. v. D.B. (PA 2006)

Genetics over birth in gestational surrogacy upheld. Surrogate took physical custody of triplets. Court ruled that no law permits genetically unrelated surrogate to have custody.

2.6.4.3 Johnson v. Calvert (CA 1993)

Couple with intent to parent are the parents. Couple entered agreement with a surrogate, and court ruled that where there is a tie between giving birth and a genetic connection, the court will look at the intent to procreate in deciding parentage.

2.6.4.4 Re Buzzanca (CA 1998)

Couple with intent to parent are the parents. Couple utilized egg donor, sperm donor, and gestational surrogate and husband later claimed nonparent status because there was no genetic connection. Court ruled that intent justified his responsibility.

2.6.5 *Disposition of Frozen Genetic Material*

(laws vary by state)

2.6.5.1 Litowitz v. Litowitz (WA 2002)

Consent document options are critical in disposition. Embryos remained after using donor egg IVF. Couple separated with wife desiring another child and husband choosing donation of the embryos to third party. Court ruled embryos would be destroyed as noted on the consent document.

2.6.5.2 Roman v. Roman (TX 2006)

Courts look to consent forms in the event of a dispute. Married couple with three frozen embryos. In divorce proceedings, the wife sought use of frozen embryos to have a child on her own. Husband wanted embryos discarded. Court ruled consent option of disposition in the event of divorce as enforceable.

2.6.5.3 A.Z.v.B.Z. (MA 2000)

Consent documents must be administered properly. Cryopreservation document stated that, in the event of separation, the wife could use the cryopreserved embryos. Consent document was not properly administered to husband. After divorce, husband wanted to prevent use of the embryos and court ruled that involuntary parenthood was not enforceable.

2.6.5.4 Davis v. Davis (TN 1992)

When there is no consent, there is a right to not procreate. Divorced couple with frozen embryos, wife wanted to donate to third party and husband chose to discard. No consents. Court ruled without consent there is a right to not procreate.

2.6.6 *Same-Sex Issues*

(laws vary by state)

2.6.6.1 K.M. v. E.G. (CA 2005)

Same-sex cases pose unique intent, birth test and genetic questions. Same-sex female couple with K.M. donating the egg to E.G. who carried the child. EG refused to allow KM visitation after breakup. K.M. had signed donor form relinquishing rights as a parent. Court deemed both K.M. and E.G. as "mother."

2.6.6.2 Chambers v. Chambers (DE 2002)

Nongenetic same sex partner can be held responsible. A biological mother who used donor sperm to conceive a child with former nonbiological intended "mother" sued for support. Court held that, despite absence of genetic connection, the ex-partner's actions constituted a symbolic act of procreation and intended parenthood.

2.6.6.3 Re Parentage of A/B. (IN 2004)

Nongenetic same-sex partner can obtain parental rights. Former nongenetic partner sued for parental rights and was granted these rights.

2.6.6.4 Kamierazak v. Query (FL 1999)

Nonbiological partner refused parental rights. In a custody dispute between lesbian partners, the court held that since no statute allowed nonbiological partners parental rights, she would not be allowed custody.

2.6.6.5 Re Adoption of A.W., J.W. and M.R. (IL 2003)

Nonbiological partner refused parental rights. Former lesbian copartner refused parental rights to children born during the relationship because the nonbiological partner had no standing.

2.6.6.6 Jacob v. Shultz-Jacob and Frampton (NY 2007)

Three-way parenthood ruling. A sperm donor who fathered two children, voluntarily contributed financial support and interacted in their lives was found to be a biological father with obligations to the children which their rearing mothers could not waive. Case ensued after separation of the same sex-couple.

2.6.7 *Posthumous Use of Genetic Material*

(laws vary by state)

2.6.7.1 Estate of Woodward v. Comm of Social Services (MA 2000)

Wife delivered child conceived with sperm from deceased husband. Social Security benefits denied for offspring.

2.6.7.2 Gillett-Netting v. Barnhart (AZ 2004)

Husband banked sperm secondary to cancer for later use. Husband confirmed desire to father child after death using his frozen sperm. Wife had twins and applied for Social Security benefits on behalf of children. Benefits denied by Social Security because children were not dependent of husband at the time of death. Court found that Social Security should provide benefits.

2.6.7.3 In the Matter of Martin B, 2007 NY Slip Op (NY 2007)

Two children born to their widowed mother conceived from her deceased husband's sperm are considered his children and as such, are entitled to inherit from their grandfather's estate.

The ASRM has clearly defined guidelines on posthumous donation summarized in Table 2.7 [8]. Case law relevant to assisted reproduction can be found at: http://www.asrm.org/Media/LegallySpeaking/legally_index.html

2.6.8 *Uniform Laws*

In addition to regulations affecting a fertility practice, a number of Uniform Laws affect our practice. It is not unreasonable to view the practice of assisted reproduction as one of the most regulated medical specialties in the world. The Uniform Parentage Act (UPA) and Uniform Status of Children of Assisted Conception Act (USCACA) establishes regulatory guidelines by which our specialty operates (Table 2.8).

Table 2.7 Posthumous donation

Many programs for assisted reproduction have consent forms that stipulate the disposition of gametes and embryos, including disposition after death of one or both gamete donors or after a certain period of time. If donation after death is declined, this should be honored. Whether a time limit should be put on how long after death such gametes or embryos might still be used is problematic. It is not clear how the interval between death and use would affect the process and the outcome, but the general presumption is that such use should occur within an interval of no more than a few years. Programs are urged to insist that donors make their wishes known. If no decision on disposition after death has been made, one would expect that in most instances this would preclude any posthumous use.
A request by a husband or wife for use of stored gametes or embryos to override a prior denial of posthumous reproduction by the deceased spouse should not be honored. A spouse's request that sperm or ova be obtained terminally or soon after death without the prior consent or known wishes of the deceased spouse need not be honored. Such requests pose judgmental questions that should be answered within the context of the individual circumstances and applicable state laws. Many programs stipulate that unless otherwise instructed, frozen embryos will be discarded after death of either or both partners. Sperm banks are not uniform in the way they deal with saving or discarding samples from deceased donors, and a sperm bank may or may not know of a donor's death if all testing of the donor to exclude infection already has been performed.

Ethics Committee of the ASRM. Posthumous donation. Fertil Steril 2004; 82; S260–S262

Table 2.8 Uniform Parentage Act Summary (1973)

Husband and wife must provide written consent for donor insemination. Furthermore, the donor must sign a consent to act solely as a donor. The Donor is not considered the father but the intended father is assigned this right. Section 7 (2000 amendment) extends the act to include assisted reproduction including IVF and addresses death and divorce. Section 8 applies to gestational agreements and allows a written agreement between the gestational mother, her husband, donor and intended parents. No limitations are placed on an egg donor's or gestational carrier's right to make decisions regarding their own health and/or the health of the embryo or fetus. The intended parents must be married and both must sign the agreement. The court is to be petitioned for validation of the agreement. The court will validate the agreement, only if: the couple have lived in the state for 90 days; there is a medical necessity; a home study has been performed; the intended parents, gestational carrier; and donor, if any, have all entered into the written agreement; a provision is made for all reasonable health care expenses, but insurance is not required; a reasonable compensation is allowed for the gestational carrier. The intended parents must file notice with the court within 30 days of birth.

2.7 Resolving Problems

Recent establishment of the FDA's Good Tissue Practices regulations (Section 361 Public Health Services Act 21 CFR 1271.160) regarding egg and sperm donors and surrogacy arrangements, require that each center establish and maintain a quality program which is designed to prevent, detect, and correct deficiencies that could lead to the risk of introduction, transmission, or spread of communicable diseases.

As noted previously in Optimizing Practice Outcomes: Quality Improvement, practices are now required to have an active quality improvement program which includes training and education; resource management; equipment management and upkeep; supplier and client issues; process control; documents and record management including software validation; deviation, nonconformance, and adverse (error) event management; internal and external assessment (audits); process improvement through corrective and preventative actions; and facilities management and safety programs. Supervisors of academic, free-standing or provider/hospital-based clinics must assume these responsibilities and insure that an effective and functional program is operational. Analysis of processes and identification of problems and their causes are key components of ART quality improvement programs. A brief familiarization with analysis techniques is instructive.

2.7.1 Six Sigma

Six Sigma is a quality improvement methodology to reduce errors in manufacturing originally formulated by Bill Smith, a senior engineer at Motorola in 1986 [9].

Six Sigma provided Motorola the ability to address manufacturing quality concerns and support functions throughout its organization, from manufacturing to support functions. The application of Six Sigma also contributed to Motorola winning the Malcolm Baldrige National Quality award in 1988. The impact of the Six Sigma process on improving business performance has been dramatic and applicable to other organizations, such as General Electric, Allied Signal, and Citibank.

Six Sigma methodology is increasingly considered a mission-critical best practice, among mid-sized and smaller firms. Motorola claims over 20 years a $17 billion dollar (US) in savings as of 2006, which they attribute to the program.

Six Sigma asserts the following guiding principles:

1. Continuous efforts to reduce variation in process outputs is key to success.
2. Healthcare and laboratory processes can be measured, analyzed, improved and controlled.
3. Succeeding in achieving a sustained quality improvement requires commitment from the entire organization, particularly from top-level management.

The applicability of this quality manufacturing methodology has been modified for retail and healthcare applications. The method has two techniques DMAIC (Table 2.9) and DMADV (Table 2.10) which were inspired by W. Edward Deeming's Plan-Do-Act-Check cycle [10]. DMAIC is used to improve the business process and DMADV is used to develop new successful processes. Critics of the program report that a number of large companies have failed to realize the benefits noted by Motorola and that it is designed to fix existing processes and doesn't help define new, innovative methodologies. Regardless of the potential weaknesses in the program, it has shown success in the laboratory-based medical service industry.

Training in these techniques is available through Motorola University online and in regional classes. (http://www.motorola.com/motorolauniversity.jsp?ref=modules)

Table 2.9 DMAIC improves processes

DMAIC consists of the following five steps to improve processes in medical practices
Define the process improvement goals that are consistent with the mission, vision and values of the practice
Measure the current processes and collect data for future comparisons
Analyze to verify various relationships and causalityof factors. Determine what the relationships are, and attempt to consider all factors
Improve or optimize the process based upon the analysis using a variety of enhancement techniques
Control to ensure that variations in standard processes are corrected. Set up simulations to establish process capacity and standardization. After implementation continue to monitor the process

Some managers have added DMAICR (**R**ealize). Critics contend that focusing on the financial gains realized through Six Sigma is counterproductive and that financial gains are only by products of a good process improvement

Table 2.10 DMADV develops new processes

DMADV involves the following five steps in developing new processes:
Define the goals of the design activity that are consistent with the mission, vision and values of the practice
Measure and identify CTQs (critical to quality), desired outcomes, process capabilities, and risk assessments
Analyze to develop and design process and outcome alternatives, create high level process and outcome design and evaluate the designed process capacity to obtain desired outcomes
Design details, optimize the process, and plan for process/outcome verification. This phase requires simulations
Verify the process/outcome, perform simulations, and finally implement the process

2.7.2 Root Cause Analysis

In the analysis phase, useful techniques include Root Cause [11] and Ishikawa Fishbone Analysis [12].

The goal of a Root Cause Analysis is to find out

- What happened
- Why did it happen
- What to do to prevent it from happening again.

Root Cause Analysis is a tool for identifying prevention strategies utilized within a culture of safety and beyond the culture of blame. In Root Cause Analysis, basic and contributing causes are discovered in a process similar to diagnosis of disease – with the goal always in mind of preventing recurrence.

Root Cause Analysis is a process that is:

- Inter-disciplinary and involves experts from the frontline services
- Involves all who are the most familiar with the situation
- Layered, and continually digs deeper by asking why, why, why at each level of cause and effect
- Reformative, and identifies changes that need to be made to systems
- Impartial and avoids the assignment of blame

Root Cause Analysis must include the:

- Determination of human and other factors
- Determination of related processes and systems
- Analysis of underlying cause and effect systems through a series of why questions
- Identification of risks and their potential contributions
- Determination of potential improvement in processes or systems including evidence-based information

The Five Whys used in Root Cause Analysis are an analysis tool that doesn't involve data segmentation, hypothesis testing, regression or other advanced statistical tools, and in many cases can be completed without a data collection plan thus making it useful in all situations, with or without a Six Sigma project. Through repeatedly asking the question "Why" (five is not an absolute rule), organizations can peel away the layers of symptoms which can lead to the root cause of a problem. Not infrequently, the reason for a problem will lead to another question (Table 2.11).

2.7.3 Ishikawa Fishbone Analysis

An Ishikawa fishbone (cause and effect) diagram (Fig. 2.7) helps groups explore visually all potential or real causes that result in a problem or process failure. Major inputs to the

Table 2.11 The five whys

1. Writing down the specific problem. Identifying the problem helps the assembled team to formalize the problem, describe it completely, and focus specifically on the same problem.
2. The facilitator asks: "Why did the problem happen?" and writes the answer down below the problem.
3. If the answer provided doesn't clearly identify the root cause of the problem written in Step 1, ask "Why?" again and write that answer down.
4. Loop back to step 3 until the team agrees that the problem's root cause has been identified. This may take fewer or more than five "Whys?".

Problem statement: Patients are unhappy because they are waiting too long for ultrasounds performed for ovulation induction and IVF

1. *Why* are the ultrasounds taking so long? Because turnover in the ultrasound rooms has been delayed by 7–20 min per room according to a recent time/flow study compared to a previous study.
2. *Why* did the time/flow study change? Because the MA is less efficient in bring the patients back to the room and we don't get the patient out after the ultrasound as quickly as we previously did.
3. *Why* is the MA less efficient? Why is there a delay "post scan – out of room time"? Because we have changed the time retrievals are performed to coincide with ultrasound monitoring scheduling which diverts the attention of the MA to other duties associated with the post-retrieval process and not the ultrasounds. One new physician has increased in room consultation time with the patients rather than diverting that conversation to the consult room, thus slowing turnover in the ultrasound rooms.
4. *Why* did we move retrieval time to coincide with ultrasounds? Why does the physician consult immediately after the ultrasound? Because the clinic manager wanted to control overtime costs associated with retrievals performed outside of routine business hours. The retrieval times were simultaneously scheduled during morning ultrasound hours. Because the physician feels "better care" is provided with immediate consultation rather than consult room consultation.

Resolution: A time/flow study showed the staffing ratio and ultrasound machine availability to still be adequate. It suggested the "distraction" of the MAs (only a few minutes, but cumulatively up to 1 h) associated with the help they provided in post-retrieval recovery could be eliminated by having them carry an office pager that would page them each time a patient arrived for an ultrasound study with the patient's name. Once they had brought the patient back to the room they would erase that page. A survey to patients over 1 week revealed that patients did appreciate physician attention, but in fact, would rather dress and discuss them in the consult office. All physicians were advised that it was policy to complete the ultrasound and say, "Please dress now and we will discuss your findings and plan in the consultation room." Physicians were advised of the need to complete the ultrasound examination within 5 min. Implementation and re-implementation of these practices resulted in the previous time/flow patterns that accommodated the clinic volume and improved patient satisfaction with only a $90 dollar per month cost increase and the complete elimination of the previous overtime expenditures for "outside of normal business hour" retrievals.

development of the problem can be established on the fishbone such as: People; Policies; Procedures; and Technology and then the participants use the Five Whys technique to drill down to the root causes.

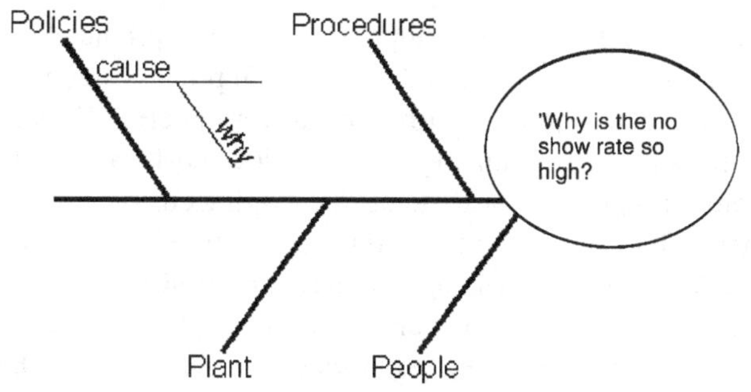

Fig. 2.7 Ishikaura fishbone diagram

To create a fishbone diagram, start with stating the problem as a question, such as "Why is the no show rate so high?" The team should agree on the statement of the problem and then place this question in a box at the "head" of the fishbone. Posing it as a "why" question will help in brainstorming, as each root cause idea answers the question.

The rest of the fishbone then consists of one line drawn across the page, attached to the problem statement, and several lines, or "bones," coming out vertically from the main line. These branches are labeled with different categories. The categories you use are up to you to decide. There are a few standard choices: people, policies, procedures, and technology.

2.7.4 Lean Process

In 1913, Henry Ford integrated interchangeable parts and defined work tasks with conveyors to create what he called "flow production." The revolutionary "assembly line" concept provided simultaneous delivery of perfectly fitting components directly to line side. The problem with his system was limited variety of the product.

To provide variety, automobile production systems regressed toward process areas with much longer throughput times. More efficient machines lowered costs per process step, but in most cases increased throughput times and inventories. Furthermore, more robust information management systems were required.

In the late 1940s, Kiichiro Toyoda and Taiichi Ohno, and others at Toyota determined that a series of simple innovations, known as the Toyota Production System, would provide both continuity in process flow and a wide variety of products. This system changed focus from individual machines and their utilization, to the flow of the product through the process. By right-sizing machines for the actual volume, introducing self-monitoring machines to ensure quality, lining the machines up in process sequence, pioneering quick machine setups so each could produce small volumes of many parts, and having each process step notify the previous step of its current needs for materials, it would be possible to obtain high quality, low cost variety with rapid throughput in order to meet changing customer preferences. The process of LEAN was outlined in the book The Machine That Changed the World (1990) by James P. Womack, Daniel Roos, and Daniel T. Jones. ISBN-10: 0743299795 (Fig. 2.8). Subsequently, the same authors distilled the lean process into five key principles adjusted for medical processes in Lean Thinking (1996), ISBN-13: 9780684810355 (Fig. 2.9).

Lean Process principles:

- Specify the value(s) desired by the patient
- Identify the process stream for each product that provides the specified value and challenge all of the wasted steps in that process
- Make the process flow around the patient adding value-added steps
- Introduce points where continuous flow is possible
- Manage toward perfection so that the number of steps and the amount of time and information needed to serve the customer continually falls

Tables 2.12 and 2.13 provide overviews for determining value and the Lean Process, respectively.

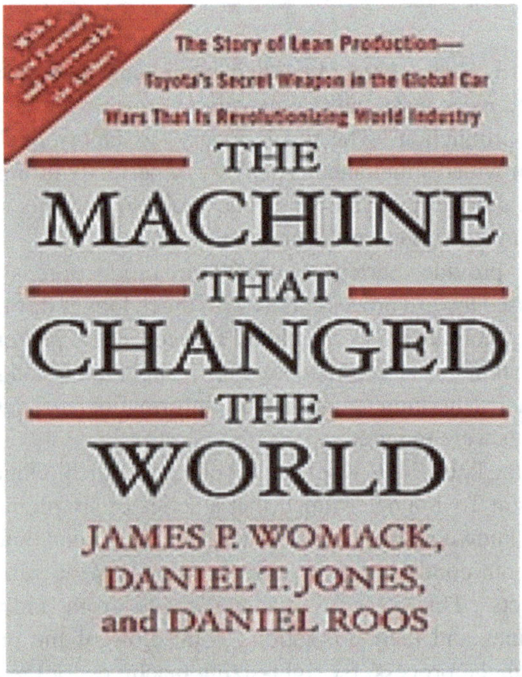

Fig. 2.8 The Machine That Changed the World (1990) by James P. Womack, Daniel Roos, and Daniel T. Jones. (ISBN-10:0743299795)

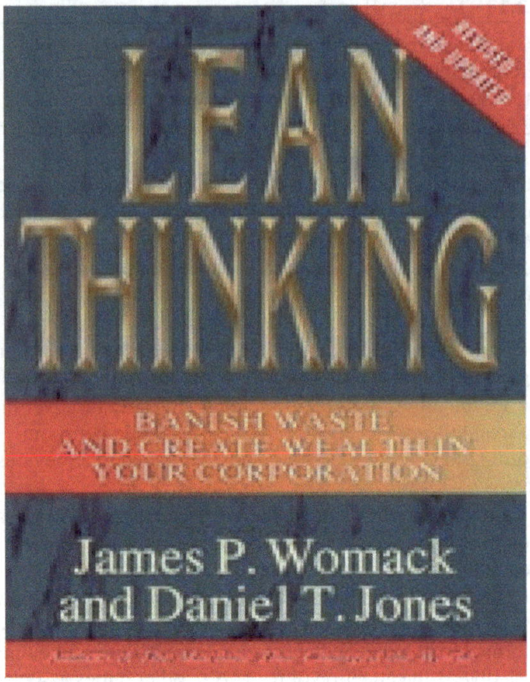

Fig. 2.9 Lean Thinking (1996) by James P. Womack, Daniel Roos, and Daniel T. Jones. (ISBN-13:9780684810355)

2.8 Capital, Capital Management and Capital Expenditures

Capital is defined as any asset, tangible or intangible, that is held as a long-term investment. Capital, combined with operating cash flows is the currency that allows practices to fulfill their missions of clinical care, education and in academic settings, research. Capital allows the practice to expand, buy equipment, add staff and faculty, finance receivables, conduct preliminary research with the goal of obtaining extramural funding, and build reserves.

Every medical practice must deal with capital and capitalization issues on a continuous basis. Three types of capital and their management are required:

- Investment Capital: comes from your institution, department or division in an academic setting, individual physicians/embryologists, and/or an investor or donor. If you are in a University setting and you have created a site of service 11 clinic /private clinic, some combination of the above is likely. Capitalizing the operation is like buying stock in a publicly traded firm, except the investments made these small medical practices differ from other investments because there is no after-market for the contribution. Therefore, you typically won't get your invested capital out until you sell the clinic. For this reason investment capital is commonly kept as low as possible. This is particularly true in the University setting, even if the

Table 2.12 Determining value in the lean process

In the lean process, every step within every activity in your practice – from the check-in to the rooming processes, to ultrasound monitoring, to discussion of medication use, to medication dispensing – should add value for your patients. While, some steps or processes may not be directly valuable to patients they may be essential to operating your business. The point of the lean process is to make the patient's experience as value-added as possible. When you create a value-added experience for the patient, you also create a more efficient, and effective practice.

To understand what is truly important to your patients, there are several ways of collecting their views. Surveys regarding specific processes and open ended questionnaires elicit needed changes. Mock patient visits are also enlightening. Periodic phone calls to your own practice will demonstrate scheduling, patient service issues and are often available through the institution (Mystery Shopping). Having a monitor/patient advocate sit through patient your processes from registration to discharge will be uniquely informative. (See the Dartmouth workbook and turn to the "Through the Eyes of Your Patients" worksheet for help in conducting a walk-through.) Stepping back and simply observing the flow of your care process will also provide additional insights. A tool for these observations is the "Gaining Customer Knowledge" worksheet, found at http://cms.dartmouth.edu/images/PDF%20Files/GainCustKnowWrksht.pdf.

The Picker Institute has identified eight dimensions of patient-centered care: (1) respect for their values, preferences and needs, (2) information, communication and education, (3) access to care, (4) emotional support, (5) involvement of family and friends, (6) continuity of care and seamless transitions, (7) physical comfort and (8) coordination and integration of care. Details on the eight dimensions can be found at: http://nrcpicker.com/Default.aspx?DN=112,22,2,1,Documents.

Once you understand what your patients want and need from your practice, you can select one aspect of care delivery (e.g., IVF consults with physicians and nursing, new infertility visits, follicle monitoring, sonohysterography, hysteroscopy, IVF retrievals) that you will focus on first. The process you select should be based on your assessment of patients' needs. Identify who will be involved in improving the process and how you intend to go about it. A key principle of lean design is that those who do the work should design the work based on their personal knowledge of the patients' needs. You next examine the processes, also called "value streams," with the goal of eliminating all steps that do not add value.

Table 2.13 Lean process overview

1. *Map the current state.* Determine the beginning and ending points of the process from the patient's perspective. Map all the main steps. To insure accuracy, walk the process, considering how, when and where people move and act during the process. Determine who the customers and providers are, when and how information is recorded and exchanged and what technologies are applied, sequencing of the steps, what triggers each work activity, and how much time is spent at each step, and for the entire process including waiting time. Stay focused on high-level steps and focus on the usual process, not on the exceptions.
2. *Identify waste.* Next, identify any flow problems and/or any steps that do not add value. These flow constraints and value-devoid activities are the waste in your process. Lean design identifies seven categories of waste, which can be applied to the practice setting:

   Overproduction involves completing any work that isn't needed for an encounter, this could include discussing unproven adjuvant to therapeutic regimens with no proven benefit.

   Motion refers to any unnecessary movement of patients, staff or physicians. This can be associated with inadequate space planning for high utilization periods or lack of equipment (ultrasound).

   Material movement refers to any unnecessary transfers of materials or information, such as the hand-off of patient intake forms from the front office to the back office to the physician. Chart and paper shuffling are common material movement waste areas.

   Waiting refers to any delays or idle time involving the patient, physician or staff, such as patients waiting for an exam room to be readied, physician or staff waiting for a report to be faxed, physicians waiting for equipment or disposables.

   Inventory involves any information or materials waiting to be used, such as sonohysteroscopy catheters, a stack of unread laboratory reports or piles of patient booklets sitting in the waiting area.

   Inappropriate processing refers to handling work in a way that is excessive, such as completing all paperwork in triplicate or scheduling separate visits for various evaluations when one visit would suffice. These inappropriate processing encounters are often driven by our payer systems.

   Rework involves any unnecessary work required because of an error, such as sending the patient back to the laboratory because a lab order was incomplete.
3. *Plan the future state.* As plan the new process, build in the changes that will eliminate waste problems and maximize value. Some design features to consider in rebuilding the process include the following:

   Bring work to the patient.

   Eliminate needless work. Eliminate handoffs or outdated steps you're completing out of obsolete routines.

   Do all possible to make the physician more effective with the patient.

   Make sure your process involves direct communication between parties.

   Employ technology to improve your process.

   Create broad work roles so your staff can complete their work more efficiently and reduce the number of handoffs.
4. *Test and revise the new process.* With the redesigned process map, test it. Identify your test procedures, who will be involved, duration of the test, and how you will measure efficacy. There are a number of excellent resources for using the plan-do-study-act cycle for rapidly testing and implementing change.

clinic is a site 11 clinic/private clinic, the University is the ultimate owner and the proceeds of sale would typically be property of the University.

To capitalize in a University setting, the practice could propose investment by the university medical group with or without a return on investment. Another option is to tax departmental or divisional revenues to create an investment reserve. Additionally, the practice could request departmental tax reductions to increase cash flow for investment. Last, gifts from donors are a potential source of capitalization. Gifts from donors are usually given for a specific purpose, but not always. The donor should be approached with a business plan and the return on investment terms to using their donation for capitalization. These funds could be granted or borrowed with some return. The communications should be documented in writing and coordinated through the University Development Office.

- Retained Earnings: represents the profit made that is left in the clinic, after all expenses have been paid, including physician compensation, for strategic initiatives; growth, staff, clinical expansion, research, or educational endeavors. This earned income must be transparent and on the table for discussion within the academic setting. Institutions that cannot create a balance sheet showing annual direct earnings will have difficulty growing this service line and retaining quality faculty. Both supervising institutions and bankers appreciate seeing retained earnings on your balance sheet, perhaps even more than investment capital because it conveys two things: (1) your medical practice operates profitably; (2) there is fiscal responsibility in the organization which looks to future strategic plans rather than immediate distribution. In a University setting, there are not tax disincentives to Retained Earnings as there are in the for profit setting where Retained Earnings are taxed in addition to distributions made to owners. This advantage allows the practice to keep the profit margin to reinvest in the strategic mission.
- Borrowed Funds: are used to capitalize new space, equipment, faculty, staff, or other capital expenditures which are borrowed from a bank, individual, or in the university setting, the division, department, institution, or an individual donation based on institutional guidelines. Debt is the most common way to capitalize your practice. Debt never sleeps or takes a holiday and must be serviced creating an incremental drain on the practice's liquidity. The cash flow of the practice must be capable of making these payments. Debt should be used as a tool, along with the other capitalization mechanisms to meet the initiative and goals of the practice.

To determine the clinic's capital requirements your financial advisor and clinic directors must know projected volumes and reimbursements and how much is required to operate the clinic. A clear estimate of how long it will take you to collect, and the terms of payment for purchases will be required to plot a financial operating timeline. The timeline will initially reveal negative numbers on startup of a clinic and often with major capital expenditures and identify new capital required monthly.

Some common sense rules are instructive in allocating capital. First, don't deplete operating cash to purchase large capital items when interest rates are low. Second, avoid borrowing money for operating expenses. Third, the long-term goal of the clinic should be to fund growth more from retained earnings and less from debt.

Every dollar of profit left in the clinic as retained earnings is a step toward financial security and the power to move nimbly on strategic initiatives determined by your group. Retained earnings is the working capital that you don't have to borrow from the bank, institution, individual, and dilute your ownership stake with other investors. It is the safety net required for uncertain economic times that may dramatically affect volumes in a medical clinic providing primarily nonreimbursed medical procedures. Having said that, most clinics need growth capital faster than profits will generate in retained earnings. Thus, the risk/benefit discussions and analyses that require professional business management combined with supervising physician/embryologist input.

2.8.1 Capital Expenditures

Capital expenditure analyses are required not only in the initial practice plan, but with each major capital expenditure in all medical clinics. There are multiple project valuation methods including payback, average return on book value, internal rate of return and the most comprehensive: the Net Present Value (NPV) analysis. This calculation estimates the project's impact on the clinic's overall valuation and whether this number will be positive or negative long-term. Three steps are required for the NPV analysis: first, a forecast of Net Cash Flow (after taxes if a for-profit organization); second, a determination of the present value of each year's cash flow by discounting cash flows; and finally, subtraction of the project's up-front cost from the discounted cash flows.

For the net cash flow analysis, a number of questions should be considered regarding the incremental revenues and costs. When considering incremental volumes and revenues, one should determine whether if the service is offered by competitors; how current practice patterns will impact utilization whether new technology will eventually render the project useless; how present and future payer mix will affect reimbursement; and whether reimbursement will remain stable over time. The incremental cost analysis includes consideration of the additional staff requirements; the additional supply and equipment required; depreciation; and, expected increases in the incremental expenses.

Net Income
+ Interest Expense
+ Depreciation and Amortization
- Capital Expenditures
- Working Capital
Net Cash Flow

The time value of money assumes that money earned today can earn interest and money earned tomorrow is of less value due to inflation. Therefore, future cash flows projected for the capital expenditure analysis must be discounted resulting in a Present Value for each year's cash flow. The discount rate for most projects is 8–12% and is based on the riskiness of the project and the opportunity cost of investing the money in the project. Revenues, expenses and resulting cash flows are calculated for 5 or 10 years. Beyond that a residual year calculation is used. Residual calculations are determined by taking the cash flow of the last year, adding back the working capital investment and dividing by a cap rate (difference between the discount and inflation rate). The final step of the analysis subtracts the up-front project costs from the Present Value determination.

Present Value (Project Period + Residual Year) — Initial Investment = Net Present Value

2.9 Employee Requirements

To maximize the success of treatments that involve the laboratory handling and manipulation of human gametes and embryos, the American Society for Reproductive Medicine (ASRM) has established guidelines for personnel within the ART practice [13] (Table 2.14).

2.10 Conclusion

Studies estimate that 42% of practice-generated denials are attributable to a failure to set up the patient's insurance correctly and 88% of patient-generated errors are due to inaccurate personal information. Thus, insurance verification and updated information from the patient at each encounter are critical steps in the revenue cycle. The dollar amount of claims denied for registration/insurance related reasons as a percentage of total denied dollars may be used to assess registration function. Healthcare providers in best practices submit the encounter form, commonly called a superbill, within 24 h of the encounter. Monitoring strategies include nightly reconciliation of missing encounter forms with schedules documenting "arrived" patients. Charge entry after a patient encounter should be completed within 48 h. Within 24 h after the encounter, the superbills are collected and batched. In the next 24 h period, the charges should be entered. Best practices reconcile missing charges daily to weekly. Submission of claims and subsequent payments are improved by the use of a clearinghouse that filters the claim for errors or through the use of a claim scrubber. Claim scrubbers allow the provider to utilize the same software payers use to deny claims and hold reimbursements longer. Furthermore, practices can identify undercoding in services. Analysis/assessment tools include practice metrics and reports that will flag difficulties with the revenue cycle. Useful metrics include: accounts receivable (AR); claim denials; write-offs; collection rates; patient complaints; volume of unanswered payer and patient correspondence; claim edits; timely submission of charges; lag days; missing charges; and turnover in revenue cycle employees. Of all improvements that can be recommended for revenue cycle processes, standardization is proven to benefit not only revenue, but quality and patient satisfaction.

Employee files should contain personal information (name, address, Social Security number, date of birth and education); job application and resume; licenses or certifications required for the job; a signed employee handbook receipt or employment contract; attendance and leave records; payroll records; performance appraisals, commendation letters, merit awards; disciplinary records; and, job description, title, location and schedule. Employees can examine this file once per year in the presence of a designated representative. The employee has the right to request a correction or a deletion or write a statement of disagreement with any item in the file in the presence of a designated representative. The employee may not remove any item from the file. Employers can require a written request to view the file. Exempted information regarding personnel files include potential job assignment information, and the prediction of any future salary or career path information. It is recommended that personnel file be kept for 4–7 years after an employee leaves the practice.

Employee discipline should provide, where possible, advance notice of the consequences of misconduct; written documentation; and actions that are timely, consistent and impartial. In the articulation of a disciplinary policy reserve the right to choose the level of discipline, up to and including termination without resorting to less severe measures. There should be a nonexhaustive list of the types of infractions that will result in immediate termination. If your policy includes progressive discipline, it is mandatory that it is followed to avoid a breach of contract or discrimination action. Disciplinary actions including warnings and counseling should be documented in the personnel file. Future expectations should be written and state clearly, "we expect that you will…".

Table 2.14 ASRM guidelines for personnel within the ART practice

Personnel

There should be a backup system in place for all personnel essential to a program. A single individual may fulfill the requirement for expertise in one or more areas. An ART program must include the following personnel:

A designated overall practice director, medical director, and laboratory director. One individual may fulfill more than one of these positions, but the medical director must be a licensed physician.

An individual with training and experience in reproductive endocrinology, particularly in the use of ovulation-inducing agents and hormonal control of the menstrual cycle. An individual who has completed an American Board of Obstetrics and Gynecology (ABOG)-approved fellowship in reproductive endocrinology and infertility fulfills this requirement.

An individual with experience in laparoscopic and ultrasound-guided oocyte retrieval techniques.

An individual with specialized training and experience in gynecologic sonography who provides the monitoring of follicular .development.

An individual experienced in male reproduction (andrology) with special competence in semenology. If this individual is not a urologist, a consultant urologist with expertise in reproductive surgery should be available.

An embryology laboratory director with personal experience in the organization and maintenance of a clinical embryology laboratory and in tissue culture techniques.

A consultant/mental health professional with expertise in reproductive issues.

An individual with specialized training and experience in gamete and embryo cryopreservation techniques, when gamete and/or embryo cryopreservation is offered.

An individual with specialized training in gamete biology and micro-operative techniques, if oocyte and/or embryo micro-operative techniques are offered.

Appropriate personnel to perform hormonal assays. An outside laboratory that has demonstrated adequate competence, quality control, and service, may be used for rapid assays of all the necessary reproductive hormones (including estradiol and progesterone). Such hormone assays should be performed by a laboratory that meets Clinical Laboratory Improvement Amendments of 1988 (CLIA) standards.

Appropriate nursing support.

An individual or consultant with specialized expertise in genetics or genetic counseling.

ASRM Practice Committee. Revised minimum standards for ART programs. Fertil Steril 2006; 86, S53–S56.

Laboratory director

An earned doctorate degree (Ph.D.) from an accredited institution in a chemical, physical, or biological science as the major subject, or a medical degree (M.D. or D.O.) from an accredited institution, or have qualified as a laboratory director prior to July 20, 1999.

Effective January 1, 2006, all new laboratory directors should hold High Complexity Laboratory Director (HCLD) or American Board of Bioanalysis Embryology Laboratory Director (ABB-ELD) certification or its equivalent. Laboratory directors grandfathered in are strongly encouraged to seek HCLD or ELD certification.

Expertise and/or specialized training in biochemistry, cell biology, and physiology of reproduction with experience in experimental design, statistics, and problem solving.

Experience in formulating laboratory policies and protocols and communication with the medical director regarding patient progress and protocols as they affect the laboratory aspects of treatment.

Two years of documented pertinent experience in a program performing IVF-related procedures. This experience should include:

1. Familiarity with laboratory quality control, inspection, and accreditation procedures.
2. Detailed knowledge of cell culture and ART and andrology procedures performed in mammalian systems.

A period of training of at least 6 months (may be concurrent with documented experience) and have completed at least 60 ART procedures under supervision. A procedure is defined as a combination of the examination of follicular aspirates, insemination, documentation of fertilization, and preparation for embryo transfer. Satisfactory completion of this period of training should be documented by a signed letter from the laboratory director of the training practice.

12 h of annual accredited continuing education in assisted reproductive technology or clinical laboratory practice.

Demonstration of technical competence in the embryology laboratory by documenting performance of specific procedures and results that are within acceptable standards for that program.

Specific responsibilities of the embryology laboratory director include:

Providing accessibility for on-site, telephone or electronic consultations as needed.

Ensuring that the physical plant (space, facilities, and equipment) and environmental conditions of the laboratory are appropriate and safe.

Maintaining aseptic conditions in the laboratory.

Ensuring that patient confidentiality is maintained throughout the laboratory ART process.

Providing an approved procedural manual to all laboratory personnel and establishing and maintaining a laboratory quality assurance program.

Providing consultation to physicians and others, as appropriate, regarding laboratory aspects of treatment.

Employing a sufficient number of qualified laboratory personnel to perform the work of the laboratory. At a minimum, there should be two qualified embryologists. The table below provides minimum staff sizes for the volume of cycles (retrievals and cryopreservation cycles). Additional laboratory staff may be required if andrological and/or endocrinological duties are also assigned.

Ensuring that all personnel receive appropriate training for the ART laboratory procedures to be performed, obtain the required number of annual continuing education hours, and demonstrate continued competence for the ART laboratory procedures performed.

(continued)

Table 2.14 (continued)

Laboratory cycles and embryologists

Number of laboratory cycles	Minimum number of embryologists
1–150	2
151–300	3
301–600	4
>600	1 additional embryologist per additional 200 cycles

Off-site embryology laboratory director

An "off-site" laboratory director supervises another physical facility, which has a separate identification number (SART number) and medical director.

An off-site director has the same responsibilities as the on-site director and can direct no more than five separate laboratories of any type.

While the laboratory is actively treating patients, the off-site director must physically visit the laboratory at a frequency that ensures the proper patient care during ART.

The "off-site" director should visit no less than once per month, while the lab is active.

The lab director should be available at all times by fax, phone, or email for any issues that may arise.

The off-site director must be present on site for any accreditation or certification procedures.

ASRM Practice Committee. Revised minimum standards for ART programs. Fertil Steril 2006; 86, S53–S56.

Embryology laboratory supervisor

Embryology laboratory supervisors, under the direction of the embryology laboratory director, and as authorized in writing, provide day-to-day supervision of laboratory personnel performing ART procedures. If the medical director is also the laboratory director, there should be a designated laboratory supervisor. If the embryo laboratory director is located off-site, there should be a designated laboratory supervisor. The embryology laboratory supervisor should either meet the qualification requirements designated for laboratory director, or fulfill both of the following requirements:

Have an earned bachelor's or master's degree in chemical, physical, biological, medical technology, clinical, or reproductive laboratory science from an accredited institution.

Have documented training, which includes performing, at a minimum, at least 60 ART procedures under supervision.

In addition to meeting these requirements, the embryology laboratory supervisor should:

Obtain at least 12 h of accredited continuing education annually in assisted reproductive technology or clinical laboratory practice.

Perform at least 20 ART procedures per year.

Responsibilities of the embryology laboratory supervisor include the day-to-day supervision and oversight of the embryo laboratory and laboratory director responsibilities as authorized in writing by the embryology laboratory director.

Embryology laboratory technologist

Embryology laboratory technologists who perform ART laboratory procedures should either meet the qualification requirements for laboratory supervisor, or fulfill both of the following requirements:

Have an earned bachelor's or master's degree in chemical, physical, biological, medical technology, clinical, or reproductive laboratory science from an accredited institution.

Have documented training, which includes performing, at a minimum, at least 30 ART procedures under continuous supervision of the laboratory director or supervisor.

In addition to meeting these requirements, the embryology laboratory technologist should:

Annually obtain at least 12 h of accredited continuing education in ART or clinical laboratory practice.

Perform at least 20 ART procedures per year.

Experience and documented training in cell culture, sperm-egg interaction, or related areas of animal reproduction are desirable.

Programs for the appropriate training of embryology laboratory technologists should be in place with documentation of completion for each employee.

ASRM Practice Committee. Revised minimum standards for ART programs. Fertil Steril 2006; 86, S53–S56.

Medical director

As of January 1, 2000, a new program's medical director must be board-certified in reproductive endocrinology and infertility by the ABOG, be an active candidate for the same, or be grandfathered as a medical director, provided the individual has training and experience equivalent to a board-certified reproductive endocrinologist.

Practice director

The practice director is responsible and accountable for the activity of the practice relating to ART, and is responsible for officially communicating with the Society for Assisted Reproductive Technology (SART) and ensuring that the practice follows SART requirements for membership.

Physician performing oocyte retrievals

Each physician performing oocyte retrievals should have performed at least 20 follicular aspirations under direct supervision within a practice that meets these standards. Satisfactory completion of this training should be documented by a signed letter from the practice director.

Each physician should continue performing a minimum of 20 aspirations per year.

(continued)

Table 2.14 (continued)

It is recommended that the physicians involved in the supervision of the follicular recruitment and oocyte retrieval procedures be responsible for the ultrasound monitoring of follicular development.
Physicians responsible for ultrasound follicular monitoring should have familiarity with basic ultrasound physical principles and equipment and should have evidence of training and the requisite competence to adequately perform diagnostic ultrasound examinations.
Nursing
The registered nurse in the ART setting provides education, counseling, support, and nursing care to patients seeking assistance with conception. This role requires structured orientation to the clinical setting and demonstrated competence in the specialty.
Other staff
Other roles in the ART setting may include unlicensed assistive personnel such as Medical Assistants with specialized training in patient care management and technical procedures for the infertile patient.
ASRM Practice Committee. Revised minimum standards for ART programs. Fertil Steril 2006; 86, S53–S56.

Comparing states with mandated insurance coverage to nonmandated states shows a significant increase in available providers, and higher utilization rates. The same study shows a positive correlation between the number of physicians in a fertility center and the number of cycles performed by each physician, encouraging a group model for physicians desiring a robust REI practice.

At present, designation as a freestanding or provider-based clinic affects the dollar value of the professional fee received and whether a facility fee is to be paid. Specifically, in free standing clinics, the physicians receive a full Medicare RBRV payment rate but no separate facility fee since the full RBRV payment includes a practice expense payment component. In the provider/hospital-based clinic, the physicians receive a reduced Medicare professional fee (meant to cover work and malpractice expenses and a reduced practice expense component). The hospital in a provider/hospital-based clinic model receives a separate facility fee from Medicare (i.e., practice expense reimbursement). The provider/hospital-based clinic receives a significantly higher amount when both the professional and facility fee are combined compared to the free-standing clinic model. Despite this fact, many services, including ART practices find that a detailed analysis of reimbursement flow of funds, and governance shows a distinct advantage to the free-standing clinic model.

Many academic medical centers have found it useful to evaluate the potential advantages/disadvantages of site of service designation, in a clinic-by-clinic fashion, using a detailed analysis of patient billing information that includes CPT codes, CPT code volumes, and location of service for all Medicare and third party payer charges. The patient level data must be categorized based on APCs, and relative values units calculated under both the freestanding and provider-based scenarios and adjusted by the various third party payer contracted rates.

Potential benefits of provider/hospital-based clinics include: a significantly higher combined Medicare reimbursement which likely does not affect an REI clinic; higher reimbursement from selected payers; opportunity for joint hospital-physician management; and, potentially greater flexibility to finance/grow physician practices through increased hospital revenue sharing. The potential disadvantages of provider/hospital-based clinics include: higher practices costs related to the hospital's employment wage and benefit rates, costly facilities and less efficient cost control; greater governance complexities and regulatory burdens and their associated inefficient bureaucracies; compliance issues related to hospital-based clinic standing, and the negative impact of split billings.

Advantages found in free-standing clinics include include: a practice expense payment component which in the case of many REI practices outweighs the Medicare-based reimbursement model; a higher reimbursement from selected payers determined through an analysis of codes and reimbursements; the opportunity to solely manage the operation without restriction imposed on the provider-based model; and greater flexibility and freedom in directing profit margins solely to the practice. Disadvantages include capitalization of the practice including clinic, equipment (ultrasounds, laboratory, furnishings, supplies), and staff; assuming responsibility for employment and discipline and other human resource management issues; assuming responsibility for all regulatory burdens associated with the practice including the College of American Pathologists (CAP); Certified Laboratory Improvement Amendments (CLIA), Society for Assisted Reproductive Technology (SART); and Food and Drug Administration regulations. Regardless of the site of service designation utilized, transparency and clear communication regarding the facts surrounding the individual practice must be visible and understood by departmental, hospital and school of medicine leadership in order to perpetuate the successful union of academia and ART.**

Recent establishment of the Food and Drug Administration's Good Tissue Practices regulations (Section 361 Public Health Services Act 21 CFR 1271.160) regarding egg and sperm donors and surrogacy arrangements mandate the development of standard operating procedures (SOPs) for the following the organization's quality improvement program; training and education; resource management; equipment management and upkeep; supplier and client issues; process control; documents and record management; deviation, nonconformance, and adverse (error) event management; internal and external assessment (audits); process improvement through corrective and preventative actions; and facilities management and safety programs. Furthermore, any software that is part of the center must be validated (installation, operational, and product qualification). In the past, the majority of these regulations could be managed through the andrology/embryology component of the fertility center. However, the broad reach of the regulations now applicable requires the full participation and adherence of both REI and andrology/embryology supervisors and staff. The embryology laboratory is required to maintain a policies and procedures manual and personnel employment, training, evaluations, and continuing education. Employees who handle gametes and embryos during a cycle must be documented. The ART practice requires competent legal counsel in developing appropriate informed consent and disposition documents.

Public Health Services Act 21 CFR 1271.160 regarding egg and sperm donors and surrogacy arrangements, require that each center establish and maintain a quality program which is designed to prevent, detect, and correct deficiencies that could lead to the risk of introduction, transmission, or spread of communicable diseases.

Six Sigma asserts the following guiding principles:

- Continuous efforts to reduce variation in process outputs is key to success.
- Healthcare and laboratory processes can be measured, analyzed, improved and controlled.
- Succeeding in achieving a sustained quality improvement requires commitment from the entire organization, particularly from top-level management.

The goal of a Root Cause Analysis is to find out

- What happened
- Why did it happen
- What to do to prevent it from happening again.

Root Cause Analysis is a tool for identifying prevention strategies utilized within a culture of safety and beyond the culture of blame. In Root Cause Analysis, basic and contributing causes are discovered in a process similar to diagnosis of disease – with the goal always in mind of preventing recurrence.

Root Cause Analysis is a process that is:

- Inter-disciplinary and involves experts from the frontline services
- Inclusive of all who are the most familiar with the situation
- Layered, and continually digs deeper by asking why, why, why at each level of cause and effect
- Reformative, and identifies changes that need to be made to systems
- Impartial and avoids the assignment of blame

Root Cause Analysis must include the:

- Determination of human and other factors
- Determination of related processes and systems
- Analysis of underlying cause and effect systems through a series of why questions
- Identification of risks and their potential contributions
- Determination of potential improvement in processes or systems including evidence-based information.

By repeatedly asking the question "Why" (five is not an absolute rule), organizations can peel away the layers of symptoms which can lead to the root cause of a problem. Not infrequently the reason for a problem will lead to another question (Table 2.11). An Ishikawa fishbone (cause and effect) diagram (Fig. 2.7) helps groups explore visually all potential or real causes that result in a problem or process failure. Major inputs to the development of the problem can be established on the fishbone such as: People; Policies; Procedures; and Technology and then the participants use the five Whys technique to drill down to the root causes.

Lean Process principles:

- Specify the value(s) desired by the patient
- Identify the process stream for each product that provides the specified value and challenge all of the wasted steps in that process
- Make the process flow around the patient adding value-added steps
- Introduce points where continuous flow is possible
- Manage toward perfection so that the number of steps and the amount of time and information needed to serve the customer continually falls

Tables 2.12 and 2.13 provide overviews for determining value and the Lean Process, respectively.

References

1. Lundeen JM, Souba WW, Hollenbeak CS (2003) Sources of error in delayed payment of physician claims. Fam Med 35(5):355–359
2. Fix your denial problems (April 2004) Accessed at www.physicianspractice.com
3. Altman JA (1996) St. Anthony's reengineering the medical practice. St. Anthony's Publishing Inc, Reaston, VA
4. Hammoud AO, Gibson M, Stanford J, White G, Carrell DT, Peterson M (2009) In vitro fertilization availability and utilization in the United States: a study of demographic, social, and economic factors. Fertil Steril 91(5):1630–1635
5. Soules MR (2005) Assisted reproductive technology has been detrimental to academic reproductive endocrinology and infertility. Fertil Steril 84(3):570–572
6. American Society for Reproductive Medicine (2004) Guidelines for advertising by ART programs. ASRM Practice Committee Report, Birmingham, AL
7. Mastroianni L (2001) Risk evaluation and informed consent for ovum donation: a clinical perspective. Am J Bioeth 1(4):28–29

8. Ethics Committee of the ASRM (2004) Posthumous donation. Fertil Steril 82:S260–S262
9. Six Sigma. Accessed at http://www.motorola.com/motorolauniversity.jsp?ref=modules
10. Deeming DE (2000) The new economics for industry, government, education, 2nd edn. MIT Press, Cambridge, MA
11. Ohno T (1988) Toyota production system: beyond large-scale production. Portland, OR, Productivity Press.
12. Ishikawa K (1990) Introduction to quality control. Productivity Press, Cambridge, MA
13. ASRM Practice Committee (2006) Revised minimum standards for ART programs. Fertil Steril 86:S53–S56

Appendix

Business operations require close attention to detail. Most billing systems have the ability to extract significant amounts of data. The organization of the data is critical, to ensure appropriate and maximum oversight of the financial health of your practice.

The Operational Indicator (see figure 2.2 for example of full report) has been designed to provide a visual overview of the financial status of your practice. This picture gives access to allow for review of the most immediate month's data, trending for 13 months, benchmarking and variances – all at a quick glance. This important review can be completed quickly and efficiently. Concerns are readily identified to allow the implementation of timely corrective action. The operational indicator provides a view of financial issues. By having this information reported consistently it allows you to recognize problems and make adjustments quickly. With relevant, understandable data you can ensure that your goals are being met.

The following is a step by step review of the data, shows the importance of the assessment of the data, and gives detailed examples of areas that should be given additional review.

Please note that for best data review the indicators should allow for 13 months of data. Figure 2.2, section 1 reflects 3 months in the interest of space. You will want to include the most current month that has closed and 12 prior months.

1-1. **Charges** – Gross charges keyed into your billing system for that specific month.
You will want to ensure consistency in productivity and posting.

1-2. **Payments** – Gross payments, prior to refunds posted in that specific month.
It is important to remember that post dates have no correlation to the date of service, or the date the charge was posted in the system; especially when it relates to insurances and payment plans. A charge could be posted in April for a March date of service. A payment may be posted in April for a January date of service, etc.

1-3. **Net Payments** – Gross payments less refunds

1-4. **Contractual Adjustments** – This is the amount that has been negotiated with contracted payers and must be written off.
If you have contractually agreed to $1000 reimbursement for a specific code(s), you may bill any amount you wish.

Billed Amount	$ 1500
Allowed	$ 1000
	$ 500 **

*** This is a contractual adjustment that must be credited, and may not be billed to the patient or secondary insurances. Watch for unanticipated spikes by specific payers in their contractual adjustments. This could indicate changes in their bundling and other payer policies.*

1-5. **Refunds** – Money returned to insurances and/or patients. Refunds are costly. Are there billing practices that are contributing such as continuous submission of claims instead of actual follow up? The Federal Payers expect timely processing of refunds.
The following measures are basic but critical to the health of your practice.

1-6. **Work RVU** – Is a measurement that is used for productivity. Most CPT codes are assigned a relative value unit. An office consult 99243 has a 1.88 wrvu value, while an established patient 99203 is 1.34. The wrvu is a fairly consistent number that allows for the month to month, and year to year trending on productivity in your practice.

1-7. **Total Discounts** – Provides you with a roll up total of adjustments for hardship, bankruptcy, administrative, etc. If this number increases, further evaluation of why is important.

-------------------- 13 month Comparison --------------------

	2007/Apr	2008/Mar	2008/Apr	12 Mo Total
1-1 Charges	$ 516,065	$ 587,332	$ 445,066	$ 4,805,934
1-2 Payments	$ 241,785	$ 280,658	$ 274,525	$ 2,317,468
1-3 Net Payments	$ 239,779	$ 278,667	$ 270,568	$ 2,296,101
1-4 Contract Adj	$ 182,506	$ 243,076	$ 258,305	$ 1,665,848
1-5 Refunds	$ 2,006	$ 1,991	$ 3,958	$ 21,367
1-6 Work RVU	$ 3,730.18	$ 4,371.16	$ 3,367.12	$ 41,471.43
1-7 Total Discounts	$ 24,348	$ 20,170	$ 9,204	$ 177,087

Figure 2.2 section 1

				2-1	2-2	2-3	2-4	2-5	2-6	2-7
Measures										
	2007/Apr	2008/Mar	2008/Apr	12 Mo Total	Prev 12 Mo Tot	12 Mo Tot Var	12 Mo Avg	CM Var	PFYTD	FYTD	FY Var
Charges	$516,065	$ 587,332	$445,066	4,804,934	1,450,482	$3,355,092	$400,494	$44,571	1173455	4,274,286	3,100,830
Payments	$241,785	$ 280,658	$274,525	2,317,468	$ 873,820	$1,443,647	$193,122	$81,403	$ 682,573	2,099,792	1,417,249
Net Payments	$239,779	$ 278,667	$270,568	2,296,101	$ 851,197	$1,444,905	$191,342	$79,226	$ 663,281	2,079,504	1,416,224
Contract Adj	$182,506	$ 243,076	$258,305	1,665,848	$ 517,881	$1,147,966	$138,821	$119,484	$ 404,273	1,546,604	1,142,332
Refunds	$ 2,006	$ 1,991	$ 3,958	$ 21,367	$ 22,624	($1,257)	$ 1,781	$2,177	$ 19,293	$ 20,288	$995
Work RVU	3,730.18	4,371.16	3,367.12	41,471.43	12,545.59	28,925.84	3,455.95	(88.83)	10,118.74	36,277.79	26,159.05
Total Discounts	$ 24,348	$ 20,170	$ 9,204	$177,087	$19,456	$157,632	$14,757	($5,553)	$16,740	$167,563	$150,824

Figure 2.2 section 2

This section provides trending for the measures in figure 2.2.1. On a landscape report the above information would be to the immediate right (see figure 2.2 for example of full report).

2-1. **Previous 12 Month Total** allows a comparison between two complete 12 month time periods. This compares seasonality, conferences, etc. between years.
2-2. **12 Month Variance** shows the difference between the two 12 month periods.
2-3. **12 Month Average** allows you to identify the one month average for the last 12 months of information.
2-4. **Current Month Variance** show the difference between the most current month and the 12 month average. In this example the last complete month was April. Charges were $445,066. (See figure 1) When compared to the 12 month average of $400,494 **(2.3)** you can quickly see the operation has a gain of $44,571 in charges. Each measure from figure 1 can be quickly reviewed with this structure.
2-5. **Prior Fiscal Year to Date** allows an exact month(s) review compared to the exact number of months in the current fiscal year. For this example, the fiscal year begins in July. By April there would be a total of seven months reported. 2-5 looks at the seven months of the prior fiscal year and compares them to the seven months of this fiscal year.
2-6. **Fiscal Year to Date** as explained above looks at where the operation stands at the end of seven months.
2-7. **Fiscal Year Variance** provides a quick snapshot of whether the operation is above or behind at this same period in the fiscal year (seven months).

Collection agency/bad debt is an area that must be tracked to ensure consistent review of aged self-pay and appropriate transfer to bad debt (Figure 2.2. section 3). Are self pay accounts being reviewed monthly? Are broken payment plans for non responsive patients being sent monthly to collections? This type of A/R has your lowest return on staff time and effort and should be managed accordingly.

Figure 2.2 section 4 captures your patient population payer information. Self-Pay in this category reflects patients registered as uninsured. Process review of front desk demographic capture may be necessary. You may also have a referral problem – more than your share of uninsured patients, or you may be providing services that insurances do not cover.

COLLECTION AGENCY ACTIVITY		2008 March	2008 April	12 Month Total
TO COLLECTIONS	$ 11,979	$ 6,289	$ 12,784	$ 119,879

Figure 2.2 section 3

									4-1	4-2	4-3
ORIGINAL INSURANCE INFO CAPTURED				12 Mo Totals	12 Mo Avg	Mix 12 Mo	Prev 12 Mo Tot	Prev 12 Mo Mix	Mix CM	Mix PYTD	Mix FYTD
BLUE SHIELD	$ 93,326	$ 122,022	$ 134,471	$ 1,097,872	$ 91,489	22.84%	$ 372,628	25.68%	30.21%	26.57%	22.83%
COMMERCIAL INS	$ 3,253	$ 5,761	$ 1,759	$ 46,191	$ 3,849	0.96%	$ 19,659	1.36%	0.40%	0.87%	0.93%
CONTRACTS	$ 143,248	$ 161,619	$ 109,720	$ 1,410,186	$ 117,516	29.34%	$ 548,134	37.78%	24.65%	38.65%	27.80%
MEDICAID	$ 156,184	$ 166,431	$ 111,425	$ 1,309,426	$ 109,119	27.25%	$ 351,728	24.24%	25.04%	22.66%	27.76%
MEDICARE	$ 542	$ 3,912	$ 358	$ 17,699	$ 1,475	0.37%	$ 4,764	0.33%	0.08%	0.41%	0.33%
MISC GOVT	$ 18,941	$ 18,580	$ 14,582	$ 131,397	$ 10,950	2.73%	$ 35,577	2.45%	3.28%	2.39%	2.94%
OOS MEDICAID	$ 24,582	$ 10,037	$ 8,688	$ 103,897	$ 8,658	2.16%	$ 30,351	2.09%	1.95%	2.25%	2.16%
SELF PAY	$ 75,989	$ 98,971	$ 64,063	$ 689,266	$ 57,439	14.34%	$ 88,001	6.07%	14.39%	6.21%	15.25%

Figure 2.2 section 4

4-1. **Mix** Current Month lets you know the population mix for the most current post month.
4-2. Mix Prior Year to Date allows you to compare last prior year (exact same number of months) to the current fiscal year.
4-3. Mix Fiscal Year to Date allows you to look and see if you are trending up or down of the last prior year's insurance category.

The difference between Original Insurance information capture vs. Payer, is the Payer section reflects what percentage of your collections is paid by which Insurance Company. The measures and columns work the same as above.

If you compare the original insurance information captures in Fig 2.2 section 4 to payer category in Fig 2.2 section 5, you can ensure that you do not have a payer category that is significantly behind on payments.

Look at Blue Shield in 4-3 you will see the current mix is 22.83%. Compare this to Blue Shield the payer in 5-3, and you will see Blue Shield comprises 24.16% of the total collections.

Self-pay (figure 4-3) represented 15.25% of the original insurance charges but only 8% of the total collections. Reasons may include that many of the invoices initially reflect no insurance information and subsequently insurance is identified, billed and paid. The difference and primary concern would be the actual amount you must adjust off to bad debt – see figure 3.

Comprehensive data compilation of your outstanding accounts receivable (A/R) allows you to review the specific performance of your revenue cycle processes. If you generate a large month of billings, did it ultimately get collected? Is it being collected timely? Do you have payer/rejection issues? Do you have a billing office performance issue? How are we doing compared to others? All questions you can answer quickly with the data capture and organization indicated below in section 6 and 7.

Section 6 provides a succinct summary of aging of your outstanding A/R, whereas section 7 expands it to payer category. You may want to expand to payer – the report is much longer. The key area here to focus on is the aged A/R. If your percent of A/R > 20 is higher than the benchmarks (section 6-5 to 6-7) you wish to compare your practice to, then you need to begin the process of drilling down data and processes to identify the reasons for the aging. With complete data you can determine on what and where you want to focus your business office resources.

Benchmarking reflected in 6-5 through 6-7 is Faculty Practice Solutions (FPSC). This is appropriate if you are an academic institution. Another good source is Medical Group Management (MGMA). Also, some societies provide specific numbers based on surveys of their members.

The categories listed in 7-2 through 7-5 are standard A/R breakouts. For space purposes the first two categories of A/R 0-30 and 31-60 were removed. An important note – A/R is a good thing. You have to have it to collect it. It is the age of the A/R that must be managed carefully.

In this example, April reflects 37.63% (section 6.4;100-[17.96+13.12+10.51+20.79=62.38]) of total A/R outstanding is 0-30 days old. The corresponding benchmark indicates that the majority of members reported they have about 50% in this category 0-30. The first few categories is where you

PAYER MIX				5-1 Mix CM	5-2 Mix PYTD	5-3 Mix FYTD
BLUE SHIELD	$ 66,414	$ 68,320	$ 57,137	21.00%	26.08%	24.16%
COMMERCIAL INS	$ 1,321	$ 3,046	$ 1,463	0.54%	0.66%	0.96%
CONTRACTS	$ 77,682	$ 91,017	$ 69,635	25.59%	43.37%	34.23%
MEDICAID	$ 67,049	$ 79,316	$ 83,450	30.67%	16.61%	27.33%
MEDICARE	$ 619	$ 230	$ 2,110	0.78%	0.15%	0.35%
MISC GOVT	$ 6,850	$ 4,654	$ 9,208	3.38%	2.06%	2.57%
OOS MEDICAID	$ 6,740	$ 9,115	$ 14,846	5.46%	1.30%	2.23%
SELF PAY	$ 13,827	$ 22,023	$ 34,270	12.59%	9.77%	8.17%

Figure 2.2 section 5

OUTSTANDING ACCOUNTS RECEIVABLE						
CURRENT INSURANCE	FEB	MAR	APR	FPSC BENCHMARKS 6-5	6-6	6-7
A/R 31-60 Days	$ 182,719	$ 159,963	$ 141,606			
% A/R 31-60 Days	21.30%	17.83%	17.96%	15.29%	6.70%	34.00%
A/R 61-90 Days	$ 76,879	$ 127,462	$ 103,444			
% A/R 61-90 Days	8.96%	14.20%	13.12%	8.80%	4.90%	14.40%
A/R 91-120 Days	$ 78,029	$ 62,194	$ 82,893			
% A/R 91-120 Days	9.09%	6.93%	10.51%	6.34%	3.80%	12.50%
A/R >120 Days	$ 121,490	$ 172,324	$ 163,937			
% of AR > 120	14.16%	19.20%	20.79%	18.76%	3.30%	52.30%

Figure 2.2 section 6

7-1	7-2	7-3	7-4	7-5	7-6
CURRENT FSC	91-120 DAYS	121-150 DAYS	151-180 DAYS	> 180 DAYS	TOTAL AR
BLUE SHIELD	$ 2,284	$ 2,330	$ 496	$ 272	$ 123,507
% OF BLUE SHIELD	1.85%	1.89%	0.40%	0.22%	100.00%
COMMERCIAL INSURANCE	$ 405	$ 509	$ 118	$ 1,461	$ 13,167
% OF COMMERCIAL INS	3.08%	3.87%	0.90%	11.09%	100.00%
CONTRACTS	$ 10,971	$ 4,261	$ 4,698	$ 9,799	$ 160,320
% OF CONTRACTS	6.84%	2.66%	2.93%	6.11%	100.00%
MEDICAID	$ 11,165	$ 8,693	$ 4,685	$ 12,632	$ 108,126
% OF MEDICAID	10.33%	8.04%	4.33%	11.68%	100.00%
MEDICARE	$ 151	99	$ 164	$ 2,724	$ 4,068
% OF MEDICARE	3.71%	2.44%	4.03%	66.97%	100.00%
MISC GOVERNMENT	$ 2,039	$ 236	$ 2,571	$ 694	$ 25,643
% OF MISC GOVERNMENT	7.95%	0.92%	10.03%	2.71%	100.00%
OOS MEDICAID	$ 4,980	$ 901	$ 5,244	$ 19,798	$ 45,819
% OF OOS MEDICAID	10.87%	1.97%	11.44%	43.21%	100.00%
RESPONSIBLE PARTY	$ 50,897	$ 22,908	$ 32,102	$ 26,625	$ 308,072
% OF RESPONSIBLE PARTY	16.52%	7.44%	10.42%	8.64%	100.00%
TOTAL AR	$ 82,893	$ 39,936	$ 50,078	$ 73,923	$ 788,640
% OF TOTAL	10.51%	5.06%	6.35%	9.37%	100.00%

Figure 2.2 section 7

want the majority of you're A/R. Aged accounts receivable is usually due to rejections, pending appeals, and self-pay.

A/R over 90 days identifies some potential problem areas. The second section breaks out the A/R by category. The category should be able to be drilled down to specific insurance company.

The aging category information allows you to quickly see where the largest areas of concern lies. Self pay, by its nature, will trend older. If an account has insurance, the insurance will be billed, paid (perhaps 2-3 months later), account will be 3-4 months old as it comes into the self-pay category.

By Looking at Total A/R column on the far right you can see that Self Pay is 39% of total A/R $308,072/$788,640. The second highest is all contracted payers, and in third place is Medicaid.

In reviewing the aging self pay. We know it makes up 39% of total A/R for this practice. Again, that in itself is not problematic. How old is it? 43% is greater than 90 days [16.52+7.44+10.42+8.64=43]. Is this a problem? Could be. If you allow 2 year payment contracts, then perhaps not. Knowing what your team is doing with self-pay collections is important. This isn't captured in the report, but the report lets you decide what assessments you do need to have completed by your team. Questions like – did staff collect all appropriate point of service collections? Are accounts without payment arrangements being routinely transferred to collections? What amount of self-pay was created by incorrect insurance information at point of service? Etc.

Contracted payers generally are expected to pay within a 30-60 day time period for clean claims. This is a category that you would expect to be more timely than self pay.

In this example A/R still listed as outstanding for Contracted Payers is 20.33% of all my outstanding accounts receivable. Of the 20.33%, 18.5% [6.84+2.66+2.93+6.11 =18.5] is over 90 days. According to the FPSC benchmarks above the other practices surveys showed their A/R over 90 was about 15% (8.8% and 6.34%). Is this due to rejections, information requests, poor follow up by staff or by insurance? Some of these questions can be answered in the next section under rejections, others may require an analysis focusing on different payers.

Rejections are costly. Having to touch a claim several times takes staff time and possibly physician time. Ignoring rejections allows insurances to not fulfill their contractual obligation and in fact increases your "free care". Rejections must be managed in a timely manner. In addition to working the rejections you need to know what and why you are receiving them.

The data in section 8 is grouped into three categories. This allows you to break out where the problem may be occurring and what resources are necessary to fix process. The three categories we established are Coding (8-1), Registration (8-2) and Follow Up (8-3).

- Coding (8-1) allows you to potential documentation and coding practices that are not in alignment with payer policies.

8-1 TOP 5 REJECTIONS-OP CODING	Chg	2007/Apr	2008/Jan	2008/Feb	2008/Mar	2008/Apr	FYTD
97-SERVICE NOT PAID SEPARATELY	Chg Amt	$ 262	$ 1,049	$ 1,455	$ 387	$ 799	$ 6,134
	Rej Count	5	9	8	2	9	63
11-DIAGNOSIS SUBMITTED INCONSISTENT WITH PROCEDURE	Chg Amt	$ 16	$ 82	$ 82	$ 92	$ 164	$ 1,791
	Rej Count	2	1	3	7	2	28
7-INVALID PROC CODE INCONSISTENT WITH PT GENDER	Chg Amt	$ -	$ -	$ -	$ -	$ 151	$ 151
	Rej Count	-	-	-	-	1	1
50-NOT MEDICALLY NECESSARY	Chg Amt	$ -	$ 151	$ -	$ 359	$ 547	$ 1,057
	Rej Count	-	1	-	2	1	4
112-SVC NOT DOCUMENTED	Chg Amt	$ -	$ -	$ -	$ -	$ (85)	$ -
	Rej Count	-	-	-	-	1	2
8-2 CLIENT NOT ELIGIBLE ON DATE OF SERVICE	Chg Amt	$ 1,889	$ 1,650	$ 2,395	$ 568	$ 2,824	$ 13,521
	Rej Count	13	15	11	6	21	97
49-NON COVERED SERVICE IN CONJUNCTION WITH ROUTINE	Chg Amt	$ 1,205	$ 328	$ 1,064	$ 257	$ 857	$ 5,424
	Rej Count	10	4	8	2	5	46
L10-PROVIDE DATE OF LMP/ONSET OF ILLNESS	Chg Amt	$ 1,642	$ 113	$ 2,114	$ 1,805	$ 1,599	$ 13,297
	Rej Count	11	1	7	7	5	67
31-INVALID ID NUMBERUNABLE TO IDENTIFY INSURED	Chg Amt	$ -	$ -	$ 151	$ -	$ 509	$ 874
	Rej Count	-	-	1	-	4	7
27-COVERAGE TERMINATED BEFORE DOS	Chg Amt	$ 660	$ 233	$ 233	$ 793	$ 747	$ 4,432
	Rej Count	5	2	2	6	3	29
8-3 FOLLOW UP	**Chg**	**Apr**	**2008/Jan**	**2008/Feb**	**2008/Mar**	**2008/Apr**	**FYTD**
96-NON-COVERED CHARGES	Chg Amt	$ 692	$ 1,199	$ 6,216	$ 1,823	$ 2,854	$ 15,574
	Rej Count	6	10	27	12	17	104
D6-INS REQUESTS COPY OF REPORT	Chg Amt	$ -	$ -	$ -	$ 372	$ 2,896	$ 5,281
	Rej Count	-	-	-	2	15	30
18-DUPLICATE CLAIM	Chg Amt	$ 2,844	$ 878	$ 1,613	$ 883	$ 1,453	$ 14,963
	Rej Count	10	2	11	9	10	100
16-ADDITIONAL INFO NEEDED	Chg Amt	$ 2,188	$ 164	$ 360	$ 269	$ 151	$ 4,545
	Rej Count	5	1	1	2	5	26
17-ADDITIONAL INFO NEEDED-REQ INFO INSUFFICIENT OR INCOMPLETE	Chg Amt	$ 82	$ -	$ 943	$ 442	$ 1,071	$ 2,538
	Rej Count	1	-	2	2	4	9

Figure 2.2 section 8

				9-1	9-2	9-3	9-4	9-5	9-6
	2008/Feb	2008/Mar	2008/Apr	12 Mo Total	12 Mo Avg	CM Var	PFYTD	FYTD	% Change
9-A Charges	$ 516,065	$ 587,332	$ 445,066	$ 4,805,934	$ 400,494	$44,571	$ 1,173,455	$ 4,274,286	264.25%
9-B Charges Rejections	$ 7,279	$ 10,239	$ 8,301	$ 54,883	$ 4,574	$3,728	$ 14,483	$ 48,111	232.19%
Coding Rej %	1.41%	1.74%	1.87%	1.14%	1.14%	0.72%	1.23%	1.13%	−0.11%
Follow up Rej	$ 41,437	$ 21,390	$ 41,300	$ 267,783	$ 22,315	$18,985	$ 82,567	$ 251,896	205.08%
Follow up Rej %	8.03%	3.64%	9.28%	5.57%	5.57%	3.71%	7.04%	5.89%	−1.14%
Registration Rej	$ 13,504	$ 7,386	$ 14,368	$ 95,382	$ 7,949	$6,420	$ 40,455	$ 84,663	109.28%
Registration Rej %	2.62%	1.26%	3.23%	1.98%	1.98%	1.24%	3.45%	1.98%	−1.47%
Total Rejections	$ 62,220	$ 39,015	$ 63,970	$ 418,049	$ 34,837	$29,132	$ 137,505	$ 384,671	179.75%
Total Rejections %	12.06%	6.64%	14.37%	8.70%	9.06%	5.32%	11.72%	9.00%	−2.72%

Figure 2.2 section 9

- Registration (8-2) are generally rejections that may have been avoided with better point of service processes.
- Follow Up (8-3) are often issues with payers. They may be requesting additional information, which if not sent, claim will not be paid. Payers may have system constraints so they are not reading modifiers, and denying claims as duplicates – again requiring an appeal with documentation.

The data captured in section 9 provides greater trending then figure 8. This section provides comparisons between the months and years. Rejections are calculated as a percent of charges. So if charges (9A) have gone up, either through fee schedule increases or increased productivity, it will reflect on the % of change in this row. When you review the Coding Category (9B) of rejections – the dollar amount of change between fiscal years is up 232% (9-6), but because charges were up 264% the actual change in coding rejections is actually down as a percent of total charges (.11%).

The key to this data and any other that you are reviewing is to ensure you understand the parameters of the data you are analyzing so that it provides accurate and valid information. Insufficient or flawed data will impact your responsiveness and accurate resolution of issues.

Whether you call it your financial analysis, dashboard, scorecard or operational indicator; the final objective is to have timely, manageable data in a format that allows you to monitor and manage your business. It must provide you a tool to process and manage key information to support your strategic growth and operational decisions.

Chapter 3
Collaboration Within the Reproductive Endocrinology and Infertility Practice: Integration of Laboratory and Clinic Operations

Vincent W. Aoki and Douglas T. Carrell

Abstract The quality of patient care in the reproductive medicine clinic hinges on effective integration of laboratory and clinic operations. The reproductive endocrinology and infertility (REI) practice represents a truly unique niche, intimately partnering the laboratory and clinic in overall patient treatment and management paradigms. As such, to deliver optimal patient care, there are a number of unique challenges an REI clinic faces in effectively integrating the two arenas. This chapter discusses these challenges and outlines methods by which REI practitioners may better integrate clinic and laboratory operations to deliver high quality care to patients. Specific areas of focus include patient care and management, quality management programs, regulatory affairs, risk management, continuing education, and professional development.

Keywords ART • Laboratory organization • Clinic organization • Leadership • Integration • Management

3.1 Introduction

The quality of patient care in the reproductive medicine clinic hinges on effective integration of laboratory and clinic operations. The reproductive endocrinology and infertility (REI) practice represents a truly unique niche, intimately partnering the laboratory and clinic in overall patient treatment and management paradigms. As such, there are a number of unique challenges an REI clinic faces in effectively integrating the two arenas and achieving optimal quality of care.

Other chapters in this book highlight the complexities and multi-disciplinary coordination involved in the treatment of the infertility patient. Reproductive endocrinologists provide evaluation of couples seeking fertility treatment, coordinate diagnostic procedures, and offer clinical treatments based on diagnosis. While the reproductive endocrinologist treats the infertile female, andrologists and urologists provide evaluation and treatment of the infertile male. Each of these clinicians relies on the andrology, endocrine, and in vitro fertilization (IVF) laboratories for diagnostic procedures and treatment therapies. Each of these specialists must interact effectively if the couple is to be treated well throughout the diagnostic and therapeutic stages.

In most REI practices, the clinic and laboratory are integrated in the same facility, but integrating the diverse set of specialties and services can be difficult in the scenario of separate facilities, practices, or departments. The maintenance of a healthy and collaborative environment and working relationship between physicians, nurses, clinical support personnel, and laboratory technicians is critical for the successful delivery of patient care and one of more unique challenges facing a reproductive endocrinology practice.

This chapter is dedicated to discuss these challenges and outlines methods by which the REI practitioners may better integrate clinic and laboratory operations to deliver high quality care to their patients. Specific areas of discussion include patient care, diagnostic testing and treatment management, quality management programs, regulatory affairs, risk management, continuing education, and professional development.

3.2 Developing an Integrated Practice

3.2.1 *Patient Care and Management*

Optimal patient care requires multiple levels of coordination and communication between the laboratory, clinic personnel, and physicians. In particular, diagnostic testing and treatment therapies require the timely delivery of accurate testing requisitions from clinic staff to the laboratory. Similarly, the

V.W. Aoki
Eastside Fertility Laboratory, Bellevue, WA, USA

D.T. Carrell (✉)
Departments of Surgery (Urology), Obstetrics and Gynecology, and Physiology, University of Utah School of Medicine, Salt Lake City, UT, USA
e-mail: douglas.carrell@hsc.utah.edu

D.T. Carrell and C.M. Peterson (eds.), *Reproductive Endocrinology and Infertility: Integrating Modern Clinical and Laboratory Practice*,
DOI 10.1007/978-1-4419-1436-1_3, © Springer Science+Business Media, LLC 2010

laboratory must provide accurate and rapid reporting of laboratory results and therapeutic outcome summaries. In the intimate setting of the reproductive clinic, procedures must be developed which prevent informal orders or spurious changes to requisitions and treatment plans [1]. The clinic must therefore adopt a formal and effective platform to ensure the proper execution of this communication.

With technology advancing, reliable Electronic Medical Record (EMR) systems now provide a convenient and effective tool in communicating patient testing requisitions and treatment plans [2–4]. Additionally, these network-based platforms offer an effective mode of laboratory result reporting [5]. Used properly, the EMR can help the laboratory ensure patient results, and summaries are delivered accurately to the referring physician and with minimal turnaround time. An additional benefit of many specialized reproductive EMR platforms stems from the ability of clinicians and laboratory personnel to access all areas of patient treatment with minimal delay, may in the future allow patients direct access to their ART records [6, 7].

Given the close relationship between physicians, nurses, and laboratory staff, the implementation of frequent assisted reproductive technologies (ART) case and cycle reviews provide a simple effective means of delivering the highest quality patient care. Frequently, complex infertility cases may present themselves and communication across departments enhances the delivery of effective treatment strategies through multidisciplinary collaboration. These activities help to ensure the most effective treatment plans conveyed to patients. A regular case conference is the best way to ensure that these reviews take place and should involve appropriate personnel, including physicians, laboratory professionals, and clinic staff.

A particular important role of clinic staff is the coordination of cycle management and planning for IVF patients. Nurses often serve as the primary contacts for patients and transmit therapeutic treatment plans directed by the physician [8]. The laboratory and the clinic must have an effective mechanism to ensure nurses and laboratory staff participate in active communication regarding cycle plans. Furthermore, given the significant role the ART laboratory plays in patient treatment, laboratory personnel input must also be integrated into the cycle plans. A weekly IVF meeting between laboratory technicians and nurse coordinators is an effective and efficient tool ensuring proper coordination between the clinic and laboratory in upcoming IVF cycles [9].

The daily operating schedules of the REI clinic and associated laboratories are integrated necessitating daily coordination between the two areas. Thus, proper communication modalities must also be developed to ensure smooth patient flow through practice. EMR-based platforms provide real-time delivery of patient scheduling information to all areas of the clinic. For clinics providing IVF services, daily rounds meeting between cycle stimulation monitoring physicians, nurses, and IVF laboratory personnel are an effective means of promoting the integrity of daily patient scheduling.

3.2.2 Quality Management

Rigorous quality management programs are critical for ensuring the delivery of high quality patient care [10]. Quality management in the REI practice involves all facets of clinic operation and must be maintained on a strict schedule. Collectively these quality management programs must involve daily quality control (QC) processes, weekly maintenance activities, monthly, quarterly, and annual quality assurance (QA) reviews [11]. Used effectively, these collective activities help to ensure the REI clinic meets its responsibility in ensuring proper quality improvement (QI) objectives are established and achieved [12]. Overall strategic planning in the REI practice should also rely upon these quality management activities.

The laboratory and clinic must have a documented quality management program to systematically evaluate the quality and appropriateness of patient services (See chapter by Keel). The program should be designed to identify and resolve important problems related to patient care and identify areas and opportunities where patient care may be improved. Effective integration of laboratory and clinic quality management programs will ensure the quality improvement process that is contiguous throughout the entire practice. The quality management program should include key indicators, such as test order accuracy, therapeutic treatment accuracy, diagnostic testing turnaround times, customer satisfaction summaries, staff satisfaction surveys, and ART outcome measures.

Analytic QC is used in the clinic and laboratory to ensure the reliability of patient treatment and laboratory testing results [13]. The overall QC program must be documented with the clear assignment of responsibilities. In addition to delineating the frequency and type of controls, the QC program must also define clear tolerance limits for daily controls and corrective actions that must be taken when these controls fall outside of those limits [14].

Regular quality assurance programs that serve to systematically review quality data must also be established. Reproductive clinics should establish responsible quality assurance officers and a quality assurance committee to review these data on a regular basis. The most effective structure involves both the clinical staff and laboratory personnel presenting and reviewing key indicators related to analytic laboratory testing, treatment outcomes, and clinic operational aspects. Laboratory preanalytic variables should be reviewed, such as test requisition accuracy, specimen integrity, and quality of phlebotomy services. Postanalytic variables should also be evaluated, including laboratory result turnaround times, accuracy of result reports, and clinic charting mechanisms. Patient and staff satisfaction reviews are also important elements for consideration. Most importantly, treatment outcome reviews should focus on key outcome measures to evaluate clinic performance and identify areas for quality improvement.

3.2.3 Regulatory Affairs

The reproductive clinic and laboratory are subject to increasing regulatory oversight. Two examples of these regulatory sources include the Food and Drug Administration (FDA) (*See* Chapter 6 by Latash) and the Clinical Laboratory Improvement Act of 1988 (CLIA) (*See* Chapter 5 by Keel and Schalue). In order to ensure compliance, extensive coordination and collaboration must exist between the clinic and the laboratory. An integrated compliance committee is useful to ensure regulatory compliance.

Recent guidance by the FDA places regulations on the processing and donation of human cell and tissue based products (HCT/P). These regulations require extensive coordination between physicians, laboratory staff, nurses, and third-party coordinators in order to ensure donor sperm, oocytes, and embryos meet eligibility requirements. Extensive and well-documented processes, which afford rapid response to changes in these regulations as well as the development, coordination, and execution of clinic and laboratory operating procedures, must be developed.

A committee-based approach involving physicians, nurses, third-party coordinators, and laboratory staff is essential to maintaining compliance. The committee should develop procedures for screening and testing of gamete and embryo donors, determining donor eligibility determination, providing effective education to staff members regarding the regulations, performing and documenting personnel training, ensuring physician approval of the donor eligibility determination, providing effective delivery of valid summary of screening and testing records, and ensuring adequate laboratory processes management, including donor eligibility verification, valid labeling schema, and good tissue practices. Additionally, the clinic should maintain comprehensive EMR systems (discussed above) and may find use in outsourcing to consultants who are experts in the regulations.

With respect to CLIA regulations, the ultimate responsibility for CLIA certification rests with the laboratory. However, a number of areas in the clinic are subject to those regulations and consequently require the integration of laboratory and clinic operations. Specifically, information technology sectors, phlebotomy procedures, patient diagnostic testing procedures and treatment therapy requisitions, quality management programs, safety programs, and facilities requirements necessitate collaborative efforts between clinic and laboratory personnel.

3.2.4 Risk Management

As the looming threat of malpractice liability increases, the REI practice must be responsible and diligent in matters related to the risk management. Larger clinics may benefit from a committee-based approach with a sole purpose to continually evaluate clinic and laboratory operations susceptible to liability issues. Specifically, the clinic should standardize incident reporting, coordinate integrated and regularly scheduled review of those reports, evaluate the integrity of standard operating procedures to avoid systemic liability issues, and define individual cases that constitute a significant risk to the practice.

3.2.5 Education and Professional Development

Optimal patient care in the REI practice also requires an understanding of the various disciplines involved in the treatment process. Thus, cross-educational activities should be initiated in an effort to expand the knowledge of clinic and laboratory personnel. These continuing education activities provide the impetus for improving the appreciation of each other's roles within the clinic and fostering good working relationships between physicians, clinic staff, and laboratory professionals [15].

Clinic and laboratory leadership should ensure continuing education programs, which involve all clinical and laboratory staff, are implemented into practice operations. In the REI practice, it is useful for nurses and physicians to understand what processes are involved in the reproductive laboratory, and the laboratory staff should learn about clinical activities involved in the treatment of infertility patient. Shadowing activities also provide a useful tool to allow staff to obtain first-hand understanding of operations in other departments. Additionally, laboratory professionals and reproductive endocrinologists should present recent medical findings and emerging technologies to improve appreciation of state-of-the-art treatment modalities [16].

Other opportunities may exist to foster the professional development of staff in an integrated fashion within the REI practice. Key personnel should attend focused meetings and workshops aimed at improving management and leadership skills. In addition to national meeting, and workshops, the

REI practice may also benefit from integrating these activities into practice, such as a leadership discussion group. These focus groups provide an opportunity for staff to share their ideas, learn from their colleagues, and support the overall professional development within practice.

3.2.6 Effective Leadership

Perhaps, the most obvious ingredient, and yet the most difficult to describe, in developing a truly integrated practice is strong, supportive leadership. The director(s) of the clinic and laboratories must develop and maintain a genuine respect and support each other, which will set a positive example for relationships throughout the practice. This simple concept has been demonstrated numerous times, both in positive and negative manners. Additionally, the directors must show respect to all staff. Developing a respectful and supportive management style includes the ability to minimize harsh criticism, the development of appreciation for the roles played by all staff, and the display of appreciation for those within the clinic.

3.3 Conclusions

Reproductive medicine is a unique niche, intimately partnering the reproductive laboratory and clinic in overall patient treatment and management paradigms. As such, to achieve optimal results, there are a number of unique challenges an REI clinic faces in effectively integrating the two arenas. In order to ensure proper delivery of high quality patient care the clinic and laboratory must work together in areas of diagnostic testing and patient treatment management, quality management programs, regulatory requirements, medical liability risk, and professional development of its staff.

References

1. Valenstein PN, Howanitz PJ (1995) Ordering accuracy. A College of American Pathologists Q-Probes study of 577 institutions. Arch Pathol Lab Med 119(2):117–122
2. Renner K (1996) Electronic medical records in the outpatient setting (Part 2). Med Group Manage J 43(3):52, 54, 56, 57 passim
3. Renner K (1996) Electronic medical records in the outpatient setting (Part 2). Med Group Manage J 43(4):60–65 82
4. Adler KG (2004) Why it's time to purchase an electronic health record system. Fam Pract Manag 11(10):43–46
5. Brown EV (2008) Back to the lab. As more practices implement EMRs, a measure of effectiveness is the ability to interface with the lab and the LIS. Health Manag Technol 29(5):22, 4–6
6. Timmers T, Pierik F, Steenbergen M, et al. (1995) ARIS: integrating multi-source data for research in andrology. Proceedings / the Annual Symposium on Computer Application [sic] in Medical Care 445–448
7. Tuil WS, Verhaak CM, Braat DD, de Vries Robbe PF, Kremer JA (2007) Empowering patients undergoing in vitro fertilization by providing Internet access to medical data. Fertil Steril 88(2): 361–368
8. Morris EJ (2001) The role of infertility nurses in ovulation induction programmes. Human Fertil (Camb) 4(1):14–17
9. Kennedy R (2003) Meeting of persons responsible and senior staff of IVF units. Human Fertil (Camb) 6(3):97–99
10. Alper MM, Brinsden PR, Fischer R, Wikland M (2002) Is your IVF programme good? Hum Reprod 17(1):8–10
11. Curtis G (2004) Quality management. In: Hudson J (ed) Principles of clinical laboratory management: a study guide and workbook. Pearson, Prentice Hall, Upper Saddle River, NJ
12. Frydman N, Fanchin R, Le Du A, Bourrier MC, Tachdjian G, Frydman R (2004) Improvement of IVF results and optimisation of quality control by using intermittent activity. Reprod Biomed Online 9(5):521–528
13. Gardner DK, Reed L, Linck D, Sheehan C, Lane M (2005) Quality control in human in vitro fertilization. Semin Reprod Med 23(4):319–324
14. Mayer JF, Jones EL, Dowling-Lacey D et al (2003) Total quality improvement in the IVF laboratory: choosing indicators of quality. Reprod Biomed Online 7(6):695–699
15. Bahn D (2007) Reasons for post registration learning: impact of the learning experience. Nurse Educ Today 27(7):715–722
16. Hills LS (2007) How the medical practice employee can get more from continuing education programs. J Med Pract Manage 22(4): 230–233

Chapter 4
Informed Consent in Advanced Reproductive Technology

Kirtly Parker Jones

Abstract Informed consent is a process in which clinicians educate patients in a manner that allows the patients to make an educated decision providing permission to undergo a procedure. This chapter reviews the necessity of real education in the process and practical tools to improve informed consent in the clinic.

Keywords Informed consent • Risks • Patient education • Guidelines • Regulations

Informed consent for research participants in ART poses some important issues, as does the area of Advanced Directives for the future use of cryopreserved gametes and embryos. For successful collaboration between reproductive endocrinologists and andrologist/embryologists, the informed consent document creation process must be a shared effort. Hopefully, this chapter will provide some clarification, as well as pose new areas for discussion in the broad area of informed consent in ART.

4.1 Introduction

Informed consent is a process, not a document. Although the culmination of the process may be a document signed by the parties involved, the process is informed by the ethical standards of medical practice. These foundations of medical ethics are autonomy, beneficence, non-malfeasance, justice, and veracity. The clinical and research participants of advanced reproductive technology (ART) deal with these principles on a daily basis, but the autonomy of individuals providing them the moral right to understand the procedures they are about to encounter is the foundation of informed consent.

The following chapter will deal with informed consent in ART. The issues of consent for standard IVF will be discussed, as well as issues of consent for minors in the area of fertility sparing procedures, the troublesome concept of futility and how it is perceived by patients and clinicians will be presented. Also important are the domains of uncertainty with respect to possibly very rare risks (imprinting disorders) that may be a consequence of ART, and what the standards of the informed consent process should be when the possible risks are rare and uncertain. Decision making when informed consent is impossible (posthumous donation), will be discussed.

K.P. Jones (✉)
Utah Center for Reproductive Medicine, Department of Obstetrics and Gynecology, University of Utah School of Medicine, Salt Lake City, UT, USA
e-mail: Kirtly.jones@hsc.utah.edu

4.2 Informed Consent for IVF/ICSI

The informed consent document confirms the counseling that has occurred prior to signing the document. The document may be inclusive of all the individual parts of the IVF process: screening, ovarian preparation and suppression, ovulation induction, oocyte retrieval, the laboratory processes involved with in vitro fertilization and possible ICSI, embryo transfer, and the post procedure issues of ovarian hyperstimulation syndrome (OHSS), pregnancy test outcome and first trimester/pregnancy outcome issues. There may be an overview of the process and specific consents with required signatures taken for each part separately (consents for ovulation induction, consents for ooctye retrieval, consents for IVF/ICSI, consents for embryo transfer). However, as each ART program chooses to divide up the counseling and consent, it should be realized that the amount of information is overwhelming even to the medically sophisticated. Understanding is variable and retention is poor. For this reason, the counseling process should be provided in several media (oral, written, and visual) and repeated throughout the process, even if the consent form has already been signed. It is reasonable and often required by some hospitals that the invasive procedures, such as oocyte retrieval, have a separate counseling and consent process.

There are very few randomized trials of informed consent processes and information retention in ART. Randomized trials in other specialties are few, and the results are varied. One randomized study on the use of written summaries

D.T. Carrell and C.M. Peterson (eds.), *Reproductive Endocrinology and Infertility: Integrating Modern Clinical and Laboratory Practice*,
DOI 10.1007/978-1-4419-1436-1_4, © Springer Science+Business Media, LLC 2010

of risk in otologic surgery compared a verbal summary of risk and a written handout to a verbal summary only [1]. Recall of risks at the time of a telephonic interview about 20 days later was 51% in the handout and verbal summary group and 54% in the verbal group. Some very significant risks were more clearly remembered (88% for facial nerve paralysis and hearing loss). Other risks (dizziness, change in taste) were less well recalled in both groups (30%).

There is evidence that less of the information shared during the consent process is retained than is ideal. Most programs use a combination of oral and written information. A study on informed consent for coronary angiography and angioplasty tested the content retention of 108 consecutive patients [2]. All of the patients had previously read the standard written information sheet and were given eight multiple choice questions. Then they were shown a video of the same content and tested again. The percentage of correct answers increased from 39 to 77% while the "don't know" answers decreased from 53 to 10%. Whether the improved retention of information regarding the techniques and risks of the procedure was due to the video or because of repetition cannot be concluded, but clearly there was a very significant improvement. A randomized study of video versus pamphlet provided information on patient knowledge about surveillance and cancer risk in ulcerative colitis was performed on 124 patients [3]. The participants completed a questionnaire before being randomized to pamphlet or video. There was a 71% improvement in scores from patients randomized to video versus 47% improvement in those given pamphlets. After one month, the knowledge levels decreased in both groups to 55% in the video group and 36% in the pamphlet group. The decrease in delayed recall is informative to ART in that many couples have their consultation for ART several months before the actual procedure.

A Cochrane review of the use of audio-visual presentation for informed consent for participation in clinical trials showed small effects [4]. Another Cochrane review was of the use of "decision aids" (handouts, audiovisual aids) for people facing health treatment or screening decisions. This review of 87 decision aids, of which 23 had been evaluated in 24 randomized trials, shows some improvement in enhancing knowledge and realistic expectations of benefits and harms, but no increase in the satisfaction with the process or with the decision [5]. The very complex issue of "personalized risk" communication is important in communicating expectations in ART, but informed consent documents personalizing risk may not increase informed decision. Clearly, the expectations of a successful pregnancy in a 44-year-old woman undergoing IVF with her own ova are quite different from a 28-year-old couple undertaking the same process. Whether the informed consent document should be specifically designed for each couple's diagnosis and prognosis is not clear. Also, whether personalized risk/benefit documents enhance information retention and satisfaction in the informed consent process is not clear. A separate Cochrane review of personalized risk communication for informed decision making suggested that these interventions had only a limited effect on informed decision making by patients [6]. The effort to create a content and method for informed consent for IVF stresses each ART center. There are standardized patient handouts available from some ART organizations (ASRM) regarding the risks of IVF/ICSI. The Society for Advanced Reproductive Technology of the ASRM has developed a 20 page universal informed consent that ART centers can use when offering IVF, ICSI, assisted hatching, and embryo cryopreservation. This form is available to SART members and includes the risks of medications, egg retrievals, embryo culture, and embryo transfer. It addresses the ethical, legal, and psychosocial issues of ART and discusses alternatives. Standardized documents may help decrease the burden of informed consent document creation, and standardized patient handouts on techniques, risks, and benefits and be helpful. However, the actual face-to-face informed consent process and assessment of the patients' understanding will always be time consuming.

Much more difficult informed consent processes are experienced with couples for whom language and culture are barriers. The importance of a professional translator familiar with medical terminology and comfortable with translating personal reproductive and sexual issues cannot be overstressed. In some areas, the numbers in a particular ethnic and linguistic community may be relatively small, and therefore the likelihood that the couple may know their translator may be large. In the very personal issue of sperm or ovum donation, or the cultural taboos on discussing issues of sexuality and infertility, a known translator, even a professional, may not be acceptable. Translators available via national phone services may be the only option.

Although for each couple for each IVF cycle, the outcome will be a pregnancy or no pregnancy, in the informed consent process, the chances of outcome are usually defined as a percent of all patients (of that age, and with that diagnosis) or a fraction. For some patients with limited understanding of fractions or percents, or those from cultures where "chance" is not understood, the presentation of possible results can be difficult. A picture of 100 figures, with the percent of figures with a specific outcome highlighted or colored can be useful for patients in whom the numerical information is poorly processed. This visual representation (the "Paling Palette") can be used to display medical risks with a probability higher than 1 in 1,000 [7]. An evidence-based resource on informed decision making in reproductive issues (specifically hormonal contraception, but the tools and processes are similar) is available through the Association of Reproductive Health Professionals (ARHP) [8].

4.2.1 Specific Informed Consent Domains

4.2.1.1 Procedure

The specific procedures should be discussed in some detail with pictures or videos of the unstimulated ovary, the hyper-stimulated ovary, the transvaginal ultrasound guided egg retrieval, the embryo culture, the intracytoplasmic sperm injection, and the embryo transfer. Extensive resources of varying reliability are available to patients on the internet, and often sites are sponsored by specific ART programs. Each ART facility should decide to sponsor specific web-based information, or develop its own website. It is appropriate to ask couples if they have already investigated IVF/ICSI procedures on the internet and what they understand before discussing the procedures in detail. Sources on the internet change rapidly as do the procedures and outcomes for IVF/ICSI so a regular update of referred sources or program website is indicated.

4.2.1.2 Reasons

The specific nature of the couple's problem and the indications for IVF should be discussed and documented. Specifically, the indications for the use of ICSI should be discussed and documented.

4.2.1.3 Expectations

The expectation will be a pregnancy, but not all pregnancies lead to a term birth. The expectations should include chemical pregnancy, spontaneous abortion, ectopic pregnancy, heterotopic pregnancies, and preterm/previable birth (particularly in the setting of high order multiple gestations). The expectations for Preimplantation Genetic Diagnosis (PGD) or Preimplantation Genetic Screening (PGS) may be quite different than just a term birth (see PGD/PGS).

4.2.1.4 Probabilities

A shared dialogue between the clinicians and the laboratory staff should create the probability of pregnancy for different diagnoses and ages. All the clinicians, embryologists, and educators should use the same source for the program's pregnancy rates and it should be up-to-date. In the United States, programs that participate in the Centers for Disease Control data collection for IVF may choose to use their most recent data which is posted on the CDC website [9]. Because patients often access this website to review and compare pregnancy rates for the program in which they are receiving their care, it would be appropriate to use those data.

The more complex ethical question in the informed consent process is whether a discussion about IVF center outcomes disparities should be initiated. There is a very broad range of pregnancy rates in the CDC center specific outcomes website. Do physicians have an ethical duty to inform patients about the success rates of their center compared to other centers? This question has been raised for surgeons who infrequently perform a given procedure and their complication rates compared to surgeons who perform more of the given procedure. Significant center-specific outcomes in conditions varying from cancer care to cystic fibrosis management have been documented. In obstetrics and gynecology, there are data that women having surgery for ovarian cancer have a higher survival rate if referred to a regional center with gynecologic oncologists compared to surgery performed at a community hospital.

There are very real trends in increasing pregnancy rates and birth rates in IVF centers with higher volume. What is the role of the clinician in discussing these issues [10]? As informed consent is seen as the right of the patient and the obligation of the physician, outcomes data for an individual IVF center must be discussed. Although some couples may travel to seek care in a center with a higher pregnancy rate, it is not clear that all couples would. In research regarding hospital outcomes disparities and patient choice for a Whipple procedure, 45 out of 100 patients would not travel to a distant center if their risk of operative mortality was doubled at their local hospital. A significant number of people would not travel to a distant center if their risk of operative mortality was six times greater in their local hospital [11]. The reality is that patients will be making the decision to choose one center over another for many reasons, but the principle of shared decision making and disclosure of center specific pregnancy rates allows the couple access to the information to make their autonomous decisions.

The alternative concern in shared decision making and center-specific pregnancy rates is that centers with a relatively high pregnancy rate will use those numbers to discourage patients from a choice to seek care in a center with lower costs or one closer to home. Alternatively, physicians may refer some "high risk" patients (older patients or patients with a diagnosis that leads to a lower pregnancy risk) to another center, and keep "low risk" patients at their center. The issue of outcome disparities could be discussed in the part of the informed consent process, that includes probabilities of achieving a pregnancy, or the part that includes the alternatives.

Of course, the real challenges in discussing the probability of achieving a viable pregnancy with a couple lie in the fact that each couple is unique in their combination of ages, causes of infertility, previous pregnancy history, and previous experience with ART. As noted above, the issue of "personalized" informed consent is very important in the informed consent process, but whether a unique informed consent document should be created for each couple is not clear. In reality, the complex combination of age, ovarian reserve, uterine factors, and semen quality issues occurring in the same couple make specific evidence-based outcomes for that specific couple with several problems quite difficult.

4.2.1.5 Alternatives

Alternatives for family building (or the choice not to pursue fertility therapy or adoption) should be discussed. Alternatives are not usually added to the informed consent document, but are a very important part of the informed consent process. The issues of whether the couple has considered adoption, donor oocytes or sperm, or surrogacy should be discussed. For some couples, the personal availability of some options creates conflict. Donor oocytes may not be an option for some women with very diminished ovarian reserve even if the partner would consider that choice (the same is true for donor sperm). When conflict is apparent in the discussion of options and alternatives, the use of a counselor or psychologist familiar with the issues of infertility and ART is invaluable. Conflicts arising at the beginning of the IVF process regarding preferred alternatives predict future difficulties.

4.2.1.6 Risks

Risks of procedures should be explained as a function of their frequency and severity. Bruising from venipuncture is highly prevalent but of no significance. It is always mentioned in research consent forms, and often in IVF consent forms, but is rarely highlighted in discussion. The risk possibly attributed to IVF of known imprinting disorders such as Beckwith–Wiedemann or Angelman's Syndrome is extremely rare (less than 1 in 1,000) [12] but the consequences are very large to a family. The possibility of an increase in imprinting disorders is discussed in the Patient Fact Sheet: Risks of In Vitro Fertilization (IVF) from the American Society of Reproductive Medicine (ASRM) [12].

The risks of OHSS will vary from center to center and by the age of the patient and the response to gonadotropins. Each center should know what the incidence of OHSS in their program and modify that frequency by the individual age, history, and previous response. Part of the informed consent process is outlining for the patient the conditions under which an IVF cycle will be terminated. It is not uncommon for a patient to insist on proceeding ahead with the egg retrieval or embryo transfer in the face of hyperstimulation. Patients have a very difficult time understanding the physical and financial risk of severe OHSS and the possibility of cancellation of a cycle or freezing all fertilized ova should be clearly discussed in advance. The clinician must use the informed consent process to examine situations in which medical judgment requires termination of the cycle.

The risk of laboratory malfunction is unknown but probably rare. It should be discussed with the patients and mentioned in the informed consent document.

The discussion of risks of procedures for IVF or for neonatal outcomes should always be framed in terms of absolute or attributable risks. Particularly in the perinatal literature, risks related to multiple gestations are framed in relative risk compared to singleton births (risks of preterm birth, risks of cerebral palsy). The term "increased risk" is not informative to the patients as they begin to process the risks of IVF. Visual communication of risks in genetics and other operative risks can be enhanced through the use of the "Paling Palette" [7].

A highly recommended resource for outcomes after ART is the Joint Society of Gynaecologists of Canada (SOGC) and the Canadian Fertility and Andrology Society Guideline: Pregnancy Outcomes After Assisted Reproductive Technology [13]. The evidence collected from the Cochrane Library and MEDLINE was reviewed by the Genetics Committee and the Reproductive Endocrinology Infertility Committee of SOGC. The quality of the information was quantified using the Evaluation of Evidence Guidelines developed by the Canadian Task Force on the Periodic Health Examination. This guideline gives the absolute percent of various outcomes and relative risks for obstetrical complications and perinatal outcomes for singletons from ART and spontaneous conceptions. Of the noted obstetrical outcomes of gestational hypertension, placenta previa, placental abruption, induction of labor and cesarean delivery, the only significant difference between ART singletons and spontaneous singletons was gestational hypertension (range in studies reviewed 1–11% in ART, 0.7–8% in spontaneous pregnancies, r.r.1.8). Attitudes regarding the attractiveness of elective single embryo transfer improved markedly after patients were presented with accurate risk information about twin versus singleton outcomes (33–75%) [14].

The issue of structural congenital anomalies is mentioned in the ASRM Patient Information on Risks in ART but no specific numbers are given. The SOGC Guideline gives specific incidence of any major malformation as well as categories of cardiovascular, gastrointestinal, urogenital, musculoskeletal, and central nervous system abnormalities from IVF, IVF/ICSI, and spontaneous pregnancy.

The incidence of any chromosomal disorder in births and pregnancy terminations after adjusting for maternal age and parity are similar in IVF and spontaneous conceptions (0.7% vs. 0.2%) [12]. These numbers should be specifically adjusted for the age of the mother (with consideration of the age of the oocyte in donor cycles). The risk of any chromosomal defect is somewhat higher in IVF/ICSI compared to spontaneous cycles (1.0% vs. 0.2%). Although these numbers are significantly different statistically, to the couple it may be perceived as not clinically different. It is recommended that couples considering IVF/ICSI should be counseled and offered prenatal diagnosis should they conceive. The fact sheet from ASRM noted above can be useful as a printed adjunct to the discussion and the consent form.

4.2.1.7 Expenses

This will vary from center to center but the expectation of payment (amount, timing, and insurance coverage) should be discussed and information provided in writing.

4.2.2 Special Issues for Informed consent in IVF/ICSI

4.2.2.1 Futility

The concept of "futility" – pursuing a medical course of action in the face of exceedingly small chances of success – became an issue of discussion in the medical literature in the early 1990s. The issues have certainly existed long before this with questions of ongoing support of patients in a vegetative state, heroic cancer therapies for terminally ill cancer patients, and resuscitation of extremely premature infants. The first generation of the futility debate attempted to come to the answer of what to do when outcomes are uniformly poor by defining futility: "When physicians conclude (either through personal experience, experiences shared with colleagues, or consideration of published empiric date) that in the last 100 cases a medical treatment has been useless, they should regard that treatment as futile [15]. This framework gave clinicians a number after which to deny medical intervention, but did not address the needs of patients and families. As the concept has evolved in the literature, the second generation of processing a futility debate emphasizes consensus with the patients/family/clinicians. The American Medical Association endorsed the following statement: "Since definitions of futile care are value laden, universal consensus on futile care is unlikely to be achieved. Rather, the American Medical Association Council on Ethical and Judicial Affairs recommends a process-based approach to futility recommendations" [16]. This process included families and clinicians, hospital administrators, and ultimately judges. It still has the potential to put the patients and the clinicians in conflict. The third option is the communication and negotiation. This process uses standard dispute resolution techniques in solving the problems of patients request for futile therapy [17].

All clinicians in the field of ART are faced with patients who have exceedingly small chances of success with the procedure requested. The most common is probably the patient in her late 40s who requests IVF using her own ova, but included in this group are women with very significant uterine problems and men with no viable sperm. The following questions arise:

1. When is an ART procedure futile and who gets to decide?
2. Are there outcomes other than a live birth that are of consequence to the patient?
3. How does a clinician create an informed consent process when the risks are known, but the measurable benefits are nonexistent?

A common response from the patient whose chance of a successful pregnancy is extremely small (or zero) is frequently, "I know I have no chance of success, but I just need to try". In this scenario, the patient's autonomy could direct the clinician to move toward performing the ART procedure with the understanding that the "benefit" would be the ability to "try" and the movement toward possible emotional closure when the patient does not succeed. The procedure must certainly be relatively low risk. Fortunately, IVF is usually relatively low risk except in some very high risk patients whose medical problems or pelvic anatomy make the IVF process more risky.

The Ethics Committee of the ASRM has a report, which addresses the issue of "Fertility Treatment when the prognosis is very poor or futile" [18]. The summary is as follows:

1. For the purposes of this statement, "Futility" refers to treatment (e.g., and IVF cycle) that has a 0 or less than 1% chance of achieving a live birth; "very poor prognosis" refers to a treatment for which the odds of achieving a live birth are very low but not nonexistent (more than 1% but less than about 5% per cycle).
2. Clinicians may refuse to initiate a treatment option they regard as futile providing they have informed the patient that they regard the option as futile.
3. Clinicians may refuse to initiate a treatment option they regard as having a very poor prognosis providing they fully inform the patient about referrals, if appropriate. Decisions about refusing to treat patients should always be patient-centered.
4. Protecting fertility center success rates is not an ethical basis for refusing to treat patients with very poor prognosis.
5. Upon request, clinicians may treat patients in cases of futility or very poor prognosis provided the clinician has assessed some benefit and informed the patient of low odds of success.
6. Thorough discussions are advisable at the beginning of the patient/physician interaction when the patient has indicators of futility or very poor prognosis.
7. Programs should develop polices to guide decisions about treating patients with futile or very poor prognosis.

Using these guidelines in the informed consent process may enhance the satisfaction of the patients and the clinicians when the outcome of pregnancy is extremely unlikely.

4.2.2.2 Impaired Decision Makers

There is no significant literature about the frequency that patients who have cognitive or developmental delay attempt to access ART. Whether a person who has significant cognitive dysfunction by virtue of developmental disabilities or thought disorder (poorly controlled schizophrenia or manic depressive disorder) should have access to help with reproduction is a complex assessment of rights that is not the discussion here. However, if someone who has impaired decision making requests ART, and the ART team agrees to provide the services, the issues of informed consent become complex.

It is possible that the mother or guardian of a patient who has severe developmental delay may request ART services. How to evaluate the knowledge of the patient, and the process of informed consent may be quite difficult and beyond the scope of the ART clinic. The use of reproductive psychologists for evaluation and recommendation can be very helpful. Also, in the case of a patient who has post traumatic or hypoxic brain damage, or a poorly controlled thought disorder, the psychologist may be helpful in accessing further evaluation and treatment that can be initiated prior to accepting or denying the patient access and going through the informed consent process.

4.2.2.3 Precautionary Principle

The precautionary principle is based on the premise that action should be taken when there is evidence that not to do so would cause harm [19]. It is thought of as being a primary principle in public health – when there is a suggestion of data that something is harmful, action should be taken until further research completely illuminates the issue. The areas of uncertainty that bring the precautionary principle into ART are issues of long term effects of embryo culture [20, 21]. The parts of the precautionary principle that apply in ART are transparency and inclusiveness in decision-making, action in the face of uncertainty, and accountability.

There is increasing understanding of the field of epigenetics – modifications of the human genome after fertilization that affect the organism in future life. The ASRM has raised the issue of epigenetic risks from ART in their patient hand out on risks of IVF and embryo culture when the issue of imprinting diseases (Beckwith–Wiedemann and Angelman Syndrome) is discussed. The clinician counseling the couple as part of the informed consent process may or may not discuss this complex issue of epigenetics with the patients, and they may not understand if it were discussed. Also, the increased risk of "extremely rare" and it is difficult to know what level of frequency risks should be added to informed consent. What should be discussed is the fact that embryo culture is relatively new and reproductive endocrinologists, embryologists, and geneticists do not know all of the changes in the developing embryo that might be different in laboratory culture from in vivo. This acknowledgment to the patients, with the option of including the patients in the face of this uncertainty could be considered an important part of the informed consent process and may be added to an informed consent document. The reassurance that the vast majority of children who are the result of successful ART procedures and blastocyst culture are normal may be part of the discussion. However, acknowledgement of uncertainty in this domain is part of the transparency of the informed consent process.

4.3 Informed Consent Issues for Preimplantation Genetic Diagnosis and Preimplantation Genetic Screening

The Society of Advanced Reproductive Technology (SART) has developed a Practice Committee Opinion on the important elements if informed consent for preimplantation diagnosis and preimplantation screening [22]. The techniques for preimplantation diagnosis for well defined diseases which can be diagnosed with single cell genetic methods have been used for almost two decades. The key elements in the informed consent counseling are as follows:

1. The risks associated with IVF procedures.
2. The option of choosing not to proceed with IVF and PGD.
3. The risks associated with embryo biopsy and extended culture.
4. For carriers of autosomal and X-linked disorders, the relevant patterns of inheritance and the impact of the disorder on the quality of life for an effected child.
5. For carriers of balanced chromosomal translocations or other structural chromosomal abnormalities, a review of the possible patterns of segregation during meiosis and the increased risk for conceiving offspring having an unbalanced chromosomal composition.
6. The technical limitations and pitfalls of PGD, including the risk for misdiagnosis, (the actual probability, when known) and the need for subsequent prenatal diagnostic testing via chorionic villus sampling or amniocentesis to confirm the results obtained with PGD.

7. Options relating to prenatal diagnostic testing and their associated risks:
   (a) Chorionic villus sampling
   (b) Amniocentesis
   (c) Ultrasonography with or without additional blood tests
   (d) No prenatal testing
8. The possibilities that no embryos may be transferred if all are affected, and that unaffected embryos which carry the recessive or X-linked disorder may be transferred.
9. The disposition of embryos for which testing yields no conclusive result.
10. The disposition of embryos not transferred (e.g., discard, cryopreservation, research, or donation) as and when appropriate.
11. Alternative methods for avoiding risk of disease (e.g., use of donor gametes).

Though PGD has been used clinically for many years, PGS is only recently developing and continues with controversy regarding the role of PGS and improving the ability to choose embryos most likely to yield a successful pregnancy. Techniques for PGS are evolving very rapidly and the ability to check for aneuploidy of all 23 chromosome pairs may be available soon. Also, whole genome hybridization may allow entire genome screening not only for common mutations and aneuploidy, but also mutations that are more rarer and possibly polymorphisms that predict disease. Clearly, the ethical issues of "babies by design" are beyond the scope of this chapter, and it is important to note that the informed consent process for these new technologies will also be rapidly evolving.

Having noted that, the ASRM Practice Committee does have guidelines on counseling and informed consent issues for PGS which should include;

1. The risks associated with IVF.
2. The option of choosing not to proceed with IVF and PGS.
3. The risks associated with embryo biopsy and extended culture.
4. The possibility of a false positive result that may lead to the discard of a normal embryo.
5. The possibility of a false negative result that may lead to the transfer of an abnormal embryo.
6. The possibility that testing may yield inclusive results.
7. The possibility that no embryos may be transferred if all appear abnormal.
8. Options relating to prenatal diagnostic testing and their associated risks.
   (a) Chorionic visual sampling
   (b) Amniocentesis
   (c) Ultrasonography with or without additional blood tests
   (d) No prenatal testing
9. The nature and quality of the available evidence with regard to live birth rates after IVF with PGS.
10. The disposition of embryos not transferred (e.g., discard, cryopreservation, research, or donation) as and when appropriate.

In as much as all physicians who provide obstetrical care are required by standard to inform patients of screening techniques available for various populations, in the future it may be the standard the ART clinicians may be required to inform patients of PGS techniques, whether or not they are able to perform them at their center.

4.4 Informed Consent for Egg Donations

The process for informed consent for oocyte donors is somewhat more complex because the "risk versus benefit" is different. For identified donors, the "benefit" may be a social one of increased satisfaction for a process that improves the relationship between the donor and the recipient. The clinician who is charged with assessing and educating the donor should be quite convinced that there are no elements of coercion in the relationship between the recipient and the donor. In the case of anonymous donation, the "benefits" are either altruistic or financial or both. It is difficul to enumerate and weigh altruistic benefits, but financial benefits must be clearly outlined and documented. The circumstances under which a cycle would be cancelled and donor remunerated in these circumstances should also be discussed in advance and documented.

The risks for donors are known (risks of ovarian stimulation and oocyte retrieval) and unknown (long term physical and psychological risks). The known risks of ovulation induction and oocyte retrieval are in the literature [23]. The cumulative rate of serious complications (OHSS requiring hospitalization, ovarian torsion, infection requiring hospitalization, rupture of ovarian cyst requiring hospitalization) was 6 out of 886 retrievals (0.7%). The incidence of complications requiring office visits (mild to moderate OHSS, intraabdominal bleeding, and others) was 75 out of 866 retrievals (8.5%). The incidence of cycle cancellation (poor response, high risk of OHSS, health issues, pregnancy, positive screening tests, medication errors, and donor withdrawal) was 8.9% of anonymous donor cycles and 9.5% of identified donor cycles. Another report of a large series of oocyte donations (4,052 oocyte retrievals) suggested that the complication rate of ooctye retrieval was 0.4% (hemorrhage, torsion, severe pain) [24]. The risk of OHSS requiring hospitalization was 0.4%.

How medical complications will be handled and how cancellations will be managed or compensated must be discussed in advance and documented. Also, disclosure about the possible uses of donor oocytes is also part of informed consent [25]. If the left over oocytes are used for research, the donors must know in advance the research involved and consent [26]. Finally, however, situations compromising the long term anonymity of the donor may arise, or there may be a legal requirement to reveal the donor's identity. This possibility must be discussed and documented with the donor.

4.5 Oocyte and Ovary Tissue Cryopreservation

The ASRM Practice Committee created a very useful report on the essential elements of informed consent for elective oocyte cryopreservation [27]. The report reflects the very significant unknowns about the techniques for freezing, the techniques for thawing, the techniques for in vitro maturation, and the outcomes of fertilization. The report suggests the following elements be in the informed consent process and document:

1. The standard risks of ovarian stimulation and oocyte retrieval must be outlined as with routine IVF, including the probability of retrieving significant numbers of ova and the costs
2. The methods for oocyte cryopreservation should be discussed. Although the new techniques that promise the fertilization possibilities are still small new techniques may be available in the future.
3. Annual storage fees and where tissues should be stored should be discussed.
4. The possible requirement for extensive screening and testing of the patient if oocytes are to be stored or transported or donated in the future.
5. The expected freeze-thaw survival rate for the oocytes using the available technology. The technologies are still limited with respect to the outcome and it may be possible that no ooctyes may survive, mature, or fertilize.
6. The requirement for future ICSI and the costs and expected fertilization rates.
7. Clinic specific outcomes data should be given if available. If the clinic is new at the techniques and fertilization and live births have not been achieved, this should be acknowledged.
8. The possibility that the patient may never need these ova because she retains her spontaneous fertility in the future or decides never to become pregnant, or dies before she can use them.
9. The plan for disposition of ova if they are not used by the patient by a given age or if the patient dies.
10. The possibility of the clinic retrieving the ova and storing them may call for their transfer to another facility in the future.

The American College of Obstetrics of Gynecology also has a committee opinion on ovarian tissue and oocyte cryopreservation, outlining the same issues [28]

4.6 Informed Assent for Minors

Minors cannot give consent by the principle that they are probably unable to fully appreciate the risks and benefits of medical interventions. The term given to the process by which minor agree to a procedure is "assent" and the parents or guardians give "consent." The situations under which minors might be involved with ART procedures are primarily for obtaining and storing gametes in the setting of an adolescent undergoing fertility ending treatments. These interventions are intended to preserve the option of future fertility, but currently they are also experimental. Substantial care should be taken in the assent and consent process to acknowledge the limitations of techniques and understanding of the reproductive consequences of fertilization of cryopreserved mature or immature ova and mature or immature sperm.

The ethical issues in fertility preservation for adolescent cancer survivors have been well described [29, 30]. The following issues must be discussed in the informed assent/consent process:

1. The intervention should not dangerously postpone cancer treatment.
2. Cancer cells in the tissue removed should be at very low risk of reintroducing the cancer to the patient when tissue or oocytes are used in the future.
3. There is very limited experience as to what the cryopreservation process does to immature ova and outcomes of future ovarian tissues, oocytes, and fertilized oocytes is not completely known. Similarly, although cryopreservation of mature spermatozoa is standardized with excellent pregnancy outcomes, cryopreservation of immature testicular tissue has no standard technique or known outcome.
4. The issue of preserving fertility is often a very serious concern of the parents, but not a serious or immediate concern of the very ill adolescent. Though the parents may seek out care and give consent, obtaining assent from the child is still very important.
5. There should be a discussion about the patient's future rights to the gametes.
6. There should be clear advanced directives about disposition of gametes if the child dies. It should be quite clear to the parents that the retrieval and cryopreservation are for the benefit of the child, and not for the benefit of or for future use by, the parents.

The ESHRE Taskforce on Ethics and Law also created a statement on ethical considerations of cryopreservation of gametes and reproductive tissues for self use which outlines the ethical principles and informed consent issues for males and females which stressed the importance of interdisciplinary consulting (the oncologists, pediatricians, reproductive specialists, psychologists, and counselors) in the decision-making process [31].

4.7 Embryo Cryopreservation: Advanced Directives and Intent

A very important focus of the informed consent for embryo cryopreservation is the process of counseling regarding advanced directives. Advanced directives are thought to be part of directing actions when a person is no longer alive or able to act on his/her own. Similarly, advanced directives as part of the informed consent process for embryo cyropreservation were designed to allow the ART center to treat cryopreserved embryos in a manner that the persons for whom they were created would wish in the event that they could not act on their own. Problems arising over the past years of cryopreservation which include divorce, death of one spouse, inability to contact in the event of closure of a center, and failure to use the embryos within a certain age span have increased the possible use of advanced directives. Over the past years, the options for disposition have increased from "discard or donate for research" to include options for donation for other known couples, donation to organization for distribution to anonymous couples, or placement in a gestational surrogate. Undoubtedly, more options will arise in the future.

In the informed consent process, the clinician with the persons for whom the embryos are being made should discuss in detail as many of the possible situations that might arise that may make disposition of embryos necessary. These advanced directives are part of the informed consent document and are not a binding legal contract, but courts have used these documents as a sign of intent when the embryos were made if a couple come to disagree about the use of embryos in the future. Each couple may have scenarios that are more pressing than others and may require their own special consent form. Couples in which one member is very ill and not expected to live to use the embryos should very clearly have the issue of advanced directives discussed. Unmarried couples (heterosexual or homosexual) must clearly outline the nature of "ownership" of the embryos, especially when oocytes or sperm are donated in the creation of the embryos. Couples for whom discarding the embryos would never be an option and who may want to donate embryos in the future will need to be counseled about the importance of screening tests within the legal constructs of each country (FDA mandated screening for acceptance of embryos in transfer from one center to another). The persons for whom the embryos were created can change the directives in the future, but discordance of opinion in the future may make actual disposition very difficult and legally challenging.

Ideally, the informed consent process that includes advanced directives should include many of the scenarios that might arise with the given person or persons for whom the embryos are created. The counseling should be thoughtful and patient specific. The person/persons for whom the embryos are created should have ample time at home and in the clinic to consider their individual situation and preferable option. Finally, persons who have not used their cryopreserved embryos over several years should be contacted to determine if their situation or wishes have changed so that they can create a new advanced directive document. There have been very significant difficulties experienced by programs around the world when patients have not been able to be contacted over years. Centers should include the disposition scenario in which there is inability to find the owners of the cryopreserved embryos in the case of non-payment for storage, or dissolution of the practice [32]. The informed consent process may stress the responsibility of the couple to keep in regular contact with the center, and should consider a list of alternative contacts if the owners of the embryos cannot be located.

4.8 Posthumous Donation: When There Can Be No Informed Consent

Most ART centers have cryopreservation consents with advanced directives that allow for posthumous donation should the couple (in the case of an embryo) or the person (in the case of cryopreserved sperm or cryopreserved ova) predecease the use of the embryos or gametes. In these conditions, the persons have clearly documented their intent for the use of their embryos or gametes in the future. They have given consent.

A more complex issue arises when there is a request to "harvest" sperm or ova from a patient who is perimortem or immediately postmortem, or in a persistent vegetative state and has not given consent. The ethical considerations for retrieving sperm, testicular tissue, or oocytes from a premortem or recently deceased patient are complex, involving the rights of a body not to be disturbed (electroejaculation, testicular biopsy, or postmortem harvest of testicular tissue or ooctyes), the rights of the family to direct the use of tissue in the event that there are no specific directives (organ donation), and the rights of the future child. Without specific directives, it is common to assume that patients would not prefer to have their organs harvested for the purposes of procreation. A survey of a random computer-generated sample of Utah residents assessed willingness to posthumously donate oocytes to create a pregnancy. The survey revealed that 57% of women were willing to donate their ova after death to create a child. Similarly, 52% of people who were the guardians of a potential patient whose ova might be harvested were willing to use the ova to create a child [33]. Although this is a relatively high rate of acceptance, it still leaves almost 50% who would not choose to have their ova used to create a child. The rate of acceptance of posthumous donation might be very different in the setting of a married couple who had been in the process of attempting a pregnancy when the question for posthumous egg or sperm donation arose.

A critique of the issues of gamete harvest without consent questions whether this is fundamentally different from other organ donation. It is common for families to decide whether to allow organ harvest without prior consent for patients who are to be taken off life support. Should gametes be any different than a heart or a kidney [34]? If there is clear evidence from the family and the partner that the patient was planning children with this partner, then consent might be implied and the gametes used to create a child with the partner. Given that the parents would never have been partners in the creation of a child with the patient, the parents' wishes are not part of what may have been the original intent with the patient. They might, however, provide substantiating evidence for the partner's wish to harvest gametes.

In Israel, guidelines were published in 2003 for posthumous sperm retrieval for the purpose of future insemination or IVF by the surviving female partner. This was in response to an increase in requests for posthumous sperm donation by partners and parents of deceased men. The guidelines suggested a two step procedure which allowed for the urgency of the sperm harvest under premortem or perimortem conditions, and the thoughtful considerations of their future use at a later date under less time pressure. Requests for sperm harvest were to be honored when made by the patient's wife or partner. Requests from parents were not accepted. Sperm harvest did not necessarily authorize its use, and the decision to use the sperm was made after some later decision making processes [35].

The European Society of Human Reproduction and Embryology (ESHRE) created a task force on this issue with guidelines published in 2006 [36]. This document recognizes that the majority of requests for posthumous donation arise in the setting of an existing "parental project." In this framework, the gametes can only be used by the surviving partner and parents or other family members have no rights for request. The partner can only use the gametes for his or her reproduction. A minimum waiting period of one year should be imposed before the partner can begin therapy to use the gametes after thorough counseling of the partner during the waiting and decision making period.

This request for posthumous donation is often made with great urgency, and in the presence of considerable familial grief and conflict. ART centers that will consider offering these services should have very clear policies and procedures in place in advance that are well known to all members of the team so when these emergency requests are made, the process is clear.

4.9 Storage of Informed Consent Documents

There are no "best practices" of numbers of copies of informed consent documents and who should keep them and how they should be kept. It is prudent to have one copy for the clinicians, one copy for the embryologists and one copy for the patient/patients. There are no clear guideline of how long these documents should be kept, where they should be kept, and where they should go in the case of dissolution of the ART center. In the absence of clear guidelines and in the face of considerable uncertainty, they should be kept indefinitely, in either paper or electronic form.

4.10 Conclusion

The informed consent process is time consuming, complex, and varies from patient to patient. Patients need to feel that their requests for information and guidance have been heard. Clinicians need to feel that their information regarding risks and possible outcomes have been processed and retained. A document signed by the parties involved should reflect these issues. A well conceived and timely informed consent process, and, shared decision making that is repeated throughout the ART procedures is most likely to lead to satisfaction on the part of the patients and the clinicians, whatever the outcomes of the procedure itself.

4.11 Summary

There are standardized patient handouts available from some ART organizations (ASRM) regarding the risks of IVF/ICSI. The Society for Advanced Reproductive Technology of the ASRM has developed a 20 page universal informed consent that ART centers can use when offering IVF, ICSI, assisted hatching, and embryo cryopreservation. This form is available to SART members and includes the risks of medications, egg retrievals, embryo culture, and embryo transfer. It addresses the ethical, legal, and psychosocial issues of ART and discusses alternatives. Standardized documents may help decrease the burden of informed consent document creation, and standardized patient handouts on techniques, risks, and benefits and be helpful. However, the actual face-to-face informed consent process and the assessment of the patients' understanding will always be time consuming.

The "Paling Palette" can be used to display medical risks with a probability higher than 1 in 1,000 [7]. An evidence-based resource on informed decision making in reproductive issues (specifically hormonal contraception but the tools and processes are similar) is available through the Association of Reproductive Health Professionals (ARHP) [8].

The specific ART procedures should be discussed in some detail with pictures or videos of the unstimulated ovary, the hyperstimulated ovary, the transvaginal ultrasound guided egg retrieval, the embryo culture, the intracytoplasmic sperm injection, and the embryo transfer. Extensive resources of varying reliability are available to patients on the internet, and often sites are sponsored by specific ART programs. Each ART facility should decide to sponsor specific web-based information, or develop its own website.

A shared dialogue between the clinicians and the laboratory staff should create the probability of pregnancy for different diagnoses and ages. All the clinicians, embryologists, and educators should use the same source for the program's pregnancy rates and it should be up-to-date. In the United States, programs that participate in the Centers for Disease Control data collection for IVF may choose to use their most recent data which is posted on the CDC website [9].

The more complex ethical question in the informed consent process is whether a discussion about IVF center outcomes disparities should be initiated. There is a very broad range of pregnancy rates in the CDC center specific outcomes website.

Do physicians have an ethical duty to inform patients about the success rates of their center compared to other centers? There are very real trends in increasing pregnancy rates and birth rates in IVF centers with higher volume. What is the role of the clinician in discussing these issues [10]? As informed consent is seen as the right of the patient and the obligation of the physician, outcomes data for an individual IVF center must be discussed.

Alternatives for family building (or the choice not to pursue fertility therapy or adoption) should be discussed. Alternatives are not usually added to the informed consent document, but are a very important part of the informed consent process. Risks of procedures should be explained as a function of their frequency and severity. A highly recommended resource for outcomes after ART is the Joint Society of Gynaecologists of Canada (SOGC) and the Canadian Fertility and Andrology Society Guideline: Pregnancy Outcomes After Assisted Reproductive Technology [13]. "Since definitions of futile care are value laden, universal consensus on futile care is unlikely to be achieved. Rather, the American Medical Association Council on Ethical and Judicial Affairs recommends a process-based approach to futility recommendations" [16].

The precautionary principle is based on the premise that action should be taken would cause harm when there is evidence that not to do so [19]. It is thought of as being a primary principle in public health – when there is a suggestion of data that something is harmful, action should be taken until further research completely illuminates the issue. The areas of uncertainty that bring the precautionary principle into ART are issues of long term effects of embryo culture [20, 21]. The parts of the precautionary principle that apply in ART are transparency and inclusiveness in decision making, action in the face of uncertainty, and accountability. What should be discussed is the fact that embryo culture is relatively new and reproductive endocrinologists, embryologists, and geneticists do not know all of the changes in the developing embryo that might be different in laboratory culture from in vivo. This acknowledgment to the patients, with the option of including the patients in the face of this uncertainty could be considered an important part of the informed consent process and may be added to an informed consent document.

The ESHRE Taskforce on Ethics and Law also created a statement on ethical considerations of cryopreservation of gametes and reproductive tissues for self use which outlines the ethical principles and informed consent issues for males and females which stressed the importance of interdisciplinary consulting (the oncologists, pediatricians, reproductive specialists, psychologists, and counselors) in the decision-making process [31].

A very important focus of the informed consent for embryo cryopreservation is the process of counseling regarding advanced directives. Advanced directives are thought to be part of directing actions when a person is no longer alive or able to act on his/her own. Similarly, advanced directives as part of the informed consent process for embryo cyropreservation were designed to allow the ART center to treat cryopreserved embryos in a manner that the persons for whom they were created would wish in the event that they could not act on their own.

The request for posthumous donation is often made with great urgency, and in the presence of considerable familial grief and conflict. ART centers that will consider offering these services should have very clear policies and procedures in place in advance that are well known to all members of the team, that so when these emergency requests are made, the process is clear.

The informed consent process is time consuming, complex, and varied from patient to patient. Patients need to feel that their requests for information and guidance have been heard. Clinicians need to feel that their information regarding risks and possible outcomes have been processed and retained. A document signed by the parties involved should reflect these issues. A well conceived and timely informed consent process and shared decision making that is repeated throughout the ART procedures is most likely to lead to satisfaction on the part of the patients and the clinicians, whatever the outcomes of the procedure itself.

References[1]

1. Brown TE, Massoud E, Bance M (2003) Informed consent in otolotic surgery: prospective study of risk recall by patients and impact of written summaries of risk. J Otolaryngol 32(6):368–372
2. Steffenino G, Viada E, Marengo B, Canale R (2007) Effectiveness of video-based patient information before percutaneous cardiac interventions. J Cardiovasc Med (Hagerstown) 8(5):348–353
3. Eaden J, Abrams K, Shears J, Mayberry J (2002) Randomized controlled trial comparing the efficacy of a video and information leaflet versus information leaflet alone on patient knowledge about surveillance and cancer risk in ulcerative colitis. Inflamm Bowel Dis 8(6):407–412
4. Ryan RE, Prictor MJ, McLlaughlin KJ, Hill SJ (2008) Audio-visual presentation of information for informed consent for participation in clinical trails. Cochrane Database Syst Rev 9101: CD003717
5. Oconnor AM, Stacey D, Rovner D, Holmes-Rovner M, Tetroe J, Llewellyn-Thomas H, Entwhistle V, Rostom A, Fiset V, Barry M, Jones J (2001) Decision aids for people facing health treatment or screening decisions. Cochrane Database Syst Rev (3):CD001431
6. Edwards AG, Evans R, Dundon J, Haigh S, Hood K, Elwyn GJ (2006) Personalized risk communication for informed decision making about taking screening tests. Cochrane Database Syst Rev (4):CD001865
7. Paling J (2003) Strategies to help patients understand risks. BMJ 327:745–748
8. www.arhp.org/publications-and-resources/clinical-proceedings/riskproject
9. www.cdc.gov/ART/
10. Housri H, Weil RJ, Shalowitz DI, Konaris LG (2008) Should informed consent for cancer treatment include a discussion about hospital outcome disparities? PLoS Med 5(10):e24
11. Finlayson SR, Birkmeyer JD, Tosteson AN, Nease RF (1999) Patient preferences for location of care: implication for regionalization. Med Care 37:204–209
12. www.asrm.org/Patients/FactSheets/fact.html Patient Fact Sheet: Risks of In Vitro Fertilization (IVF)
13. The Society of Obstetricians and Gynaecologists of Canada (2006) Pregnancy outcomes after assisted reproductive technology. J Obstet Gynaecol Can 28(3):220–233
14. Newton CR, McBride J, Feyles V, Tekpetey F, Power S (2007) Factors affecting patients' attitudes toward single- and multiple-embryo transfer. Fertil Steril 87:269–278

[1]References 7, 12, 13, 22, 27, and 36 are key references for useful informed consent guidelines.

15. Schneiderman LJ, Jecker NS, Jonsen AR (1990) Medical futility: its meaning and ethical implications. Ann Intern Med 112:949–954
16. Plows CW, Tenery RM, Hartford A et al (1999) Medical futility in end-of-life care – report of the council on ethical and judicial affairs. JAMA 276:571–574
17. Burns JP, Druog RD (2007) Futility: a concept in evolution. Chest 132:1987–1993
18. The Ethics Committee of ASRM (2004) Fertility treatment when the prognosis is very poor or futile. Fertil Steril 82:806–810
19. Kurland J (2002) The heart of the precautionary principle in democracy. Public Health Rep 117:498–586
20. Lawrence LT, Moley KH (2008) Epigenetics and assisted reproductive technologies: human imprinting syndromes. Semin Reprod Med 26(2):143–152
21. Watkins AJ, Papengrock T, Fleming TP (2008) The preimplantion embryo: handle with care. Semin Reprod Med 26(2):175–185
22. The Practice Committee of the Society of Assisted Reproductive Technology and the Practice Committee of the American Society fro Reproductive Medicine (2007) Preimplantation genetic testing: a Practice Committee opinion. Fertil Steril 88(6):1497–1504
23. Maswell KA, Cholst IN, Rosenwaks Z (2008) The incidence of both serious and minor complications in young women undergoing oocyte donatation. Fertil Steril 90(6):2165–2171 Epub 2008 Feb 4
24. Bodri D, Guillen JJ, Polo A, Trullenque M, Esteve C, Coll O (2008) Complications related to ovarian stimulation and oocyte retrieval in 4052 ooctye donor cycles. Reprod Biomed Online 17(2):237–243
25. Kalfoglou AL, Geller G (2000) A follow-up study with oocyte donors exploring their experiences, knowledge, and attitudes about the use of their oocytes and the outcome of the donation. Fertil Steril 74:660–667
26. Levens ED, DeCherney AH (2008) Human oocyte research: the ethics of donation and donor protection. JAMA 300(18):2174–2176
27. Practice Committee of Society for Assisted Reproductive Technology; Practice Committee of American Society for Reproductive Medicine (2008) Essential elements of informed consent for elective oocyte cryopreservation: a practice committee opinion. Fertil Steril 90(5 Suppl):S134–S135
28. ACOG committee Opinion No.405 (2009) Ovarian tissue and oocyte cropreservation. Obstet Gynecol 111:1255–1256
29. Dudinski DM (2004) Ethical issues in fertility preservation for adolescent cancer survivors: oocyte and ovarian tissue cryopreservation. J Pediatr Adolesc Gynecol 17(2):97–102
30. Patrizio P, Butts S, Caplan A (2005) Ovarian tissue preservation and future fertility: emerging technologies and ethical considerations. J Natl Cancer Inst Monogr 34:107–110
31. The ESHRE Task Force on Ethics and Law (2004) Taskforce 7: ethical considerations for the cryopreservation of gametes and reproductive tissues for self use. Hum Reprod 19(2):460–462
32. Pennings G (2002) The validity of contract to dispose of frozen embryos. J Med Ethics 28:295–298
33. Mizukami A, Peterson CM, Huang I, Cook C, Boyack LM, Emery BR, Carrell DT (2005) The acceptability of posthumous human ovarian tissue donation in Utah. Hum Reprod 20:3560–3565
34. Strong C, Gingrich JR, Kutteh WH (2000) Ethics of postmortem sperm retrieval. Hum Reprod 15:739–745
35. Landau R (2004) Posthumous sperm retrieval for the purpose of later insemination or IVF in Israel: and ethical and psychological critique. Hum Reprod 19:1952–1956
36. ESHRE Task Force on Ethic and Law (2006) ESHRE Task for on Ethics and Law 11: posthumous assisted reproduction. Hum Reprod 21:3050–3053

Chapter 5
Reproductive Laboratory Regulations, Certifications and Reporting Systems

Brooks A. Keel and Tammie K. Schalue

Abstract The assisted reproductive technology (ART) laboratory must conform to a myriad of rules and regulations, including Clinical Laboratory Improvement Amendments of 1988 (CLIA), the Fertility Clinic Success Rate and Certification Act of 1992 (FCSRCA), also known as the Wyden Bill, and the Food and Drug Administration (FDA). In addition, laboratory inspections, personnel certification requirements, and ART data registry systems exist which can make the day to day activity in the ART laboratory complex. This chapter will attempt to provide sufficient background information on all of these rules, regulations, certifications, and registry systems to aid ART laboratory personnel in circumnavigating through this regulatory minefield.

Keywords Assisted Reproductive Technology Laboratory • Andrology laboratory • Embryology laboratory • Personnel certification • Laboratory accreditation • Data registry systems

5.1 Introduction

Although it may appear that the laboratory component of assisted reproductive technologies (ART) is heavily regulated in the US, with exception of a few State regulations, virtually all of the standards put forth for regulating the ART laboratory are voluntary and carry no sanctions for noncompliance [1, 2]. The ART laboratory has avoided regulatory oversight for many reasons, but, they center around one primary point of contention: the definition of the term *clinical laboratory* as it relates to ART, and the subtle differences between the practice of medicine (therapy), which is essentially devoid of legislative oversight, versus laboratory testing (diagnosis), which is heavily regulated. Many view the procedures carried out in the embryology laboratory, including oocyte isolation, fertilization, embryo development and transfer, as part of the patient's therapy and that no useful diagnostic information is gleaned from these procedures. Thus, according to the argument, the embryologist is involved in the patient's therapy (i.e., the practice of medicine) and the oversight mechanisms that govern diagnostic testing do not apply to this "laboratory." However, with the advent of newly codified Food and Drug Administration (FDA) [3] rules (see below), the regulatory landscape of the ART laboratory is quickly becoming treacherous.

In contrast to the embryology laboratory, the testing performed in the andrology laboratory, such as the counting of sperm, the assessment of motility and forward progression, and the determination of morphology, all are clearly diagnostic procedures in nature, and as such, are covered by Federal mandatory oversight. However, it is when these procedures are performed as an integral part of the ART procedure that the lines delineating what is considered diagnostic testing (i.e., mandatory oversight) and therapeutic procedures (i.e., voluntary oversight) become blurred. Even though the embryologist may be evaluating sperm using the exact same procedures employed by the andrologist, many feel that these procedures should not be covered by the existing mandatory Federal oversight because of their therapeutic nature. Thus, for the most part, Federal oversight of the andrology laboratory is mandatory while oversight of the embryology laboratory is voluntary even though these two "laboratories" may be housed in the same room, and the "embryologist" and the "andrologist" are often the same person.

There are three laws which either directly or indirectly regulate the ART laboratory in the United States; the Clinical Laboratory Improvement Amendments of 1988 (CLIA) [4] and subsequent final rule [5], the Fertility Clinic Success Rate and Certification Act of 1992 (FCSRCA), also known as the Wyden Bill [6], and the FDA [7]. The authors have provided detailed overviews of these regulations as they pertain to ART laboratories elsewhere [1, 2, 8–10], and the reader will no doubt notice similarities between this chapter

B.A. Keel (✉)
Departments of Biological Sciences and Research and Economic Development, Louisiana State University, Baton Rouge, LA, USA
e-mail: bkeel@lsu.edu

T.K. Schalue
Birenbaum and Associates, St. Louis, MO, USA

D.T. Carrell and C.M. Peterson (eds.), *Reproductive Endocrinology and Infertility: Integrating Modern Clinical and Laboratory Practice*,
DOI 10.1007/978-1-4419-1436-1_5,

and previous reviews. However, FDA regulations have changed drastically very recently, and the impact on the ART laboratory is still being gauged.

In January of 2003, the Centers for Disease Control and Prevention [11] and the Centers for Medicare and Medicaid Services [12] published final laboratory regulations (i.e., "CLIA"), that became effective from April 24, 2003. CLIA is the federal law which sets the standards for essentially all clinical laboratory testing in the United States except forensic laboratories, research laboratories, and drug-testing laboratories. Although some individual states have passed laws which govern laboratory testing within their respective boundaries, these State laws are based upon, and must be at least as strict, as CLIA. FCSRCA is aimed specifically at "embryo laboratories," and does not address andrology testing per se, or classical laboratory testing. Whereas compliance with CLIA is mandatory, and there are strict penalties for noncompliance, compliance with FCSRCA is completely voluntary, and there are no sanctions for noncompliance. The premise behind the creation of what may appear to be duplicative regulatory laws relates to the long-standing disagreement mentioned above over whether the activities which take place in the ART laboratory provide an actual diagnosis, and therefore come under CLIA, or instead constitute therapy, and therefore require separate and distinct regulatory language (hence, FCSRCA) [2].

In 1997, the FDA announced plans to regulate human cellular and tissue based products under the communicable disease provisions of the Public Health Service Act (Section 361). Later the term human cells, tissues, and cellular and tissue-based products (HCT/Ps) were implemented which clarified the terminology without changing the scope of FDA's purpose. This comprehensive plan of regulation for HCT/Ps included establishment registration, donor-suitability requirements, good tissue practice requirements, and other regulations. The plan was to protect public health with as minimal governmental regulation as necessary to accomplish this goal.

The plan was implemented by regulation in a tiered fashion. The establishment registration subpart became effective 75 days after publication in January 2001. Reproductive establishments were required to register by March 2004. The portion of the rule that covers donor eligibility was published in May 2004, and became effective from May 25, 2005. On May 24, 2005, the FDA published the Interim Final Rule for Donor Eligibility, with requirements for implementation on May 25, 2005. The final tier of the plan, which considered good tissue practices, was published in November 24, 2004. However, as of the writing of this edition, except for small sections, the Current Good Tissue Practices portion of the plan does not apply to the majority of reproductive establishments.

5.2 The Clinical Laboratory Improvement Amendments

CLIA defines a laboratory as "a facility for the biological, microbiological, serological, chemical, immunohematological, hematological, biophysical, cytological, pathological, or other examination of materials derived from the human body for the purpose of providing information for the diagnosis, prevention, or treatment of any disease or impairment of, or the assessment of the health of, human beings" [4]. Under CLIA, all laboratory tests are categorized as being Waived, Moderate Complexity or High Complexity. All laboratories must meet minimal standards based on the complexity categorization of the specific test [13], which depends upon many factors primarily related to the degree of difficulty and interpretation required for successful test performance. It should be noted that even if the laboratory performs only a single high complexity test, then this laboratory must meet all of the requirements for high complexity testing. The vast majority of ART laboratories performing diagnostic testing fall under the requirements of high complexity testing, and we will therefore limit our discussion in this chapter to requirements for this category.

In general, CLIA provides standards for six main aspects of laboratory testing: proficiency testing (PT), patient test management, quality control (QC), personnel requirements and responsibilities, quality assessment (QA) and inspections and sanctions.

5.2.1 Proficiency Testing

PT is a process of external, inter-laboratory quality control whereby simulated patient samples are tested by participating laboratories, and the performance of the individual laboratory is compared with the collective performance of all participants [14]. All laboratories in the United States engaged in high complexity testing are required to enroll in a government approved PT program, if such a program is available, and failure to achieve satisfactory performance in PT may result in sanctions against the laboratory [8]. Currently, the American Association of Bioanalysts (AAB) [15] and the College of American Pathologists (CAP) [16] are the only government approved PT programs offering PT in andrology and embryology. The results of the AAB PT program in embryology [17] and andrology [18] have previously been reported. These results, and other such reports [19, 20], indicate an urgent need for improvement in the quality of andrology testing.

5.2.2 Patient Test Management

Patient test management is one of the most important aspects of CLIA, especially as it relates to the handling of gametes. Standards associated with patient test management help to ensure that a specimen is properly collected, labeled, processed, analyzed, and that accurate results are reported. To accomplish this goal, CLIA divides clinical testing into three main processes: specimen receiving (i.e., preanalytic), specimen testing (i.e., analytic) and result reporting (i.e., postanalytic).

Positive identification of the patient and his/her specimen is maintained throughout these three processes to ensure proper chain of custody of the specimen from the time of collection, through testing, to accurate reporting of test results. The preanalytic standards ensure that patients are properly informed about specimen collection; that adequate labeling, preservation, transportation and processing of the specimen take place and that the laboratory only performs tests which are requested by authorized individuals. The analytic standards ensure that the actual testing is performed in such a way as to provide accurate and reliable results. A major part of this process is laboratory QC (see below). The postanalytic standards ensure that laboratory tests are reported in a timely manner; that the test report form itself is accurate and meaningful; that test results are only reported to authorized individuals; and that the reporting process protects the patient's confidentiality. The definition of an "authorized individual" to whom test results may be reported is typically defined by State law. Most States define this individual as the person who ordered the test, who is usually a physician or health care worker. Some States do, however, allow "direct access testing," where the patient him/herself can order laboratory tests on themselves. In these States, laboratory test results may be provided directly to the patient without a health care worker acting as an intermediary.

5.2.3 Quality Control

QC, according to CLIA, involves a more broad approach to laboratory testing than merely including a known positive and negative sample in each assay. It is a comprehensive program that covers all aspects of the laboratory, including facilities, test methods, equipment, instrumentation, reagents, materials and supplies; procedure manual, establishment and verification of method performance specifications; equipment maintenance and function checks; calibration and calibration verification procedures; assay control procedures; remedial action; and QC records [8]. QC in the ART may seem problematic, especially in the andrology laboratory. However, several novel approaches have been proposed [21–23]. Another unique aspect of the embryology laboratory involves the need, or lack thereof, for quality control testing of media [24]. Controversy exists as to whether media used for oocyte/embryo culture needs to be QC tested in light of the fact that most commercial medial now is pre-tested prior to shipment. CLIA does allow the laboratory to use manufacturer's control checks of media provided the manufacturer's product insert specifies that the manufacturer's quality control checks meet the national standards for media quality control. The laboratory must document that the physical characteristics of the media are not compromised and report any deterioration in the media to the manufacturer. The laboratory must follow the manufacturer's specifications for using the media and be responsible for the test results.

5.2.4 Personnel Requirements and Responsibilities

Laboratories performing high complexity testing must identify five qualified individuals to assume the responsibilities of the director, clinical consultant, technical supervisor, general supervisor, and testing personnel. One single individual may assume the role of one or more of these positions. In fact, a single individual, if qualified, may assume the role of all five. This is not unusual in small laboratories. Each individual assuming these positions must meet certain well defined qualifications based on formal education, training and experience. In general, to qualify for the Director, an individual must either be: (1) a board certified pathologist or a licensed physician with 2 years experience in directing or supervising testing; or (2) posses an earned doctoral degree in science with 4 years experience in clinical laboratory testing, 2 years of which must be at the level of supervisor of director. In addition, as of December 31, 2000, the non-physician director must obtain board certification by one of several government approved certification boards (see Sect. 5.7 below).

The responsibilities of the director are numerous, broad, and all-encompassing [8]. In general, the director is responsible for the overall operation and administration of the laboratory, including the employment of personnel who are competent to perform test procedures, record and report test results promptly, accurately and proficiently and for assuring compliance with the applicable regulations [8]. Although some of the duties of the director may be delegated to others, he/she must maintain the responsibility. There are several duties for which the director must maintain direct oversight [25]. The director must ensure that:

- Testing systems in the laboratory provide quality services in all aspects of test performance, i.e., the preanalytic, analytic, and postanalytic phases of testing and are appropriate for your patient population.
- Physical and environmental conditions of the laboratory are adequate and appropriate for the testing performed.
- The environment for employees is safe from physical, chemical, and biological hazards and safety and biohazard requirements are followed.
- A general supervisor (high complexity testing) is available to provide day-to-day supervision of all testing personnel and reporting of test results as well as provide on-site supervision for specific minimally qualified testing personnel when they are performing high complexity testing.
- Sufficient numbers of appropriately educated, experienced, and/or trained personnel who provide appropriate consultation, properly supervise, and accurately perform tests and report test results in accordance with the written duties and responsibilities specified by the director, are employed by the laboratory.
- New test procedures are reviewed, included in the procedure manual and followed by personnel.
- Each employee's responsibilities and duties are specified in writing.

The director must be accessible to the laboratory at all times, but this accessibility may be achieved through telephone or electronic means. However, a single director may direct up to five individual laboratories, even at distinct and distant geographical sites.

The clinical consultant is responsible for assisting the laboratory's clients in ordering appropriate tests and interpreting test reports. The technical supervisor carries a number of responsibilities including selection and verification of test methodologies, enrollment in PT, establishing QC programs, resolving technical problems, and identifying training needs and evaluating competency of testing personnel. The general supervisor is responsible for providing the day-to-day supervision of high complex test performance by the testing personnel, and the testing personnel's primary responsibility is performing accurate testing.

5.2.5 Quality Assessment

CLIA requires each laboratory to establish and follow written policies and procedures for a comprehensive QA program designed to monitor and evaluate the ongoing and overall quality of the total testing process [8]. QA attempts to address all aspects of the preanalytic, analytic and postanalytic processes in a continuous fashion. It is a system which monitors not just how well an incubator holds temperature, or the accuracy and precision of an internal assay control, but also considers other relevant things such as communication with physician clients and continuing education of laboratory employees. This process is usually best monitored by a periodic (i.e., monthly) QA meeting which includes the laboratory personnel and if possible, the ordering physician and his/her staff. Specifically, CLIA requires the laboratory to address several things, including:

- Monitoring all aspects of patient test management mentioned earlier, including criteria established for patient preparation, sample collection, quality control, test requisition and test reporting.
- Documenting problems that occur as a result of breakdowns in communication between the laboratory and the authorized individual who orders or receives the results of test procedures. Furthermore, corrective actions taken to resolve the problems and minimize communications breakdowns must be documented.
- Documenting all complaints and problems reported to the laboratory. Investigations of complaints must be made, when appropriate, and as necessary corrective actions instituted, with ongoing monitoring to minimize reoccurrences.
- Documenting of all QA activities including problems identified and corrective actions taken.

5.2.6 Inspections and Sanctions

The United States Government Department of Health and Human Services (DHHS) [26] ensures laboratory compliance with CLIA standards by performing on-site inspections at least once every 2 years. The actual entity which performs the inspection, on behalf of DHHS, depends upon the State in which the laboratory is located and the type of certificate the laboratory has requested. Laboratories have the option of being inspected by representatives of their respective State Department of Health, or requesting that inspections be conducted by one of several private accrediting agencies. The most common of these is the CAP, the Commission on Office Laboratory Accreditation (COLA) [27], and the Joint Commission on Accreditation of Health Care Organizations (JCAHO) [28]. For practical reasons, the vast majority of these on-site inspections are announced, rather than surprise unannounced visits. These inspectors typically use detailed checklists to determine if the laboratory is in compliance with all of the CLIA standards. If deficiencies are noted, the laboratory is given an opportunity to correct these problems. Failure to correct the noted deficiencies, or other violations of CLIA may result in a range of sanctions, which may include suspension, limitation or revocation of the laboratory's certificate, civil suit against the laboratory, or imprisonment or fine for any person convicted of intentional violation of CLIA requirements [8]. Fines can range from $50 to $10,000 per day. In addition, the Secretary of DHHS is required to publish annually, a list of all laboratories that have been sanctioned during the preceding year. Thus, participation in CLIA is not a matter of choice, and failure to comply with these standards carry stiff penalties.

5.3 The Fertility Clinic Success Rate and Certification Act of 1992

In 1988, in response to consumer concerns about the conduct of ART programs and the apparent lack of uniform information relating to the pregnancy success rates, Congressman Ron Wyden conducted public hearings to address these concerns [29, 30]. Later that same year, a survey was sent to the directors of all ART programs to determine clinic specific success rates, and the results of this survey were released at a second hearing held in 1989. Congressman Wyden held a press conference on June 21, 1990 and introduced the Fertility Clinic Success Rate and Certification Act (FCSRCA) of 1992, which became widely known as the Wyden bill [29]. The final version of the Wyden bill was passed into law on October 24, 1992 [6].

The FCSRCA was intended to provide the public with comparable information concerning the effectiveness of infertility services and to assure the quality of such services by providing for the certification of embryo laboratories [6, 31]. Basically, FCSRCA consists of two components. The first component prescribed a mechanism whereby each clinic performing ART in the United States would report its clinic-specific pregnancy rates on an annual basis, and this will be discussed in more detail below (see Sect. 5.8).

The second component of FCSRCA called for the Secretary of DHHS, through the CDC, to develop a model program for the certification of embryo laboratories to be administered by the individual States [31]. In developing such a model, the CDC consulted with various consumer (i.e., RESOVLE) [32] and professional groups (i.e., the ASRM, SART and the AAB) who had expertise and interest in ART laboratory services. The standards that were to be developed include standards to assure consistent performance of laboratory procedures; a standard for QA and QC; standards for the maintenance of all laboratory records (including laboratory tests and procedures performed, as well as personnel and equipment records); and a standard for personnel qualifications [6, 31]. Interestingly, these standards were prohibited from establishing any such regulation, standard or requirement that has the effect of exercising supervision or control over the practice of medicine in ART programs [6]. Furthermore, compliance with the standards set forth by FCSRCA is completely voluntary, and no sanctions were prescribed for noncompliance.

After several years of consultation and planning, the final notice of the model program for embryo laboratory certification was published in July 1999 [31]. The model laboratory program defined an Embryo laboratory as a "facility in which human oocytes and sperm, or embryos, are subjected to ART laboratory procedures" [31]. It further defined ART laboratory procedures as:

> All laboratory procedures for handling and processing of human oocytes and sperm, or embryos, with the intent of establishing a pregnancy. These procedures include, but are not limited to, the examination of follicular aspirates, oocyte classification, sperm preparation, oocyte insemination, assessment of fertilization, assessment of embryo development, preparation of embryos for embryo transfer, and cryopreservation of specimens.

The model program for laboratory certification consists of four main sections: Personnel Qualifications and Responsibilities, Facilities and Safety, Quality Management, and Maintenance of Records.

5.3.1 Personnel Qualifications and Responsibilities

The FCSRCA states as a guideline that the embryo laboratory should employ one fully trained individual for every 90–150 ART cycles performed annually, and at least two qualified individuals should be available to provide appropriate services. According to the model program, the embryo laboratory must identify three key laboratory individuals: Director, Supervisor and Reproductive Biologist. If qualified, one individual may assume the responsibilities and role of more than one position. In order to qualify as a Director, the individual must: (1) possess a doctoral degree (2) have 2 years' pertinent experience including 6 months' training in an ART laboratory (3) document 1.2 continuing education units (CEUs) in ART or clinical laboratory activity annually and (4) if actively doing ART procedures, perform at least 20 procedures annually. The FCSRCA does provide a "grandfather clause" for nondoctoral directors provided they were serving as a director prior to July 20, 1999. In order to qualify as a Supervisor, the individual must possess at least a bachelor degree and demonstrate similar experience and training to that of the Director. Qualifications for Reproductive Biologists are similar to Supervisors except that these individuals are only required to have previously performed 30 ART procedures

In general, the director is responsible for the overall operation, administration, and technical and scientific oversight of the ART laboratory, and is charged with hiring qualified personnel to perform the ART laboratory procedures. The director does not have to be physically present during procedures, but must be accessible to the laboratory to provide on-site consultations by telephone or electronic means as needed. The supervisor, as the name implies, is responsible for providing day-to-day supervision and oversight of the embryo laboratory operation and the personnel performing ART laboratory procedures. The supervisor must be accessible to the laboratory to provide on-site, telephone or electronic consultation to resolve technical problems. It is this individual who is charged with the responsibility of ensuring proper training of all laboratory personnel. The reproductive biologist, synonymous with CLIA defined "testing personnel," is responsible for performing the ART laboratory procedures and for recording and reporting procedural outcomes. This individual is limited to independently performing only those procedures in which training has been documented. All other procedures must be performed under direct and constant supervision.

5.3.2 Facilities and Safety

The model program states that the lab must provide adequate space and appropriate environmental conditions to ensure safe working conditions and quality performance of ART laboratory procedures. These standards not only provide for aseptic conditions required for successful ART procedures, but also ensure a safe working environment for employees. It further mandates that all Federal, State and local regulations be followed regarding the use of human and animal materials and hazardous chemicals.

5.3.3 Quality Management

The model program spells out standards for a comprehensive quality management program that is designed to monitor and evaluate the ongoing ART laboratory procedures performed and services provided. The program contains standards for the make-up of the ART laboratory procedure manual which are similar in scope to those outlined in CLIA. The program provides standards for proper maintenance and calibration of all equipment used in the ART laboratory, including 24 h monitoring of applicable equipment and emergency backup in the event of power failure. The standards state that the laboratory must maintain records of the batch or lot number, date of receipt and date placed in use of all reagents and media, and must also verify that materials which come in contact with sperm, oocytes and embryos have been tested and found to be nontoxic either by the ART laboratory or by the manufacturer.

The model program standards, in keeping with the spirit of CLIA, stipulate that the laboratory must obtain written or electronic requests from an authorized person (usually a physician) before performing any procedure on patient's gametes or embryos. Any additional applicable information, including verification of informed consent, must also be obtained before performing procedures. The laboratory must establish written procedures and criteria for: (1) evaluation and assessment of oocyte morphology and maturity, fertilization, and embryo quality (2) insemination schedule relative to oocyte maturity (3) the volume, numbers and quality of sperm used for insemination of each oocyte (4) disposition of oocytes with an abnormal number of pronuclei, as well as disposition of excess oocytes (5) the time period following insemination for examination of fertilization (6) micromanipulation of oocytes and embryos (7) re-insemination of oocytes (8) length of time embryos are cultured prior to transfer, and medium and protein supplementation used for transfers (9) types of catheters available, and circumstances when each should be used (10) methods of transfer and techniques for checking the catheters posttransfer for retained embryos and (11) disposition of all excess embryos. Similarly, the model plan contains standards requiring detailed records on the outcome of each of the above mentioned steps, including the identity of the individual performing each step. The standards require duplicate log books or files for cryopreserved samples.

Prior to implementing any procedure in the ART laboratory, appropriate performance measures of the procedure must be verified and documented. For each batch of culture media prepared in-house, the quality of the media, including pH, osmolality and culture suitability using an appropriate bioassay system, must be confirmed. The model program standards allow the laboratory to accept quality control procedures performed by the manufacturer if commercially prepared media are used.

Lastly, the model program stipulates that the ART laboratory must establish and follow a written quality assurance (i.e., "assessment") program aimed at monitoring the quality of ART laboratory services provided, and to resolve problems identified. The details of this QA program are virtually identical to that described in CLIA, with the inclusion of ART-specific standards including the requirement to track and evaluate fertilization rates, cleavage rates and embryo quality.

5.3.4 Maintenance of Records

The model program provides standards for the retention of records of all of the laboratory's policies and procedures; personnel employment, training, evaluations and continuing education activities, and quality management activities. The laboratory must maintain these records for a period of time specified by Federal, State and local laws or for 10 years beyond the final disposition of all specimens obtained during each patient's ART cycle, whichever is later. The standard requires that all records must be maintained on-site for at least 2 years.

5.3.5 Sanctions and Enforcement

The Secretary of DHHS is instructed to publish annually a list of laboratories who have not complied with the standards of FCSRCA, but, the noncompliant laboratory is free to continue to offer ART laboratory services. The final rule stated that while it was anticipated "that the costs of Federal and State monitoring and oversight of embryo laboratories would be covered by the fees paid by participating laboratories, participation by embryo laboratories is voluntary and laboratories not willing to pay these fees would not be limited in their ability to operate" [31]. So far, embryo laboratories in the US have "not indicated they would opt into such a voluntary program" [31]. The final ruling further stated that "while the model certification program for embryo laboratories does not provide for a Federal oversight role, we do believe that this model provides an excellent resource for States that wish to develop their own programs and professional organizations with an interest in establishing or adopting standards for the embryo laboratory" [31]. Thus, the major difference between the laboratory standards spelled out in CLIA and the FCSRCA is that compliance with CLIA is mandatory while FCSRCA is voluntary.

5.3.6 American Society for Reproductive Medicine Guidelines

The Practice Committees of the American Society for Reproductive Medicine [33] and the Society for Assisted Reproductive Technology (SART) [34] have recently published updated and revised guidelines for human embryology and andrology laboratories [35]. While completely voluntary, these guidelines have become the gold standard for many embryology laboratories, and are adhered to by many, if not all, active SART clinical programs. Essentially, these Guidelines follow the recommendations set down by the FCSRCA with a few differences and refinements. First, the Guidelines provide more definitive recommendations for staffing levels, with the minimum number of embryologists set at two, three and four for 1–150, 151–300 and 301–600 ART cycles per year, respectively (1 additional embryologist is recommended per additional 200 cycles above 600). Second, while acknowledging that a single director may direct as many as five separate laboratories, the Guidelines recommend that while the laboratory is actively treating patients, the off-site director is required to physically visit the laboratory at a frequency of no less that one visit per month. Finally, and perhaps the most significant, the Guidelines state that with effect from February 1, 2006, all new laboratory directors should hold High Complexity Laboratory Director (HCLD) or Embryology Laboratory Director (ELD) certifications from the American Board of Bioanalysis (see Sect. 5.7 below). Furthermore, the Guidelines strongly encourage all laboratory directors, even those "grandfathered," to seek the HCLD or ELD certifications.

5.4 FDA

Oocyte, sperm, and embryo donation in the United States are regulated as human cell, tissue, and cellular and tissue-based products (HCT/Ps) by the FDA's Center for Biologics Evaluation and Research (CBER) branch under regulation 21 CFR part 1271. This regulation is comprised of six parts (Part A, B, C, D, E, and F) and was implemented in a tired fashion between 2001 and 2005. This regulation applies to all tissues recovered after May 25, 2005. The goal of 21 CFR 1271 is to increase protection of public health while, in the words of the FDA, "minimizing regulatory burden." The FDA does not regulate oocytes, sperm, and embryos collected prior to May 25, 2005.

21 CFR 1271 regulates tissues in addition to oocytes, sperm, and embryos. This chapter is concerned solely with the regulation as it relates to oocytes, sperm, and embryos. The reader is cautioned that the regulation differs significantly for nonreproductive tissues types. In addition, situations that may occur within infertility facilities but are not typical, such as recovery of tissue from donors who are deceased, sick, or who have undergone transfusions will not be discussed in this section. Finally, due to size constraints this chapter will not fully cover every aspect of the regulation. For the full regulation, the reader should see 21CFR 1271 regulation in its entirety [36].

21 CFR 1271 regulations, unlike some regulations governing infertility centers and laboratories, come with stiff penalties for noncompliance. The FDA has the authority to close donor programs which they feel, do not adequately protect public safety. In addition, individuals in violation of the regulation may be imprisoned for up to 1 year and fined up to $250,000 [37] for noncompliance with the regulation.

5.4.1 General Provisions and Establishment Registration

The first tier of the regulation implemented on January 19, 2001, comprised Subpart A (General Provisions) and Subpart B (Procedures for Registration and Listing) [37]. These regulations provided insight into the remainder of the regulation scheduled for implementation in the coming years. It provided a list of definitions many of which were unfamiliar to infertility centers, at least in the manner of usage by the FDA; it explained what entities are required to comply with the regulation and it provided information and instructions for registration with the FDA.

In Subpart A, infertility centers across the country learned that, in the eyes of the FDA, they were "establishments," and instead of assisting subfertile couples to conceive a family, they were "manufacturing" preembryos and embryos. In later releases of 21 CFR 1271, infertility centers accepted the logic that an embryo was not a single piece to donor tissue, but a culmination of donor tissue from two separate and distinct donors. A whole new vocabulary emerged in infertility centers; couples were to become known as Sexually Intimate Partners or "SIPs" for short, and with the new terminology a new way of looking at the couple or SIP also emerged. SIPs, while exempt for many of the requirements of the regulation, are donors in the eyes of the FDA. This was a whole new way of viewing the typical couple treated by infertility centers.

Facilities are required to register with the FDA if they are involved in any step of the manufacture of HCT/P's regulated solely under section 361 of the PHS Act. Reproductive tissues meet regulation criteria for section 361 of the PHS Act. Typically, all full service infertility centers are required to comply with 21 CFR 1271. However, there are exemptions that may apply to some limited providers of infertility treatment. Centers that solely perform intrauterine inseminations (IUIs) or embryo transfers utilizing cryopreserved samples obtained elsewhere are not required to comply. Likewise, surgery centers or physician offices that recover and immediately relinquish control of the tissue to registered facilities for tissue processing and donor eligibility determination elsewhere, are not required to register with FDA, but must comply with all other parts of the regulation. Finally, although it is unlikely such centers exist any longer, centers that perform ONLY gamete intrafallopian transfer (GIFT) for SIPs are also exempt.

Subpart B outlined registration requirements. Establishments must register with the FDA within five days after beginning operation and must update the registration annually, in December. In addition, registrations must be updated in the event of a change of location or ownership with five days of the change. The registration must include the establishment name, address, and the signature of the reporting official. It must also include a list of all HCT/Ps that are recovered, processed, stored, labeled, packaged, distributed, and for which donor screening or donor testing is conducted. Any time the list of HCT/Ps changes, the establishment is required to provide an updated list to FDA. The updated list must be provided to FDA in June or December, depending on which month occurs first, or at the time of the change.

Upon registration acceptance, the FDA will assign each facility a permanent registration number. Unlike accrediting organizations, the issuance of a registration number does not constitute FDA's approval of the facility, compliance of the facility with the regulation, or the approval of the HCT/Ps produced by the facility.

5.4.2 Donor Eligibility and Specimen Labeling

Subpart C was implemented on May 25, 2004 [38] and is the subpart that has had the greatest affect on reproductive facilities. Some of the requirements of this subpart were very familiar, at least to the laboratory component of the reproductive facility, while others were unfamiliar and initially difficult to grasp.

Procedures are required for all facets of the donor eligibility determination process including all recovery, processing, storage, labeling, packaging, distribution, donor screening, and donor testing. These procedures must be reviewed and signed by a responsible person prior to implementation and they must be kept in an area readily accessible by personnel using the procedures. Any departure from the procedure must be within the scope of the regulation and must be documented at the time of the departure. In addition, a responsible person must review all departures prior to a donor eligibility determination to assure that the departure did not increase the risks of communicable disease transmission by the HCT/P.

Records for HCT/Ps must be indelible, legible, and readily available for inspection by the FDA for at least 10 years after the HCT/P has been distributed, or disposed. A copy of the HCT/Ps summary of records must "accompany" the HCT/P throughout the process from recovery to distribution or disposal. In the case of anonymous donations, the records must include a unique identifier and may not include the name or social security of the donor. The accompanying records when complete include the donor eligibility determination and the summary of records used to make the donor eligibility determination. The donor eligibility must include a statement that the testing was conducted by a laboratory certified to perform clinical testing under CLIA; a list and interpretation of all tests; the name and address of the FDA registered facility; the signature of the person who made the determination of eligibility and if the donor is determined to be ineligible, a statement noting the reason for the determination along with all the proper warning labels to be discussed later in this section.

Prior to donor eligibility determination, all HCT/Ps must be held in quarantine. All quarantine HCT/Ps must be stored in a location that clearly identifies the HCT/Ps as in quarantine. This may be accomplished in a number of ways (e.g., separate incubator shelves clearly marked, separate dewer canisters, or even separate cryopreservation tanks).

The accompanying records must include a donor identifier and state that the donor eligibility has not been determined and therefore the HCT/P cannot be transferred until completion of the donor eligibility determination. An HCT/P in quarantine may be shipped to another location as long as the accompanying paper work is shipped with the HCT/P.

With the exception of SIP donors, all donors must be screened [39] for risk factors, and clinical evidence of relevant communicable disease agents or disease. Currently for reproductive tissues, collected as most infertility centers perform collections in the US, this list includes:

- Human immunodeficiency virus (including HIV group O)
- Hepatitis B virus
- Hepatitis C virus
- Human transmissible spongiform encephalopathy
- *Treponema pallidum* (syphilis)
- Disease risks associated with xenotransplantation
- West Nile virus
- Sepsis
- Vaccinia
- *Chlamydia trachomatis*
- *Neisseria gonorrhea*
- Human T-lymphotropic virus (sperm donors only)

Testing is required for directed and anonymous oocyte donors within 30 days prior to retrieval. Testing for directed and anonymous sperm donors is required within 7 days before or after collection and again after 6 months storage for anonymous sperm donors prior to donor determination. Testing must be performed using FDA approved or cleared tests and in accordance with the manufacturer's instructions. A list of current FDA acceptable tests may be found on the CBER/Tissues web page under the Safety heading of Donor Screening Tests [40].

With the exception of SIP donors, all donors must be tested for evidence of infection due to relevant communicable disease agents. Given the collection techniques used by most fertility centers in the US, the current list of FDA required tests includes:

- HIV type 1 and type 2 or combination (including NAT testing). Testing for HIV type O is optional at this time if screening is preformed.
- HBV
- HCV
- *Treponema pallidum*
- *Chlamydia trachomatis*
- *Neisseria gonorrhea*
- Human T-lymphotropic virus types I and II (sperm donors only)
- Cytomegalovirus (sperm donors only)

Donors who are determined to be at risk for, or who are reactive for a communicable disease are ineligible. Ineligible donors may be used for tissue donation in the instance of a known or SIP donation. Paperwork for HCT/Ps from ineligible donors must contain the biohazard legend and contain the warning "WARNING: Advise recipient of communicable disease risks" and "WARNING: Reactive test results for (name the disease agent or disease)."

As mentioned earlier, sexually intimate partners are exempt from the donor eligibility determination requirement. However, these HCT/Ps must be labeled "NOT EVALUATED FOR INFECTIOUS SUBSTANCES" and "WARNING: Advise recipient of communicable disease risks." In addition, even thought a donor eligibility determination is not required, if it is known that the donor is at risk for or is reactive for a communicable disease, the HCT/P must be labeled with the biohazard legend and "WARNING: Reactive test results for (name the disease agent or disease)."

It is not unusual for couples to produce and cryopreserve embryos, with the intent to use the embryos, only to later decide that they no longer want them. FDA allows the use of the embryos as either a known or an anonymous donation. The embryos should remain in storage for 6-months. After this period, the oocyte and sperm donor (the original SIPs) should be screened and tested if possible (although it is not required) and a donor eligibility determination completed. If the donors in this instance are tested after recovery, but prior to transfer, the paperwork for the embryo(s) must be labeled "Advise recipient that screening and testing of the donors were not performed at the time of cryopreservation of the reproductive cells or tissue, but have been performed subsequently." If testing indicated one or both of the donors were reactive for a communicable disease agent or disease, the paperwork must also be labeled with the biohazard legend and "WARNING: Reactive test results for (name the disease agent or disease)." If the donors are not able to be tested, the FDA allows the use of the HCT/P but the paperwork must contain the label "WARNING: Advise recipient of communicable disease risks" and "NOT EVALUATED FOR INFECTIOUS SUBSTANCES."

5.4.3 Current Good Tissue Practice and Inspections

Subparts D, E, and F were implemented from November 24, 2004, and comprised the current good tissue practice; adverse reaction reporting; and inspection and enforcement regulations [41]. Subpart E does not currently apply to reproductive HCT/Ps; Subpart D has only limited applicability to reproductive HCT/Ps while Subpart F fully applies to reproductive HCT/Ps.

Reproductive facilities and those involved in the recovery, processing, storage, labeling, packaging, distribution, or who perform donor screening or donor testing must meet the manufacturing arrangement requirements of Subpart D (21 CFR 1271.150(c)). Each establishment involved in the process must assure that other involved establishments comply with all requirements applicable to the manufacturing steps under their control. Typically, for infertility centers, an example of an entity for which an agreement would be necessary is the testing laboratory that performs their disease agent testing. However, depending on the facility, it could include other parties such as a donor center that provides screening for potential donors. In these instances, the infertility center must assure that the testing center (or donor provider, etc.) is compliant with all regulation and if it becomes known that they are not compliant, attempt to bring them into compliance, or terminate the agreement.

Subpart F outlines the FDA's right to conduct inspections and how these inspections may be conducted; regulations for the import of HCT/P's and orders of retention. FDA investigators may conduct inspections without prior notice and at a frequency the FDA chooses. The investigators may observe procedures, take samples, and review and copy any required records.

In instances in which the FDA determines a facility is not in compliance with the regulation to a degree that public health or safety may be affected, they may issue a cessation of manufacturing order. If specific HCT/Ps are determined to be involved, the FDA may issue a recall of all HCT/P not yet transferred to a recipient and the retention of these HCT/Ps. The FDA has determined it will not issue destruction orders for reproductive tissues regardless of the threat the HCT/Ps may pose to public health.

5.5 The College of American Pathologists Reproductive Laboratory Accreditation Program

The College of American Pathologists (CAP) is a private organization which has offered inspection and accreditation of clinical laboratories in the United States for many years. The CAP is one of several private accrediting agencies recognized by the Federal government as meeting or exceeding the standards of CLIA. Thus, laboratories who choose CAP as a vehicle for accreditation can meet the standards set down by Federal law. As early as 1991, the members of the ASRM began collaborations with the CAP toward the development of a voluntary accreditation program specific for ART laboratories [29]. This collaboration took advantage of the ART expertise of the ASRM along with the years of experience of CAP in performing on-site inspections and accreditation of clinical laboratories. Out of this collaboration developed the Reproductive Laboratory Accreditation Program (RLAP). The RLAP also provides a mechanism by which the individual States could, on a voluntary basis, implement the model certification program prescribed by FCSRCA [31].

5.5.1 Performance Standards and Checklist

By using an extensive checklist, the RLAP inspects and subsequently accredits ART laboratories through a process involving on-site inspectors who evaluate the laboratory in the areas of test methodologies, reagents, control media, equipment, specimen handling, procedure manuals, test reporting, record keeping, PT, personnel qualifications, facilities, safety and overall laboratory management. Failure to meet the criteria described in the checklist results in a deficiency, and the laboratory is provided with an opportunity to document corrective actions to address these deficiencies. Accreditation is granted by CAP when the laboratory has documented correction of all deficiencies and has responded to all of the recommendations of the CAP.

5.5.2 Inspections and Accreditation

Inspectors are assigned by one of several regional commissioners. Inspections are performed by a peer process. The inspectors, recognized experts in the areas of embryology and andrology and typically practicing laboratory directors and supervisors, are not employed by CAP, and volunteer their services for this purpose. The CAP is "deemed" by CLIA as an approved accrediting agency, which is to say that the criteria by which CAP uses to accredit laboratories is at least as strict as the standards set down in CLIA. ART laboratories opting to use CAP as its accrediting agency meet the Federal mandatory oversight requirement for the andrology laboratory, as well as voluntary oversight of the embryology laboratory. Currently, SART requires the ART laboratories associated with its member clinics to become accredited as a contingency of membership. The CAP/ASRM and JCAHO are two private accrediting agencies recognized by SART as meeting this membership requirement. This has had a positive effect regarding oversight of ART laboratories in the United States, resulting in a large increase in ART laboratories seeking accreditation. However, although the majority of ART programs in the United States are currently members of SART, the absolute number of centers offering ART services to patients in this country is unknown because registering ART clinics is not required and membership in SART is voluntary.

5.6 The Joint Commission Accreditation Program for Assisted Reproductive Technology Laboratories

The Joint Commission (formerly the Joint Commission on Accreditation of Healthcare Organizations) has been evaluating and accrediting hospital laboratory services since 1979 and freestanding laboratories since 1995 [42]. Today, the Joint Commission accredits almost 2,000 organizations providing laboratory services. This represents almost 3,200 CLIA-certified laboratories, including freestanding laboratories, such as reference labs and ART labs, and those connected with other health care organizations such as ambulatory surgical centers and long term care facilities. The Joint Commission, like CAP, is recognized by the federal government as meeting or exceeding the CIIA standards.

There are many similarities between the CAP and JCAHO system of accreditation [2]. They both emphasize professional review for compliance with established performance standards and, through education, seek to improve overall patient care and safety within the laboratory setting. However, there are slight differences in the way the two organizations accomplish their goals. The JCAHO uses full-time paid inspectors ("surveyors") for the inspection process instead of professional peers from within the same field, as does CAP. The reasoning behind this from JCAHO's prospective is that a professional inspector adds consistency to the inspection process. Like CAP, the JCAHO uses a list of questions to aid the inspector in determining whether a particular laboratory has met all of the requirements. However, unlike CAP where each question will result in an all or none response (i.e., a deficiency or no deficiency), the JCAHO system may use several questions to determine the final score in a section.

5.6.1 Standards

The Joint Commission survey of laboratories is conducted using the *Comprehensive Accreditation Manual for Laboratory and Point-of-Care Testing (CAMLAB)* [42]. The standards emphasize the results a laboratory should achieve, instead of the specific methods of compliance, and were developed with input from professional laboratory organizations. In compliance with CLIA regulations, Joint Commission standards address processes that follow laboratory specimens through the laboratory from specimen collection to result reporting focusing on the provision of high quality, safe laboratory services. These standards highlight the essential nature of laboratory services on the actual care and service delivery processes that contribute to and support the overall health care delivery system.

5.6.2 Survey Process

Joint Commission accreditation process emphasizes the laboratory's operational systems that are critical to the safety and quality of patient care. The objective of the survey is not only to evaluate the laboratory, but to provide education and "good practice" guidance that will help staff continually improve the laboratory's performance. In 2004, the Joint Commission initiated a new survey process which focused the surveyor on evaluating actual service processes by tracing patients through the care, treatment and services they received [42]. In addition to these patient "tracers," surveyors conduct systems tracers to analyze key operational systems that directly impact the quality and safety of patient care. Through the Priority Focus Process, surveyors use presurvey information to conduct a more organization-specific and consistent survey. The new process has shifted the emphasis from "survey preparation" to more "continuous improvement" of the laboratory's operational systems that contribute directly to improved delivery of safe, quality care and reduction in medical errors.

Joint Commission surveyors use scoring guidelines to assist them in making judgments about standards compliance in specific performance areas. Following the on-site survey, the organization receives an accreditation report that outlines the survey findings and any requirements for improvement, supplemental findings and organizational strengths. Before it can be accredited, the laboratory must address all requirements for improvement by submitting evidence of standards compliance.

5.7 Laboratory Personnel Certification

CLIA requires that all laboratory directors, with some exceptions, be certified by a national certifying board. At present, there are eight approved certification boards for clinical consultants and directors of high complexity testing in the United States, and these are the: American Board of Medical Microbiology [43], American Board of Clinical Chemistry [44], American Board of Medical Laboratory Immunology [43], American Board of Bioanalysis (ABB) [45], American Board of Medical Genetics [46], American Board of Histocompatibility and Immunogenetics [47], American Board of Forensic Toxicology [48], and the National Registry of Certified Chemists [49]. Currently, the ABB is the only approved board offering certifications in the specialties of andrology and embryology.

The ABB evaluates, through the certification process, individuals who wish to enter, continue or advance in the clinical laboratory profession [45]. ABB identifies, on a non discriminatory basis, individuals who meet ABB's requirements for clinical laboratory directors, consultants, and supervisors. ABB certification is done on the basis of an individual's education, experience, and knowledge of the laboratory field in which certification is granted.

In 1968, the American Board of Bioanalysis was established by the American Association of Bioanalysts (AAB) [15] in response to the passage of the Medicare regulations (1966) and the original Clinical Laboratories Improvement Act of 1967 (CLIA '67), which defined the qualifications for a laboratory director. In 1972, ABB's certification program was expanded to include supervisors, in 1982 to include managers (subsequently discontinued in July 1, 2005), and in 1993 to include clinical consultants. The 1974 Medicare regulations for independent laboratories recognized ABB as a certifying agency. At that time, ABB revised its standards for director certification, creating three levels: Bioanalyst Clinical Laboratory Director (BCLD), Clinical Laboratory Director (CLD), and Bioanalyst Laboratory Director (BLD). With the advent of the CLIA regulations first promulgated in 1988, ABB again revised its certification standards and classifications. Currently, ABB certifies directors in the following two categories: Bioanalyst Clinical Laboratory Director (BCLD) and High-complexity Clinical Laboratory Director (HCLD). The regulations implementing the Clinical Laboratory Improvement Amendments of 1988 [4, 5] also recognize ABB as a certifying agency for laboratory directors and clinical consultants. In addition, most state laboratory regulatory programs recognize ABB's director certification.

In 2002, ABB added a certification category for Embryology Laboratory Directors (ELDs). The ELD certification resembles the director qualifications contained in the minimum standards for assisted reproductive technologies of the ASRM's Practice Committee [35] and the CDC's model program for the certification of embryology laboratories under the FCSRCA [6, 31]. It is important to note, however, that individuals who are certified as an ELD at present may or may not meet CLIA requirements since embryology laboratories per se are not recognized by CLIA.

5.8 Laboratory and Clinic Data Reporting Systems

In 1988, SART began publishing annual reports of ART activities, termed the National IVF/ET Registry [50]. The Secretary of DHHS charged the Centers for Disease Control (CDC) with the responsibility for collecting, analyzing and reporting pregnancy data through the FCSRCA [6, 31]. The CDC initially contracted with SART to use the registry system that they had in place to voluntarily collect clinic-specific pregnancy data from member clinics. With the passage of the FCSRCA [6, 31], SART's voluntary registry system became mandated by law. Currently, in the United States, all clinics performing ART procedures are required to submit their clinic-specific pregnancy data to SART for subsequent reporting to the CDC.

SART initially published the results from the Registry survey representing ART procedures performed from 1985 to 1994 [50–58], and the CDC began publishing surveillance reports on the basis of this information in 1997, representing ART cycles performed in 1995 [59]. SART, in cooperation with the CDC, has continued to publish the results of this survey, representing ART cycles performed from 1985 to 2005 [50–58, 60–66]. These survey results show a (not surprising) dramatic increase in the number of ART cycles from 3,921 cycles performed by 30 clinics in 1985 to 134,260 cycles performed by 422 clinics in 2005 (Table 5.1) [50–58, 60–66]. Concomitant with the increase in cycles, the number of live deliveries associated with ART procedures has also increased from 260 to 38,910 in this same time period (Table 5.1).

Canadian ART centers reported their data in conjunction with the SART database in 1991–1995. The Canadian Assisted Reproductive Technologies Register (CARTR) was first established in 1999 for the collection of treatment cycles from Canadian ART centers [67]. The first report from this registry presented data from the calendar year 2001 [68], and reports from calendar years 2002 [67] and 2003 [69] have also been published. In the latest report, CARTR published results from 24 ART centers performing 10,656 total cycles, and resulting in 3,107 infants born.

The SART/CDC ART data registry is perhaps the most comprehensive, but not the only system in the world for reporting results of ART programs. Several other countries have implemented various forms of reporting systems. Australia and New Zealand report their ART data through the Australian Institute of Health and Welfare Perinatal Statistics Unit [70]. In 2002, the Australian and New Zealand Assisted Reproduction Database (ANZARD) was introduced as a means of collecting and reporting data from all fertility centers operating in Australia and New Zealand. Comprehensive data are available for 1991–2005 (Table 5.2), and show a similar increase in ART activity [71–81].

In 1999, the European Society for Human Reproduction and Embryology (ESHRE) invited representatives from all European national ART data registers to a joint effort to establish an ART data collection program for Europe, termed the European IVF-monitoring programme (EIM) [82]. The EIM first reported ART data collected from the year 1997 and included information on more than 200,000 cycles from 482 clinics and 18 countries (Table 5.3). The number of clinics and countries participating steadily increased over the next 6 years [82–88] with data obtained from the year 2003

Table 5.1 Report of clinics participating in the ASRM/SART ART Registry[a]

Year	Number of clinics	Number of cycles	Number of retrievals	Number of deliveries
1985	30	3,921	2,941	260
1986	41	4,867	3,504	381
1987	96	14,647	10,818	1,858
1988	135	22,649	17,753	2,627
1989	163	24,183	20,404	3,472
1990	180	25,744	22,077	3,951
1991	212	33,001	28,410	5,699
1992	249	37,955	33,237	7,355
1993	267	43,975	35,570	8,741
1994	249	42,509	29,729	9,573
1995	281	59,142	39,756	11,631
1996	300	65,863	42,594	14,702
1997	335	73,069	47,385	17,311
1998	360	81,899	53,578	20,241
1999	360	88,077	57,298	21,904
2000	383	99,989	72,096	25,394
2001	385	108,130	77,911	29,585
2002	391	115,392	83,166	33,141
2003	399	122,872	88,874	35,785
2004	411	127,977	92,064	36,760
2005	422	134,260	NA	38,910

[a]Data obtained from assisted reproductive technology (ART) clinics in the United States (1985–2005) and Canada (1991–1995). See text for references

Table 5.2 ART data reported from centers in Australia and New Zealand[a]

Year	Number of clinics	Number of cycles	Number of live births
1991	NA	16,809	NA
1992	27	17,874	2,344
1993	28	18,765	2,484
1994	28	20,706	2,875
1995	29	22,303	3,095
1996	33	24,121	3,418
1997	35	25,766	3,732
1998	NA	NA	4,182
1999	38	26,579	4,740
2000	41	27,067	5,275
2001	45	28,797	NA
2002	58	36,483	6,816
2003	64	39,720	7,479
2004	66	41,904	7,913
2005	74	47,459	NA

[a]Data obtained from assisted reproductive technology (ART) clinics in Australia and New Zealand as reported to the Australian Institute of Health and Welfare, National Perinatal Statistics Unit. *NA* data not available. See text for references

Table 5.3 Report of European ART clinics participating in the EIM Monitoring Program for ESHRE[a]

Year	Number of clinics	Number of countries	Number of cycles
1997	482	18	203,893
1998	521	18	232,443
1999	538	22	258,460
2000	569	22	279,267
2001	579	23	289,690
2002	631	25	324,238
2003	725	28	365,103

[a]Data obtained from assisted reproductive technology (ART) clinics in the Europe participating in the European IVF-monitoring system for the European Society of Human Reproduction and Embryology (ESHRE). See text for references

representing 725 clinics from 28 countries and more than 365,000 cycles (Table 5.3).

Lastly, an attempt at collecting ART statistics from across the world has been reported through the International Committee for Monitoring Assisted Reproductive Technology (ICMART), and the first world report has been published [89]. Data were collected form a total of 1,429 clinics in 49 countries, representing more than 475,044 ART procedures. This report provides the most comprehensive perspective on the practice of ART in the world in 2000 and allows for some general international comparisons [89].

References

1. Keel B, Schalue T (2004) Accreditation of the ART laboratory: the North American perspective. In: Gardner D et al (eds) Textbook of assisted reproductive techniques. Laboratory and clinical perspectives. Martin Dunitz, Ltd, London, pp 41–50
2. Keel B, Schalue T (2001) Accreditation of the ART laboratory: the North American perspective. In: Gardner D et al (eds) Textbook of assisted reproductive techniques. Laboratory and clinical perspectives. Martin Dunitz, Ltd, London, pp 35–45
3. United States Food and Drug Administration. 2008 (cited 2008 March 19); Available from: http://www.fda.gov/
4. Code of Federal Register (1992) Clinical laboratory improvement amendments of 1988: final rule. Fed Regist 57:7002
5. Code of Federal Register (2003) Medicare, Medicaid, and CLIA programs; laboratory requirements relating to quality systems and certain personnel qualifications. Final rule. Fed Regist 68: 3639–3714
6. PL. 102-493 (1992) The fertility clinic success rate and certification act of 1992. 102nd Congress, Second Session
7. Food and Drug Administration. Human cells, tissues, and cellular and tissue-based products. 2008 (cited 2008 March 20); Available from: http://www.access.gpo.gov/nara/cfr/waisidx_07/21cfr1271_07.html
8. Keel B (1998) The assisted reproductive technology laboratories and regulatory agencies. In: May J (ed) Infertility and reproductive medicine clinics of North America. W.B. Saunders Co, Philadelphia, pp 311–330
9. Keel B (2000) Clinical laboratory improvement amendments of 1988 (CLIA'88): a review. In: Keel B, May J, DeJong C (eds) Handbook of the assisted reproduction laboratory. CRC Press, Boca Raton, FL, pp 327–357
10. Keel B (2000) The physician-laboratory relationship. In: Keel B, May J, DeJong C (eds) Handbook of the assisted reproduction laboratory. CRC Press, Boca Raton, FL, pp 359–366
11. Centers for Disease Control and Prevention. 2008 (cited 2008 March 19); Available from: http://www.cdc.gov/
12. Centers for Medicare and Medicaid Services. 2008 (cited 2008 March 19); Available from: http://www.cms.hhs.gov/
13. College of American Pathology (1992) CLIA'88 final rules: a summary of major provisions of the final rules implementing the clinical laboratory improvement amendments of 1998. The College of American Pathologists, Northfield, IL
14. Stull TM, Hearn TI, Hancock JS, Handsfield JH, Collins CL (1998) Variation in proficiency testing performance by testing site. JAMA 279:462–467
15. American Association of Bioanalysts. 2008 (cited 2008 March 19); Available from: http://www.aab.org/
16. College of American Pathologists. 2008 (cited 2008 March 19); Available from: http://www.cap.org/apps/cap.portal
17. Quinn P, Keel B, Serafy NTJ, Serafy NTS, Schmidt CF, Hortsman FC (1998) Results of the American Association of Bioanalysts (AAB) embryology proficiency testing (PT) program. Proceedings of the 55th Annual Meeting of the American Society for Reproductive Medicine, S100
18. Keel B, Quinn P, Schmidt CF, Serafy NTJ, Serafy NTS, Schalue T (2000) Results of the American association of bioanalysts national proficiency testing programme in andrology. Hum Reprod 15: 680–686
19. Keel B (2004) How reliable are results from the semen analysis? Fertil Steril 82:41–44
20. Keel B, Stembridge T, Pineda G, Serafy NTS (2002) Lack of standardization in performance of the semen analysis among laboratories in the United States. Fertil Steril 78:603–608
21. Tomlinson M, Barratt C (2000) Internal and external control in the andrology laboratory. In Keel B, DeJong C, May J (eds) Handbook of the assisted reproduction laboratory. CRC Press, Boca Raton, FL, p 269
22. Keel B (2002) Quality control, quality assurance, and proficiency testing in the andrology laboratory. Arch Androl 48:417–431
23. Johnson C, Kellum T, Boldt J et al (2000) Quality assurance in the embryology, andrology and endocrine laboratories. In Keel B, DeJong C, May J (eds) Handbook of the assisted reproduction laboratory. CRC Press, Boca Raton, FL, p 279
24. Go K (2000) Quality control: a framework for the ART laboratory. In: Keel B, DeJong C, May J (eds) Handbook of the assisted reproduction laboratory. CRC Press, Boca Raton, FL, pp 253–268
25. Centers for Medicare and Medicaid Services. Clinical Laboratory Improvement Amendments (CLIA) Laboratory Director Responsibilities. 2006 (cited 2008 March 20); Available from: http://www.cms.hhs.gov/CLIA/downloads/brochure7.pdf
26. United States Department of Health and Human Services. 2008 (cited 2008 March 19); Available from: http://www.hhs.gov/
27. Commission on Office Laboratory Accreditation. 2008 (cited 2008 March 19); Available from: http://www.cola.org/
28. The Joint Commission. 2008 (cited 2008 March 19); Available from: http://www.jointcommission.org/
29. Visscher R (1991) Partners in pursuit of excellence: development of an embryo laboratory accreditation program. Fertil Steril 56: 1201–1202
30. Lawrence L, Rosenwaks Z (1993) Implications of the fertility clinic success rate and certification act of 1992. Fertil Steril 59:288–290
31. Code of Federal Register (1999) Implementation of the fertility clinic success rate and certification Act of 1992 – a model program for certification of embryo laboratories. Fed Regist 64: 39374–39392
32. RESOLVE. 2008 (cited 2008 March 19); Available from: http://www.resolve.org/site/PageServer?pagename=homepage
33. American Society for Reproductive Medicine. 2008 (cited 2008 March 19); Available from: http://www.asrm.org/
34. Society for Assisted Reproductive Technology. 2008 (cited 2008 March 19); Available from: http://www.sart.org/
35. American Society for Reproductive Medicine (2006) Revised guidelines for human embryology and andrology laboratories. Fertil Steril 86(Suppl.4):S57–S72
36. Food and Drug Administration. 21CFR1271: Human cells, tissues, and cellular and tissue-based products. 2007 (cited 2008 March 20); Available from: http://www.access.gpo.gov/nara/cfr/waisidx_07/21cfr1271_07.html
37. Food and Drug Administration (2001) Human cells, tissues, and cellular and tissue-based products; establishment registration and listing. Fed Regist 66:5447–5469
38. Food and Drug Administration (2004) Eligibility determination for donors of human cells, tissues, and cellular and tissue-based products. Fed Regist 69:29786–29834
39. Food and Drug Administration. Guidance for industry: eligibility determination for donors of human cells, tissues, and cellular and

tissue-based products (HCT/Ps). 2004 (cited 2008 March 20); Available from: http://www.fda.gov/cber/gdlns/tissdonor.pdf
40. Food and Drug Administration. Center for biologics evaluation and research. 2008 (cited 2008 March 20); Available from: http://www.fda.gov/cber/tiss.htm
41. Food and Drug Administration (2004) Current good tissue practice for human cell, tissue, and cellular and tissue-based product establishments; inspection and enforcement. Fed Regist 69: 68612–68688
42. The Joint Commission. Facts about Laboratory Accreditation. 2008 (cited February 22, 2008); Available from: http://www.jointcommission.org/AccreditationPrograms/LaboratoryServices/lab_facts.htm
43. American College of Microbiology. 2008 (cited 2008 March 19); Available from: http://www.microbiologycert.org/
44. American Board of Clinical Chemistry. 2008 (cited 2008 March 19); Available from: http://apps.aacc.org/abcc/
45. American Board of Bioanalysis. 2008 (cited February 20, 2008); Available from: http://www.aab.org/abb%20home%20page.htm
46. American Board of Medical Genetics. 2008 (cited 2008 March 19); Available from: http://www.abmg.org/
47. American Board of Histocompatibility and Immunogenetics. 2008 (cited 2008 March 19); Available from: http://www.ashi-hla.org/abhi/
48. American Board of Forensic Toxicology. 2008 (cited 2008 March 19); Available from: http://www.abft.org/
49. National Registry of Certified Chemists. 2008 (cited 2008 March 19); Available from: http://www.nrcc6.org/
50. Society for Assisted Reproductive Technology (1988) In vitro fertilization/embryo transfer in the United States: 1985 and 1986 results from the National IVF/ET Registry. Fertil Steril 49:212–215
51. Society for Assisted Reproductive Technology (1996) Assisted reproductive technology in the United States and Canada: 1994 results generated from the American Fertility Society/Society for Assisted Reproductive Technology Registry. Fertil Steril 66:697–705
52. Society for Assisted Reproductive Technology (1995) Assisted reproductive technology in the United States and Canada: 1993 results generated from the American Fertility Society/Society for Assisted Reproductive Technology Registry. Fertil Steril 64:13–21
53. Society for Assisted Reproductive Technology (1993) Assisted reproductive technology in the United States and Canada: 1991 results from the Society for Assisted Reproductive Technology generated from the American Fertility Society Registry. Fertil Steril 59:956–962
54. Society for Assisted Reproductive Technology (1992) Assisted reproductive technology in the United States and Canada: 1992 results generated from the American Fertility Society/Society for Assisted Reproductive Technology generated Registry. Fertil Steril 62:1121–1128
55. Society for Assisted Reproductive Technology (1992) In vitro fertilization-embryo transfer (IVF-ET) in the United States: 1990 results from the IVF-ET registry. Fertil Steril 57:15–24
56. Society for Assisted Reproductive Technology (1991) In vitro fertilization-embryo transfer (IVF-ET) in the United States: 1989 results from the IVF-ET registry. Fertil Steril 55:14–22
57. Society for Assisted Reproductive Technology (1990) In vitro fertilization-embryo transfer in the United States: 1988 results from the National IVF-ET registry. Fertil Steril 53:13–20
58. Society for Assisted Reproductive Technology (1989) In vitro fertilization/embryo transfer in the United States: 1987 results from the National IVF-ET registry. Fertil Steril 51:13–19
59. Centers for Disease Control and Prevention (1997) 1995 assisted reproductive technology success rates. Centers for Disease Control and Prevention, Atlanta, GA
60. Society for Assisted Reproductive Technology (2007) Assisted reproductive technology in the United States: 2001 results generated from the American Fertility Society/Society for Assisted Reproductive Technology Registry. Fertil Steril 87:1253–1266
61. Society for Assisted Reproductive Technology (2004) Assisted reproductive technology in the United States: 2000 results generated from the American Fertility Society/Society for Assisted Reproductive Technology Registry. Fertil Steril 81:1207–1220
62. Society for Assisted Reproductive Technology (2002) Assisted reproductive technology in the United States: 1999 results generated from the American Fertility Society/Society for Assisted Reproductive Technology Registry. Fertil Steril 78:918–931
63. Society for Assisted Reproductive Technology (2002) Assisted reproductive technology in the United States: 1998 results generated from the American Fertility Society/Society for Assisted Reproductive Technology Registry. Fertil Steril 77:18–31
64. Society for Assisted Reproductive Technology (2000) Assisted reproductive technology in the United States: 1997 results generated from the American Fertility Society/Society for Assisted Reproductive Technology Registry. Fertil Steril 74:641–653
65. Society for Assisted Reproductive Technology (1999) Assisted reproductive technology in the United States: 1996 results generated from the American Fertility Society/Society for Assisted Reproductive Technology Registry. Fertil Steril 71:798–807
66. Society for Assisted Reproductive Technology (1998) Assisted reproductive technology in the United States and Canada: 1995 results generated from the American Fertility Society/Society for Assisted Reproductive Technology Registry. Fertil Steril 69: 389–398
67. Gunby J, Daya S (2005) Assisted reproductive technologies (ART) in Canada: 2001 results from the Canadian ART Register. Fertil Steril 84:590–599
68. Centers for Disease Control and Prevention (2004) Assisted reproductive technology surveillance – United States, 2001. MMWR 53
69. Gunby J, Daya S (2007) Assisted reproductive technologies (ART) in Canada: 2003 results from the Canadian ART Register. Fertil Steril 88:550–559
70. AIHW National Perinatal Statistics Unit. 2008 November 23, 2007 (cited 2008 March 19). Available from: http://www.npsu.unsw.edu.au/NPSUweb.nsf/page/home
71. Waters A-M, Dean J, Sullivan E (2003) Assisted reproduction technology in Australia and New Zealand 2003. AIHW National Perinatal Statistics Unit, Sydney
72. Wang Y, Dean J, Sullivan E (2007) Assisted reproduction technology in Australia and New Zealand 2005. AIHW National Perinatal Statistics Unit, Sydney
73. Wang Y, Dean J, Grayson N, Sullivan E (2006) Assisted reproduction technology in Australia and New Zealand. AIHW National Perinatal Statistics Unit, Sydney
74. Lancaster P, Shafir E, Hurst T, Huang J (1997) Assisted conception Australia and New Zealand, 1994 and 1995. AIHW National Perinatal Statistics Unit, Sydney
75. Lancaster P, Shafir E, Huang J (1995) Assisted conception, Australia and New Zealand, 1992 and 1993. AIHW National Perinatal Statistics Unit, Sydney
76. Hurst T, Shafir E, Lancaster P (1999) Assisted conception Australia and New Zealand 1997. AIHW National Perinatal Statistics Unit, Sydney
77. Hurst T, Shafir E, Lancaster P (1997) Assisted conception, Australia and New Zealand 1996. AIHW National Perinatal Statistics Unit, Sydney
78. Hurst T, Lancaster P (2001) Assisted conception Australia and New Zealand 1999 and 2000. AIHW National Perinatal Statistics Unit, Sydney
79. Hurst T, Lancaster P (2001) Assisted conception Australia and New Zealand 1998 and 1999. AIHW National Perinatal Statistics Unit, Sydney
80. Dean J, Sullivan E (2003) Assisted conception Australia and New Zealand 2000 and 2001. AIHW National Perinatal Statistics Unit, Sydney

81. Bryant J, Sullivan E, Dean J (2002) Assisted reproduction technology in Australia and New Zealand. AIHW National Perinatal Statistics Unit, Sydney
82. Nygren K, Andersen AN (2001) Assisted reproductive technology in Europe, 1997. Results generated from European registers by ESHRE. Hum Reprod 16:384–391
83. Nygren K, Andersen AN (2002) Assisted reproductive technology in Europe, 1999. Results generated from European registers by ESHRE. Hum Reprod 17:3260–3274
84. Nygren K, Andersen AN (2001) Assisted reproductive technology in Europe, 1998. Results generated from European registers by ESHRE. Hum Reprod 16:2459–2471
85. Andersen AN, Goossens V, Gianaroli L, Felberbaum R, De Mouzon J, Nygren K (2007) Assisted reproductive technology in Europe, 2003. Results generated from European registers by ESHRE. Hum Reprod 22:1513–1525
86. Andersen AN, Gianaroli L, Nygren K (2004) Assisted reproductive technology in Europe, 2000. Results generated from European registers by ESHRE. Hum Reprod 19:490–503
87. Andersen AN, Gianaroli L, Felberbaum R, De Mouzon J (2006) Assisted reproductive technology in Europe, 2002. Results generated from European registers by ESHRE. Hum Reprod 21:1680–1697
88. Andersen AN, Felberbaum R, de Mouzon J, Nygren K (2005) Assisted reproductive technology in Europe, 2001. Results generated from European registers by ESHRE. Hum Reprod 20:1158–1176
89. Adamson G, de Mouzon J, Lancaster P, Nygren K, Sullivan E, Zegers-Hochschild F (2006) World collaborative report on in vitro fertilization, 2000. Fertil Steril 85:1586–1622

Chapter 6
Successfully Integrating the FDA Regulations into Your Practice

Wendy D. Latash

Abstract The fertility field has had its challenges with regard to state and federal regulations over the past 20 years. In 2005, ART programs were faced with a new regulatory challenge – the Food and Drug Administration. The ruling entitled "21 CFR Part 1271 Human Cells, Tissues, and Cellular and Tissue-Based Products" regulates non-vascularized human tissues including reproductive tissues and touches on donor and non-donor tissues affecting the clinical, as well as the laboratory areas of an ART program. This chapter examines the history of ART regulation, defines the scope of what is regulated for ART programs, and describes the most important aspects of the ruling that medical and laboratory directors need to know for compliance. In addition, practical "field-tested" information from a fertility perspective is given on how to develop and maintain a compliance program specifically focused on dealing with the 21 CFR Part 1271 ruling. Finally, case examples from real donor situations are described in order to test the reader's knowledge and comprehension of the regulations as applied to an ART program.

Keywords Fertility • Reproductive tissue • FDA regulations • 21 CFR Part 1271 • Donor eligibility determination • Current Good Tissue Practice • Relevant communicable disease • Human Cells Tissues and Cellular and Tissue Based Products (HCT/Ps)

6.1 Introduction

6.1.1 History of 21 CFR Part 1271

The fertility field has, for many years, been the focus of public debate. As with many debates, the fertility field eventually came under the regulatory spotlight in the early 1990s [1] such that now, Assisted Reproductive Technology (ART) programs must do their best to become compliant with what have become commonly known in the field as the "FDA regulations" – referring to the 21 CFR Part 1271 ruling [2–11]. Contrary to popular thought, the fertility field is not a stranger to regulations from governmental agencies. Like many physicians' practices, embryology laboratories had to comply with the Clinical Laboratory Improvement Amendments of 1988 when implemented in 1992 [12, 13]. However, unlike other medical practices, fertility clinics were also faced with the "Implementation of the Fertility Clinic Success Rate and Certification Act of 1992: A Model Program for the Certification of Embryo Laboratories" as administered by the Department of Health and Human Services through the Centers for Disease Control and Prevention [14]. This continued for approximately 10 years until the first portions of 21 CFR Part 1271 were published, which added another regulatory concern and changed the regulatory landscape for reproductive tissue.

Many believe that the impetus for regulating donor tissue began with "the LifeNet incident" of 1985 [1]. LifeNet Transplant Services, a tissue procurement agency, had procured 61 organs and tissue grafts from a donor who had originally tested HIV-negative twice in 1985, and these had been transplanted into various recipients. It was only afterwards, during a retrospective analysis performed in 1991 using better testing methodologies, that it was discovered that the donor tested positive for HIV. After this finding, although the bank initiated the search for the tissue recipients, only 34 out of the 40 recipients were identified and located because hospitals and physicians had poor recordkeeping practices. Seven had contracted AIDS and three had died.

Reproductive tissue came into the spotlight in the context of communicable disease during congressional testimony by New York state officials in 1993 [1]. These officials testified that before 1989, when New York state instituted stricter sperm bank standards, a good portion of New York's sperm banks (1) utilized semen from untested donors, (2) were located out of physician's offices, and (3) had personnel that lacked the necessary screening and testing expertise for

W.D. Latash (✉)
Jade Tree Solutions, LLC, PO Box 1302, Northbrook, IL, 60062, USA
e-mail: wendy.latash@jadetreesolutions.com

D.T. Carrell and C.M. Peterson (eds.), *Reproductive Endocrinology and Infertility: Integrating Modern Clinical and Laboratory Practice*,
DOI 10.1007/978-1-4419-1436-1_6, © Springer Science+Business Media, LLC 2010

sperm donors. Furthermore, the owners of two sperm banks were leading their clients to believe that their banks had released semen from more than a dozen donors, when actually it was sperm from themselves.

As a result, the FDA published interim regulations in 1993 that placed most banked human tissue, except for reproductive tissue, under the same controls and communicable disease testing as blood banks. In response, the American Society of Reproductive Medicine (ASRM) and the American Association of Tissue Banks (AATB) established guidelines for anonymous donor sperm banking practices in an effort to encourage self-regulatory practices [15]. Reproductive tissue was initially exempt from the interim rules set forth in 1993. However, this did not last. The first FDA documents to address reproductive tissue were published about 10 years later. The FDA continues to release publications concerning reproductive tissue and is likely to continue to do so.

Many ART programs have expressed concern and displeasure regarding these regulations. They have questioned whether a public health issue exists with regard to the possibility of passing on communicable disease through reproductive tissues, especially embryos. Currently, no published documentation exists to indicate that embryos created through ART procedures could have the potential to pass on communicable disease. Despite these concerns, the fact remains that the FDA has both the mandate and the authority to take action if it deems it necessary. ART programs must take the regulations seriously and are required to comply. Moreover, the FDA has little tolerance for willful noncompliance.

6.1.2 Scope of the Regulations for ART Programs

For any industry that is newly regulated by a governmental agency, it is usually a challenge to ensure that the field being regulated and the agency enacting the regulations understand each other. Misunderstandings may often occur. Each entity may have a different definition, or alternative interpretations of the same term, or even be unaware of definitions used by the other. As a result, in order to understand the regulations and to become and remain FDA compliant, it is essential that a regulated establishment understand the basic document structures that the FDA uses to communicate its intentions to industry.

There are two basic types of documentation: "rulings" and "guidances". An FDA "ruling" is a set of obligations published in the Federal Register that outlines specific, legally-enforceable rules with regard to a particular set of operations within an industry or field. These rulings are also known as "regulations." An FDA "guidance", on the other hand, is the FDA's current thinking on a particular topic that usually relates directly to a ruling or to a part of a ruling. A "guidance" is used to assist a field or industry in developing measures to comply with a specific ruling. Although the FDA states that a guidance is a *recommendation* and is not legally enforceable, it is essential to remember that if an establishment chooses not to follow the recommendations in the guidance, it must first obtain FDA approval for its alternative approach. Otherwise, the guidance recommendations must be followed.

Moreover, there are many times that the FDA will publish more than one guidance for a particular ruling – either during the initial implementation phase of compliance measures by an industry, or as an addition or a change to the FDA's current thinking. The guidance document is the primary method that the FDA uses to communicate its interpretation of the ruling to the regulated field or industry. It is important, therefore, for an establishment to monitor the publication of relevant FDA documents closely to ensure that it employs the most recent compliance measures.

The challenge of dealing with multiple, and sometimes confusing, ruling documents also pertains to 21 CFR Part 1271 for which ruling documents and guidances have been published since its inception. Table 6.1 lists the different ruling documents and guidances that are essential for ART programs and the dates they were published.

Finally, it is crucial for ART programs to know the scope of the regulations as not all of 21 CFR Part 1271 is applicable to reproductive tissue *at this point*. The following portions of the regulation apply to ART programs:

- All of Subpart A – General Provisions
- All of Subpart B – Registration & Listing
- All of Subpart C – Donor Eligibility
- Two subsections of Subpart D – Good Tissue Practices
- §1271.150(c) – Manufacturing Arrangements
- §1271.155 – Exemptions & Alternatives
- Subpart F – Inspection & Enforcement

Note that ART programs are exempt from the rest of Subpart D (except for the two subsections just listed) [1271.150(c)(3)] and all of Subpart E [1271.330], but this exemption may change. The FDA has indicated that these exemptions for ART programs are only temporary. Also note that for the purposes of this chapter, any reference to specific sections of 21 CFR Part 1271 will be given in brackets with the appropriate subsection listed – i.e., [1271.75(a)(1)(i)].

Finally, it must be emphasized that the regulations affecting ART Programs took effect as of May 25, 2005. This means that the FDA expects that ART programs were compliant with the regulations *as of May 25, 2005*. As per the writing of this chapter, which is several years into the life of the regulation, ART programs are expected to have had ample opportunity to become compliant.

Table 6.1 Ruling and guidance documents important for ART programs

Type of document	Title	Date published
Federal Register publication	Human cells, tissues, and cellular and tissue-based products; CFR correction to 1271.22 [6]	1/18/08
Guidance for Industry	Regulation of human cells, tissues, and cellular and tissue-based products (HCT/Ps) – small entity compliance guide [35]	8/24/07
Guidance for Industry	Eligibility determination for donors of human cells, tissues, and cellular and tissue-based products [16]	8/8/07
Federal Register publication	Human cells, tissues, and cellular and tissue-based products; donor screening and testing, and related labeling; final rule [11]	6/19/07
Guidance for Industry	Certain human cells, tissues, and cellular and tissue-based products (HCT/Ps) recovered from donors who were tested for communicable diseases using pooled specimens or diagnostic tests [29]	1/23/07
Guidance for Industry	Compliance with 21 CFR Part 1271.150(c)(1) – manufacturing arrangements [25]	9/8/06
Federal Register publication	Eligibility determination for donors of human cells, tissues, and cellular and tissue-based products; correction [8]	3/24/06
Federal Register publication	Human cells, tissues, and cellular and tissue-based products; donor screening and testing, and related labeling; interim final rule; opportunity for public comment [7]	5/25/05
Federal Register publication	Current good tissue practice for human cell, tissue, and cellular and tissue-based product establishments; inspection and enforcement; final rule [10]	11/24/04
Federal Register publication	Eligibility determination for donors of human cells, tissues, and cellular and tissue-based products; final rule and notice [9]	5/25/04
Federal Register publication	Human cells, tissues, and cellular and tissue-based products; establishment registration and listing; interim final rule; correction [5]	2/4/04
Federal Register publication	Human cells, tissues, and cellular and tissue-based products; establishment registration and listing; interim final rule; opportunity for public comment [3]	1/27/04
Federal Register publication	Human cells, tissues, and cellular and tissue-based products; establishment registration and listing; final rule; delay of effective date [2]	1/21/03
Federal Register publication	Human cells, tissues, and cellular and tissue-based products; establishment registration and listing; final rule [4]	1/19/01

6.2 Overview of the 21 CFR part 1271 Regulations

The regulations governing donor eligibility for ART programs exist in three different sections: Registrations Final Rule [2–6]; Donor Eligibility Final rule [7–9, 11]; and Current Good Tissue Practices [7, 10, 11]. Furthermore, there are six subparts lettered A through F. While each subpart has a different purpose, all of them must be taken together to understand how they interact with one another.

Constant vigilance over developments in guidance and ruling documents published by the FDA is not only a good idea, but it is also essential for ART programs to remain compliant. Simply put, for 21 CFR Part 1271, *there is no steady state.* Information on this regulation – FDA interpretations, current FDA inspection emphasis – has changed on a fairly consistent basis. Moreover, ART programs must monitor changes through professional publications and industry meetings to ensure that their own compliance status is as up to date as possible.

Finally, it must be emphasized that for every section of the regulations that apply, it is essential that an ART program has formal, approved, detailed, written policies, and procedures. The lack of clearly written policies and procedures that have been approved by a "Responsible Person" will automatically put an ART program at risk for violations during an FDA inspection. As one ART program laboratory director so aptly put it: "If you stand on your head while administering the screening questionnaire, then you must write it in your procedure!"

6.2.1 Registrations Final Rule

6.2.1.1 Subpart A: General Provisions. Sections 1271.1, 1271.3, 1271.10, 1271.15, 1271.20

Subpart A discusses general information regarding the regulations. The purpose and scope of the regulations are stated [1271.1] and important terms defined by the FDA [1271.3]. This section also discusses the conditions under which certain HCT/Ps are regulated in Section 361 of the Public Health Service (PHS) Act and 21 CFR Part 1271 [1271.10], and the exceptions to the requirements and who qualifies for these exceptions [1271.15]. Section 1271.20 discusses which regulations apply in the event that the criteria outlined in 1271.10 are not met, but the HCT/Ps in question do not qualify for any exceptions in 1271.15.

In general, all ART programs performing in vitro fertilization techniques are subject to the regulations and must be registered with the FDA. Additionally, commercial sperm banks, egg banks, clinical testing laboratories, and long-term cryostorage facilities that store reproductive tissue for release to other establishments are also subject to the regulations and must be registered. The definitions section, 1271.3, is particularly important for ART programs to incorporate, since (1) this is the terminology the FDA uses with regards to HCT/Ps during inspections, and (2) the definitions used *may or may not* be consistent with the same terms generally accepted by the fertility field. Other important terms that are crucial to know: "Manufacture", "Directed reproductive donor", "Donor medical history interview", "Quarantine", "Relevant communicable disease agent or disease", "Relevant medical records", "Distribution", "HCT/P deviation", and "Processing". It is initially apparent that terms such as "Manufacture" and "Processing" do not appear to apply to ART program practices. ART programs do not "Manufacture" anything per se and "Processing" would not necessarily be the term a clinician or embryologist would use when culturing embryos. However, this is the terminology the FDA stipulates for these regulations and it is the responsibility of ART programs to know this in order to interpret the regulations correctly. Finally, it is important to note that the only OBGYN practices required to register with the FDA are those practices that perform donor inseminations from sperm whose donor eligibility determination was NOT performed by an FDA registered and compliant facility.

Important Guidance(s) Information for this Section

Currently, there is one guidance published that is important for this Subpart: "Guidance for Industry: Regulation of Human Cells, Tissues, and Cellular and Tissue-Based Products (HCT/Ps)" ("DED Guidance") [16]. The most important information in this guidance concerns the scope of the regulation for ART programs and what applied before and after May 25, 2005.

6.2.1.2 Subpart B: Procedures for Registration and Listing. Sections 1271.21, 1271.22, 1271.25, 1271.26, 1271.27, 1271.37

This subpart more specifically addresses the actual registration and HCT/P listing requirements. It discusses when registration and registration updates must occur [1271.21], where and how to register (including the different methods of registration) [1271.22, 1271.26], what information must be provided [1271.25], how the FDA identifies a tissue establishment in their system [1271.27] and how to obtain registration and listing information on a particular tissue establishment [1271.37].

ART programs must register and provide a list of HCT/Ps manufactured within 5 days after donor program procedures have begun and must be renewed annually every December by the establishment. The renewal is not automatically performed by the FDA. Any change in information, i.e., a change in office location, must be updated with the FDA either at the time the change occurred or the following June or December; whichever arrives first. Registration may be accomplished either by fax, e-mail, or on the internet and must use Form FDA 3356. The registration must include: (1) the legal contact name and location information (including multiple locations if applicable), (2) name, contact information, job title, and dated signature of the person responsible for registering the establishment, (3) all HCT/Ps that are "manufactured" currently by the FDA's definition [1271.3(e)], and (4) indications of any changes compared to the last registration – including HCT/Ps handled. After submission, the FDA then assigns a registration number called the "Federal Establishment Identifier" (FEI) number that distinguishes the establishment. ART program registrations are publicly available over the internet, and copies of FDA Form 3356 are available on the FDA's website.

6.2.2 *Donor Eligibility Final Rule*

6.2.2.1 Subpart C: Donor Eligibility. Sections 1271.45, 1271.47, 1271.50, 1271.55, 1271.60, 1271.65, 1271.75, 1271.80, 1271.85, 1271.90

This subpart delves into the complex process of donor eligibility, introducing the concept of a "donor eligibility determination" along with the screening/testing and documentation requirements that ensue. It states requirements for establishing policies and procedures for donor eligibility [1271.45, 1271.47], how donors are to be screened and tested [1271.75, 1271.80, 1271.85], how to determine a donor's eligibility [1271.50], and how quarantine, labeling, storage, shipping/receiving and non-clinical uses of tissues should be handled [1271.60, 1271.65, 1271.90]. Recordkeeping requirements [1271.55] and exemptions from donor eligibility requirements [1271.90] are also noted. For ART programs, this subpart has perhaps the greatest affect on day to day operations due to the current scope of 21 CFR Part 1271. Therefore, for most ART programs, this section will have the most associated policies and procedures.

To address this section in the most logical fashion for compliance, it has been divided into the following sections: Donor Program Offerings, Donor Screening, Donor Testing, Donor Eligibility Determination, Records and

Recordkeeping, Laboratory section: Labeling, Quarantine, Storage, Shipping/Receipt & Non-Clinical Uses, and Departures from Procedures & Deviations.

Important Guidance(s) Information for this Section

- Several guidances essential to understanding donor eligibility compliance will be discussed and referred to when the corresponding information is discussed. The most current relevant guidances can be found in Table 6.1.

Donor Program Offerings

When approaching these regulations to determine what an ART program needs to do in order to become compliant, one of the first questions to consider is "What donor programs will be offered?" The answer to this question will determine the scope of which written policies and procedures are needed. Most programs offer some form of oocyte and sperm donation; however, not all programs offer embryo donation, traditional surrogacy, or a gestational carrier program.

Most ART programs currently outsource some portion of the donor eligibility process to other establishments such as: commercial sperm banks, egg donor agencies, embryo donation agencies, or gestational carrier agencies. Some of these agencies may currently be required to register with the FDA and establish compliance; some may not. Knowing which agencies are registered and FDA compliant is essential for an ART program's compliance under 1271.150(c) (see Subpart D).

Donor Screening [1271.75]

The FDA requires that any reproductive tissue donor be screened for relevant communicable disease agents and diseases (RCDADs) as defined in 1271.3(r) and in the DED Guidance [16]. The current list of RCDADs for reproductive tissue screening is listed in Table 6.2.

Definition of terms is critically important. In discussions of donor screening, the terms "screening" and "testing" are commonly used interchangeably. It is important to note that the FDA *does not* use these terms interchangeably. For example, the phrase "screening test" has been commonly used to refer to the actual FDA licensed and approved (or cleared) test for "donor screening". This can be a source of confusion, because the FDA views "donor screening" and "donor testing" as two separate processes of performing a donor eligibility determination [(1271.3(e)]. To clarify this issue, we will discuss the usage of these two separate terms.

"Donor screening" involves the review of donor medical records for: (1) "Risk factors for, and clinical evidence of, relevant communicable disease agents and diseases" and (2) "Communicable disease risks associated with xenotransplantation" [1271.75(a)]. The DED Guidance describes in great detail how to screen a donor for RCDADs. From a practical standpoint for this ruling, donor screening means: (1) administration and review of a donor medical history questionnaire, (2) performing and/or review of a recent donor physical assessment, and (3) reviewing past relevant donor medical records if available. "Donor testing" is the process by which blood or other physical samples are taken from a potential donor and tested. The tests are those which are indicated for "donor screening" and which have been FDA-licensed and approved, or cleared, if approved tests are not available.

The donor situation under consideration is important for determining whether the donor needs to be screened. All anonymous and directed (or known) donors of reproductive tissue are required to undergo screening except for a sexually intimate partner (SIP) of the recipient. Special attention should be paid to "Directed reproductive donor" [(1271.3(l)] situations, since an ART program has the responsibility to evaluate whether the donation relationship meets the definition, intent, and spirit of the FDA regulations *and* those of the ART program itself. The challenge for an ART program with this definition is to define appropriately what it considers to be "known", since this is not defined by the FDA and because it is inherently important to characterizing the donor/recipient relationship. Most importantly, regardless of whether the donor situation is anonymous or directed, the donor *must* be screened. From the FDA standpoint, the distinction between an anonymous and directed donor only matters when a donor is determined ineligible (see "Donor Eligibility Determination").

A full donor screen must be completed for every donor within six months before the donation. The screen must include a donor medical history, a donor physical and a clinical evidence review of relevant and available donor medical records. If a donor repeats a donation within that 6 month period, the ART program is allowed to perform an abbreviated screen that should include updates to the donor's medical history and a documented reminder to the donor of the risks that could make the donor ineligible. Note that any information regarding the screening process must be documented appropriately throughout and that policies and procedures exist describing these processes.

A donor medical history must at least include a series of questions administered to or reviewed with the donor through a live interaction. These questions are very detailed, contain specific time elements, and require a thorough understanding by both the donor and the person administering the questions of what the questions mean. The questions must adequately screen for risk factors for, or clinical evidence of RCDADs. The DED Guidance has a complete list of risk factors and conditions that must be considered in accordance with

Table 6.2 Current list of relevant communicable disease agent or disease (RCDAD) required for donor screening

Relevant communicable disease agent or disease (RCDAD)	Section of ruling or guidance	Females or males
Human immunodeficiency virus (HIV)	1271.75(a)(1)(i)	Both
Heptatitis B Virus (Hep B)	1271.75(a)(1)(ii)	Both
Hepatitis C Virus (Hep C)	1271.75(a)(1)(iii)	Both
Human transmissible spongiform encephalopathy, including Cretzfeldt-Jakob disease ("Mad-Cow")	1271.75(a)(1)(iv)	Both
Treponema pallidum (Syphilis)	1271.75(a)(1)(v)	Both
Communicable disease risks associated with xenotransplantation	1271.75(a)(2)	Both
Chlamydia trachomatis[a]	1271.75(c)(1)	Both
Neisseria gonorrhea[a]	1271.75(c)(2)	Both
Human T-lymphotropic virus (HTLV)	1271.75(b)	Males only
West Nile virus (WNV)	DED guidance; IIID p.5–6	Both
Sepsis[b]	DED guidance; IIID p.6	Both
Vaccinia (from small-pox vaccination)	DED guidance; IIID p.6–7	Both

[a]Screened for these RCDADs are required unless "the reproductive cells or tissues are recovered by a method that ensures freedom from contamination of the cells or tissue by infectious disease organisms that may be present in the genitourinary tract" [1271.75(c)]

[b]As noted in the DED guidance "If a living donor appears healthy, the donor usually does not need to be evaluated for sepsis" [20]

1271.75 [17]. Most ART programs have additional screening questions that go beyond the scope of the FDA ruling. In particular, these include questions about personal history, family history (including genetic background), physical/mental attributes, and occupation. It is important to note that these questions required de facto by the ART program must be accounted for in the policies and procedures.

A donor physical must also be performed every six months. However, an ART program may depend on a donor exam report generated by another health care professional as long as (1) the clinician performing the physical is trained and qualified to do so, and (2) the ART program is assured that the donor has been screened appropriately. To adequately screen for physical evidence of relevant communicable diseases, ART programs should follow the physical parameters listed in the DED Guidance [18]. Once again, as with the medical history, proper documentation is absolutely essential.

The final part of the screening process involves a review of relevant donor medical records for clinical evidence of or high-risk behaviors associated with RCDADs. This process requires obtaining any previous relevant donor medical records and looking for specific groups of symptoms or conditions previously recorded in the donor's records that could indicate the presence of any of the RCDADs. The DED Guidance provides examples of clinical evidence of relevant communicable disease for HIV, Hepatitis, Syphilis, *Chlamydia trachomatis*, *Neisseria gonorrhea*, Vaccinia (smallpox vaccination), West Nile Virus, Sepsis, and HTLV [19]. All of these diseases are important for a clinical evidence review. However, since ART programs work with living donors, the DED Guidance states that "… if a living donor appears healthy, the donor usually does not have to be evaluated for sepsis" [20]. As with the other recommendations listed in the DED Guidance, an ART program should incorporate these examples into a documented process for reviewing these records.

Another important concept for donor screening is dealing with "relevant medical records" [(1271.3(s)]. An ART program should attempt to obtain and review these records if the records were available in time for the donor eligibility determination. For example, egg donor profiles from egg donor agencies or previous IVF cycle information often contains crucial information important for an ART program to cross-reference with its own screening information on the donor (i.e., country of origin, social behaviors, etc). In these cases, the current treating ART program should make a documented attempt to obtain these records, if they are available, and review them before the donor eligibility determination [21].

Donor Testing (1271.80; 1271.85)

The FDA requires that any reproductive tissue donor be tested for RCDADs, although the RCDADs tested are different than those for screening since some RCDADs do not yet have tests that have been approved (or cleared) for this purpose (i.e., Creutzfeldt-Jakob disease). Table 6.3 depicts the current list of RCDADs for donor testing. Additionally, these donors must be tested "using appropriate FDA-licensed, approved, or cleared donor screening tests, in accordance with the manufacturer's instructions, to adequately and appropriately reduce the risk of transmission of relevant communicable disease agents or diseases"[(1271.80(c)]. Table 6.4 lists the current types of tests that should be performed [22]. ART programs are also allowed to perform additional or more stringent tests in addition to what is required. However, if this is done, then results of these tests must be documented, maintained, reviewed, and considered when performing a donor eligibility determination [23].

All donors subject to testing must have their specimens for testing obtained within a defined period of time. For egg donors, samples must be obtained within 30 days *before* egg retrieval, and for sperm donors, seven days *before* or *after* semen collection. These timing requirements may present

Table 6.3 Current list of relevant communicable disease agent or disease (RCDAD) required for *donor testing*

Relevant communicable disease agent or disease (RCDAD)	Section of ruling or guidance	Females or males
Human Immunodeficiency Virus (HIV) type 1	1271.85(a)(1)	Both
Human Immunodeficiency Virus (HIV) type 2	1271.85(a)(2)	Both
Heptatitis B Virus (Hep B)	1271.85(a)(3)	Both
Hepatitis C Virus (Hep C)	1271.85(a)(4)	Both
Treponema pallidum (Syphilis)	1271.85(a)(5)	Both
Chlamydia trachomatis[a]	1271.85(c)(1)	Both
Neisseria gonorrhea[a]	1271.85(c)(2)	Both
Human T-lymphotropic virus (HTLV)	1271.85(b)(1)	Males only
Cytomegalovirus (CMV)	1271.85(b)(2)	Males only

[a]Testing for these RCDADs is required unless "the reproductive cells or tissues are recovered by a method that ensures freedom from contamination of the cells or tissue by infectious disease organisms that may be present in the genitourinary tract" [1271.85(c)]

Table 6.4 Current types of RCDAD tests recommended by the FDA

Relevant communicable disease agent or disease (RCDAD)	Type of tests
Human immunodeficiency virus (HIV) type 1	FDA-licensed screening test either for anti-HIV-1 or combined with anti-HIV-2[a]
	FDA-licensed HIV-1 screening NAT[b] test or combination test
Human immunodeficiency virus (HIV) type 2	FDA-licensed screening test either for anti-HIV-1 or combined with anti-HIV-2
Heptatitis B virus (HBV)	FDA-licensed screening test for HBV surface antigen (HBsAg)
	FDA-licensed screening test for HBV core antigen (anti-HBc)
Hepatitis C virus (HCV)	FDA-licensed screening test for anti-HCV
	FDA licensed HCV screening NAT test or combination test
Treponema pallidum (Syphilis)	FDA-cleared screening test for syphilis or FDA-cleared diagnostic serologic test for Syphilis[c]
Chlamydia trachomatis	FDA-licensed, approved or cleared diagnostic test labeled for the detection of these organisms in an asymptomatic, low-prevalence population. NAT tests are recommended.[d]
Neisseria gonorrhea	FDA-licensed, approved or cleared diagnostic test labeled for the detection of these organisms in an asymptomatic, low-prevalence population. NAT tests are recommended.[d]
Human T-lymphotropic Virus (HTLV)	FDA-licensed screening test for anti-HTLV I/II
Cytomegalovirus (CMV)	FDA-cleared screening test for anti-CMV (total IgG and IgM)

[a]If the HIV test utilized does not test for HIV group O antibodies, then the RTE must also screen these donors for HIV group O risk factors [36]

[b]NAT = Nucleic acid test

[c]For more information regarding syphilis testing, see DED Guidance; "Discussion of Syphilis Assays", p 32–33

[d]These particular test recommendations are made is because currently there are no FDA-licensed, approved or cleared tests for donor screening of *Chlamydia trachomatis or Neisseria gonorrhea*

Note: The FDA may change these recommendations in the future "due to technological advances or evolving scientific knowledge." [37]

some unique challenges to an ART program, since the donor eligibility process can take place over a period of months and may involve physical/mental health and financial considerations for the recipient. A balance must be struck between obtaining as many of the results as possible before the IVF cycle, and the costs to the recipient, all within the context of maintaining FDA compliance.

Typically, first-time egg donors are tested twice, because the 30-day testing time frame occurs after the matching of the donor and recipient. The first round is usually made when the donor enters the program or during preliminary screening. The second and most crucial round, due to the 30-day window requirement, usually occurs around or before the initiation of gonadotropins for ovarian stimulation. At this point, if the donor tests positive or reactive for an RCDAD, the cycle must be canceled. However, for repeat egg donors, who have both demonstrated their commitment and who have previously tested negative for any RCDADs, the question is whether it is necessary to test them more than the required 30-day window testing round. An ART program may determine that the risk of the donor testing positive before egg retrieval is lower, therefore a first round of testing is not necessary. The costs and benefits of an additional round of testing outside of the required timeframe should be weighed appropriately and a decision made *before* the matching process begins.

Although the time frame for male donor testing is the 7 days before or after semen collection, there are distinctions between anonymous and directed sperm donors concerning quarantine and retesting. Anonymous donors must be tested initially within seven days of the first donation. They must then be retested after the quarantining of their sperm for six months from the date of the *last semen collection*. Only after these two testing periods, can the donor's sperm be released for distribution. Additionally, since most anonymous sperm donors are repeat donors, ART programs are not required to collect a donor specimen for testing at the time of each semen donation [1271.80(b)(2)]. However, it is important to note that each new batch of sperm must be quarantined for 6 months from the date of the first test before being released for distribution.

Conversely, directed sperm donors do not have the six-month quarantine and retest requirement. However, they must be tested with every single donation within seven days, before or after semen collection. Alternatively, ART programs have the option of treating directed donors like anonymous sperm donors, in which case this action would not affect compliance [24].

ART programs have particular responsibilities for donor testing that may or may not be immediately obvious. Most ART programs outsource their donor testing to special testing laboratories that provide clinical and diagnostic testing services. Under 1271.150(c), if an ART program engages "another establishment (e.g., a laboratory to perform communicable disease testing, or…), under a contract, agreement, or other arrangement, to perform any step in manufacture for you [the ART program], that establishment is responsible for complying with requirements applicable to that manufacturing step" [1271.150(c)(1)(ii)]. In other words, clinical testing laboratories performing donor tissue testing must comply with all applicable regulations under this ruling, and the ART program is responsible for ensuring this [25].

Other ART programs' responsibilities concerning testing include the following: (1) ensuring and documenting that the correct FDA-approved or cleared tests for donor screening are ordered and used; (2) maintaining documentation verifying that specimen collection and storage requirements are observed; and (3) checking that results are interpreted properly. This requires a commitment of time on the part of the ART program, but it is absolutely essential to do. There have been anecdotal reports of samples being ruined and not tested because of faulty handling and storage. It is important to pay close attention to where and how the specimens for testing are stored between collection and pickup by a testing laboratory courier. For example, ART programs will often place specimens at the end of a work day in a "drop box" located within or immediately outside the controled environment of the facility. Location of the drop box is important in terms of security and temperature. Room temperature is obviously dependent on the building temperature, weather conditions, time of day, proximity to sunlight, etc. and may fluctuate depending on the seasons. Conducting specimen pick-up procedures in this manner would not be in compliance with most manufacturer's test kit package inserts and, therefore, would not be FDA compliant.

Two additional issues for ART programs include CMV testing for males and plasma dilution. The FDA requires that an ART program "must test a specimen from the donor of viable, leukocyte-rich cells or tissue for evidence of infection due to cytomegalovirus (CMV), to adequately and appropriately reduce the risk of transmission. You [an ART program] must establish and maintain a standard operating procedure governing the release of an HCT/P from a donor whose specimen tests reactive for CMV" [1271.85(b)(2)]. Notice that this statement does not indicate what this policy and procedure must include – only that an ART program must have one and adhere to it. While on the surface this appears simple, the implications can be more complex, depending on what the ART program's policy is regarding the release of CMV positive tissue – i.e., an IgG positive/IgM negative vs. IgG negative/IgM positive donor. The clinical implications of utilizing CMV positive sperm for inseminations or IVF are beyond the scope of this chapter. Furthermore, the author acknowledges that multiple CMV policies exist among ART programs. Finally, it is crucial for an ART program that orders sperm from commercial sperm banks to be aware of each banks' policies regarding release of CMV positive sperm and how it relates to its own CMV policy.

Plasma dilution occurs when there is "a decrease in the concentrations of the donor's plasma proteins and circulating antigens or antibodies resulting from the transfusion of blood or blood components and/or infusion of fluids" [1271.3(p)]. If a donor has had a transfusion or infusion of any kind within 48 h before the blood draw for infectious disease testing, the test results may be affected. Therefore, the simplest solution is to ask the potential donor at the time of the blood draw if they have had a transfusion or infusion within the past 48 h. If so, the donor should be instructed to return no earlier than 48 h following the infusion/transfusion. If this cannot be done, the program must consult the plasma dilution sections of the DED Guidance [26, 27].

Finally, ART programs must always keep in mind that the field of donor testing is always changing with advances in technology and the knowledge of infectious disease. As new, more sensitive, more accurate methods for infectious disease testing are developed and approved, it is likely that the FDA will require additional testing for tissue donors in the future. Therefore, ART programs must keep up with the current FDA's thinking on particular testing topics and pay attention to any new testing guidances as they are published.

Donor Eligibility Determination (1271.45; 1271.50; 1271.65; 1271.75; 1271.80; 1271.90)

The "Donor Eligibility Determination" represents the decision point at which a donation may occur; and if so, under what conditions. If all screening and testing have been performed correctly, then the donor eligibility determination is straightforward. It requires only that a responsible person review the completed records and decide as to whether the prospective donor is "eligible" or "ineligible" to donate tissue.

For purposes of preparing for the review, it is important to have a clear understanding of which prospective donors require a donor eligibility determination and which are exempt. There are a number of specific donor situations that should be discussed here. All anonymous and directed oocyte and sperm donors that are not sexually intimate with a recipient MUST have a donor eligibility determination performed [1271.45(b)]. There are significant exemptions *for fresh tissue* from this requirement, namely for (1) autologous cells and tissues (note: the FDA does *not* consider sperm, testicular biopsy tissue, or embryos as "autologous"; 1271.3(a)) and (2) reproductive tissue from a sexually intimate partner (SIP) [1271.90(a)(1) & (2)].

Additionally, there are two more exemptions for *cryopreserved* tissue which should be clarified here. The first cryopreserved tissue exemption [1271.90(a)(3)] must meet *all* of the following criteria: (1) the cryopreserved cells or tissue are either oocytes, sperm, ovarian tissue, or testicular tissue; (2) the tissue is already exempt under the first exemption #1 and #2 above; and (3) the tissue is now intended for directed donation from a donor who cannot make further donations due to the health or infertility of the donor and measures are taken to screen and test the donor before transfer to the recipient. The second cryopreserved tissue exemption deals with embryos [1271.90(a)(4)]. The following conditions are required for embryos to be exempt: (1) the cryopreserved embryos are originally exempt under #2, since they are from sexually intimate partners; (2) the embryos are intended for directed or anonymous donation; and (3) appropriate measures, when possible, are taken to screen and test the semen and oocyte donors before transfer of the embryo to the recipient. These examples and further explanation of these exemptions are detailed in the DED Guidance [28] and will also be covered under "Cases" in this chapter.

The basics of performing a donor eligibility determination should be rather simple at this point if *all screening and testing procedures have been followed and results obtained.* The process of performing a donor eligibility determination is depicted in Fig. 6.1. The eligibility determination must be performed before transfer of tissue occurs

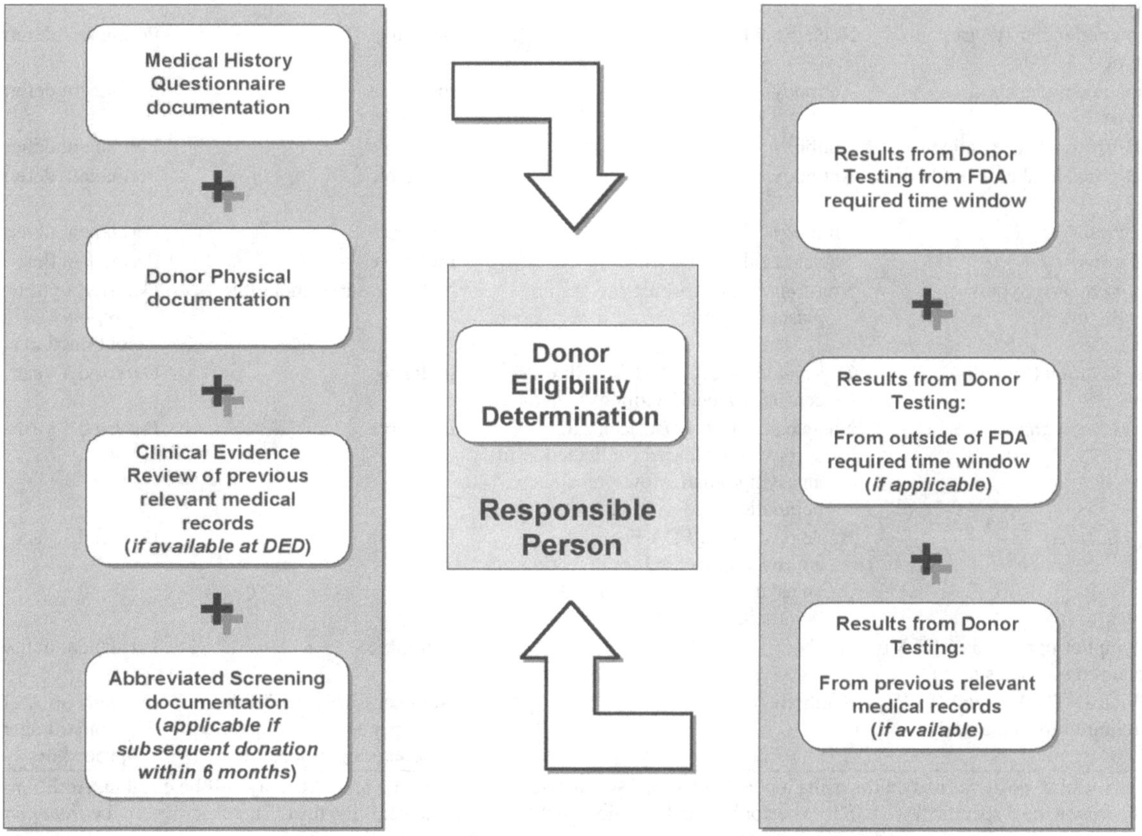

Fig. 6.1 The process of performing a donor eligibility determination (DED)

except for cases of urgent medical need [1271.60(d)(1)]. In general, however, the FDA generally does not consider reproductive tissue to fall under the definition of urgent medical need [1271.3(u)]. The responsible person performing the donor eligibility determination reviews the screening and testing results and reaches a conclusion as to whether the donor is "eligible" or "ineligible" to donate based on these results.

A donor is "eligible" only if (1) donor screening indicates that the donor "(a) is free from risk factors for, and clinical evidence of, infection due to relevant communicable disease agents and diseases; and (b) is free from communicable disease risks associated with xenotransplantation"; and (2) donor testing for all RCDADs indicates that the donor is "negative or nonreactive, except as provided in Sect. 1271.80(d)(1)" (syphilis).

From a practical standpoint, it is fairly straightforward to determine a donor's eligibility based on test results (see Table 6.5) because if testing was performed correctly *and* clear results were obtained, the results are usually objective and accurate indications of a donor's infectious disease status. However, there are situations when "false-positive" or "inconclusive" results may be obtained. From a clinical perspective, these types of results do not necessarily mean that the donor has an ultimate *diagnosis* of the particular disease; follow-up testing with the same or different testing methodologies may indicate that the donor is negative clinically. However, *from an FDA standpoint*, the only point at which a donor is considered "eligible" is when the donor clearly tests negative or non-reactive. All other test results render a donor "ineligible," regardless of resolving a false-positive or inconclusive test to a negative outcome.

There have been cases in which the FDA has made very limited exceptions to this rule; however, these exceptions are very narrow in scope and deal with specific testing issues. A separate guidance published by the FDA deals with testing pooled blood samples from tissue donors (not supposed to occur) and the use of diagnostic tests instead of tests indicated for donor screening [29].

Table 6.5 Eligibility of donors based on RCDAD test results

Relevant communicable disease agent or disease (RCDAD)	Testing methodology	Eligibility of donor with positive or reactive results	Deferral status
Human immunodeficiency virus (HIV) type 1	Antibody	Ineligible	Permanent deferral
Human immunodeficiency virus (HIV) type 1	Nucleic acid Test	Ineligible	Permanent deferral
Human immunodeficiency virus (HIV) type 2	Antibody	Ineligible	Permanent deferral
Heptatitis B Virus, surface antigen	Antibody	Ineligible	Permanent deferral
Heptatitis B virus, total core antibody (IgG/IgM)	Antibody	Ineligible	Permanent deferral
Hepatitis C virus	Antibody	Ineligible	Permanent deferral
Hepatitis C virus	Nucleic acid test	Ineligible	Permanent deferral
Treponema pallidum (Syphilis)	Non-*treponemal* specific (i.e., rapid plasma reagin)	Not necessarily ineligible[a]	Deferred until results from *treponemal*-specific test obtained to confirm[a]
Treponema pallidum (Syphilis)	*Treponemal*-specific test (i.e., fluorescent *Treponemal* antibody)	Ineligible[a]	Deferred 1 year[a] pending
Chlamydia trachomatis	Nucleic acid test; FDA licensed, approved or cleared for detection in an asymptomatic, low-prevalence population	Ineligible	Deferred 1 year
Neisseria gonorrhea	Nucleic acid test; FDA licensed, approved or cleared for detection in an asymptomatic, low-prevalence population	Ineligible	Deferred 1 year
Human T-lymphotropic Virus (HTLV) I, II (required for males only)	Antibody	Ineligible	Permanent deferral
Cytomegalovirus (CMV) Total (IgG/IgM) (required for males only)	Antibody	Not necessarily ineligible; depends on RTE standard operating procedure	Depends on ART program standard operating procedure

[a]Note: Donors testing positive for syphilis using a non-*treponemal* specific screening test (i.e., an RPR) may still be eligible. Additional testing in the form of a *treponemal*-specific test MUST be performed to determine final eligibility status. If the results are negative on the *treponemal*-specific test, the donor may still be considered "eligible" and the donation can continue. If the results are positive, the donor is considered "ineligible" and must be deferred for at least 1 year

Making a donor eligibility determination based on screening results is a different issue. Screening results are more subjective. The clinician(s) performing the separate screening steps and the responsible person conducting the donor eligibility determination must interpret the information contained in the DED Guidance. In general, if the donor exhibits any risks of or clinical evidence of any RCDAD, the donor is usually considered "ineligible". However, the exact questions asked of the donor, as well as all pertinent physical and clinical evidence are beyond the scope of this chapter. For details concerning basic eligibility statements, where screening information is obtained for a particular RCDAD, and deferral information for screening results, see Table 6.6.

If a donor is determined to be "ineligible" based on screening and/or testing, then the next step in the process depends on the relationship between the donor and recipient. If the donor/recipient relationship is anonymous, then the tissue *cannot be transferred under any circumstances* [1271.45(c)]. However, if the relationship is one of a directed reproductive donor or if the donation is for "allogeneic use in a first-degree or second-degree blood relative" [1271.3(l)], then the tissue can be donated with the following provisions: (1) the HCT/Ps must be labeled properly [1271.65(b)(2)] and (2) it must be documented by the ART program that "manufactured" the tissue that the physician transferring the tissue was notified of the results of screening and testing [1271.65(b)(3)]. In practice, this means that the recipient and the donor must be aware of the risks associated with transfer of the tissue, advised as to the labeling, and know that the consent is documented. One of the more common misconceptions concerns directed donors and the use of ineligible tissue. If an ART program has determined a directed donor to be ineligible, the donor is ineligible. Seeking an alternative solution, such as receiving a signed consent from the recipient,

Table 6.6 Eligibility of donors based on RCDAD screening results

Relevant communicable disease agent or disease (RCDAD)	Screening results from:	Eligibility of donor if risk/clinical evidence of RCDAD is found	Deferral status
Human immunodeficiency virus (HIV) type 1,2; subtype O	Medical history, physical exam; medical records review	Ineligible	Permanent deferral
Hepatitis B or C virus	Medical history, physical exam; medical records review	Ineligible	Permanent deferral
Human transmissible spongiform encephalopathy, including Cretzfeldt-Jakob disease ("Mad-Cow")	Medical history, medical records review	Ineligible	Permanent deferral
Treponema pallidum (Syphilis)	Medical history, physical exam; medical records review	Ineligible	Deferred 1 year from date of exposure/diagnosis plus evidence of successful treatment for re-entry
Chlamydia trachomatis[a]	Medical history, physical exam; medical records review	Ineligible	Deferred 1 year from date of exposure/diagnosis plus evidence of successful treatment for re-entry
Neisseria gonorrhea[a]	Medical history, physical exam; medical records review	Ineligible	Deferred 1 year from date of exposure/diagnosis plus evidence of successful treatment for re-entry
Human T-lymphotropic virus (HTLV)	Medical records review	Ineligible	Permanent deferral
West Nile virus (WNV)	Medical history, medical records review	Ineligible	Deferred 120 days from diagnosis, previous positive test result or onset of illness (whichever is later)
Sepsis	Medical history, physical exam; medical records review (*if a living donor appears healthy, sepsis usually does not apply*)	Ineligible	No deferral criteria mentioned by FDA for living donors if this occurs
Communicable disease risks associated with xenotransplantation	Medical history, medical records review	Ineligible	Permanent deferral
Vaccinia (from small-pox vaccination)	Medical history, physical exam; medical records review	Ineligible	Deferred 14 days to 3 months; dependent on status of lesion and/or complications

does not reverse the donor's ineligibility. A donor's ineligibility cannot change, unless the donor was ineligible for an RCDAD which has an associated time-related deferral.

Records and Recordkeeping (1271.55)

Documentation of all steps of the donor eligibility process is vital for an ART program's compliance with 21 CFR 1271. The FDA has established specific requirements regarding the types of records to maintain, which records must accompany the HCT/P(s) and the retention time of those records. The FDA requires that all records pertaining to screening, testing, and donor eligibility determination [1271.55(d)(i–iii)] be (1) "accurate, indelible and legible" [1271.55(d)(2)], (2) made available *upon request* during an FDA inspection [1271.55(d)(3)] and (3) retained for at least 10 years after the date the HCT/P was used (transferred, distributed, disposed, donated to research, or other final disposition) or expired – whichever occurs last.

Additionally, there are types of records termed "accompanying records" and "summary of records" that have specific requirements and can be a major source of negative observations during an FDA inspection. For a breakdown of these requirements, see Fig. 6.2. These accompanying records must "accompany" the corresponding HCT/Ps at all times after a donor eligibility determination has been made [1271.55(a)] and must not contain any personally identifying information of the donor unless the donation is directed where both parties are known to each other.

Laboratory Section: Labeling, Quarantine, Storage, Shipping/Receipt, and Non-Clinical Uses (1271.60; 1271.65; 1271.90; 1271.370(b)(4)[1])

It may appear that the bulk of this ruling affects the clinical side of an ART program. This is primarily due to the fact that currently, the FDA has temporarily exempt ART programs from the rest of the Current Good Tissue Practices (CGTPs). Even so, ART programs are still covered by portions of the ruling requiring compliance measures and adoption of practices. This section focuses specifically on how the ruling affects an ART laboratory. As noted before, specific policies and procedures that describe these processes *must* be established and maintained.

Labeling: 1271.90; 1271.370(b)(4)

For an ART laboratory, the labeling required of reproductive tissue can be a confusing process. Questions that are the main source of confusion include: which tissue is subject to labeling, how labeling is physically performed, and which textual labels are required. The ruling requires that all tissue in an ART laboratory has labeling that will "accompany" the tissue at all times, regardless of whether it is exempt or not from the donor eligibility determination requirement [1271.90(b)]. This means that although sexually intimate partners (SIPs) are exempt from the donor eligibility determination requirement [1271.90(a)(2)], their tissue must be labeled as outlined in section 1271.90(a)(1)–(6). This also includes tissue for

Accompanying Records

- Distinct and unique identification code affixed to container[1]
- A statement detailing whether the donor is "eligible" or "ineligible"
  - Include responsible person name/signature + date
- ***Summary of records***
  - *See next column*

Summary of Records

- Statement that the testing was performed by a CLIA[2] (or equivalent[3]) certified lab
- Listing and interpretation of ***all*** RCDAD test results
- Name & address of establishment that performed the DED
- If ineligible based on screening, then must state reason

1. *In accordance with 1271.55(a)(1), the identification code must relate to the donor, but must NOT include their name, social security number of medical record number; unless it is a directed donation (including first or second-degree blood relatives).*
2. *Clinical Laboratory Improvement Amendments (CLIA) of 1988*
3. *Equivalent requirements as set by the Centers for Medicare and Medicaid Services*

Fig. 6.2 "Important elements for accompanying records" and "summary of records"

[1]Note: see "Subpart E: Additional requirements" for explanation on how 1271.370 is important for labeling

Table 6.7 Warnings required for FDA compliant labeling of HCT/Ps

Required label	Applicable situation(s)	Section of ruling
"For autologus use only"	For autologous use[a]	1271.90(b)(1)
"Not evaluated for infectious substances"	Required screening and/or testing is incomplete or not been performed according to the ruling[b]	1271.90(b)(2)
"Warning: Advise recipient of communicable disease risks"	(1) DED is not performed or not completed; (2) If screening or testing results indicate presence of RCDs and/or risk factors or clinical evidence of RCDADs. Not utilized in cases of autologous use.	1271.90(b)(3)
Biohazard legend (note that this symbol must be in orange)	Screening or testing shows presence of RCDs and/or risk factors or clinical evidence of RCDADs.	1271.90(b)(4) (symbol shown in 1271.3(h))
"Warning: Reactive test results for (*insert name of disease agent or disease*)"	Positive or reactive test results (for any tissue – donor or non-donor)	1271.90(b)(5)
"Advise recipient that screening and testing fo the donor(s) were not performed at the time of cryopreservation of the reproductive cells or tissue, but have been performed subsequently"	All conditions must apply: (1) For embryos fulfilling the exemption in 1271.90(a)(4) or gametes fulfilling the exemption in 1271.90(a)(3); (2) Intent indicated for donation, and (3) Oocyte and/or sperm contributors have had ALL required screening and testing.	1271.90(b)(6)
"For non-clinical use only"	Use with the *Biohazard legend* for ineligible tissue designated for non-clinical use (i.e., donation to research or training)	1271.65(c)
Other types of labels required (or helpful)		
Label or some other clear indication that tissue is in quarantine	(1) A DED is required on the donor, and (2) A DED is not complete by the time of tissue collection.	1271.60(b)
Statement indicating that the tissue "… must not be implanted, transplanted, infused or transferred until completion of the donor-eligibility determination, except…" in cases of documented urgent medical need (as referred to in 1271.60(d))	Tissue is to be shipped in quarantine	1271.60(c)(3); 1271.60(d)

[a]For reproductive tissue, this label is ONLY used for oocytes (or ovarian tissue) being cryopreserved for future autologous use; this does NOT apply to embryos or sperm (or testicular tissue)

[b]ALL screening and testing described under sections 1271.75, 1271.80 and 1271.85 must be performed (including the more specific information given in the DED Guidance) for this label NOT to apply. Also, this label does not apply to cryopreserved embryos as described in section 1271.90(a)(4). However, labeling under 1271.90(b)(6) MAY apply to embryos in 1271.90(a)(4)

Note: Labeling requirements are not just required for donors – they extend to ALL tissue in an ART program

autologous use [(1271.90(a)(1)], cryopreserved gametes [1271.90(a)(3)], and embryos [1271.90(a)(4)] originally meant for self use and subsequently intended for donation. The labels required for the different situations that arise in an ART laboratory is listed in Table 6.7. Although the bulk of the labeling generated is usually for SIPs undergoing IVF procedures, the ART laboratory must still consider *any* test results for RCDs from either SIP for labeling.

An ART laboratory must know the following three important pieces of information in order to label tissue accurately: (1) whether a donor eligibility determination was required, (2) the complete (or incomplete) results, if it was required, and (3) if it was *not* required, then the results of any screening or testing that was performed. Furthermore, the ART laboratory must also know the collection date of the tissue to determine if a "quarantine" indication is appropriate (see the next section on "Quarantine). Each one of these important pieces of information will be discussed.

If a donor eligibility determination was required, this means that the situation is considered to be a non-exempt donor situation in which ALL the necessary screening and testing should have been completed. If a completed eligibility determination indicates the donor was "eligible", no special labeling applies beyond the requirements for accompanying and summary of records [1271.55]. However, if screening and/or testing indicates that the donor had any risk factors/clinical evidence of, or had tested positive for, a RCDAD, then specific warnings must be included in the labeling. These warnings are dependent on the reason for ineligibility. If an eligibility determination was not required, for instance, in cases of SIPs undergoing IVF, the laboratory still needs to know the kind of testing and screening that was done and the results in order to determine the warnings that are appropriate for the tissue. All these warnings and other types of required or helpful labeling are included in Table 6.7.

Finally, there are three more instances where labeling is required – two concerning quarantined tissue and one regarding non-clinical use of ineligible tissue. The FDA requires that tissue deemed ineligible for donation to a recipient and instead designated for non-clinical use must be labeled with the warning "FOR NON-CLINICAL USE ONLY" and the *Biohazard legend* [1271.65(c)]. The other two cases are addressed in the next section on "Quarantine".

Quarantine: 1271.60(a),(b)

The FDA definition of "quarantine" for HCT/Ps is "the storage or identification of an HCT/P, to prevent improper release, in a physically separate area clearly identified for such use, or through use of other procedures, such as automated designation" [1271.3(q)]. Understanding what this definition is and how it is applied is essential for compliance, since the FDA definition is somewhat different from the definition commonly used by ART laboratories.

The basic purpose of this requirement is to ensure that any tissue collected from a donor requiring an eligibility determination is kept from distribution until the determination has been completed. Tissue exempt from the eligibility requirement does not fall into this category. The ART laboratory "must clearly identify as quarantined an HCT/P that is in quarantine pending completion of a donor-eligibility determination" and "must be easily distinguishable from HCT/Ps that are available for release and distribution" [1271.60(b)]. Note that much of the emphasis the FDA places on quarantine concerns *identification and distinction* from other tissues. Therefore, the ART laboratory must develop a documented system to ensure that all personnel are aware when tissue is in quarantine and that quarantined tissue must not be transferred in any way to the recipient until the donor eligibility determination is completed and meets all other requirements for use. This requires the development of written procedures that acknowledge the FDA's definition of quarantine and that detail how the ART program will fulfill the definition during "Processing," i.e., culturing of embryos, sperm preparation, and during tissue storage. In practice, this process should not be difficult, since well-run laboratories understand that there are few things as important as correctly identifying samples for use.

Additionally, the FDA has specific requirements for shipping tissue that is in quarantine [1271.60(c)]. First, the donor tissue must have records accompanying the tissue that (1) identify the donor (i.e., ID code) and (2) state that the donor eligibility determination has not been made and that the tissue cannot be transferred until the eligibility determination process has been completed (see Table 6.7). The only exception is for cases of "urgent medical need" [1271.60(d)]. Note, however, that reproductive tissue generally does not meet the definition of "urgent medical need" [1271.3(u)]; therefore, this exception does not apply to ART programs.

Storage: 1271.65(a)

Meeting the requirements for tissue storage according to 1271.65(a) has often vexed ART laboratory personnel, as interpretation of compliance varies widely. The ART laboratory "must store or identify HCT/Ps from donors who have been determined to be ineligible in a physically separate area clearly identified for such use" or may impart other measures to ensure donor tissue is not improperly released (such as "automated designation") [1271.65(a)]. The key phrases to focus on are ineligible and physically separate area. The main requirement is that any ineligible tissue that is stored must be designated and separated *in some way* from all other tissue. How this is accomplished can vary. A physically separate area can mean a completely separate tank or a canister within a tank specifically designated for only storing ineligible tissue. However, the *spirit* of the ruling implies that all tissue storage should have written policies and procedures that describe the process of storing and accounting for all tissue.

Shipping (and Receipt): 1271.60(c); 1271.55

The last area of ART laboratory-specific requirements concerns shipping and receipt of tissue. The only section that specifically mentions shipping requirements for tissue has already been addressed in the section on *Quarantine* – records requirements for shipping tissue in quarantine. On first glance, this seems to be the only issue regarding shipping of tissue that needs attention. However, from a realistic standpoint, this is not the case. There has also been discussion of the terms "accompanying records" and "summary of records" in this chapter (see section on "Records and Recordkeeping" above). Note the wording of 1271.55(a): "Once a donor-eligibility determination has been made, the following must accompany the HCT/P *at all times*". This means that not only these "accompanying records" must be with the tissue while in use or in storage at a given ART laboratory, but they must also *accompany* the tissue when it is *shipped to other locations*. This same line of reasoning would also apply to appropriate labeling as well. Additionally, then any tissue *received* from another ART program must also have these records and should be checked and documented.

Departures from Procedures and Deviations (1271.47(d))

This next section focuses on another important area – the responsibilities of an ART program when issues arise. Even the most efficient and meticulous of ART programs will find itself in the position of confronting problems. Sometimes, these events are unexpected and after the fact. Other times, they may be known beforehand, when there is time to do something about it.

The FDA requires that all ART programs document any departures from procedures performed. Furthermore, FDA requires that ART programs cannot transfer tissue under a departure from procedure unless a responsible person has "determined that the departure does not increase the risks of communicable disease transmission through the use of the HCT/P" [1271.47(d)]. It is essential to understand what the FDA means by "departures from procedures" in order to employ the concept properly. The meaning is not intuitively obvious. The FDA considers a departure from procedure "to be an intended change from an established procedure, including a standard operating procedure (SOP), which occurs before the HCT/P is distributed, and is consistent with applicable regulations and standards" [30]. For example, an ART laboratory may use different culture media because the media listed in the procedure was not available at the time oocytes were collected. In this case, the change was intended to happen and is consistent with the regulations. By contrast, a deviation is "an event that is *inconsistent* with applicable regulations, standards, or established specification, or is *unexpected or unforeseeable*" [1271.3(dd)]. An example of a deviation is a situation in which embryos from an anonymous oocyte donor/male SIP partner's sperm is transferred to the female SIP, and it is discovered after the fact that the oocyte donor has been erroneously determined eligible when the donor is, in fact, ineligible. Departures from procedures are required to be documented by the ART program. Currently, however, ART programs are not required to document or report deviations to the FDA under 1271.350(b) – a part of the ruling from which ART programs are temporarily exempt.

6.2.3 *Current Good Tissue Practice: Final Rule*

6.2.3.1 Subpart D: Current Good Tissue Practice: Sections 1271.145–1271.320

Subpart D establishes what are called the Current Good Tissue Practice (CGTP) requirements. These requirements are meant to reduce the potential of communicable disease transmission during the multiple steps of tissue "manufacturing": recovery, donor screening, donor testing, processing, storage, labeling, packaging, and distribution. The elements of Subpart D are listed in Table 6.8. Only the currently applicable sections will be discussed here.

At present, ART programs are exempt from most of the CGTPs, *except for the following*: (1) 1271.150(c)(1–3): Compliance with applicable requirements; and (2) 1271.155: Exemptions and alternatives. 1271.150(c) discusses the roles and responsibilities of a tissue establishment during the process of evaluating and entering into manufacturing arrangements with other establishments that are required to comply with any part of 21 CFR Part 1271. 1271.155 states that tissue establishments may request an exemption or an alternative in order to meet any of the Subpart C or D requirements. Currently, it is understood that this exemption for ART programs is only *temporary* and that eventually the FDA will apply the CGTPs to reproductive tissue – in some form. If, or more likely when, ART programs are required to become compliant with the CGTPs, there probably will be a tremendous impact on ART laboratories from both a practice and documentation standpoint.

Table 6.8 Section breakdown of subpart D: current good tissue practice

Section	Topic
1271.145	Prevention of the introduction, transmission, or spread of communicable diseases.
1271.150	Current good tissue practice requirements.
1271.155	Exemptions and alternatives.
1271.160	Establishment and maintenance of a quality program.
1271.170	Personnel.
1271.180	Procedures.
1271.190	Facilities.
1271.195	Environmental control and monitoring.
1271.200	Equipment.
1271.210	Supplies and reagents.
1271.215	Recover.
1271.220	Processing and process controls.
1271.225	Process changes.
1271.230	Process validation.
1271.250	Labeling controls.
1271.260	Storage.
1271.265	Receipt, predistribution shipment, and distribution of an HCT/P.
1271.270	Records.
1271.290	Tracking.
1271.320	Complaint file.

1271.150(c) has the largest impact on ART programs of Subpart D and should play an important part in the overall compliance plan and practices of an ART program. Due to the importance of this section, there is a separate part of this chapter which discusses these issues ("Manufacturing Arrangements"). The FDA has published a separate guidance regarding this topic ("Guidance for Industry: Compliance with 21 CFR Part 1271.150(c)(1) – Manufacturing Arrangements") [25].

Manufacturing Arrangements (1271.150(c)(1))

As mentioned earlier, it is the responsibility of a registered ART program to ensure that any establishment regulated under 21 CFR 1271 with which it has manufacturing arrangements is FDA compliant [1271.150(c)(1)]. This portion of the regulation states that an ART program or an establishment with whom the ART program contracts need only comply with the parts of the regulation that are "applicable to the operations" performed [1271.150(c)(1)(i)] or with "requirements applicable to that manufacturing step" [1271.150(c)(1)(ii)]. Additionally, ART programs are required to ensure that the contracted establishment "complies with all applicable CGTP requirements" BEFORE it enters into any contract or understanding with the contracted establishment, and DURING the course of the relationship. If the ART program ever finds that the contracted establishment is not in compliance, it must take "reasonable steps" to ensure compliance. If this effort is unsuccessful, the ART program must terminate the relationship [1271.150(c)(1)(iii)].

From the perspective of an ART program, the challenge is to determine "reasonable steps" to take to ensure compliance. The Manufacturing Arrangements Guidance makes several suggestions about how to accomplish this: (1) conducting an initial audit; (2) reviewing standard operating procedures; (3) reviewing the establishment's compliance history [31]. Another suggestion would be to have mechanisms in place to detect compliance problems from information received, i.e., documenting receipt of the Accompanying and Summary of Records information each time tissue is received by the ART program. Figure 6.3 depicts "red flags" that could indicate compliance issues with a contracted establishment.

There are several actions an ART program should take to verify compliance of a contracted establishment: verify the FEI number (Federal Establishment Identifier number that is generated during the course of registration with the FDA), verify current registration, interview the contracted establishment, and ask specific questions designed to gauge its working knowledge of the regulations and obtain recent copies of all relevant certifications (CLIA, CAP, state certifications).

Finally, it is highly recommended that the ART program sign a contractual agreement with the establishment, even if it is a vendor relationship and not an exclusive one. The contract should establish the responsibilities of both parties, and indicate that sufficient notification, with a specified time range, should be given when changes to established policies and procedures are made that affect the ART program. The agreement should also contain language indicating that, if an activity affecting an ART program's donor was found to be out of compliance, then the establishment would be responsible for notifying the ART program within a reasonable period of time and set consequences for non-compliance. The ART program may also want to consider other elements in the agreement with legal guidance.

- *Failure to re-register for the coming year*
- *Repeated failure to send accompanying records with tissue or there are incorrect or missing required elements*
- *Improper screening (i.e. sending an oocyte donor who is automatically ineligible)*
- *Suspect test results—i.e. inordinate number of "inconclusive" or "positive" results*
- *Incomplete testing, use of a non-FDA registered testing laboratory, or use of non-FDA approved/cleared tests*
- *Testing methodology changes without sufficient notification*

Fig. 6.3 "Red flags" indicating a potential compliance issue with a contracted establishment

6.2.3.2 Subpart E: Additional Requirements for Establishments Described in Sect. 1271.10; Sections 1271.330, 1271.350 and 1271.370

The requirements presented in this subpart deal with the necessity of reporting certain information to the FDA and with additional labeling requirements. For ART programs, this is another section that is not yet applicable, as set forth in 1271.330. However, one labeling aspect is important to note due to the physical nature of cryopreserved tissue [1271.370]. The small size of the containers used for reproductive tissue makes it difficult or impossible to include all the necessary labeling on the container itself. The FDA has made allowances for this in the Interim Final Rule, published May 25, 2005, and finalized on June 19, 2007 (7, 11). The altered ruling states that "If it is not physically possible to include these warnings [in reference to sections 1271.60(d)(2), 1271.65(b)(2) and 1271.90(b)] on the label, the warning must, instead, accompany the HCT/P" [1271.370(b)(4)]. This means that these warnings can be placed on, or included separately with, documentation that accompanies the tissue, i.e., in a "sticker" format or as a separate labeling sheet.

6.2.3.3 Subpart F: Inspection and Enforcement of Establishments Described in Sect. 1271.10; Sections 1271.390, 1271.400, 1271.420 and 1271.440)

Finally, the last part of the applicable ruling deals with FDA inspections and enforcement. The four different areas of this subpart deal with, in the order of numbers listed above: (1) Applicability, (2) Inspections, (3) HCT/Ps offered for import, and (4) Orders of retention, recall, destruction, and cessation of manufacturing. The first two sections establish that the FDA can inspect at any time, announced or unannounced, during normal business hours, and inspect the ART program's "establishment, facilities, equipment, finished and unfinished materials, containers, processes, HCT/Ps, procedures, labeling, records, files, papers, and controls" [1271.400(a)]. The FDA inspector will ask for the most responsible person available at the time of the inspection and can take samples and review records [1271.400(d)]. Note that the FDA will not expose names or other identifying information of donors or recipients if any information is made public. Financial and personnel records are not required to be shown during an inspection. The FDA can order the cessation of manufacturing of an establishment, but CANNOT order the destruction of reproductive tissue or carry out the destruction itself [1271.440(f)].

6.3 Summary: Evidence-Based Guidelines

6.3.1 Implementation of Compliance Measures

Achieving and maintaining compliance with the FDA regulations may appear to be a daunting task. It will be if approached in a haphazard fashion. However, there are ways to approach designing and implementing a compliance system that can serve to achieve and maintain FDA compliance as well as elevate an ART program's overall standards of care.

Once it is decided that compliance measures are necessary, the ART program should take the following actions:

1. Determine who has authority for decisions and actions

ART programs commonly have organizational structures and responsibility assignments for personnel that may differ from other fields. Regardless of the structure, it is crucial that the senior management of an ART program understands absolutely that FDA compliance is a serious matter and communicates this to personnel. If the Medical and Laboratory Director are not firmly committed to compliance, neither will their personnel be committed to it. A well-coordinated, team approach is important to achieving compliance. Definition and delegation of roles and responsibilities according to specific areas of expertise is a critical component of a successful compliance program. A joint sense of ownership among the staff in the compliance effort is essential. Finally, it is vitally important to designate the ultimately "responsible person" as well as the specific areas and levels of authority and responsibility of other personnel.

2. Develop an action plan

Establishing an action plan is one of the most effective ways of completing the design and implementation of a compliance system. Details include: (a) key action steps to be taken, (b) personnel responsible for enacting each step, and (c) specific, reasonable, and *enforceable* deadlines. Furthermore, an action plan is dependent upon the current level of compliance of an establishment.

3. Putting the action plan into practice

After development and approval, the plan should be implemented systematically with enforceable deadlines. The most responsible person is ultimately at fault for non-compliance and, therefore, should drive the process, obtaining updates, and providing guidance and leadership when appropriate.

- *Decide high level policies FIRST—generally, procedures are determined from policy decisions and forms are used as tools to document procedures*
- *When writing the manual, clarity is essential–FDA inspectors will be attempting to understand the donor program from the manual*
- *Organization and modularization is key for ease of use and updating the manual when necessary*
  - *Decide on a numbering system for all policies, procedures and forms*
  - *Include document control information on all documents (version/date)*
- *Proper signage/dating is essential*
- *Directly address overlap between the clinic and the laboratory*
- *Remember the policies and procedures manual is a "lives"—it must be updated when policies and processes change*

Fig. 6.4 Helpful hints for designing an effective policies and procedures manual

The following elements should be the fundamental first steps in initiating a plan for an ART program:

(a) Design and completion of the ART program's policies and procedures manual. *This is the most essential compliance tool for an ART program.* This manual contains all policies, procedures, and forms appropriate to cover the scope of the regulations. The manual may also include quality assurance information such as auditing, corrective, and preventative action (CAPA) programs, FDA inspection information, reference information, communication logs, contracts etc. See Fig. 6.4 for helpful hints in designing an effective policies and procedures manual.
(b) Training of necessary personnel. Employees must be trained in the policies, procedures, and forms appropriate to their position and training must be documented;
(c) Formal implementation of all policies and procedures (final release); and
(d) Conducting audits.

6.3.2 Putting It All Together: The FDA Compliance Cycle and How It All Fits

After the policies and procedures manual is approved, personnel are trained, and compliance procedures are in place, the program is not yet finished. Compliance comprises not only what is written in the policies and procedures manual, but it also, and most importantly, includes what is practiced. Compliance is not a single event. A "compliance

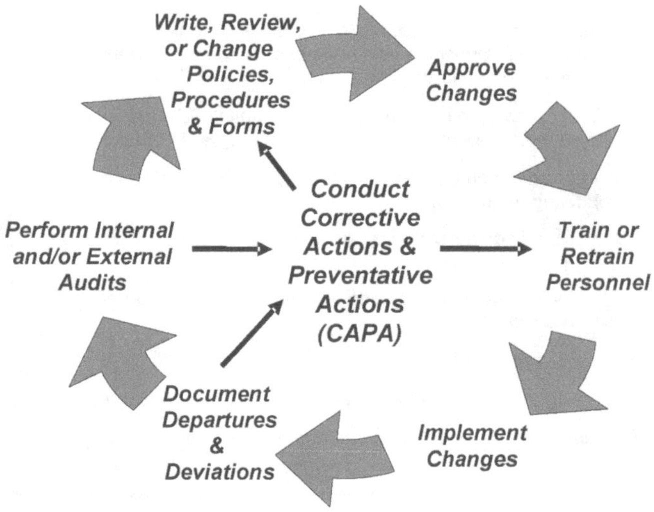

Fig. 6.5 The compliance cycle

cycle" essentially never ends, but exists in a dynamic state (see Fig. 6.5).

If personnel do not implement the policies, procedures, and forms *according to what is written in the manual*, the establishment is out of compliance and at risk during an FDA inspection. Internal and/or external audits must be conducted to ensure that everything in the policies and procedures manual has been *and continues to be* implemented properly. There have been cases in which an establishment found a serious breach, documented and attempted to correct it *prior to an FDA inspection*, and thus avoided an inspectional observation. However, the best way of dealing with potential violations is to prevent them from happening.

In order for an ART program to prevent the recurrence of problems, it must put in place a functioning plan of corrective and preventative actions. Corrective actions address violations that have occurred, i.e., correcting signage of a document, rescreening or testing of a donor or correcting a chart notation. After corrective actions have been taken, preventative actions must be employed to decrease the likelihood of these issues recurring. This may include enacting new policies and retiring old ones, modifying procedures or forms, changing existing documentation in the compliance manual and retraining of personnel.

6.3.3 Handling an FDA Inspection

When an ART program finds itself in the unhappy position of facing an FDA inspector at its door for the first time or yet again, it will realize that an inspection can be extremely disruptive – especially for those directly involved in the inspection. In dealing with the anxiety of an inspection, it is important for ART program professionals to keep several points in mind:

First, there are several levels of enforcement that the FDA can take. These include an untitled letter, a warning letter, orders of retention, recall, destruction, and cessation of manufacturing, and prosecution [31]. To this date, only a handful of establishments have been subject to any of these measures [32] and the regulation states that the "FDA will not issue an order for the destruction of reproductive tissue … nor will it carry out such destruction itself "[1271.440(f)].

Second, as discussed earlier, ART programs are currently subject to only the following portions of 21 CFR Part 1271: Subparts A, B, C, and 21 CFR 1271.150(c)(1) and 1271.155 of Subpart D [31]. Other sections are not applicable at this time.

Third, ART programs are not required to show financial and personnel records during an inspection [31].

Fourth, there are certain "hot spot" issues for the FDA that have been particular areas of concern [32, 33]. The majority of these areas are listed in Table 6.9.

The best way of dealing with an FDA inspection is to be prepared beforehand. The policy and procedure manual must be completed and personnel must be trained on the sections appropriate to them. All personnel, including those at the reception desk, have a role to play during an inspection. It is imperative that personnel know their individual roles and responsibilities when the time comes – from when the inspector first arrives, to when he or she finally leaves. Regular and consistent internal and/or external audits can make a tremendous difference in discovering and correcting any breaches before the FDA arrives. Finally, mock inspections should be

Table 6.9 Some "Hot Spot" issues for FDA inspectors

Frequent inspection/audit issues found[a]	Regulation cited
Failure to establish, maintain, document, review or revise donor eligibility procedures	1271.47(a)
Failure to perform a donor eligibility determination; not determined by a responsible person	1271.50(a)
Donors not screened appropriately for risk factors or clinical evidence through review of medical records	1271.75(a)
Failure to perform abbreviated donor screen when required	1271.75(e)
Incorrect timing of specimen collection	1271.80(b)
Failure to use FDA licensed/approved/cleared test kits for testing or failure to follow manufacturer's instructions	1271.80(c)(
Failure to ensure compliance of establishments performing manufacturing steps under contract or other agreement	1271.150(c)(1)(iii)
Failure to complete all testing before determining donor eligibility	1271.50
Failure to determine donors ineligible after positive test results	1271.80(d)(1)
Failure to test for all relevant communicable diseases	1271.85(c)

[a]Adapted from FDA presentations [32, 33]

performed to test the compliance measures the ART program has put in place and to determine how personnel respond under realistic conditions.

6.4 Case Studies

The successful application of the regulations to daily practice is the ultimate goal. Often, the best way to illustrate this is to address various donor-related situations and describe how each is managed in terms of donor eligibility steps and handling of tissue. Several theoretical cases typical of ART programs are outlined in the following section. These cases illustrate typical situations and how to handle them in a successful and compliant manner.

6.4.1 Example 1: Anonymous Oocyte Donor

6.4.1.1 Donor Situation

- A sexually intimate couple used an anonymous oocyte donor and the male SIP's sperm to create embryos for a fresh IVF cycle.
- The anonymous oocyte donor was fully screened: a donor medical history questionnaire and a donor physical. No medical records were supplied.
- The donor had initial infectious disease testing prior to the 30-day window before oocyte retrieval. This round of testing *did not include* HIV-1/Hepatitis C NAT testing. All tests returned negative or non-reactive results.
- The donor did have infectious disease testing at the start of her stimulation medications that included all necessary tests (including HIV-1/Hep C NAT) that were required within 30 days of oocyte retrieval.
- *At the time of oocyte retrieval, not all test results were received (HIV-1/HCV NAT results). However, negative results were obtained before the transfer.*
- The male SIP was not screened (the FDA regulations do not require it) and was tested for HIV-1&2 Ab, Hep B Surface Antigen, and Hep C Ab. Results were negative.
- Extra embryos were available for cryopreservation and the SIP couple chose to store these embryos for future use.

Table 6.10 Selected FDA web resources

FDA web resource	URL
Center for biologics evaluation and research: tissues	http://www.fda.gov/cber/tiss.htm
Guidances & rulings	http://www.fda.gov/cber/tissue/docs.htm
Registration documents	http://www.fda.gov/cber/tissue/tisreg.htm
Registered establishment search	http://www.fda.gov/cber/tissue/tissregdata.htm
Listserve to sign up for updates	http://www.fda.gov/cber/pubinfo/elists.htm
Donor screening tests for testing HCT/P donors	
Includes Chlamydia, Gonorrhea CMV and Syphilis tests	http://www.fda.gov/cber/tissue/prod.htm
Other living donors	http://www.fda.gov/cber/products/testkits.htm

6.4.1.2 Donor Eligibility/Transfer/Labeling/Tissue Handling

- A donor eligibility determination was performed on the anonymous oocyte donor; the male SIP was exempt.
- Since the HIV-1/HCV NAT test results were not yet obtained, a donor eligibility determination could not be performed at retrieval. Therefore, the resulting oocytes (and embryos) were put into Quarantine.
- As soon as the test results were obtained, the donor was determined "eligible", the embryos were released from quarantine and the transfer performed.
- Extra embryos that were cryopreserved were labeled with the following: (1) "NOT EVALUATED FOR INFECTIOUS SUBSTANCES"; and (2) "Warning: Advise recipient of communicable disease risks" (both due to the male SIP).

6.4.2 Example 2: Directed Sperm Donor

6.4.2.1 Donor Situation

- A sexually intimate couple used the female SIP's oocytes and a directed donor's sperm (relationship: brother to male SIP) to create embryos for a fresh IVF cycle.
- The directed sperm donor was fully screened: donor medical history questionnaire and a donor physical administered by the donor's primary care physician. Previous medical records were supplied for review.
- The donor produced a backup sperm sample before the start of the IVF cycle; he was subjected to full infectious disease testing at the time he produced his semen sample. All results were negative, except that the donor tested positive/reactive for Hepatitis B Surface Antigen and CMV total.
- Additional follow-up CMV testing was performed that specified the donor was CMV IgG positive/IgM negative.
- The donor was tested again for all infectious diseases within 7 days prior to producing his fresh semen sample on the day of the recipient's oocyte retrieval. All results

were received before embryo transfer and were negative, except for Hepatitis B Surface Antigen, and CMV total which were again positive.

- The female SIP was not screened according to FDA regulations, and she was only tested for HIV-1&2 Ab, for which results were negative.
- Extra embryos were available for cryopreservation and the SIP couple chose to store these embryos for future use.

6.4.2.2 Donor Eligibility/Transfer/Labeling/Tissue Handling

- A donor eligibility determination was performed on the directed sperm donor. Medical records were reviewed. The female SIP was exempt.
- At the time the donor produced *either* of his semen samples, the samples were put into Quarantine until all screening and testing results were returned.
- According to the ART program's SOP on CMV, the donor was eligible to donate since follow-up CMV testing indicated the donor was CMV IgG positive *only*.
- The donor was determined "ineligible" due to the positive Hepatitis B Surface Antigen test and the embryos were released from quarantine.
- The female recipient was subjected to the informed consent process and gave documented consent before the embryos were transferred.
- Extra cryopreserved embryos were labeled as follows: (1) "NOTEVALUATEDFORINFECTIOUSSUBSTANCES" (due to female recipient); (2) "Warning: Advise recipient of communicable disease risks" (due to female recipient and directed sperm donor); (3) the Biohazard legend (due to directed sperm donor); and (4) "Warning: Reactive Test Results for *Hepatitis B Surface Antigen*" (due to directed sperm donor). NOTE: The FDA does not consider CMV a relevant communicable disease Therefore, no labeling relating to CMV was required.

6.4.3 Example 3: Gestational Carrier/ Anonymous Oocyte Donor; Fresh Cycle

6.4.3.1 Donor Situation

- A sexually intimate couple from England wanted to pursue a fresh IVF cycle with a known gestational carrier from an agency, but they needed to use an anonymous oocyte donor. They wanted to use the male SIP's sperm.
- The anonymous oocyte donor was fully screened and tested with all negative results obtained *before* oocyte retrieval. The donor was determined to be eligible.
- The male SIP, now considered a directed sperm donor, was fully screened and tested. Test results were obtained and results were negative. All screening results were acceptable, except one indicating a risk for Creutzfeldt-Jacob Disease (CJD).
- Extra embryos were available for cryopreservation.

6.4.3.2 Donor Eligibility/Transfer/Labeling/Tissue Handling

- A donor eligibility determination was not required of the gestational carrier.
- A donor eligibility determination was required for both the anonymous oocyte donor and the male SIP (directed sperm donor) since the intent was to transfer the resulting embryos to a gestational carrier.
- After the male SIP (directed sperm donor) produced his semen sample, it was put into Quarantine until all screening and testing results were returned.
- The anonymous oocyte donor was determined "eligible". However, the male SIP (directed sperm donor) was determined "ineligible" since the FDA has deemed England is unacceptable as country of origin due to the occurrence of Bovine Spongiform Encephalitis (BSE), which includes risks for CJD. This reason was noted on the eligibility form.
- Since the relationship of the gestational carrier (recipient) to the male SIP (directed sperm donor) was known and the male SIP was ineligible, the ART program explained to the carrier the risks associated with CJD and obtained from the carrier informed consent to allow the embryo transfer. After consent was obtained, the embryo transfer *did occur*.
- Any extra embryos cryopreserved were labeled as follows: (1) "Warning: Advise recipient of communicable disease risks" (due to the male SIP/directed sperm donor); and (2) the Biohazard legend (due to the male SIP/directed sperm donor).
- *Notes and variations on this case*: Note that if the gestational carrier/male SIP relationship were not "directed" (meaning "known"), then the male SIP would have been considered an anonymous sperm donor and the embryo transfer *could not have occurred*.

6.4.4 Example 4: Embryo Donation; Third-party Mixed Embryos

6.4.4.1 Donor Situation

- An SIP couple had cryopreserved embryos from a previous IVF cycle. They had used an anonymous oocyte donor and the male SIP's sperm with the female SIP as the recipient. They wanted to donate their embryos anonymously.

- The anonymous oocyte donor was fully screened and tested with all negative results obtained and was determined "eligible" for the cycle the embryos were created.
- The male SIP was tested originally for HIV-1&2 and Hepatitis B Surface Antigen using a non-FDA registered laboratory; results were negative. He had no further tests and was not screened at the time of the cycle.

6.4.4.2 Donor Eligibility/Transfer/Labeling/Tissue Handling

- A donor eligibility determination per se *was not* required for this situation. However, appropriate measures should have been taken to screen and test the male SIP.
- The male SIP was later screened and tested, but for one exception. In this case, ART programs are not required to test for *Chlamydia trachomatis* or *Neisseria gonorrhea* since the FDA has determined that testing for these diseases at this point "... would not provide information about the status of the donor(s) for these agents at the time of the earlier cryopreservation" [34]. All results were negative.
- The embryo labeling was changed to: "Advise recipient that screening and testing of the donors were not performed at the time of cryopreservation of the reproductive cells or tissue, but have been performed subsequently."
- The recipient was notified that the anonymous oocyte donor, had been screened and tested at the time of the cycle and the label ONLY applied to the male SIP.

6.5 Conclusions

The regulatory environment, like the field of medicine, is forever changing. New guidances, interpretations, and issues will continue to develop over time. As mentioned in this chapter, although ART programs are not presently subject to most Current Good Tissue Practices and Additional Requirements (Subparts D and E of 21 CFR 1271), it is expected that these parts of the regulations will eventually be required – at least in some form. Additionally, it is possible that the regulations may be extended or have additions in the areas of screening and testing of gestational carriers. Finally, as more diseases are found to be "relevant" by the FDA, they will undoubtedly be added to the list of communicable diseases for which screening or testing may be required of donors.

In the short term, some ART programs have decided to limit their donor program offerings, based on the complicated and time-consuming nature of implementing an FDA compliant program. This may limit access to treatment for some patients. Others have retained their programs but have limited the number of donor cycles they perform. Still, others have not decreased their volume at all and continue as before. In the long term, it is uncertain how the regulations will ultimately affect ART programs. What is certain is that the FDA regulations are here to stay. The regulatory environment for ART programs has been changed forever.

References

1. Henkel J (1994) Safeguarding human tissue transplants. FDA Consum 28(7):9–13
2. U.S. Department of Health and Human Services; Food and Drug Administration (2003) 21 CFR part 1271: human cells, tissues, and cellular and tissue-based products; establishment registration and listing; final rule; delay of effective date. Fed Regist 68(13):2689–2691
3. U.S. Department of Health and Human Services; Food and Drug Administration (2004) 21 CFR part 1271: human cells, tissues, and cellular and tissue-based products; establishment registration and listing; interim final rule; opportunity for public comment. Fed Regist 69(17):3823–3826
4. U.S. Department of Health and Human Services; Food and Drug Administration (2001) 21 CFR parts 207, 807, and 1271: human cells, tissues, and cellular and tissue-based products; establishment registration and listing; final rule. Fed Regist 66(13):5447–5469
5. U.S. Department of Health and Human Services; Food and Drug Administration (2004) 21 CFR part 1271: human cells, tissues, and cellular and tissue-based products; establishment registration and listing; correction. Fed Regist 69(23):5272
6. U.S. Department of Health and Human Services; Food and Drug Administration (2008) 21 CFR part 1271: human cells, tissues, and cellular and tissue-based products; CFR correction to 1271.22. Fed Regist 73(13):3387
7. U.S. Department of Health and Human Services; Food and Drug Administration (2005) 21 CFR part 1271: human cells, tissues, and cellular and tissue-based products; donor screening and testing, and related labeling; interim final rule; opportunity for public comment. Fed Regist 70(100):29949–29952
8. U.S. Department of Health and Human Services; Food and Drug Administration (2006) 21 CFR part 1271: eligibility determination for donors of human cells, tissue, and cellular and tissue-based products; correction. Fed Regist 71(57):14798
9. U.S. Department of Health and Human Services; Food and Drug Administration (2004) 21 CFR parts 210, 211, 820, and 1271: eligibility determination for donors of human cells, tissues, and cellular and tissue-based products; final rule and notice. Fed Regist 69(101):29786–29834
10. U.S. Department of Health and Human Services; Food and Drug Administration (2004) 21 CFR parts 16, 1270, and 1271: current good tissue practice for human cell, tissue, and cellular and tissue-based product establishments; inspection and enforcement; final rule. Fed Regist 69(226):68612–68688
11. U.S. Department of Health and Human Services; Food and Drug Administration (2007) 21 CFR part 1271: human cells, tissues, and cellular and tissue-based products; donor screening and testing, and related labeling; final rule. Fed Regist 72(117):33667–33669
12. Department of Health and Human Services (1992) Medicare, Medicaid and CLIA programs; regulations implementing the

Clinical Laboratory Improvement Amendments of 1988 (CLIA) – HCFA. Final rule with comment period. Fed Regist 57(40): 7002–7186
13. Department of Health and Human Services (1993) Medicare, Medicaid and CLIA programs; regulations implementing the Clinical Laboratory Improvement Amendments of 1988 (CLIA) and Clinical Laboratory Improvement Act Program fee collection – HCFA. Final rule with comment period. Fed Regist 58(11): 5215–5237
14. Department of Health and Human Services; Centers for Disease Control and Prevention (1999) Implementation of the fertility clinic success rate and certification act of 1992 – a model program for the certification of embryo laboratories; notice. Fed Regist 64(139): 39374–39392
15. Critser J (1998) Current status of semen banking in the USA. Hum Reprod 13(Suppl. 2):55–67 Discussion 68–9
16. U.S. Department of Health and Human Services; Food and Drug Administration; Center for Biologics Evaluation and Research (2007) Guidance for industry: eligibility determination for donors of human cells, tissues, and cellular and tissue-based products (HCT/Ps).
17. U.S. Department of Health and Human Services; Food and Drug Administration; Center for Biologics Evaluation and Research (2007) Guidance for industry: eligibility determination for donors of human cells, tissues, and cellular and tissue-based products (HCT/Ps). 14–21
18. U.S. Department of Health and Human Services; Food and Drug Administration; Center for Biologics Evaluation and Research (2007) Guidance for industry: eligibility determination for donors of human cells, tissues, and cellular and tissue-based products (HCT/Ps). 24–5
19. U.S. Department of Health and Human Services; Food and Drug Administration; Center for Biologics Evaluation and Research (2007) Guidance for industry: eligibility determination for donors of human cells, tissues, and cellular and tissue-based products (HCT/Ps). 21–4
20. U.S. Department of Health and Human Services; Food and Drug Administration; Center for Biologics Evaluation and Research (2007) Guidance for industry: eligibility determination for donors of human cells, tissues, and cellular and tissue-based products (HCT/Ps). 23
21. U.S. Department of Health and Human Services; Food and Drug Administration; Center for Biologics Evaluation and Research (2007) Guidance for industry: eligibility determination for donors of human cells, tissues, and cellular and tissue-based products (HCT/Ps). 13
22. U.S. Department of Health and Human Services; Food and Drug Administration; Center for Biologics Evaluation and Research (2007) Guidance for industry: eligibility determination for donors of human cells, tissues, and cellular and tissue-based products (HCT/Ps). 31–7
23. U.S. Department of Health and Human Services; Food and Drug Administration; Center for Biologics Evaluation and Research (2007) Guidance for industry: eligibility determination for donors of human cells, tissues, and cellular and tissue-based products (HCT/Ps). 33–4
24. U.S. Department of Health and Human Services; Food and Drug Administration; Center for Biologics Evaluation and Research (2007) Guidance for industry: eligibility determination for donors of human cells, tissues, and cellular and tissue-based products (HCT/Ps). 37–8
25. U.S. Department of Health and Human Services; Food and Drug Administration; Center for Biologics Evaluation and Research (2006) Guidance for industry: compliance with 21 CFR Part 1271.150(c)(1) – manufacturing arrangements.
26. U.S. Department of Health and Human Services; Food and Drug Administration; Center for Biologics Evaluation and Research (2007) Guidance for industry: eligibility determination for donors of human cells, tissues, and cellular and tissue-based products (HCT/Ps). 28–31
27. U.S. Department of Health and Human Services; Food and Drug Administration; Center for Biologics Evaluation and Research (2007) Guidance for industry: eligibility determination for donors of human cells, tissues, and cellular and tissue-based products (HCT/Ps). 58–61
28. U.S. Department of Health and Human Services; Food and Drug Administration; Center for Biologics Evaluation and Research (2007) Guidance for industry: eligibility determination for donors of human cells, tissues, and cellular and tissue-based products (HCT/Ps). 40–2
29. U.S. Department of Health and Human Services; Food and Drug Administration; Center for Biologics Evaluation and Research (2007) Guidance for industry: certain human cells, tissues, and cellular and tissue-based products (HCT/Ps) recovered from donors who were tested for communicable diseases using pooled specimens or diagnostic tests.
30. U.S. Department of Health and Human Services; Food and Drug Administration; Center for Biologics Evaluation and Research (2007) Guidance for industry: eligibility determination for donors of human cells, tissues, and cellular and tissue-based products (HCT/Ps). 7
31. U.S. Department of Health and Human Services; Food and Drug Administration; Center for Biologics Evaluation and Research (2007) Guidance for industry: regulation of human cells, tissues, and cellular and tissue-based products (HCT/Ps); small entity compliance guide. 11
32. Malarkey M. HCT/P Compliance update. 2008 Jan 10 [cited 2008 Feb 25]. Available from: http://www.fda.gov/cber/summaries/hctp010808mm.pdf
33. Wells M FDA update: relevant to reproductive establishments. 2007 Sep 17 [cited 2008 Feb 29]. Available from: http://www.fda.gov/cber/tissue/aatb091707mw.pdf
34. U.S. Department of Health and Human Services; Food and Drug Administration; Center for Biologics Evaluation and Research (2007) Guidance for industry: eligibility determination for donors of human cells, tissues, and cellular and tissue-based products (HCT/Ps). 41
35. U.S. Department of Health and Human Services; Food and Drug Administration; Center for Biologics Evaluation and Research (2007) Guidance for industry: regulation of human cells, tissues, and cellular and tissue-based products (HCT/Ps); small entity compliance guide.
36. U.S. Department of Health and Human Services; Food and Drug Administration; Center for Biologics Evaluation and Research (2007) Guidance for industry: eligibility determination for donors of human cells, tissues, and cellular and tissue-based products (HCT/Ps). 19
37. U.S. Department of Health and Human Services; Food and Drug Administration; Center for Biologics Evaluation and Research (2007) Guidance for industry: eligibility determination for donors of human cells, tissues, and cellular and tissue-based products (HCT/Ps). 31

Chapter 7
Psychosocial Consequences of Infertility and Treatment

Lone Schmidt

Abstract Infertility, besides being a medical condition, is a social situation. Infertility is a low-control, chronic stressor with severe long-lasting negative social and psychological consequences. Achieving a pregnancy/delivery after assisted reproduction technology treatment is associated with increased mental well-being. Treatment failure is associated with increased levels of anxiety and depression during the treatment period and after end of treatment. It is still unclear whether depression and/or fertility problem stress is related to treatment outcome. Some infertile couples experience marital benefit, i.e., that the infertility brings the partner closer together and strengthens their marriage. Appraisal-oriented coping strategies including emotional coping are predictors of lower fertility problem stress. Long-term studies among involuntary childless women in previous unsuccessful treatment show that although most adjusted well psychologically the childlessness was a major life theme. Fertility patients are, in general, satisfied with fertility treatment. However, the satisfaction ratings are in general higher with the medical care than with the patient-centered care. Fertility patients express a need for oral and written information about treatment as well as psychosocial consequences of infertility and for improvements in patient-centered care and access to professional psychosocial services if needed. Drop-out rates of treatment are high and are mostly related to the psychological burden. In order to decrease drop-out rates, and hence increase delivery rates after fertility treatment, it is important to further develop user friendly treatment programs.

Keywords Psychosocial aspects of infertility • Self-esteem • Relationship • Depression • Anxiety • Coping strategies • Marriage

L. Schmidt (✉)
Institute of Public Health, University of Copenhagen, 5 Øster Farimagsgade, P.O. Box 2099, Copenhagen DK-1014, Denmark
e-mail: L.Schmidt@pubhealth.ku.dk

7.1 Introduction

The far majority of young people intend to become parents in the future. Some of them will later experience infertility in one or more periods in their life, and on average 56% (range 42–76.3%) of infertile couples in developed countries have sought medical advice [1]. For most couples, the infertility is unexpected. For many couples, infertility causes a serious strain on their interpersonal relationship, as well as personal distress, reduced self-esteem, and loss of the meaning with life [2]. Besides being a medical condition, infertility is also a social situation. One of the important challenges infertile couple faces is learning how to manage infertility and treatment in relation to oneself, with the partner and in the different social arenas (family, friends, coworkers) [3]. As some of the psychological consequences of infertility and its treatment are different in different cultures [4, 5], this chapter focuses on studies from industrialized, Western countries.

7.2 Distress and Marital Benefit

7.2.1 Fertility Problem Stress

Fertility problem stress is related to the strains infertility and its treatment produce in the personal, social, and marital domains [2, 3, 6, 7]. In order to measure stress specifically related to infertility, it is therefore important to use instruments specifically developed to measure this specific stressor, e.g., the instruments developed by Abbey et al. [6]; Newton et al. [8]; Schmidt [3].

Infertility and its treatment are low-control stressors; that is, stressful situations in which the infertile couple can do little or nothing to influence the nature or the outcome of their situation [9]. Further, infertility is a chronically stressful situation, a nonevent transition [10]. Chronic stressors develop slowly as continuous and problematic conditions in our social conditions or social roles [11].

D.T. Carrell and C.M. Peterson (eds.), *Reproductive Endocrinology and Infertility: Integrating Modern Clinical and Laboratory Practice*,
DOI 10.1007/978-1-4419-1436-1_7, © Springer Science+Business Media, LLC 2010

Jacob et al. [12] compared fertility-specific stress in a population-based sample among US women. Self-identification as infertile was the largest source of fertility-specific stress when compared to women with other fertility problems.

7.2.2 *Anxiety and Depression*

7.2.2.1 Before Treatment

Studies using standardized measures of general psychological distress have shown that either clinical samples of infertile couples differ moderately from norms overall, or they differ on subscales related to interpersonal sensitivity and depression [2]. A more recent review covering the last 25 years research on women in IVF-treatment [13] showed that before treatment, in general, female fertility patients did not differ from norm groups with respect to depression levels. Some studies showed elevated levels of state anxiety among women starting IVF, while other studies found no difference when comparing to norm groups. Fekkes et al. [14] measured both general and infertility-related emotional problems and found no differences when comparing with norm groups on the general instruments, but a higher level of emotional complaints for the fertility-related measures. Further, an intense focus on having a child was related to less optimal emotional and psychosocial functioning. In Newton et al.'s study [8] among couples referred to fertility treatment, symptoms of depression were more highly associated with social, sexual, and relationship concerns than with the need for parenthood.

Most studies measuring anxiety among infertile couples are based only on couples who had sought fertility treatment. However, King [15] reported, from a representative population-based sample, that subfecund women were having significantly more symptoms of anxiety. This association did not change when analyses were controlled for having sought medical treatment recently.

7.2.2.2 During and After Treatment

Among women undergoing their first IVF treatment attempt, emotional well-being after the treatment attempt was worse among those who had not achieved pregnancy when compared with those who became pregnant [16]. On the basis of a review of longitudinal studies among women in IVF treatment with pre- and posttreatment measures of depression and anxiety, Verhaak et al. [13] reported that depression levels increased after one or more unsuccessful treatment cycles with a significant interaction effect between time and treatment outcome. On the other hand, Boivin et al. [17] reported, on the basis of a cross-sectional study, that women with high amounts of treatment failures reported less stress than women with a moderate amount of treatment failures.

Only one prospective cohort study among women and their partners in IVF-treatment investigated anxiety and depression during treatment and 6 months after their last treatment cycle [18]. Women showed an increase in both anxiety and depression after treatment without having achieved a pregnancy and showed no recovery at the 6-months follow-up. At this point in time, >20% of the women showed subclinical forms of depression and/or anxiety. Women who achieved a pregnancy after treatment reported a decrease in anxiety and depression levels. Men showed no significant changes in anxiety and/or depression during treatment and at 6-months after end of treatment either among the successful or unsuccessful group.

7.2.2.3 Depression and Treatment Outcome

It is still not clear whether depressive symptoms among women in treatment are a predictor of a lower chance of achieving a delivery after fertility treatment. According to a recently published review, many studies, but not all, have found that depressive symptoms may decrease success rates of assisted reproduction treatment [19]. On the other hand, de Klerk et al. [20] found that women less negative at baseline at start of treatment had a decreased chance of a live birth after first IVF cycle when compared to women with more pronounced negative feelings.

7.2.3 *Marital Benefit*

Previous qualitative interview studies have shown that infertility can bring the partners closer together and strengthen the marriage [21–23]. We have termed this positive effect of infertility among couples as a marital benefit. Among 2,250 people initiating fertility treatment, 25.9% of the women and 21.1% of the men reported high marital benefit [24]. Longitudinal analyses at 1-year follow-up among those who had not become parents after ART treatment showed among men that high use of meaning-based coping (e.g., have grown as a person in a good way, think about the infertility problem in a positive light) was a significant predictor of high marital benefit. Significant predictors of low marital benefit were not disclosing infertility to others, having difficulties in partner communication, and high use of active-avoiding coping (e.g., turning to work or substitute activity to take mind off things). No significant predictors among women were identified. Similarly, Holter et al. [16] found among couples in IVF/ICSI treatment, a majority reporting that treatment had affected their partner relationship to the better.

7.3 Predictors of Stress

7.3.1 Coping

The use of different coping strategies and its effect on fertility problem stress or distress in general have been studied both in short-term and long-term longitudinal studies with pre- and posttreatment measurements of the coping strategies used. Terry and Hynes [9] found among women in IVF treatment that problem-appraisal coping strategies (e.g., trying to step back and be more objective, trying to see the positive side of the situation) were predictive of better adjustment, and approach-oriented coping (including problem-focused coping, emotional processing, and expression) were related to lower distress [25]. Schmidt et al. [26] found that among men, active-confronting coping (e.g., letting feelings out somehow, accept sympathy and understanding from someone, ask others for advice, talk to someone about emotional reactions) was a significant predictor of low fertility problem stress in the marital domain.

Conversely, longitudinal studies have shown that avoidance or escape coping was a predictor of poor adjustment to infertility [9] and of increased stress after one treatment attempt [25]. Further, high use of active-avoidance coping (e.g., avoiding being with pregnant women, leaving when people are talking about pregnancies and deliveries, turn to work or substitute activity to take mind off things) among men and women initiating fertility treatment was at 1-year follow-up a significant predictor of high fertility problem stress in the personal domain and the social domain [26].

Peterson et al. [27] found among couples seeking fertility treatment that both women and men who engaged in a disproportionate degree of escape/avoidance, coping and accepting responsibility for infertility, were more vulnerable to symptoms of depression. Further, these coping strategies were positively associated with infertility stress [28]. In line with this, Lechner et al. [29] found among definite childless couples that a passive coping style was positively associated with health complaints, depression and anxiety.

7.3.2 Infertility-Related Communication

7.3.2.1 To Other People

Most infertile people talk to other people about their situation and women disclose to more people than men [3, 30–32].

Van Balen and Trimbos-Kemper [31] found in a cross sectional study that among men, nondisclosure was associated with lower well-being. On the other hand, Schmidt et al. [26] found in a longitudinal study that neither among men nor women keeping the infertility a secret at inclusion of the study was a predictor of high fertility problem stress at the 1-year follow-up among those not having achieved a pregnancy or delivery after ART. Disclosure when initiating treatment was in Schmidt's study [3] separated in a formal strategy when only formal information were shared with others (e.g., kind of treatment, number of eggs retrieved) and an open-minded strategy when both formal information and emotional reactions of the infertility experience were shared. When comparing the formal strategy with the open-minded strategy at start of treatment with odds ratios of reporting high fertility problem stress at 1-year follow-up, these odds ratios were in all three domains (personal, marital, social) for both men and women insignificantly above 1.00. This indicated a consistent pattern of an increased risk of high fertility problem stress among those participants who did talk to other people but without communicating how they experienced the emotional consequences of infertility and its treatment [26].

7.3.2.2 To the Partner

Most people in fertility treatment do not find it difficult to talk with their partner about infertility and its treatment [3, 16]. However, at start of treatment, 26.9% of the women and 22.0% of men reported difficulties in infertility-related partner communication in a large prospective cohort study [3]. Difficulties in partner communication was in the longitudinal analyses a significant predictor of having high fertility problem stress in both the personal, the marital, and the social domain at 1-year follow-up [26]. Pasch et al. [33] found that it was the husbands' involvement alone that predicted wives seeing an overall negative effect of infertility on the marriage. Husbands, who saw having children as important and were involved in trying to have a baby, expressed less negative effect on marital communication, and wives perceived then a more positive effect of infertility on their marriage.

One of the important functions of marriage is giving and receiving emotional support. Abbey et al. [34] showed that increased received emotional support from the partner was related to increased marital life quality for both men and women. Studies using standardized measures for marital satisfaction tended to find high marital satisfaction among infertile couples in treatment or even higher measures when compared to noninfertile groups [2].

7.3.3 Treatment Failure

As mentioned earlier, longitudinal studies with pre- and posttreatment measurements find that not achieving a pregnancy after a treatment attempt is a predictor of increased levels of anxiety and depression and a decreased level of lower emotional well-being [16, 35]. The negative effects of unsuccessful treatment on well-being is either most pronounced among women when compared with the men [16] or only identified among women [18]. A recent study compared the psychological impact of treatment failure among women in mild vs. standard IVF treatment [36]. Women experiencing treatment failure after a standard IVF treatment reported significantly more symptoms of depression 1 weak after treatment termination when compared with women with treatment failure after mild IVF treatment. A randomized study comparing mild IVF treatment with standard IVF treatment showed no differences in 1-year cumulative rates of term live births [37].

7.4 Stress and Treatment Outcome

It is still not clear whether high level of fertility problem stress is a predictor of lower chance of achieving a pregnancy after fertility treatment. Boivin and Schmidt [38] found that higher levels of fertility problem stress at start of treatment was a predictor among both women and men for poorer treatment outcome. This effect was most pronounced for fertility problem stress in the marital and social domain. On the other hand, other studies have found no association between level of stress and treatment outcome [39, 40]. Smeenk et al. [41] studied the association between the concentration of urine adrenalin and self-reported stress levels. They found that urine adrenalin level was positive, associated with the level of depressive symptoms, and suggested that this hormone could be a link between the complex pattern between psychosocial stress and treatment outcome. Further, a recent review of mood disorders and fertility [19] suggested that fertility treatment independently may "influence mood through their effects on estrogen and progesterone, which have been shown to influence mood on their actions on serotonin." It is concluded that future studies are necessary in order to investigate the complex relations between mood disorders and fertility.

7.5 Social Stigmatization

Stigma is a negative sense of social difference from others. Infertility is potentially stigmatizing [32, 42, 43]. In general, infertile people find that most other people are supportive, but infertile women have also reported their experiences of receiving unsupportive reactions from others [42]. Mindes et al. [44] showed in cross sectional analyses that receiving infertility-specific unsupportive responses were positively associated with poorer psychological adjustment. However, in the longitudinal analyses, the unsupportive reactions predicted depressive symptoms and overall psychological distress only among those women who remained infertile at the follow-up 6–12 months later.

The perceptions of stigma for both men and women are related to low social support [32]. For men, stigma was linked to disclosure and support and to higher fertility-related and generic stress. Disclosure was not associated with increased support. For women, more disclosure was a predictor of higher generalized stress.

7.6 Mental Well-Being after Having Achieved Pregnancy/Delivery

Short time longitudinal studies reported that emotional well-being increased both among women and men when the woman had achieved a pregnancy after treatment [16]. On the other hand, Verhaak et al. [18] reported a decrease in anxiety and depression only among the women who achieved an ART-pregnancy and no changes in anxiety and/or depression were observed among the men.

Repokari et al. [45] conducted a large 1-year follow-up study comparing couples with IVF/ICSI singletons with couples having spontaneous singleton pregnancies when the children were 2 months (T2) and 12 months old (T3). There were no between-group differences in dyadic cohesion or marital satisfaction. However, dyadic cohesion deteriorated between T2 and T3 among control women, and depression during pregnancy was only a predictor of deteriorated marital relations in the control group. Further, sexual affection was low among control men at T2. The authors concluded that successful ART did not constitute a risk factor for infertility, and that the shared stress of infertility may even stabilize marital relationships. These findings support the previous findings in some studies that infertile couples initiating treatment report higher levels of marital satisfaction when compared with norm groups [2], indicating that there could be a selection bias in that infertile couples having strong marriages, to a larger extent, seek medical treatment.

7.7 Long-Term Adjustment to Childlessness

Those couples who had longed for parenthood and who had tried to achieve pregnancy and delivery with fertility treatment maybe for many years will sense a loss. Lechner et al. [29] investigated women and men who had acknowledged their definite involuntary childlessness. Involuntarily childless women reported more health complaints, more anxiety and depression symptoms, and more complicated grief when compared with the general population.

In a study investigating women 2–3 years after they having ceased IVF treatment [46], the women who had not achieved a delivery scored significantly lower on satisfaction with life when compared to the women who had become mothers. There were no differences between the groups regarding marital satisfaction or general health.

Peddie et al. [47] interviewed women who had decided to end fertility treatment after not having achieved a pregnancy after IVF treatment. It was difficult for the women to accept that their infertility remain unresolved and many felt vulnerable to the pressures of the media and society. Daniluk [48] interviewed prospectively with 10-months intervals infertile couples who had stopped to trying to get pregnant. She found that in the beginning, the couples experienced a relief having stopped treatment. Later, the couples attempted to make sense of their lost years and began to reenvision their lives. Thirty-two months after having ended the unsuccessful treatment, most of the participants were more comfortable with themselves and with their relationships. Nearly 40% had decided to remain childless, while 60% had decided to adopt a child.

Verhaak et al. [35] investigated couples in IVF treatment from start of treatment to the final fourth data collection 3–5 years after last treatment cycle. Results among those women not having achieved a live born child showed that anxiety and depression at the last follow-up returned to baseline values. Those women who focused on new life goals showed lower levels of anxiety and depression when compared with those women who persisted to become pregnant.

Wirtberg et al. [49] interviewed involuntary childless women 20 years after their unsuccessful fertility treatment. For all participants, the childlessness had a strong impact on the women's lives and was a major life theme. Nearly all the women reported that they had: felt inferior to other women, lacked self-esteem, and felt socially isolated during the years they had tried to conceive. For half of the women, the feeling of social isolation had persisted. The feeling of isolation became stronger as their peer group reached grand-parenthood. In all but one, sexual life was affected in a negative and long-lasting way. Sundby et al. [50] reported in a study among women in IVF treatment 10 years earlier, that two-thirds of the female participants experienced infertility as one of the worst and most stressful episodes in their life. Ten years posttreatment, 82% of the participants were living with and responsible for one or more children, and around 50% reported that infertility was now something in the past. However, most of the women still found it difficult to talk about this period in their life.

7.8 Fertility Patients' Needs

7.8.1 Expectations to Treatment

Expectations to treatment have been measured in a large consecutive sample ($n=2{,}250$) of new fertility couples immediately before initiating the first treatment cycle [51]. Almost all participants rated medical care as explanation of test results and in person explanations of treatment options as important. Most women and men (82.0% vs. 75.7%) found it important to receive written treatment information. Further, most women and men found patient-centered care important (clinical staff showing concern and understanding) and around half of the participants rated it as important to receive written information about the psychosocial aspects of infertility and its treatment. Among women 9–19% would have attended specifically professional psychosocial services if these services had been available (a course about childlessness; a support group; individual sessions with a psychologist or with a sex therapist), whereas 4–9% of the men would have attended these services. Both among women and men, higher levels of fertility problem stress was significantly associated with higher importance ratings of patient-centered care and professional psychosocial services.

Glover et al. [52] asked 29 men attending a specialist male infertility clinic about their expectations and motivations for seeking treatment. The most important reason was to increase their partner's chance of conceiving. Further, 75–88% of men expected general information as well as information about their specific problem, discussion of possible alternatives, having their questions answered, and help with decision-making. Finally, 52% found it important to be able to discuss their feelings about their infertility and the way in which it was treated.

7.8.2 Evaluation of Treatment

A study among women having delivered after ART treatment [53] found that the women wished to be treated with respect and dignity and given appropriate information and support. The women wanted their distress to be recognized, to feel cared for and to have confidence in health professionals in situations where outcomes are uncertain. In line with this, Malin et al. [54] reported that among women in previous fertility treatment, the most positive treatment experience was respectful, empathic and personal care from the doctor. Leite et al. [55] investigated women's interaction with their physician during an infertility consultation. Four physicians' communicative behaviors showed significant differences in the general satisfaction scores: introducing oneself, setting the main reason for the visit, providing information about the treatment procedures, and asking whether the patient had other issues or concerns.

Medical care includes, for example the staff's technical skills and preparation for examinations and treatment. In general, both men and women are satisfied with the quality of medical care at the fertility clinics [56]. Having achieved a treatment-related pregnancy and/or delivery was associated with greater satisfaction ratings [46, 56, 57]. Souter et al. [58] reported that only a third of women in fertility treatment had received any written information and 78% would like receiving more literature.

Patient-centered care is the routine psychosocial care provided by all members of the staff, for example that staff listen to the patient [59]. In the largest and most recent prospective satisfaction study [56], satisfaction ratings with both medical care and patient-centered care were high. In both men and women, high marital benefit was a significant predictor of higher satisfaction ratings. Among women, a high level of fertility problem stress was a significant predictor of lower satisfaction ratings.

In all other studies, satisfaction ratings with patient-centered care were lower than ratings with medical care. Infertile couples expressed the wish for a more couple-centered approach [22, 58, 60], for more emotional advice and support [46, 57, 58], for counseling about when to stop treatment [46], and information about alternative ways to become parents (e.g., adoption) [22, 61, 62].

7.9 Drop-Out of Fertility Treatment

It has been shown that couples in fertility treatment frequently decide to end treatment while treatment options still exist. In a study from Sweden, where fertility treatment is subsidized 54% of the couples decided to discontinue subsidized treatment of their own will [63]. In UK also, up to three attempts are offered on National Health Service Funding, even though drop-out rates were 25% after the first treatment cycle and 33% after the second cycle [64]. The psychological burden and lack of success are important self-reported reasons for discontinuation of treatment [63–65]. In a prospective cohort study among women in IVF/ICSI treatment [66], treatment drop-out was also related to psychological factors. Further, the group that discontinued treatment after their first treatment cycle showed higher scores pretreatment on depression and anxiety.

It is of importance to decrease high drop-out rates in order to increase the probability for the couple to achieve a delivery as multiple attempts improve the pregnancy rate. One of the possibilities is to further develop user friendly treatment guides in order to lower the psychosocial stress related to ART.

7.10 Effects of Psychosocial Interventions

In a review of psychosocial interventions in infertility, Boivin [67] identified 25 independent evaluation studies. Psychosocial interventions were more effective in reducing negative affect than in changing interpersonal functioning. Further, group interventions that emphasized education and skills training were significantly more effective in producing positive changes than counseling interventions emphasizing emotional expression and support and/or discussion of infertility-related thoughts and feelings. Schmidt et al. [68] evaluated a communication and stress management training program for couples in fertility treatment, and found that the participant perceived improvement in their competence to actively manage changes in marital communication and in communication in different social arenas.

De Liz and Strauss [69] conducted a review of 22 intervention studies with psychotherapy. They concluded that group as well as individual/couple psychotherapy reduced anxiety and depression for infertile couples.

7.11 Clinical Recommendations

On the basis of the empirical literature, it is recommended that fertility clinic staff:

- Treat the couple, not only one partner, as infertility is a problem related to a couple
- Offer high quality medical and patient-centered care
- Medical care is defined as the personal explanation of test results and treatment options including written treatment information from a respectful, empathic caregiver. Four behaviors were considered critical to patient satisfaction: introducing oneself, establishing the primary purpose of the visit, providing information about the treatment procedures, and asking whether the patient has other issues or concerns.
- Patient-centered care is the routine psychosocial care provided by all members of the staff and active listening and addressing specific concerns is considered foremost in this effort.
- Inform the couple both verbally and in writing about the treatment as well as the psychosocial consequences of infertility and treatment
- Inform the couples about coping strategies and communication strategies that are predictors of high/low fertility problem stress and of high/low marital benefit
- Further develop user friendly treatment in order to reduce treatment drop-out and hence increase chances of achieving a delivery after treatment

- Provide access through referral or in-house professional psychosocial services if the couple have a need for this service
- Initiate termination of treatment after sufficient but unsuccessful treatment and initiate discussions regarding future possibilities for achieving parenthood or future life goals other than parenthood

References

1. Boivin J, Bunting L, Collins JA, Nygren KG (2007) International estimates of infertility prevalence and treatment-seeking: potential need and demand for infertility medical care. Hum Reprod 22:1506–1512
2. Greil AL (1997) Infertility and psychological distress: a critical review of the literature. Soc Sci Med 45:1679–1704
3. Schmidt L (2006) Infertility and assisted reproduction in Denmark: epidemiology and psychosocial consequences. [Medical Dissertation]. Dan Med Bull 53:390–417. http://www.danmedbul.dk/Dmb_2006/0406/0406-disputatser/DMB3808.htm
4. Inhorn MC (2004) Privacy, privatization, and the politics of patronage: ethnographic challenges to penetrating the secret world of Middle Eastern, hospital-based in vitro fertilization. Soc Sci Med 59:2095–2108
5. Dyer SJ (2007) The value of children in African countries – insights from studies on infertility. J Psychosom Obstet Gynaecol 28:69–77
6. Abbey A, Andrews FM, Halman LJ (1991) Gender's role in responses to infertility. Psychol Women Q 15:295–316
7. Tjørnhøj-Thomsen T (2005) Close encounters with infertility and procreative technology. In: Steffen V, Jenkins R, Jessen H (eds) Managing uncertainty. Ethnographic studies of illness, risk and the struggle for control. Museum Tusculanum Press, University of Copenhagen, Copenhagen, pp 71–91
8. Newton CR, Sherrard W, Glavac I (1999) The Fertility Problem Inventory: measuring perceived infertility-related stress. Fertil Steril 72:54–62
9. Terry DJ, Hynes GJ (1998) Adjustment to a low-control situation: reexaming the role of coping responses. J Pers Soc Psychol 74: 1078–1092
10. Koropatnick S, Daniluk J, Pattinson HA (1993) Infertility: a non-event transition. Fertil Steril 59:163–171
11. Wheaton B (1999) Social stress. In: Aneshensel CS, Phelan JC (eds) Handbook of the sociology of mental health. Kluwer Academic/Plenum Publishers, New York, pp 277–300
12. Jacob MC, McQuillan J, Greil AL (2007) Psychological distress by type of fertility barrier. Hum Reprod 22:885–894
13. Verhaak CM, Smeenk JMJ, Evers AWM, Kremer JAM, Kraaimaat FW, Braat DDM (2007) Women's emotional adjustment to IVF: a systematic review of 25 years of research. Hum Reprod Update 13:27–36
14. Fekkes M, Buitendijk SE, Verrips GHW, Braat DDM, Brewaeys AMA, Dolfing JG, Kortman M, Leerentveld RA, Macklon NS (2003) Health-related quality of life in relation to gender and age in couples planning IVF treatment. Hum Reprod 18:1536–1543
15. King RB (2003) Subfecundity and anxiety in a national representative sample. Soc Sci Med 56:739–751
16. Holter H, Anderheim L, Bergh C, Möller A (2006) First IVF treatment – short-term impact on psychological well-being and the marital relationship. Hum Reprod 21:3295–3302
17. Boivin J, Takefman JE (1995) Stress level across stages of in vitro fertilization in subsequent pregnant and non-pregnant women. Fertil Steril 64:802–810
18. Verhaak CM, Smeenk JMJ, Van Minen A, Kremer JAM, Kraaimat FW (2005) A longitudinal, prospective study on emotional adjustment before, during and after consecutive fertility treatment cycles. Hum Reprod 20:2253–2260
19. Williams KE, Marsh WK, Rasgon NL (2007) Mood disorder and fertility in women: a critical review of the literature and implications for future research. Hum Reprod Update 6:607–616
20. de Klerk C, Hunfeld JAM, Heijnen EMEW, Eijkemans MJC, Fauser BCJM, Passchier J, Macklon NS (2008) Low negative affect prior to treatment is associated with a decreased chance of live birth from a first IVF cycle. Hum Reprod 23:112–116
21. Greil AL, Leitko TA, Porter KL (1988) Infertility: his and hers. Gend Soc 2:172–199
22. Schmidt L (1996) Psykosociale konsekvenser af infertilitet og behandling [Psychosocial consequences of infertility and treatment, in Danish, PhD-thesis]. FADL's Publishers, Copenhagen
23. Tjørnhøj-Thomsen T (1999) Tilblivelseshistorier. Barnløshed, slægtskab og forplantningsteknologi i Danmark [Genesis. Childlessness, kinship, and reproductive technology in Denmark, in Danish, PhD-thesis]. University of Copenhagen, Copenhagen
24. Schmidt L, Holstein BE, Christensen U, Boivin J (2005) Does infertility cause marital benefit? An epidemiological study of 2250 women and men in fertility treatment. Patient Educ Couns 59:244–251
25. Berghuis JP, Stanton AL (2002) Adjustment to a dyadic stressor: a longitudinal study of coping and depressive symptoms in infertile couples over an insemination attempt. J Consult Clin Psychol 70:433–438
26. Schmidt L, Holstein BE, Christensen U, Boivin J (2005) Communication and coping as predictors of fertility problem stress: cohort study of 816 participants who did not achieve a delivery after 12 months of fertility treatment. Hum Reprod 20:3248–3256
27. Peterson BD, Newton CR, Rosen KH, Skaggs GE (2006) The relationship between coping and depression in men and women referred for in vitro fertilization. Fertil Steril 85:802–804
28. Peterson BD, Newton CR, Rosen KH, Skaggs GE (2006) Gender differences in how men and women who are referred for IVF cope with infertility stress. Hum Reprod 21:2443–2449
29. Lechner L, Bolman C, Van Dalen A (2007) Definite involuntary childlessness: associations between coping, social support and psychological distress. Hum Reprod 22:288–294
30. Abbey A, Andrews FM, Halman LJ (1991) The importance of social relationships for infertile couples' well-being. In: Stanton AL, Dunkel-Schetter C (eds) Infertility. Perspectives from stress and coping research. Plenum Press, New York, pp 61–86
31. Van Balen F, Trimbos-Kemper TCM (1994) Factors influencing the well-being of long-term infertile couples. J Psychosom Obstet Gynecol 15:157–164
32. Slade P, O'Neill C, Simpson AJ, Lashen H (2007) The relationship between perceived stigma, disclosure patterns, support and distress in new attendees at an infertility clinic. Hum Reprod 22:2309–2317
33. Pasch LA, Dunkel-Schetter C, Christensen A (2002) Differences between husbands' and wives' approach to infertility affect marital communication and adjustment. Fertil Steril 77:2141–2147
34. Abbey A, Andrews FM, Halman LJ (1995) Provision and receipt of social support and disregard: what is their impact on the marital life quality of infertile and fertile couples. J Pers Soc Psychol 68:455–469
35. Verhaak CM, Smeenk JMJ, Nahuis MJ, Kremer JAM, Braat DDM (2007) Long-term psychological adjustment to IVF/ICSI treatment in women. Hum Reprod 22:305–308
36. de Klerk C, Macklon NS, Heijnen EMEW, Eijkemans MJC, Fauser BCJM, Passchier J, Hunfeld JAM (2007) The psychological impact of IVF failure after two or more cycles of IVF with a mild versus standard treatment strategy. Hum Reprod 22:2554–2558
37. Heijnen EMEW, Eijkemans MJC, Polinder S, Beckers NGM, Klinkert ER, Broekmans FJ, Passchier J, Te Velde ER, Macklon NS, Fauser BCJM (2007) A mild strategy for in-vitro fertilisation: a randomised non-inferiority trial. Lancet 369:743–749

38. Boivin J, Schmidt L (2005) Infertility-related stress in men and women predicts treatment outcome 1 year later. Fertil Steril 83: 1745–1752
39. Anderheim L, Holter H, Bergh C, Möller A (2005) Does psychological stress affect the outcome of in vitro fertilization? Hum Reprod 20:2969–2975
40. Panagopoulou E, Vedhara K, Gaintarzti C, Tarlatzis B (2006) Emotionally expressive coping reduces pregnancy rates in patients undergoing in vitro fertilization. Fertil Steril 86:672–677
41. Smeenk JM, Verhaak CM, Vingerhoets AJ, Sweep CG, Merkus JM, Willemsen SJ, van Minnen A, Straatman H, Braat DD (2005) Stress and outcome success in IVF: the role of self-reports and endocrine variables. Hum Reprod 20:991–996
42. Miall CE (1986) The stigma of involuntary childlessness. Soc Probl 33:268–282
43. Whiteford LM, Gonzalez L (1995) Stigma: the hidden burden of infertility. Soc Sci Med 40:27–36
44. Mindes EJ, Ingram KM, Kliewer W, James CA (2003) Longitudinal analysis of the relationship between unsupportive social interactions and psychological adjustment among women with fertility problems. Soc Sci Med 56:2165–2180
45. Repokari L, Punamäki R-L, Unkila-Kallio L, Vilska S, Poikkeus P, Sinkkonen J, Almqvist F, Tiitinen A, Tulppala M (2007) Infertility treatment and marital relationships: a 1-year prospective study among successfully treated ART couples and their controls. Hum Reprod 22:1481–1491
46. Hammarberg K, Astbury J, Baker HWG (2001) Women's experience of IVF: a follow-up study. Hum Reprod 16:374–383
47. Peddie VL, van Teijlingen E, Bhattacharya S (2005) A qualitative study of women's decision-making at the end of IVF treatment. Hum Reprod 20:1944–1951
48. Daniluk JC (2001) Reconstructing their lives: a longitudinal, qualitative analysis of the transition to biological childlessness for infertile couples. J Couns Dev 79:439–449
49. Wirtberg I, Möller A, Hogström L, Tronstad S-E, Lalos A (2007) Life 20 years after unsuccessful infertility treatment. Hum Reprod 22:598–604
50. Sundby J, Schmidt L, Heldaas K, Bugge S, Tanbo T (2007) Consequences of IVF among women: 10 years post-treatment. J Psychosom Obstet Gynaecol 28:115–120
51. Schmidt L, Holstein BE, Boivin J, Sångren H, Tjørnhøj-Thomsen T, Blaabjerg J, Hald F, Nyboe Andersen A, Rasmussen PE (2003) Patients' attitudes to medical and psychosocial aspects of care in fertility clinics: findings from the Copenhagen Multi-centre Psychosocial Infertility (COMPI) Research Programme. Hum Reprod 18:628–637
52. Glover L, Gannon K, Platt Z, Abel PD (1999) Male subfertility clinic attenders' expectations of medical consultation. Br J Health Psychol 4:53–61
53. Redshaw M, Hockley C, Davidson LL (2007) A qualitative study of the experience of treatment for infertility among women who successfully became pregnant. Hum Reprod 22:295–304
54. Malin M, Hemminki E, Räikkönen O, Sihvo S, Perälä M-L (2001) What do women want? Women's experiences of infertility treatment. Soc Sci Med 53:123–133
55. Leite RC, Makuch MY, Petta CA, Morais SS (2005) Women's satisfaction with physicians' communication skills during an infertilæity consultation. Patient Educ Couns 59:38–45
56. Schmidt L, Holstein B, Boivin J, Tjørnhøj-Thomsen T, Blaabjerg J, Hald F, Rasmussen PE, Nyboe Andersen A (2003) High ratings of satisfaction with fertility treatment are common: findings from the Copenhagen Multi-centre Psychosocial (COMPI) Research Programme. Hum Reprod 18:2638–2646
57. Sundby J, Olsen A, Schei B (1994) Quality of care for infertility patients. An evaluation of a plan for a hospital investigation. Scand J Soc Med 22:139–144
58. Souter VL, Penney G, Hopton JL, Templeton AA (1998) Patient satisfaction with the management of infertility. Hum Reprod 13:1831–1836
59. Boivin J, Kentenich H (eds) (2002) Guidelines for counselling in infertility. ESHRE Monographs, Oxford University Press, Oxford
60. Wirtberg I (1992) His and her childlessness. Dissertation, Karolinska Institute, Stockholm
61. Sabourin S, Wright J, Duschesne C, Belisle S (1991) Are comsumers of modern fertility treatment satisfied? Fertil Steril 56: 1084–1090
62. Halman LJ, Abbey A, Andrews FM (1993) Why are couples satisfied with infertility treatment? Fertil Steril 59:1046–1054
63. Olivius C, Friden B, Borg G, Bergh C (2004) Why do couples discontinue in vitro fertilization treatment? A cohort study. Fertil Steril 81:258–261
64. Rajkhowa M, Mcconnell A, Thomas GE (2006) Reasons for discontinuation of IVF treatment: a questionnaire study. Hum Reprod 21:358–363
65. Domar AD (2004) Impact of psychological factors on dropout rates in insured infertility patients. Fertil Steril 81:271–273
66. Smeenk JMJ, Verhaak CM, Stolwijk AM, Kremer JAM, Braat DDM (2004) Reasons for drop-out in an in vitro fertilization/intracytoplasmic sperm injection programme. Fertil Steril 81:262–268
67. Boivin J (2003) A review of psychosocial interventions in infertility. Soc Sci Med 57:2325–2341
68. Schmidt L, Tjørnhøj-Thomsen T, Boivin J, Nyboe Andersen A (2005) Evaluation of a communication and stress management training programme for infertile couples. Patient Educ Couns 59:252–262
69. de Liz TM, Strauss B (2005) Differential efficacy of group and individual/couple psychotherapy with infertile couples. Hum Reprod 20:1324–1332

Chapter 8
A Live Baby or Your Money Back: The Marketing of In Vitro Fertilization Procedures

David C. Schmittlein and Donald G. Morrison

Abstract Many clinics that offer in vitro fertilization (IVF) have begun to market the following options to couples: (1) an a la carte program where the couple pays $7,500 per attempt regardless of the outcome; or (2) a money-back-guarantee program where the couple pays a $15,000 fee that covers up to three attempts, however, if after three cycles there is no live-birth delivery, then the full $15,000 is refunded.

We assess the a la carte versus the money-back-guarantee programs, and find the surprising result that the money-back-guarantee program appears (for the patients) to be "too good to be true." That is, the money-back guarantee yields a substantial *negative* expected profit per couple for the clinics. More importantly, from the patients' perspective, the money-back guarantee is the better option for all couples with less than 0.5 success probability per cycle. Virtually, all traditional IVF patients have had per-cycle success probabilities below 0.5.

A detailed analysis of the key variables – i.e., success rate per attempt heterogeneity of couples' rates of success, individual couples' "learning" on successive attempts, and cost to the clinic per attempt – shows that these money-back guarantees are unprofitable for the clinics. Since presumably, clinics are not in business to lose money, the standard analysis must be missing something major. We suggest that the marketing of money-back guarantees is inducing couples who would previously have used – successfully – other less invasive procedures with fewer side effects and less risk of multiple births to decide to proceed directly to IVF, and that this scenario makes the money-back guarantees profitable for the clinics.

The implications of earlier use of IVF are then considered from an overall public policy point of view. Just as mothers everywhere tell their children, "When something looks too good to be true, then it is too good to be true!"

D.C. Schmittlein (✉)
MIT Sloan School of Management, E52-473, 50 Memorial Drive, Cambridge, MA 02142, USA
e-mail: dschmitt@mit.edu

D.G. Morrison
Anderson Graduate School of Management,
University of California at Los Angeles, Los Angeles, CA, USA

(Marketing; In Vitro; Assisted Reproduction; Health Care Marketing)

Keywords Marketing • Performance • Risk • Cost • IVF success • Cost effectiveness

Proof Note This chapter was published under the same title in Management Science, INFORMS 49 (12) Dec. 2003, pp 1617–1635, and included with permission in this text because of its thoroughness in addressing money-back guarantees. While pregnancy rates, live-birth rates and charges have increased the principles have application in today's environment. Patient's can benefit from the information provided when weighing individual clinic payment options.

8.1 Introduction

In the two decades since the first "test tube" baby, in vitro fertilization (IVF) has become the "last best hope" for a child for hundreds of thousands of infertile couples. Typically, such a couple has already attempted natural conception, the use of fertility-enhancing drugs, and intrauterine insemination without success (see Fig. 8.1). Because IVF is rarely covered by health insurance in the United States [1, 2], assisted reproductive technology (ART) clinics are typically chosen by the couple, which would expect to pay between $7,000 and $10,000 for each in vitro attempt [3, 4]. The chance of a live healthy birth from that procedure has been 20–25%. While the ART clinics may not use the language of marketing strategy, the evolution of this competitive service environment has led them to focus on two of the four major marketing decision variables: Product performance, and price. The other two marketing variables – promotion and place (distribution) – are important but have remained more stable and are managed consistently with other medical procedures. That is, promotional activities include relationships with hospitals and physicians, and brochures, informational presentations, and so on. Distribution decisions trade-off the customer convenience of multiple locations with

DOI 10.1007/978-1-4419-1436-1_8,

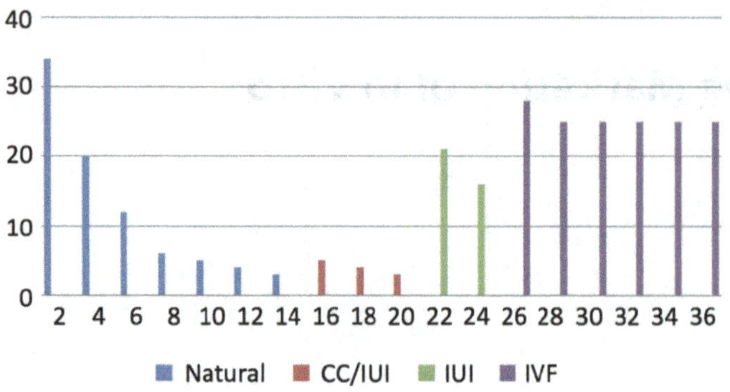

Fig. 8.1 Typical progression of assisted reproduction treatment. Conception rate (percent) per cycle using various treatments. (Note: conception rate does not equal live-delivery rate.) In later cycles the live-delivery rate is approximately 20% lower than the conception rate. Data from Hull, MGR. Infertility treatment: Relative effectiveness of conventional and assisted conception methods. Human Reproduction 1992; 7:785–96

economies of scale with service provision from one or a few central locations.

From the customer (patient) standpoint, the most important product performance measure is the live-birth probability per initiated IVF cycle. One of our goals in this paper is to show what such performance measures say (and do not say) about a couple's prospects for success with a particular clinic. To our knowledge, this kind of analysis has not been undertaken to date. We find that clinics do substantially differ from each other in the success rates that one can expect them to experience in the future. One-year success performance, however, provides a useful guide for the future for only about half the North American clinics. For the remainder, the average performance across all clinics would be a better guide to their future than the clinic's experience to date.

Price, the second marketing variable, has received even more attention. Since 1997, many ART clinics have begun to offer as an option to patients "money-back guarantees" – i.e., "a live baby or your money back," in addition to the option of paying per cycle as above. For example, one Minnesota clinic has offered three IVF tries for approximately $15,000 with a guarantee to refund the fee if a live birth does not occur via these three attempts. More than 60 clinics are believed to offer similar incentives to prospective customers [5].

Understandably, this pricing innovation has attracted significant attention from consumers. In light of the medical decision context the complicated economic incentives for the ART clinics, the asymmetry in information between these clinics and prospective patients, the amounts of money involved, and the emotional state of some infertile couples, this pricing "innovation" has also generated controversy in professional publications [3, 6, 7] and in popular media [2, 5, 8].

In this paper, we show how to estimate the economic consequences of these guarantees for any clinic. Doing so requires knowledge of this clinic's overall success rate and a stochastic model of IVF success for any given couple on successive IVF attempts. The latter model will incorporate both heterogeneity in success rate across couples and the learning effect observed to occur across IVF cycles. Models to date in the literature have not captured these two effects.

We also analyze factors that affect the economics of the new money-back policies for clinics. Some of these factors are compatible with the goals of patients and others are not. Prospective patients may, through specific questioning, infer which factors are driving the pricing policy of a certain clinic. For clinic managers, our analyses provide a mechanism for integrating cost and history information to set a sensible pricing program.

Using an analysis of clinic performance statistics, and of patients' success rates on successive IVF cycles, we show that these guarantees are "too good to be true." Our analysis suggests that guarantees of the sort described above are made economically viable for clinics by pursuit of less-infertile couples who are in the beginning stages of fertility assistance, rather than using IVF as a "last resort" as had been the case previously. Specifically, we conclude that

1. These guarantees – which are typically offered to all customers virtually – are not economically viable for the average clinic and the average couple.
2. The guarantees, in fact, are not viable for most of the "better" clinics either and, in practice, are currently being offered by many "average" performing clinics.
3. The guarantees are not made viable by the "economies of scale" in addition to the current customer base of a clinic.
4. The guarantees are viable if new, relatively fertile couples are induced to proceed directly to IVF instead of trying natural conception or less invasive procedures. For these couples, on standard economic bases, these IVF "guarantees" are not a good deal.

The next section describes the practice of IVF. This is followed by a straightforward economic assessment of the "money-back guarantee" for a typical clinic. Next, we examine two factors that might be imagined to explain such offers: Heterogeneity in clinic performance, and heterogeneity/learning effects for couples making successive IVF attempts. Finally, we consider the factor that does appear to be responsible for these offers: Targeting a new customer base characterized by higher IVF success rates.

8.2 The Prevalence and Practice of IVF

8.2.1 The Scope and Scale of IVF

During its 20 years of experience, IVF has gone from an expensive procedure available in a handful of clinics whose success rate was extremely low to one that is expensive, widely accepted, available in numerous clinics, with a modest success rate. This, of course, can be seen as a glass either "half empty" or "half full." In 1996, when the money-back guarantees at issue in this paper were being initiated, the approximate 300 clinics in the United States and Canada that performed IVF accounted for about 45,500 "standard" IVF cycles, i.e., cycles using fresh, nondonor eggs [9]. The number of babies born as a result was about 10,000 in 1996. Thus, more than 35,000 of the 45,500 IVF cycles failed to produce a live birth; but approximately 10,000 couples achieved at least one child – an outcome highly unlikely in the absence of the IVF procedure. (The natural-conception birth rate per cycle for couples classified as infertile is about 1.6% [10].)

8.2.2 IVF Decision Process for Patients: High Risk, High Return, and When to Stop?

The most meaningful measure of success for each in vitro cycle started is the live-birth probability. This success rate has increased from 6% in the early 1980s to about 22% in 1996 when money-back guarantees were being planned by clinics to 25% by 1999, the most recent data available [9, 11–13]. Taking into account the typical number of IVF cycles pursued by a couple, however, more than half of them complete their attempts at IVF without taking a child home.

Accompanying each IVF cycle's uncertain outcome is a substantial cost typically in the range of $7,000–$10,000. Couples often pursue multiple IVF cycles if needed, so a total cost in the range of $10,000–$30,000 is common. In some European countries, national health insurance pays for a certain number of IVF tries, but coverage of IVF by U.S. health insurers is usually limited (e.g., one cycle) or more often nonexistent [14–16]. As a result, most U.S. couples considering IVF are placing the largest-scale single economic gamble of their lives. That is, they may make a few investment decisions involving more money (e.g., a home purchase) but none whose "payoff" is so random and stark (i.e., about a 50–50 chance of a genetically related child versus losing the entire investment with no benefit).

In addition to the economic risk above, other factors also make IVF decisions difficult for patients. These include the risk of multiple conception (twins, triplets, and so on) with attendant health risks for the fetuses or infants, and risk to the female of hyperstimulation and other possible long-term health risks [17, 18]. They also include the difficulty in deciding when to stop IVF attempts, a decision faced after each (failed) IVF cycle. Couples typically want to feel that they did "all they could" to conceive [16, 19, 20], but success rates for IVF do not appear to substantially drop after several failures for a particular couple. Clinics report this finding to those considering an additional cycle [21] making it difficult to stop.

8.2.3 IVF Decision Process for Clinics

IVF represents a large and growing service opportunity. In 1994, the amount spent on such procedures in the United States and Canada was approximately $300 million. IVF procedures are likely to continue to grow in popularity, because it is estimated that 10–15% of all married couples in the reproductive age group are infertile [22]. To the extent that couples are paying for the procedure themselves, opportunities to "lock in" patients through the emerging relationships in the healthcare market are minimized, leaving at least the potential for regional competition across clinics. Indeed, metropolitan areas are generally now served by at least two such clinics.

8.3 Money-Back Guarantees: Economics for a Typical Patient and Clinic

The money-back guarantees for IVF are largely standard: The patient pays about $15,000 for up to three IVF attempts as needed to produce a live-birth delivery. If after three attempts the couple has not succeeded, the $15,000 is refunded. Alternatively, the patient is offered the choice of paying "a la carte," about $7,500 per attempt.

We initially will analyze the economic effects for clinics and patients as of the time that money-back guarantees were being created as marketing programs, i.e., 1996. (Later, we will note that the basic economic conclusions had not changed by 2002.) A clinic's average cost per IVF cycle was estimated to be $5,000 in 1988 [23]. By 1996, a 2% annual nominal cost increase would lead to an IVF cost per cycle of $6,000. This cost figure, combined with the recent past's a la carte price of $7,500, leads to a return on investment (ROI) (actually return on cost) of 25%. This is a high return in light of the competition between clinics and, accordingly, we conclude that cost per cycle in 1996 has risen to at least $6,000 per cycle.

With notation C=clinic's cost per cycle, p=success probability on any IVF attempt π=clinic's profit (or loss), and G=the patient's payment for the guarantee, the clinic's expected profit resulting from the guarantee is:

$$E[\pi] = G - C - C(1-p) - C(1-p)^2 - G(1-p)^3. \quad (8.1)$$

With C=6,000, G=15,000, p=0.22 (as noted in Sect. 2), expected profit for the clinic is minus $6,448 per patient. Via this calculation, the money-back guarantee is not close to break even. To put this in perspective, recall that ROI was 25% for patients paying a la carte (with C=6,000). Under the guarantee, the expected number of IVF cycles that a patient will undergo is 2.4, so the average incurred cost is 2.4 times $6,000 or $14,400. Accordingly, the return on cost under the guarantee is –6,448/14,400 or minus 45%.

Our simple equation (8.1) assesses financial outcomes only for the IVF cycles themselves. A particular new patient at an IVF clinic may also undergo some testing, whose cost is separate from the guarantee (and nonrefundable). Discussion with clinic operators suggests that such testing could approach \$4,000, and a generous estimate of the profit on such testing is \$3,000. So to be conservative in our assessment of a clinic's loss on the money-back guarantee, we will reduce the \$6,448 loss from the previous paragraph by a \$3,000 gain on testing; leaving an expected loss per IVF patient of \$3,448.

To see a clinic's difficulty another way, note that setting $C=6{,}000$ and $G=15{,}000$, and assuming a \$3,000 profit from testing as above, the success percentage per attempt p would have to be 31% (rather than 22%) to break even. It would need to be 40% to generate a 20% return on expected cost.

While altruism on a grand scale or gross mismanagement could explain this conundrum, we are interested in examining other explanations for the guarantee policy. We deal with four here, and then turn to the ones that require a more serious examination of clinic performance statistics and patient success dynamics.

8.3.1 Marginal Cost vs. Average Cost

One might posit that the clinic's marginal cost of conducting one more IVF cycle is more relevant in calculating profitability, and that marginal cost would be much lower than average cost. In this case, however, several factors undermine such a notion, specifically:

1. Only 10% of the clinic cost is equipment or location [24] and the trend is to individualize equipment (e.g., incubator) to the specific patient.
2. Of the total IVF clinic costs, 40% is material/lab tests/drugs [24], which are not subject to many economies of scale.
3. Of total clinic costs, 50% is personnel [24], and clinics were already operating at an efficient economic scale, doing on average over 100 IVF procedures a year, each cycle requiring 4–6 office visits.
4. Clinics offering the guarantee are finding that a substantial fraction of patients take it making average cost more relevant than marginal cost.

8.3.2 Patient Selection: Aggressive Screening

Another possible enhancement to profit is limiting the guarantee program to patients whose likelihood of IVF success is "high." Clinics generally make such restrictions public, and many do limit the age of the female to less than 40 years, and some also eliminate couples with a male infertility factor. Based on clinic performance data [12], these two restrictions raise the IVF success probability by three percentage points. Beyond this, clinics claim that they do not "discriminate" and, indeed, the available studies have not succeeded in identifying additional observable factors that predict IVF success [25–27]. We will, as a result, assume that patient screening adds only three percentage points to the clinic's success rate.

8.3.3 Breakthrough in IVF Success Rates

A third possible explanation for the guarantee's financial loss is a breakthrough in IVF success rates since 1996 that was well anticipated by clinics as they launched money-back guarantees in 1997 and 1998. This is unlikely for two reasons. First, to go from 22% to 40% in just a year or two would mean a significant breakthrough and the medical literature points to no such advance during this period. Second, IVF success, summarized in Fig. 8.2, shows a slow and steady increase through 1996. Indeed, that slow steady pace is now known to have persisted through 1999. The rate of success, in fact increased only from 22% to 25% between 1996 and 1999, quite consistent with the historical trend [9, 13].

8.3.4 Risk Transfer

Another approach to improve the financials for the guarantee is to shift the balance between minimizing risk of the IVF procedure and maximizing the probability that a live birth occurs. This means transferring additional risk to the patient

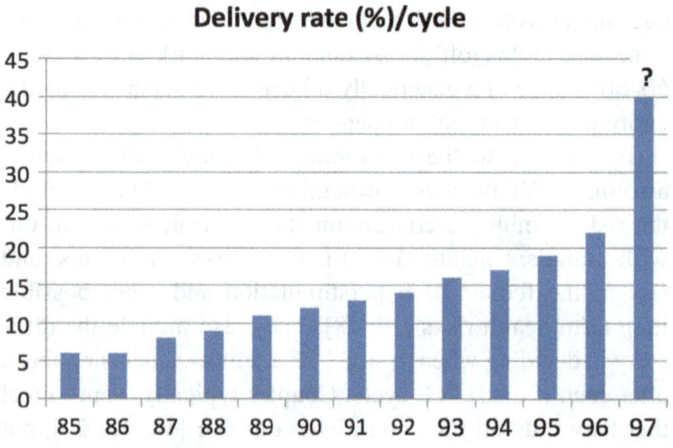

Fig. 8.2 Historical trend in IVF success rate, North America. Source: Dawood (1996), SART (1996), US Centers for Disease Control and Prevention (1999)

and could be accomplished in multiple ways. For instance, the drug regimen can be increased to stimulate production of more eggs. This also increases the risk of hyperstimulation, a potentially serious health consequence for the female [18]. The success rate can also be increased by using more viable embryos [18]. This also increases the risk of multiple conception, and higher order multiples carry both health risks for the infants (prenatal death, cerebral palsy low birth weight) and for the mother (preeclampsia, hydramnios varicosities, anemia) [17, 18]. Clinics claim that they do not do these things [16] and, indeed, these kinds of activities and their negative outcomes are reasonably observable. In short, risk transfer to patients would likely become public, and we assume that this does not occur on a significant scale.

In summary the four factors considered here are estimated, collectively to increase the probability of success by a total of three percentage points from the baseline level of 22% in the 1996 data. That is, those clinics that do screen on age (<40 years) and male factor infertility can achieve a 25% chance of a live birth per IVF cycle in 1997 – well under the 40% chance required for break even on the guarantee.

8.3.5 Heterogeneity

Staying within the framework of our profitability equation (8.1), there are really only two additional factors to consider, and they both involve heterogeneity. First equation (8.1) implicitly assumes that all clinics have the same success rate, and second, it assumes that this success rate does not differ from cycle to cycle for an individual customer.

Regarding the first of these factors, if clinics differ reliably in their success rates, the "better" ones may be able to afford the guarantee and, indeed, such a guarantee might signal a strong clinic to a prospective patient. In the next section, we analyze this across-clinic heterogeneity.

Our second source of heterogeneity concerns the repeated experiences of a single patient. Heterogeneity across patients in seriousness of infertility will tend to drive down success probability across repeated cycles. That is, the "healthier" patients will tend to have success on the early IVF cycles, leaving them out of the sample for later cycles. On the other hand, useful information is acquired during the IVF cycles, which can counteract this negative effect of heterogeneity Specifically, the drug regimen used may be optimized to a particular patient on later IVF cycles, or some patients may be counseled out of additional IVF attempts when previous cycles suggest that IVF will not work for them [21]. To examine both heterogeneity across patients and learning across repeated attempts will require some new probability modeling. We will turn to such a model after the next section's summary of heterogeneity across clinics.

8.4 Variation in Performance Across IVF Clinics

We consider the extent to which clinics differ in prospects for IVF success by examining the 1994 clinic performance data reported to SART for the U.S. eastern region [9, 11, 12]. (Clinic-specific reports for 1995–1999, the most recent data available, collapse IVF with other ART procedures, such as zygote intrafallopian transfer (ZIFT) and gamete intrafallopian transfer (CIFT), and so are not as valuable for considering guarantees that apply only to IVF.) The leading infertility support organization in the United States, RESOLVE, promotes these statistics to couples considering IVF [28]. This information includes the number of live deliveries per IVF cycle started, for each of the 101 reporting clinics. In total, these clinics began 14,322 IVF cycles and had 2,646 deliveries, for a delivery rate of 0.185. During 1994, the average number of IVF cycles was 142 per clinic. We noted earlier that age and presence of a male infertility factor are sometimes used to exclude patients from the guarantee programs. Accordingly, we focus our analysis on the 8,714 IVF cycles for which the female was under age 40 and there was no male infertility factor.

In any 1 year, the success rate does greatly vary from clinic to clinic. The top two panels of Fig. 8.3 highlight this, showing the "top 5" and "bottom 5" clinics. From the standpoint of both patients and clinic managers, of course, the relevant quantity is not the observed success rate in some previous year. Rather, it is the best estimate, based on history, of future success for that clinic. For this purpose, the historical success rates are deficient estimators, due to the influence of sampling variation. Indeed, clinics that are observed to be outliers will tend to be those that happened to do few cycles, irrespective of long-run success rates. This is evident in Fig. 8.3, all five of the "worst" clinics and four of the five "best" clinics did very few IVF cycles.

Let p denote a particular clinic's long-run success probability, and x denote the number of live-birth deliveries arising from n IVF cycles started in some time period. We are interested in estimating p from x and n – or specifically from the observed success rate x/n. In doing so, we adopt the empirical Bayes approach of estimating both the sampling variance for successes x, and the real variance in success probability p across clinics [29]. The estimate for p is then a combination of this clinic's historical success rate (x/n) and the observed average success across clinics ($E[p]$).

Specifically, we assume that the clinic-specific probability of success p is distributed beta across clinics and, accordingly, births x at a specific clinic follow the well-known beta-binomial (BB) model. This model has been highly effective for representing heterogeneous Bernoulli processes in marketing and in other social science applications, including biomedical research [30–32]. On the basis of its two beta

Original "Top 5"

Rank	Original Observation	Updated Probability
1	2/4=0.5	0.235
2	11/27= 0.407	0.285
3	8/20=0.4	0.270
4	15/39=0.385	0.292
5	69/182=0.346	0.346

Updated "Top 5"

Rank	Original Observation	Updated Probability
1	69/182=0.379	0.346
2	169/480=0.352	0.340
3	55/166=0.331	0.306
4	15/39=0.385	0.292
5	26/77=0.338	0.291

Original "Bottom 5"

Rank	Original Observation	Updated Probability
5	1/28=0.036	0.144
4	0/1=0.000	0.207
3	0/4=0.000	0.194
2	0/5=0.000	0.190
1	0/24=0.000	0.138

Updated "Bottom 5"

Rank	Original Observation	Updated Probability
5	3/39=0.077	0.149
4	1/28=0.036	0.144
3	0/24=0.000	0.138
2	23/213=0.108	0.126
1	23/222=0.104	0.122

Fig. 8.3 Assessing heterogeneity in clinic performance

distribution parameters a and b, the expected future success rate for a clinic that was observed to experience x successes in n IVF attempts is

$$E[p \mid x, n, a, b] = \frac{n}{a+b+n} \cdot \frac{x}{n} + \frac{a+b}{a+b+n} \cdot \frac{a}{a+b'} \tag{8.2}$$

which represents a weighted average of the clinic's observed success rate (x/n) and the average success rate for all clinics ($a/(a+b)$).

Maximum likelihood estimates of the model parameters for this set of 101 clinics are ($a=9.44$; $b=35.15$), which corresponds to a mean and standard deviation of real long-run success rates across clinics of ($E[p]=0.212$; $\sigma_p=0.0605$). Accordingly, using the one- and two-sigma heuristics, two-thirds of clinics have a true delivery rate between 15% and 27% (one sigma) and 95% of clinics have a true delivery rate between 9% and 33%. These results rule out heterogeneity in clinics as a contributor to the viability of IVF money-back guarantees. Virtually none of the clinics have a stable success rate that is even at break even (31%). We focused here on eastern region clinics to help remove geographic differences. However, the same beta-binomial model estimated with all 244 North American clinics resulted in MLEs $a=8.41$ and $b=32.04$, which produce the same kind of confidence interval results as above.

As (8.2) makes clear, expected future success is driven not only by observed success rate (x/n), but by the number of IVF cycles performed (n) relative to the sum of the two beta distribution parameters $a+b$. This is highlighted in Fig. 8.3. Note how our "top 5" and "bottom 5" clinics' expectations are changed when an empirical Bayes updated probability is calculated for each clinic. In the bottom half of Fig. 8.3, we provide the updated "top 5" and "bottom 5" clinics, i.e., clinics ranked on the probability of success on future IVF attempts. Only three have expected probability greater than 0.3 and none exceed 0.35. Because about 60 of 300 North American clinics are offering the IVF guarantee, again, we see that differential clinic performance is not the explanation.

Of course, there are real differences in clinic performance that should persist and matter to patients. Clinics in the top third of real performance (p) are about twice as likely to experience a live-birth delivery as those in the bottom third. The challenge for a patient is to see a large enough base of experience to "tell" the strong performers from the weak.

8.5 Patient Outcomes Across Successive IVF Attempts

Our equation (8.1) for economics of the money-back guarantee assumed that all of a clinic's patients have the same success probability p, and that this success probability for a single couple does not vary across successive IVF attempts. Neither assumption is likely to well represent the IVF process, nor can each greatly affect the expected financial outcome. First, we will discuss the effect of patient heterogeneity under the simplifying assumption that p-values remain stationary for each patient across successive attempts. Then, we will incorporate nonstationarity in the patient probabilities, and estimate a formal model that captures both phenomena.

A couple that succeeds on IVF cycle t naturally does not progress to cycle $t+1$, i.e., the only couples who attempt to enter cycle $t+1$ are those unsuccessful thus far. When success probabilities differ from couple to couple, those entering cycle $t+1$ will tend to be the ones who started out with relatively low p-values. In short, the success rates observed for a random set of patients for successive cycles should decline from cycle to cycle, as a result of this adverse selection effect. This effect of heterogeneity was not reflected in (8.1) and is, in fact, detrimental to the economics of the IVF guarantee. Recall that the assumption of homogeneity across patients in (8.1) produced a net loss of \$3,448 per patient including a profit from testing. Imagine the extreme case of patient heterogeneity with the same average success rate $p=0.22$ as assumed earlier. That is, imagine that 22% of patients have an IVF success rate on any cycle of 100%, and the remaining 78% of patients have a success rate of 0. Using the same arithmetic as in (8.1), the clinic will net \$15,000 − \$6,000 from 22% of the patients (who succeed on the first try), and will "net" \$15,000 − 3 × \$6,000 − \$15,000 from the remaining 78%, who do not succeed even after three tries. The expected loss per patient under this complete heterogeneity scenario is minus \$12,060, 3.5 times greater than the loss of \$3,448 if patients are homogeneous in success rates. Heterogeneity scenarios between these two extremes examined here will produce losses between \$3,448 and \$12,060. In short, heterogeneity makes the guarantee programs, which "push" all patients through three tries if they need them, even more economically disadvantageous for the clinics.

There is, however, a potentially countervailing effect related to successive IVF attempts. While our heterogeneity across patients scenario above assumes that the success rate for any individual patient does not change from attempt to attempt, anecdotal reports suggest that the prospects for success can be increased for a particular couple from attempt to attempt. This "learning" effect stems from two kinds of sources. First, information on the body's response to the drug regimen, sperm, egg, and embryo quality can be used to help improve the chances for success on later IVF attempts, at least for a while. So, the actual "p-value" for a patient is not constant from attempt to attempt but may instead increase. Second, the information gleaned from initial cycles will sometimes reveal that the prospects for IVF success are remote, and the couple can be counseled to move on to another therapy (donor egg, intracytoplasmic sperm injection (ICSI)) or to adoption. This second learning effect helps remove low p-value patients from later cycles and, thus, runs directly counter to heterogeneity's adverse selection effect discussed above. Of course, only the former of these two learning effects would actually benefit a clinic offering a money-back guarantee. We will not be able to differentiate between these two possible learning effects, but we will be able to estimate the combined effect from historical data, placing an upper limit on the learning effect's benefit for clinics offering the guarantee.

Which of these two countervailing effects, heterogeneity depressing success rates across cycles or learning increasing them, is larger? Many studies have provided data concerning success prospects on successive attempts, though none have incorporated both learning and heterogeneity effects [21, 26, 27, 33–36].

Let p_1 denote a particular couple's success probability on the first IVF attempt. To incorporate learning in this model, we rewrite this cycle 1 success probability p_1 as

$$p_1 = \frac{x}{x+y'} \quad x>0, y>0, \tag{8.3}$$

which, of course, can be done without loss of generality. It is useful to think of x as representing the impact of success factors, and y as representing the factors making the IVF cycle likely to fail. The probability p is then the result of the relative magnitude of these two sets of factors as in (8.3). Now, if learning occurs, this couple's success probability should be higher on later attempts, which can be accomplished by replacing x in (8.3) with $x+\lambda\ (\lambda \geq 0)$. This approach would, however, restrict learning to a "one-shot" effect, i.e., no incremental learning after IVF cycle 1. Our proposed model for learning assumes more generally that there may, indeed, be learning on each IVF cycle, but that the magnitude of this learning may decline across cycles. As a result, the formula for the couple's success probability on attempt t ($t \geq 2$) is

$$p_t = \frac{x+\sum_{i=2^{\lambda} i}^{t}}{x+y+\sum_{i=2^{\lambda} i}^{t}}, \quad \lambda_i \geq 0, \tag{8.4}$$

Where λ_i represents the incremental learning effect for attempt i based on the learning on attempt, I – 1. On the first IVF attempt (8.4) simply reduces to (8.3). On the second attempt, the numerator "success" factor increases from x to $x+\lambda_2$, so λ_2 represents the contribution of learning from the first cycle. On the third IVF attempt, the numerator is $x+\lambda_2+\lambda_3$.

To incorporate heterogeneity across patients, we allow the baseline success factor x, baseline failure factor y, and learning effects λ_1 to vary across patients. Specifically, each of these three factors is assumed to follow an (independent) gamma distribution with idiosyncratic shape parameters and a common scale parameter.

$$f(x \mid r_x, \alpha) = \frac{\alpha^{r_x}}{\Gamma(r_x)} x^{r_x - 1} e^{-ax},$$

$$f(y \mid r_y, \alpha) = \frac{\alpha^{r_y}}{\Gamma(r_y)} y^{r_y - 1} e^{-\alpha y},$$

$$f(\lambda_t \mid r_{\lambda_t}, \alpha) = \frac{\alpha^{r_{\lambda_t}}}{\Gamma(r_{\lambda_t})} \lambda_t^{r_{a_t} - 1} e^{-a\lambda_t}.$$

For each of these gamma distributions, the mean is its shape parameter divided by the scale parameter, i.e., *r/a*. So, the average magnitude of the positive effects x and λ_1, and of the negative effect y, is proportional to the respective distribution's shape parameter. We will assume that the average size of the incremental learning effect decreases geometrically with repeated IVF attempts, and with rate $1 - K$ $(0 \leq K \leq 1)$. That is, because $K \leq 1$ the learning effect due to the information from the second IVF cycle will not generally be as great as learning from the first cycle. To capture this phenomenon, the shape parameter for each learning effect's gamma distribution is specified as

$$r_{\lambda t} = r_\lambda K^{t-2} \quad \text{for } t = 2,3 \tag{8.5}$$

If K is close to 1, the incremental learning dies out only slowly across cycles. For example, imagine that $r_\lambda = 1$ and $K = 1/2$. Then, on the second IVF attempt in addition to the positive effect x (whose mean is r_x/α), we have a learning effect in the numerator and denominator of (8.4), but now the average size of the incremental effect is only $Kr_\lambda/\alpha = r_\lambda/2\alpha$, i.e., half the size of the learning effect for the second cycle. With $K = 1/2$, the incremental learning effect for the fourth cycle would again drop by half, to only 1/4, what it was on the second cycle, and so on.

These assumptions mean that for any IVF attempt the success probability is distributed beta across patients [40]. For the first attempt (no learning), success probabilities are simply distributed beta (r_x, r_y), with mean $E[p] = r_x/(r_x + r_y)$. For the second attempt, we have to reflect both the effects of heterogeneity and learning. The latter is already specified above. The effect of heterogeneity is easy to assess: Given that the first attempt failed, we must update the beta distribution for success probability as in any BB model. That is, the parameter r_y is updated by one unit for each observed IVF failure [31, 37]. So, on the second IVF attempt we replace r_y with $r_y + 1$. As a result, for patients entering the second IVF attempt the probability of success is distributed beta $(r_x + r_\lambda, r_y + 1)$, with mean $E[p] = (r_x + r_\lambda)/(r_x + r_\lambda + r_y + 1)$. In the same way for the *t*th attempt given that the first $t-1$ attempts failed, the expected success probability is

$$E[p_t \mid r_x, r_y, r_\lambda, K] = \frac{r_x + r_\lambda \sum_{i=2}^{t} K^{i-2}}{r_x + r_y + (t-1) + r_\lambda \sum_{i=2}^{t} K^{i-2}} \tag{8.6}$$

In the absence of any learning $(r_\lambda = 0)$, (8.6) is simply the success probability for attempt t (conditional on failure through attempt $t-1$) for the beta-geometric (BG) model, i.e., the waiting time version of the BB model. With the learning effect as specified above, we will call the formulation equation (8.6) the beta-geometric with learning (BGL) model. Equation (8.4) provides the basis for estimating the parameters (r_x, r_y, r_λ, K) via maximum likelihood, from a histogram of success rates on successive IVF attempts.

The most promising such histogram appears to have been published by [33]. In this case, all 3,824 patients who began an initial IVF cycle at one particular clinic were tracked through successive IVF attempts. The number of patients entering each successive attempt was recorded, along with the number that achieved a live-birth delivery. The Tan et al. [33] data are particularly valuable because of the large number of patients tracked, and because the outcome measure is live births. Many of the studies examining successive IVF attempts [26, 34, 36] look instead at "ongoing pregnancies" as a "success," yet often about 20% of those pregnancies do not result in deliveries, and this percentage can vary substantially.

For the Tan et al. [33] data, the maximum likelihood estimates of the BGL model are

$$r_x = 0.263,\ r_y = 2.247,\ \{r_\lambda = 0.130, \text{ and } K = 0.510$$

These parameters tell an interesting story about the effects of learning and heterogeneity and about the trade-off between them. First, consider just the learning effect. Because r_λ is about half the size of r_x, on the second IVF attempt the learning effect increases the positive factors for IVF success by about half. A further increase accrues for the third attempt but because K is approximately 0.5, the contribution from learning on the second IVF cycle is only half as valuable as the learning from the first cycle. The incremental learning from the third cycle is only 1/4 $(= 0.5^2)$ what it was from the first cycle, and so on.

Now, we add in the effect of heterogeneity. Recall that failure on an IVF cycle increases de facto the parameter by 1 for succeeding cycles. Neither heterogeneity nor learning operate on the first cycle, for which the average probability of success was $r_x/(r_x + r_y) = 0.105$. For patients who do not succeed on the first attempt what happens on the second try? Via (8.6), the net positive factors $(r_x + r_\lambda)$ increase by 50% relative to attempt, 1 (i.e., 0.263 + 0.130) due to learning. But because of heterogeneity, our updated sense of this patient's success rate (having failed at attempt 1), adds 1 to the negative factors parameter r_y, thus, increasing it from 2.247 to 3.247, i.e., also an increase of essentially 50%. In short then, for the second IVF cycle, the effects of learning and heterogeneity offset and the overall probability of success remains unchanged from what it was on cycle 1. Learning has succeeded in counteracting adverse selection.

On later cycles, this balance between learning and adverse selection is, of course, not maintained. The incremental learning effect decreases (decaying by approximately half at each cycle). The negative effect of adverse selection, by comparison, remains constant from cycle to cycle. So, by IVF cycle 4, 5, and so on, the probability of success falls.

Figure 8.4 illustrates this set of results. (Fig. 8.4 data cover patients who began treatment between 1984 and 1990. This is why the success rate is less than the 22% figure that was relevant as guarantee programs were launched. The pattern on successive cycles, which is of primary interest, is not affected by this downward shift in success rates.) The top half shows the fit of the BG (i.e., no learning) model to patients' delivery rates on successive IVF cycles. It clearly cannot represent the slight uptick in success observed on the second IVF cycle. Further, when the learning effect diminishes and the effect of adverse selection takes over on cycles 4 and 5, the BG cannot capture this phenomenon either. By contrast, the BGL is able to represent both phenomena.

This general pattern of interaction between learning and heterogeneity effects is not a fluke in the Tan et al. [33, 38] data. While the specifics of the histograms do differ across studies, we also estimated the BGL model on four other published repeat cycle data sets that covered different clinics, time periods, and outcome measures (pregnancy versus live birth) [21, 26, 34, 36]. The average BGL parameter values across these four data sets are

$$r_x = 0.057,\ r_y = 0399,\ r_\lambda = 0.125, \text{and } K = 0646.$$

Note that the average size of the learning effect (r_λ) and the decay rate for this effect (indicated by K) are similar to our results for the Tan et al. [33, 38] data. (The parameters r_x and r_y differ more from the values earlier due to the different time periods and outcome measures in these studies.) One other qualitative conclusion here matches that observed earlier. Namely, in moving to the second IVF cycle, the impact of learning and the impact of heterogeneity essentially cancel, leaving the probability of success essentially the same as it was on attempt 1. Beyond cycle 3, however, the effect of heterogeneity (adverse selection) takes over and success rates drop. Figure 8.5 shows the success rate on repeated IVF attempts for the expanded set of studies reporting such histograms.

This analysis of IVF success dynamics allows us to draw several conclusions. First, learning and adverse selection (heterogeneity) are each substantial influences on the success prospects for patients who continue IVF attempts. Second, across the initial three IVF cycles that are most relevant for our money-back-guarantee scenario, these two influences cancel and success prospects can be viewed as constant across these cycles, as our BB analysis of clinic heterogeneity assumed in the previous section. Further, the constant success probability across cycles 1–3 represents both "good news" and "bad news" for clinics that offer a money-back guarantee. The good news is that adverse selection does not represent an additional financial drawback to the guarantee, over and above our calculation in (8.1). The bad news is that while learning does counter adverse selection, it does not manage to add anything to our analysis in (8.1). In short, the financial viability of the money-back guarantee remains unexplained.

A third conclusion from our analyses here concerns success prospects beyond the third IVF attempt. Across a variety of studies, our analyses suggest that success prospects begin to decline for such later attempts. In the next section, we leave the framework of (8.1) and investigate in great detail these later IVF cycles: What may happen after the money is refunded for a third (failed) IVF attempt?

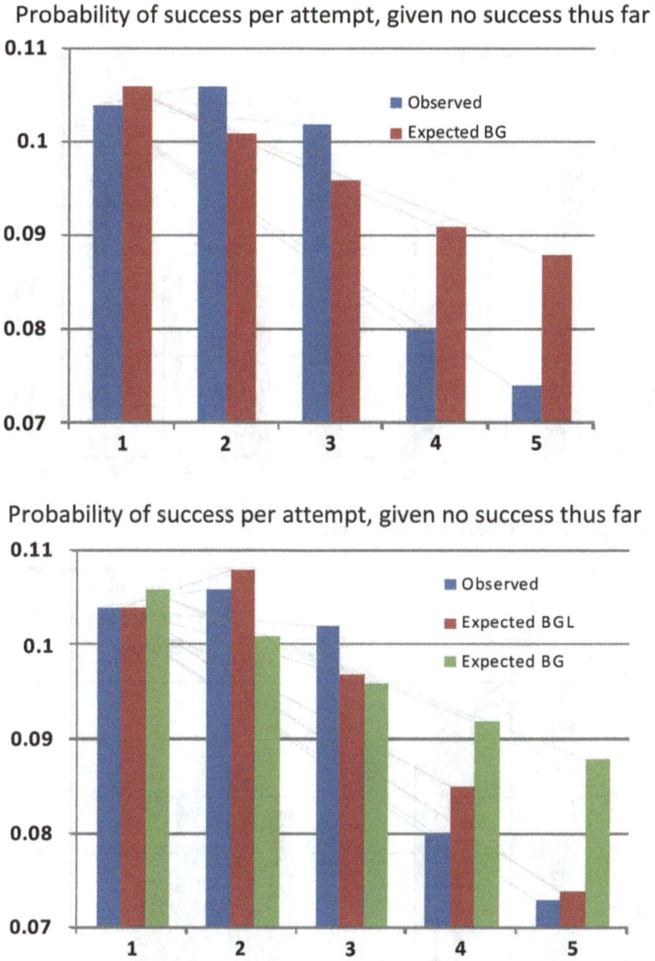

Fig. 8.4 Modeling the likelihood of success on repeated IVF attempts

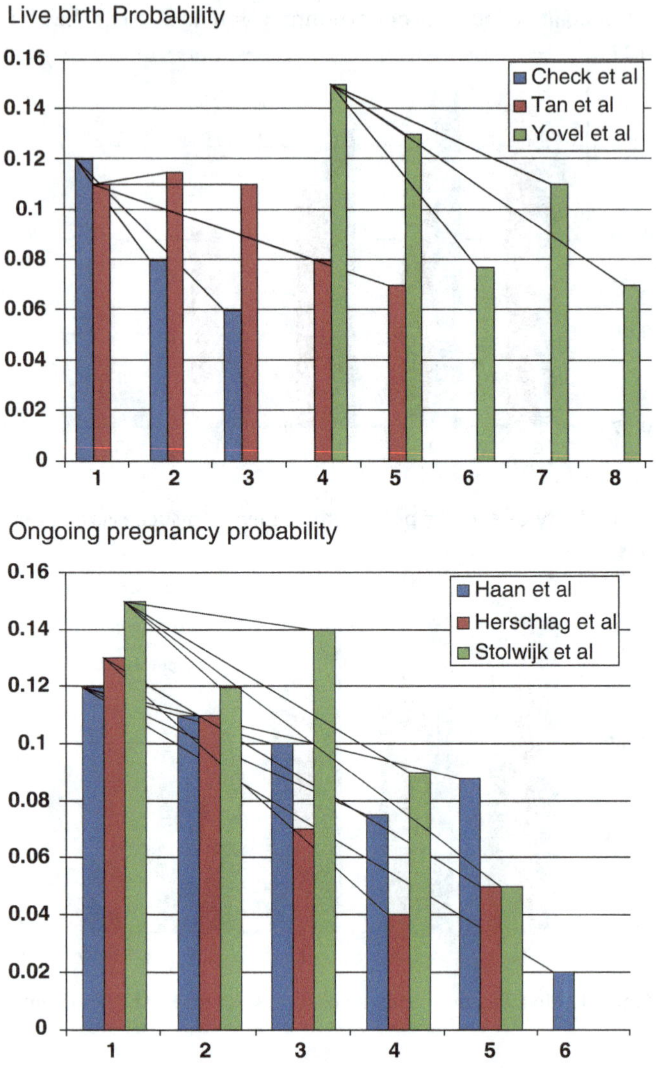

Fig. 8.5 Outcome probability on successive IVF attempts in various empirical studies

8.6 Perseverance and the House Money Effect

For a typical IVF clinic offering the standard money-back guarantee, our analysis so far has been able to reduce the expected loss per patient from $3,448 (shown in Sect. 3; based on (8.1) and the clinic's potential profit from testing) to $2,203. The latter figure arises simply by substituting $p=0.25$ in (8.1), i.e., the increase of three percentage points in the per-cycle IVF success rate that stemmed from patient screening.

In this section, and in the next, we explore ways to close the remaining gap by examining factors that lie outside the framework of (8.1). In that formula (and the ensuing sections), we have examined the outcomes of the guarantee across the three possible IVF attempts that it covered. In this section, we look ahead at "what comes after" the refund of a couple's $15,000. It is easy to describe the options. A couple can conclude their attempts at assisted reproduction, or the couple can continue with IVF, paying a la carte for additional cycles. Of course, the refund can also provide cash for such attempts.

One might think that it is highly unlikely that a couple, after three failures, would elect to continue pursuing IVF cycles (and paying for them), but the empirical evidence to date suggests otherwise. Looking at the pattern of behavior prior to the offering of money-back guarantees – i.e., when all couples not covered by insurance were paying for each attempt – the inclination to continue IVF cycle after cycle is striking. Pooling results from three empirical studies, Fig. 8.6 shows that approximately 60% of those who fail on an IVF cycle go on to the next cycle, and this statistic remains virtually constant across the first eight IVF cycles.

Under the money-back guarantee, what will happen after a third failure/refund? Certainly, clinic managers did not know how to institute the guarantee. But they did have the access to the empirical pattern of Fig. 8.6. Indeed, for several reasons, the 60% perseverance rate seems a good working assumption. These reasons stem from the decision process a patient is likely to use considering whether to continue on to the next IVF attempt. First, the 60% rate has been robust to the actual decision process the patient is likely to be using. One might imagine that the first attempt after refund "feels" like the decision an a la carte patient faces after failure on the "first for pay" attempt. That is, this is the first time a couple really have to make a decision about going further.

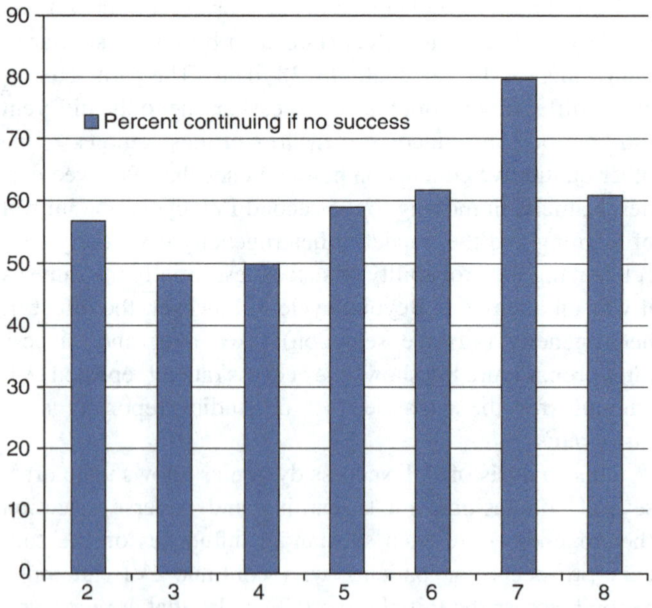

Fig. 8.6 The propensity to continue IVF after failed attempts. Sources: Check (1994), Tar (1994), Yovel (1994)

This would suggest that the perseverance rate for refund receivers would be similar to the rate historically observed for a la carte patients after their first IVF failure. On the other hand, it might act more like a failure on the "third IVF attempt overall," because this is the number of failures the refund receivers actually experienced. But based on the empirical evidence for a la carte patients in Fig. 8.6, such distinctions have not mattered, i.e., the 60% perseverance has been a constant across cycles.

Second, the refund receivers have just obtained a check for roughly $15,000, which can be expected to lead to a "house money" effect [39]. That is, the decision-process literature predicts a heightened proclivity to gamble with the "found money" just obtained. Note that it will take at least 6 months for a couple to exhaust their initial three IVF attempts, so the $15,000 refund is likely to have been viewed as "new" (found) money. Acting counter to the house money effect is a possible framing effect of the guarantee itself. That is, setting the refund at three IVF failures may suggest the couple that three is the "right" number of attempts to represent "all that I can do." Certainly, there is anecdotal evidence that couples find it difficult to establish such a benchmark without some external criterion [16, 20]. On the other hand, clinics provide data indicating a roughly constant success rate on repeated attempts [21]. This encourages couples to go on regardless of this kind of benchmark, i.e., the odds of pregnancy are presumably no worse on the next try than on the last. In fact this kind of logic, and the powerful desire for a genetically related child, pushes some patients to pursue more than 20 IVF attempts [20].

So, we assume that 60% of patients who experience a failure will go on to the next IVF cycle, for cycles 4–8 following the refund. There may, of course, be additional cycles beyond the eighth, but even with the 60% perseverance, the number of such cycles is so small that it can be ignored. To calculate the consequences of cycles 4–8, we need to know the IVF success rate on these cycles, because success also removes the patient from later cycles. Based on the BCL model parameters reported in the last section (using the Tan et al. data [33, 38]), the success probability is essentially constant across the first three IVF attempts. We denote this probability p_{1-3}, and set it equal to 0.25, as discussed earlier. Again, using the BGL parameters from the Tan et al. [33, 38] data in (8.6), we calculate the proportionate drop in the success probability for each of attempts 4–7, compared to the average success probability on attempts 1–3. Applying this proportionate drop to the value $p_{1-3} = 0.25$, the success probabilities on cycles 4–7 become 0.204, 0.180, 0.159, and 0.142, respectively.

With this parameter set, 60% of those receiving a refund will go on to pay a la carte for IVF cycle 4. Of this 60%, approximately 20.4% are expected to succeed on cycle 4, so 79.6% of the 60% (i.e., 48%) of the refund receivers will go on to fail on cycle 4. And of these, again 60% (i.e., 29% of all the refund receivers) will go on to attempt IVF cycle 5, and so on. The number of patients going on from cycle to cycle after the refund, therefore, decays with retention rate $(0.6)(1-p_t)$ for each cycle t.

Later, the economic consequence of these a la carte cycles for a clinic is then easy to calculate, because the typical contribution margin per cycle is (price cost) = $7,500 − $6,000 = $1,500. Considering only IVF cycles 4–8, with the failure/perseverance pattern described above, the average number of additional a la carte cycles pursued by a refund receiver is 1.13 cycles. Multiplying this figure by the $1,500 contribution per cycle means an additional $1,695 economic contribution per refund receiver.

This last figure must be adjusted before tallying it against the current $2,203 loss per patient described at the beginning of this section. The only patients who may proceed to a la carte are those who receive a refund, so the $1,695 figure must be reduced by that proportion. With $p = 0.25$, approximately 42.2% of couples will fail through three tries and receive the refund. So, the economic contribution of a la carte cycles 4–8 per patient who begins the guarantee program is $1,695 × 0.422 = $715. This positive amount reduces the per-patient loss from the guarantee to $2,203 − $715 = $1,488.

The money-back guarantee still does not make money without one last factor.

8.7 Abandoning the "No First Use" Policy

We noted at the outset of the paper that IVF has become the "last best hope" for many infertile couples. Figure 8.1 highlighted the treatments that typically have preceded IVF: 6–12 months attempting natural conception, drug therapy and intrauterine insemination (IUI) being common. Doctors would tend to recommend IVF only after these options for two reasons. First IVF is more invasive and carries some risks (including greater risk of multiples). Second, IVF is expensive and not often covered by insurance in the United States. While this sequencing of treatment may minimize health risks and economic cost, it has not minimized emotional costs for the patient. While Fig. 8.1 shows that across the entire sequence preceding IVF, many couples can achieve a child without needing in vitro, in fact incurring "failure" month after month can be emotionally debilitating [19]. Further, during the time that patients pursue these treatments, they may be concerned about their own aging, e.g., a 38-year-old couple sees background pregnancy rates that virtually fall off the table for 40- to 44-year-old couples relative to ages 35–39.

Enter into this process the IVF money-back guarantee with mass media advertising directed toward patients rather than doctors. For those willing to spend \$15,000, it emphasizes the complete lack of (economic) risk. It holds the promise of a baby now, rather than (maybe) a few years from now. It minimizes the emotional cost in repeated failure. It is being marketed no longer as the "last hope" but instead, with the positioning: Why wait? For infertility clinics that offer the IVF guarantee, accessing the large pool of patients in earlier stages of treatment – who are more fertile than IVFs traditional patients – can, in fact make the money-back guarantee programs earn money. The assumptions we require for this calculation may not apply to all clinics, but they are reasonable and provide an explanation for the guarantees that have, until now, been absent. Consider the following scenario for earlier use of IVF in infertility treatment:

1. Couples wishing a child pursue natural conception for 6 months.
2. If no natural conception in 6 months, half the couples pursue drug therapy (the common progression, see Fig. 8.1) and half take the IVF guarantee.
3. For those pursuing drug therapy if no success in two attempts, half pursue IUI (the common historical progression) and half take the IVF guarantee.
4. For those pursuing IUI, if no success in two attempts, half pursue IVF. The other half pursue some other option (e.g., adoption).

This sequence is illustrated in Fig. 8.7. Of course, other assumptions are possible. IVF clinic guarantees may attract couples even earlier in the natural conception process. The IVF guarantee may take more than half the drug/IUI patients – after all, the latter treatments may cost some patients, offer a lower probability of success and, accordingly a high likelihood of emotional distress, and delay the arrival of a child. Finally, less than 50% may choose to pursue IVF, either due to counseling regarding the source of infertility or because of the \$15,000 cost under the guarantee. Each of these alternative assumptions will increase the clinic's economic reward for pursuing infertility patients earlier. So in this sense, the calculation below is a conservative estimate of the payoff.

We need one more assessment to calculate the financial implications here: The success rate for IVF per cycle in the more fertile populations. In this assessment, it is useful to consider the steps required for an ongoing pregnancy i.e., production of viable egg and sperm, egg fertilization, embryo implantation, and sustained ongoing pregnancy. In couples who could conceive via natural conception or drug/IUI therapy, by far, the weakest link in this chain of events is fertilization. On the other hand, fertilization is the strong point of IVF. As Fig. 8.8 clarifies, two-third of couples using IVF produce at least one fertilized, growing embryo. For these relatively infertile couples, the weak point of IVF is implantation – this is the stage where more than half the IVF cycle failures arise. Implantation for such patients is often difficult due to the source of infertility, e.g., endometrial dysfunction. Yet, this is a relatively successful stage for more fertile couples, i.e., those who could conceive via natural conception or IUI.

Specifically, we assume that couples who would have pursued 6–12 months of natural delivery (after 6 months without a conception) would have an IVF success rate of 50% per cycle. For couples who do not conceive naturally and would have pursued drug/IUI therapy, we assume a 40% per cycle IVF success rate.

To calculate the effect of pursuing infertility patients earlier, let N represent the number of couples that complete 6 months of natural conception without a pregnancy. The sequence of reproductive procedures chosen by the couples, and outcomes experienced, are illustrated in Fig. 8.7. Prior to the IVF guarantee programs, the statistics in Fig. 8.1 indicate that about $0.274N$ would achieve a delivery during an additional 6 months of natural conception attempts. We imagine that the IVF guarantee would capture 50% of these patients, or $0.137N$ ("Group 3" in Fig. 8.7).

This leaves $0.726N$ patients who complete 12 months without a delivery and go on to drug/IIJI therapy. Again, via the statistics in Fig. 8.1, after four attempts, an additional $0.282N$ would have had a baby – and we assume that the IVF guarantee captures 50% of them or $0.141N$ ("Group 2" in Fig. 8.7). Finally, $0.726N - 0.282N = 0.444N$ would not achieve a birth after the drug/IUI sequence, and we assumed that half of these – or $0.222N$ – go on to IVF ("Group 1" in Fig. 8.7).

Under the guarantee, with the impact of attracting infertility patients earlier, the clinic's population of IVF-guarantee patients is, therefore, composed of three groups:

1. Group 1, of size $0.222N$, is the "usual" IVF patients who have repeatedly failed to conceive naturally or with drug/IUI therapy and who, accordingly have success probability on IVF cycles 1–3 of 0.25 (with success on later cycles 4–8 as described in the previous section).
2. Group 2, of size $0.141N$, is composed of patients who have repeatedly failed to conceive naturally and who would have conceived via drug/IUI therapy but elect to go to IVF instead, and who, accordingly have success probability $=0.4$ on each of IVF cycles 1–3.
3. Group 3, of size $0.137N$, is composed of patients who did not conceive in 6 months of natural conception, but who would have conceived in another 6 months of such attempts, but who elect to go with the IVF guarantee instead, and who, accordingly, have success probability $=0.5$ on each of IVF cycles 1–3.

For Groups 2 and 3, the success probability on each of cycles 4–7 is envisioned to fall off relative to cycles 1–3 by the same proportionate decline as for Group 1, using the

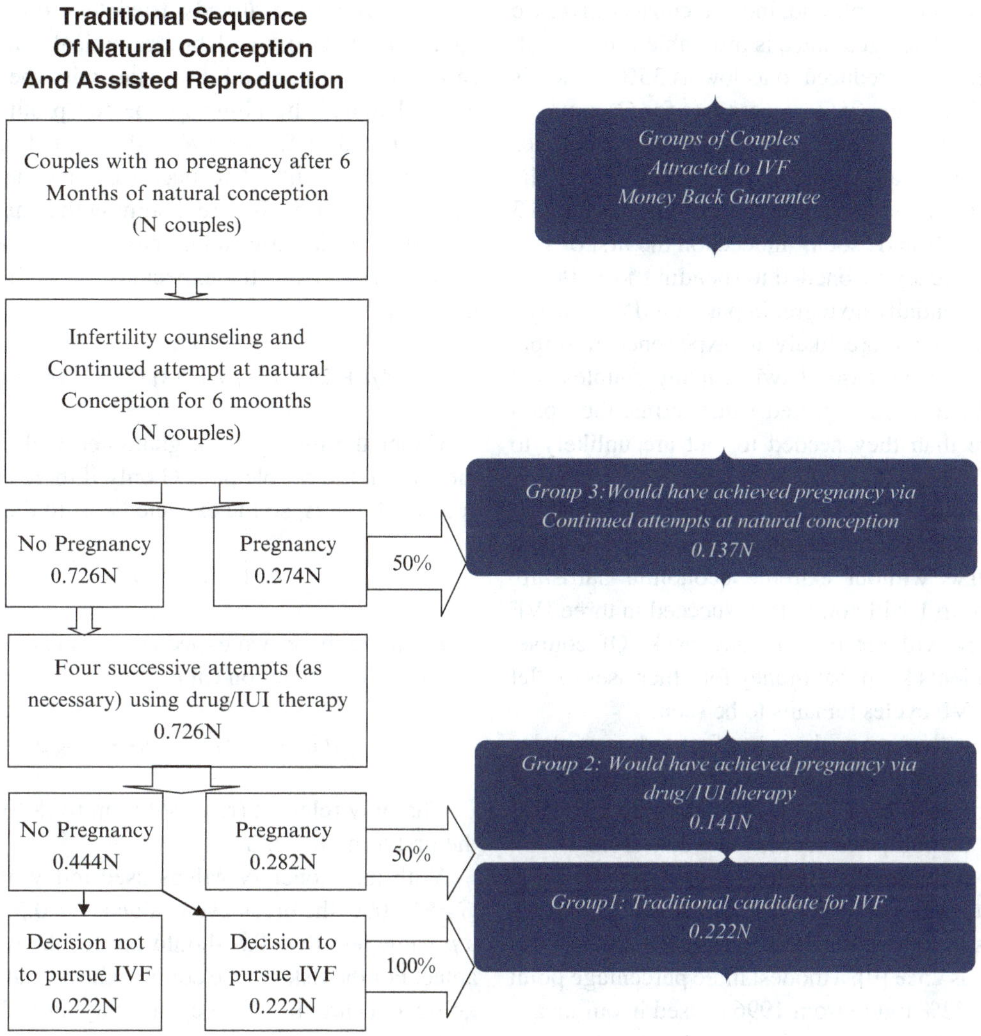

Fig. 8.7 Event tree for use of assisted reproductive procedures

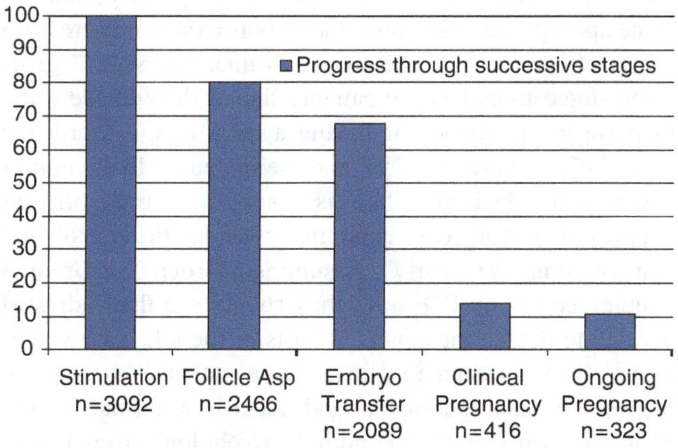

Fig. 8.8 Patient progress through successive stages within and IVF cycle. Source: Adapted from Haan et al. (1991)

BGL model and parameters as in the last section. Then, for each group, the per-patient profit (or loss) from the IVF guarantee (including the possibility of IVF cycles 4–8) can be calculated as in the last section (para 6 of Sect. 6 above), together with (8.1). Doing so, the average return per patient for each group is: Group 1: –$1,488, Group 2: +$3,328, and Group 3: +$5,802.

The economic consequence of the IVF guarantee is then just the weighted average of the within-group returns, the weights being the relative sizes of the three groups listed above. (Group 1 accounts for 44% of IVF patients, Groups 2 and 3 account for 28% and 27%, respectively) With our scenario for attracting patients to IVF earlier, in their fertility treatment this overall return is positive at last at $1,844 per patient (approximately a 13% return on average cost). The key to a positive economic return is obviously the high IVF success rate for both Group 2 and Group 3 couples. While we believe that the success rates assumed (Group 3 = 50%;

Group 2 = 40%) are reasonable and, indeed, conservative, we note that the money-back guarantee is profitable even if both groups' success rates are reduced to as low as 35%, which is a 10% "premium" over the 25% success rate for Group 1.

The financial effect of pursuing these more-fertile couples is obviously dramatic and positive for clinics. From the patients' standpoint, most of the members of Groups 2 and 3 will conceive via IVF, and "soon," indeed, on the first or second try. They are already reconciled to spending $15,000 for a child, so have essentially no regret in pursuing IVF "early." They, as a group, are more likely to experience multiple births, but at least in the case of twins, many couples will view this as a "bonus." In expected value terms, they paid collectively more than they needed to, but are unlikely to complain.

What about Group 1? These are the couples who historically made it to IVF. The money-back guarantee lets them pursue this course without extreme economic hardship. About half of Group 1 will not, in fact, succeed in three IVF attempts, but they will get their money back. Of course, whether these patients keep that money for other uses or "let it ride" on more IVF cycles remains to be seen.

Finally, we note that our analysis has focused on explaining the economic viability of money-back guarantees for IVF as they were becoming widely available, i.e., in 1997 and 1998 (based on published success rate data from 1996). This is not, however, simply a historical exercise. In 2002, the most recent IVF success rates published for North American clinics cover the year 2000, during which the overall success rate was 25% [9], a modest three percentage point increase over the 22% figure from 1996 is used in our analysis. The additional three percentage points do not, of course, explain the continued viability of money-back guarantees for these clinics, and the clinics have persisted in offering the guarantees during this period. In short, our analysis and conclusions regarding the guarantees is now as applicable as it was in 1997–1998 when they were being launched.

8.8 Conclusion

We conclude by examining the implications of our analysis for patients, clinics, and regulatory agencies, or public policy advocates.

8.8.1 Patients

For the Group 1 patients (typical IVF patients pre-money-back guarantees), the implications are clear. If they pursue IVF, they should take the money-back guarantee. For these patients who have already tried less invasive procedures, their expected cost will be dramatically less than the a la carte option. To see this, we start with the same model [1] that calculated the clinic's expected profit. Under the a la carte method of $\$A$ per cycle, the patient pays A if the first cycle is successful, $2A$ if success occurs on the second cycle, and $3A$ otherwise. (We are assuming that the couple deciding between the a la carte and money-back guarantee commits to three cycles.) Thus, the expected cost to the patient under a la carte is

$$Ap + 2Ap(1-p) + 3A[1-p-p(1-p)].$$

Under the money-back guarantee with an up-front payment of G, the couple pays G only if there are not three consecutive failures, so the expected cost to the patient is

$$G[1 - \{(1-p)^3\}].$$

Equating these two expected costs and rearranging terms give the cubic equation (in p)

$$(Gp - A)(\{p^2\} - 3p + 3) = 0.$$

The only relevant (real) solution to (8.6) is the root from the first term: $p = A/G$.

With the monetary values used today of $A = \$7{,}500$ and $G = \$15{,}000$, the break even value is $p = 0.5$. Any couple with a p-value less than 0.5 should opt for the money-back guarantee. For the risk-averse couple who would be very unhappy going a la carte for three cycles, paying $22,500 and getting no baby, the break even p-value will be even higher than 0.5. In any event, the typical Group 1 traditional patient for IVF should most definitely take the money-back guarantee. Their best guess p-values will be far below the nonrisk adverse break even value of 0.5.

The typically younger and less infertile Group 2 and Group 3 patients need to assess their personal p-value to some appropriate level above the Group 1 value. (There is no single obviously correct way to do this, but Sect. 7 gives some suggestions.) These patients should then decide if the increase in the chance of having a baby now is worth the potential side effects of IVF and the increased likelihood of having multiple births. This is a subjective trade-off, but couples should at least explicitly consider these pros and cons of doing IVF "early". Assuming a Group 2 or Group 3 couple decides on IVF now, they should use their adjusted p-value to decide the expected costs of the a la carte versus money-back guarantee option. Those patients who opt for the money-back guarantee and receive a refund should explicitly consider the economic, psychological, and side-effect costs yet again before treating that refund as "house money."

Of course, all of the above is predicated on patients gaining as much information as possible on the success rates for the IVF clinics that are geographically feasible for them. They should be especially wary of high success rates based on small sample sizes or high success rates where the prevalence of multiple births is above average. The couple should also find out on how aggressively each clinic screens its patients as much as possible, i.e., what kind of patient pool produced the clinic's historical success rate.

8.8.2 Clinic Managers

The clinic manager needs to estimate the overall success rate per cycle for patients the clinic is currently attracting, and this is especially true if the clinic offers the money-back guarantee. The clear-cut economic questions should be addressed via (8.1). The key ethical considerations for a clinic follow. Are patients given data that are appropriate for their particular situations? Are the downsides of IVF vis-à-vis less invasive procedures adequately addressed? Are the patients who receive their money back being pressured to "let it ride" on additional a la carte IVF attempts?

8.8.3 Public Policy Advocates

Organizations such as SART and RESOLVE that provide information to infertility patients play an important role, that is increasingly challenging with new payment options and expanded competition. The data, model, projection, and scenario analyses in this paper can help patient education and, indeed, a menu-driven interactive computer version of this work would be valuable for patients. It is also important to expand the monitoring of clinics. Some of the key variables, e.g., success rate by age, incidence of multiple births, have been comprehensively collected. Other key variables, e.g., success rates by previous infertility treatment history, pricing policy, and number of IVF attempt for the patient, are not available clinic by clinic. This information would add incentive for the clinics to "do the right thing."

8.8.4 The Simple Model Works

Finally, we stress the need for formal probabilistic models to analyze the existing IVF data. These models give insights not available with the usual summary statistics. But perhaps the best news from our efforts is that the simplest possible model, (8.1), "works." That is, assuming that each patient has the same baseline success probability (wrong) and that this probability stays unchanged on successive cycles (wrong) leads to a good economic analysis of the money-back guarantee. The heterogeneity of these base rates across patients (who drive down the aggregate probability of success on repeated attempts) is counterbalanced by the individual patient "learning" (which drives up the aggregate probability of success on repeated attempts), at least for the first three cycles. Clinics know their cost per cycle, C, and both the clinics and the patients know the up-front money-back guarantee fee, G, and the a la carte price, A. Because the homogeneous (Bernoulli) model in (8.1) provides a good approximation to reality, the clinics need to know only their overall success rate p to see if the money-back guarantee will be profitable.

For those deciding between the a la carte and money-back guarantee, only A, G, and their personal p-value matter. The break even p-value is just A/G. By coaching the couple, their personal p-value can be estimated. Even just telling the couples the A/G break even point and a p-value for "couples like them" would improve on current patient education.

Acknowledgments The authors appreciate helpful comments contributed by Eric Bradlow, Barbara Kalm, Mary Frances Luce, and the participants of the 1998 UCLA Winter Marketing Camp.

References

1. Davis K (1996) The agonizing price of infertility. In: Kiplinger Online, www.kiplinger.com, pp 1–7
2. Freudenheim M (1998) Aetna is reducing fertility benefits: advanced treatment coverage is eliminated by a pioneer. The New York Times, 1998 January 10; Sect. 1–11
3. Robertson JA, Schneyer TJ (1997) Professional self-regulation and shared-risk programs for in vitro fertilization. J Law Med Ethics 25(4):283–291, 231
4. Rubin AJ, Zitner A (2000) Infertility cases spur an illicit drug market. Los Angeles Times, 2000; Sect. 20, 2
5. Traftord A (1997) Medicine's money back warranty. The Washington Post, 1997 August 5; Sect. 06
6. Hyman DA, Silver C (1998) Letter to the Editor. J Law Med Ethics : 94–95
7. Murray TH (1997) Money-back guarantees for 1 W: an ethical critique. J Law Med Ethics 25:292–294
8. Norris P (1997) The many lives made miserable by a low-down high-roller. The New York Times, 1997 March 9; Sect. 7
9. U.S. Centers for Disease Control and Prevention (2009) Assisted Reproductive Technology (ART) Report: National Summary and Fertility Clinic Reports. http://apps.nccd.cdc.gov/ART/Marquee.aspx
10. Gleicher N, VanderLaan B, Pratt D, Karande V (1996) Background pregnancy rates in an infertile population. Hum Reprod 11(5):1011–1012
11. (1996) Assisted reproductive technology in the United States and Canada: 1994 results generated from the American Society for Reproductive Medicine/Society for Assisted Reproductive Technology Registry. Fertil Steril 66(5):697–705
12. Society for Assisted Reproductive Technology, American Society for Reproductive Medicine (1996) Clinic specific report for 1994. ASRM, Birmingham, AL

13. U.S. Centers for Disease Control and Prevention (2009) Assisted Reproductive Technology (ART) Report: National Summary and Fertility Clinic Reports. http://apps.nccd.cdc.gov/ART/Marquee.aspx
14. Friedler S, Mashiach S, Laufer N (1992) Births in Israel resulting from in-vitro fertilization/embryo transfer, 1982–1989: National Registry of the Israeli Association for Fertility Research. Hum Reprod 7(8):1159–1163
15. Haan G, Rutten F (1989) No cure, no pay: an acceptable way of financing fertility treatments? Health Policy 13:239–249
16. Strictly Business (1997) "The Newshour With Jim Lehrer: Monday, January 27, 1997", Overland Park, KS: Strictly Business
17. Dawood MY (1996) In vitro fertilization, gamete intrafallopian transfer, and superovulation with intrauterine insemination: efficacy and potential health hazards on babies delivered. Am J Obstet Gynecol 174(4):1208–1217
18. (1996) Infertility revisited: the state of the art today and tomorrow. The ESHRE Capri Workshop. European Society for Human Reproduction and Embryology. Hum Reprod 11:1779–1807
19. Golombok S (1992) Psychological functioning in infertility patients. Hum Reprod 7(2):208–212
20. Stolberg SG (1997) For the infertile, a high-tech treadmill. The New York Times, 1997; Sect. 1, 36
21. Haan G, Bernardus RE, Hans MG et al (1991) Selective drop-out in successive in-viro fertilization attempts: the pendulum danger. Hum Reprod 6(7):939–943
22. Diczfalusy E, Crosignani PG (1996) Introduction: from reproductive endocrinology to reproductive health. The short history of a new departure by ESHRE. European Society for Human Reproduction and Embryology. Hum Reprod 11(8):1776–1777
23. Wagner MG, St Clair PA (1989) Are in-vitro fertilisation and embryo transfer of benefit to all? Lancet 2(8670):1027–1030
24. Haan G, van Steen R (1992) Costs in relation to effects of in-vitro fertilization. Hum Reprod 7(7):982–986
25. Hann G, Bernardus RE, Hollanders JMG, Leerentveld RA, Prak FM, Naaktgeboren N (1991) Results of IVF from a prospective multicenter study. Hum Reprod 6(6):805–810
26. Stolwijk AM, Hamilton CJ, Hollanders JM, Bastiaans LA, Zielhuis GA (1996) A more realistic approach to the cumulative pregnancy rate after in-vitro fertilization. Hum Reprod 11(3):660–663
27. Zhou H, Weinberg CR, Wilcox AJ, Baird DD (1996) A random-effects model for cycle viability in fertility studies. J Am Stat Assoc 91(436): 1413–1422
28. RESOLVE (1997) *RESOLVE National Newsletter*. Volume 22, No.1 (Winter). Somerville, MA: RESOLVE
29. Maritz J (1970) Empirical Bayes methods. Methuen, London, UK
30. Griffiths DA (1973) Maximum likelihood estimation for the beta-binomial distribution and an application to the household distribution of the total number of cases of a disease. Biometrics 29(4):637–648
31. Greene JD (1982) Consumer behavior models for non-statisticians. Praeger, New York
32. Crowder MJ (1978) Beta-binomial ANOVA for proportions. Appl Stat 27(1):34–37
33. Tan SL, Doyle P, Maconochie N et al (1994) Pregnancy and birth rates of live infants after in vitro fertilization in women with an without previous in vitro fertilization pregnancies: a study of eight thousand cycles at one center. Am J Obstet Gynecol 170(1 Pt 1):34–40
34. Hershlag A, DeCherney AH, Kaplan EH, Lavy G, Loy RA (1991) Heterogeneity in patient populations explains differences in in vitro fertilization programs. Fertil Steril 56:913–917
35. Check JH, Lurie D, Callan C, Baker A, Benfer K (1994) Comparison of the cumulative probability of pregnancy after in vitro fertilization-embryo transfer by infertility factor and age. Fertil Steril 61(2):257–261
36. Alsalili M, Yuzpe A, Tummon I et al (1995) Cumulative pregnancy rates and pregnancy outcome after in-vitro fertilization: >5000 cycles at one centre. Hum Reprod 10(2):470–474
37. Schmittlein DC (1989) Surprising inferences from unsurprising observations: do conditional expectations really regress to the mean? Am Stat 43(3):176–183
38. Tan SL, Maconochie N, Doyle P et al (1994) Cumulative conception and live-birth rates after in vitro fertilization with and without the use of long, short, and ultrashort regimens of the gonadotropin-releasing hormone agonist buserelin. Am J Obstet Gynecol 171(2):513–520
39. Thaler RH, Johnson EJ (1990) Gambling with the house money and trying to break even: the effects of prior outcomes on risky choice. Manage Sci 36:643–660
40. Johnson, NL, Kotz, S (1970) Continuous univariate distributios - 2. Wiley, New York

Part II
Female Reproductive Physiology and Medicine

Chapter 9
Ovulation: A Molecular View

Mats Brännström, Anna Karin Lind, and Pernilla Dahm-Kähler

Abstract Ovulation is a complex process that after initiation by LH involves cascades of several pathways that interact within cell types and between cell compartments. Major functions of these pathways are to promote permeability and increased blood flow, to accelerate ECM remodelling leading to degradation of the follicular apex and restructuring of the cystic follicle into a solid corpus luteum, to induce expansion within the cumulus granulosa cells, to modify steroidogenesis within granulosa and theca cells toward secretion of progesterone, and to maintain a positive intra-follicular pressure so the follicular wall eventually ruptures and that the cumulus-enclosed oocyte is expelled.

Keywords Ovulation • Luteinizing hormone surge • Granulosa cells • Eicosanoids • Corpus luteum

9.1 Introduction

Ovulation, the central episode of the ovarian cycle, is a complex and multifaceted process that ultimately leads to rupture of the exterior follicle wall with a release of fertilizable oocyte. The intra-ovarian regulation of the ovulatory process has been a major area in reproductive research for a long time. In this review, the older biochemical-oriented research on ovulation will be integrated into the modern molecular-oriented research, which has made tremendous advances with the availability of methods for wide genomic analysis and genetically modified animal models. Most studies of molecular pathways in ovulation are derived from studies in rodents, and only few studies in this area have, due to natural reasons, been conducted in nonhuman primates and humans. Since the ultimate clinical goal of research in this area is to increase the knowledge of the human ovulatory process for fertility regulation purposes, the research in human and nonhuman primates will be included and discussed in this review, even if the results of these studies are less complete regarding proof of function for any proposed ovulatory mediator.

In general, the ovulatory process includes profound changes in gene expression in the theca cells, the mural granulosa cells, the cumulus granulosa cells, the oocyte, and invading leukocytes, which are the main cellular compartments of the follicle. A coordinated array of signals in all these compartments leads to changes in the oocyte toward oocyte maturation, in the follicular apex toward rupture, and within the granulosa and theca cells toward luteinization.

9.2 Dynamics of Ovulation

This review is primarily focused on the molecular events of ovulation. However, when looking at the ovulatory process from a scientific standpoint, it may be beneficial to be able to identify the dynamic macro and microscopic changes in the follicular apex during the ovulatory interval. This will help the researcher to understand the entire process and could also give ideas about possible molecular changes that may occur and that can be tested in properly designed experiments.

Our group has performed cinematographic and intravital microscopic studies of ovulation in rabbit and rat. In experiments on the in vitro perfused rabbit [1] and rat [2] ovary, typical features during the ovulatory interval could be observed. However, the results of these in vitro observations may not directly be pertinent to the conditions in vivo since several important components such as blood supply, nervous influence, and lymphatic drainage are missing during in vitro perfusion. In follow-up studies, we were able to capture ovulation in vivo both in rat [2] and in rabbit [3] in experimental setups in which the ovary was exteriorized but connected to the animal that was under anaesthesia. The main findings of these studies were that of a gonadotropin-induced change in the shape of the follicle, which was followed by alterations in the microcirculation over the apex. Vasomotion was first seen, but the blood flow then gradually disappeared to leave an avascular zone over the apex. Within minutes before rupture,

M. Brännström (✉), A.K. Lind, and P. Dahm-Kähler
Department of Obstetrics and Gynecology, Sahlgrenska Academy at University of Gothenburg, Göteborg, Sweden
e-mail: mats.brannstrom@obgyn.gu.se

D.T. Carrell and C.M. Peterson (eds.), *Reproductive Endocrinology and Infertility: Integrating Modern Clinical and Laboratory Practice*,
DOI 10.1007/978-1-4419-1436-1_9,

a cone-shaped stigma was formed, and the major rupture of the thinned exterior follicle wall was in most instances accompanied by profuse bleeding. This bleeding stopped within minutes, but the extrusion of granulosa cells went on for several minutes after the oocyte had been expelled. Some typical features are shown in Fig. 9.1.

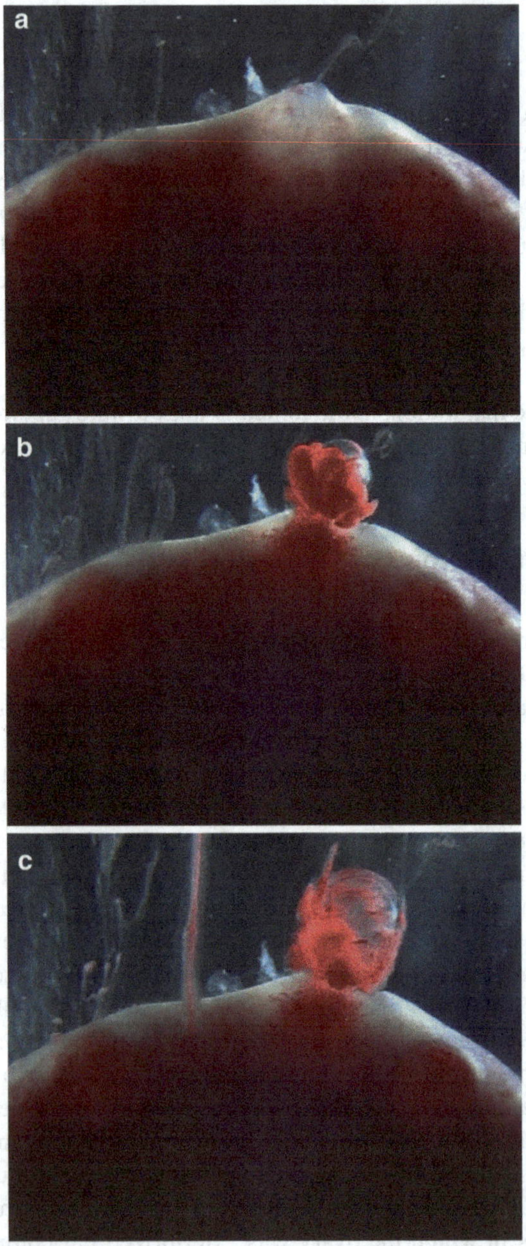

Fig. 9.1 Ovulation in vivo in rabbit ovary. The shape of the follicle is changed during the ovulatory process (**a**) with the rupture accompanied by initial bleeding (**b**) followed by expulsion of granuolsa cells and the oocyte (**c**)

9.3 Endocrine Signal and Second Messengers

The mid-cycle gonadotropin surge of luteinizing hormone (LH) and follicle-stimulating hormone (FSH) from the pituitary is the initiator of ovulation. The LH component of the gonadotropin surge is the major trigger, (Fig. 9.2) but FSH has a specific role on the cumulus granulosa cells to induce mucification [4, 5]. It should be pointed out that older studies in rat demonstrated that purified FSH by itself can induce ovulations [6, 7], although not as effectively as LH.

Several studies clearly show that LH is the physiological trigger of ovulation by binding to the LH receptor. The LH receptors are present in high density on theca cells and on mural granulosa cells, but the density on the cumulus granulosa cells is substantially lower [8]. The importance of activation of the LH receptor for ovulation is shown by findings in LH receptor null mice, which do no ovulate [9] and the observed impaired ovulation in estradiol receptor beta null mice, which have considerably reduced number of LH receptors [10].

Several separate intracellular signalling pathways have been implicated as further mediators of LH action to alter transcriptional complexes that mediate upregulation in expression of ovulatory genes and down-regulation in expression of genes that counteract ovulatory changes. The LH-receptor, which is a G-protein-coupled-receptor, activates membrane-associated adenylate cyclase leading to generation of cyclic AMP. An activation of cAMP-dependent protein kinase A (PKA) occurs and downstream of that the cAMP response element-binding protein (CREB) becomes phosphorylated [11]. A rapid consequence of cAMP-PKA activation is additional activation of the extracellular regulated kinase (Erk) pathway [12, 13]. Other second messenger pathways for LH action involve phosphoinositide production [14] and phospholipase C activity [15].

9.4 Transcriptional Regulation

The signalling pathways that are induced by the LH surge alter transcriptional regulation mainly in the follicular cells that carry a high density of LH-receptors, such as the mural granulosa cells and theca cells, but also in the cumulus granulosa cells with lower levels of LH-receptors. Indirect regulation of transcription by LH seems to occur in invading leukocytes. The reprogramming of gene expression leads to that a large number of genes become markedly upregulated. However, there is also a downregulation of several genes, and this negative regulation may also be important.

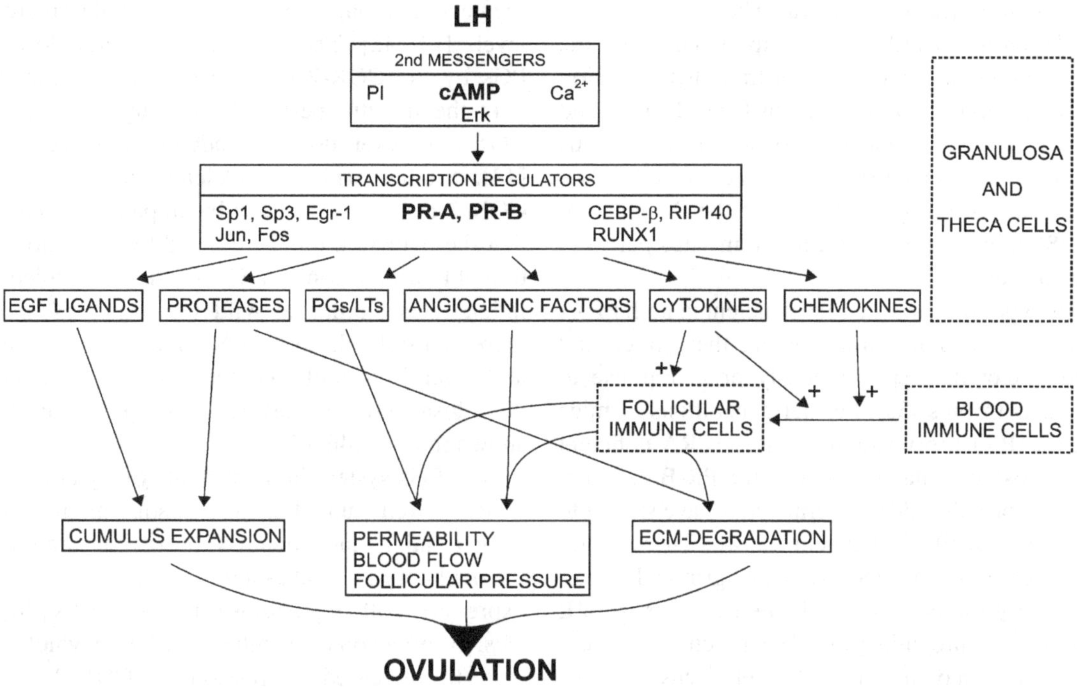

Fig. 9.2 Schematic overview of the mediators of ovulation and their role in the ovulatory process. The granulosa and theca cells are the sites for LH binding and action through 2nd messengers, transcription regulators and several factors that directly promote changes that lead to ovulation. Immune cells are drawn into the follicle from the blood by action of chemokines, are activated by cytokines and are rich sources of several ovulatory mediators

Taken together, the net effect of these changes in gene transcription is that the processes of degradation of the follicular apex, induction of oocyte maturation, and luteal transition of the steroid-producing cells get initiated and proceed undisturbed during the ovulatory interval. This interval spans over about 12–15 h in rodent animals [16] and about 32–40 h in human [17] and primates [18].

The serum response factors 1 and 3 (SP1, SP3) have key roles as transcriptional activators in the granulosa cells during ovulation. These transcription factors are constitutively expressed in granulosa cells, but show an increased binding to several gene promoters after LH induction [11]. This leads to induction of secondary transcription factors with specific roles to regulate transcription of a number of ovulatory genes. Examples of these transcription factors, with major roles in the ovulatory process, are Jun, Fos [19], and early growth response-1 (Egr-1) [11]. Major effects on transcription during ovulation are also carried out by various transcriptional regulators. The nuclear receptor coregulator RIP140 [20, 21], CEPB beta [22], and RUNX1 [23] are expressed in granulosa cells at high levels after LH in rats and regulate the transcription of numerous genes.

9.5 Progesterone

The most central transcription regulator in ovulation is the progesterone receptor (PR). The PR is primarily induced by the cAMP-PKA system, and further by binding of SP1-SP3 to GC-box elements in the PR promoter [24]. The PR has two transcriptional starting sites producing two distinct isoforms of the receptors, PR-A and PR-B. The PR can function both as a classical transcription factor by binding to DNA, but also as a co-regulatory factor [25]. The expression of the two isoforms, PR-A and PR-B, varies between tissues and species. In rodent granulosa cells, PR-A seems to be the predominant form [26]. The two PR isoforms have differential effects on expression [27].

Experiments in monkeys have revealed that PR-B is the predominant form in the ovary, with a localization also in the theca [28]. In human ovaries, both PR-A and PR-B isoforms are found in granulosa and theca cells, but with PRA found at higher levels [29].

At the same time, as the LH-induced increase in PR expression is seen in the follicular cells, there is a substantial amplification in P synthesis within the follicle. It has been known for a long time that P plays a central role in ovulation.

This was first demonstrated in the rat where P antiserum inhibited ovulation in vivo [30]. Later experiments with the in vitro perfused rat ovary could demonstrate that ovulation was inhibited by suppression of ovarian P production and that this ovulatory block could be reversed by exogenous addition of P [31]. It was later shown that the effects of P on ovulation was carried out by the PR, since the PR receptor blocker RU 486 inhibited ovulation in the in vitro perfused rat ovary preparation [32].

Subsequent experiments with mice deficient in both PR-A and PR-B demonstrated infertility among these mice and that they did not ovulate spontaneously or in reponse to exogenous gonadotropins [33]. Further generations of mice deficient in either PR isoforms showed that the PRA-deficient mouse were almost anovulatory and that the PR-B deficient mouse ovulated normally [34]. Several genes have shown to be down-regulated in PR-A deficient mouse. These genes include the proteases ADAMTS-1 (a disintegrin and metalloproteinase with thrombospondin-like repeat), cathepsin L [35] as well as amphiregulin [36]. The function of these PR-regulated factors in ovulation are further discussed in the following lines.

The essential ovarian role of P in ovulation has also been demonstrated in the non-human primate macaque, in which a steroidogenic inhibitor blocked ovulation, with this blockage being reversed by exogenous P [37]. Such experiments have of natural reasons not been conducted in the human. However, an in vitro study on incubated pieces of the human follicular wall indicated that P promoted the breakdown of the follicular apex since the presence of this steroid decreased incorporation of proline into collagen [38].

9.6 Eicosanoids

Eicosanoids are autocrine and paracrine mediators that derive from arachidonic acid (AA) mobilized from the cell membranes. Cyclooxygenase (COX) enzymes metabolize AA into prostaglandins (PGs) and thromboxanes. Lipoxygenases metabolize AA into leukotrienes (LTs) and hydroxyeicosatetranoic acids.

Several studies have shown that PGs and LTs are instrumental in the intraovarian events of ovulation. More than 30 years ago, it was demonstrated that PGs may play a role in ovulation as shown by inhibition of ovulation in rat by various unselective blockers of COX [39]. Further studies showed that the COX-1 enzyme is constitutively expressed in the theca cells, and that COX-2 is induced in the granulosa cells by LH [40]. This induction of COX-2 results in major increases of the follicular levels of PGs, and in rat, a 50-fold increase of PGF2alpha levels were seen at ovulation, with a somewhat smaller increase in PGE2 levels [41, 42]. The importance of granulosa cell-derived PGs by the COX-2 enzyme was demonstrated by studies with the in vitro perfused rat ovary, in which a selective COX-2 blocker dose-dependently reduced ovulation rate [43]. Studies with gene-deleted mice demonstrated that COX-2 deficient mice exhibit impaired ovulation [44] and that the ovulation rate is restored by exogenous administration of PGE2. In contrast, COX-1 deficient mice display ovulation rates similar to wild type mice [45]. There is an increased follicular production rate of PGs during ovulation and several types of receptors for PGE2 are induced in the granulosa cell compartment during ovulation, as clearly shown in mice [46, 47].

The PGs system in the primate ovary at ovulation is particularly well studied in the macaque monkey, in which PG concentrations in follicular fluid rise during the last 10 h of the ovulatory interval as a result of a previous rise in COX-2 expression both in granulosa and theca cells [48]. In this species, the effect on PG synthesis by LH may not only be attributed to increased expression of COX-2 since also the cytosolic enzyme phospholipase A2, which promotes AA release from the cell membrane, is induced in granulosa cells by LH [49]. In the human, nonselective COX inhibitors block ovulation [50], and a selective COX-2 inhibitor delays follicular rupture [51]. The important PG in the human seems to be PGE2, which is secreted by human granulosa cells [52] that also express the EP-2 receptor [53].

Several LTs are induced in the ovary by the preovulatory gonadotropin surge [54], and pharmacological inhibitors of lipoxygenases reduce the ovulation rate [55]. Especially, LTB4 has been ascribed a facilitating role in ovulation since a specific LTB4 receptor antagonist inhibits ovulation in rat both when given intrabursally in vivo and when administered in the perfusion media of in vitro perfused rat ovaries [56].

The exact roles of the eicosanoids in ovulation are not fully understood, but effects on the vasculature to promote permeability and promotion of connective tissue degradation have been suggested as important.

9.7 Angiogenic Factors

The ovary is a highly vascularized organ with dramatic changes during the ovarian cycle. The ovarian blood flow is increased within minutes after the LH surge [57], and at the same time, there is a redistribution of blood flow around the preovulatory follicle so that more blood is directed toward the base of the follicle and less to the apex of the follicle [58]. Simultaneously, there is an increase in the vascular permeability of the capillaries [59, 60] that are abundant in the theca layer [61]. It is proposed that angiogenesis, increased blood flow and the augmented permeability are important for follicular rupture to occur.

Several vasoactive mediators have been shown to contribute to the ovulatory process and may be responsible for these changes. These vasoactive mediators include eicosanoids [59], nitric oxide [62, 63], angiotensin II [64], vascular endothelial growth factor [65], endothelin-2 [66], and angiopoetin [65].

9.8 Epidermal Growth Factor like Factors

During recent years, it has become evident that the epidermal growth factor receptors (EGFRs) – ligands epiregulin, amphiregulin, and betacellulin–exert effects on the ovulatory process. These factors are rapidly induced by LH in the mouse ovary, and they trigger meiosis and cumulus expansion in follicles in vitro [67]. Further studies in rat have confirmed these roles in ovulation but also shown that the EGFR ligands are important for expression of several ovulation-associated genes and that an EGFR kinase receptor inhibitor attenuates hCG-induced ovulation [68]. Both amphiregulin and epiregulin are induced by LH in human granulosa-lutein cells [69].

9.9 Proteases and Their Inhibitors

The extracellular matrices (ECMs) of the theca externa, the overlying stroma, and the tunica albuginea as well as the two basal membranes of the exterior wall of the preovulatory follicle are rich in collagens [70]. These fibrils and networks of collagens as well as the other components of the ECM make up the tensile strength of the follicle wall that can balance the positive intrafollicular pressure [71].

A tight regulation of ECM remodeling in these compartments seems to be a requirement for ovulation. Modulation of cell-matrix communication takes place through the action of proteinases that are not only responsible for protein degradation but also control signals produced by other matrix molecules. The proteinases that have been most extensively studied in relation to ovulation are the matrix metalloproteinases (MMPs) [72–76], the plasmin/plasminogen activator (PA) system [72, 77], and the ADAMTS family [78, 79]. The experimental evidence for their role in the ovulatory process is summarized in the following lines.

9.9.1 Matrix Metalloproteinases

The MMPs are zinc-dependent, neutral endopeptidases that synergistically degrade the major ECM components, in particular collagens and proteoglycans [80]. The MMP family is subdivided into collagenases, gelatinases, stromelysins, matrilysins, membrane-type MMPs (MT-MMPs) based on their substrate specificity and molecular structure [81]. It is assumed that their major role in ovulation is to degrade the fibrils and networks of collagen that make up the tensile strength of the follicular wall and thereby facilitate rupture.

The MMPs are strictly regulated on multiple levels, including gene transcription as well as post-translational influences such as activation of proMMPs and regulation by humoral inhibitors like α2-macroglobulin and particularly endogenous inhibitors of the family tissue inhibitors of metalloproteinases (TIMPs). The four types of TIMPs (TIMP-1, -2, -3 and -4) are major regulators of ECM remodelling in several organs [82–85]. Recent studies have concluded that TIMPs also exhibit growth factor-like activity and inhibitory action on angiogenesis [84], activities that seem to be independent of an inhibitory activity on the MMPs.

A great number of studies have been conducted in rodents to explore the role and the temporal expression patterns of the various MMPs and TIMPs. By use of inhibitors of varying selectivity for specific MMPs, ovulation in rat ovary was inhibited both in vivo [86] and in vitro [87].

The gelatinases (MMP-2, 9) may play key roles in degradation of the basal lamina separating the granulosa and theca layers as well as to further hydrolyze denatured fibrillar collagens following their initial cleavage by the collagenases. In the rat ovary, MMP-2 mRNA expression is stimulated by LH, while MMP-9 expression is unchanged throughout the periovulatory period [88]. Certain species differences seem to exist also in rodents since in the mouse ovary MMP-9 mRNA increases after LH-stimulus, whereas MMP-2 is unchanged [35, 89]. However, even if results of the two studies in the mouse suggest a role for MMP-9 in the remodelling events during ovulation, gene-deletion experiments have indicated that MMP-9 by itself does not seem to have an essential role in ovulation [90]. The lack of effect of could be explained by a redundancy in the system so that other MMPs could compensate for the lack of functional MMP-9. A key regulator in regulation of the gelatinases within the ovary may be the cytokine interleukin (IL) -1, since IL-1β dose-dependently induced secretion of MMP-9 in cultures of whole ovarian dispersates [91]. The cytokine IL-1β furthermore inhibits PA activity in cultured rat granulosa cells [92], suggesting that IL-1 interacts with both the MMP and PA system.

The inhibitors TIMP-1 and TIMP-2 are capable of inhibiting the activities of most MMPs and as such play key roles in maintaining the balance between ECM deposition and degradation [83]. TIMP-1 and TIMP-2 are secreted as glycoproteins and bind to the active form of many MMPs, especially to MMP-9 and MMP-2, respectively. Ovarian expression of TIMP-2 mRNA was not changed during ovulation in rat [93] or in mouse [94]. The study in the rat indicated that mRNA for TIMP-1 is localized to the stroma and theca of developing follicles [93] and that the expression is markedly increased after hCG stimulus [95]. The mRNA levels of TIMP-1 are maximally increased at late proestrus in the natural estrous cycle of the mouse [94]. In more detailed temporal studies in immature eCG-primed rodent models, an increase of TIMP-1 mRNA was seen after hCG both in rat [96, 97] and mouse [89]. The localization of TIMP-1 during ovulation in the rat switches from thecal origin to a granulosa cell-derived pattern [93]. A redundancy in the role of different TIMPs in ovulation is suggested by that the deletion of the gonadotropin-induced TIMP-1 gene in mice does not change the phenotype of the animals in regards to ovulatory frequency and fertility [98]. The modulation of TIMP-1 on other components of the MMP-TIMP network is suggested by the reduced levels of ovarian TIMP-2 and TIMP-3 expression in the TIMP-1-deficient mice [98]. The role of granulosa cell-derived TIMP-1 may not only be to regulate MMP activity. Several studies point towards that TIMP-1 regulates steroidogenesis within the granulosa cells. Thus, a TIMP-1 like protein was reported to stimulate P production in rat granulosa cells [99]. Moreover, recombinant human TIMP-1 stimulates estradiol production in cultured mouse granulosa cells [98], while mice deficient in TIMP-1 exhibit reduced blood levels of estradiol [100] and P [100]

Membrane type 1-matrix metalloproteinase (MT1-MMP) has been identified in vitro as an activator of pro-MMP-2, carried out by formation of a complex with TIMP-2 [101]. The MT1-MMP-associated MMP-2 activation increases in rat ovary in response to an ovulatory dose of hCG [102] indicating that MT1-MMP mRNA may be an important part of a mechanism required for efficient production of active MMP-2 during the ovulatory process.

The MMP-TIMP system does also seem to be functional in the ovary during ovulation in nonhuman primates and the human. The gelatinases are expressed in the preovulatory follicle of the macaque monkey with the mRNA levels of MMP-9 only slightly increased just prior to follicular rupture, but a greater increase of MMP-2 mRNA is seen already after 12 h into the ovulatory interval [103]. In this species, MMP-1 seems to be the major MMP since it is highly upregulated in granulosa cells during ovulation [103]. On the other hand, TIMP-1 mRNA is maximally increased at the preovulatory stage in the natural menstrual cycle of the macaque monkey [104]. The local regulation of expression of MMP-1 and TIMP-1 in the nonhuman primate ovary seems to be carried out by both P and PGs [105].

In the human, initial findings of increased collagenolytic activity within human follicular fluid at ovulation [106] and of a higher collagenase activity in ovarian tissue of menstruating women compared to after menopause [107] suggested a role for the MMP-TIMP system in the follicular ECM remodelling during ovulation. Our group has examined the expression patterns of the gelatinases and their respective inhibitors in and around the human follicle during precise stages of hCG-induced ovulation in natural cycles. In the perifollicular stroma, there was a significant increase during ovulation of both mRNA and protein levels of TIMP-1 [108]. A study on material from IVF-cycles shows that human granulosa lutein cells contain mRNA for TIMPs [109] and high levels of TIMP-1 protein is present in follicular fluid of IVF [110]. In our studies, we saw also an almost 100-fold increase of TIMP-1 mRNA in the granulosa cells during ovulation and a somewhat smaller increase in the theca cell compartment (unpublished observations). We have also identified a large increase of MMP-9 mRNA in both the granulosa and theca cell compartments, and clear immunostainings for both TIMP-1 and MMP-9 in both the granulosa and theca cells are seen with an increase during ovulation (our unpublished results). Proteins for MMP-2 and MMP-9 have been found in follicular fluid of IVF patients [110]. A role for the MMP/TIMP system in regulation of steroidogenesis also in the human ovary is suggested by the fact that the MMP-2/TIMP ratio in cultures of human luteinized granulosa cells is inversely related to P levels [111].

9.9.2 The Plasmin/Plasminogen Activator System

The key components of the plasmin/PA system are the proteolytic activators, tissue-type PA (tPA) and urokinase-type PA (uPA), the proenzyme plasminogen and its enzymatically active degradation product, plasmin, together with the central inhibitors of this system, PA inhibitor-1 and -2 (PAI-1, PAI-2) [72]. This system is activated by the release of tPA or uPA from specific cells, initiated by external signals such as cytokines, growth factors, and hormones [112]. Plasmin, the end product of the PA cascade, is able to cleave ECM proteins, regulate growth factor activity and to convert some proMMPs into active MMPs.

The expression and secretion of PAs and PAIs during ovulation is induced in a cell-specific and time-coordinated manner by gonadotropins as demonstrated in several species such as rat [113], the mouse [114], the pig [115], and the rhesus monkey [116]. Thus, in rat, tPA expression in granulosa and theca-interstitial cells was induced by gonadotropins, and PAI-1 was up-regulated in the theca-interstitial cells and the surrounding stroma 6 h before follicular rupture [113]. By comparison, uPA, expressed by granulosa cells, appears to be the most abundant and most noticeably up-regulated PA during the ovulatory process in the mouse [114]. There was also a synchronized up-regulation of tPA in theca-interstitial tissue, also in the mouse [114]. Moreover, in the macaque monkey, high tPA expression in granulosa cells was seen during ovulation, and this was accompanied by a decline in theca-derived PAI-1, resulting in a shift in the balance of substrate and inhibitor, which may assist in the breakdown of the follicular wall [116]. The PA-system has not been extensively investigated during ovulation in the human. A limited number of studies have been performed on granulosa-lutein cells from IVF-cycles showing relative abundance of PAI, yet little or no PA [117, 118].

Even though a considerable body of indirect evidence obtained from different species has indicated that the PA-system plays a role in ovulation, studies on knockout (KO) mice with single deficiencies for either of the components of the PA system, as well as on tPA/uPA double deficient mice, have shown that these mice are fertile although the ovulation rate was reduced to some degree in the double KO mouse [119, 120]. Taken together, this indicates that the PA-system may be of less importance for follicular rupture, but at the same time, it is likely that a great redundancy has been built in this very important reproductive process, so that other pathways may be able to compensate for the deficiency of one pathway.

9.9.3 ADAMTS

The ADAMTS enzymes are functionally grouped according to their substrate specificity and today the family includes 19 members. Concerning the ovary, ADAMTS-1 has attracted most attention. It has clearly been shown that ADAMTS-1 expression is selectively induced by LH in mural and cumulus granulosa cells of the preovulatory follicle of the mouse [35], rat [121], and horse [122]. This upregulation of ADAMTS-1 is brought about by an effect on PR [25, 35]. Functionally associated family members such as ADAMTS-4 and ADAMTS-5 have been studied in the mouse ovary wherein ADAMTS-4 was induced by LH in mural and cumulus granulosa cells and ADAMTS-5 was expressed in granulosa cells of all healthy follicles [123].

It is known that ADAMTS-1 proteolytically can process large proteoglycans indicating a potential role in ECM turnover in the ovary during ovulation. The proteoglycan versican is synthesized by the mural granulosa cells and participates in the organization of the cumulus ECM by binding hyaluronic acid [124]. During ovulation, ADAMTS-1, mostly secreted by the mural granulosa cells, concentrate to the matrix of the expanding cumulus and cleave versican during this process [125]. Selective induction of ADAMTS-4 in theca cells by the LH surge may coordinate with ADAMTS-1 to cleave proteoglycans such as versican of the basal lamina prior to ovulation [123]. This ADAMTS-mediated versican cleavage may be required for matrix organization during the large expansion of the inter-cellular space of the cumulus-oocyte complexes, and in addition, ADAMTS-1 may modulate the release or efficacy of specific growth factors [126].

ADAMTS-1 null mice have exhibit markedly reduced ovulation rates and show oocytes retained within luteinised follicles [127] as well as follicle dysgenesis, ranging from focal disruption in ECM integrity to complete loss of follicular structure during folliculogenesis [128]. This subfertile phenotype is similar but not identical to the ovarian phenotype of PR-null mice [35]. This points towards that ADAMTS-1 partly mediates its biological functions via PR. Compensation in ADAMTS-1 null mice may be carried out by other components, such as ADAMTS-4 and ADAMTS-5, which also are expressed in granulosa cells and share enzymatic properties with ADAMTS-1 [129].

ADAMTS-1 is highly expressed in luteinized granulosa cells of the nonhuman primate ovary follicle [130], but its regulation is till date unknown. In the human ovary, ADAMTS-16 was shown to be expressed in the mural granulosa cells of preovulatory follicles and experiments with cultured granulosa-lutein cells revealed stimulation by FSH but not LH [131].

9.10 Immune Cells

Certain subtypes of immune cells are drawn into the preovulatory follicle as a consequence of the LH-induced changes in follicular gene-expression. These immune cells seem to be actively engaged in the changes that bring about follicular rupture since leukocyte supplementation increased the LH-induced ovulation rate in the perfused rat ovary [132].

There seems to be a selectivity in the accumulation of immune cells in the preovulatory follicle at ovulation. In rat ovary, predominantly macrophages and neutrophils are found in the theca layer of the follicle after the LH-surge [133]. Evidence for a functional role of macrophages in ovulation are that mice with extremely low monocyte/macrophage counts, because of a mutation within the macrophage-colony stimulating factor (M-CSF) gene, exhibit markedly reduced ovulation rate [134]. Likewise, administration of clondronate liposome or M-CSF neutralizing antibodies into the ovarian bursa of eCG/hCG primed rats, to deplete the ovary from macrophages, results in decreased ovulation rate [135]. Interactions between monocyte integrins and endothelial adhesion molecule -1

(ICAM-1) of the follicular microvasculature mediate firm adhesion of the monocytes and enable their migration between the endothelial cells into the ovary [136] and further differentiation into macrophages. A role for neutrophils in ovulation is suggested by that neutrophil-depletion from the peripheral blood decreases the ovulation rate in rat [137].

Several studies exist on the presence of leukocytes in the human ovary at ovulation. Studies on human follicular fluid of IVF patients revealed existence of a number of leukocyte subtypes in the fluid at different concentrations [138]. The number of leukocytes in human follicular fluid does not correlate to the numbers of erythrocytes in the fluid, implying that the leukocytes are selectively drawn into the follicle [138]. The most abundant leukocytes subtype in the human ovary seems to be the macrophage [139, 140]. A fairly large population of macrophages has been identified close to the capillaries in the stroma of the human ovary [141], and a raise in macrophage density in the tunica albuginea and the theca layer of the human follicle is seen just prior to ovulation [139]. Moreover, an increasing number of macrophages was seen in the perifollicular stroma during hCG-induced human ovulation of natural cycles from well defined ovulatory stages. Upon activation in the tissue, the macrophage produces an array of biologically active substances including ECM remodelling enzymes (see above) and cytokines (see in the following section).

9.11 Cytokines and Chemokines

Cytokines belong to a group of more than 100 proteins with a large number of overlapping functions to carry out autocrine/paracrine regulation of immune cells and also other type of cells. The family of cytokines includes members such as interleukins (IL), tumour necrosis factors (TNFs), interferons (IFNs), colony stimulating factors (CSFs), and chemokines.

Many cytokines have been linked to the ovulatory process by demonstrations of increased mRNA expression or protein levels within the ovary after an LH stimulus or by direct demonstrations of functional roles in ovulation. Most of these ovulation-associated cytokines are produced by the activated macrophage, and these cytokines are also expressed in granulosa and theca cells.

Interleukin-1 is a central regulator of ovulation as first demonstrated by that recombinant IL-1 potentiated the LH-induced ovulatory rate in the perfused rat ovary preparation [142]. In a similar in vitro system, the natural occurring IL-1 antagonist was shown to suppress ovulation [143]. This cytokine has effects on several pathways of the ovulatory cascade such as P synthesis [143], induction of gelatinases [91], and nitric oxide synthase activity [144]. The cytokine IL-1 is present human follicular fluid, albeit at fairly low concentrations [145]. The other major proinflammatory cytokine, TNF-α may also carry a functional role in ovulation since it induces ovulation in the perfused rat ovary [146] and intrafollicular injection of TNFα antiserum blocks ovulation in the sheep ovary [147]. This cytokine is also present in human follicular fluid and may have effects to stimulate cell proliferation and PG production [148].

The cytokine macrophage-CSF (M-CSF) increase the number of macrophages in rat ovary and as a consequence of this induce a higher ovulation rate [149]. In the same study, administration of an anti-M-CSF antibody inhibited ovulation. Another CSF with effects on macrophages is granulocyte-macrophage-CSF (GM-CSF), which is produced in large quantities at ovulation in rat [150]. Mice with gene deficiency in the GM-CSF gene exhibit similar ovulation rate as control animals, but the ovaries produce less P and contain fewer leukocytes [151]. The cytokine GM-CSF is present in human ovaries, and the levels in follicular fluid increases during hyperstimulation [152].

Cytokines, with mainly chemotactic activity on leukocyte populations, are named chemokines. Based on the position of their cysteine residues, the chemokines are divided into four subgroups (CC, CXC, C, and CXC3). The two major chemokine families are the CC-chemokines with activity towards monocytes/macrophages, basophils and T-cells and the CXC-chemokines with activity towards T-lymphocytes and neutrophils. Interleukin-8 and GROα are examples of chemokines that belong to the CXC-chemokine family. Monocyte chemotactic protein (MCP), monocyte inflammatory protein (MIP), and RANTES (regulated upon activation normal T-cell expresses and secreted) belong to the CC-chemokine family.

Chemokines act by binding to specific cell surface recptors that signal through G-binding proteins [153]. In the human, eight CC chemokine receptors (CCR) and 4 CXC chemokine receptors (CXCR) have been identified [153]. A concentration gradient of chemotaxis is maintained within the tissue by the clearance of chemokines from the circulation by the erythrocyte chemokine receptor DARC (Duffy antigen receptor for chemokines) and neutralization of the chemokines in ECM by binding to heparin sulphate and other proteoglycans. The net effect is a concentration gradient of chemokines in the tissue which ensures the leukocytes to migrate towards the chemotactic gradient [153]. The proinflammatory cytokines IL-1 and TNFα, are the main stimuli for chemokine production, but also interferon-γ (IFNγ) and IL-4 synergize with IL-1 and TNFα to stimulate chemokine secretion [153].

Several studies report chemokines to be upregulated during the ovulatory process. Thus, MCP-1, MCP-3, and GROα are induced in rat ovary during ovulation [154], and the CC-chemokine TECK (thymus expressed chemokine) shows a more than 100-fold induction in the mouse ovary 10–12 h after hCG [155].

In the human ovary, the chemokines IL-8 [156–159] and M-CSF [160] were found at significant concentrations. Concerning IL-8, the follicular fluid levels were more than tenfold higher at ovulation as compared to the follicular phase and gonadotropins stimulated human granulosa cells of natural cycles to IL-8 synthesis [158]. The CC-chemokine RANTES was detected in cultures of human granulosa cells and the proinflammatory cytokine TNFα potentiated RANTES production [161].

The chemokine which seems to be most essential for the intraovarian events of ovulation is MCP-1, which in the human consists of 76 amino acids [162]. This mediator is produced by a number of cell types, such as epithelial and endothelial cells, fibroblasts, chondrocytes and tumour cells, but the major source of MCP-1 is the monocyte/macrophage [163]. Expression of MCP-1 is stimulated by IL-1β, TNFα, M-CSF, and IFNγ, but production in the absence of stimuli has also been reported [164]. The receptor for MCP-1 is CCR2, which is expressed on monocytes, T-cells, natural killer cells, and basophils [153]. The major effect of MCP-1 is recruitment of circulating monocytes into different tissues, with secondary roles being stimulation of migration of T-lymphocytes, proliferation of vascular smooth muscle cells, cytotoxic activity of T/NK-cells as well as synthesis of proinflammatory cytokines by macrophages [165]. This latter activating effect of MCP-1 on monocytes/macrophages also involve induction of respiratory burst, expression of the β_2-integrins, and production of IL-1 and IL-6 [163]. Thus, this dual effect to attract and activate the macrophage may be important to allow early activation of an attracted macrophage at ovulation.

Much interest has been focused on the mechanisms behind the attraction of monocytes/macrophages into the preovulatory follicle during the inflammation-like ovulatory process. In an investigation of the expression patterns in the mouse ovary during the periovulatory interval, a substantial upregulation of MCP-1 was seen during ovulation [166]. In rat ovary, an 18-fold upregulation of MCP-1 was seen when the preovulatory levels were compared with the levels 6 h after administration of an ovulatory gonadotropin stimulus [154]. Concerning the human ovary, MCP-1 levels were found to be higher in follicular fluid of hyperstimulated IVF-cycles than in peripheral blood [167–169], indicating a substantial local production of this cytokine in the ovary. The concentrations of MCP-1 in human follicular fluid were markedly higher as compared to blood plasma in menstrual cycles [169], with a 3-fold difference during follicular phase and a 25-fold difference during the late ovulatory phase.

In vitro experiments with cultured human granulosa cells showed synthesis of MCP-1 with IL-1 and TNFα being stimulatory [167, 170]. The chemokine MCP-1 is also produced in other cellular compartments within the human follicle since MCP-1 mRNA levels were increased in the perifollicular stroma around the preovulatory follicle after an ovulatory injection of hCG had been given [171]. In the latter study, a large number of macrophages were seen at this site immediately outside the theca layer and the MCP-1 receptor (CCR2) were found in increasing concentrations as ovulation proceeded. It may well be that there is a requirement of high local concentrations of MCP-1 in the follicle for a full ovulatory response with oocyte maturation, degradation of the follicular apex, and luteinization, since a correlation exists between protein levels of MCP-1 in follicular fluid and the probability of a follicle containing a mature oocyte in IVF cycles. [170]

References

1. Lofman CO, Janson PO, Kallfelt BJ, Ahren K, LeMaire WJ (1982) The study of ovulation in the isolated perfused rabbit ovary. II. Photographic and cinematographic observation. Biol Reprod 26(3):467–473
2. Lofman CO, Brannstrom M, Holmes PV, Janson PO (1989) Ovulation in the isolated perfused rat ovary as documented by intravital microscopy. Steroids 54(5):481–490
3. Dahm-Kahler P, Lofman C, Fujii R, Axelsson M, Janson PO, Brannstrom M (2006) An intravital microscopy method permitting continuous long-term observations of ovulation in vivo in the rabbit. Hum Reprod 21(3):624–631
4. Shimada M, Nishibori M, Isobe N, Kawano N, Terada T (2003) Luteinizing hormone receptor formation in cumulus cells surrounding porcine oocytes and its role during meiotic maturation of porcine oocytes. Biol Reprod 68(4):1142–1149
5. Hillensjo T, Magnusson C, Svensson U, Thelander H (1981) Effect of luteinizing hormone and follicle-stimulating hormone on progesterone synthesis by cultured rat cumulus cells. Endocrinology 108(5):1920–1924
6. Tsafriri A, Lieberman ME, Koch Y et al (1976) Capacity of immunologically purified FSH to stimulate cyclic AMP accumulation and steroidogenesis in Graafian follicles and to induce ovum maturation and ovulation in the rat. Endocrinology 98(3):655–661
7. Sogn JH, Curry TE Jr, Brannstrom M et al (1987) Inhibition of follicle-stimulating hormone-induced ovulation by indomethacin in the perfused rat ovary. Biol Reprod 36(3):536–542
8. Peng XR, Hsueh AJ, LaPolt PS, Bjersing L, Ny T (1991) Localization of luteinizing hormone receptor messenger ribonucleic acid expression in ovarian cell types during follicle development and ovulation. Endocrinology 129(6):3200–3207
9. Rao CV, Lei ZM (2002) Consequences of targeted inactivation of LH receptors. Mol Cell Endocrinol 187(1–2):57–67
10. Couse JF, Yates MM, Deroo BJ, Korach KS (2005) Estrogen receptor-beta is critical to granulosa cell differentiation and the ovulatory response to gonadotropins. Endocrinology 146(8):3247–3262
11. Russell DL, Doyle KM, Gonzales-Robayna I, Pipaon C, Richards JS (2003) Egr-1 induction in rat granulosa cells by follicle-stimulating hormone and luteinizing hormone: combinatorial regulation by transcription factors cyclic adenosine 3′, 5′-monophosphate regulatory element binding protein, serum response factor, sp1, and early growth response factor-1. Mol Endocrinol 17(4): 520–533
12. Maizels ET, Mukherjee A, Sithanandam G et al (2001) Developmental regulation of mitogen-activated protein kinase-

activated kinases-2 and -3 (MAPKAPK-2/-3) in vivo during corpus luteum formation in the rat. Mol Endocrinol 15(5):716–733
13. Das S, Maizels ET, DeManno D, St Clair E, Adam SA, Hunzicker-Dunn M (1996) A stimulatory role of cyclic adenosine 3′, 5′-monophosphate in follicle-stimulating hormone-activated mitogen-activated protein kinase signaling pathway in rat ovarian granulosa cells. Endocrinology 137(3):967–974
14. Davis JS, West LA, Farese RV (1984) Effects of luteinizing hormone on phosphoinositide metabolism in rat granulosa cells. J Biol Chem 259(24):15028–15034
15. Gudermann T, Birnbaumer M, Birnbaumer L (1992) Evidence for dual coupling of the murine luteinizing hormone receptor to adenylyl cyclase and phosphoinositide breakdown and Ca^{2+} mobilization. Studies with the cloned murine luteinizing hormone receptor expressed in L cells. J Biol Chem 267(7):4479–4488
16. Tanaka N, Espey LL, Kawano T, Okamura H (1991) Comparison of inhibitory actions of indomethacin and epostane on ovulation in rats. Am J Physiol 260(2 Pt 1):E170–E174
17. Andersen AG, Als-Nielsen B, Hornnes PJ, Franch Andersen L (1995) Time interval from human chorionic gonadotrophin (HCG) injection to follicular rupture. Hum Reprod 10(12):3202–3205
18. Stouffer RL, Zelinski-Wooten MB (2004) Overriding follicle selection in controlled ovarian stimulation protocols: quality vs. quantity. Reprod Biol Endocrinol 2:32
19. Sharma SC, Richards JS (2000) Regulation of AP1 (Jun/Fos) factor expression and activation in ovarian granulosa cells. Relation of JunD and Fra2 to terminal differentiation. J Biol Chem 275(43):33718–33728
20. Tullet JM, Pocock V, Steel JH, White R, Milligan S, Parker MG (2005) Multiple signaling defects in the absence of RIP140 impair both cumulus expansion and follicle rupture. Endocrinology 146(9):4127–4137
21. White R, Leonardsson G, Rosewell I, Ann Jacobs M, Milligan S, Parker M (2000) The nuclear receptor co-repressor nrip1 (RIP140) is essential for female fertility. Nat Med 6(12):1368–1374
22. Pall M, Hellberg P, Brannstrom M et al (1997) The transcription factor C/EBP-beta and its role in ovarian function; evidence for direct involvement in the ovulatory process. EMBO J 16(17):5273–5279
23. Jo M, Curry TE Jr (2006) Luteinizing hormone-induced RUNX1 regulates the expression of genes in granulosa cells of rat periovulatory follicles. Mol Endocrinol 20(9):2156–2172
24. Sriraman V, Sharma SC, Richards JS (2003) Transactivation of the progesterone receptor gene in granulosa cells: evidence that Sp1/Sp3 binding sites in the proximal promoter play a key role in luteinizing hormone inducibility. Mol Endocrinol 17(3):436–449
25. Doyle KM, Russell DL, Sriraman V, Richards JS (2004) Coordinate transcription of the ADAMTS-1 gene by luteinizing hormone and progesterone receptor. Mol Endocrinol 18(10):2463–2478
26. Natraj U, Richards JS (1993) Hormonal regulation, localization, and functional activity of the progesterone receptor in granulosa cells of rat preovulatory follicles. Endocrinology 133(2):761–769
27. Conneely OM, Mulac-Jericevic B, Lydon JP, De Mayo FJ (2001) Reproductive functions of the progesterone receptor isoforms: lessons from knock-out mice. Mol Cell Endocrinol 179(1–2):97–103
28. Duffy DM, Wells TR, Haluska GJ, Stouffer RL (1997) The ratio of progesterone receptor isoforms changes in the monkey corpus luteum during the luteal phase of the menstrual cycle. Biol Reprod 57(4):693–699
29. Stouffer RL (2003) Progesterone as a mediator of gonadotrophin action in the corpus luteum: beyond steroidogenesis. Hum Reprod Update 9(2):99–117
30. Mori T, Suzuki A, Nishimura T, Kambegawa A (1977) Inhibition of ovulation in immature rats by anti-progesterone antiserum. J Endocrinol 73(1):185–186
31. Brannstrom M, Janson PO (1989) Progesterone is a mediator in the ovulatory process of the in vitro perfused rat ovary. Biol Reprod 40:1170–1178
32. Brannstrom M (1993) Inhibitory effect of mifepristone (RU 486) on ovulation in the isolated perfused rat ovary. Contraception 48(4):393–402
33. Lydon JP, DeMayo FJ, Funk CR et al (1995) Mice lacking progesterone receptor exhibit pleiotropic reproductive abnormalities. Genes Dev 9(18):2266–2278
34. Mulac-Jericevic B, Conneely OM (2004) Reproductive tissue selective actions of progesterone receptors. Reproduction 128(2):139–146
35. Robker RL, Russell DL, Espey LL, Lydon JP, O'Malley BW, Richards JS (2000) Progesterone-regulated genes in the ovulation process: ADAMTS-1 and cathepsin L proteases. Proc Natl Acad Sci USA 97(9):4689–4694
36. Shimada M, Hernandez-Gonzalez I, Gonzalez-Robayna I, Richards JS (2006) Paracrine and autocrine regulation of epidermal growth factor-like factors in cumulus oocyte complexes and granulosa cells: key roles for prostaglandin synthase 2 and progesterone receptor. Mol Endocrinol 20(6):1352–1365
37. Hibbert ML, Stouffer RL, Wolf DP, Zelinski-Wooten MB (1996) Midcycle administration of a progesterone synthesis inhibitor prevents ovulation in primates. Proc Natl Acad Sci USA 93(5):1897–1901
38. Tjugum J, Dennefors B, Norstrom A (1984) Influence of progesterone, androstenedione and oestradiol-17 beta on the incorporation of [3H]proline in the human follicular wall. Acta Endocrinol (Copenh) 105(4):552–557
39. Armstrong DT (1981) Prostaglandins and follicular functions. J Reprod Fertil 62(1):283–291
40. Morris JK, Richards JS (1995) Luteinizing hormone induces prostaglandin endoperoxide synthase-2 and luteinization in vitro by A-kinase and C-kinase pathways. Endocrinology 136(4): 1549–1558
41. Bauminger A, Lindner HR (1975) Periovulatory changes in ovarian prostaglandin formation and their hormonal control in the rat. Prostaglandins 9(5):737–751
42. LeMaire WJ, Leidner R, Marsh JM (1975) Pre and post ovulatory changes in the concentration of prostaglandins in rat graafian follicles. Prostaglandins 9(2):221–229
43. Mikuni M, Pall M, Peterson CM et al (1998) The selective prostaglandin endoperoxide synthase-2 inhibitor, NS-398, reduces prostaglandin production and ovulation in vivo and in vitro in the rat. Biol Reprod 59(5):1077–1083
44. Davis BJ, Lennard DE, Lee CA et al (1999) Anovulation in cyclooxygenase-2-deficient mice is restored by prostaglandin E2 and interleukin-1beta. Endocrinology 140(6):2685–2695
45. Langenbach R, Morham SG, Tiano HF et al (1995) Prostaglandin synthase 1 gene disruption in mice reduces arachidonic acid-induced inflammation and indomethacin-induced gastric ulceration. Cell 83(3):483–492
46. Segi E, Haraguchi K, Sugimoto Y et al (2003) Expression of messenger RNA for prostaglandin E receptor subtypes EP4/EP2 and cyclooxygenase isozymes in mouse periovulatory follicles and oviducts during superovulation. Biol Reprod 68(3):804–811
47. Takahashi T, Morrow JD, Wang H, Dey SK (2006) Cyclooxygenase-2-derived prostaglandin E(2) directs oocyte maturation by differentially influencing multiple signaling pathways. J Biol Chem 281(48):37117–37129
48. Duffy DM, Stouffer RL (2001) The ovulatory gonadotrophin surge stimulates cyclooxygenase expression and prostaglandin production by the monkey follicle. Mol Hum Reprod 7(8):731–739
49. Duffy DM, Seachord CL, Dozier BL (2005) An ovulatory gonadotropin stimulus increases cytosolic phospholipase A2 expression and activity in granulosa cells of primate periovulatory follicles. J Clin Endocrinol Metab 90(10):5858–5865

50. Killick S, Elstein M (1987) Pharmacologic production of luteinized unruptured follicles by prostaglandin synthetase inhibitors. Fertil Steril 47(5):773–777
51. Pall M, Friden BE, Brannstrom M (2001) Induction of delayed follicular rupture in the human by the selective COX-2 inhibitor rofecoxib: a randomized double-blind study. Hum Reprod 16(7):1323–1328
52. Chandras C, Ragoobir J, Barrett GE et al (2004) Roles for prostaglandins in the steroidogenic response of human granulosa cells to high-density lipoproteins. Mol Cell Endocrinol 222(1–2):1–8
53. Harris TE, Squires PE, Michael AE, Bernal AL, Abayasekara DR (2001) Human granulosa-lutein cells express functional EP1 and EP2 prostaglandin receptors. Biochem Biophys Res Commun 285(5):1089–1094
54. Higuchi Y, Yoshimura T, Tanaka N, Ogino H, Sumiyama M, Kawakami S (1995) Different time-course production of peptidic and nonpeptidic leukotrienes and prostaglandins E2 and F2 alpha in the ovary during ovulation in gonadotropin-primed immature rats. Prostaglandins 49(3):131–140
55. Mikuni M, Yoshida M, Hellberg P et al (1998) The lipoxygenase inhibitor, nordihydroguaiaretic acid, inhibits ovulation and reduces leukotriene and prostaglandin levels in the rat ovary. Biol Reprod 58(5):1211–1216
56. Matousek M, Mitsube K, Mikuni M, Brannstrom M (2001) Inhibition of ovulation in the rat by a leukotriene B(4) receptor antagonist. Mol Hum Reprod 7(1):35–42
57. Janson PO (1975) Effects of the luteinizing hormone on blood flow in the follicular rabbit ovary, as measured by radioactive microspheres. Acta Endocrinol (Copenh) 79(1):122–133
58. Brannstrom M, Zackrisson U, Hagstrom HG et al (1998) Preovulatory changes of blood flow in different regions of the human follicle. Fertil Steril 69(3):435–442
59. Abisogun AO, Daphna-Iken D, Reich R, Kranzfelder D, Tsafriri A (1988) Modulatory role of eicosanoids in vascular changes during the preovulatory period in the rat. Biol Reprod 38(4): 756–762
60. Gerdes U, Gafvels M, Bergh A, Cajander S (1992) Localized increases in ovarian vascular permeability and leucocyte accumulation after induced ovulation in rabbits. J Reprod Fertil 95(2):539–550
61. Murakami T, Ikebuchi Y, Ohtsuka A, Kikuta A, Taguchi T, Ohtani O (1988) The blood vascular wreath of rat ovarian follicle, with special reference to its changes in ovulation and luteinization: a scanning electron microscopic study of corrosion casts. Arch Histol Cytol 51(4):299–313
62. Mitsube K, Mikuni M, Matousek M, Brannstrom M (1999) Effects of a nitric oxide donor and nitric oxide synthase inhibitors on luteinizing hormone-induced ovulation in the ex-vivo perfused rat ovary. Hum Reprod 14(10):2537–2543
63. Mitsube K, Zackrisson U, Brannstrom M (2002) Nitric oxide regulates ovarian blood flow in the rat during the periovulatory period. Hum Reprod 17(10):2509–2516
64. Mitsube K, Mikuni M, Matousek M, Zackrisson U, Brannstrom M (2003) Role of the angiotensin II system in regulation of ovulation and blood flow in the rat ovary. Reproduction 125(3):425–435
65. Xu F, Hazzard TM, Evans A, Charnock-Jones S, Smith S, Stouffer RL (2005) Intraovarian actions of anti-angiogenic agents disrupt periovulatory events during the menstrual cycle in monkeys. Contraception 71(4):239–248
66. Ko C, Gieske MC, Al-Alem L et al (2006) Endothelin-2 in ovarian follicle rupture. Endocrinology 147(4):1770–1779
67. Park JY, Su YQ, Ariga M, Law E, Jin SL, Conti M (2004) EGF-like growth factors as mediators of LH action in the ovulatory follicle. Science 303(5658):682–684
68. Ashkenazi H, Cao X, Motola S, Popliker M, Conti M, Tsafriri A (2005) Epidermal growth factor family members: endogenous mediators of the ovulatory response. Endocrinology 146(1):77–84
69. Freimann S, Ben-Ami I, Dantes A, Ron-El R, Amsterdam A (2004) EGF-like factor epiregulin and amphiregulin expression is regulated by gonadotropins/cAMP in human ovarian follicular cells. Biochem Biophys Res Commun 324(2): 829–834
70. Lind AK, Weijdegard B, Dahm-Kahler P, Molne J, Sundfeldt K, Brannstrom M (2006) Collagens in the human ovary and their changes in the perifollicular stroma during ovulation. Acta Obstet Gynecol Scand 85(12):1476–1484
71. Matousek M, Carati C, Gannon B, Brannstrom M (2001) Novel method for intrafollicular pressure measurements in the rat ovary: increased intrafollicular pressure after hCG stimulation. Reproduction 121(2):307–314
72. Ny T, Wahlberg P, Brandstrom IJ (2002) Matrix remodeling in the ovary: regulation and functional role of the plasminogen activator and matrix metalloproteinase systems. Mol Cell Endocrinol 187(1–2):29–38
73. Smith MF, Ricke WA, Bakke LJ, Dow MP, Smith GW (2002) Ovarian tissue remodeling: role of matrix metalloproteinases and their inhibitors. Mol Cell Endocrinol 191(1):45–56
74. Curry TE Jr, Osteen KG (2003) The matrix metalloproteinase system: changes, regulation, and impact throughout the ovarian and uterine reproductive cycle. Endocr Rev 24(4):428–465
75. Goldman S, Shalev E (2003) The role of the matrix metalloproteinases in human endometrial and ovarian cycles. Eur J Obstet Gynecol Reprod Biol 111(2):109–121
76. Curry TE Jr, Smith MF (2006) Impact of extracellular matrix remodeling on ovulation and the folliculo-luteal transition. Semin Reprod Med 24(4):228–241
77. Liu YX (2004) Plasminogen activator/plasminogen activator inhibitors in ovarian physiology. Front Biosci 9:3356–3373
78. Sternlicht MD, Werb Z (2001) How matrix metalloproteinases regulate cell behavior. Annu Rev Cell Dev Biol 17:463–516
79. Somerville RP, Oblander SA, Apte SS (2003) Matrix metalloproteinases: old dogs with new tricks. Genome Biol 4(6):216
80. Birkedal-Hansen H, Moore WG, Bodden MK et al (1993) Matrix metalloproteinases: a review. Crit Rev Oral Biol Med 4(2):197–250
81. Visse R, Nagase H (2003) Matrix metalloproteinases and tissue inhibitors of metalloproteinases: structure, function, and biochemistry. Circ Res 92(8):827–839
82. Brew K, Dinakarpandian D, Nagase H (2000) Tissue inhibitors of metalloproteinases: evolution, structure and function. Biochim Biophys Acta 1477(1–2):267–283
83. Gomez DE, Alonso DF, Yoshiji H, Thorgeirsson UP (1997) Tissue inhibitors of metalloproteinases: structure, regulation and biological functions. Eur J Cell Biol 74(2):111–122
84. Lambert E, Dasse E, Haye B, Petitfrere E (2004) TIMPs as multifacial proteins. Crit Rev Oncol Hematol 49(3):187–198
85. Woessner JF, Nagase H (2000) Matrix metalloproteinases and TIMPs. Oxford University Press, New York
86. Reich R, Tsafriri A, Mechanic GL (1985) The involvement of collagenolysis in ovulation in the rat. Endocrinology 116(2):522–527
87. Brannstrom M, Woessner JF Jr, Koos RD, Sear CH, LeMaire WJ (1988) Inhibitors of mammalian tissue collagenase and metalloproteinases suppress ovulation in the perfused rat ovary. Endocrinology 122(5):1715–1721
88. Curry TE, Komar CM, Burns PD, Nothnick WB (2000) Periovulatory changes in ovarian metalloproteinases and tissue inhibitors of metalloproteinases (TIMPS) following indomethacin treatment. In: Adashi EY, Serono Symposia USA (eds) Ovulation: evolving scientific and clinical concepts. Springer, New York, pp 265–276

89. Hagglund AC, Ny A, Leonardsson G, Ny T (1999) Regulation and localization of matrix metalloproteinases and tissue inhibitors of metalloproteinases in the mouse ovary during gonadotropin-induced ovulation. Endocrinology 140(9):4351–4358
90. Vu TH, Shipley JM, Bergers G et al (1998) MMP-9/gelatinase B is a key regulator of growth plate angiogenesis and apoptosis of hypertrophic chondrocytes. Cell 93(3):411–422
91. Hurwitz A, Dushnik M, Solomon H et al (1993) Cytokine-mediated regulation of rat ovarian function: interleukin-1 stimulates the accumulation of a 92-kilodalton gelatinase. Endocrinology 132(6):2709–2714
92. Hurwitz A, Finci-Yeheskel Z, Dushnik M et al (1995) Interleukin-1-mediated regulation of plasminogen activation in pregnant mare serum gonadotropin-primed rat granulosa cells is independent of prostaglandin production. J Soc Gynecol Investig 2(5):691–699
93. Curry TE Jr, Song L, Wheeler SE (2001) Cellular localization of gelatinases and tissue inhibitors of metalloproteinases during follicular growth, ovulation, and early luteal formation in the rat. Biol Reprod 65(3):855–865
94. Inderdeo DS, Edwards DR, Han VK, Khokha R (1996) Temporal and spatial expression of tissue inhibitors of metalloproteinases during the natural ovulatory cycle of the mouse. Biol Reprod 55(3):498–508
95. Mann JS, Kindy MS, Edwards DR, Curry TE Jr (1991) Hormonal regulation of matrix metalloproteinase inhibitors in rat granulosa cells and ovaries. Endocrinology 128(4):1825–1832
96. Chun SY, Popliker M, Reich R, Tsafriri A (1992) Localization of preovulatory expression of plasminogen activator inhibitor type-1 and tissue inhibitor of metalloproteinase type-1 mRNAs in the rat ovary. Biol Reprod 47(2):245–253
97. Curry TE Jr, Komar CM, Burns PD, Nothnick WB (2000) Periovulatory changes in ovarian metalloproteinases and tissue inhibitors of metalloproteinases (TIMPS) following indomethacin treatment. In: Adashi EY (ed) Ovulation: evolving scientific and clinical concepts. Springer-Verlag, New York
98. Nothnick WB, Soloway P, Curry TE Jr (1997) Assessment of the role of tissue inhibitor of metalloproteinase-1 (TIMP-1) during the periovulatory period in female mice lacking a functional TIMP-1 gene. Biol Reprod 56(5):1181–1188
99. Boujrad N, Ogwuegbu SO, Garnier M, Lee CH, Martin BM, Papadopoulos V (1995) Identification of a stimulator of steroid hormone synthesis isolated from testis. Science 268(5217): 1609–1612
100. Nothnick WB (2003) Tissue inhibitor of metalloproteinase-1 (TIMP-1) deficient mice display reduced serum progesterone levels during corpus luteum development. Endocrinology 144(1):5–8
101. Strongin AY, Collier I, Bannikov G, Marmer BL, Grant GA, Goldberg GI (1995) Mechanism of cell surface activation of 72-kDa type IV collagenase. Isolation of the activated form of the membrane metalloprotease. J Biol Chem 270(10):5331–5338
102. Jo M, Thomas LE, Wheeler SE, Curry TE Jr (2004) Membrane type 1-matrix metalloproteinase (MMP)-associated MMP-2 activation increases in the rat ovary in response to an ovulatory dose of human chorionic gonadotropin. Biol Reprod 70(4):1024–1032
103. Chaffin CL, Stouffer RL (1999) Expression of matrix metalloproteinases and their tissue inhibitor messenger ribonucleic acids in macaque periovulatory granulosa cells: time course and steroid regulation. Biol Reprod 61(1):14–21
104. Young KA, Hennebold JD, Stouffer RL (2002) Dynamic expression of mRNAs and proteins for matrix metalloproteinases and their tissue inhibitors in the primate corpus luteum during the menstrual cycle. Mol Hum Reprod 8(9):833–840
105. Duffy DM, Stouffer RL (2003) Luteinizing hormone acts directly at granulosa cells to stimulate periovulatory processes: modulation of luteinizing hormone effects by prostaglandins. Endocrine 22(3):249–256
106. Puistola U, Salo T, Martikainen H, Ronnberg L (1986) Type IV collagenolytic activity in human preovulatory follicular fluid. Fertil Steril 45(4):578–580
107. Postawski K, Rechberger T, Jakimiuk AJ, Skorupski P, Bogusiewicz M, Jakowicki JA (1999) Interstitial collagenase (MMP-1) activity in human ovarian tissue. Gynecol Endocrinol 13(4):273–278
108. Lind AK, Dahm-Kahler P, Weijdegard B, Sundfeldt And K, Brannstrom M (2006) Gelatinases and their tissue inhibitors during human ovulation: increased expression of tissue inhibitor of matrix metalloproteinase-1. Mol Hum Reprod 12(12):725–736
109. Curry TE Jr, Mann JS, Estes RS, Jones PB (1990) Alpha 2-macroglobulin and tissue inhibitor of metalloproteinases: collagenase inhibitors in human preovulatory ovaries. Endocrinology 127(1):63–68
110. D'Ascenzo S, Giusti I, Millimaggi D et al (2004) Intrafollicular expression of matrix metalloproteinases and their inhibitors in normally ovulating women compared with patients undergoing in vitro fertilization treatment. Eur J Endocrinol 151(1):87–91
111. Ben-Shlomo I, Goldman S, Shalev E (2003) Regulation of matrix metalloproteinase-9 (MMP-9), tissue inhibitor of MMP, and progesterone secretion in luteinized granulosa cells from normally ovulating women with polycystic ovary disease. Fertil Steril 79(Suppl 1):694–701
112. Myohanen H, Vaheri A (2004) Regulation and interactions in the activation of cell-associated plasminogen. Cell Mol Life Sci 61(22):2840–2858
113. Peng XR, Hsueh AJ, Ny T (1993) Transient and cell-specific expression of tissue-type plasminogen activator and plasminogen-activator-inhibitor type 1 results in controlled and directed proteolysis during gonadotropin-induced ovulation. Eur J Biochem 214(1):147–156
114. Hagglund AC, Ny A, Liu K, Ny T (1996) Coordinated and cell-specific induction of both physiological plasminogen activators creates functionally redundant mechanisms for plasmin formation during ovulation. Endocrinology 137(12):5671–5677
115. Politis I, Srikandakumar A, Turner JD, Tsang BK, Ainsworth L, Downey BR (1990) Changes in and partial identification of the plasminogen activator and plasminogen activator inhibitor systems during ovarian follicular maturation in the pig. Biol Reprod 43(4):636–642
116. Liu YX, Liu K, Feng Q et al (2004) Tissue-type plasminogen activator and its inhibitor plasminogen activator inhibitor type 1 are coordinately expressed during ovulation in the rhesus monkey. Endocrinology 145(4):1767–1775
117. Jones PB, Muse KN, Wilson EA, Curry TE Jr (1988) Expression of plasminogen activator (PA) and a PA inhibitor in human granulosa cells from preovulatory follicles. J Clin Endocrinol Metab 67(4):857–860
118. Jones PB, Vernon MW, Muse KN, Curry TE Jr (1989) Plasminogen activator and plasminogen activator inhibitor in human preovulatory follicular fluid. J Clin Endocrinol Metab 68(6):1039–1045
119. Leonardsson G, Peng XR, Liu K et al (1995) Ovulation efficiency is reduced in mice that lack plasminogen activator gene function: functional redundancy among physiological plasminogen activators. Proc Natl Acad Sci USA 92(26):12446–12450
120. Ny A, Leonardsson G, Hagglund AC et al (1999) Ovulation in plasminogen-deficient mice. Endocrinology 140(11):5030–5035
121. Espey LL, Yoshioka S, Russell DL, Robker RL, Fujii S, Richards JS (2000) Ovarian expression of a disintegrin and metalloproteinase with thrombospondin motifs during ovulation in the gonadotropin-primed immature rat. Biol Reprod 62(4):1090–1095
122. Boerboom D, Russell DL, Richards JS, Sirois J (2003) Regulation of transcripts encoding ADAMTS-1 (a disintegrin and metalloproteinase with thrombospondin-like motifs-1) and progesterone

receptor by human chorionic gonadotropin in equine preovulatory follicles. J Mol Endocrinol 31(3):473–485
123. Richards JS, Hernandez-Gonzalez I, Gonzalez-Robayna I et al (2005) Regulated expression of ADAMTS family members in follicles and cumulus oocyte complexes: evidence for specific and redundant patterns during ovulation. Biol Reprod 72(5):1241–1255
124. Russell DL, Ochsner SA, Hsieh M, Mulders S, Richards JS (2003) Hormone-regulated expression and localization of versican in the rodent ovary. Endocrinology 144(3):1020–1031
125. Russell DL, Doyle KM, Ochsner SA, Sandy JD, Richards JS (2003) Processing and localization of ADAMTS-1 and proteolytic cleavage of versican during cumulus matrix expansion and ovulation. J Biol Chem 278(43):42330–42339
126. Park PW, Reizes O, Bernfield M (2000) Cell surface heparan sulfate proteoglycans: selective regulators of ligand-receptor encounters. J Biol Chem 275(39):29923–29926
127. Mittaz L, Russell DL, Wilson T et al (2004) Adamts-1 is essential for the development and function of the urogenital system. Biol Reprod 70(4):1096–1105
128. Brown HM, Dunning KR, Robker RL, Pritchard M, Russell DL (2006) Requirement for ADAMTS-1 in extracellular matrix remodeling during ovarian folliculogenesis and lymphangiogenesis. Dev Biol 300(2):699–709
129. Ohnishi J, Ohnishi E, Shibuya H, Takahashi T (2005) Functions for proteinases in the ovulatory process. Biochim Biophys Acta 1751(1):95–109
130. Young KA, Tumlinson B, Stouffer RL (2004) ADAMTS-1/METH-1 and TIMP-3 expression in the primate corpus luteum: divergent patterns and stage-dependent regulation during the natural menstrual cycle. Mol Hum Reprod 10(8):559–565
131. Gao S, De Geyter C, Kossowska K, Zhang H (2007) FSH stimulates the expression of the ADAMTS-16 protease in mature human ovarian follicles. Mol Hum Reprod 13(7):465–471
132. Hellberg P, Thomsen P, Janson PO, Brannstrom M (1991) Leukocyte supplementation increases the luteinizing hormone-induced ovulation rate in the in vitro-perfused rat ovary. Biol Reprod 44(5):791–797
133. Brannstrom M, Mayrhofer G, Robertson SA (1993) Localization of leukocyte subsets in the rat ovary during the periovulatory period. Biol Reprod 48(2):277–286
134. Cohen PE, Zhu L, Pollard JW (1997) Absence of colony stimulating factor-1 in osteopetrotic (csfmop/csfmop) mice disrupts estrous cycles and ovulation. Biol Reprod 56(1):110–118
135. Van der Hoek KH, Maddocks S, Woodhouse CM, van Rooijen N, Robertson SA, Norman RJ (2000) Intrabursal injection of clodronate liposomes causes macrophage depletion and inhibits ovulation in the mouse ovary. Biol Reprod 62(4):1059–1066
136. Wu R, Van der Hoek KH, Ryan NK, Norman RJ, Robker RL (2004) Macrophage contributions to ovarian function. Hum Reprod Update 10(2):119–133
137. Brannstrom M, Bonello N, Norman RJ, Robertson SA (1995) Reduction of ovulation rate in the rat by administration of a neutrophil-depleting monoclonal antibody. J Reprod Immunol 29(3):265–270
138. Smith MP, Flannery GR, Randle BJ, Jenkins JM, Holmes CH (2005) Leukocyte origin and profile in follicular aspirates at oocyte retrieval. Hum Reprod 20(12):3526–3531
139. Brannstrom M, Pascoe V, Norman RJ, McClure N (1994) Localization of leukocyte subsets in the follicle wall and in the corpus luteum throughout the human menstrual cycle. Fertil Steril 61(3):488–495
140. Best CL, Pudney J, Welch WR, Burger N, Hill JA (1996) Localization and characterization of white blood cell populations within the human ovary throughout the menstrual cycle and menopause. Hum Reprod 11(4):790–797
141. Takaya R, Fukaya T, Sasano H, Suzuki T, Tamura M, Yajima A (1997) Macrophages in normal cycling human ovaries; immunohistochemical localization and characterization. Hum Reprod 12(7):1508–1512
142. Brannstrom M, Wang L, Norman RJ (1993) Ovulatory effect of interleukin-1 beta on the perfused rat ovary. Endocrinology 132(1):399–404
143. Peterson CM, Hales HA, Hatasaka HH, Mitchell MD, Rittenhouse L, Jones KP (1993) Interleukin-1 beta (IL-1 beta) modulates prostaglandin production and the natural IL-1 receptor antagonist inhibits ovulation in the optimally stimulated rat ovarian perfusion model. Endocrinology 133(5):2301–2306
144. Ellman C, Corbett JA, Misko TP, McDaniel M, Beckerman KP (1993) Nitric oxide mediates interleukin-1-induced cellular cytotoxicity in the rat ovary. A potential role for nitric oxide in the ovulatory process. J Clin Invest 92(6):3053–3056
145. Wang LJ, Norman RJ (1992) Concentrations of immunoreactive interleukin-1 and interleukin-2 in human preovulatory follicular fluid. Hum Reprod 7(2):147–150
146. Brannstrom M, Bonello N, Wang LJ, Norman RJ (1995) Effects of tumour necrosis factor alpha (TNF alpha) on ovulation in the rat ovary. Reprod Fertil Dev 7(1):67–73
147. Gottsch ML, Van Kirk EA, Murdoch WJ (2000) Tumour necrosis factor alpha up-regulates matrix metalloproteinase-2 activity in periovulatory ovine follicles: metamorphic and endocrine implications. Reprod Fertil Dev 12(1–2):75–80
148. Wang LJ, Brannstrom M, Robertson SA, Norman RJ (1992) Tumor necrosis factor alpha in the human ovary: presence in follicular fluid and effects on cell proliferation and prostaglandin production. Fertil Steril 58(5):934–940
149. Nishimura K, Tanaka N, Ohshige A, Fukumatsu Y, Matsuura K, Okamura H (1995) Effects of macrophage colony-stimulating factor on folliculogenesis in gonadotrophin-primed immature rats. J Reprod Fertil 104(2):325–330
150. Brannstrom M, Norman RJ, Seamark RF, Robertson SA (1994) Rat ovary produces cytokines during ovulation. Biol Reprod 50(1):88–94
151. Jasper MJ, Robertson SA, Van der Hoek KH, Bonello N, Brannstrom M, Norman RJ (2000) Characterization of ovarian function in granulocyte-macrophage colony-stimulating factor-deficient mice. Biol Reprod 62(3):704–713
152. Jasper MJ, Brannstrom M, Olofsson JI et al (1996) Granulocyte-macrophage colony-stimulating factor: presence in human follicular fluid, protein secretion and mRNA expression by ovarian cells. Mol Hum Reprod 2(8):555–562
153. Luster AD (1998) Chemokines–chemotactic cytokines that mediate inflammation. N Engl J Med 338(7):436–445
154. Wong KH, Negishi H, Adashi EY (2002) Expression, hormonal regulation, and cyclic variation of chemokines in the rat ovary: key determinants of the intraovarian residence of representatives of the white blood cell series. Endocrinology 143(3):784–791
155. Zhou C, Wu J, Borillo J et al (2005) Transient expression of CC chemokine TECK in the ovary during ovulation: its potential role in ovulation. Am J Reprod Immunol 53(5):238–248
156. Arici A, Oral E, Bukulmez O, Buradagunta S, Engin O, Olive DL (1996) Interleukin-8 expression and modulation in human preovulatory follicles and ovarian cells. Endocrinology 137(9):3762–3769
157. Runesson E, Bostrom EK, Janson PO, Brannstrom M (1996) The human preovulatory follicle is a source of the chemotactic cytokine interleukin-8. Mol Hum Reprod 2(4):245–250
158. Runesson E, Ivarsson K, Janson PO, Brannstrom M (2000) Gonadotropin- and cytokine-regulated expression of the chemokine interleukin 8 in the human preovulatory follicle of the menstrual cycle. J Clin Endocrinol Metab 85(11):4387–4395
159. Buscher U, Chen FC, Kentenich H, Schmiady H (1999) Cytokines in the follicular fluid of stimulated and non-stimulated human

ovaries; is ovulation a suppressed inflammatory reaction? Hum Reprod 14(1):162–166
160. Shinetugs B, Runesson E, Bonello NP, Brannstrom M, Norman RJ (1999) Colony stimulating factor-1 concentrations in blood and follicular fluid during the human menstrual cycle and ovarian stimulation: possible role in the ovulatory process. Hum Reprod 14(5):1302–1306
161. Machelon V, Nome F, Emilie D (2000) Regulated on activation normal T expressed and secreted chemokine is induced by tumor necrosis factor-alpha in granulosa cells from human preovulatory follicle. J Clin Endocrinol Metab 85(1):417–424
162. Callard R, Gearing A (1994) The Cytokine. Academic Press Limited, London, Great Britain
163. Baggiolini M, Dewald B, Moser B (1994) Interleukin-8 and related chemotactic cytokines–CXC and CC chemokines. Adv Immunol 55:97–179
164. Cushing SD, Fogelman AM (1992) Monocytes may amplify their recruitment into inflammatory lesions by inducing monocyte chemotactic protein. Arterioscler Thromb 12(1):78–82
165. Arefieva TI, Kukhtina NB, Antonova OA, Krasnikova TL (2005) MCP-1-stimulated chemotaxis of monocytic and endothelial cells is dependent on activation of different signaling cascades. Cytokine 31(6):439–446
166. Zhou C, Borillo J, Wu J, Torres L, Lou YH (2004) Ovarian expression of chemokines and their receptors. J Reprod Immunol 63(1):1–9
167. Arici A, Oral E, Bukulmez O, Buradagunta S, Bahtiyar O, Jones EE (1997) Monocyte chemotactic protein-1 expression in human preovulatory follicles and ovarian cells. J Reprod Immunol 32(3):201–219
168. Kawano Y, Kawasaki F, Nakamura S, Matsui N, Narahara H, Miyakawa I (2001) The production and clinical evaluation of macrophage colony-stimulating factor and macrophage chemoattractant protein-1 in human follicular fluids. Am J Reprod Immunol 45(1):1–5
169. Dahm-Kahler P, Runesson E, Lind AK, Brannstrom M (2006) Monocyte chemotactic protein-1 in the follicle of the menstrual and IVF cycle. Mol Hum Reprod 12(1):1–6
170. Kawano Y, Fukuda J, Itoh H, Takai N, Nasu K, Miyakawa I (2004) The effect of inflammatory cytokines on secretion of macrophage colony-stimulating factor and monocyte chemoattractant protein-1 in human granulosa cells. Am J Reprod Immunol 52(2):124–128
171. Dahm-Kähler P, Ghahremani M, Lind AK, Sundfeldt K, Brännström M (2009) Monocyte chemotactic protein-1 (MCP-1), its receptor and macrophages in the perifollicular stroma during the human ovulatory process. Fertil Steril 91(1):231–9

Chapter 10
Clinical Evaluation of Female Factor Infertility

Yulian Zhao, Lisa Kolp, Melissa Yates, and Howard Zacur

Abstract An infertility evaluation is designed to detect problems responsible for preventing pregnancy and is traditionally divided into male and female evaluations. The purpose of this chapter is to discuss the clinical evaluation of female infertility. Causes of female infertility include failure to have or release oocytes, failure to possess a patent reproductive tract receptive to an embryo, or a coexisting medical condition affecting all or some of the above. The evaluation to be performed to detect these causes, such as medical history and physical examination, assessment of oocyte reserve, assessment of patency of the female reproductive tract, assessment of endometrial receptivity, and assessment of the abdominal pelvic cavity, is discussed in this chapter. Improvement in the success rates of the assisted reproductive technology procedure of IVF will continue to influence the evaluation of infertility. The balance between the necessity for certain clinical evaluations and financial expenses incurred for the patients must be weighed by both the infertile couple and treating physician.

Keywords Female factor infertility • Ovulation assessment • Reproductive tract patency • Endometrial receptivity • Clinical evaluation • Sonohysteroscopy • Hysteroscopy • Fragile X syndrome • Diminished ovarian reserve • Luteal phase defect • Pregnanediol-3 alpha-glucuronide • Laparoscopy

10.1 Introduction

In order for human pregnancy to occur in vivo a male gamete (spermatozoa) that is able to travel through the female reproductive tract to encounter and fertilize a female gamete (oocyte) must exist. Following fertilization, the newly formed embryo must then travel to and implant itself within a receptive uterine cavity where it will grow and develop. Following implantation, the trophoblast created by the embryo within the uterine cavity begins to secrete human chorionic gonadotropin (hCG), which can be detected within seven days after ovulation using sensitive research hormone assays [1, 2]. At this stage of life, this gestation is now known as a "biochemical pregnancy". Clinical research studies have revealed that, on average, there is a 24% chance of a clinically detectable pregnancy (pregnancy diagnosed by physician or conventional pregnancy test) occurring during each month of unprotected intercourse in women attempting to conceive [3]. Research studies using sensitive urinary HCG assays have also demonstrated a 22% loss in pregnancies before they are detected clinically [3, 4]. This would mean that there is approximately a 30–31% chance of pregnancy occurring during each month of unprotected intercourse. In 1982, investigators in France reported on the result of artificial insemination in 2,193 nulliparous women whose husbands were azoospermic [5]. In this study, using frozen donor semen samples, the cumulative pregnancy success rates after 12 months ranged from 74.1% in women younger than 31 years of age to 53.6% for women older than 35 years of age (Fig. 10.1). Due to data such as this, infertility is usually defined as the inability to conceive after one year of unprotected intercourse. This definition has been criticized as being imprecise because of the fact that couples defined as being "infertile" are still able to become pregnant after 12 months of trying without any treatment at rates approaching those for couples given treatment [6]. The definition of infertility becomes important when determining when to perform a clinical evaluation. An infertility evaluation may be performed only after a few months of being unable to conceive in older couples, while in younger couples waiting longer than one year to perform a clinical evaluation is also appropriate. In keeping with this view, the Practice Committee of the American Society for Reproductive Medicine recently defined infertility as a disease and indicated that evaluation and treatment for infertility is warranted after 6 months of inability to conceive in women over age 35 years [7].

Y. Zhao, L. Kolp, M. Yates, and H. Zacur (✉)
Division of Reproductive Endocrinology and Infertility in the Department of Gynecology and Obstetrics at the Johns Hopkins University School of Medicine, Johns Hopkins at Green Spring Station, Lutherville, MD, USA
e-mail: hzacur1@jhmi.edu

D.T. Carrell and C.M. Peterson (eds.), *Reproductive Endocrinology and Infertility: Integrating Modern Clinical and Laboratory Practice*,
DOI 10.1007/978-1-4419-1436-1_10,

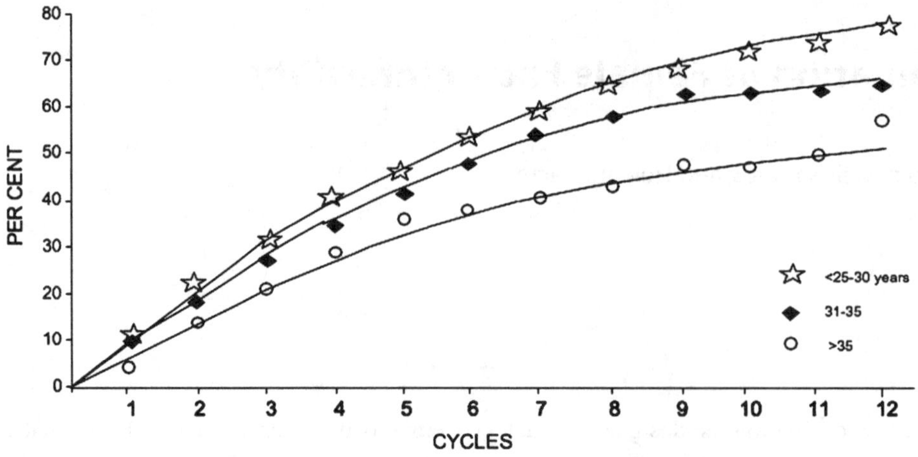

Fig. 10.1 Theoretical cumulative pregnancy success rates in the different age groups. The three curves differ significantly ($p<0.01$). Group of less than 30 years old differs significantly from those of two older groups ($p<0.03$ for those 31–35, and $p<0.001$ for those over 35) (Adapted from Schwartz D and Mayaux BA, N Engl J Med 1982)

A formal infertility evaluation is designed to detect problems responsible for preventing pregnancy and is traditionally divided into male and female evaluations. It will be the purpose of this chapter to discuss the clinical evaluation of female infertility. Causes of female infertility include failure to have or release oocytes, failure to possess a patent reproductive tract receptive to an embryo, or a coexisting medical condition affecting all or some of the above. The evaluation to be performed to detect these causes will be discussed below in this chapter. A brief summary of the optimal evaluation of the infertile female has been created by The Practice Committee of the American Society for Reproductive Medicine (ASRM) in 2006, and readers may refer to this for reference [8]. When appropriate, comparisons will be made in this chapter to the recommendations made by the practice committee for the ASRM. It should be mentioned that these recommendations are currently undergoing review.

10.2 Medical History and Physical Examination

As the initial step in an infertility evaluation, an appropriate medical history should be taken with both partners present if possible. This should include a comprehensive gynecologic and obstetric history. The duration of infertility should be defined as the total duration of time over which sexual intercourse without contraception has occurred without conception. Frequency of intercourse, use of lubricants with intercourse, all of which are either spermicidal or inhibitors of sperm motility [9] as well as any difficulties with intercourse should be discussed. Age at menarche, menstrual cycle interval, duration of menstrual blood flow, and presence or absence of dysmenorrhea should be inquired about. Past history of abdominal or pelvic surgery, pelvic infections and/or sexually transmitted diseases, and abnormal pap smears should be requested as well as any past history of serious medical illnesses. Cigarette smoking, alcohol consumption, and caffeine intake should be determined as cigarette smoking, alcohol consumption of more than four drinks per week, and caffeine intake of greater than 250 mg daily have all been associated with a decrease in fertility [10]. Past use of contraceptive methods should be obtained along with a history of current medication use. It is also extremely important to obtain the history relevant to preconception counseling by identifying any family history of genetic defects, birth defects, or other serious medical illnesses. While trying to conceive, the female partner should be taking at least 0.4 mg of folic acid daily at least one month prior to conceiving and then for three months after conception to reduce the risk of having a child born with a neural tube defect. Determination of the female partner's blood type should be made so that in the case of any future obstetric event it will be known if administration of Rho (D) immune globulin should be administered to avoid Rh immunization. When appropriate, couples should be offered screening for transmittable genetic disorders such as cystic fibrosis or Tay-Sachs and immunity to the Rubella virus should be determined.

Physical and pelvic examinations should be performed with particular attention to identifying thyroid enlargement or nodules, breast nipple fluid discharges, and signs of androgen excess. Pelvic examination with attention to identifying any vaginal or cervical abnormality should take place. If available in the office, transvaginal pelvic ultrasound is useful to image the uterus and adnexal structures. In the absence of pelvic ultrasound, bimanual examination to determine uterine size and shape and the presence or absence of any adnexal abnormalities should be performed.

10.3 Assessment of Oocyte Reserve

Oocytes must be present within the ovary of the female partner in order for pregnancy to occur. A clinical history of normal secondary sexual development followed by vaginal bleeding at regular intervals (every 21–35 days) provides evidence for the presence of oocytes, but does not give an indication of the number of oocytes remaining within the ovaries. Vaginal bleeding occurring at regular intervals suggests that ovulation is taking place but does not prove it. Vaginal bleeding occurring more frequently than every 21 days or less frequently than every 35 days suggests that ovulation may not be occurring.

At birth there are approximately two million oocytes within each ovary [11] and no new oocytes are created within the ovaries after birth. Throughout a woman's life, only about 500 of these oocytes will be released into the pelvis through the process of ovulation and the remainder will undergo atresia. With each passing year, fewer oocytes will remain in each ovary and the loss of all oocytes within the ovaries results in menopause. Menopause usually occurs between 50 and 51 years of age and is defined as the absence of vaginal bleeding for one calendar year. During reproductive life there is a rise in the basal serum FSH level associated with increasing age [12]. This is associated with a decline in serum concentrations of inhibin B indicating that this may be the result of fewer early stage (primordial to antral) follicles [13]. During the human menstrual cycle, the serum concentration of FSH is lowest during the first week of the cycle with the normal ranges for FSH during the different phases of the menstrual cycle provided by the laboratory performing the hormonal measurement. Serum concentration of FSH, which exceeds the normal range early in the menstrual cycle, implies that ovarian oocyte reserve could be diminished and could serve as a warning that attempts to conceive should take place sooner rather than later. In addition, the measurement of an elevated level of FSH early in the menstrual cycle in women younger than 40 years of age may indicate premutation carrier status of Fragile X necessitating screening [14].

Fragile X syndrome is the most common inherited form of mental retardation and is transmitted in a X-linked recessive manner. Expansion of the trinucleotide DNA segment (cytosine-guanine-guanine) of the affected X chromosome results in altered transcription of the fragile X mental retardation 1 (FMR1) gene. The number of trinucleotide repeats has been correlated with the risk of developing mental retardation. If there are fewer than 40 repeats, the individual is considered normal. If there are repeats between 41 and 60 the individual is classified as being in the "grey zone". If there are trinucleotide repeats between 61 and 200, an individual is phenotypically normal but is characterized as having a premutation. If more than 200 trinucleotide repeats are identified, then the individual has the full mutation resulting in full expression of the fragile X syndrome in males with variable expression in females depending upon the extent of X inactivation. Women carrying the premutation for the fragile X gene have a higher risk (20–30%) of premature ovarian failure and are therefore at increased risk for having a higher than normal FSH early in the menstrual cycle [15].

That a correlation between the FSH concentration early in the menstrual cycle and oocyte reserve exists is generally agreed upon, but whether this hormone measurement indicates anything about the "quality" of the oocytes remains to be determined. Several studies have clearly shown that the measurement of the FSH concentration performed on the third day of the menstrual cycle is predictive of the success of an in vitro fertilization (IVF) attempt if done during that same cycle [16, 17]. Women whose FSH concentration exceeds a particular value as determined by each infertility center (usually a concentration above10 mIU/ml) on the third day of the menstrual cycle generally do not become pregnant if IVF is attempted during that particular cycle. Some infertility centers have argued that the chance of pregnancy taking place during any IVF attempt during any menstrual cycle in women previously found to have an elevated menstrual cycle day 3 FSH level will be compromised [18] while other centers have argued that the chance of conceiving with IVF is not compromised if the IVF is done during a cycle in which the menstrual cycle day 3 FSH level is below the elevated value set by the center. The prognostic value of an elevated menstrual cycle day 3 FSH is less clear in younger women having menses at regular intervals [19]. If the concentration of serum FSH measured early in the menstrual cycle is associated with pregnancy success, is this association an indication of oocyte quantity or quality? If it is quality, is this association applicable to all remaining oocytes within the ovary or does this association pertain only to the oocytes undergoing further development during that particular menstrual cycle? This remains to be determined. Also a precise explanation for the inability of IVF to succeed during a menstrual cycle in which the FSH is elevated also remains to be presented. If it were primarily an oocyte problem, then one would suspect that all subsequent attempts at pregnancy with IVF would be compromised. If, however, there was another explanation, such as an endometrial problem which could change from cycle to cycle, this might explain why some IVF cycles would be successful and others would not be. Lastly, a correlation also exists between menstrual cycle day 3 serum FSH levels, and chance of pregnancy success in women who are ovulatory and who are attempting to become pregnant with levels higher than 8 IU/L associated with a decreased probability of spontaneous pregnancy success [20].

It is clear that pregnancy success is inversely correlated with age whether one attempts to conceive naturally or through the use of assisted reproductive technologies.

From the rates of pregnancy success reported in women undergoing IVF with donated oocytes, it is also clear that the reason for the inverse correlation with age does not result from the age of the uterus. Women of advance reproductive age still have an excellent chance of successful pregnancy using donated oocytes from a younger woman. Evaluation of the oocyte as part of the evaluation of female infertility may become possible in the future. Until then, the clinician is limited in his or her ability to adequately assess ovarian reserve as part of the clinical evaluation of female infertility. At the present time, the evaluation consists of measuring a menstrual cycle day 3 serum concentration of FSH. If the value is elevated in a woman younger than 40 years of age, that woman should be screened for a premutation for the fragile X gene. If that screening is negative, then the clinical evaluation of the infertile female should proceed rapidly as an elevated menstrual cycle day 3 FSH level could imply diminished oocyte reserve with an increased risk of premature ovarian failure.

10.4 Assessment of Ovulation

Vaginal bleeding occurring at regular intervals (21–35 days) usually implies that ovulation is taking place as previously mentioned, but this does not "prove" that ovulation is occurring. In a study involving 550 couples trying to conceive, 410 were judged to be eumenorrheic with predictable menstrual cycles of 25–35 days. Out of this group, 96.3% were found to have luteal phase serum progesterone concentrations exceeding 15 nmol/L consistent with ovulation [21]. At the beginning of the menstrual cycle, follicles within the ovaries will begin the process of recruitment and development. Approximately, after the seventh day of the menstrual cycle a "dominant" follicle will be selected to undergo further growth ultimately leading to a 20–24 mm in diameter pre-ovulatory follicle [22]. The development of the follicle is associated with a progressive rise in the circulating serum concentration of estradiol, which is being secreted by the granulosa cells of the follicle. Increasing concentrations of estradiol will eventually stimulate the hypothalamus and pituitary causing the pituitary to begin to secrete increasing amounts of the protein hormone luteinizing hormone (LH). The LH surge triggers the process of ovulation and luteinization of the granulosa cells of the follicle that releases the oocyte which then begin to secrete the steroid hormone progesterone. This hormone in turn affects the brain's temperature regulating center resulting in a mild elevation (approximately 0.3°F) of the basal body temperature and also stimulates the uterine endometrium to become "secretory" in its histological appearance.

Ovulation may be inferred by measuring the basal body temperature throughout the menstrual cycle as well as by measuring the levels of the hormones LH and progesterone throughout the cycle. Use of serial pelvic ultrasonography to document ovarian follicle growth and subsequent follicle rupture accompanied by changes in the appearance of the endometrial stripe has also been used to infer that ovulation has occurred. Lastly, biopsy of the endometrium of the uterus to detect secretory endometrium may be employed to detect ovulation as well.

Any thermometer may be used to measure body temperature and detect the changes that infer that ovulation is taking place. While it has been traditional to recommend taking the oral temperature immediately upon awakening in the morning as the most sensitive method to detect changes in the basal temperature, measuring the oral temperature at any time during the day as long as it is done at the same time each day will provide the information needed to prove that a shift in basal temperature has happened (Fig. 10.2). Temperature readings are recorded on a chart and a sustained upward shift in temperature (usually about 0.3°F for 3 days) infers that progesterone is now being synthesized and released into the circulation as a result of ovulation [23]. There have been many attempts to correlate the pattern of the biphasic temperature changes observed each month in an ovulatory woman with the chance of pregnancy success, but this has proven to be unsuccessful [24]. The exact time of ovulation in relation to the changes in the basal body temperature has also been investigated with most (69.5%) but not all follicle ruptures taking place 24 h or more following the rise in the basal temperature [25]. There have also been reports that a rise may be seen in the basal body temperature without follicle rupture and without a rise in the serum progesterone level during some menstrual cycles suggesting that basal body temperature charting is not a definitive proof that oocyte release has occurred.

Prior to ovulation the serum progesterone concentration is less than 3 ng/ml. After ovulation, the serum progesterone level will exceed 3 ng/ml, often rising to 15 ng/ml or more during the middle of the luteal phase of the cycle. As with basal body temperature monitoring when serum progesterone measurements have been taken while performing serial pelvic ultrasonography a rise in the serum progesterone level may be seen without evidence of follicle collapse. This is known as a luteinized unruptured follicle and appears to occur infrequently, occurring in only 4.9% of 183 cycles monitored in 66 regularly cycling women [26]. Measurement of the serum progesterone level, while suggestive of ovulation, is therefore not a definitive proof that it has occurred. Measurement of the serum progesterone concentration during the middle of the luteal phase of the menstrual cycle to provide additional information about the cause of infertility will be discussed later in this chapter.

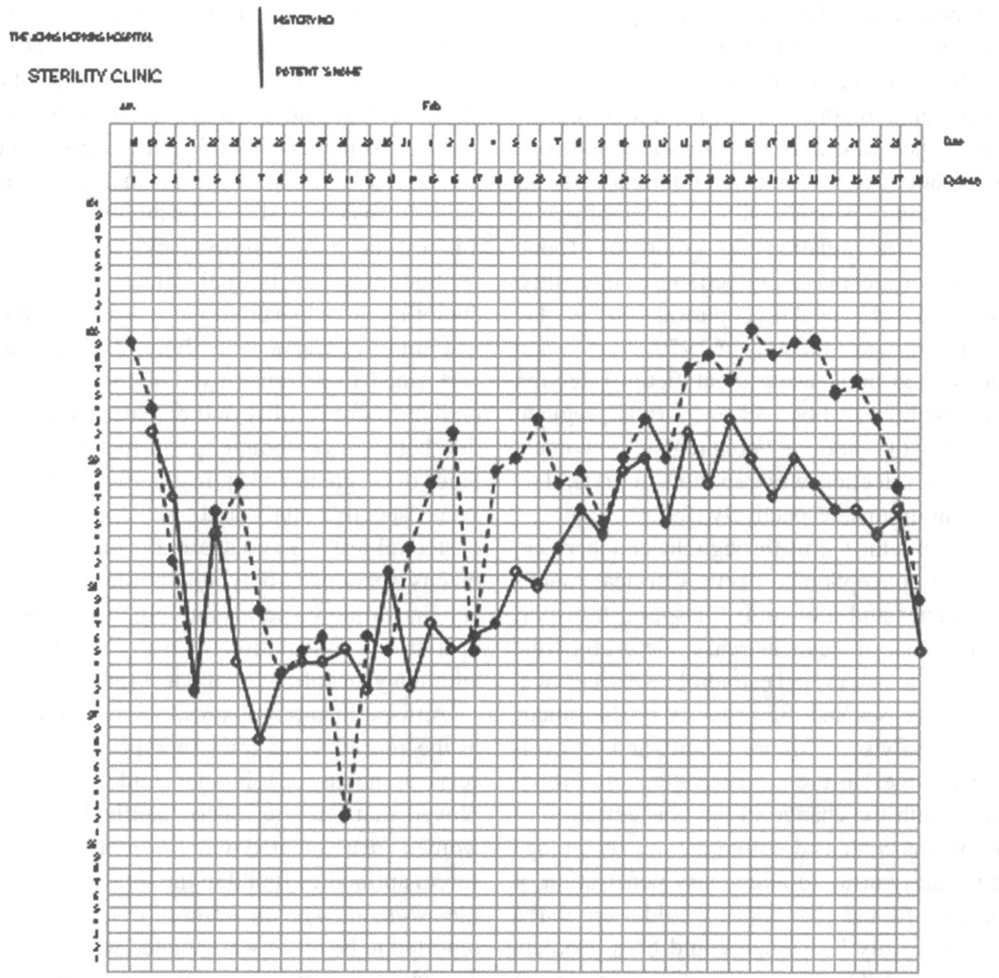

Fig. 10.2 Daily basal body temperature changes during menstrual cycle. Oral temperatures were taken in the morning (o—o) and afternoon (•---•) each day for over 38 days by the same woman. Temperature readings were recorded on the chart and shift in temperature ranged from 96.2 to 100 °F during the cycle

Serial measurement of serum LH levels, either directly in the bloodstream or indirectly via urinary excretion, has been used as an indirect method to infer that ovulation is taking place. Chemically prepared test sticks or dip sticks may be purchased over the counter for use in detecting ovulation. These sticks are exposed to midmorning and not first morning voided urine samples. Color indicators exist to inform the patient that a surge in LH has been detected informing the patient that ovulation is imminent [27].

Ascertainment that ovulation is occurring and is taking place at predictable time periods provides the patient and her physician with the knowledge that failure to release oocytes is not likely to be the cause of infertility. If anovulation or oligo-ovulation is detected or suspected as a result of this evaluation, treatment may be instituted to correct this cause of infertility.

10.5 Assessment of Patency of the Female Reproductive Tract

To conceive, the spermatozoa and oocyte must be able to come into contact with each other. This is achieved via an open passageway through the vagina, cervical os and endocervical canal, uterine cavity, and fallopian tubes. Abnormalities at any level of the female reproductive tract may prevent sperm from meeting the oocyte and will result in infertility.

Speculum examination at the time of the pelvic examination should provide the clinician with information concerning the existence of a vaginal infection, the position of the cervix relative to the cylindrical axis of the vagina and whether cervical scarring and/or stenosis of the os exists. Existence of mucopurulent cervicitis should prompt the culture for Neisseria gonorrhea and Chlamydia trachomatis and institution of antibiotic coverage. Whether to routinely obtain a cervical culture for mycoplasma and ureaplasma is debatable. In 1984, Gump et al. reported on the results of infertility studies in 205 women who were infertile for at least one year [28]. While isolation of mycoplasma hominis was significantly more common in patients with a history of pelvic inflammatory disease, no relationship could be found between mycoplasma or ureaplasma infection and infertility. The authors concluded that genital mycoplasmas do not play a role in causing infertility. Similarly, in 1979, Nagata and colleagues demonstrated ureaplasma urealyticum infection in 63% of patients with infertility, 68% of normal pregnant women, and 62% of normal nonpregnant women. Mycoplasma hominis infection was reported in 10%, 1%, and 6% of the patient groups, respectively [29].

Passage of sperm into the uterus through the endocervical canal is essential for conception to occur. Cervical mucus serves as both a barrier and a conduit for sperm transport depending upon the phase of the menstrual cycle. At the time of ovulation, in response to elevated estradiol levels, cervical mucus production increases and the property of the mucus changes, becoming less viscous, more elastic, and less cellular. Due to the changes in the concentration of sodium chloride associated with the change in the concentration of serum estradiol, mucins contained within the mucus arrange themselves in an orderly array to allow easy penetration of sperm [30]. Because of these changes, it would seem that a possible cause of infertility in women could be a problem with cervical mucus. In 1868, the postcoital examination of cervical mucus was described by Sims [31], and in 1913 the postcoital test as a routine part of the infertility evaluation was mentioned by Huhner [32]. This test involves obtaining cervical mucus from the female partner of the infertile couple following intercourse. Unfortunately, despite its long standing use in the evaluation of the infertile couple, this test has never been standardized nor validated. Depending upon the reference used, cervical mucus is to be removed from the cervical os using either a bulb syringe, an lcc tuberculin syringe without a needle, or a small syringe with an intravenous catheter. The mucus is to be collected following intercourse, which may have taken place minutes to hours previously. Results are reported either in terms of characteristic of the mucus itself (i.e., volume, viscosity, spinnbarket or cellularity) or in terms of the number and motility of the sperm found in the mucus.

In a comprehensive review on the clinical approach to the evaluation of sperm-cervical mucus interactions published in 1977, it was mentioned that physicians develop standards by which the results of the test can be judged through their own experience [33]. After evaluating the world literature (published in English using Medline) on the postcoital test, Griffith and Grimes in 1990 [34] found the sensitivity of the test (the ability to detect infertility) to range from 0.09 to 0.71, with specificity (the ability to detect fertility) to range from 0.62 to 1.00, with a predictive value of an abnormal test (likelihood that an abnormal test predicts an infertile couple) to range from 0.56 to 1.00, and the predictive value of a normal test (likelihood that a normal test predicts fertility) to range from 0.25 to 0.75. The authors concluded that because this test has poor validity, lacks standardization in terms of methodology and normal values, and has unknown reproducibility, it lacks validity as a test for infertility. A prospective study in Canada involving 355 infertility couples was performed to determine the ability of the postcoital test to predict future fertility and revealed no independent association between postcoital sperm motility and the later occurrence of pregnancy [35]. In contrast, in the Netherlands using a retrospective study and simplifying the test result of the postcoital test (i.e., no spermatozoa is present in the cervical mucus specimen, only nonmotile spermatozoa is present, and one or more sperms moving forward is present), resulted in a strong association with the ability to predict fertility within a year following the test [36].

Antisperm antibody (ASA) may be present in the blood or in the reproductive tract secretions, such as seminal fluid, cervical mucus, or follicular fluid [37]. Convincing evidence proved that stronger sperm antibody responses in men or women are associated with lowered fertility. Among the antisperm antibodies found in the sera of immunologically infertile women, sperm immobilizing antibodies have been reported to be closely associated with female infertility [38]. The incidence of infertile women with sperm immobilizing antibodies in their sera has been shown to be approximately 3% when it is tested on their first visit to an infertility outpatient clinic [39].

Numerous methodologies are used to detect ASA. Each has distinct advantages and disadvantages as reviewed by Mazumdar and Levine [40]. Commercially available ASA assays either directly measure ASA bound to sperm or indirectly measure ASA in solution (serum, semen, vaginal or cervical secretion, or follicular fluid). These assays include immunobead assays (IBD), mixed antiglobulin reaction (MAR) test, ELISA, tray agglutination tests (TAT), sperm immobilization assay tests, flow cytometry, and radiolabeled agglutinin assays. Routine ASA screening in couples with unexplained infertility is limited since there is no well accepted consensus about which assay should be used. Assessment of in vitro sperm-mucus interaction by means of the capillary (Kremer) test and /or the semen/cervical mucus contact test (SCMCT) may suggest the likely presence of sperm antibodies in cervical mucus, even though circulating antibodies are weak or undetectable. The presence of high cervical mucus antibody levels and associated negative or low titres of circulating antibodies suggests a good prognosis for the treatment of the couple by intrauterine artificial insemination [41]. In contrast, the presence of high antibody concentrations or titres both locally and systemically suggests a poor prognosis.

The study of ASA and the improvement in their detection advanced rapidly from 1970s to early 1990s, but has not advanced as rapidly during the last decade. This is, in large part, because of the observation that intracytoplasmic sperm injection (ICSI) could be used as an effective treatment for circumventing immunoinfertility [42]. This technique bypasses most of the steps in conception that are adversely affected by antisperm antibodies and may allow some couples to avoid fertilization failure secondary to an autoimmune mechanism. Lahteenmaki et al. [43] treated 29 infertile ASA-positive couples with ICSI, after 22 of them previously demonstrated a poor fertilization rate (6%) during IVF. After ICSI the fertilization and cleavage rate for ASA-positive group (79% and 89% respectively) were similar to the ASA-negative group (68% and 93% respectively). It is notable that 46% of the pregnancies occurring in the ASA-positive group ended in spontaneous pregnancy loss compared with none in the ASA-negative group. However, a study by Clarke et al. [42] showed no evidence of an increased incidence of first-trimester pregnancy loss in sperm antibody-positive patients treated by ICSI. A retrospective analysis of a cohort of 33 infertile couples with ASA in 47 IVF treatment cycles concluded that couples with high mixed antiglobulin reaction (MAR) ASA titres had a lower fertilization rate than those with lower ASA titres [44]. After controlling for the fertilization rate, ASA titres did not affect the pregnancy rate.

The epidemiology of ASA interference in ART is widely reported in literature. The large majority of studies have been retrospective. A thorough evaluation of the literature by Chamley and Clarke [41] led to a conclusion that stronger sperm antibody responses are associated with lowered fecundity. However, it is important for clinicians to appreciate that variables, such as antibody specificity, immunoglobulin class, and dose, come into the equation when evaluating patient's results. Thus, a positive sperm antibody screening result alone without further assessment should not be accepted as necessarily indicative of immunoinfertility. There is a general understanding that the presence of ASAs, even when in high titre, in the absence of additional causes of infertility, does not generally cause complete infertility. High antibody titres more likely produce impaired fertility. There is sufficient evidence to support the hypothesis that ASA play a role in selected couples with unexplained infertility. Both the prevalence and magnitude of this role remains controversial. Also questions remain about which method of ASA testing is best, which isotypes (generally IgM, IgA, or IgG) are most relevant to infertility and what levels of ASAs are significant.

Use of gas to determine tubal patency was suggested by Malgaigne as long ago as 1849 [45]. Determination of the patency of the uterus and fallopian tubes using a gas was initially described by Rubin in 1920 and this test soon became to be known as the "Rubin" test [46]. While Rubin used oxygen as the gas in his initial studies, carbon dioxide was soon substituted. In this procedure, a cannula is used to infuse carbon dioxide gas into the uterine cavity under controlled flow and pressure. Using a stethoscope, bubbles are heard to escape from the tubal ends into the abdominal pelvic cavity signaling patency. Verification of transtubal passage of carbon dioxide gas is made at the conclusion of the test when the patient is asked to stand to determine if referred pain is experienced in one or both shoulders from diaphragmatic irritation by the gas. Both falsenegative and falsepositive results have been reported using this test, and it is no longer used clinically.

Use of a radiopague medium to image the uterine cavity and fallopian tubes at the time of abdominal pelvic x-ray was initially described by Rindfleisch in 1910 [47] and then by Carey in 1914 [48] and by Rubin as well [49]. Because of patient discomfort from the infusion of the radiopaque solutions in use at that time as well as the risk from radiation exposure, the hysterosalpinogram or HSG for many years was usually recommended in order to confirm a Rubin test suggesting tubal obstruction and when surgical correction was being contemplated [50]. Following the introduction of iodized oil and then radiopaque water-soluble dyes coupled with improvements in x-ray imaging devices, the HSG became the standard test to use to image the uterine cavity and fallopian tubes [51]. It is recommended that the procedure be performed under fluoroscopy after menses have ended and before ovulation has occurred. A small amount of water soluble contrast media (8–16 ml) is slowly injected into the uterine cavity through the cervix using either a rigid or balloon tipped flexible catheter. Infusion of the contrast medium is performed under fluoroscopic monitoring, and one to three x-ray films are taken to image the uterine cavity and fallopian tubes during this process (Fig. 10.3). Mild pelvic cramps may be experienced during the procedure which may be lessened by prior use of nonsteriodal anti-inflammatory drugs taken orally 30–60 min prior to the procedure. The procedure is usually well tolerated, and while the risks of infection and allergic reaction are possible, they are very rarely encountered. Radiation exposure during HSG is minimal and estimated to be 1 millisievert (mSV) which is roughly equivalent to natural background radiation experienced over a period of 4 months. The HSG is used to assess the uterine cavity to determine if there is uterine cavity filling defects, such as foreign bodies, adhesions, polyps or leiomyomata, which could adversely affect fertility. Tubal filling with contrast coupled with spill from the fimbriated end of the tube is also evaluated (Fig. 10.3). Three common technical errors to avoid in performing hysterosalpingography are: (1) Failure to remove the speculum prior to performing the

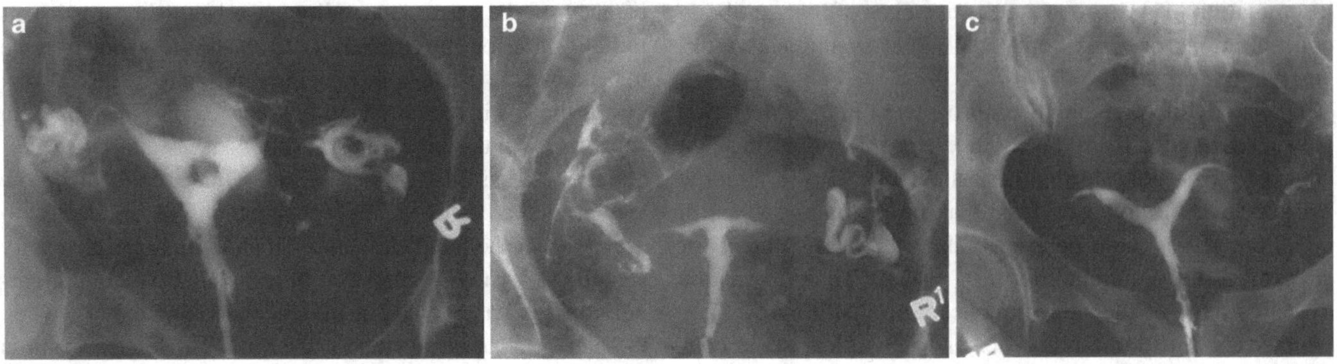

Fig. 10.3 Hysterosalpingogram showing uterine cavity and fallopian tubes. (**a**) Filling defect; (**b**) T shaped uterus; (**c**) Septate or bicornuate uterus

imaging, (2) failure to evaluate the lower uterine cavity when using an intrauterine catheter by not removing it and taking an additional image, and (3) failure to place adequate traction on the cervix of an anteverted or retroverted uterus to permit adequate visualization of the long axis (fundus to cervix) of the uterine cavity [52].

Evaluation of the uterine cavity and the fallopian tubes may also be performed by infusing saline, Ringer's lactate or glycine into the uterine cavity while imaging with ultrasonography performed either abdominally or vaginally but most often transvaginally [53]. The technique of "echohysteroscopy" was first described by Nannini et al. in 1981[54] while Parsons mentioned the term sonohysterography when infusing saline into the uterine cavity during sonographic imaging [55]. Use of Doppler color flow is believed to be of value in assessing fallopian tube patency, especially when combined with contrast media [56].

Sonohysterography performed to image the uterine cavity of an infertile patient should be performed after menses and before ovulation to avoid the insertion of a catheter into a gravid uterine cavity. Using a speculum, a specialized catheter which may or may not have an occlusive balloon is inserted through the endocervical canal into the uterine cavity. The imaging solution to be used, usually saline, is flushed through the catheter prior to its insertion to remove air bubbles. The speculum is then removed and normal saline is slowly injected into the uterine cavity (less than 5 ml/min) after the ultrasound probe has been inserted into the vagina. The uterus is scanned in the longitudinal plane from one corner to the other and then in the transverse plane from fundus to cervix. No more than 20 ml of saline should be needed to accomplish the imaging [53, 57].

Proximal tubal obstruction (at the uterotubal conjunction) identified either by HSG or sonohysterogram may result not only from a disease process but also from cornual muscular spasm. Repeating the HSG after administration of antispasmolytics such as glucagon, diazepam, terbutaline, and isoxuprine has been recommended along with performing the HSG under general anesthesia [58–61]. Additional evaluation of tubal patency may be performed at the time of laparotomy or laparoscopy by chromotubation or by transcervical fallopian tube cannulation done under fluoroscopy or at the time of hysteroscopy when performed simultaneously with laparoscopy [62].

When abnormalities are reported within the uterine cavity following either an HSG or a sonohysterogram, hysteroscopy is used to identify them. Hysteroscopy is the direct visualization of the uterine cavity using an endoscope known as a hysteroscope and a distending medium. The hysteroscope may be flexible or rigid and the distending medium either a gas (most commonly carbon dioxide) or a liquid such as normal saline or 3.3% glycine [63]. Visualization through the hysteroscope is best when the procedure is done following menses and prior to ovulation. Hysteroscopy may be performed in the office using a micro or flexible hysteroscope under local anesthesia with a paracervical block or without any anesthesia, or may be done in an outpatient operating room where an appropriate level of sedation and/or anesthesia may be provided. During the procedure, the cervix and endocervical canal are inspected, followed by the inspection of the uterotubal ostia followed by inspection of the anterior, posterior, and lateral uterine walls looking for adhesions, polyps, leiomyotata and any abnormal irregularities of the surfaces of the uterine walls. Hysteroscopy may be performed alone or may be performed in conjunction with a laparoscopy. Comparisons between findings at HSG, sonohysterogram, and hysteroscopy in infertility patients have only been infrequently performed and have generally found the HSG and sonohysterogram to provide comparable information agreeing with the findings at hysteroscopy 70–90% of the time. Neither technique provides as much information about the uterine cavity as the hysteroscopy does [64, 65]. Fallopian tube patency is better judged by HSG than sonohysterogram at the present time but may improve in the future with the development and use of specialized contrast media [57]. Hysteroscopy, while the "gold standard" for evaluating the uterine cavity, cannot be used to assess tubal patency as well as the HSG or sonohysterogram.

10.6 Assessment of Endometrial Receptivity

Approximately, seven days following ovulation and fertilization of the human oocyte the embryo is within the uterine cavity and ready to implant [66]. From the pioneering work of Noyes, Hertig, and Rock [67], distinctive histological changes of the human endometrium can be identified from ovulation until menstruation as a result of the actions of the steroid hormones estradiol and progesterone produced by the ovaries. The inability of the endometrium to allow successful implantation was suspected to be a possible cause of infertility, but a means to diagnose this did not exist until Dr. Georgeanna Seegar Jones in 1949 suggested that diagnosis of corpus luteum insufficiency could be made through the use of a properly timed endometrial biopsy [68]. In order to perform a properly timed endometrial biopsy, an endometrial tissue sample must be obtained using an endometrial sampling curette after the 26th day of the human menstrual cycle or within three days of the onset of the subsequent menses [69]. The first day of the next menses is arbitrarily defined as cycle day 28 and the presumed menstrual cycle day at the time of the endometrial biopsy is determined by counting backwards from day 28. For example, if the endometrial biopsy was done on January 31st and the first day of menses took place on February 2nd, menstrual cycle day 28 would be assigned to February 2nd and menstrual cycle day 26 would be assigned to January 31st even though those dates may not correspond to the actual cycle dates. The endometrial biopsy tissue is submitted to pathology and then fixed and dated according to the criteria of Noyes, Hertig, and Rock. If the biopsy is found to be two or more days out of phase, then a luteal phase defect would be suspected indicating inadequate progesterone effect upon the endometrium. A second out of phase endometrial biopsy is required to be taken in a subsequent cycle in order for the diagnosis of a luteal phase defect to be finally made [69]. In the example given above, an out of phase endometrial biopsy would have been reported as cycle day 23 or earlier instead of the expected day 26.

Controversy about the diagnosis as well as the method used to make the diagnosis of a luteal phase disorder as a cause of infertility existed as soon as the concept was suggested in 1949 and has continued until the present time. As Dr. Jones mentioned in her 1976 Fertility and Sterility article on the topic of luteal phase defect, failure to accept the diagnostic approach that she proposed was most likely based on either the inability of the involved clinician to perform an endometrial biopsy or upon the inability of the pathology lab to accurately date the endometrial sample taken. Because of these limitations, alternatives to diagnose luteal phase problems as a cause of infertility were proposed. These included detection of a lower than normal luteal phase serum progesterone concentration identified in a menstrual cycle with a normal interval from ovulation to menstruation which was called an "inadequate luteal phase" [70]. Alternatively, a "short luteal phase" was defined as the luteal phase duration of eight days or less established by knowing the actual time from ovulation to menstruation as determined by measuring the midcycle LH surge [71].

In an effort to resolve the controversy surrounding the usefulness of a timed endometrial biopsy in the clinical evaluation of the infertile female, the National Institute of Child Health and Human Development (NICHD) sponsored a multicenter prospective clinical study designed to assess the ability of histological dating to discriminate between women of fertile and infertile couples [72]. Prior to this study, use of a timed endometrial biopsy to identify a luteal phase defect had not undergone rigorous testing comparing results between fertile and infertile couples. Almost uniformly, studies reporting the existence of a luteal phase defect involved only infertile couples. The original publication of Dr. Georgeanna Jones showed that in 206 menstrual cycles, 35 or 17% were found to have a luteal phase defect diagnosed either by endometrial biopsy or by lowered luteal phase basal body temperature [68]. In her later report, Dr. Jones mentioned that using only a timed endometrial biopsy, a luteal phase defect was found to be an etiologic factor for infertility in 3.5% of cases [69]. In the NICHD study, 287 women of infertile couples were compared to 332 women of fertile couples. Each woman underwent endometrial biopsy performed either during the midluteal phase (menstrual cycle day 21–22) as defined by designating the day of urinary LH surge as cycle day, 14, or performed late in the menstrual cycle (days 26–27) again as defined by the urinary LH surge. The biopsy was reported to be out of phase biopsies if more than a two day difference existed between the menstrual cycle day determined by the urinary LH surge and the determination of pathologist based on the histological criteria of Noyes et al. [67]. Results demonstrated that out of phase biopsies discriminated poorly between women from fertile or infertile couples. For midluteal phase biopsies, the prevalence of an out of phase biopsy was 49.4% in women from fertile couples contrasted to 43.2% in women from infertile couples. For late luteal phase biopsies, the prevalence of out of phase biopsies from women of fertile couples was 35.3% contrasted to 23.0% from women of infertile couples [72]. It could be argued that these results were different from those expected due to the fact that the timing for the endometrial biopsy was based upon a urinary LH surge and not upon trying to perform the biopsy within 3 days of expected menses and then counting the day of menses as day 28 and counting backwards. However, in a much smaller study involving five regularly menstruating women of proven fertility who underwent a total of 39 endometrial biopsies performed in this manner, it was reported that if a two day difference was the criterion, the incidence for a single out of phase biopsy was 51.4% while the incidence of a sequential out of phase biopsy (biopsy performed on a subsequent cycle) was 26.7%. If a three day difference was used, then the incidence for out of phase biopsies done either singly or sequentially would be 31.4% and 6.6%, respectively [73]. These results while obtained only from fertile women agree with the incidence of out of phase biopsies reported for infertile women in previous studies and also agree with the results of the NICHD study. As a result, it would be difficult to refute the conclusion from the NICHD study that the timed endometrial biopsy followed by histological dating of the endometrium provides no clinically useful information as a screening test and that it is recommended that this test be abandoned as a diagnostic tool for the routine evaluation of the infertile couple [72]. It should be emphasized that the results of the NICHD study, however, do not invalidate the concept of a luteal phase defect but only dispute that the timed endometrial biopsy is the "gold standard" for diagnosis of it.

Measurement of pregnanediol-3 alpha-glucuronide (PdG) in first morning voided urine samples provides a means of hormonally monitoring the luteal phase of the human menstrual cycle without performing an endometrial biopsy. In studies involving regularly menstruating women, as well as nonbreastfeeding and breastfeeding women postpartum, differences in the timing of the resumption of ovulation were observed as well as abnormalities in the area under the curve for PdG in the luteal phases of the first three postpartum menstrual cycles (Fig. 10.4) [74, 75]. Delay in the resumption of ovulation postpartum in breastfeeding mothers as well as decreased risk for pregnancy during this time is well known. Changes observed in the hormonal profile of PdG during the luteal phase following the initial resumption of ovulation in these women may perhaps in part account for this [75]. Recommending measuring PdG in daily first morning voided urine samples as the test to perform in order to diagnose a luteal phase defect would need to be validated in a study similar to the one funded by NICHD. Given the lack of technology of easily measuring PdG in first morning urine samples coupled with the inconvenience of doing this would mean that the likelihood of this type of test being used clinically to diagnose a luteal phase defect would be remote.

Treatment for a luteal phase defect involves the administration of exogenous progesterone. This is routinely provided during almost all forms of assisted reproductive technologies used in infertile women. Unless another type of luteal phase defect is identified requiring a different form of treatment, the indication for evaluation of the luteal phase of the menstrual cycle in infertile women for the purposes of diagnosing this as a cause for infertility would be for research purposes and not for general clinical practice.

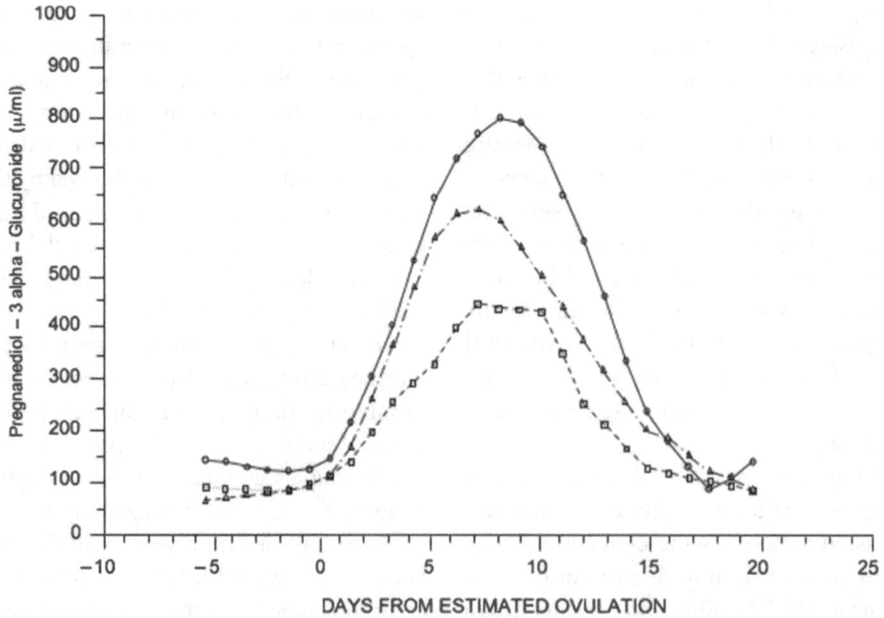

Fig.10.4 Mean daily luteal phase urinary pregnanediol glucuronide (PdG) excretion (first morning urine) in a series of postpartum cycles with a normal luteal phase. Data from 3 first postpartum cycles (o—o), 10 s postpartum cycles (Δ-··-Δ), and 4 third postpartum cycles (λ---λ), are shown (Gray et al., JCEM 1987)

10.7 Assessment of the Abdominal Pelvic Cavity

A simple and safe technique for inspection of the abdominal pelvic cavity to identify fallopian tube and/or peritoneal causes for infertility has recently become available. In 1902, Georg Kelling used a cystoscope to examine the abdomen of a living dog using room air [76], and in 1910 Jacobaeus published his report on endoscopic inspection in the human, and he called this procedure, laparoscopy [77]. In the United States, Bernheim used a protoscope to perform the first laparoscopy in 1911 [78]. Since those early days, the technique of laparoscopy has evolved to employ the use of sophisticated endoscopic equipment coupled with gas infusion systems which safely insufflate the abdominal pelvic cavity with carbon dioxide gas. Laparoscopy was first widely used in England and then in the United States in the 1960s and 1970s as a method for tubal sterilization [79, 80].

Before being replaced by laparoscopy in the 1960s and 1970s, culdoscopy was the endoscopic procedure employed to evaluate the abdominal-pelvic cavity. This technique was reported by Albert Decker in 1944 and involved first placing the patient in a knee chest position after which a pneumoperitoneum was created by passing gas through a needle placed in the cul-de-sac [81]. To assess tubal function, a Foley catheter was inserted into the uterine cavity with the culdoscope in place and indigo carmine was then infused through the foley and spill of dye from the distal ends of the tubes looked for under direct vision [82].

Since the 1970s in the United States, laparoscopy has been performed as part of a standard infertility evaluation to directly observe tubal patency following the administration of indigo carmine dye through the uterine cervix. In addition, laparoscopy has been used as a method to identify tubal disease or peritoneal factors that could adversely affect fertility, such as fimbrial phimosis, peritubal adhesions, and endometriosis. In addition to diagnosing these tubal and/or peritoneal disorders, treatment by lysis of adhesions or destruction of endometrial implants could also be provided simultaneously. It is now known, however, that infertility believed to be due to tubal and/or peritoneal factors may be successfully treated using assisted reproductive technologies. Given the marked improvement in the success of achieving pregnancy with the assisted reproductive technology of in vitro fertilization, questions are now being asked as to the precise role that laparoscopy should play in the evaluation of the infertile female. Specifically, should laparoscopy always be recommended as part of the evaluation of the infertile woman no matter what her age or if she gives no history to suggest pelvic infection, pelvic adhesions or endometriosis and her hysterosalpinogram is entirely normal? Some have suggested that laparoscopy should be omitted as part of the routine workup in otherwise unexplained infertility and that ovarian stimulation coupled with intrauterine insemination be tried first [83].

One report has suggested that operative laparoscopy to treat endometriosis following a failed attempt with IVF in 29 patients resulted in 22 of these patients becoming pregnant in a subsequent attempt [84]. Unfortunately, this was a retrospective case series and the relationship between the diagnosis of endometriosis and infertility has been extremely controversial with some investigators indicating that no matter what the initial stage of endometriosis is found to be that the chances of pregnancy occurring following either medical or surgical treatment is similar if the patients are followed long enough [85]. In addition, other investigators have indicated that whether endometriosis is treated medically or not the chance for pregnancy success is comparable [86].

Whether a laparoscopy that should be performed prior to intrauterine insemination after a normal hysterosalpingogram had been done was recently questioned in a prospective randomized clinical trial [87]. The authors concluded that laparoscopy performed after six cycles of unsuccessful IUI did not detect more abnormalities with clinical consequences compared with those performed prior to IUI treatment and questioned the value of routinely performing a laparoscopy prior to IUI treatment. A need for more randomized clinical trials to answer questions about the value of routinely performing a laparoscopy prior to assisted reproductive technology treatment is clearly needed as it has been noticed by others [88].

10.8 Conclusions

Sufficient data exist to justify requesting a couple with infertility to have a semen analysis performed and to undergo a hysterosalpingogram. Absence of sperm or blockages of both fallopian tubes are clear examples of the cause(s) of infertility. Cervical mucus abnormalities or defects in endometrial receptivity to an embryo may also be the causes of infertility, but accurate diagnostic tests to detect these causes remain to be developed. As documented in this chapter neither the post coital test nor timed endometrial biopsy has been shown to be valid diagnostic tests for infertility. Routine performance of a laparoscopy prior to treatment with IUI or IVF in a woman younger than 35 years of age who has no other gynecological complaint other than infertility, whose husband's semen analysis is normal and, whose, hysterosalpingogram is normal may be questioned. Prospective randomized clinical trials to address this issue are needed. Use of the term 'fecundibility' defined as the chance of becoming pregnant per menstrual cycle with lower fecundibility rates being described as subfertility as opposed to use of the term 'sterility' where there is no chance of becoming pregnant should be emphasized in discussing the results of an infertility evaluation to patients [89]. This is important because a young couple with unexplained infertility whose monthly conception rate is low (3%)

as compared to a "normal" couple whose monthly conception rate is high (20%) will still be able to conceive but at a slower rate and thus be subfertile. For example, it may only take 2 months of trying for the "normal" couple to have a 49% chance of conceiving as compared to 24 months of trying for the subfertile couple to have a 52% chance of becoming pregnant. These concepts have utility in evaluating the impact of chronological age on fertility since the monthly conception rate will decline with increasing age increasing the time interval for pregnancy success. Subfertility, as a term, will also be of value in evaluating the impact of an elevated menstrual cycle day 2 or 3 FSH level in a younger woman who desires to conceive but is having difficulty. Improvement in the success rates of the assisted reproductive technology procedure of IVF will continue to influence the evaluation of the infertile couple. Why should patients undergo unnecessary clinical evaluations for infertility or receive treatments for infertility whose value is questioned prolonging their duration of infertility and increasing their financial expense when pregnancy may be rapidly and less expensively achieved with IVF? Whether this conclusion will be agreed upon by all physicians treating patients with infertility and insurers providing the coverage for the evaluation and treatment of infertility remain to be seen.

References[1]

1. Armstrong EG, Ehrlich PH, Birken S, Schlatterer JP, Siris E, Hembree WC, Canfield RE (1984) Use of a highly sensitive and specific immunoradiometric assay for detection of human chorionic gonadotropin in urine of normal, nonpregnant, and pregnant individuals. J Clin Endocrinol Metab 59:867–874
2. O'Connor JF, Schlatterer JP, Birken S, Krichevsky A, Armstrong EG, McMahon D, Canfield RE (1988) Development of highly sensitive immunoassays to measure human chorionic gonadotropin, its beta-subunit, and beta core fragment in the urine: application to malignancies. Cancer Res 48:1361–1366
3. Wilcox AJ, Weinberg CR, O'Connor JF, Baird DD, Schlatterer JP, Canfield RE, Armstrong EG, Nisula BC (1988) Incidence of early loss of pregnancy. N Engl J Med 319:189–194
4. Hakim RB, Gray RH, Zacur HA (1995) Infertility and early pregnancy loss. Am J Obstet Gynecol 172:1510–1517
5. Schwartz D, Mayaux MJ (1982) Female fecundity as a function of age: results of artificial insemination in 2,193 nulliparous women with azoospermic husbands: Federation CECOS. N Engl J Med 306:404–406
6. Collins JA, Wrixon W, Janes LB, Wilson EH (1983) Treatment-independent pregnancy among infertile couples. N Engl J Med 309:1201–1206
7. Practice Committee of the American Society for Reproductive Medicine (2008) Definitions of infertility and recurrent pregnancy loss. Fertil Steril 89:1603
8. The Practice Committee of the American Society for Reproductive Medicine (2006) Optimal evaluation of the infertile female. Fertil Steril 86(Suppl. 4):S264–S267
9. Goldenberg RL, White R (1975) The effect of vaginal lubricants on sperm motility in vitro. Fertil Steril 26:872–873
10. Barbieri RL (2001) The initial fertility consultation: recommendations concerning cigarette smoking, body mass index, and alcohol and caffeine consumption. Am J Obstet Gynecol 185:1168–1173
11. Sadler TW (1985) Medical embryology. In: Langman (ed) Medical embryology, 5th edn. Williams and Wilkins, Baltimore, p 11
12. Reyes FI, Winter JS, Faiman C (1977) Pituitary-ovarian relationships preceding the menopause. Am J Obstet Gynecol 129:557–564
13. Klein NA, Illingworth PJ, Groome NP, McNeilly AS, Battaglia DB, Soules MR (1996) Decreased inhibin B secretion is associated with the monotropic RSH rise in older ovulatory women: a study of serum and follicular fluid levels of dimeric inhibin A and B in spontaneous menstrual cycles. J Clin Endocriol Metab 81:2742–2745
14. American College of Obstetricians and Gynecologists (2006) Screening for fragile X syndrome. ACOG committee opinion number 338. Obstet Gynecol 107:1483–1485
15. Welt CK, Smith PC, Taylor AE (2004) Evidence of early ovarian aging in fragile X permutation carriers. J Clin Endocrinol Metab 89:4569–4574
16. Muasher SJ, Oehninger S, Simonetti S, Matta J, Ellis LM, Liu HC, Jones GS, Rosenwaks Z (1988) The value of basal and/or stimulated serum gonadotropin levels in prediction of stimulation response and in vitro fertilization outcome. Fertil Steril 50:298–307
17. Scott RT, Toner JP, Muasher SJ, Oehninger S, Robinson S, Rosenwaks Z (1989) Follicle-stimulating hormone levels on cycle day 3 are predictive of in vitro fertilization outcome. Fertil Steril 51:651–654
18. Scott RT, Hofmann GE, Oehninger SO, Muasher SJ (1990) Intercycle variability of day 3 follicle-stimulating hormone levels and its effect on stimulation quality in in vitro fertilization. Fertil Steril 54:297–302
19. Barnhart K, Osheroff J (1999) We are overinterpreting the predictive value of serum follicle-stimulating hormone levels. Fertil Steril 72:8–9
20. van der Steeg JW, Steures P, Eijkemans MJ, Habbema JD, Hompes PG, Broekmans FJ, Bouckaert PX, Bossuyt PM, van der Veen F, Mol BW (2007) Predictive value and clinical impact of basal follicle-stimulating hormone in subfertile, ovulatory women. J Clin Endocrinol Metab 92:2163–2168
21. Malcolm C, Cumming DC (2003) Does anovulation exist in eumenorrheic women? Obstet Gynecol 102:317–318
22. Hodgen GD (1982) The dominant ovarian follicle. Fertil Steril 38:281–300
23. McCarthy JJ, Rockette HE (1983) A comparison of methods to interpret the basal body temperature graph. Fertil Steril 39:640–646
24. Newill RG, Katz M (1982) The basal body temperature chart in artificial insemination by donor pregnancy cycles. Fertil Steril 38:431–438
25. Leader A, Wiseman D, Taylor P (1985) The prediction of ovulation: a comparison of the basal body temperature graph, cervical mucus score, and real-time pelvic ultrasonography. Fertil Steril 43:385–388
26. Kerin JF, Kirby C, Morris D, McEvoy M, Ward B, Cox LW (1983) Incidence of the luteinized unruptured follicle phenomenon in cycling women. Fertil Steril 40:620–626
27. Nielsen MS, Barton S, Hatasaka HH, Stanford JB (2001) Comparison of several one-step home urinary luteinizing hormone detection test kits to OvuQuick. Fertil Steril 76(384):387
28. Gump DW, Gibson M, Ashikaga T (1984) Lack of association between genital mycoplasmas and infertility. N Engl J Med 310:937–941

[1]**Key references: 7, 8, 14, 69, 72.**

29. Nagata Y, Iwasaka T, Wada T (1979) Mycoplasma infection and infertility. Fertil Steril 4:392–395
30. Gould KG, Ansari AH (1983) Chemical alteration of cervical mucus by electrolytes. Am J Obstet Gynecol 145:92–99
31. Sims JM (1868) Illustrations of the value of the microscope in the treatment of the sterile condition. Br Med J 2:465
32. Huhner M (1913) Sterility in the male and female, and its treatment. Rebman, New York
33. Blasco L (1977) Clinical approach to the evaluation of sperm-cervical mucus interactions. Fertil Steril 28:1133–1145
34. Griffith CS, Grimes DA (1990) The validity of the postcoital test. Am J Obstet Gynecol 162:615–620
35. Collins JA, So Y, Wilson EH, Wrixon Casper RF (1984) The postcoital test as a predictor of pregnancy among 355 infertile couples. Fertil Steril 41:703–708
36. Eimers JM, te Velde ER, Gerritse R, van Kooy RJ, Kremer J, Habbema JD (1994) The validity of the postcoital test for estimating the probability of conceiving. Am J Obstet Gynecol 171:65–70
37. Marin-Briggiler CI, Vazquez-Levin MH, Gonzalez-Echeverria F, Blaquier JA, Miranda PV, Tezon JG (2003) Effect of antisperm antibodies present in human follicular fluid upon the acrosome reaction and sperm-zona pellucida interaction. Am J Reprod Immunol 50:209–219
38. Isojima S, Li TS, Ashitaka Y (1968) Immunologic analysis of sperm immobilizing factor found in sera of women with unexplained sterility. Am J Obstet Gynecol 101:677–683
39. Isojima S (1983) Recent advances in reproductive immunology. Asia Oceania J Obstet Gynecol 9:15–26
40. Mazumdar S, Levine AS (1998) Antisperm antibodies: etiology, pathogenesis, diagnoses, and treatment. Fertil Steril 70:799–810
41. Chamley LW, Clarke GN (2007) Antisperm antibodies and conception. Semin Immunopathol 29:169–184
42. Clarke GN, Bourne H, Baker HWG (1997) Intracytoplasmic sperm injection for treating infertility associated with sperm autoimmunity. Fertil Steril 68(1):112–117
43. Lahteenmaki A, Reima I, Hovatta O (1995) Treatment of severe male immunological infertility by intracytoplasmic sperm injection. Hum Reprod 10:2824–2828
44. Lahteenmaki A (1993) In-vitro fertilization in the presence of antisperm antibodies detected by the mixed antiglobulin reaction (MAR) and the tray agglutination test (TAT). Hum Reprod 8:84–88
45. Malgaigne, JF (1849) Du Catheterisme de la trompe de fallope pour remedier a la sterilite, par le docteur. Tyler Smyth. Rev Med Chir 6:113
46. Rubin IC (1920) Subphrenic pneumoperitoneum produced by insufflation of oxygen as a test of patency of the fallopian tubes in sterility and allied gynecological conditions. Am J Roentgenology 120–128
47. Rindfleisch W (1910) Darstellung des Cavum Uteri Klin. Wochenschr 4:780
48. Carey WH (1914) Note on determination of patency of fallopian tubes by the use of Collargol and X-ray shadow. Am J Obstet Dis Women Child 69:462
49. Rubin IC (1914) Rontgendiagnostik der Uterustumoren mit Hilfe von intrauterinen Collargolinjecktionen. Zentralbl Gynaekol 18:658
50. Novak ER, Jones GS, Jones HW (1970) Infertility and abortion. In: Novak ER, Jones GS, Jones HW (eds) Textbook of gynecology, 8th edn. Williams and Wilkins Co., Baltimore, p 561
51. Baramki TA (2005) Hysterosalpingography. Fertil Steril 83:1595–1606
52. Hofmann GE, Scott RT, Rosenwaks Z (1992) Common technical errors in hysterosalpingography. Int J Fertil 37:41–43
53. Lindheim SR, Adsuar N, Kushner DM, Pritts EA, Olive D (2003) Sonohysterography: a valuable tool in evaluating the female pelvis. Obstet Gynecol Surv 58:770–784
54. Nannini R, Chelo E, Branconi F, Tantini C, Scarselli GF (1981) Dynamic echohysteroscopy: a new diagnostic technique in the study of female infertility. Acta Eur Fertil 12:165–171
55. Parsons AK, Lense JJ (1993) Sonohysterography for endometrial abnormalities: preliminary results. J Clin Ultrasound 21:87–95
56. Deichert U, Schlief R, van de Sandt M, Daume E (1992) Transvaginal hysterosalpingo-contrast sonography for the assessment of tubal patency with gray scale imaging and additional use of pulsed wave Doppler. Fertil Steril 57:62–67
57. Goldstein SR (1996) Saline infusion sonohysterography. Clin Obstet Gynecol 39:248–258
58. Winfield AC, Pittaway D, Maxson W, Daniell J, Wentz AC (1982) Apparent cornual occlusion in hysterosalpingography: reversal by glucagon. AJR Am J Roentgenol 139:525–527
59. Page EP (1968) Use of isoxuprine in uterosalpingography and uterotubal insufflation. Am J Obstet Gynecol 101:358–364
60. Thurmond AS, Novy M, Rosch J (1988) Terbutaline in diagnosis of interstitial fallopian tube obstruction. Invest Radiol 23:209–210
61. World Health Organization (1983) A new hysterographic approach to the evaluation of tubal spasm and spasmolytic agents. Fertil Steril 39:105–107
62. Novy MJ, Thurmond AS, Patton P, Uchida BT, Rosch J (1988) Diagnosis of cornual obstruction by transcervical fallopian tube cannulation. Fertil Steril 50:434–440
63. Zacur HA, Murray D (1992) Techniques and instrumentation of operative hysteroscopy. In: Azziz R, Murphy AA (eds) Practical manual of operative laparoscopy and hysteroscopy. Springer-Verlag, New York, pp 151–165
64. Bartkowiak R, Kaminski P, Wielgos M, Bobrowska K (2006) The evaluation of uterine cavity with saline infusion sonohysterography and hysteroscopy in infertile patients. Neuro Endocrinol Lett 27:523–528
65. Soares SR, Barbosa dos Reis MM, Camargos AF (2000) Diagnostic accuracy of sonohysterography, transvaginal sonography, and hysterosalpingography in patients with uterine cavity diseases. Fertil Steril 73:406–411
66. Psychoyos A (1973) Hormonal control of ovoimplantation. Vitam Horm 31:201–256
67. Noyes RW, Hertig AT, Rock J (1950) Dating the endometrial biopsy. Fertil Steril 1:3–25
68. Jones GES (1949) Some newer aspects of the management of infertility. JAMA 141:1123–1129
69. Jones GS (1976) The luteal phase defect. Fertil Steril 27:351–356
70. Moszkowski E, Woodruff JD, Jones GES (1962) The inadequate luteal phase. Am J Obstet Gynecol 83:363–372
71. Strott CA, Cargille CM, Ross GT, Lipsett MD (1970) The short luteal phase. J Clin Endocrinol Metab 30:246–251
72. Coutifaris C, Myers ER, Guzick DS, Diamond MP, Carson SA, Legro RS, Mcgovern PG, Schlaff WE, Carr BR, Steinkampf MP, Silva S, Vogel DL, Leppert PC (2004) Histological dating of timed endometrial biopsy tissue is not related to fertility status. Fertil Steril 82:1264–1272
73. Davis OK, Berkeley AS, Naus GJ, Cholst IN, Freedman KS (1989) The incidence of luteal phase defect in normal, fertile women, determined by serial endometrial biopsies. Fertil Steril 51:582–586
74. Gray RH, Campbell OM, Zacur HA, Labbok MH, MacRae SL (1987) Postpartum return of ovarian activity in nonbreastfeeding women monitored by urinary assays. J Clin Endocrinol Metab 64:645–650
75. Gray RH, Campbell OM, Apelo R, Eslami SS, Zacur H, Ramos RM, Gehret JC, Labbok MH (1990) Risk of ovulation during lactation. Lancet 335:25–29
76. Kelling G (1902) Uber Oesphagoskopie: Gastroskopie und Koelioskopie. Munch Med Wochenschr 49:21–24
77. Jacobaeus HC (1910) Uber die Moglichkeit die Zystoskopie bei Untersuchung seroser Hohlungen anzuwenden. Munch Med Wochenschr 57:2090–2092
78. Bernheim BM (1911) Organoscopy: IV: cystoscopy of the abdominal cavity. Ann Surg 53:764–767
79. Steptoe PC (1967) Laparoscopy in gynecology. E. & S. Livingstone, Edinburgh

80. Wheeless CR Jr (1972) Outpatient laparoscopic sterilization under local anesthesia. Obstet Gynecol 39:767–770
81. Decker A, Cherry T (1944) Culdoscopy: a new method in diagnosis of pelvic disease: preliminary report. Am J Surg 64:40–44
82. Jones GS (1976) Culdoscopy. Clini Obstet Gynecol 19:299–306
83. Fatum M, Laufer N, Simon A (2002) Investigation of the infertile couple: should diagnostic laparoscopy be performed after normal hysterosalpingography in treating infertility suspected to be of unknown origin? Hum Reprod 17:1–3
84. Littman E, Giudice L, Lathi R, Berker B, Milki A, Nezhat C (2005) Role of laparoscopic treatment of endometriosis in patients with failed in vitro fertilization cycles. Fertil Steril 84:1574–1578
85. Hoeger KM, Guzick DS (1997) Classification of endometriosis. Obstet Gynecol Clin North Am 24:347–359
86. Olive DL, Pritts E (2001) Treatment of endometriosis. N Engl J Med 345:266–275
87. Tanahatoe SJ, Lambalk CB, Hompes PG (2005) The role of laparoscopy in intrauterine insemination: a prospective randomized reallocation study. Hum Reprod 20:3225–3230
88. Bosteels J, Van Herendael B, Weyers S, D'Hoogh T (2007) The position of diagnosticlaparoscopy in current fertility practice. Hum Reprod Update 13:477–485
89. Penzias AS (2005) Subfertility, fecundability, and the impact of laparoscopy on conceptionrates. Fertil Steril 84:1579–1580

Chapter 11
Polycystic Ovary Syndrome

Catherine J. Wheeler, William R. Keye, and C. Matthew Peterson

Abstract This chapter reviews Polycystic Ovary Syndrome.

11.1 Introduction

Arguably, one of the most commonly diagnosed endocrinopathies in women is polycystic ovary syndrome (PCOS). The combination of hyperandrogenism, menstrual dysfunction, and weight control issues are the traditional criteria used to establish the diagnosis. Today, the obesity epidemic has accelerated consideration of this disorder to an even younger population of women and the recent inclusion of ultrasound diagnostic criteria increases the population considered for the diagnosis of PCOS. PCOS is a disorder comprising multiple clinical variants and apparent genetic propensities grouped together into the "PCOS phenotype." The diagnostic criteria-based subcategorization of PCOS will hopefully assist in unmasking the multiple unique phenotypes as well as their genetic origins. Future texts will likely have detailed descriptions of the genetic origins, environmental triggers, specific treatments, and outcomes of the different clinical entities that we now comingle as "PCOS."

11.2 Polycystic Ovary Syndrome: Diagnostic Criteria

Stein-Leventhal syndrome, the association of amenorrhea with bilateral polycystic ovaries and obesity was first described in 1935 by Stein and Leventhal [1]. Its complex genetic origins are likely polygenic and/or multifactorial [2]. Diagnostic criteria have been established by the modified consensus of the National Institutes of Health and Child Health and Human Development (1990) and/or by consensus criteria established during the ESHRE/Rotterdam Conference in (2003) (Table 11.1).

In the NIH schema, there are only two major criteria for the diagnosis of PCOS: anovulation and the presence of hyperandrogenism documented by clinical and/or laboratory evidence. These criteria alone are necessary after other pathologies for hyperandrogenism (congenital adrenal hyperplasia, nonclassic congenital adrenal hyperplasia, adrenal or ovarian neoplasm, Cushing syndrome) or anovulation (hypo- or hypergonadotropic disorders, hyperprolactinemia, thyroid disease) are excluded. Minor NIH criteria add subtype categorization. The Rotterdam Diagnostic Criteria requires two of the three criteria for the diagnosis of PCOS. In essence, it adds two new groups: ovulatory women with hyperandrogenemia and polycystic ovaries by ultrasound, as well as anovulatory women with polycystic ovaries on ultrasound, but no hyperandrogenemia.

Recently published data confirm that women with regular cycles and polycystic ovaries share many of the biochemical features of PCOS [3]. Familial PCOS studies find that the sisters of women with classical symptoms of PCOS (anovulation and hyperandrogenism), may be equally hyperandrogenemic, but demonstrate polycystic ovaries [4], and regular menstrual cyclicity [5, 6]. Of interest is the fact that women with polycystic ovaries, hyperandrogenism, and regular cycles, are less likely to have insulin resistance and hyperinsulinemia than those who demonstrate chronic anovulation [7–9]. This linkage of a metabolic abnormality to anovulation suggests that follicular growth may be intimately associated with key metabolic pathway(s) and/or product(s). These subtle differentiators, now recognized by investigators, may help unravel the genetic susceptibilities and environmental effectors that will explain the various PCOS manifestations.

The second category now included in PCOS by Rotterdam Criteria are anovulatory women with polycystic ovaries on ultrasound, but no hyperandrogenemia. This inclusion appears to be a small numerical addition to the PCOS population, at large. In a small series of 84 patients with anovulation and polycystic ovaries, less than half the patients were

C.J. Wheeler
Department of Obstetrics and Gynecology, University of Utah School of Medicine, Salt Lake City, UT, USA

W.R. Keye and C.M. Peterson (✉)
University Center for Reproductive Medicine, Department of Obstetrics and Gynecology, University of Utah School of Medicine, Salt Lake City, UT 84132, USA
e-mail: c.matthew.peterson@hsc.utah.edu

D.T. Carrell and C.M. Peterson (eds.), *Reproductive Endocrinology and Infertility: Integrating Modern Clinical and Laboratory Practice*,
DOI 10.1007/978-1-4419-1436-1_11,

Table 11.1 PCOS diagnostic criteria

NIH Criteria – both required
Chronic anovulation
Clinical or biochemical signs of hyperandrogenism
Minor NIH Criteria
Insulin resistance
Perimenarchal onset of hirsutism and obesity
Elevated LH-to-FSH ratio
Intermittent anovulation associated with hyperandrogenemia (elevated free testosterone and/or DHEAS)
Ultrasound evidence of polycystic ovaries
Rotterdam Criteria – two of three required
Oligo and/or anovulation
Clinical or biochemical signs of hyperandrogenism
Polycystic ovaries

hirsute, and only 3% had no biochemical features to support the diagnosis of PCOS (elevated serum concentrations of testosterone, androstenedione, and/or LH) [10]. Further study of this subtype with well- characterized and validated androgen assays and clinical assessments will assist in defining or eliminating this newly included group.

While critics have labeled the Rotterdam criteria as more inclusive and necessarily less precise, an alternative viewpoint opines that utilizing subtype categorization will allow more precise characterization of the various phenotypes, genotypes, epigenetic markers, and environmental factors that create the total PCOS population.

11.3 Classical Clinical Manifestations of PCOS

The routine *menstrual dysfunction* found in PCOS arises from anovulation or oligoovulation and ranges from amenorrhea to oligomenorrhea. Regular menses in the presence of anovulation in PCOS is uncommon, though one report found that among hyperandrogenic women with regular menstrual cycles, the rate of anovulation was 21% [11]. Classically, the disorder is lifelong, characterized by abnormal menses from puberty with acne and hirsutism arising in the teens. It also, however, may arise in adulthood, concomitant with the emergence of obesity, presumably because this is accompanied by increasing hyperinsulinemia [12].

11.4 Pathology

Macroscopically, ovaries in women with diagnosed with PCOS are two to five times the normal size. Histopathologic sections of the ovary reveal a white, thickened cortex with multiple cysts usually less than one centimeter in diameter. Microscopically, the superficial cortex is fibrotic and hypocellular with prominent blood vessels. There is an increase in the number of follicles with luteinized theca interna as well as atretic follicles. The stroma contains luteinized stromal cells [13].

11.4.1 Radiologic Studies in PCOS

Ultrasonographic examination of PCOS women reveals an increase in ovarian size and an increased number of immature follicles. The Rotterdam criteria include enlarged ovaries measuring >10 cm^3 and/or more than 12 follicles measuring 2–9 mm in diameter [14, 15].

11.4.2 Pathophysiology and Laboratory Findings

Hyperandrogenism and anovulation in PCOS may be attributed to endocrine abnormalities in (a) the ovaries, (b) the adrenal glands, (c) the periphery (fat), and (d) the hypothalamus-pituitary compartment. Pathophysiologic mechanisms in each compartment are reviewed. *Ovarian dysregulation of CYP17*, the androgen-forming enzyme in both the adrenals and the ovaries, is thought to play a significant role in mechanisms underlying hyperandrogenism in PCOS [16]. First, PCOS ovaries appear to be more sensitive to gonadotropic stimulation, possibly as a result of CYP17 dysregulation [16]. Second, the ovarian stroma, theca, and granulosa, are stimulated by LH, and excess secretion may result in hyperandrogenemia [17]. In fact, total and free testosterone levels correlate with LH levels [18]. Third, when a gonadotropin-releasing hormone (GnRH) agonist is administered in PCOS patients, serum testosterone and androstenedione levels are suppressed [19], however, even larger doses are required for estrogen suppression [20]. For the above reasons, elevated testosterone levels in patients with PCOS appear to be predominantly ovarian in origin. The serum total testosterone levels may be within normal limits or no more than twice the upper normal range (20–80 ng/dL). In ovarian hyperthecosis, values may reach 200 ng/dL or more [21].

The adrenal compartment also plays a role in the development of PCOS. Although the hyperfunctioning CYP17 androgen-forming enzyme coexists in both the ovaries and the adrenal glands, DHEAS is increased in only about 50% of patients with PCOS [22, 23]. The hyperresponsiveness of DHEAS to stimulation with ACTH [21], the onset of symptoms around puberty, and the observation that 17,20-lyase activation (one of the two CYP17 enzymes) is a key event in adrenarche have led to the hypothesis that *PCOS may arise as an exaggeration of adrenarche.*

In the peripheral compartment (skin and the adipose tissue), the activity of 5α-reductase in the skin determines the presence or absence of hirsutism [24, 25]. Aromatase and 17β-hydroxysteroid dehydrogenase activities are increased in fat cells [26], and increased peripheral aromatization parallels increased body weight [27]. Obesity decreases the metabolism of estrogens through reduced 2-hydroxylation and 17α-oxidation, resulting in an increased E1 to E2 ratio [28]. The E1 levels are increased due to the peripheral aromatization of androstenedione [29]. As a result of the reversed E1-to-E2 ratio, a chronic hyperestrogenic state is created.

The hypothalamic-pituitary compartment also contributes to the development of PCOS. As a result of an increased GnRH pulse frequency, the LH pulse frequency is increased compared to normal follicular phase levels [30]. This hypothalamic activity is the cause of the frequently noted LH to FSH reversal. FSH is not elevated perhaps because of the GnRH pulse frequency and the chronic hyperestrogenic state. To date, a clear pathogenic relationship between hypothalamic-pituitary system and insulin resistance in polycystic ovary syndrome remains elusive. Controversy over essential diagnostic criteria continue in PCOS, and although LH/FSH ratio >2 has been considered to be a useful diagnostic criteria, this is now under question as significant heterogeneity is now recognized based on the varying PCOS subtypes. A recent study demonstrated that the LH/FSH ratio was not a characteristic attribute of all PCOS women and was detected in a subpopulation smaller than 50%. The PCOS women with normal gonadotropin ratios belonged to a group of patients suffering from hyperinsulinemia and obesity. Thus, patients with hyperinsulinemia and excess of LH may constitute a distinct subgroup possessing increased adrenal androgenic activity. Additional studies will characterize and determine the utility of the LH/FSH ratio for various subtypes of the PCOS disorder [31]. In as many as 25% of PCOS patients, prolactin levels are elevated, which also may be a result of abnormal estrogen feedback on the pituitary. In one study, bromocriptine reduced LH levels and resulted in ovulation [32].

11.5 Long-Term Risks OF PCOS

In chronic anovulatory patients with PCOS, persistent estrogen stimulation, unopposed by progesterone, increases the risk of endometrial carcinoma [33]. The majority of these endometrial cancers are well-differentiated, stage I lesions with a cure rate of more than 90%. Endometrial biopsy should be considered in all PCOS patients, as they may occasionally harbor these cancers early in their reproductive years. Abnormal bleeding, increasing weight, duration of symptoms, and age are factors that lower the threshold for endometrial sampling. Preventing endometrial cancer is a primary management goal for patients with PCOS. If individualized management does not induce regular ovulation (e.g., clomiphene) or introduce continuous progestation influence (e.g., oral contraceptives or progestin-containing intrauterine device), regular secrectory transformation should be induced with periodic administration of a progestational agent. Additionally, a hyperestrogenic state in PCOS is associated with an increased risk of breast cancer [34] as well as a two to threefold increase in ovarian cancer [34, 35]. The risks are greater in nonobese women and patients who have not been taking OCs.

The incidence of insulin resistance in PCOS women is 25–70% [36, 37]. A recent meta-analysis regarding pregnancy outcomes in PCOS patients showed a nearly threefold higher rate of gestational diabetes mellitus among women with PCOS (OR, 2.94; 95% CI, 1.72–5.08) [38]. While some consider this increased risk to be associated with a higher level of obesity in PCOS women, a number of other studies confirm PCOS itself is associated with an increased risk of developing gestational diabetes [38].

When considering pregnancy complications and neonatal outcomes, a recent meta-analysis of eight studies demonstrates a significantly higher risk of pregnancy-induced hypertension in PCOS women (OR, 3.67; 95% CI, 1.98–6.81), and a higher risk of preterm delivery (OR, 1.75; 95% CI 1.16–2.62) [38]. The relationship between birth weight and PCOS is not clear. Analysis of multiple studies shows no significant increase in the incidence of macrosomia or growth retardation in PCOS women [38]. Because pregnancy complications are increased in PCOS women (preeclampsia, preterm birth, gestational), studies also document a higher rate of admission to newborn ICUs in babies born of PCOS mothers compared to controls (OR, 2.31; 95% CI, 1.25–4.26) [38]. Despite the prenatal and neonatal concerns, there does not appear to be any increased risk of neonatal malformations in infants born to women with PCOS [39–41].

In women with PCOS, the rate of early pregnancy loss has been reported to be as high as 40% [42]. Studies of control populations suggest an early pregnancy loss rate of 14.3% in normal fertile women, and 23% in pregnancies that have been preceded by subfertility [43]. The early pregnancy loss rate in women with PCOS has been attributed to elevated LH concentrations [44], higher androgen levels [45, 46], insulin resistance [47], and obesity. A recent meta-analysis of 13 studies demonstrated a significant difference in miscarriage rate in obese PCOS women compared with nonobese PCOS women (OR, 3.05; 95% CI, 1.45–6.44) [48]. While the general perception is that PCOS does increase the rate of miscarriage, evidence to support this is marginal.

11.6 Genetic Origins

PCOS is presently considered a complex genetic disorder such as schizophrenia, asthma, and type 2 diabetes [49]. Multiple factors in gene discovery efforts for such complex genetic disorders render the labors problematic: (1) multiple genes likely contribute to the disease, each with a small magnitude of effect – thus necessitating very large sample sizes in order to have adequate power to detect each gene's role; (2) environmental and lifestyle factors which are difficult to quantify and study and also contribute to risk of disease; (3) multiple gene/gene and gene/environment interactions, which participate in the manifestation of the disease; (4) the heterogeneity of severity in various phenotypic clinical presentations such that various genes may be important in various phenotypes and not others and the possibility that various genetic combinations may result in the same phenotype; (5) inappropriate selection of candidate genes for study; and the fact that (6) PCOS has ability to impair fertility, which may limit family based genetic studies (Fig. 11.1).

To date, over 150 publications and 100 candidate genes have been evaluated [50–55]. Candidate gene studies have targeted loci in four general areas:

- Steroid biosynthesis and action
- Gonadotropin synthesis and action
- Weight and energy regulation
- Insulin secretion and action

Table 11.2 lists promising PCOS candidate genes.

Table 11.2 Promising PCOS candidate genes

CYP19 aromatase
D19S884 chromosome 19 microsatellite (in gene for fibrillin-3)
IL6 – Interleukin 6
IRS1 – Insulin receptor substrate 1
SHBG – Sex hormone binding globulin

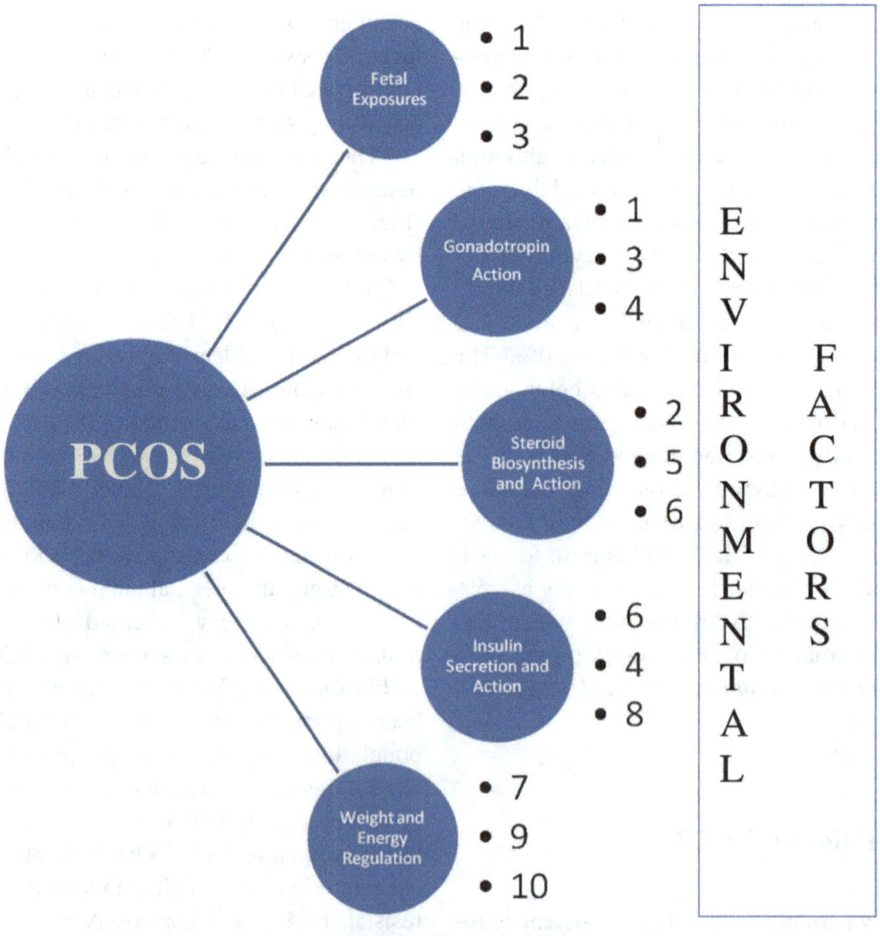

Fig. 11.1 Multiple genotypes may result in a common pathway to the phenotypic presentation of PCOS. In this illustration, a number of underlying genes (1 through 10) and environmental factors on the right, may lead to various pathophysiologic events (*small blue circles*) resulting in the common phenotype of PCOS on the left. The heterogeneity of genetic, environmental and pathophysiologic origins challenges specific gene discovery research, particularly in PCOS. Clinicians and scientists approach from the clinical presentation of PCOS with great uncertainty regarding the combination(s) of genes and environmental factors and subsequent pathophysiological events which lead to the diagnosis of the PCOS phenotype

11.6.1 Cautions Regarding the Genetic Studies of PCOS

In candidate gene studies of PCOS thus far, results are often based on less than 200 affected women, which may result in false positive results. One cause of false positive results is population stratification. Population stratification occurs when there are unidentified genetic differences between cases and controls that are not related to the disease. An example of this would be a genetic ancestry that differs significantly between cases and controls. Because the genetic ancestry is different, there may be a genetic variance, which is more common in the cases, but it actually has no causal relationship with the disease. The majority of PCOS studies have not addressed the problem of population stratification. Addressing this issue would require genotyping of ancestry informative markers. Ancestry informative markers are alleles that demonstrate substantial variances between ethnic groups. An additional complication of candidate gene studies is the evaluation of only one or two variants in each gene, which provides only partial information on whether a gene may be associated with PCOS. Genotyping of only one or two single-nucleotide polymorphisms (SNPs) yields inadequate coverage of a candidate gene. If a study does not evaluate multiple variants and results in negative findings, this discourages further investigation of that candidate gene, which may, in reality, be promising. When positive results are noted, they require confirmation in subsequent studies, which requires a significantly larger sample size [56].

Family studies, which are not affected by population stratification, appear to be a promising tool in the determination of genes associated with PCOS. Such studies have resulted in one of the most promising loci in the field, the DS19S884 microsatellite in the fibrillin-3 gene [57–59]. Another promising area of research is the use of expression differences in tissue samples from affected individuals [60]. In experiments conducted to date utilizing ovarian tissues, genes associated with altered expression patterns include transcription factors, immune response, apoptosis, Wnt signaling pathway, retinoic acid biosynthesis, cell adhesion/extracellular matrix, and cell proliferation genes. An additional pursuit is genome-wide analysis in PCOS subjects.

11.7 The Mevalonate Pathway and PCOS

Research suggests that the mevalonate pathway may potentially play a role in PCOS. The mevalonate pathway starts from acetyl-coenzyme A (acetyl-CoA) leading to the formation of farnesyl pyrophosphate (FPP). FPP acts as a substrate for a multitude of biologically important precursors, including: cholesterol, isoprenylated proteins, ubiquinone (coenzyme Q), and dolichols [61, 62] (Fig. 11.2).

Dolichols mediate the maturation of insulin and type 1 IGF-1 receptors [63]. The rate-limiting step in the mevalonate pathway is a conversion of HMG-CoA to mevalonate by HMG-CoA reductase. This enzyme (HMG-CoA reductase) is reversibly blocked by statins. The inhibition of mevalonate production leads to a decrease in downstream precursors, including FPP and geranylgeranyl pyrophosphate (GGPP). Potent posttranslational modifications of these proteins (FPP and GGPP), referred to collectively as isoprenylation, have significant downstream effects [64]. Isoprenylation is required for membrane attachment and function of multiple proteins, including Ras and Ras-related guanosine triphosphate (GTP)-binding proteins (GTPases) and protein kinases, all of which act as critical cellular membrane proteins that modulate proliferation, apoptosis, and the functional activities of various cells. Thus, interference with isoprenylation has significant cellular and metabolic downstream effects. Isoprenylation also impacts the generation of reactive oxygen species. Because activities of the mevalonate pathway correlate with sites of insulin action, including ovarian steroidogenesis, protein isoprenylation, and ovarian theca-interstitial cell proliferation [65–69], its role in PCOS is being ellucidated.

11.7.1 Statin Effects on Ovarian Function

Ovarian theca interstitial cells treated with statins demonstrate decreased cell proliferation, testosterone production, expression of steroidogenic enzymes, expression of NADPH oxydase subunits, and MAPK-dependent phosphorylation [70–80]. Thus, statins may result in a decreased thecal hyperplasia, hyperandrogenism, and oxidative stress.

11.7.2 Clinical Trials of Statins in PCOS

A recent randomized perspective clinical trial investigated the use of simvastatin (HMG-CoA reductase inhibitor) on women with PCOS [81, 82]. In that study of laboratory and clinical parameters, the effects of simvastatin and a combined oral contraceptive pill versus an oral contraceptive pill alone were evaluated. They found a reduction in total and free testosterone levels, hirsutism score, LH, total cholesterol, LDL, and CRP in simvasatin/OCP treated patients compared to those on OCPs alone for treatment. This study demonstrated the potential metabolic and endocrine benefits of HMG-CoA reductase inhibitor therapy for women with PCOS. However, statins are listed as category X medications because of their potential teratogenicity. Thus, extreme care must be taken to avoid the use of statins in any woman at risk of, or desiring pregnancy.

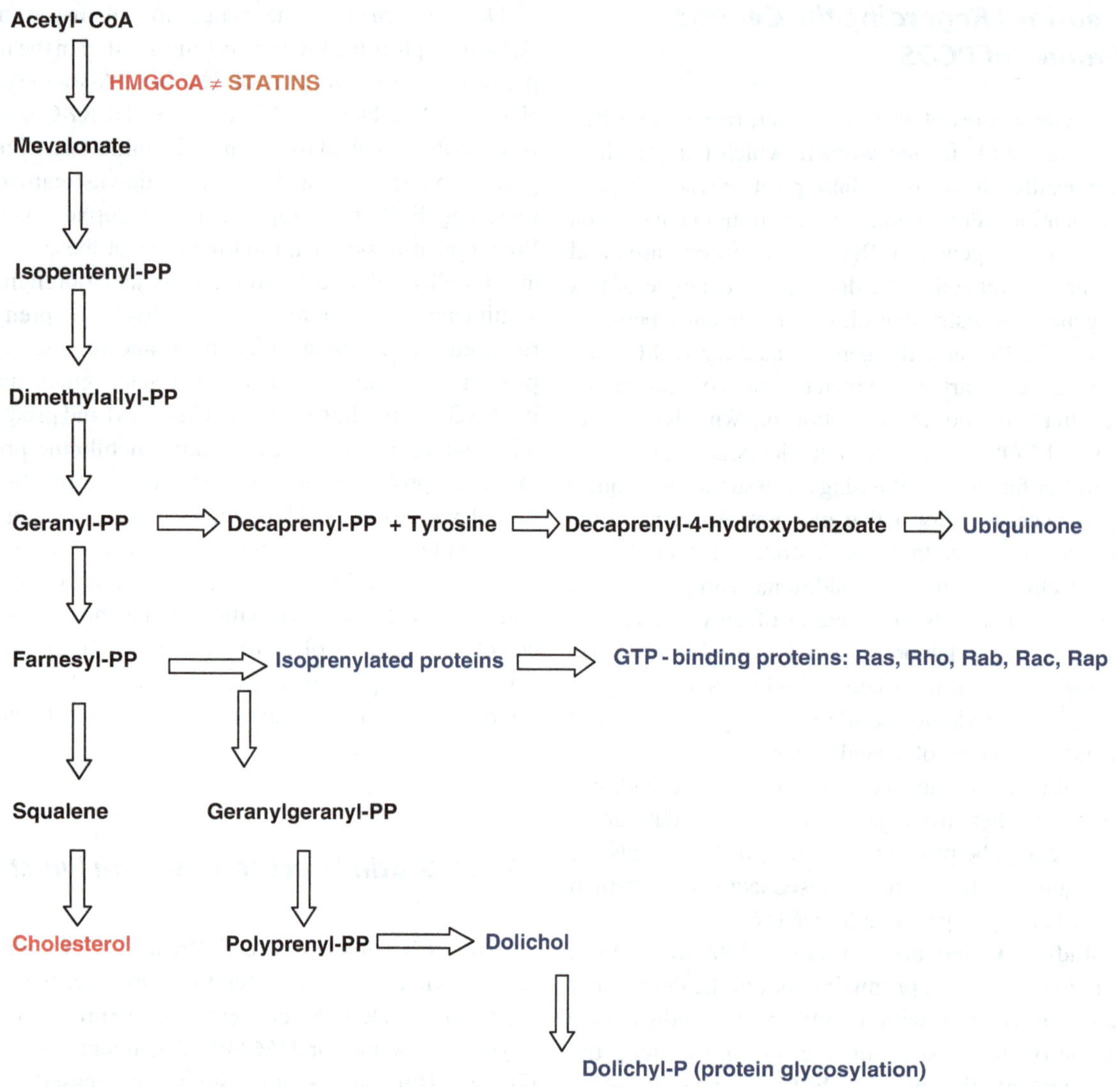

Fig. 11.2 Mevalonate pathway. Cholesterol is a major structural component of all cell membranes. In addition to its role in the control of cell osmolarity, it plays a pivotal role in the process of pinocytosis and in the activities of membrane-associated proteins such as ionic pumps, immune responses, and cell-growth. Cholesterol is derived from endogenous synthesis or from exogenous sources, principally delivered by plasma low-density-lipoproteins (LDL), which enter the cells by receptor-mediated endocytosis. Both pathways are functional in rapidly growing cells. If cholesterol synthesis is inhibited, cell growth is blocked. 3-hydroxy-3-methylglutaryl CoA (HMG-CoA) reductase (the rate-limiting reaction in cholesterol biosynthesis) is the enzyme which catalyzes the conversion of HMG-CoA to mevalonic acid. Mevalonic acid (mevalonate) is important in cell proliferation. All cells require a minimum of two products synthesized from mevalonate in order to proliferate. Cholesterol is one, and the other(s) are yet to be determined. Other mevalonate-derived products with significant roles in cellular function include the dolichols, the cofactor ubiquinone, and isopentenyladenosine derivatives (GTP-binding proteins: Ras, Rho, Rab, Rac, Rap), etc. The development of cholesterol-synthesis-inhibiting drugs, used to lower plasma cholesterol levels, has mainly been focused on the control of HMG-CoA reductase activity (STATINS). Because mevalonic acid is a precursor for many metabolic products, any reduction of HMG-CoA reductase activity may result in other effects. Statins are now being evaluated as potential pharmacological tools in a number of mevlonate pathway dependent cellular functions found in PCOS

In summary, there is accumulating evidence that statins may help correct dyslipidemia, reduce systemic inflammation, improve endothelial function and reduce oxidative stress in women with PCOS. Additionally, there is an indirect reduction in steroidogenesis and cellular proliferation. These effects may ultimately deliver positive cardiovascular benefits to women with PCOS.

11.8 Insulin Resistance in PCOS

Insulin resistance and hyperinsulinemia participate in the ovarian steriodogenic dysfuction of PCOS. Insulin has been shown to alter ovarian steroidogenesis independent of gonadotropin secretion in PCOS. Both insulin and insulin-like growth factor I (IGF-I) receptors are present in the ovarian stromal cells. Diminished autophosphorylation in insulin receptor-mediated signaling has been identified in 50% of women with PCOS [83]. *Insulin resistance*, diagnosed by an impaired glucose tolerance (IGT), is found in nearly one-third of obese PCOS patients, and 7.5–10% exhibit type 2 diabetes mellitus [84]. Nonobese PCOS women show a 10% prevalence of IGT, and 1.5% display diabetes [85], compared with 7.8% IGT and 1% diabetes, respectively, in the general population of the United States [86].

While the most common cause of insulin resistance and compensatory hyperinsulinemia is obesity, obesity alone does not completely explain this association in PCOS [32]. Additionally, the insulin resistance associated with PCOS is not solely the result of hyperandrogenism. In general, hyperinsulinemia is not characteristic of hyperandrogenism [87]. Furthermore, suppressing ovarian steroidogenesis in women with PCOS with GnRH analogs does not change insulin levels or insulin resistance [7]. Finally, studies of patients with hyperthecosis, hyperinsulinemia, and hyperandrogenemia who had undergone oophorectomy revealed no change in insulin resistance, despite a drop in androgen levels [88].

Acanthosis nigricans, a pigmented, velvety skin lesion most often found on the vulva, axilla, nape of the neck, below the breast, or on the inner thigh, is a reliable marker of insulin resistance [89]. The HAIR-AN syndrome [83, 90], acronym finds its origin in the constellation of hyperandrogenism (HA), insulin resistance (IR), and acanthosis nigricans (AN). These patients often have fasting insulin levels of greater than 25 μIU/mL (normal <20–24 μIU/mL), and maximal serum insulin responses to glucose load (75 g) exceeding 300 μIU/mL (normal is <160 μIU/mL at 2 h post-glucose load).

11.8.1 Screening Strategies for Diabetes and Insulin Resistance in PCOS

Multiple testing/screening schema have been proposed to assess hyperinsulinemia and hence insulin resistance. In one, the fasting glucose-to-insulin ratio is determined, and values less than 4.5 indicate insulin resistance. Using the 2-h GTT with insulin levels, 10% of nonobese and 40–50% of obese PCOS women have impaired glucose tolerance (IGT = 2 h glucose level ≥140≤199 mg/dL) or overt Type II diabetes mellitus (any glucose level >200 mg/dL). Peak insulin levels of over 150 mcIU/mL or a mean level of over 84 mcIU/mL over the three blood draws of a 2-h GTT may be used as criteria to diagnose hyperinsulinemia in research settings. Tables 11.3 and 11.4 detail normal, impaired and type II diabetes diagnostic glucose levels after a glucose load.

Unfortunately, documenting hyperinsulinemia with a glucose to insulin ratio <4.5 or the 2-h GTT with insulin levels is problematic. It has been shown that the glucose-to-insulin ratio does not always accurately portray insulin resistance when compared to the gold standard for measuring insulin resistance, the hypeinsulinemic-euglycemic clamp. Additionally, in hyperglycemic states, a relative insulin secretion deficit is present. This deficit of insulin secretion exacerbates the effects of insulin resistance and renders the measurement inaccurate. For the reasons noted, routine insulin level measurements may not be particularly useful. However, testing for glucose intolerance is uniformly recommended. A woman with PCOS can be advised that her risk of cardiovascular disease correlates with this finding. The recommended frequency for such screening depends on her age, body mass index and waist circumference, all of which increase her risk.

Obesity is found in 50% of patients with PCOS (BMI > 30 kg/m^2). Centripedal (android) obesity, with a higher waist-to-hip ratio is associated with insulin resistance, and suggests an increased risk of diabetes mellitus and cardiovascular disease [91].

Impaired glucose tolerance may be significantly improved with weight reduction, which may also reduce hyperandrogenism and restore ovulatory function [92]. As evidence, caloric restriction resulting in a 10-kg weight loss will yield a 40% decrease in insulin levels [93]. Similarly, a 10-kg weight loss results in a 35% reduction in testosterone levels [94]. The addition of exercise also reduces insulin resistance, independently from any associated weight loss.

Recognition of the importance of insulin resistance/hyperinsulinemia as a risk factor for cardiovascular disease led to the publication of criteria for diagnosing the Metabolic Syndrome X (ICD-9 Code: 277.7) (Table 11.5). The more criteria present, the higher the level of insulin resistance and its downstream consequences. Three criteria confirm the diagnosis and identify candidates for treatment with an insulin-lowering agent.

Table 11.3 Two-hour GTT glucose levels (WHO criteria, after 75 gm glucose load)

Fasting	64–128 mg/dL
1 h	120–170 mg/dL
2 h	70–140 mg/dL

Table 11.4 Two-hour glucose values for impaired glucose tolerance and type II diabetes (WHO criteria, after 75 gm glucose load)

Normal (2 h) < 140 mg/dL
Impaired (2 h) = 140–199 mg/dL
Type II DM (2 h) ≥ 200 mg/dL

Table 11.5 Metabolic syndrome diagnostic criteria

Female waist > 35 in.
Triglycerides > 150 mg/dL
HDL Chol < 50 mg/dL
BP > 130/85 mmHg
Fasting Glucose: 110–125 mg/dL
2 h pp Glucose (75 gm): 140–199 mg/dL

At risk individuals include those with: cardiovascular disease; hypertension; polycystic ovary syndrome; hyperandrogenemia, insulin resistance and acanthosis nigricans (HAIR-AN); nonalcoholic steatohepatosis (NASH); a family history of Type II DM; gestational diabetes; impaired glucose tolerance; non-Caucasian; sedentary lifestyle; BMI > 25; and Age > 40 year. (National Cholesterol Education Program expert panel on Detection, Evaluation, and Treatment of High Blood Cholesterol in Adults (ATP III).

The *Metabolic Syndrome* (MBS) has a twofold higher prevalence in PCOS compared to age-matched women in the general population [95]. A significant proportion of those with PCOS and MBS demonstrate *abnormal lipoproteins* including: elevated total cholesterol, triglycerides, and low-density lipoproteins (LDL), and low levels of high-density lipoproteins (HDL) and apoprotein A-I [91, 96]. A decrease in $HDL_{2\alpha}$ levels is characteristic of the PCOS population [97]. Additional findings in PCOS include impaired fibrinolysis demonstrated by elevated circulating levels of plasminogen activator inhibitor [98], an increased incidence of hypertension progressing to a 40% prevalence by perimenopause [96], a greater prevalence of atherosclerosis and cardiovascular disease [99, 100], and an estimated sevenfold increased risk for myocardial infarction [101].

11.9 Hyperandrogenism in PCOS

Hyperandrogenism most often presents as hirsutism, which is a result of androgen excess originating from the ovary and/or adrenal glands, or constitutive increase in expression of androgen effects at the level of the pilosebaceous unit, or a combination of these activities. Virilization is rare compared to hirsutism. It indicates marked elevations in androgen levels, and is commonly caused by an ovarian or adrenal neoplasm.

11.9.1 Hirsutism

Hirsutism is defined as excessive growth of terminal hair in a male distribution. Hirsutism is relative, and is based on ethnic variation in skin sensitivity to androgens and cultural acceptability. Androgen-dependent hair (excluding pubic and axillary hair), or hirsutism, occurs in only 5% of premenopausal Caucasian women and is considered abnormal by North American white women. In contrast, facial and male pattern hair in other areas may be more common and socially acceptable in groups such as the Inuit and Mediterranean women. Hirsutism in PCOS women shows ethnic diversity and is likely based on differences in skin 5α-reductase activity [24, 25]. Hirsutism is found in approximately 70% of PCOS patients in the United States [102] and in only 10–20% of Japanese patients with PCOS [103].

In determining the extent of hirsutism, a culturally sensitive and tactful approach by the physician is mandatory. It is instructive to ellicit should include descriptions of the use and frequency of shaving and/or chemical or mechanical depilatories.

Typically, clinical evaluation of the degree of hirsutism is quite subjective, with most classifying the degree of hirsutism as mild, moderate, or severe. Objective assessment is helpful, however, especially to aide in the evaluation of therapy. A hirsutism scoring scale of androgen-sensitive hair in nine body areas rated on a scale of 0–4 has been used [104] (Fig. 11.3). Scores higher than 8 are defined as hirsutism.

A family history should be obtained to disclose evidence of idiopathic hirsutism, PCOS, congenital or adult onset adrenal hyperplasia (CAH or AOAH), diabetes mellitus, and cardiovascular disease. A history of drug use should also be obtained. In addition to drugs that commonly cause hypertrichosis, anabolic steroids and testosterone derivatives may cause hirsutism and even virilization (Table 11.6).

During the physical examination, attention should be directed to obesity, hypertension, galactorrhea, male-pattern baldness, acne (face and back), and hyperpigmentation. With virilization, the presence of an androgen-producing ovarian neoplasm or Cushing's syndrome must be considered. In many cases of Cushing's syndrome, dissection of the patient's presenting symptoms reveal that hirsutism and proximal muscle weakness were primary complaints. Cushing's syndrome may masquerade as AOAH and PCOS. Each evaluation of hirsutism should include inspections for the physical signs of Cushing's syndrome, such as proximal muscle weakness, "moon face," plethora, purple striae, dorsocervical and supraclavicular fat pads. The usual preservation or even enhancement of the radial musculature in non-Cushing's, hyperandrogenic disorders is a useful tip for this differential diagnosis.

Hirsutism most commonly occurs in midline hair, side burns, mustache, beard, chest or intermammary hair, as well as inner thigh and midline lower back hair entering the intergluteal area. These androgen responsive areas transforms vellus hair (fine, non pigmented, short) into terminal hair (coarse, stiff, pigmented, and long).

Androgen responsiveness relates to body regions. Lanugo, eyebrow, and eyelashes show no androgen responsivity. Hair of the limbs and portions of the trunk exhibits minimal androgen sensitivity. Pilosebaceous units of the axilla and pubic region are highly sensitive to low levels of androgens. In these area, the weak adrenal origin androgens elicit a notable expression of terminal hair. Follicles in the distribution associated with male patterns of facial and body hair (midline, facial, inframammary) require higher levels of androgens, such as those seen with normal testicular function or abnormal ovarian or adrenal androgen production. Scalp hair is inhibited by gonadal androgens, to varying degrees. The variations are determined by age and the genetic determination of follicular responsiveness. Clinically, this

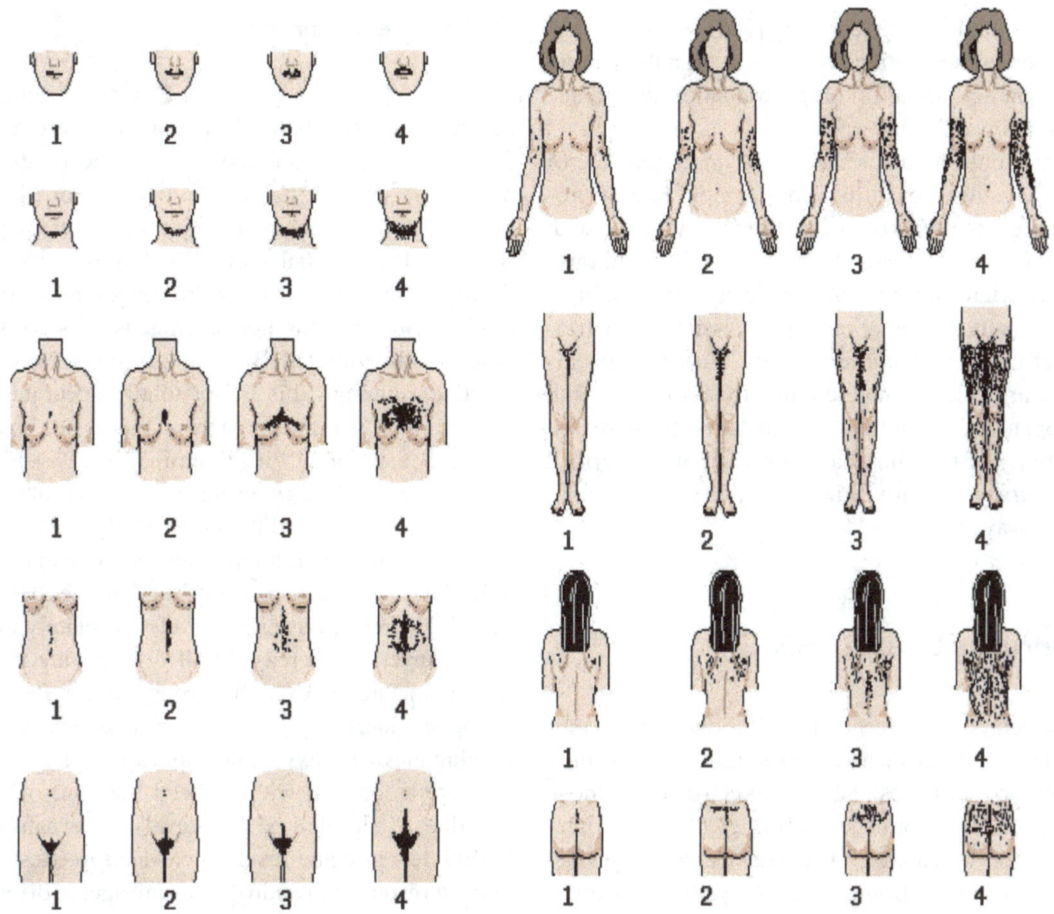

Fig. 11.3 Modified Ferriman-Gallway Scoring. Hirsutism is the presence of excess terminal hairs in androgen-dependent areas on a female, and can be measured objectively using a scoring system such as the modified Ferriman-Gallway (mF-G) score. This test is done by adding hair scores (0 = none, 4 = frankly virile) in nine body locations. A total score >8 is considered hirsute. When making the assessment personal hair removal activities prior to assessment should be ascertained to improve accuracy. Reprinted with permission from Hatch R, Rosenfield RL, Kim MH, Tredway D (1981) Hirsutism: implications, etiology, and management. Am J Obstet Gynecol 140:815–830

Table 11.6 Drugs causing hypertrichosis

Acetazolamide
Corticosteroids
Cyclosporine
Diazoxide
Interferon
Minoxidil
Phenytoin
Streptomycin

results in the common frontal-parietal balding seen in some males and in virilized females. Hirsutism results from both increased androgen production and skin sensitivity to androgens. Skin sensitivity depends on the genetically determined local activity of 5α-reductase, the enzyme that converts testosterone to dihydrotestosterone (DHT), the bioactive androgen in hair follicles.

Hair demonstrates dyssynchronous, cyclic activity between growth (anagen), involution (catagen), and resting (telogen) phases. The durations of the growth and resting phases vary according to region of the body, genetic factors, age, and hormonal effects. When synchronous entry into telogen phase is triggered by major metabolic/endocrine events, such as pregnancy, delivery, or severe illness, transient and notable hair loss may occur in the following months (telogen effluvium).

11.9.2 Hypertrichosis and Virilization

Two conditions should be distinguished from hirsutism. Hypertrichosis refers to androgen-independent terminal hair in nonsexual areas, such as the trunk and extremities. This condition may be the result of an autosomal-dominant congenital disorder, metabolic disorders (such as anorexia nervosa, hyperthyroidism, porphyria cutanea tarda), or medications (Table 11.6). Virilization is a markedly global masculine transformation that includes coarsening and deepening of the voice, increase in muscle mass, clitoromegaly (normal clitoral dimensions ± SD are 3.4 + 1 mm width by 5.1 + 1.4 mm length) and defeminization (loss of breast volume and body fat contributing to feminine body contour) [105]. Although hirsutism accompanies virilization, virilization signals a more serious condition and should prompt evaluation to exclude ovarian or adrenal neoplasm.

The history should focus on the age of onset and rate of progression of hirsutism or virilization. A rapid rate of progression of androgen effects or virilization is associated with a more severe degree of hyperandrogenism, and should raise suspicion of ovarian and adrenal neoplasms or Cushing's syndrome. This is true whether rapid progression or virilization occurs before, during or after puberty. Hirsutism occurring with regular cycles is more commonly associated with normal androgen levels, and thus is attributed to increased genetic sensitivity of the pilosebacesous unit, and is termed *idiopathic hirsutism.* When virilization is present, anovulation virtually always occurs.

11.9.3 Androgen Biosynthesis

Androgens as well as their precursors are produced by a combination of adrenal and ovarian synthesis in response to their respective trophic hormones, adrenocorticotropic hormone (ACTH) and luteinizing hormone (LH) (Fig. 11.4). The rate-limiting conversion of cholesterol to pregnenolone by side-chain cleavage enzyme begins the biosynthetic activity. Pregnenolone then undergoes a two-step conversion to the 17-ketosteroid dehydroepiandrosterone (DHEA) along the Δ-5 steroid pathway. CYP17, an enzyme with both 17α-hydroxylase and 17,20-lyase activities, performs this conversion. In a parallel fashion, progesterone undergoes transformation to androstenedione in the Δ-4 steroid pathway. The metabolism of Δ-5 to Δ-4 intermediates is accomplished through Δ-5-isomerase, 3β-hydroxysteroid dehydrogenase (3β-HSD).

11.9.3.1 Adrenal 17-Ketosteroids

Adrenal 17-ketosteroid synthesis rises prepubertally and is independent of pubertal maturation of the hypothalamic-pituitary-ovarian axis. This increase in adrenal steroid secretion is termed adrenarche, which signals a change in the response of the adrenal cortex to ACTH as well as the preferential secretion of Δ-5 steroids, including 17-hydroxypronenolone, DHEA, and dehydroepiandrosterone sulfate (DHEAS). This increased responsitivity to ACTH and focused steroid synthesis beginning in adrenarche is attributed to the increase in the zona reticularis and in the increased activity of the 17-hydroxylase and the 17,20-lyase enzymes (CYP 17). The increased adrenal androgen production in adrenarche accounts for significant increases in pubic and axillary hair, and sweat production by the axillary pilosebaceous units.

11.9.3.2 Testosterone

The peripheral conversion of secreted androstenedione accounts for one-half of a woman's serum testosterone. Direct ovarian and adrenal secretion accounts for the other half of the serum testosterone. Both the ovaries and adrenal glands contribute about equally to testosterone production in women. The adrenal's contribution is achieved primarily through secretion of androstenedione. Approximately 66–78% of circulatory testosterone is bound to sex hormone-binding globulin (SHBG) and is considered biologically inactive, although this is not totally accurate. Most of the proportion of serum testosterone that is not bound to SHBG is weakly associated with albumin (20–32%). Finally, a small percentage (1–2%) of testosterone is entirely unbound or free, and is considered the biologically active component.

The fraction of circulating testosterone that is unbound by SHBG has an inverse relationship with the SHBG concentration (high free testosterone levels correlate with low SHBG and its inverse). Increased SHBG levels are noted in conditions associated with high estrogen levels. Pregnancy, use of estrogen (including oral contraceptives), and conditions causing elevated thyroid hormone levels and cirrhosis of the liver are associated with reduced fractions of free testosterone due to elevated SHBG levels. Alternatively, levels of SHBG decrease and result in elevated free testosterone fractions in response to androgens, androgenic disorders (PCOS, adrenal hyperplasia, Cushing's syndrome), androgenic medications (progestational agents with androgenic biologic activities), danazol, and glucocorticoids, growth hormone, hyperinsulinemia, obesity, and prolactin.

It is not uncommon that total testosterone levels are well within normal limits in clinical hyperandrogenic states in women. This is due to the depression of SHBG that accompanies even mildly increased testosterone production, resulting in an increased free testosterone level but normal total testosterone level. Severe hyperandrogenism from neoplastic production of testosterone, however, is reliably detected by measures of total testosterone. Therefore, in the clinical evaluation of the hyperandrogenic patient, determination of the total testosterone level in concert with clinical assessment is frequently sufficient for diagnosis and management. If a more precise delineation of the degree of hyperandrogenism is desired, measurement or estimation of free testosterone levels can be undertaken. Although such measurements are not necessary in evaluating the majority of patients, they are common in clinical research studies and may be useful in some clinical settings. Because many practitioners measure some form of testosterone level, a rudimentary understanding of the methods and accuracy of various techniques for these measurements is useful. *Equilibrium dialysis for the measurement of testosterone* is the gold standard for measuring free testosterone, but, it is an expensive and complex

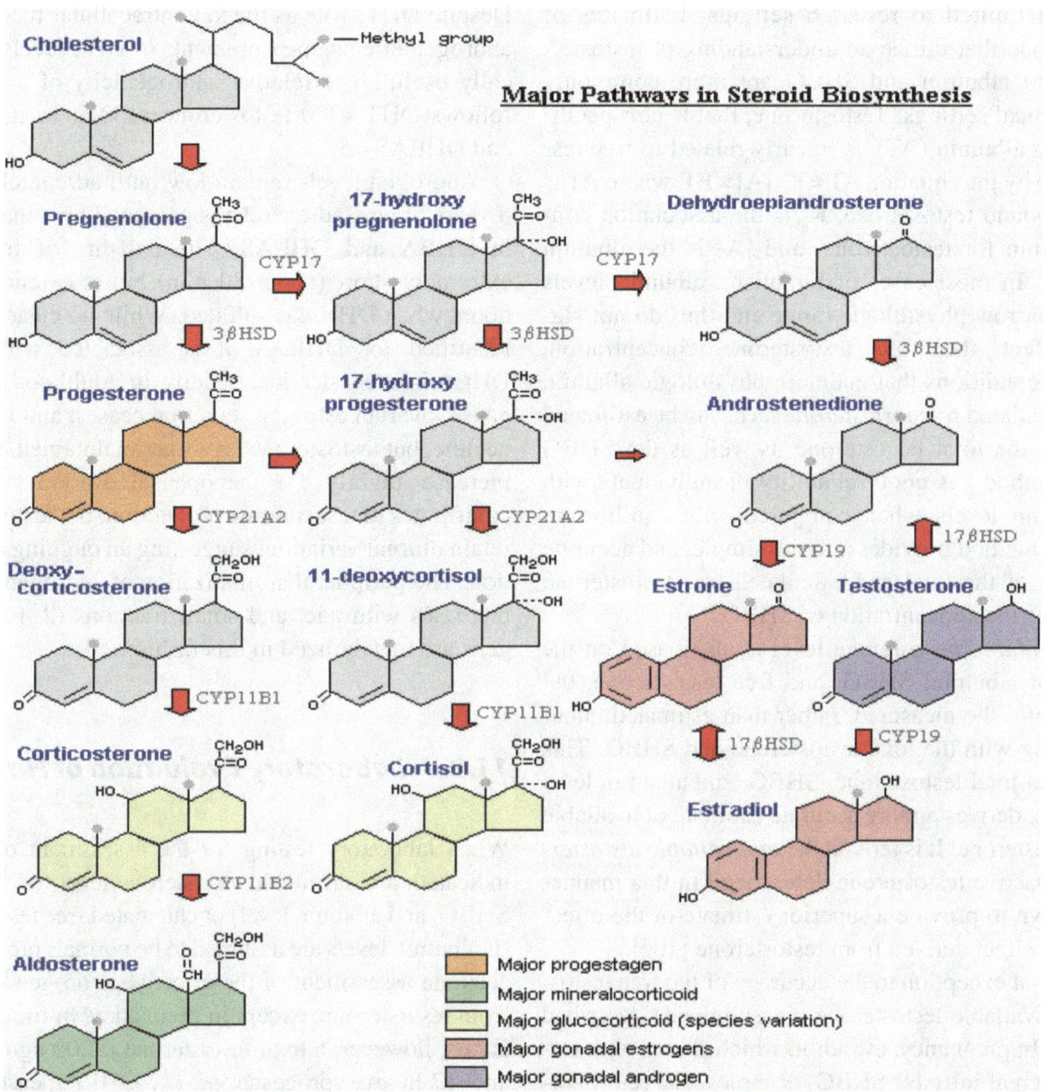

Fig. 11.4 Major Pathways in Steroid Biosynthesis: Steroid hormones are derivatives of cholesterol synthesized by a variety of tissues, most prominently the adrenal gland and gonads. The cholesterol precursor comes from: intracellular synthesis from acetate; cholesterol ester stores in intracellular lipid droplets; or, from uptake of cholesterol-containing low density lipoproteins. The basic cyclopentanoperhydrophenanthrene ring structure and carbon numbering system of all steroid hormones is depicted below, using pregnenolone as an example. Pregnenolone is an example of what is called a "C-21 steroid" because it has 21 carbons. Similarly, a steroid such as testosterone is referred to as a "C-19 steroid" and estrogen a "C-18 steroid."

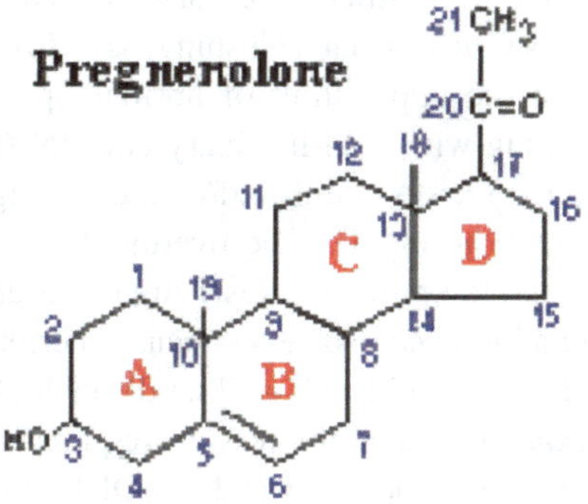

The rate-limiting step in this process is the transport of free cholesterol from the cytoplasm into mitochondria. Within mitochondria, cholesterol is converted to pregnenolone by an enzyme in the inner membrane called CYP11A1. Pregnenolone itself is not a hormone, but is the immediate precursor for the synthesis of all of the steroid hormones. The table below delineates the enzymes required to synthesize the major classes of steroid hormones depicted in the diagram above

Common name	"Old" name	Current name
Side-chain cleavage enzyme; desmolase	$P450_{SCC}$	CYP11A1
3 beta-hydroxysteroid dehydrogenase	3 beta-HSD	3 beta-HSD
17 alpha-hydroxylase/17,20 lyase	$P450_{C17}$	CYP17
21-hydroxylase	$P450_{C21}$	CYP21A2
11 beta-hydroxylase	$P450_{C11}$	CYP11B1
Aldosterone synthase	$P450_{C11AS}$	CYP11B2
Aromatase	$P450_{aro}$	CYP19

Fig 11.4, Pregnenolone and Table on this page modified and printed with permission from Richard Bowen, DVM, PhD at Colorado State University

determination limited to research settings. Estimates of free testosterone that utilize an understanding of testosterone binding to albumin and SHBG are more commonly applied in clinical settings. Testosterone, that is nonspecifically bound to albumin (AT), is linearly related to free testosterone (FT) by the equation $AT = K_a [A] \times FT$, where AT is the albumin-bound testosterone, K_a is the association constant of albumin for testosterone, and [A] is the albumin concentration. In most cases of hirsutism, albumin levels are within a narrow physiologic range and thus do not significantly affect the free testosterone concentration. Therefore, in conditions that maintain physiologic albumin levels, the calculated *free testosterone level* can be estimated by measuring the total testosterone as well as the SHBG level. This method has good reliability in individuals with normal albumin levels when compared with equilibrium dialysis. This method provides a rapid, simple, and accurate determination of the total and calculated free testosterone level as well as the concentration of SHBG.

The *bioavailable testosterone* level is also based on the relationship of albumin, SHBG, and free testosterone, but also incorporates the measured, rather than estimated, albumin level along with the total testosterone and SHBG. This combination of total testosterone, SHBG, and albumin level measurements, derives a more accurate estimate of available bioactive testosterone. It is termed the *bioavailable testosterone level.* Bioactive testosterone determined in this manner has been shown to provide a superior estimate of the effective androgen effect derived from testosterone [106].

An important exception to the accuracy of the free testosterone or bioavailable testosterone measurements described is pregnancy. In pregnancy, estradiol, which shares with testosterone a high affinity for SHBG, occupies a large proportion of SHBG binding sites, so that measurement of SHBG levels overestimate the binding capacity of SHBG for testosterone. Therefore, derived estimates of free testosterone are inaccurate during pregnancy. Testosterone measurements in pregnancy are primarily of interest when autonomous secretion by tumor or luteoma is in question, and for these, the total testosterone determination provides sufficient information for diagnosis.

The enzyme 5α-reductase, a cytosolic enzyme that reduces testosterone and androstenedione, converts testosterone into its active metabolite, DHT, resulting in biological effects. Two isozymes of 5α-reductase exist: type 1, located predominately in the skin, and type 2, or acidic 5α-reductase, found in the liver, prostate, seminal vesicles, and genital skin. The type 2 isozyme possesses a 20-fold higher affinity for testosterone than type 1. In males, both type 1 and 2 deficiencies result in ambiguous genitalia. Both isozymes may play a role in androgen effects on hair growth. Dihydrotestosterone is more potent than testosterone because of its higher binding affinity and slower dissociation from the androgen receptor. Despite DHTs role as the key intracellular mediator of most androgen effects, measurements of DHT levels are not clinically useful. The relative androgenicity of androgens is as follows: DHT = 300, testosterone = 100, androstenedione = 10, and DHEAS = 5.

Androgen levels remain low until adrenarche. At around 8 years of age, adrenarche is preceded by a marked increase in DHEA and DHEAS. The half-life of free DHEA is extremely short (about 30 min) but is extended to several hours when DHEA is sulfated. While no clear role has been identified for DHEAS, it is associated with stress, and DHEAS levels decline steadily in adulthood. After menopause, ovarian estrogen secretion ceases, and DHEAS levels decline, but testosterone levels are maintained, and may even increase slightly. Postmenopausal ovarian steroidogenesis contributes to testosterone production, but testosterone levels retain diurnal variation, suggesting an ongoing adrenal secretion. The peripheral aromatization of androgens to estrogens increases with age, and small fractions (2–10%) of androgens are metabolized in this fashion.

11.9.4 Laboratory Evaluation of Hirsutism

When laboratory testing for the assessment of hirsutism is indicated, a bioavailable testosterone level (total testosterone, SHBG, and albumin level) or calculated free testosterone level (if albumin levels are assumed to be normal) provides the most accurate assessment of the effective androgen effect derived from testosterone, except in pregnancy. In most clinical situations, however, a total testosterone (≤200 ng/mL), DHEAS, and 17-hydroxyprogesterone (17-OHP) measurements will screen for the conditions that require additional evaluation. When amenorrhea or irregular cycles accompany the presentation, LH, follicle-stimulating hormone (FSH), prolactin, and thyroid-stimulating hormone (TSH) values are required to determine the diagnosis of the ovulatory disorder. Hypothyroidism and hyperprolactinemia may result in reduced levels of SHBG and may increase the fraction of unbound testosterone levels, occasionally resulting in hirsutism. Elevated LH-to-FSH ratios are noted in some women with PCOS, but are neither necessary, nor sufficient for the diagnosis. In cases of suspected Cushing's syndrome (DHEAS elevated > twice the upper limit of normal), patients should undergo screening with a 24-h urinary cortisol (most sensitive and specific) assessment and/or an overnight dexamethasone suppression test. For the overnight dexamethasone suppression test, the patient takes 1 mg of dexamethasone at 11:00 PM, and a blood cortisol assessment is performed at 8:00 AM the next day. Cortisol levels of 2 ug/dL or higher after the overnight dexamethasone suppression require an evaluation for Cushing's syndrome. Elevated 17-OHP levels identify patients with adult onset adrenal hyperplasia (AOAH), and are found in 1–5% of hirsute women. 17-OHP levels vary significantly in the cycle, increasing in the periovulatory period and luteal phase, and may be modestly elevated in PCOS. Standardized testing requires evaluation in the morning during the follicular phase. Normal AM, baseline follicular phase 17-OHP levels are less than 200 ng/dL (6 nmol/L). When levels are greater than 200 ng/dL but less than 800 ng/dL (24 nmol/L), ACTH testing should be performed to distinguish between PCOS and AOAH. Levels greater than 800 ng/dL (24 nmol/L) are virtually diagnostic of AOAH due to 21-hydroxylase deficiency (Fig. 11.5).

Some hirsute women manifest total testosterone levels above normal (20–80 ng/dL [0.723 nmol/L]). Recalling that increased testosterone production is not reliably reflected by total testosterone levels, a clinician may choose to rely on typical male pattern hirsutism as confirmation of its presence, or may elect measures that reflect levels of free or unbound testosterone (bioavailable or calculated free testosterone levels). The total testosterone level does function reliably as a marker for testosterone producing neoplasms. Total testosterone levels >200 ng/dL should prompt a workup for ovarian or adrenal tumors and DHEAS levels greater than twice the upper limit of normal should prompt evaluation for adrenal neoplasm. Both should be measured in the presence of virilization.

In the past, testing for androgen conjugates (e.g., 3α-androstenediol G [3α-diol G] and androsterone G [AOG] as markers for 5α-reductase activity in the skin) was advocated.

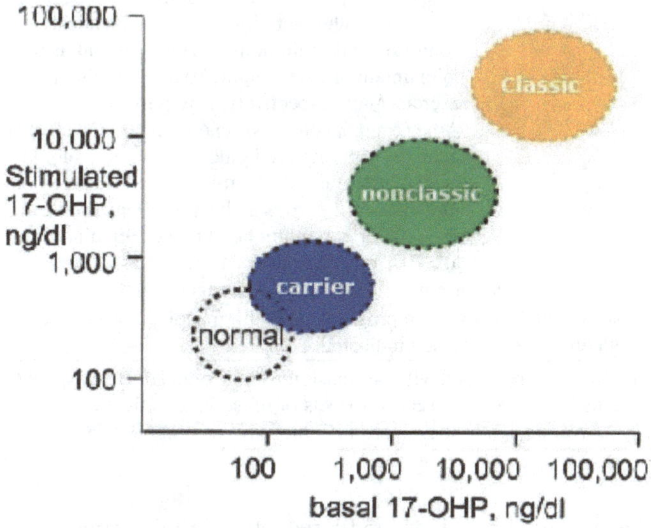

Fig. 11.5 Normogram for comparing 17-OHP levels before and 60 min after a 0.25 mg iv bolus of cosyntropin in subjects with or without 21-hydroxylase deficiency. The values for normals and heterozygotes (carriers) overlap. Therefore, DNA testing and other hormone tests may also be used to confirm the diagnosis. Reprinted with permission from Speiser and White (2000) Congenital adrenal hyperplasia due to 21-hydroxylase deficiency. Endocr Rev 21(3):245–291

However, routine determination of androgen conjugates to assess hirsute patients is not recommended, because hirsutism itself is an excellent bioassay of free testosterone action on the hair follicle and because these androgen conjugates arise from adrenal precursors and are likely markers of only adrenal steroid production [107].

For most laboratories, the upper limit of a DHEAS level is 350 μg/dL (9.5 nmol/L). A random sample suffices because the level of variation is minimized due to the long half-life of this sulfated steroid. A normal level essentially rules out adrenal disease, and moderate elevations are a common finding in the presence of PCOS *and* obesity. As a general guideline, a DHEAS level of over twice the upper limit of normal, 700 ug/dL (20 nmol/L), indicates the need to rule out an adrenal tumor or Cushing's syndrome. Absolute ceilings for this threshold vary significantly by age, as levels decline steadily after a peak around age 20. Therefore, laboratories commonly provide reference levels for age. Only rarely, ovarian tumors are associated with high DHEAS levels.

11.10 Treatment of Hyperandrogenism and PCOS

Treatment regimens depend on a patient's goals: hormonal contraception; a reduction in the effects of hyperandrogenemia; and/or ovulation induction. In all cases where there is significant ovulatory dysfunction, a progestational intervention of unopposed estrogen effects on the endometrium is required. This can be provided through periodic luteal function resulting from ovulation induction, progestational control via contraceptive formulations, or intermittent administration of progestational agents for endometrial/menstrual regulation. Interruption of the hyperandrogenism and control of hirsutism usually can be accomplished simultaneously. An exception is those patients desiring pregnancy, in whom effective control of hirsutism may not be possible. Treatment regimens for hirsutism are listed in Table 11.7. The induction of ovulation and treatment of infertility are discussed in the chapter by Gibson.

11.10.1 Weight Reduction

Weight reduction is the primary recommendation for all patients with accompanying obesity, because it is health promoting and because it reduces insulin, SHBG and androgen levels, and may restore ovulation either alone or combined with ovulation-induction agents [93]. Weight loss of as little as 5–7% over a 6-month period can reduce the bioavailable

Table 11.7 Medical treatment of hirsutism

Treatment category	Regimens
Weight loss	Dietary and lifestyle modifications Orlisat
Hormonal suppression	Oral contraceptives
	Medroxyprogesterone
	Gonadotropin-releasing hormone analogs
	Glucocorticoids
Steroidogenic enzyme inhibitors	*Ketoconazole*
5α-reductase inhibitors	*Finasteride*
Antiandrogens	*Spironolactone*
	Cyproterone acetate
	Flutamide
Insulin sensitizer	*Metformin*
Mechanical	Temporary
	Permanent
	Electrolysis
	Laser hair removal

or calculated free testosterone level significantly and restore ovulation and fertility in over 75% of women [108]. By the age of 40 years, nearly 40% of women with PCOS in the United States will have developed type-2 diabetes or impaired glucose tolerance [92].

While prevalence of a metabolic syndrome, impaired glucose tolerance, and type 2 diabetes mellitus are elevated in PCOS [85, 109], it is unclear whether there is increased long-term cardiovascular morbidity or mortality [110]. Presently, 40–60% of women with PCOS are overweight [111]. Additionally, women with PCOS display an increased central or visceral obesity [112].

National rates of obesity have increased significantly over the last 30 years in all populations, all ages, and in all countries [113, 114]. Unfortunately, in the United States, a majority of the adult population is now either overweight or obese [115]. This obesity epidemic has been attributed to a decline in energy expenditure and the intake of calorie-dense foods [116]. As our population trends towards obesity, the incidence of diabetes also increases. Presently, type-2 diabetes affects more than 60 million Americans, or about 8% of the adult population [117]. PCOS women have a greater risk of insulin resistance secondary to obesity, and hence the rates of diabetes are also increased [85, 118]. Unfortunately, the majority of patients who are able to lose weight over time regain that weight [119]. Keys to successful weight loss include regular physical activity, behavioral management strategies, social support, and particular attention to psychological adjustments including behavior modification and stress management (Moran 17). It has been documented in women with PCOS that moderate weight loss reduces insulin resistance and hyperandrogenemia [93, 98, 120], ovarian volume and follicle number [121], and results in improved menstrual function, as well as ovulation [121–123]. Additional benefits of weight loss include a reduction in the risk of developing gestational

Table 11.8 Dietary and lifestyle interventions in PCOS

Lifestyle	Lifestyle modification includes exercise, dietary and behavioral modifications
Behavioral	Behavioral modification programs are available at minimal cost from local hospitals, the American Heart Association, and other organizations
Dietary	Reduced-energy diets (500–1000 kcal/day reduction) can reduce body weight by 7–10% over a 6–12 month period
	Diets should include:
	Dairy (low fat) 2–3 servings/day
	Bread/cereals 3 servings/day
	Fruit 2 servings/day
	Vegetables 2 cups/day
	Meat/chicken/fish (lean) 1–2 servings/day
	Fats/oils (low saturated fat) 3–4 teaspoons/day or as nuts/seeds
	<10% of calories from saturated fats
	Increased fiber, whole grains, fruits and vegetables
	Increased dietary protein or unrefined carbohydrates improve reproductive and metabolic parameters equally and may be used as diet modification options. Other diet options (increased protein, reducing glycemic index, and reduced carbohydrates) are successful in achieving and maintaining optimal weight, but long-term consequences are not well studied in PCOS, to date
Exercise	Both resistance and aerobic training are required. Resistance training: 2–3 times per week, with one set of 8–15 repetitions at moderate intensity, using 8–10 exercises that work each of the major muscle groups. Aerobic training in obese individuals should begin by increasing physical activity to a goal of 200–300 min per week (20 min increasing to 45 min/day; 3–5 h/week; ≥2,000 kcal per week). This activity can be brisk walking or other activities based on physical condition and limitations. A rule of thumb is that to maintain or lose weight, 30 and 60 min of exercise/day, respectively, is requiredThe American Diabetes Association recommends that patients with impaired glucose tolerance should have a minimum of 150 min of exercise/week of moderate to vigorous activity. (150 min/week at 50–70% of maximum heart rate or 90 min/week at >70% of maximum heart rate. Resistance training is strongly encouraged
Tobacco and alcohol use	Cessation programs and pharmacologic assistance when indicated

Modified and reprinted with permission from Moran LJ, Brinkworth G, Noakes M, Norman RJ (2006) Effects of lifestyle modification in polycystic ovarian syndrome. Reprod Biomed Online 12:569–578

diabetes mellitus [124], and a reduction in miscarriage rates [123]. Furthermore, psychological parameters including self-esteem, anxiety, mean depression scores, and general health scores are improved [125]. Dietary and lifestyle interventions are listed in Table 11.8.

Exercise alone involving large muscle groups reduces insulin resistance, and is an important component of the

Table 11.9 Health benefits of regular exercise

Cardiovascular	Improves – HDL cholesterol and triglycerides
	Decreases visceral fat
	Improves blood pressure
	Reduces incidence of cardiovascular event
Diabetes type 2	Reduces development of diabetes
	Lowers Hemoglobin A1C levels
	Improves insulin sensitivity
Obesity	Reduces adiposity, including visceral fat
	Maintains lean body mass during weight loss
	Assists in maintaining weight loss and reduces regain
Osteoporosis	Enhances bone mass deposition in adolescence
	Maintains bone mass
	Protects from fractures

nonpharmacologic, lifestyle-modifying recommendations for PCOS women. It has been shown that moderate exercise can reduce, by 25%, the rate of diabetes, if at risk individuals walk briskly for 30 min per day for at least 5 days per week [126]. Women who walk 2–3 h per week total are 34% less likely to develop diabetes [127]. In addition to a reduced risk of diabetes, moderate intensity physical activity reduces cardiovascular events [128, 129] and improves insulin sensitivity [130].

While lifestyle modifications of diet and exercise are critical to the management of PCOS, there is some preliminary evidence that certain macronutrient profiles may be optimal in achieving weight loss for individuals with insulin resistance. While weight loss drugs may be helpful in initiating a reduction in weight, there does not appear to be sustained benefit from the continued use of these drugs. Bariatric surgery may be a useful technique in morbidly obese women with PCOS. Studies in this area demonstrate improvements in hirsutism, hyperandrogenism, insulin resistance, menstrual cyclicity, and ovulation [131–133].

Beyond the benefits noted, there is significant evidence from observational perspective studies that adherence to an exercise regimen after weight loss will sustain the weight loss more significantly than sedentary behavior. The American College of Obstetricians and Gynecologists provides exercise recommendations in the management of gestational diabetes [134]. Many feel these guidelines are applicable to the PCOS population. In summary, weight reduction and regular exercise should be the initial therapy for overweight PCOS patients. Table 11.7 details the Medical Treatments of PCOS-related Hirsutism, Table 11.8 reviews Dietary and Lifestyle Interventions in PCOS and Table 11.9 the Health Benefits of Regular Exercise.

11.10.2 Oral Contraceptives

Combination OCs suppress adrenal and ovarian androgen production [135–138] and reduce hair growth in nearly two-thirds of hirsute patients. OCs offer the following benefits to PCOS patients:

- The progestin component suppresses LH, resulting in diminished ovarian androgen production.
- The estrogen increases hepatic production of SHBG, resulting in decreased free testosterone concentration [139, 140].
- Circulating androgen levels are reduced, including those of DHEAS, which to some extent is independent of the effects of both LH and SHBG [91, 141].
- Estrogens decrease conversion of testosterone to DHT in the skin by inhibition of 5α-reductase.

When choosing an OC that is used to treat hirsutism, consideration of the androgenicity of the progestin must be considered. Three progestin compounds, structurally similar to 19-nortestosterone, which are present in OCs (*norgestrel, norethindrone,* and *norethindrone acetate*) are believed to be androgen dominant [142]. Oral contraceptives containing the so-called *new progestins* (*desogestrel*, *gestodene*, *norgestimate*, and *drospirenone*) have minimized androgenic activity. There is growing evidence that there is a difference in hyperandrogenic signs and symptoms using OC use based on androgenic potency. A recent study documents the potential advantages, with regards to acne, of minimally androgenic progestins (drospirenone) [143].

The use OCs with progestins similar to 19-nortestosterone may be relatively ineffective (<10% success rate) in the treatment of hirsutism in women with PCOS [144]. Insulin resistance may also be exacerbated by OCs in these patients [145]. Therefore, unless utilizing minimally androgenic progestins in the OC, management of hirsutism with OC's will usually include coadministration of agents that impede androgen action, such as spironolactone.

11.10.3 Medroxyprogesterone Acetate

Oral or intramuscular administration of *medroxyprogesterone acetate* successfully treats hirsutism [146]. It decreases GnRH production and the release of gonadotropins, thereby reducing testosterone and estrogen production by the ovary. Despite a decrease in SHBG, total and free androgen levels are decreased significantly [147]. The recommended oral dosage is 20–40 mg daily in divided doses or 150 mg given intramuscularly every 6 weeks to 3 months in the depot form. Hair growth is reduced in up to 95% of patients [148]. Side effects of the treatment include weight gain, amenorrhea, bone mineral density loss, depression, fluid retention, headaches, and hepatic dysfunction. Before instituting an intramuscular regimen of medroxyprogesterone acetate for hirsutism, a course of oral therapy may help to determine if potential adverse effects such as weight gain will be problematic.

11.10.4 Gonadotropin-Releasing Hormone Agonists

Administration of GnRH agonists may allow the differentiation of androgen produced by adrenal sources from that of ovarian sources [20]. GnRH agonists suppress ovarian steroids, including androgens, to castrate levels in patients with PCOS [149]. Treatment with *leuprolide acetate* given intramuscularly every 28 days decreases hirsutism and hair diameter in both idiopathic hirsutism and hirsutism secondary to PCOS [150]. The addition of OC or estrogen replacement therapy to GnRH agonist treatment (add-back therapy) prevents bone loss and other side effects of menopause, such as hot flushes and genital atrophy. The hirsutism-reducing effect is retained [147, 151], but not potentiated by the addition of estrogen replacement therapy [152]. Such a regimen is rarely employed due to cost considerations.

11.10.5 Glucocorticoids

Dexamethasone may be used to treat patients with adrenal hyperandrogenism (non-classic congenital adrenal hyperplasia). Routine use for PCOS is not recommended. Doses of *dexamethasone* as low as 0.25 mg every night or every other night are used initially to suppress DHEAS concentrations to less than 400 μg/dL. *Dexamethasone* has 40 times the glucocorticoid effect of cortisol, therefore, daily doses greater than 0.5 mg every evening should be avoided to prevent the risk of adrenal suppression and severe side effects that resemble Cushing's syndrome. To avoid oversuppression of the pituitary–adrenal axis, morning serum cortisol levels should be monitored intermittently (maintain at >2 μg/dL). Reduction in hair growth rate has been reported [153], as well as significant improvement in acne associated with adrenal hyperandrogenism. The utility of short-term high dose dexamethasone in ovulation induction with clomid in PCOS is discussed in the chapter by Gibson.

11.10.6 Ketoconazole

Ketoconazole inhibits the key steroidogenic cytochromes. Administered at a low dose (200 mg/day), it can significantly reduce the levels of androstenedione, testosterone, and calculated free testosterone [154]. Ketoconazole is rarely used to treat hirsutism.

11.10.7 Spironolactone

Spironolactone is a specific antagonist of aldosterone, which competitively binds to the aldosterone receptors in the distal tubular region of the kidney. This potassium-sparing diuretic was originally used to treat hypertension. The effectiveness of *spironolactone* in the treatment of hirsutism is based on the following mechanisms:

- Competitive inhibition of DHT at the intracellular receptor level [24]
- Suppression of testosterone biosynthesis by a decrease in the CYP enzymes [155]
- Increase in androgen catabolism (with increased peripheral conversion of testosterone to estrone)
- Inhibition of skin 5α-reductase activity [24]

Both total and free testosterone levels are significantly reduced in patients with both PCOS and idiopathic hirsutism (hyperandrogenism with regular menses) after treatment with *spironolactone.* The total and free testosterone levels in patients with PCOS remain higher than those with idiopathic hirsutism (hyperandrogenism with regular menses) [156]. In both groups, SHBG levels are unaltered. A modest improvement in hirsutism can be anticipated in 70–80% of women using even the minimum of 100 mg of *spironolactone* per day for 6 months [157]. Spironolactone reduces the daily linear growth rate of sexual hair, daily hair volume, and average hair shaft diameter [158]. The most common dosage is 100–200 mg per day in a divided dosage. Women treated with 200 mg/day show a greater reduction in hair shaft diameter than women receiving 100 mg/day [159]. The maximal effect on hair growth is noted at close to 6 months but continues for 12 months. Electrolysis can be recommended 9–12 months after the initiation of *spironolactone* for permanent hair removal.

Menstrual irregularity (usually metrorrhagia), is the most common side effect of *spironolactone* and occurs in over 50% of patients with a dosage of 200 mg/day [159]. Normal menses may resume with reduction of the dosage. Other side effects such as mastodynia, urticaria, or scalp hair loss occur infrequently. Nausea and fatigue can occur with high doses [157]. Because spironolactone can increase serum potassium levels, its use is not recommended in patients with renal insufficiency or hyperkalemia. Periodic monitoring of potassium and creatinine levels is suggested. Amenorrheic patients have a return of normal menses in amenorrheic patients is reported in up to 60% of cases [156]. Patients must be counseled to use contraception while taking *spironolactone* because it theoretically can feminize a male fetus.

11.10.8 Cyproterone Acetate

Cyproterone acetate, a synthetic progestin derived from 17-OHP, has potent antiandrogenic properties. The primary mechanism of *cyproterone acetate* is the competitive inhibition of testosterone and DHT at the androgen receptor [155, 160].

This agent also induces hepatic enzymes and may increase the metabolic clearance rate of plasma androgens [161]. A European formulation of *ethinyl estradiol* with *cyproterone acetate* significantly reduces plasma testosterone and androstenedione levels, suppresses gonadotropins, and increases SHBG levels [162]. *Cyproterone acetate* also shows mild glucocorticoid activity [163] and may reduce DHEAS levels [160]. It is administered in a reverse sequential regimen (cyproterone acetate 100 mg/day on days 5–15, and *ethinyl estradiol* 30–50 mg/day on cycle days 5–26). This cyclic schedule allows regular menstrual bleeding, provides excellent contraception, and is effective in the treatment of hirsutism and acne [164]. Side effects of *cyproterone acetate* include decreased libido, fatigue, headaches, irregular bleeding, nausea, and weight gain. These symptoms occur less often when used in combination with *ethinyl estradiol*. *Cyproterone acetate* administration has been associated with liver tumors in beagles and is not approved by the U.S. Food and Drug Administration for use in the United States.

11.10.9 Flutamide

Flutamide, a pure nonsteroidal antiandrogen, is approved for treatment of advanced prostate cancer. Its mechanism of action is inhibition of nuclear binding of androgens in target tissues. Although it has a weaker affinity to the androgen receptor than spironolactone or *cyproterone acetate*, larger doses (250 mg given two or three times daily) may compensate for the reduced potency. *Flutamide* also acts as a weak inhibitor of testosterone biosynthesis. In a single, 3-month study of *flutamide* alone, most patients demonstrated significant improvement in hirsutism with no change in androgen levels [165]. Significant improvement in hirsutism with a significant drop in androstenedione, DHT, LH, and FSH levels was observed in an 8-month follow-up of *flutamide* and low-dose OCs in women who did not respond to OCs alone [166]. The side effects of *flutamide* treatment combined with a low-dose OC included breast tenderness, decreased libido, dizziness, dry skin, fatigue, headaches, hot flashes, increased appetite, liver toxicity, nausea, and breast tenderness [167]. In hyperinsulinemic hyperandrogenemic nonobese PCOS adolescents on a combination of metformin (850 mg/day) and flutamide (62.5 mg/day), the low dose OC containing drospirenone, resulted in a more effective reduction in total and abdominal fat excess more efficiently than those utilizing an OC with gestodene as the progestin [168]. Additional work has demonstrated the combination of ethinyl-drospirenone, metformin and flutamide are effective in reducing excess total and abdominal fat as well as attenuating dysadipocytokinemia in young women with the hyperinsulinemic PCOS. The use of the antiandrogen, flutamide, appeared to be critical to the effects noted [169]. Many patients taking *flutamide* (50–75%) report dry skin and/or a blue-green discoloration of urine. The risk of liver enzyme elevation may preclude flutamide as a routine option for the treatment of hirsutism. Flutamide should not be used in women desiring pregnancy. Flutamide has shown efficacy in the treatment of hirsutism but has a high incidence of adverse effects and is associated with low long-term compliance [170]. At present, flutamide is considered an investigational drug and is not approved for this indication by the FDA.

11.10.10 Cimetidine

Cimetidine is a histamine H_2 receptor antagonist with a weak antiandrogenic effect as a result of its ability to occupy androgen receptors, and inhibit DHT binding at the level of the hair follicles. Although *cimetidine* has been reported to reduce hair growth in women with hirsutism [171], two later studies show no beneficial effect [172, 173]. Its use is not recommended.

11.10.11 Finasteride

Finasteride, a specific inhibitor of type 2 5α-reductase enzyme activity, has been approved in the United States at a 5-mg dose for the treatment of benign prostatic hyperplasia and at a 1-mg dose to treat male-pattern baldness. In a study in which *finasteride* (5 mg daily) was compared with *spironolactone* (100 mg daily) [174], both drugs resulted in similar significant improvement in hirsutism despite differing effects on androgen levels. Most of the improvement in hirsutism occurred after 6 months of therapy with 7.5 mg of *finasteride* everyday [175]. The improvement in hirsutism in the presence of rising testosterone levels serves as convincing evidence that it is the binding of DHT, and not testosterone, to the androgen receptor that is responsible for hair growth. *Finasteride* does not prevent ovulation or cause menstrual irregularity. The increase in SHBG caused by OCs further decreases free testosterone levels; OCs in combination with *finasteride* are more effective in reducing hirsutism than *finasteride* alone. As with *spironolactone and flutamide, finasteride* could theoretically feminize a male fetus; therefore, both of these agents are used only with additional contraception. The use of finasteride is considered investigational and is not FDA approved.

11.10.12 Ovarian Wedge Resection

Bilateral ovarian wedge resection is associated with a transient reduction in androstenedione levels and a minimal decrease in plasma testosterone [176, 177]. In patients with hirsutism and PCOS who had wedge resection, hair growth was reduced by approximately 16% [1, 178]. Despite Stein's original report citing a pregnancy rate of 85% following wedge resection and the maintenance of ovulatory cycles, subsequent reports show much lower pregnancy rates and a concerning incidence of periovarian adhesions [179].

11.10.13 Laparoscopic Ovarian Diathermy

Laparoscopic ovarian diathermy is an alternative to wedge resection in patients with *clomiphene citrate* resistant PCOS. In a recent series [180], ovarian drilling was achieved laparoscopically with an insulated electrocautery needle, using 100-W cutting current to aid in entry and 40-W coagulating current to treat each microcyst over 2 s (8-mm needle in ovary). In each ovary, 10 to 15 punctures were created. This led to spontaneous ovulation in 73% of patients, with 72% conceiving within 2 years. Of those who had undergone a follow-up laparoscopy, 11 of 15 were adhesion-free. To reduce adhesion formation, a technique that cauterized the ovary only in four points, led to a similar pregnancy rate [181], with a miscarriage rate of 14%. Most series report a decrease in both androgen and LH concentrations and an increase in FSH concentrations [182, 183]. Unilateral diathermy has been shown to result in bilateral ovarian activity [184]. A recent Cochrane review concluded that there was no evidence of a difference in the live birth rate and miscarriage rate in women with clomiphene-resistant PCOS undergoing laparoscopic ovarian diathermy (LOD) compared to gonadotrophin treatment. The reduction in multiple pregnancy rates in women undergoing LOD enhanced consideration of this option. However, there continued to be concerns about long-term effects of LOD on ovarian function [185]. The risks of surgical intervention, adhesion formation and potential alteration of ovarian function should be discussed with the patient.

11.10.14 Physical Methods of Hair Removal

Depilatory creams remove hair only temporarily. These agents break down and dissolve hair by hydrolyzing disulfide bonds. While depilatories are effective, many women cannot tolerate these irritative chemicals. The addition of a topical corticosteroid cream may prevent contact dermatitis. *Eflornithine hydrochloride* cream, also known as *difluoromethylornithine* (*DMFO*), irreversibly blocks ornithine decarboxylase (ODC), the enzyme in hair follicles that is important in regulating hair growth. It is also effective in the treatment of unwanted facial hair [186].

Shaving is effective, and contrary to common belief, does not change the quality, quantity, or texture of hair [187]. Plucking, however, may cause inflammation and damage to hair follicles and cause them to be less amenable to electrolysis. Waxing is a grouped method of plucking in which hairs are plucked out from under the skin surface. The results of waxing last longer (up to 6 weeks) than shaving or depilatory creams [187].

Bleaching removes the hair pigment through the use of hydrogen peroxide (usually 6% strength), which is sometimes combined with ammonia. Although the hair lightens and softens during oxidation, this method is associated with hair discoloration, skin irritation, and is not always effective [186]. Electrolysis and laser hair removal are the only permanent methods of hair removal. Under magnification, a trained technician destroys each hair follicle one by one. A needle is inserted into a hair follicle and galvanic current, electrocautery, or both used in combination (blend) are applied to destroy the hair follicle. After the needle is removed, a forceps removes the hair. Hair regrowth ranges from 15 to 50%. Problems with electrolysis include scarring, pain, and pigmentation. Cost may also be an obstacle [188]. Laser hair removal destroys the hair follicle through photoablation. These methods are most effective after medical therapy has arrested further growth. Thus, these techniques can be advised 6 to 9 months after medical therapy has been initiated.

11.10.15 Insulin Sensitizers

As hyperinsulinemia appears to play a role in PCOS-associated anovulation, treatment with insulin sensitizers has been a contemporary investigation. In the chapter by Legro, he reviews in detail the role of metformin in PCOS today. The following recommendations are based on current evidence.

- Clomiphene is superior to metformin in achieving live birth in infertile women with the polycystic ovary syndrome, although multiple birth is a complication [189].
- *Metformin* (*Glucophage*) is an oral biguanide antihyperglycemic drug used extensively in noninsulin-dependent diabetes and can be considered in women showing impaired glucose tolerance and improves the chances of a successful pregnancy [190].
- Amelioration of hyperinsulinemia and hyperandrogenemia with dietary intervention or metformin treatment improves significantly the clinical features and reproductive function in overweight PCOS women [191].
- While clomiphene citrate is the first choice therapy for women with therapy naïve PCOS, in clomiphene citrate-resistant women, the combination of clomiphene citrate plus metformin is an option that may be appropriately

entertained. This combination may be rationally advised before laparoscopic ovarian diathermy or gonadotropin therapy. The combination of metformin and clomiphene increases the likelihood of ovulation (OR 4.39; 95% CI 1.94–9.96; number-needed-to-treat 3.7) and pregnancy (OR 2.67; 95% CI 1.45–4.94; number-needed-to-treat 4.6) when compared with clomiphene alone, particularly in clomiphene-resistant and obese women with polycystic ovary syndrome [192].

- Presently, there is no evidence of an improvement in live birth when adding metformin to laparoscopic diathermy or gonadotropins, Metformin use in PCOS patients undergoing IVF, reduces the risk of OHSS [193].
- Metformin does not appear to be teratogenic [194].

Metformin lowers blood glucose mainly by inhibiting hepatic glucose production and by enhancing peripheral glucose uptake. *Metformin* enhances insulin sensitivity at the post-receptor level and stimulates insulin-mediated glucose disposal [195]. The hyperandrogenism seen in PCOS is substantially relieved with metformin therapy, and leads to a drop in insulin levels and improved reproductive function [196–198]. *Metformin* (500 mg, three times daily) increases ovulation rates, both spontaneously, and when used in combination with *clomiphene citrate* in obese patients with PCOS. In this group, a 90% ovulation rate has been achieved [199]. Despite the recommendation for Clomiphene citrate as first choice therapy for women with therapy naïve PCOS, in clomiphene citrate-resistant women, the combination of clomiphene citrate plus metformin is an appropriate option to employ before laparoscopic ovarian diathermy or gonadotropin therapy. The combination of metformin and clomiphene increases the likelihood of ovulation fourfold, and pregnancy twofold when compared with clomiphene alone, particularly in clomiphene-resistant and obese women with polycystic ovary syndrome [192, 200]. The most common side effects are gastrointestinal, including bloating, diarrhea, flatulence, nausea, and vomiting. Because the drug has caused fatal lactic acidosis in men with diabetes who have renal insufficiency, baseline renal function testing is suggested [201]. The drug should not be given to women with elevated serum creatinine levels [195]. In light of the association between the dysmetabolic syndrome and PCOS, some have suggested that metformin may be an appropriate first-line agent for ovulation induction in this category. Whether metformin is used as a primary ovulation induction agent or in combination with clomid, weight loss and life style interventions should be encouraged. A prevailing concern over the increased incidence of spontaneous abortions in women with PCOS and the potential reduction afforded by insulin sensitizers suggest that insulin sensitizers may be beneficial in combination with gonadotropin therapy for ovulation induction or in vitro fertilization [202].

11.10.16 Orlistat

Current concepts regarding the role of obesity and insulin resistance/hyperinsulinemia in PCOS suggest that the primary intervention should be to recommend weight loss (5–10% of body weight). In those with an elevated BMI, *orlistat* has proven to be helpful in initiating and maintaining weight loss. A percentage of PCOS patients will respond to weight loss alone with spontaneous ovulation. In those who do not respond to weight loss alone or who are unable to lose weight, the sequential addition of *clomiphene citrate*, followed by the combination of these agents, may promote ovulation without the need to proceed to injectable gonadotropins or surgery. Orlistat administration, combined with diet, for 24 weeks, resulted in significant weight loss and improvement of insulin resistance in obese women, with or without PCOS. Moreover, T levels were significantly decreased in women with PCOS. There appeared to be a trend during the first 12-week period for greater improvement of metabolic and hormonal parameters in women with PCOS [203].

11.11 Adrenal Conditions to Be Considered When Diagnosing PCOS

Cushing's syndrome, congenital adrenal hyperplasia must be entertained in when considering the diagnosis of PCOS. While these conditions are rare compared to PCOS, the consequences of these conditions warrant prompt diagnosis. Fortunately, these conditions are accompanied by more severe symptoms and laboratory abnormalities. Thus, on occasion, the evaluation of PCOS patients may include some of the screening tests indicated below.

11.11.1 Cushing's Syndrome

The adrenal cortex produces three classes of steroid hormones-glucocorticoids, mineralocorticoids, and sex steroids (androgen and estrogen precursors). Hyperfunction of the adrenal gland can produce clinical signs of increased activity of any or all of these hormones. Increased glucocorticoid production results in nitrogen wasting and a catabolic state resulting in: atrophy of the skin with striae, ecchymoses, glucose intolerance resulting from enhanced gluconeogenesis and antagonism to insulin action, muscle weakness, nonhealing ulcerations, osteoporosis, and reduced immune resistance that increases the risk of bacterial and fungal infections.

Most patients with Cushing's syndrome gain weight, however, some lose it. Obesity is typically central, with a characteristic redistribution of fat over the clavicles, around the neck, and on the trunk, abdomen, and cheeks. Cortisol excess may lead to depression, insomnia, mood disturbances, and even overt psychosis. With overproduction of sex steroid precursors, women may also exhibit hyperandrogenism (acne, hirsutism, oligomenorrhea or amenorrhea, thinning of scalp hair). Masculinization is rare, and its presence suggests an autonomous adrenal origin, most often an adrenal malignancy. When mineralocorticoids are oversecreted, patients may manifest arterial hypertension and hypokalemic alkalosis. The associated fluid retention may cause pedal edema. Characteristic clinical laboratory findings associated with hypercortisolism are confined mainly to a complete blood count showing evidence of granulocytosis and reduced levels of lymphocytes and eosinophils. Increased urinary calcium secretion may be present.

11.11.1.1 Causes of Cushing's Syndrome

The six recognized noniatrogenic causes of Cushing's syndrome can be divided between those that are ACTH dependent and those that are ACTH independent (Table 11.10).

The ACTH-dependent causes can result from ACTH secreted by pituitary adenomas or from an ectopic source. The hallmark of ACTH-dependent forms of Cushing's syndrome is the presence of normal or high plasma ACTH concentrations with increased cortisol levels. The adrenal glands are hyperplastic bilaterally. Pituitary ACTH-secreting adenoma, or Cushing's disease, is the most common cause of Cushing's syndrome. These pituitary adenomas are usually microadenomas (<10 mm in diameter) that may be as small as 1 mm. They behave as if they are resistant, to a variable degree, to the feedback effect of cortisol. Like the normal gland, these tumors secrete ACTH in a pulsatile fashion; unlike the normal gland, the diurnal pattern of cortisol secretion is lost. Ectopic ACTH syndrome most often is caused by malignant tumors. About one-half of these tumors are small-cell carcinomas of the lung [204]. Other tumors include bronchial and thymic carcinomas, carcinoid tumors of the pancreas, and medullary carcinoma of the thyroid.

Ectopic corticotropin-releasing hormone (CRH) tumors are rare and include such tumors as bronchial carcinoids, medullary thyroid carcinoma, and metastatic prostatic carcinoma [204]. The presence of an ectopic CRH-secreting tumor should be suspected in patients whose dynamic testing suggests pituitary ACTH-dependent disease but who have rapid disease progression and very high plasma ACTH levels.

The most common cause of ACTH-independent Cushing's syndrome is exogenous or iatrogenic (i.e., superphysiologic therapy with corticosteroids) or factitious (self-induced). Corticosteroids are used in pharmacologic quantities to treat a variety of diseases with an inflammatory component. Over time, such therapy will result in Cushing's syndrome. When corticosteroids are taken by the patient but not prescribed by a physician, the diagnosis may be especially challenging. The diagnostic workup for Cushing's syndrome focuses on the ability to suppress autonomous cortisol secretion, and whether ACTH is elevated or suppressed is summarized in Fig. 11.6 and Tables 11.10–11.12 [205–211].

Table 11.10 Causes of Cushing's syndrome

Category	Cause	Relative incidence
ACTH-dependent	Cushing's syndrome	60%[a]
	Ectopic ACTH-secreting tumors	15%
	Ectopic CRH-secreting tumors	Rare
ACTH-independent	Adrenal cancer	15%
	Adrenal adenoma	10%
	Micronodular adrenal hyperplasia	Rare
	Iatrogenic/factitious	Common

ACTH, adrenocorticotropic hormone; CRH, corticotropin-releasing hormone

[a]ACTH-dependent Cushing's syndrome may be caused by pituitary adenoma, basophil hyperplasia, nodular adrenal hyperplasia, or cyclic Cushing's syndrome

11.11.1.2 Treatment of ACTH-Independent Forms of Cushing's Syndrome

Excluding cases that are of iatrogenic or factitious etiology, ACTH-independent forms of Cushing's syndrome are adrenal in origin. Adrenal cancers are usually very large by the time Cushing's syndrome is manifest. This is because the tumors are relatively inefficient in the synthesis of steroid hormones. In general, tumors are larger than 6 cm in diameter and are easily detectable by computed tomography (CT) scanning or magnetic resonance imaging (MRI). Adrenal cancers often produce steroids other than cortisol. Thus, when Cushing's syndrome is accompanied by hirsutism or virilization in women or feminization in men, adrenal cancer should be suspected.

An adrenal tumor that appears large and irregular on radiologic imaging is suggestive of carcinoma. In these cases, a unilateral adrenalectomy through an abdominal exploratory approach is preferable. In most malignant tumors, complete resection is virtually impossible. However, a partial response to postoperative chemotherapy or radiation may be achieved. Most patients with malignancy die within 1 year. When administered immediately after surgery, mitotane (O,P-DDD, adrenocorticolytic drug) may be of benefit in preventing or delaying recurrent disease [212]. Manifestations of Cushing's syndrome in these patients are controlled by adrenal enzyme inhibitors.

Adrenal adenomas are smaller than carcinomas and average 3 cm in diameter. These tumors are usually unilateral and

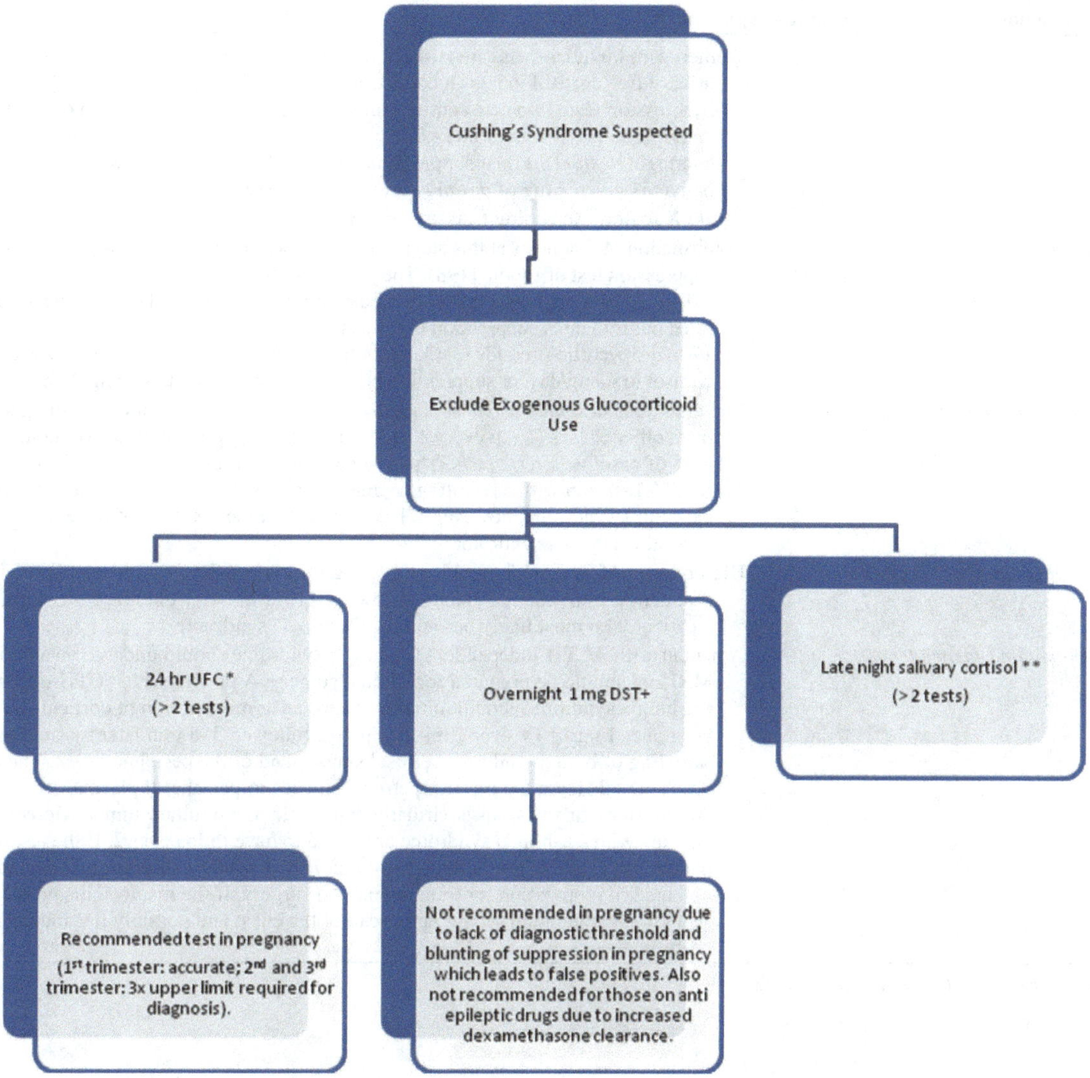

Fig. 11.6 Screening for Cushing's Syndrome. *UFC** Urinary Free Cortisol: Insure complete sample collection by discarding first morning void and collecting all subsequent voids including the first morning void of the second day. Samples should be kept refrigerated. Collectors should avoid all steroid creams including hemorrhoidal preparations. *DST** Dexamethasone Suppression Test: Phenytoin, phenobaritone, carbomazepine, rifampicin, rifapentine, ethosuximide, ploglitazone, and alcohol increase dexamethasone clearance rates. Dexamethasone metabolism is impaired by aprepitant/fosaprepitant, itraconazole, ritonavir, fluoxetine, diltiazem, cimetidine, estrogens and mitotane increase cortisol binding globulin and may falsely elevate cortisol levels. Late Night Salivary Cortisol: Salivary samples are obtained on two successive nights between 2300 and 2400. Collection occurs by passive drooling into a plastic tube or by chewing a pledget (salivette) for 1–2 min. These samples are stable for 2 weeks at room temperature. Salivary and blood cortisol correlate well. Avoid licorice, chewing tobacco or smoking when collecting sample

infrequently are associated with other steroid-mediated syndromes. Micronodular adrenal disease is a disorder of children, adolescents, and young adults. The adrenal glands contain numerous small (>3 mm) nodules, which often are pigmented and secrete sufficient cortisol to suppress pituitary ACTH. This condition can be sporadic or familial.

Surgical removal of a neoplasm is the treatment of choice [213, 214]. If a unilateral, well-circumscribed adenoma is identified by MRI or CT scanning, the flank approach may be the most convenient. The cure rate following surgical removal of adrenal adenomas approaches 100%. Because normal function of the hypothalamic-pituitary-adrenal axis is suppressed by autonomous cortisol production, cortisol replacement follows surgery and is titrated downwards over several months during which recovery of normal adrenal function is monitored.

11.11.1.3 Treatment of Cushing's Disease

Surgical Therapy

The treatment of choice for Cushing's disease is transsphenoidal resection. The cure rate is approximately 80% in patients with microadenomas who undergo surgery by an

Table 11.11 Diagnostic workup for Cushing's syndrome

Screening	Women with hirsutism who are suspected of having Cushing's syndrome should be tested for urinary free cortisol in a 24-h collection and should undergo an overnight *dexamethasone* suppression test. Two consecutive collections are recommended with creatinine determination. Normal urinary free cortisol should range from 30 to 80 μg/day. The overnight *dexamethasone* suppression test is an 8:00 AM cortisol determination after the patient is given 1 mg of *dexamethasone* at 11:00 PM the previous night. Figure X reviews screening tests and their limitations
Confirmation of diagnosis	Confirmation of diagnosis at this stage can be performed by the 2-day, low-dose *dexamethasone* suppression test of Liddle [198]. The patient is given 0.5 mg of *dexamethasone* every 6 h for 2 days. A 24-h urine specimen is collected during the second day. Cushing's syndrome is ruled out if there is suppression of urinary 17-hydroxycorticosteroids to <3 mg/24 h (or to 0% of baseline), suppression of plasma cortisol to <4 μg/day, or suppression of urinary free cortisol to <25 μg/24 h
Differentiation of Cushing's syndrome	The high-dose *dexamethasone* suppression test is used to differentiate Cushing's syndrome from other causes (2 mg every 6 h). Normally, urinary 17-hydroxycorticoids should be 40% of baseline after 2 days. This test partially suppresses adrenocorticotropic hormone (ACTH) section with a resulting decrease in cortisol production in most patients with Cushing's syndrome; however, it has no effect on the majority of patients with ectopic or adrenal Cushing's syndrome
Differentiation of ectopic ACTH syndrome	High plasma ACTH (>4.5 pmol/L or >20 pg/mL) is consistent with ectopic ACTH production from adrenal glands. A low ACTH level (<1.1 pmol/L or <5 pg/mL) identifies a patient who most likely has adrenal Cushing's syndrome
ACTH-independent and -dependent	A patient with ACTH-independent Cushing's syndrome should undergo an adrenal scan by MRI and should be prepared for adrenal surgery. A patient with ACTH-dependent Cushing's syndrome should initially receive an administration of cortical-releasing hormone (1 ug/kg IV over 1 min), which is followed 3–5 min later by simultaneous sampling of both the inferior petrosal sinuses and of the peripheral vein. The ratio of ACTH levels from the inferior petrosal sinuses to peripheral plasma is then calculated. An inferior petrosal sinus is virtually diagnostic of a pituitary tumor. Moreover, 95% of patients with Cushing's syndrome are found to have ratios over 2. If the test indicates a patient has Cushing's syndrome, a pituitary MRI with gadolinium enhancement should be obtained in preparation for transsphenoidal surgery. If the results indicate ectopic ACTH secretion, a computed tomography scan of the chest and possibly the abdomen should be performed

IV intravenous; *MRI* magnetic resonance imaging

Table 11.12 Laboratory diagnosis of Cushing's syndrome

	24 h	DEX	DEX	
Diagnosis	Urinary cortisol	Low dose	High dose	ACTH
ACTH-dependent				
Cushing's syndrome (60%)	Increased	Increased	Decreased	Normal
Pituitary adenoma				
Basophil hyperplasia				
Nodular adrenal hyperplasia				
Cyclic Cushing's syndrome				
Ectopic ACTH (15%)	Increased	Increased	Increased	Increased
Ectopic CRH (rare)	Increased	Increased	Increased or decreased	Increased
ACTH-independent				
Adrenal neoplasia	Increased	Increased	Increased	Decreased
Adenoma (10%)				
Carcinoma (15%)				
Primary adrenocorticoid nodular dysplasia (<1%)				
Pseudo-Cushing's syndrome (alcohol-related, <1%)	Increased	Increased	Decreased	Normal
Exogenous glucocorticoids/factitious (not cortisol)	Increased or decreased	Decreased	Decreased	Decreased

DEX dexamethasone; *ACTH* adrenocorticotropic hormone; *CRH* corticotropin-releasing hormone experienced surgeon [208], and is less than 50% in patients with macroadenomas [209]. Following surgery, transient diabetes insipidus and enduring compromise of anterior pituitary secretion of growth hormone, gonadotropins, and TSH, are common [210].

Radiation Therapy

High-voltage external pituitary radiation (4,200–4,500 cGy) is given at a rate not exceeding 200 cGy/day. Although only 15–25% of adults show total improvement [210], approximately 80% of children respond [211].

Medical Therapy

Mitotane can be used to induce medical adrenalectomy during or after pituitary radiation [212]. The role of medical therapy is to prepare the severely ill patient for surgery and to maintain normal cortisol levels while a patient awaits the full effect of radiation. Occasionally, medical therapy is used for patients who respond to therapy with only partial remission. Adrenal enzyme inhibitors include *aminoglutethimide*, *metyrapone*, *trilostane*, and *etomidate*.

A combination of *aminoglutethimide* and *metyrapone* may cause a total adrenal enzyme block requiring corticosteroid-replacement therapy. *Ketoconazole*, an FDA-approved antifungal agent, also inhibits adrenal steroid biosynthesis at the side arm cleavage and 11β-hydroxylation steps. The dose of *ketoconazole* for adrenal suppression is 600–800 mg/day for 3 months to 1 year [215]. *Ketoconazole* is effective for long-term control of hypercortisolism of either pituitary or adrenal origin.

Nelson's syndrome results from adenomatous progression of ACTH-secreting cells in patients with Cushing's syndrome treated by bilateral adrenalectomy. This macroadenoma that causes this syndrome produces sellar pressure symptoms of headaches, visual field disturbances, and ophthalmoplegia. Extremely high ACTH levels in Nelson's syndrome are associated with severe hyperpigmentation (melanocyte-stimulating hormone activity). The treatment is surgical removal or radiation. The offending adenomatous tissue is often resistant to complete surgical removal [216]. This syndrome reportedly complicates 10–50% of bilateral adrenalectomy cases. Nelson's syndrome is less common today, because bilateral adrenalectomy is less frequently used as initial treatment.

11.11.2 Congenital Adrenal Hyperplasia

CAH is transmitted as an autosomal recessive disorder. Several adrenocortical enzymes necessary for cortisol biosynthesis may be affected. Failure to synthesize the fully functional enzyme has the following effects:

- A relative decrease in cortisol production
- A compensatory increase in ACTH levels
- Hyperplasia of the zona reticularis of the adrenal cortex
- An accumulation of the precursors of the affected enzyme in the bloodstream

11.11.2.1 21-Hydroxylase Deficiency

Deficiency of 21-hydroxylase (CYP21A2) is responsible for over 90% of all cases of adrenal hyperplasia attributed to adrenal enzyme deficiencies. The disorder produces a spectrum of conditions congenital adrenal hyperplasia (CAH), with or without salt wasting, and milder forms that are expressed as hyperandrogenism of pubertal onset (nonclassic, late onset, cryptic, or adult-onset adrenal hyperplasia). Salt-wasting CAH, the most severe form, affects 75% of patients with congenital manifestations during the first 2 weeks of life, and results in a life-threatening hypovolemic salt-wasting crisis, accompanied by hyponatremia, hyperkalemia, and acidosis. The salt-wasting form results from a severity of enzyme deficiency sufficient to result in ineffective aldosterone synthesis. With or without salt-wasting and newborn adrenal crisis, the condition is usually diagnosed earlier in affected female newborns than in males as genital virilization (e.g., clitoromegaly, labioscrotal fusion, and abnormal urethral course) is apparent at birth.

In simple virilizing CAH, affected patients are diagnosed as virilized newborn females or as rapidly growing masculinized boys at 3–7 years of age. Diagnosis is based on basal levels of the substrate for 21-hydroxylase, 17-hydroxyprogesterone (17-OHP), in cases of congenital adrenal hyperplasia due to 21 hydroxylase deficiency. In milder forms of the disorder with manifestations later in life (acquired, late onset, or adult-onset adrenal hyperplasia), diagnosis depends upon basal and ACTH-stimulated levels of 17-OHP. Figure 11.7 reviews the effects of 21-hydroxylase deficiency (CYP21A2).

1. Basal follicular phase 17-OHP <200 ng/dL virtually excludes the disorder; no further testing is required.
2. Basal 17-OHP >500 ng/dL establishes the diagnosis; there is no need for further testing [217].
3. Basal 17-OHP >200 ng/dL and <500 ng/dL requires ACTH stimulation testing.
4. In the ACTH stimulation test, plasma levels of 17-OHP are checked 1 h following intravenous administration of a bolus of 0.25 mg ACTH 1–24 (*cosyntropin* [*Cortrosyn*]) (Fig. 25.3). 17-OHP levels after ACTH stimulation in adult-onset adrenal hyperplasia are generally >1,000 ng/dL [217] (Fig. 11.5).

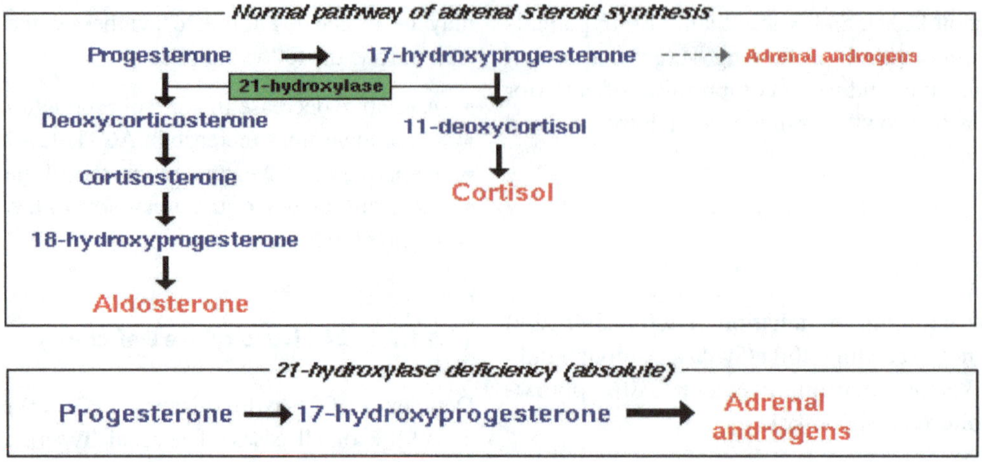

Fig. 11.7 Congenital Adrenal Hyperplasia. Congenital adrenal hyperplasias (CAH) are a group of heritable disorders associated with an inability or deficiency in the ability to produce cortisol. Approximately 90% of these disorders are due to 21-hydroxylase deficiency. Without adequate cortisol production excessive secretion of corticotropin-releasing hormone from the hypothalamus and ACTH from the anterior pituitary results in continuous stimulation of the adrenal cortex leading to hyperplasia. The deficiency in aldosterone production results in a mild to severe loss of body sodium. Because of the block in 21-hydroxylase enzyme there is an overproduction of adrenal androgens, which leads to the development of ambiguous genitalia in the female fetus during pregnancy. Modified and printed with permission from Richard Bowen, DVM, PhD at Colorado State University

5. Individuals who are heterozygous (carriers) for both adult-onset adrenal hyperplasia and CAH reveal stimulated 17-OHP values <1,000 ng/dL. In many cases, an overlap with the values seen in the normal population is observed [218] (Fig. 11.5).

11.11.2.2 Nonclassic or Adult Onset or Late Onset or Cryptic Congenital Adrenal Hyperplasia (NCCAH)

The nonclassic type of 21-hydroxylase deficiency (CYP21A2) represents partial deficiency in 21-hydroxylation, which produces a late-onset, milder hyperandrogenemia. Its occurrence depends on some degree of functional deficit resulting from mutations affecting both alleles for the 21-hydroxylase enzyme. Heterozygote carriers for mutations in the 21-hydroxylase enzyme will demonstrate normal basal, and modestly elevated stimulated levels of 17-OHP, but exhibit no abnormalities in circulating androgens. Some women with a mild gene defects in both alleles demonstrate modest elevations in circulating 17-OHP concentrations but no clinical symptoms or signs.

The hyperandrogenic symptoms of AOAH are mild and typically present at or after puberty. Following are the three phenotypic varieties [217]:

- Those with ovulatory abnormalities and features consistent with PCOS (39%)
- Those with hirsutism alone without oligomenorrhea (39%)
- Those with elevated circulating androgens but without symptoms (Cryptic) (22%)

The need for screening patients with hirsutism for nonclassic adrenal hyperplasia depends on the patient population. The frequency of some form of the disorder varies by ethnicity and is estimated at 0.1% of the general population, 1–2% of Hispanics and Yugoslavs, and 3–4% of Ashkenazi Jews [219].

Treatment of Adult-Onset Congenital Adrenal Hyperplasia (AOAH)

In adults with CAH, *dexamethasone* has been shown to suppress the hypothalamic-pituitary axis better than cortisone acetate or hydrocortisone administered in equivalent doses and to possibly induce less fluid retention than other corticosteroids. Evening administration with a dosage of 0.25–0.5 mg is most effective [220]. In some patients, alternate-day therapy using the same dosage is sufficient. Periodic evaluation of serum cortisol is recommended. If morning serum cortisol concentrations are maintained at greater than 2 μg/dL, oversuppression, with consequent impaired hypothalamic-pituitary-adrenal responsiveness to acute stress, is unlikely [221]. Many patients with AOAH undoubtedly are treated, undiagnosed, with therapies for ovarian hyperandrogenism and/or PCOS, with progestins for endometrial regulation, clomiphene or gonadotropins for ovulation induction, or progestins and antiandrogens for control of hirsutism. These therapies may be appropriate, as an alternative to glucocorticoid therapy, even when AOAH is recognized as the cause for the patient's symptoms.

Genetics of 21-Hydroxylase Deficiency

Classical congenital adrenal hyperplasia (CAH) affects one in 14,000 patients, however, mild forms of the disease may occur in one of every 100 to 1,000 individuals. Congenital adrenal hyperplasia is caused by the deficient synthesis of cortisol, with 90% of cases attributed to 21-hydroxylase deficiency. The affected enzyme can be totally or partially impaired and is altered by at least nine mutations, many of which leave the enzyme impaired but not totally inactive. The incidence of classic congenital adrenal hyperplasia is especially high in Madagascar and certain areas of Alaska. Mild congenital adrenal hyperplasia occurs more frequently in Ashkenazi Jews, and in Hispanic, Slavic and Italian populations. Approximately, 1 in 60 people in North America are carriers of Classic CAH and the frequency of LOCAH carriers may be as high as 1 in 5.

1. The 21-hydroxylase gene is located on the short arm of chromosome 6, in the midst of the HLA region.
2. The 21-hydroxylase gene is now termed *CYP21*. Its homologue is the pseudogene *CYP21P* [222].
3. Because *CYP21P* is a pseudogene, the lack of transcription renders it nonfunctional. The *CYP21* is the active gene.
4. The *CYP21* gene and the *CYP21P* pseudogene alternate with two genes called *C4B* and *C4A,* both of which encode for the fourth component (C4) of serum complement [222].
5. The close linkage between the 21-hydroxylase genes and HLA alleles has allowed the study of 21-hydroxylase inheritance patterns in families through blood HLA typing (e.g., linkage of HLA-B14 was found in Ashkenazi Jews, Hispanics, and Italians) [223].

Prenatal Diagnosis and Treatment

Women with congenital and nonclassic forms of the disorder are at a significant risk for having affected infants, owing to the high frequency of mutations in 21-hydroxylase mutations in the general population. This fact comprises an important rationale for screening hyperandrogenic women for this disorder in the event they anticipate childbearing. In families at risk for CAH, and in instances where one partner expresses the congenital or adult onset form of the disease, first-trimester prenatal screening using chorionic villus sampling is advocated [222]. Currently, the fetal DNA is used for specific amplification of the *CYP21* gene using polymerase chain reaction (PCR) amplification [224]. When there is evidence for fetal involvement, an aggressive and still controversial approach involves the use of *dexamethasone* treatment for all pregnant women at risk of having a child with CAH. The dosage of 20 mg/kg in three divided doses is administered as soon as pregnancy is recognized and no later than 9 weeks of gestation. This is done prior to performing chorionic villus sampling or amniocentesis in the second trimester. *Dexamethasone* crosses the placenta and suppresses ACTH in the fetus. If the fetus is determined to be an unaffected female or a male, treatment is discontinued. If the fetus is an affected female, dexamethasone therapy is continued. When *dexamethasone* is administered before 9 weeks of gestation and is continued to term, it effectively reduces genital ambiguity in genetic females [222]. However, at least two-thirds of treated females may still require surgical repair of the genitalia. Although prenatal treatment reduces virilization in females, the efficacy and safety to both mother and baby have not been verified. The unnecessary treatment in seven out of every eight pregnancies poses a serious ethical dilemma [225].

11.11.2.3 11β-Hydroxylase Deficiency

In a small percentage of patients with CAH, hypertension rather than mineralocorticoid deficiency develops. The hypertension responds to corticosteroid replacement [226]. Most of these patients have a deficiency in 11*β*-hydroxylase. In most populations, 11*β*-hydroxylase deficiency accounts for 5–8% of the cases of CAH, or 1 in 100,000 births [227]. A much higher incidence, 1 in 5,000 to 7,000, has been described in Moroccan Jewish immigrants [228].

Two 11*β*-hydroxylase isoenzymes are responsible for cortisol and aldosterone synthesis, respectively, CYP11-B1 and CYP11-B2. They are encoded by two genes on the middle of the long arm of chromosome 8 [229, 230].

Inability to synthesize a fully functional 11*β*-hydroxylase enzyme causes a decrease in cortisol production, a compensatory increase in ACTH secretion, and increased production of androstenedione, 11-deoxycortisol, 11-deoxycorticosterone, and DHEA. The diagnosis of 11*β*-hydroxylase-deficient late-onset adrenal hyperplasia is determined when 11-deoxycortisol levels are higher than 25 ng/mL 60 min after ACTH 1–24 stimulation [231].

Patients with 11*β*-hydroxylase deficiency may present with either a classic pattern of the disorder or symptoms of a mild deficiency. The severe, classic form is found in about two-thirds of the patients with mild-to-moderate hypertension during the first years of life. In about one-third of the patients, it is associated with left ventricular hypertrophy, with or without retinopathy, and death is occasionally reported from cerebrovascular accident [226]. Signs of androgen excess are common in the severe form and are similar to those seen in the 21-hydroxylase deficiency.

In the mild, nonclassic form, children are found to have virilization or precocious puberty but not hypertension. Adult women will seek treatment for postpubertal onset of hirsutism, acne, and amenorrhea. This enzyme mutation and others are reviewed in Table 11.13.

Table 11.13 Congenital adrenal hyperplasia due to enzyme mutations other than 21-hydroxylase

Deficiency	Incidence	Comments
11 beta-hydroxylase CYP11B1	~1 in 100,000 livebirths	Females are virilized; salt-wasting is rare
17 alpha-hydroxylase CYP17	Rare	Males are virilized; females fail to achieve puberty. Salt-wasting not observed
3 beta-hydroxysteroid dehydrogenase (3 beta-HSD)	Rare	Males are virilized; female virilization is mild. Salt-wasting may be seen
Aldosterone synthase CYP11B2	Rare	Cortisol concentrations normal and virilization not seen. Salt-wasting occurs
StAR	Rare	Males are virilized; females fail to achieve puberty. Salt-wasting occurs

11.11.2.4 3β-Hydroxysteroid Dehydrogenase Deficiency

Deficiency of 3*β*-hydroxysteroid dehydrogenase occurs with varying frequency in hirsute patients [232, 233]. The enzyme is found in both the adrenal glands and ovaries (unlike 21- and 11-hydroxylase) and is responsible for transforming Δ-5 steroids into the corresponding Δ-4 compounds, a step integral to the synthesis of glucocorticoids, mineralocorticoids, as well as testosterone and estradiol. In severe forms, cortisol and mineralocorticoids are deficient. In mild forms, elevated ACTH levels overcome these critical deficiencies, and the diagnosis of this disorder relies on the relationship of Δ-5 and Δ-4 steroids. A marked elevation of DHEA and DHEAS in the presence of normal or mildly elevated testosterone or androstenedione may be a signal to initiate a screening protocol for 3*β*-hydroxysteroid dehydrogenase deficiency using exogenous ACTH stimulation [232]. Following intravenous administration of a 0.25-mg ACTH 1–24 bolus, 17-hydroxypregnenolone levels rise significantly within 60 min in women with 3*β*-hydroxysteroid dehydrogenase deficiency compared with normal women (2,276 ng/dL compared with normal of 1,050 ng/dL). The mean poststimulation ratio between 17-hydroxypregnenolone and 17-OHP is markedly elevated (mean ratio of 11 compared with 3.4 in normal controls and 0.4 in 21-hydroxylase deficiency). Because of the rarity of this disorder, routine screening of hyperandrogenic patients is not justified [232, 233]. This enzyme mutation and others are reviewed in Table 11.13.

11.12 Androgen-Secreting Ovarian and Adrenal Tumors

Patients with severe hirsutism, virilization, or recent and rapidly progressing signs of androgen excess require careful investigation for the presence of an androgen-secreting neoplasm. In prepubertal girls, virilizing tumors may cause signs of heterosexual precocious puberty in addition to hirsutism, acne, and virilization. All patients with rapidly progressing or severe hyperandrogenism should undergo determination of levels of testosterone and DHEAS. A markedly elevated total testosterone level (2.5 times the upper normal range or over 200 ng/dL) is typical of an ovarian androgen-secreting tumor, and a DHEAS level greater than 800 μg/dL is typical of an adrenal tumor. An adrenal tumor is unlikely when serum DHEAS and urinary 17-ketosteroid excretion measurements are in the normal basal range, and the serum cortisol concentration is less than 3.3 μg/dL after dexamethasone administration [234]. The results of other dynamic tests, especially testosterone suppression and stimulation, are unreliable [235].

A vaginal and abdominal ultrasonographic examination is the first step in the evaluation of findings suggesting ovarian neoplasm. Duplex Doppler scanning may increase the accuracy of tumor diagnosis and localization [236]. CT scanning can reveal tumors larger than 10 mm (1 cm) in the adrenal gland but may not help to distinguish among different types of solid tumors, or benign incidental nodules [237]. In the ovaries, CT scanning cannot help differentiate hormonally active from functional tumors [236, 237]. MRI is comparable, if not superior, to CT scanning in detecting ovarian neoplasms, but is not more sensitive than high quality ultrasound, nor more useful in clinical decision making when ultrasound identifies likely neoplasm. Nuclear medicine imaging of the abdomen and pelvis after injection with NP-59 ((131-iodine) 6-beta-iodomethyl-19-norcholesterol), preceded by adrenal and thyroid suppression, may facilitate tumor localization [232]. In the rare circumstances when imaging fails to provide clear evidence for a neoplastic source of excess androgens, selective venous catheterization with measurement of site-specific androgen levels to identify an occult source of androgen excess may be utilized [238]. If all four vessels are catheterized transfemorally, selective venous catheterization allows direct localization of the tumor. Samples are obtained for hormonal analysis, with positive localization defined as a 5:1 testosterone gradient compared with lower vena cava values [239]. Under such circumstances, specificity approaches 80%, but this rate should be weighed against the 5% rate of significant complications such as adrenal hemorrhage and infarction, venous thrombosis, hematoma, and radiation exposure [240].

11.12.1 Androgen-Producing Ovarian Neoplasms

Ovarian neoplasms are the most frequent androgen-producing tumors. *Granulosa cell tumors* constitute 1–2% of all ovarian tumors and occur most commonly in adult postmenopausal women. Usually granulose cell tumors are associated with estrogen production, and are the most common functioning tumors in children, and lead to isosexual precocious puberty [241]. Total abdominal hysterectomy and bilateral salpingo-oophorectomy are the treatments of choice. If fertility is desired, in the absence of contralateral ovarian or pelvic node involvement, a unilateral salpingo-oophorectomy is a consideration. The malignant potential of these lesions is variable. The 10-year survival rates vary from 60 to 90%, depending on the stage, tumor size, and histologic atypia [241].

Thecomas are rare and occur most often in older patients. In one study, only 11% were androgenic, even in the presence of steroidogenic cells (luteinized thecomas) [241]. The tumor is rarely malignant and rarely bilateral. A unilateral oophorectomy is adequate treatment.

Sclerosing stromal tumors are benign neoplasms found in patients younger than 30 years [241]. A few cases with estrogenic or androgenic manifestations have been reported.

Sertoli-Leydig cell tumors, previously classified as androblastoma or arrhenoblastoma, comprise 11% of solid ovarian tumors. They contain various proportions of Sertoli cells, Leydig cells, and fibroblasts [241]. Sertoli-Leydig cell tumors are the most common virilizing tumors in women of reproductive age; however, only one-third of patients are masculinized. Bilateral tumors are found in 1.5%. In 80% of cases, it is diagnosed at stage IA [241]. A unilateral salpingo-oophorectomy is appropriate in patients with stage IA disease who desire to maintain fertility. Total abdominal hysterectomy, bilateral salpingo-oophorectomy, and adjuvant therapy, are recommended for postmenopausal women with advanced-stage disease. *Pure Sertoli cell tumors* are usually unilateral. For a premenopausal woman with stage I disease, a unilateral salpingo-oophorectomy is the treatment of choice. Malignant tumors are rapidly fatal [242].

Gynandroblastomas are benign tumors with well-differentiated ovarian and testicular elements. A unilateral oophorectomy or salpingo-oophorectomy is sufficient treatment. *Sex cord tumors with annular tubules (SCTAT)* are frequently associated with Peutz-Jeghers syndrome (gastrointestinal polyposis and mucocutaneous melanin pigmentation) [243]. Morphologic features include characteristics of both the granulosa cell and Sertoli cell tumors.

SCTAT with Peutz-Jeghers syndrome tends to be bilateral and benign. SCTAT without Peutz-Jeghers syndrome is almost always unilateral, and is malignant 20% of the time [241].

11.12.2 Steroid Cell Tumors

According to Young and Scully, steroid cell tumors are steroid-secreting cells subclassified as: stromal luteoma; Leydig cell tumors (hilar and nonhilar); and steroid cell tumors that are not otherwise specified [241]. Virilization or hirsutism is found in 75% of Leydig cell tumors, 50% of steroid cell tumors that are not otherwise specified, and in 12% of stromal luteomas.

11.12.3 Nonfunctioning Ovarian Tumors

Ovarian neoplasms not directly secreting androgens are occasionally associated with androgen excess. This is caused by excess secretion from adjacent ovarian stroma. Potential androgen secreting tumors include serous and mucinous cystadenomas, Brenner tumors, Krukenberg tumors, benign cystic teratomas, and dysgerminomas [244]. Gonadoblastomas associated with the dysgenetic gonads of patients with a Y chromosome are rarely associated with androgen and estrogen secretion [245, 246].

11.12.4 Stromal Hyperplasia and Stromal Hyperthecosis

Stromal hyperplasia is a nonneoplastic proliferation of ovarian stromal cells. Stromal hyperthecosis is defined as the presence of luteinized stromal cells at a distance from the follicles [247]. Stromal hyperplasia is usually seen in patients between 60 and 80 years of age. It may be associated with hyperandrogenism, endometrial carcinoma, obesity, hypertension, and glucose intolerance [247]. *Hyperthecosis* also is seen in a mild form in older patients. In patients of reproductive age, hyperthecosis may manifest with virilization, obesity, and hypertension. Hyperinsulinemia and glucose intolerance may occur in up to 90% of patients with hyperthecosis and may contribute to the etiology of stromal luteinization and hyperandrogenism [89]. Hyperthecosis is found in many patients with hyperandrogenemia, insulin resistance, and acanthosis nigricans (HAIR-AN syndrome). In patients with hyperthecosis, levels of ovarian androgens, including testosterone, DHT, and androstenedione are increased, usually in the male range. The predominant estrogen, as in PCOS, is estrone, which is derived from peripheral aromatization. The E_1-to-E_2 ratio is increased. Unlike in PCOS, gonadotropin levels are normal [248]. Wedge resection for the treatment of mild hyperthecosis has been successful and has resulted in resumption of ovulation and even in a pregnancy [249].

In more severe hyperthecosis with high total testosterone levels, the ovulatory response to wedge resection is transient [248]. In a study in which bilateral oophorectomy was used to control severe virilization, hypertension and glucose intolerance sometimes disappeared [250]. GnRH agonist treatment for severe hyperthecosis results in decreased ovarian androgen production [251].

11.13 Virilization During Pregnancy

Luteomas of pregnancy are often found in cases maternal and fetal masculinization. This entity is not a true neoplasm, but a reversible hyperplasia that usually regresses postpartum. The literature suggests a 30% incidence of maternal virilization and a 65% incidence of virilized female newborns in the presence of a pregnancy luteoma and maternal masculinization [252].

Other tumors causing virilization in pregnancy include (in descending order of frequency) Krukenberg tumors, mucinous cystic tumors, Brenner tumors, serous cystadenomas, endodermal sinus tumors, and dermoid cysts [241].

11.14 Virilizing Adrenal Neoplasms

The most common virilizing adrenal neoplasms are *adrenal carcinomas*. When these malignancies virilize, they are invariably associated with elevations in DHEAS and hypercortisolism. These tumors are usually large, and can often be detected on abdominal examination. The adrenals are also the site for *testosterone secreting adenomas*. A high testosterone level (in the tumor range), accompanied by normal or only moderately elevated DHEAS levels, should still prompt the physician to evaluate the adrenal gland and not the ovary.

The majority of adenomas are benign. The literature reveals that the peak age for the diagnosis of adenomas is 20–40 years, but the majority of the pure testosterone-producing adenomas occur in menopausal women. Adenomas were almost exclusively unilateral. Fifty percent were palpable abdominally in children, but none were palpable in adults [253].

11.15 Evidence-Based Guidelines in PCOS

The diagnosis of PCOS is based on:

- NIH Criteria – both required
  - Chronic anovulation
  - Clinical or biochemical signs of hyperandrogenism; or
- Rotterdam Criteria – two of three required
  - Oligo and/or anovulation
  - Clinical or biochemical signs of hyperandrogenism
  - Polycystic ovaries

All women with PCOS should be screened for glucose intolerance with a 2-h glucose level after a 75 g fasting glucose challenge. Furthermore, screening for dyslipidemia should be performed with a total cholesterol, LDL, HDL and triglyceride determination. Additional evaluations, based on clinical findings, may include a:

- TSH to detect thyroid hypofunction, which can be associated with hyperandrogenism
- Prolactin level to detect hyperprolactinemia that can be found in hyperandrogenemia
- Total testosterone, if there are concerns on the clinical exam (virilization) that suggest an ovarian or adrenal testosterone secreting tumor
- Fasting 17-OHP to screen for 21-hydroxylase deficiency
- 24 h urinary cortisol to screen for Cushing's syndrome

Table 11.14 details other conditions that can mimic PCOS as well as their incidence and workup.

Those who have three criteria qualify for the diagnosis of the metabolic syndrome and should be advised of their increased risk for diabetes, cardiovascular disease, and stroke.

Metabolic Syndrome Diagnostic Criteria
Female waist > 35 in.
Triglycerides > 150 mg/dL
HDL Chol < 50 mg/dL
BP > 130/85 mmHg
Fasting Glucose: 110–125 mg/dL
2 h pp Glucose (75 gm): 140–199 mg/dL

The *Metabolic Syndrome* (MBS) has a twofold higher prevalence in PCOS compared to age-matched women in the general population. *Obesity* is found in 50% of patients with PCOS (BMI > 30 kg/m^2). Centripedal (android) obesity, with a higher waist-to-hip ratio, is associated with insulin resistance, and suggests an increased risk of diabetes mellitus and cardiovascular disease. Weight loss should be emphasized as the primary treatment option in PCOS and in some cases insulin sensitizers may be indicated. Regular exercise (aerobic and resistance training) is a critical aspect of long term maintenance. A rule of thumb is that to maintain or lose weight, 30 and 60 min of exercise/day, respectively, is required. Hirsutism is found in approximately 70% of PCOS patients in the United States. Combination OCs suppress adrenal and ovarian androgen production and reduce hair growth in nearly two-thirds of hirsute patients. A number of other therapies may be indicated based on clinical findings and patient wishes.

Clomiphene citrate is the first choice for ovulation induction in PCOS patients seeking pregnancy. Weight loss and

Table 11.14 Conditions that can mimic PCOS

Diagnosis	Clinical findings	Evaluations	Incidence
PCOS	± irregular menses, hirsutism, obesity, infertility, diabetes, hypertension, family history of PCOS	2 h glucose after a 75 g (fasting) load, lipid profile, blood pressure, abdominal girth, BMI	82%
Hyperandrogenism, Hirsutism, Normal cycles	Regular menses, acne, hirsutism without detectable endocrine cause	Elevated androgen levels and normal serum progesterone in luteal phase	6.8%
Idiopathic Hirsutism	Regular menses, hirsutism,	Normal total testosterone, possible bioavailable testosterone abnormalities	4.7%
Hyperandrogenism,insulin-resistance and acanthosis nigricans (HAIR-AN)	Brown velvety patches of skin (acanthosis nigricans), obesity, hypertension, hyperlipidemia, family history of diabetes	Fasting glucose and 2 h glucose after 75 gm load, lipid profile, fasting insulin level not necessary with AN	3.1%
21-hydroxylase non-classic adrenal hyperplasia (late-onset CAH)	Significant hirsutism or virilization, strong family history of CAH, short stature, signs of defeminization, more common in Ashkenazi Jews and Eastern European decent	17-OHP levels after ACTH stimulation in adult-onset adrenal hyperplasia are generally >1,000 ng/dL,CYP21 genotyping before childbearing	1.6%
21-hydroxylase-deficient congenital adrenal hyperplasia (Classic and Simple-virilizing)	Hypovolemic salt-wasting crisis, hyponatremia, hyperkalemia, and acidosis Classic CAH is usually diagnosed earlier in affected female newborns than in males due to genital virilization Simple virilizing CAH is usually diagnosed as a virilized newborn female or as a rapidly masculinizing boys 3–7 years of age	Basal 17-OHP >500 ng/dL establishes the diagnosis; there is no need for further testing	0.7%
Hypothyroidism	Fatigue, weight gain, constipation, history of thyroid ablation and untreated hypothyroidism, amenorrhea	TSH, anti TPO, anti thyroglobulin antibodies if TSH elevated	0.7%
Hyperprolactinemia	Amenorrhea, galactorrhea, infertility	Prolactin, drug history, MRI as necessary	0.3%
Androgenic secreting neoplasm	Rapid-onset hirsutism or virilization, over age 30 with onset of symptoms, pelvic masses	Pelvic imaging: ultrasound or abdomen/pelvic CT scan	0.2%
Cushing's syndrome	Proximal muscle weakness, hypertension, buffalo hump, purple striae, truncal obesity	Elevated blood pressure, positive 24 h urinary free cortisol and dexamethasone suppression test	0%

Source: Azziz et al. (2004) J Clin Endocrinol Metab; and Azziz (2003) Obstet Gynecol

insulin sensitizer therapy in PCOS patients and particularly in those with the metabolic syndrome may reduce cardiovascular risk. When gonadotropins are used to induce ovulation in PCOS, low dose protocols reduce the risk of ovarian hyperstimulation. When undergoing IVF the addition of metformin reduces the risk of ovarian hyperstimulation. In chronic anovulatory patients with PCOS, persistent estrogen stimulation, unopposed by progesterone, increases the risk of endometrial carcinoma. The majority of these endometrial cancers are well-differentiated, stage I lesions with a cure rate of more than 90%. Endometrial biopsy should be considered in all PCOS patients. Preventing endometrial cancer is a primary management goal for patients with PCOS. If individualized management does not induce regular ovulation (e.g., clomiphene) or introduce continuous progestation influence (e.g., oral contraceptives or progestin-containing intrauterine device), regular secrectory transformation should be induced with periodic administration of a progestational agent. Additionally, a hyperestrogenic state in PCOS is associated with an increased risk of breast cancer as well as a two to threefold increase in ovarian cancer. The incidence of insulin resistance in PCOS women is 25–70%. A recent meta-analysis regarding pregnancy outcomes in PCOS patients showed a nearly a threefold higher rate of gestational diabetes mellitus among women with PCOS (OR, 2.94; 95% CI, 1.72–5.08). While some consider this increased risk to be associated with a higher level of obesity in PCOS women, a number of other studies confirm PCOS itself is associated with an increased risk of developing gestational diabetes. When considering pregnancy complications and neonatal outcomes, a recent meta-analysis of eight studies demonstrates a significantly higher risk of pregnancy-induced hypertension in PCOS women (OR, 3.67; 95% CI, 1.98–6.81) and a higher risk of preterm delivery (OR, 1.75; 95% CI, 1.16–2.62). Because pregnancy complications are increased in PCOS women (preeclampsia, preterm birth, gestational), studies also document a higher rate of admission to newborn ICUs in babies born of PCOS mothers compared to controls (OR, 2.31; 95% CI, 1.25–4.26). Despite the prenatal and neonatal concerns, there does not appear to be any increased risk of neonatal malformations in infants born to women with PCOS. In women with PCOS, the rate of early pregnancy loss has been reported to be as high as 40%. Studies of control populations suggest an early pregnancy loss rate of 14.3% in normal fertile women, and 23% in pregnancies that have been preceded by subfertility. The early pregnancy loss rate in women with PCOS has been attributed to elevated LH concentrations, higher androgen levels, insulin resistance, and obesity. A recent meta-analysis of 13 studies demonstrated a significant difference in miscarriage rate in obese women compared to nonobese PCOS women (OR, 3.05; 95% CI, 1.45–6.44). Regular follow-up with PCOS patients is warranted in order to intervene and have an impact on long term health.

References

1. Stein IF, Leventhal ML (1935) Amenorrhea associated with bilateral polycyctic ovaries. Am J Obstet Gynecol 29:181–191
2. Zawadzki JK, Danif A (1992) Diagnostic criteria for polycystic ovary syndrome towards a rational approach. In: Dunaif A, Givens JR, Hasetine FP et al (eds) Polycystic ovary syndrome. Blackwell Science, Cambridge, pp 377–384
3. Carmina E, Lobo RA (2001) Polycystic ovaries in Hirsute women with normal menses. Am J Med 111(8):602–606
4. Franks S, Gharani N, Waterworth D, Batty S, White D, Williamson R et al (1997) The genetic basis of polycystic ovary syndrome. Hum Reprod 12(12):2641–2648
5. Carey AH, Chan KL, Short F, White D, Williamson R, Franks S (1993) Evidence for a single gene effect causing polycystic ovaries and male pattern baldness. Clin Endocrinol (Oxf) 38(6):653–658
6. Legro RS, Driscoll D, Strauss JF III, Fox J, Dunaif A (1998) Evidence for a genetic basis for hyperandrogenemia in polycystic ovary syndrome. Proc Natl Acad Sci U S A 95(25):14956–14960
7. Dunaif A, Graf M, Mandeli J, Laumas V, Dobrjansky A (1987) Characterization of groups of hyperandrogenic women with acanthosis nigricans, impaired glucose tolerance, and/or hyperinsulinemia. J Clin Endocrinol Metab 65(3):499–507
8. Robinson S, Kiddy D, Gelding SV, Willis D, Niththyananthan R, Bush A et al (1993) The relationship of insulin insensitivity to menstrual pattern in women with hyperandrogenism and polycystic ovaries. Clin Endocrinol (Oxf) 39(3):351–355
9. Carmina E, Chu MC, Longo RA, Rini GB, Lobo RA (2005) Phenotypic variation in hyperandrogenic women influences the findings of abnormal metabolic and cardiovascular risk parameters. J Clin Endocrinol Metab 90(5):2545–2549
10. Adams J, Polson DW, Franks S (1986) Prevalence of polycystic ovaries in women with anovulation and idiopathic hirsutism. Br Med J (Clin Res Ed) 293(6543):355–359
11. Carmina E, Lobo RA (1999) Do hyperandrogenic women with normal menses have polycystic ovary syndrome? Fertil Steril 71(2):319–322
12. Peserico A, Angeloni G, Bertoli P, Marini A, Piva G, Panciera A et al (1989) Prevalence of polycystic ovaries in women with acne. Arch Dermatol Res 281(7):502–503
13. Clement PB (1994) Nonneoplastic lesions of the ovary. In: Kurman RJ (ed) Blaustein's pathology of the female genetial tract, 4th edn. Springer-Verlag, New York, pp 559–604
14. Comparetto G, Gullo D, Venezia R, Mogavero G (1982) Proposal for a purely echographic classification of the polycystic ovary syndrome. Acta Eur Fertil 13(2):79–94
15. Farquhar CM, Birdsall M, Manning P, Mitchell JM, France JT (1994) The prevalence of polycystic ovaries on ultrasound scanning in a population of randomly selected women. Aust NZ J Obstet Gynaecol 34(1):67–72
16. Rosenfield RL, Barnes RB, Cara JF et al (1990) Dysregulation of cytochrome P450-17 α as the cause of polycystic ovarian syndrome. Fertil Steril 53:785–791
17. McNatty KP, Makris A, DeGrazia C, Osathanondh R, Ryan KJ (1979) The production of progesterone, androgens, and estrogens by granulosa cells, thecal tissue, and stromal tissue from human ovaries in vitro. J Clin Endocrinol Metab 49(5):687–699
18. Lobo RA, Kletzky OA, Campeau JD, diZerega GS (1983) Elevated bioactive luteinizing hormone in women with the polycystic ovary syndrome. Fertil Steril 39(5):674–678
19. Chang RJ, Laufer LR, Meldrum DR, DeFazio J, Lu JK, Vale WW et al (1983) Steroid secretion in polycystic ovarian disease after ovarian suppression by a long-acting gonadotropin-releasing hormone agonist. J Clin Endocrinol Metab 56(5):897–903
20. Biffignandi P, Massucchetti C, Molinatti GM (1984) Female hirsutism: pathophysiological considerations and therapeutic implications. Endocr Rev 5(4):498–513
21. Rittmaster RS (1988) Differential suppression of testosterone and estradiol in hirsute women with the superactive gonadotropin-releasing hormone agonist leuprolide. J Clin Endocrinol Metab 67(4):651–655
22. Lobo RA (1991) Hirsutism in polycystic ovary syndrome: current concepts. Clin Obstet Gynecol 34(4):817–826
23. Hoffman DI, Klove K, Lobo RA (1984) The prevalence and significance of elevated dehydroepiandrosterone sulfate levels in anovulatory women. Fertil Steril 42(1):76–81
24. Serafini P, Ablan F, Lobo RA (1985) 5 alpha-Reductase activity in the genital skin of hirsute women. J Clin Endocrinol Metab 60(2): 349–355
25. Lobo RA, Goebelsmann U, Horton R (1983) Evidence for the importance of peripheral tissue events in the development of hirsutism in polycystic ovary syndrome. J Clin Endocrinol Metab 57(2):393–397
26. Lobo RA (1984) The role of the adrenal in polycystic ovary syndrome. Semin Reprod Endocrinol 2:251–264
27. Deslypere JP, Verdonck L, Vermeulen A (1985) Fat tissue: a steroid reservoir and site of steroid metabolism. J Clin Endocrinol Metab 61(3):564–570
28. Edman CD, MacDonald PC (1978) Effect of obesity on conversion of plasma androstenedione to estrone in ovulatory and anovulator young women. Am J Obstet Gynecol 130(4):456–461
29. Schneider J, Bradlow HL, Strain G, Levin J, Anderson K, Fishman J (1983) Effects of obesity on estradiol metabolism: decreased formation of nonuterotropic metabolites. J Clin Endocrinol Metab 56(5):973–978
30. Judd HL (1978) Endocrinology of polycystic ovarian disease. Clin Obstet Gynecol 21(1):99–114
31. Banaszewska B, Spaczynski RZ, Pelesz M, Pawelczyk L (2003) Incidence of elevated LH/FSH ratio in polycystic ovary syndrome women with normo- and hyperinsulinemia. Rocz Akad Med Bialymst 48:131–134
32. Hall JE, Whitcomb RW, Rivier JE, Vale WW, Crowley WF Jr (1990) Differential regulation of luteinizing hormone, follicle-stimulating

hormone, and free alpha-subunit secretion from the gonadotrope by gonadotropin-releasing hormone (GnRH): evidence from the use of two GnRH antagonists. J Clin Endocrinol Metab 70(2):328–335
33. Jafari K, Javaheri G, Ruiz G (1978) Endometrial adenocarcinoma and the Stein-Leventhal syndrome. Obstet Gynecol 51(1):97–100
34. Cowan LD, Gordis L, Tonascia JA, Jones GS (1981) Breast cancer incidence in women with a history of progesterone deficiency. Am J Epidemiol 114(2):209–217
35. Schildkraut JM, Schwingl PJ, Bastos E, Evanoff A, Hughes C (1996) Epithelial ovarian cancer risk among women with polycystic ovary syndrome. Obstet Gynecol 88(4 Pt 1):554–559
36. Dunaif A, Segal KR, Futterweit W, Dobrjansky A (1989) Profound peripheral insulin resistance, independent of obesity, in polycystic ovary syndrome. Diabetes 38(9):1165–1174
37. Legro RS, Castracane VD, Kauffman RP (2004) Detecting insulin resistance in polycystic ovary syndrome: purposes and pitfalls. Obstet Gynecol Surv 59(2):141–154
38. Boomsma CM, Eijkemans MJ, Hughes EG, Visser GH, Fauser BC, Macklon NS (2006) A meta-analysis of pregnancy outcomes in women with polycystic ovary syndrome. Hum Reprod Update 12(6):673–683
39. Urman B, Sarac E, Dogan L, Gurgan T (1997) Pregnancy in infertile PCOD patients. Complications and outcome. J Reprod Med 42(8): 501–505
40. Turhan NO, Seckin NC, Aybar F, Inegol I (2003) Assessment of glucose tolerance and pregnancy outcome of polycystic ovary patients. International Journal of Gynaecology and Obstetrics: The Official Organ of the International Federation of Gynaecology and Obstetrics 81(2):163–168
41. Sir-Petermann T, Hitchsfeld C, Maliqueo M, Codner E, Echiburu B, Gazitua R et al (2005) Birth weight in offspring of mothers with polycystic ovarian syndrome. Hum Reprod 20(8):2122–2126
42. Jakubowicz DJ, Iuorno MJ, Jakubowicz S, Roberts KA, Nestler JE (2002) Effects of metformin on early pregnancy loss in the polycystic ovary syndrome. J Clin Endocrinol Metab 87(2):524–529
43. Gray RH, Wu LY (2000) Subfertility and risk of spontaneous abortion. Am J Public Health 90(9):1452–1454
44. Homburg R, Armar NA, Eshel A, Adams J, Jacobs HS (1988) Influence of serum luteinising hormone concentrations on ovulation, conception, and early pregnancy loss in polycystic ovary syndrome. BMJ 297(6655):1024–1026
45. Okon MA, Laird SM, Tuckerman EM, Li TC (1998) Serum androgen levels in women who have recurrent miscarriages and their correlation with markers of endometrial function. Fertil Steril 69(4):682–690
46. Tulppala M, Stenman UH, Cacciatore B, Ylikorkala O (1993) Polycystic ovaries and levels of gonadotrophins and androgens in recurrent miscarriage: prospective study in 50 women. Br J Obstet Gynaecol 100(4):348–352
47. Tian L, Shen H, Lu Q, Norman RJ, Wang J (2007) Insulin resistance increases the risk of spontaneous abortion after assisted reproduction technology treatment. J Clin Endocrinol Metab 92(4):1430–1433
48. Mulders AG, Laven JS, Eijkemans MJ, Hughes EG, Fauser BC (2003) Patient predictors for outcome of gonadotrophin ovulation induction in women with normogonadotrophic anovulatory infertility: a meta-analysis. Hum Reprod Update 9(5):429–449
49. King R, Rotter J, Motulsky A (2002) The genetic basis of common diseases, 2nd edn. Oxford University Press, New York
50. Nam Menke M, Strauss JF III (2007) Genetics of polycystic ovarian syndrome. Clin Obstet Gynecol 50(1):188–204
51. Franks S, McCarthy M (2004) Genetics of ovarian disorders: polycystic ovary syndrome. Rev Endocr Metab Disord 5(1):69–76
52. Escobar-Morreale HF, Luque-Ramirez M, San Millan JL (2005) The molecular-genetic basis of functional hyperandrogenism and the polycystic ovary syndrome. Endocr Rev 26(2):251–282
53. Diamanti-Kandarakis E, Piperi C (2005) Genetics of polycystic ovary syndrome: searching for the way out of the labyrinth. Hum Reprod Update 11(6):631–643
54. Urbanek M (2007) The genetics of the polycystic ovary syndrome. Nat Clin Pract Endocrinol Metab 3(2):103–111
55. Unluturk U, Harmanci A, Kocaefe C, Yildiz BO (2007) The Genetic Basis of the Polycystic Ovary Syndrome: A Literature Review Including Discussion of PPAR-gamma. PPAR Res 2007:49109
56. Beavis WD (1998) QTL analyses: power, precision, and accuracy. In: Paterson AH (ed) Molecular dissection of complex traits. CRC Press, New York, pp 145–162
57. Urbanek M, Woodroffe A, Ewens KG, Diamanti-Kandarakis E, Legro RS, Strauss JF III et al (2005) Candidate gene region for polycystic ovary syndrome on chromosome 19p13.2. J Clin Endocrinol Metab 90(12):6623–6629
58. Urbanek M, Legro RS, Driscoll DA, Azziz R, Ehrmann DA, Norman RJ et al (1999) Thirty-seven candidate genes for polycystic ovary syndrome: strongest evidence for linkage is with follistatin. Proc Natl Acad Sci U S A 96(15):8573–8578
59. Stewart DR, Dombroski BA, Urbanek M, Ankener W, Ewens KG, Wood JR et al (2006) Fine mapping of genetic susceptibility to polycystic ovary syndrome on chromosome 19p13.2 and tests for regulatory activity. J Clin Endocrinol Metab 91(10):4112–4117
60. Hughes C, Elgasim M, Layfield R, Atiomo W (2006) Genomic and post-genomic approaches to polycystic ovary syndrome – progress so far: mini review. Hum Reprod 21(11):2766–2775
61. Goldstein JL, Brown MS (1990) Regulation of the mevalonate pathway. Nature 343(6257):425–430
62. Turunen M, Olsson J, Dallner G (2004) Metabolism and function of coenzyme Q. Biochim Biophys Acta 1660(1–2):171–199
63. Carlberg M, Dricu A, Blegen H, Wang M, Hjertman M, Zickert P et al (1996) Mevalonic acid is limiting for N-linked glycosylation and translocation of the insulin-like growth factor-1 receptor to the cell surface. Evidence for a new link between 3-hydroxy-3-methylglutaryl-coenzyme a reductase and cell growth. J Biol Chem 271(29):17453–17462
64. Zhang FL, Casey PJ (1996) Protein prenylation: molecular mechanisms and functional consequences. Annu Rev Biochem 65:241–269
65. Duleba AJ, Spaczynski RZ, Olive DL (1998) Insulin and insulin-like growth factor I stimulate the proliferation of human ovarian theca-interstitial cells. Fertil Steril 69(2):335–340
66. Goalstone ML, Leitner JW, Wall K, Dolgonos L, Rother KI, Accili D et al (1998) Effect of insulin on farnesyltransferase. Specificity of insulin action and potentiation of nuclear effects of insulin-like growth factor-1, epidermal growth factor, and platelet-derived growth factor. J Biol Chem 273(37):23892–23896
67. Goalstone ML, Draznin B (1996) Effect of insulin on farnesyltransferase activity in 3T3-L1 adipocytes. J Biol Chem 271(44): 27585–27589
68. Goalstone ML, Leitner JW, Golovchenko I, Stjernholm MR, Cormont M, Le Marchand-Brustel Y et al (1999) Insulin promotes phosphorylation and activation of geranylgeranyltransferase II. Studies with geranylgeranylation of rab-3 and rab-4. J Biol Chem 274(5):2880–2884
69. Barbieri RL, Makris A, Ryan KJ (1983) Effects of insulin on steroidogenesis in cultured porcine ovarian theca. Fertil Steril 40(2):237–241
70. Izquierdo D, Foyouzi N, Kwintkiewicz J, Duleba AJ (2004) Mevastatin inhibits ovarian theca-interstitial cell proliferation and steroidogenesis. Fertil Steril 82(Suppl 3):1193–1197
71. Kwintkiewicz J, Foyouzi N, Piotrowski P, Rzepczynska I, Duleba AJ (2006) Mevastatin inhibits proliferation of rat ovarian theca-interstitial cells by blocking the mitogen-activated protein kinase pathway. Fertil Steril 86(4 Suppl):1053–1058
72. Axel DI, Riessen R, Runge H, Viebahn R, Karsch KR (2000) Effects of cerivastatin on human arterial smooth muscle cell proliferation and migration in transfilter cocultures. J Cardiovasc Pharmacol 35(4):619–629
73. Buemi M, Allegra A, Senatore M, Marino D, Medici MA, Aloisi C et al (1999) Pro-apoptotic effect of fluvastatin on human smooth muscle cells. Eur J Pharmacol 370(2):201–203

74. El-Ani D, Zimlichman R (2001) Simvastatin induces apoptosis of cultured rat cardiomyocytes. J Basic Clin Physiol Pharmacol 12(4):325–338
75. Danesh FR, Sadeghi MM, Amro N, Philips C, Zeng L, Lin S et al (2002) 3-Hydroxy-3-methylglutaryl CoA reductase inhibitors prevent high glucose-induced proliferation of mesangial cells via modulation of Rho GTPase/ p21 signaling pathway: Implications for diabetic nephropathy. Proc Natl Acad Sci U S A 99(12):8301–8305
76. Wu CH, Lee SC, Chiu HH, Yang YC, Lian ST, Shin SJ et al (2002) Morphologic change and elevation of cortisol secretion in cultured human normal adrenocortical cells caused by mutant p21K-ras protein. DNA Cell Biol 21(1):21–29
77. Dobs AS, Schrott H, Davidson MH, Bays H, Stein EA, Kush D et al (2000) Effects of high-dose simvastatin on adrenal and gonadal steroidogenesis in men with hypercholesterolemia. Metabolism 49(9):1234–1238
78. Hernandez R, Teruel T, Lorenzo M (2001) Akt mediates insulin induction of glucose uptake and up-regulation of GLUT4 gene expression in brown adipocytes. FEBS Lett 494(3):225–231
79. Welsh GI, Hers I, Berwick DC, Dell G, Wherlock M, Birkin R et al (2005) Role of protein kinase B in insulin-regulated glucose uptake. Biochem Soc Trans 33(Pt 2):346–349
80. Piotrowski P, Kwintkiewicz J, Rzepczynska I, Duleba AJ (2005) Simvastatin and mevastatin inhibit expression of NADPH oxidase subunits: p22phox and p47phox in rat thecainterstitial cells. 52nd Annual Meeting of the Society for Gynecological Investigations, Los Angeles, 23–26 March 2005
81. Duleba AJ, Banaszewska B, Spaczynski RZ, Pawelczyk L (2006) Simvastatin improves biochemical parameters in women with polycystic ovary syndrome: results of a prospective, randomized trial. Fertil Steril 85(4):996–1001
82. Banaszewska B, Pawelczyk L, Spaczynski RZ, Dziura J, Duleba AJ (2007) Effects of simvastatin and oral contraceptive agent on polycystic ovary syndrome: prospective, randomized, crossover trial. J Clin Endocrinol Metab 92(2):456–461
83. Barbieri RL, Ryan KJ (1983) Hyperandrogenism, insulin resistance, and acanthosis nigricans syndrome: a common endocrinopathy with distinct pathophysiologic features. Am J Obstet Gynecol 147(1):90–101
84. Ehrmann DA, Barnes RB, Rosenfield RL et al (1999) Prevalence of impaired glucose tolerance and diabetes in women with polycystic ovary syndrome. Diabetes Care 22:141–146
85. Legro RS, Kunselman AR, Dodson WC, Dunaif A (1999) Prevalence and predictors of risk for type 2 diabetes mellitus and impaired glucose tolerance in polycystic ovary syndrome: a prospective, controlled study in 254 affected women. J Clin Endocrinol Metab 84(1):165–169
86. Harris MI, Hadden WC, Knowler WC, Bennett PH (1987) Prevalence of diabetes and impaired glucose tolerance and plasma glucose levels in U.S. population aged 20–74 yr. Diabetes 36(4):523–534
87. Seibel MM (1984) Toward understanding the pathophysiology and treatment of polycystic ovary disease. Semin Reprod Endocrinol 2:297
88. Dunaif A, Green G, Futterweit W, Dobrjansky A (1990) Suppression of hyperandrogenism does not improve peripheral or hepatic insulin resistance in the polycystic ovary syndrome. J Clin Endocrinol Metab 70(3):699–704
89. Nagamani M, Van Dinh T, Kelver ME (1986) Hyperinsulinemia in hyperthecosis of the ovaries. Am J Obstet Gynecol 154(2):384–389
90. Grasinger CC, Wild RA, Parker IJ (1993) Vulvar acanthosis nigricans: a marker for insulin resistance in hirsute women. Fertil Steril 59(3):583–586
91. Wild RA (1995) Obesity, lipids, cardiovascular risk, and androgen excess. Am J Med 98(1A):27S–32S
92. Dunaif A (1995) Hyperandrogenic anovulation (PCOS): a unique disorder of insulin action associated with an increased risk of non-insulin-dependent diabetes mellitus. Am J Med 98(1A):33S–39S
93. Kiddy DS, Hamilton-Fairley D, Bush A, Short F, Anyaoku V, Reed MJ et al (1992) Improvement in endocrine and ovarian function during dietary treatment of obese women with polycystic ovary syndrome. Clin Endocrinol (Oxf) 36(1):105–111
94. Pasquali R, Antenucci D, Casimirri F, Venturoli S, Paradisi R, Fabbri R et al (1989) Clinical and hormonal characteristics of obese amenorrheic hyperandrogenic women before and after weight loss. J Clin Endocrinol Metab 68(1):173–179
95. Apridonidze T, Essah PA, Iuorno MJ, Nestler JE (2005) Prevalence and characteristics of the metabolic syndrome in women with polycystic ovary syndrome. J Clin Endocrinol Metab 90(4):1929–1935
96. Dahlgren E, Johansson S, Lindstedt G, Knutsson F, Oden A, Janson PO et al (1992) Women with polycystic ovary syndrome wedge resected in 1956 to 1965: a long-term follow-up focusing on natural history and circulating hormones. Fertil Steril 57(3):505–513
97. Conway GS, Agrawal R, Betteridge DJ, Jacobs HS (1992) Risk factors for coronary artery disease in lean and obese women with the polycystic ovary syndrome. Clin Endocrinol (Oxf) 37(2):119–125
98. Andersen P, Seljeflot I, Abdelnoor M, Arnesen H, Dale PO, Lovik A et al (1995) Increased insulin sensitivity and fibrinolytic capacity after dietary intervention in obese women with polycystic ovary syndrome. Metabolism 44(5):611–616
99. Guzick DS, Talbott EO, Sutton-Tyrrell K, Herzog HC, Kuller LH, Wolfson SK Jr (1996) Carotid atherosclerosis in women with polycystic ovary syndrome: initial results from a case-control study. Am J Obstet Gynecol 174(4):1224–1229, discussion 9-32
100. Birdsall MA, Farquhar CM, White HD (1997) Association between polycystic ovaries and extent of coronary artery disease in women having cardiac catheterization. Ann Intern Med 126(1):32–35
101. Danigren E, Janson PO, Johansson S et al (1992) Polycistic ovary syndrome and risk for myocardial infarction. Acta Obstet Cynecol Scand 71:559–604
102. Goldzieher JW, Axelrod LR (1963) Clinical and biochemical features of polycystic ovarian disease. Fertil Steril 14:631–653
103. Aono T, Miyazaki M, Miyake A, Kinugasa T, Kurachi K, Matsumoto K (1977) Responses of serum gonadotrophins to LH-releasing hormone and oestrogens in Japanese women with polycystic ovaries. Acta Endocrinol (Copenh) 85(4):840–849
104. Ferrimann D, Gallway JD (1961) Clinical assessment of body hair growth in women. J Clin Endocrinol Metab 21:1440
105. Verkauf BS, Von Thron J, O'Brien WF (1992) Clitoral size in normal women. Obstet Gynecol 80(1):41–44
106. Vermeulen A, Verdonck L, Kaufman JM (1999) A critical evaluation of simple methods for the estimation of free testosterone in serum. J Clin Endocrinol Metab 84(10):3666–3672
107. Rittmaster RS (1995) Clinical relevance of testosterone and dihydrotestosterone metabolism in women. Am J Med 98(1A):17S–21S
108. Futterweit W (1994) An endocrine approach obesity. In: Simopoulos AP, Vanltallie TB, Gullo SP et al (eds) Obesity:new directions in assessment and management. Charles Press, New York, pp 96–121
109. Cussons AJ, Stuckey BG, Watts GF (2006) Cardiovascular disease in the polycystic ovary syndrome: new insights and perspectives. Atherosclerosis 185(2):227–239
110. Wild S, Pierpoint T, McKeigue P, Jacobs H (2000) Cardiovascular disease in women with polycystic ovary syndrome at long-term follow-up: a retrospective cohort study. Clin Endocrinol (Oxf) 52(5):595–600
111. Balen AH, Conway GS, Kaltsas G, Techatrasak K, Manning PJ, West C et al (1995) Polycystic ovary syndrome: the spectrum of the disorder in 1741 patients. Hum Reprod 10(8):2107–2111
112. Pasquali R, Casimirri F, Cantobelli S, Labate AM, Venturoli S, Paradisi R et al (1993) Insulin and androgen relationships with abdominal body fat distribution in women with and without hyperandrogenism. Horm Res 39(5–6):179–187
113. Kosti RI, Panagiotakos DB (2006) The epidemic of obesity in children and adolescents in the world. Cent Eur J Public Health 14(4):151–159

114. Popkin BM, Gordon-Larsen P (2004) The nutrition transition: worldwide obesity dynamics and their determinants. Int J Obes Relat Metab Disord 28(Suppl 3):S2–S9
115. Ogden CL, Carroll MD, Curtin LR, McDowell MA, Tabak CJ, Flegal KM (2006) Prevalence of overweight and obesity in the United States, 1999–2004. JAMA 295(13):1549–1555
116. Trends in leisure-time physical inactivity by age, sex, and race/ethnicity--United States, 1994–2004 (2005) MMWR Morb Mortal Wkly Rep 54(39):991–994
117. Prevalence of diabetes and impaired fasting glucose in adults – United States, 1999–2000 (2003) MMWR Morb Mortal Wkly Rep 52(35):833–837
118. Morin-Papunen LC, Vauhkonen I, Koivunen RM, Ruokonen A, Tapanainen JS (2000) Insulin sensitivity, insulin secretion, and metabolic and hormonal parameters in healthy women and women with polycystic ovarian syndrome. Hum Reprod 15(6):1266–1274
119. Anderson JW, Konz EC, Frederich RC, Wood CL (2001) Long-term weight-loss maintenance: a meta-analysis of US studies. Am J Clin Nutr 74(5):579–584
120. Moran LJ, Noakes M, Clifton PM, Tomlinson L, Galletly C, Norman RJ (2003) Dietary composition in restoring reproductive and metabolic physiology in overweight women with polycystic ovary syndrome. J Clin Endocrinol Metab 88(2):812–819
121. Crosignani PG, Colombo M, Vegetti W, Somigliana E, Gessati A, Ragni G (2003) Overweight and obese anovulatory patients with polycystic ovaries: parallel improvements in anthropometric indices, ovarian physiology and fertility rate induced by diet. Hum Reprod 18(9):1928–1932
122. Huber-Buchholz MM, Carey DG, Norman RJ (1999) Restoration of reproductive potential by lifestyle modification in obese polycystic ovary syndrome: role of insulin sensitivity and luteinizing hormone. J Clin Endocrinol Metab 84(4):1470–1474
123. Clark AM, Thornley B, Tomlinson L, Galletley C, Norman RJ (1998) Weight loss in obese infertile women results in improvement in reproductive outcome for all forms of fertility treatment. Hum Reprod 13(6):1502–1505
124. Glazer NL, Hendrickson AF, Schellenbaum GD, Mueller BA (2004) Weight change and the risk of gestational diabetes in obese women. Epidemiology 15(6):733–737
125. Galletly C, Clark A, Tomlinson L, Blaney F (1996) A group program for obese, infertile women: weight loss and improved psychological health. J Psychosom Obstet Gynaecol 17(2):125–128
126. Hu FB, Sigal RJ, Rich-Edwards JW, Colditz GA, Solomon CG, Willett WC et al (1999) Walking compared with vigorous physical activity and risk of type 2 diabetes in women: a prospective study. JAMA 282(15):1433–1439
127. Weinstein AR, Sesso HD, Lee IM, Cook NR, Manson JE, Buring JE et al (2004) Relationship of physical activity vs body mass index with type 2 diabetes in women. JAMA 292(10):1188–1194
128. Manson JE, Greenland P, LaCroix AZ, Stefanick ML, Mouton CP, Oberman A et al (2002) Walking compared with vigorous exercise for the prevention of cardiovascular events in women. N Engl J Med 347(10):716–725
129. Manson JE, Hu FB, Rich-Edwards JW, Colditz GA, Stampfer MJ, Willett WC et al (1999) A prospective study of walking as compared with vigorous exercise in the prevention of coronary heart disease in women. N Engl J Med 341(9):650–658
130. Mayer-Davis EJ, D'Agostino R Jr, Karter AJ, Haffner SM, Rewers MJ, Saad M et al (1998) Intensity and amount of physical activity in relation to insulin sensitivity: the Insulin Resistance Atherosclerosis Study. JAMA 279(9):669–674
131. Martin LF, Finigan KM, Nolan TE (2000) Pregnancy after adjustable gastric banding. Obstet Gynecol 95(6 Pt 1):927–930
132. Eid GM, Cottam DR, Velcu LM, Mattar SG, Korytkowski MT, Gosman G et al (2005) Effective treatment of polycystic ovarian syndrome with Roux-en-Y gastric bypass. Surg Obes Relat Dis 1(2):77–80
133. Escobar-Morreale HF, Botella-Carretero JI, Alvarez-Blasco F, Sancho J (2005) San Millan JL. The polycystic ovary syndrome associated with morbid obesity may resolve after weight loss induced by bariatric surgery. J Clin Endocrinol Metab 90(12):6364–6369
134. ACOG Practice Bulletin. Clinical management guidelines for obstetrician-gynecologists. Number 30, September 2001 (replaces Technical Bulletin Number 200, December 1994) (2001) Gestational diabetes. Obstet Gynecol 98(3):525–538
135. Givens JR, Andersen RN, Wiser WL, Umstot ES, Fish SA (1976) The effectiveness of two oral contraceptives in suppressing plasma androstenedione, testosterone, LH, and FSH, and in stimulating plasma testosterone-binding capacity in hirsute women. Am J Obstet Gynecol 124(4):333–339
136. Raj SG, Raj MH, Talbert LM, Sloan CS, Hicks B (1982) Normalization of testosterone levels using a low estrogen-containing oral contraceptive in women with polycystic ovary syndrome. Obstet Gynecol 60(1):15–19
137. Wiebe RH, Morris CV (1984) Effect of an oral contraceptive on adrenal and ovarian androgenic steroids. Obstet Gynecol 63(1):12–14
138. Wild RA, Umstot ES, Andersen RN, Givens JR (1982) Adrenal function in hirsutism. II. Effect of an oral contraceptive. J Clin Endocrinol Metab 54(4):676–681
139. Marynick SP, Chakmakjian ZH, McCaffree DL, Herndon JH Jr (1983) Androgen excess in cystic acne. N Engl J Med 308(17):981–986
140. Schiavone FE, Rietschel RL, Sgoutas D et al (1983) Elevated free testosterone levels in women with acne. Arch Dermatol 119:799–802
141. Amin ES, El-Sayed MM, El-Gamel BA, Nayel SA (1980) Comparative study of the effect of oral contraceptives containing 50 microgram of estrogen and those containing 20 microgram of estrogen on adrenal cortical function. Am J Obstet Gynecol 137(7):831–833
142. Goldzieher JW (1981) Polycystic ovarian disease. Fertil Steril 35(4):371–394
143. Maloney JM, Dietze P Jr, Watson D, Niknian M, Lee-Rugh S, Sampson-Landers C et al (2008) Treatment of acne using a 3-milligram drospirenone/20-microgram ethinyl estradiol oral contraceptive administered in a 24/4 regimen: a randomized controlled trial. Obstet Gynecol 112(4):773–781
144. Rittmaster RS (1995) Clinical review 73: Medical treatment of androgen-dependent hirsutism. J Clin Endocrinol Metab 80(9):2559–2563
145. Godsland IF, Walton C, Felton C, Proudler A, Patel A, Wynn V (1992) Insulin resistance, secretion, and metabolism in users of oral contraceptives. J Clin Endocrinol Metab 74(1):64–70
146. Ettinger B, Golditch IM (1977) Medroxyprogesterone acetate for the evaluation of hypertestosteronism in hirsute women. Fertil Steril 28(12):1285–1288
147. Jeppsson S, Gershagen S, Johansson ED, Rannevik G (1982) Plasma levels of medroxyprogesterone acetate (MPA), sex-hormone binding globulin, gonadal steroids, gonadotrophins and prolactin in women during long-term use of depo-MPA (Depo-Provera) as a contraceptive agent. Acta Endocrinol (Copenh) 99(3):339–343
148. Gordon GG, Southern AL, Calanog A et al (1972) The effect of medroxyprogesterone acetate on androgen metabolism in the polycystic ovary syndrome. J Clin Endocrinol Metab 35:444–447
149. Meldrum DR, Chang RJ, Lu J, Vale W, Rivier J, Judd HL (1982) "Medical oophorectomy" using a long-acting GNRH agonist–a possible new approach to the treatment of endometriosis. J Clin Endocrinol Metab 54(5):1081–1083
150. Falsetti L, Pasinetti E (1994) Treatment of moderate and severe hirsutism by gonadotropin-releasing hormone agonists in women with polycystic ovary syndrome and idiopathic hirsutism. Fertil Steril 61(5):817–822
151. Morcos RN, Abdul-Malak ME, Shikora E (1994) Treatment of hirsutism with a gonadotropin-releasing hormone agonist and estrogen replacement therapy. Fertil Steril 61(3):427–431

152. Tiitinen A, Simberg N, Stenman UH, Ylikorkala O (1994) Estrogen replacement does not potentiate gonadotropin-releasing hormone agonist-induced androgen suppression in treatment of hirsutism. J Clin Endocrinol Metab 79(2):447–451
153. Cunningham SK, Loughlin T, Culliton M et al (1973) Plasma sex hormone-binding globulin and androgen levels in the management of hirsute patients. Acta Endocrinol (Copenh) 104:365–371
154. Gal M, Orly J, Barr I, Algur N, Boldes R, Diamant YZ (1994) Low dose ketoconazole attenuates serum androgen levels in patients with polycystic ovary syndrome and inhibits ovarian steroidogenesis in vitro. Fertil Steril 61(5):823–832
155. Menard RH, Guenthner TM, Kon H, Gillette JR (1979) Studies on the destruction of adrenal and testicular cytochrome P-450 by spironolactone. Requirement for the 7alpha-thio group and evidence for the loss of the heme and apoproteins of cytochrome P-450. J Biol Chem 254(5):1726–1733
156. Cumming DC, Yang JC, Rebar RW, Yen SS (1982) Treatment of hirsutism with spironolactone. Jama 247(9):1295–1298
157. Rittmaster R (1991) Evaluation and treatment of hirsutism. Infert Reprod Med Clin North Am 2:511–545
158. Barth JH, Cherry CA, Wojnarowska F et al (1989) Spironolactone is an effective and well tolerated systemic andiandrogen therapy for hirsute women. J Clin Endocrinol Metab 68:966–970
159. Lobo RA, Shoupe D, Serafini P, Brinton D, Horton R (1985) The effects of two doses of spironolactone on serum androgens and anagen hair in hirsute women. Fertil Steril 43(2):200–205
160. Calaf-Alsina J, Rodriguez-Espinosa J, Cabero-Roura A, Lenti-Paoli O, Mora-Brugues J, Esteban-Altirriba J (1987) Effects of a cyproterone-containing oral contraceptive on hormonal levels in polycystic ovarian disease. Obstet Gynecol 69(2):255–258
161. Helfer EL, Miller JL, Rose LI (1988) Side-effects of spironolactone therapy in the hirsute woman. J Clin Endocrinol Metab 66(1):208–211
162. Miller JA, Jacobs HS (1986) Treatment of hirsutism and acne with cyproterone acetate. Clin Endocrinol Metab 15(2):373–389
163. Mowszowicz I, Wright F, Vincens M, Rigaud C, Nahoul K, Mavier P et al (1984) Androgen metabolism in hirsute patients treated with cyproterone acetate. J Steroid Biochem 20(3):757–761
164. Girard J, Baumann JB, Buhler U, Zuppinger K, Haas HG, Staub JJ et al (1978) Cyproteroneacetate and ACTH adrenal function. J Clin Endocrinol Metab 47(3):581–586
165. Marcondes JA, Minnani SL, Luthold WW, Wajchenberg BL, Samojlik E, Kirschner MA (1992) Treatment of hirsutism in women with flutamide. Fertil Steril 57(3):543–547
166. Ciotta L, Cianci A, Calogero AE, Palumbo MA, Marletta E, Sciuto A et al (1995) Clinical and endocrine effects of finasteride, a 5 alpha-reductase inhibitor, in women with idiopathic hirsutism. Fertil Steril 64(2):299–306
167. Cusan L, Dupont A, Belanger A, Tremblay RR, Manhes G, Labrie F (1990) Treatment of hirsutism with the pure antiandrogen flutamide. J Am Acad Dermatol 23(3 Pt 1):462–469
168. Ibanez L, De Zegher F (2004) Flutamide-metformin plus an oral contraceptive (OC) for young women with polycystic ovary syndrome: switch from third- to fourth-generation OC reduces body adiposity. Hum Reprod 19(8):1725–1727
169. Ibanez L, Valls C, Cabre S, De Zegher F (2004) Flutamide-metformin plus ethinylestradiol-drospirenone for lipolysis and antiatherogenesis in young women with ovarian hyperandrogenism: the key role of early, low-dose flutamide. J Clin Endocrinol Metab 89(9):4716–4720
170. Castelo-Branco C, Moyano D, Gomez O, Balasch J (2009) Long-term safety and tolerability of flutamide for the treatment of hirsutism. Fertil Steril 91(4):1183–1188
171. Vigersky RA, Mehlman I, Glass AR, Smith CE (1980) Treatment of hirsute women with cimetidine. N Engl J Med 303(18):1042
172. Lissak A, Sorokin Y, Calderon I, Dirnfeld M, Lioz H, Abramovici H (1989) Treatment of hirsutism with cimetidine: a prospective randomized controlled trial. Fertil Steril 51(2):247–250
173. Golditch IM, Price VH (1990) Treatment of hirsutism with cimetidine. Obstet Gynecol 75(6):911–913
174. Wong IL, Morris RS, Chang L, Spahn MA, Stanczyk FZ, Lobo RA (1995) A prospective randomized trial comparing finasteride to spironolactone in the treatment of hirsute women. J Clin Endocrinol Metab 80(1):233–238
175. Ciotta L, Cianci A, Marletta E, Pisana L, Agliano A, Palumbo G (1994) Treatment of hirsutism with flutamide and a low-dosage oral contraceptive in polycystic ovarian disease patients. Fertil Steril 62(6):1129–1135
176. Judd HL, Rigg LA, Anderson DC, Yen SS (1976) The effects of ovarian wedge resection on circulating gonadotropin and ovarian steroid levels in patients with polycystic ovary syndrome. J Clin Endocrinol Metab 43(2):347–355
177. Katz M, Carr PJ, Cohen BM, Millar RP (1978) Hormonal effects of wedge resection of polycystic ovaries. Obstet Gynecol 51(4):437–444
178. Goldzieher JW, Green JA (1962) The polycystic ovary. I. Clinical and histologic features. J Clin Endocrinol Metab 22:325–338
179. Adashi EY, Rock JA, Guzick D, Wentz AC, Jones GS, Jones HW Jr (1981) Fertility following bilateral ovarian wedge resection: a critical analysis of 90 consecutive cases of the polycystic ovary syndrome. Fertil Steril 36(3):320–325
180. Felemban A, Tan SL, Tulandi T (2000) Laparoscopic treatment of polycystic ovaries with insulated needle cautery: a reappraisal. Fertil Steril 73(2):266–269
181. Armar NA, Lachelin GC (1993) Laparoscopic ovarian diathermy: an effective treatment for anti-oestrogen resistant anovulatory infertility in women with the polycystic ovary syndrome. Br J Obstet Gynaecol 100(2):161–164
182. Armar NA, McGarrigle HH, Honour J, Holownia P, Jacobs HS, Lachelin GC (1990) Laparoscopic ovarian diathermy in the management of anovulatory infertility in women with polycystic ovaries: endocrine changes and clinical outcome. Fertil Steril 53(1):45–49
183. Rossmanith WG, Keckstein J, Spatzier K, Lauritzen C (1991) The impact of ovarian laser surgery on the gonadotrophin secretion in women with polycystic ovarian disease. Clin Endocrinol (Oxf) 34(3):223–230
184. Balen AH, Jacobs HS (1994) A prospective study comparing unilateral and bilateral laparoscopic ovarian diathermy in women with the polycystic ovary syndrome. Fertil Steril 62(5):921–925
185. Farquhar C, Lilford RJ, Marjoribanks J, Vandekerckhove P (2007) Laparoscopic 'drilling' by diathermy or laser for ovulation induction in anovulatory polycystic ovary syndrome. Cochrane Database Syst Rev 3:CD001122
186. Wolf JE Jr, Shander D, Huber F, Jackson J, Lin CS, Mathes BM, Schrode K; Eflornithine HCI Stydy Group. (2007) Randomized, double-blind clinical evaluation of the efficacy and safety of topical eflornithine HCl 13.9% cream in the treatment of women with facial hair. Int J Dermatol 46(1):94–98
187. Lynfield YL, Macwilliams P (1970) Shaving and hair growth. J Invest Dermatol 55(3):170–172
188. Wagner RF, Jr (1990) Physical methods for the management of hirsutism. Cutis 45(5):319–321, 25–26
189. Legro RS, Barnhart HX, Schlaff WD, Carr BR, Diamond MP, Carson SA et al (2007) Clomiphene, metformin, or both for infertility in the polycystic ovary syndrome. N Engl J Med 356(6):551–566
190. Zolghadri J, Tavana Z, Kazerooni T, Soveid M, Taghieh M (2008) Relationship between abnormal glucose tolerance test and history of previous recurrent miscarriages, and beneficial effect of metformin in these patients: a prospective clinical study. Fertil Steril 90(3):727–730

191. Qublan HS, Yannakoula EK, Al-Qudah MA, El-Uri FI (2007) Dietary intervention versus metformin to improve the reproductive outcome in women with polycystic ovary syndrome. A prospective comparative study. Saudi Med J 28(11):1694–1699
192. Creanga AA, Bradley HM, McCormick C, Witkop CT (2008) Use of metformin in polycystic ovary syndrome: a meta-analysis. Obstet Gynecol 111(4):959–968
193. Moll E, van der Veen F, van Wely M (2007) The role of metformin in polycystic ovary syndrome: a systematic review. Hum Reprod Update 13(6):527–537
194. Elizur SE, Tulandi T (2008) Drugs in infertility and fetal safety. Fertil Steril 89(6):1595–1602
195. Kim LH, Taylor AE, Barbieri RL (2000) Insulin sensitizers and polycystic ovary syndrome: can a diabetes medication treat infertility? Fertil Steril 73(6):1097–1098
196. Velazquez EM, Mendoza S, Hamer T, Sosa F, Glueck CJ (1994) Metformin therapy in polycystic ovary syndrome reduces hyperinsulinemia, insulin resistance, hyperandrogenemia, and systolic blood pressure, while facilitating normal menses and pregnancy. Metabolism 43(5):647–654
197. Nestler JE, Jakubowicz DJ (1996) Decreases in ovarian cytochrome P450c17 alpha activity and serum free testosterone after reduction of insulin secretion in polycystic ovary syndrome. N Engl J Med 335(9):617–623
198. Diamanti-Kandarakis E, Kouli C, Tsianateli T, Bergiele A (1998) Therapeutic effects of metformin on insulin resistance and hyperandrogenism in polycystic ovary syndrome. Eur J Endocrinol 138(3):269–274
199. Nestler JE, Jakubowicz DJ, Evans WS, Pasquali R (1998) Effects of metformin on spontaneous and clomiphene-induced ovulation in the polycystic ovary syndrome. N Engl J Med 338(26):1876–1880
200. Lord JM, Flight IH, Norman RJ (2003) Metformin in polycystic ovary syndrome: systematic review and meta-analysis. BMJ 327(7421):951–953
201. Hasegawa I, Murakawa H, Suzuki M, Yamamoto Y, Kurabayashi T, Tanaka K (1999) Effect of troglitazone on endocrine and ovulatory performance in women with insulin resistance-related polycystic ovary syndrome. Fertil Steril 71(2):323–327
202. Stadtmauer LA, Toma SK, Riehl RM, Talbert LM (2001) Metformin treatment of patients with polycystic ovary syndrome undergoing in vitro fertilization improves outcomes and is associated with modulation of the insulin-like growth factors. Fertil Steril 75(3):505–509
203. Panidis D, Farmakiotis D, Rousso D, Kourtis A, Katsikis I, Krassas G (2008) Obesity, weight loss, and the polycystic ovary syndrome: effect of treatment with diet and orlistat for 24 weeks on insulin resistance and androgen levels. Fertil Steril 89(4):899–906
204. Orth DN (1987) Ectopic hormone production. In: Felig P, Baster JD, Broadus AE et al (eds) Endocrinology and metabolism. McGraw-Hill, New York, pp 1692–1735
205. Liddle GW (1960) Tests of pituitary-adrenal suppressibility in the diagnosis of Cushing's syndrome. J Clin Endocrinol Metab 20:1539–1560
206. Oldfield EH, Doppman JL, Nieman LK et al (1991) Petrosal sinus sampling with and without corticotropin-releasing hormone for the differential diagnosis of Cushing's syndrome. N Engl J Med 325(13):897–905
207. Gold EM (1979) The Cushing syndromes: changing views of diagnosis and treatment. Ann Intern Med 90(5):829–844
208. Boggan JE, Tyrrell JB, Wilson CB (1983) Transsphenoidal microsurgical management of Cushing's disease. Report of 100 cases. J Neurosurg 59(2):195–200
209. Bigos ST, Somma M, Rasio E et al (1980) Cushing's disease: management by transsphenoidal pituitary microsurgery. J Clin Endocrinol Metab 50(2):348–354
210. Aron DC, Findling JW, Tyrrell JB (1987) Cushing's disease. Endocrinol Metab Clin North Am 16(3):705–730
211. Jennings AS, Liddle GW, Orth DN (1977) Results of treating childhood Cushing's disease with pituitary irradiation. N Engl J Med 297(18):957–962
212. Schteingart DE, Tsao HS, Taylor CI, McKenzie A, Victoria R, Therrien BA (1980) Sustained remission of Cushing's disease with mitotane and pituitary irradiation. Ann Intern Med 92(5):613–619
213. Orth DN, Liddle GW (1971) Results of treatment in 108 patients with Cushing's syndrome. N Engl J Med 285(5):243–247
214. Valimaki M, Pelkonen R, Porkka L, Sivula A, Kahri A (1984) Long-term results of adrenal surgery in patients with Cushing's syndrome due to adrenocortical adenoma. Clin Endocrinol (Oxf) 20(2):229–236
215. Loli P, Berselli ME, Tagliaferri M (1986) Use of ketoconazole in the treatment of Cushing's syndrome. J Clin Endocrinol Metab 63(6):1365–1371
216. Nelson DH, Meakin JW, Dealy JB et al (1958) ACTH-producing tumor of the pituitary gland. N Engl J Med 85:731–734
217. Azziz R, Zacur HA (1989) 21-Hydroxylase deficiency in female hyperandrogenism: screening and diagnosis. J Clin Endocrinol Metab 69(3):577–584
218. Dewailly D, Vantyghem-Haudiquet MC, Sainsard C et al (1986) Clinical and biological phenotypes in late-onset 21-hydroxylase deficiency. J Clin Endocrinol Metab 63(2):418–423
219. New MI, Lorenzen F, Lerner AJ et al (1983) Genotyping steroid 21-hydroxylase deficiency: hormonal reference data. J Clin Endocrinol Metab 57(2):320–326
220. Nichols T, Nugent CA, Tyler FH (1965) Diurnal variation in suppression of adrenal function by glucocorticoids. J Clin Endocrinol Metab 25:343–349
221. Boyers SP, Buster JE, Marshall JR (1982) Hypothalamic-pituitary-adrenocortical function during long-term low-dose dexamethasone therapy in hyperandrogenized women. Am J Obstet Gynecol 142(3):330–339
222. Speiser PW, Dupont B, Rubinstein P, Piazza A, Kastelan A, New MI (1985) High frequency of nonclassical steroid 21-hydroxylase deficiency. Am J Hum Genet 37(4):650–667
223. New MI (1995) Steroid 21-hydroxylase deficiency (congenital adrenal hyperplasia). Am J Med 98(1A):2S–8S
224. Speiser PW, New MI, White PC (1988) Molecular genetic analysis of nonclassic steroid 21-hydroxylase deficiency associated with HLA-B14, DR1. N Engl J Med 319(1):19–23
225. Owerbach D, Ballard AL, Draznin MB (1992) Salt-wasting congenital adrenal hyperplasia: detection and characterization of mutations in the steroid 21-hydroxylase gene, CYP21, using the polymerase chain reaction. J Clin Endocrinol Metab 74(3):553–558
226. White PC (2001) Steroid 11 beta-hydroxylase deficiency and related disorders. Endocrinol Metab Clin North Am 30(1):61–79, vi
227. White PC, Curnow KM, Pascoe L (1994) Disorders of steroid 11 beta-hydroxylase isozymes. Endocr Rev 15(4):421–438
228. Rosler A, Leiberman E, Cohen T (1992) High frequency of congenital adrenal hyperplasia (classic 11 beta-hydroxylase deficiency) among Jews from Morocco. Am J Med Genet 42(6):827–834
229. Mornet E, Dupont J, Vitek A, White PC (1989) Characterization of two genes encoding human steroid 11 beta-hydroxylase (P-450(11) beta). J Biol Chem 264(35):20961–20967
230. Taymans SE, Pack S, Pak E, Torpy DJ, Zhuang Z, Stratakis CA (1998) Human CYP11B2 (aldosterone synthase) maps to chromosome 8q24.3. J Clin Endocrinol Metab 83(3):1033–1036
231. Azziz R, Boots LR, Parker CR Jr, Bradley E Jr, Zacur HA (1991) 11 beta-hydroxylase deficiency in hyperandrogenism. Fertil Steril 55(4):733–741
232. Pang SY, Lerner AJ, Stoner E et al (1985) Late-onset adrenal steroid 3 beta-hydroxysteroid dehydrogenase deficiency. I. A cause

of hirsutism in pubertal and postpubertal women. J Clin Endocrinol Metab 60(3):428–439
233. Azziz R, Bradley EL Jr, Potter HD, Boots LR (1993) 3 beta-hydroxysteroid dehydrogenase deficiency in hyperandrogenism. Am J Obstet Gynecol 168(3 Pt 1):889–895
234. Derksen J, Nagesser SK, Meinders AE, Haak HR, van de Velde CJ (1994) Identification of virilizing adrenal tumors in hirsute women. N Engl J Med 331(15):968–973
235. Ettinger B, Von Werder K, Thenaers GC, Forsham PH (1971) Plasma testosterone stimulation-suppression dynamics in hirsute women. Am J Med 51(2):170–175
236. Surrey ES, de Ziegler D, Gambone JC, Judd HL (1988) Preoperative localization of androgen-secreting tumors: clinical, endocrinologic, and radiologic evaluation of ten patients. Am J Obstet Gynecol 158(6 Pt 1):1313–1322
237. Korobkin M (1989) Overview of adrenal imaging/adrenal CT. Urol Radiol 11(4):221–226
238. Taylor L, Ayers JW, Gross MD, Peterson EP, Menon KM (1986) Diagnostic considerations in virilization: iodomethyl-norcholesterol scanning in the localization of androgen secreting tumors. Fertil Steril 46(6):1005–1010
239. Moltz L, Pickartz H, Sorensen R, Schwartz U, Hammerstein J (1984) Ovarian and adrenal vein steroids in seven patients with androgen-secreting ovarian neoplasms: selective catheterization findings. Fertil Steril 42(4):585–593
240. Wentz AC, White RI Jr, Migeon CJ, Hsu TH, Barnes HV, Jones GS (1976) Differential ovarian and adrenal vein catheterization. Am J Obstet Gynecol 125(7):1000–1007
241. Young RH, Scully RE (1994) Sex-cord stromal steroid cell and other ovarian tumors with endocrine, paraendocrine, and paraneoplastic manifestations. In: Kurman RJ (ed) Blaustein's pathology of the female genital tract, 4th edn. Springer-Verlag, New York, pp 783–847
242. Young RH, Scully RE (1984) Ovarian Sertoli cell tumors: a report of 10 cases. Int J Gynecol Pathol 2(4):349–363
243. Young RH, Welch WR, Dickersin GR, Scully RE (1982) Ovarian sex cord tumor with annular tubules: review of 74 cases including 27 with Peutz-Jeghers syndrome and four with adenoma malignum of the cervix. Cancer 50(7):1384–1402
244. Aiman J (1991) Virilizing ovarian tumors. Clin Obstet Gynecol 34(4):835–847
245. Scully RE (1970) Gonadoblastoma. A review of 74 cases. Cancer 25(6):1340–1356
246. Ireland K, Woodruff JD (1976) Masculinizing ovarian tumors. Obstet Gynecol Surv 31(2):83–111
247. Boss JH, Scully RE, Wegner KH, Cohen RB (1965) Structural variations in the adult ovary. Clinical significance. Obstet Gynecol 25:747–764
248. Judd HL, Scully RE, Herbst AL, Yen SS, Ingersol FM, Kliman B (1973) Familial hyperthecosis: comparison of endocrinologic and histologic findings with polycystic ovarian disease. Am J Obstet Gynecol 117(7):976–982
249. Karam K, Hajj S (1979) Hyperthecosis syndrome. Clinical, endocrinologic and histologic findings. Acta Obstet Gynecol Scand 58(1):73–79
250. Braithwaite SS, Erkman-Balis B, Avila TD (1978) Postmenopausal virilization due to ovarian stromal hyperthecosis. J Clin Endocrinol Metab 46(2):295–300
251. Steingold KA, Judd HL, Nieberg RK, Lu JK, Chang RJ (1986) Treatment of severe androgen excess due to ovarian hyperthecosis with a long-acting gonadotropin-releasing hormone agonist. Am J Obstet Gynecol 154(6):1241–1248
252. Garcia-Bunuel R, Berek JS, Woodruff JD (1975) Luteomas of pregnancy. Obstet Gynecol 45(4):407–414
253. Pittaway DE (1991) Neoplastic causes of hyperandrogenism. Infert Reprod Med Clin North Am 2:531–545

Chapter 12
The Current Status for Metformin Use in Reproductive Medicine

Richard S. Legro

Abstract Metformin has been used extensively in multiple reproductive settings to ameliorate hyperandrogenism and chronic anovulation, to treat infertility, to prevent miscarriage and to prevent later pregnancy complications as well. Metformin does result in modest improvements in the PCOS phenotype with reductions in circulating insulin and testosterone levels, weight loss, and improved menstrual/ovulatory frequency. It is relatively ineffective as a solo agent to treat infertility, and further has a relative anti-fecundity compared to clomiphene alone. Clomiphene remains the first choice for infertility therapy and the gold standard for women with PCOS. Metformin may be useful in preventing OHSS when used in conjunction with gonadotropins. The use of metformin to prevent pregnancy loss or to prevent pregnancy complications is still experimental and better trials are needed to guide therapy.

Keywords Metformin • PCOS • Diabetes • Ovulation induction • Clomiphene citrate

12.1 Metformin Pharmacology

Metformin was approved for the treatment of type 2 diabetes by the FDA in 1994, but was used clinically for close to 20 years before that in other parts of the world, such that this represents one of the most widely used drugs worldwide. Metformin is a biguanide that works primarily by suppressing hepatic gluconeogenesis, but it also improves insulin sensitivity in the periphery (estimated to be ~20% of its treatment benefit in type 2 diabetes). It is not protein bound in the circulation, and is excreted unmetabolized in the urine. Gastrointestinal symptoms (diarrhea, nausea, vomiting, abdominal bloating, flatulence, and anorexia) are the most common reactions to metformin, and approximately 30% more frequent in women with metformin compared to placebo treated patients. For this reason, the dose is often escalated in a stepwise fashion to increase patient tolerance. An extended release version is available with a GI side effect profile identical to placebo with equal efficacy [1].

There is a small risk of lactic acidosis, among women taking this medication, which may be triggered by exposure to intravenous iodinated radiocontrast agents in susceptible individuals. This most commonly occurs in patients with poorly controlled diabetes and impaired renal function. Metformin is pregnancy category B with no known human teratogenic risk or no known embryonic lethality in humans. There have been no reported abnormalities associated with its use during pregnancy in women with diabetes, or to the small number of PCOS women who have conceived during treatment. The dose for reproductive medicine indications tends to be empiric as no adequately powered and designed dose ranging studies have been performed for these indications. The dose tends to range from 1,500 to 2,550 mg a day. None of the indications for metformin discussed in this chapter have received FDA approval.

12.2 Metformin and Effects on the PCOS Phenotype

Metformin has been associated with weight loss in women with PCOS in multiple trials, though metformin has failed in obesity trials and has no specific indication for obesity per se [2]. However, the consistent findings in many of the larger trials of metformin suggest that perhaps an insulin resistant or glucose intolerant population is more likely to respond with weight loss. The best example of this is the Diabetes Prevention Program where subjects who participated in the metformin only group experienced and maintained a significant weight loss from baseline over the course of the trial [3]. Similarly, in the largest multicenter trial conducted to date in women with polycystic ovary syndrome, the Pregnancy in Polycystic Ovary Syndrome Study (PPCOS), metformin was associated with a significant weight loss over the course of the trial, and in

R.S. Legro (✉)
Department of Obstetrics and Gynecology, Penn State College of Medicine, M.S. Hershey Medical Center, Hershey, PA, USA
e-mail: RSL1@psu.edu

D.T. Carrell and C.M. Peterson (eds.), *Reproductive Endocrinology and Infertility: Integrating Modern Clinical and Laboratory Practice*,
DOI 10.1007/978-1-4419-1436-1_12,

combination with clomiphene, a significant decrease in the waist hip ratio, a marker of centripetal obesity [4].

Metformin has also consistently been associated with a decrease in circulating testosterone levels. Further, some studies have shown increases in circulating sex hormone binding globulin (SHBG), which favors androgens as a substrate, and this increase is thought to ameliorate the peripheral potency of excess androgen. However, the findings on this are mixed and in the PPCOS trial, only a decrease in total testosterone was noted with a negligible effect on SHBG (Fig. 12.1). Longer term effects on hyperandrogenism, such as hirsutism and acne and androgenic alopecia, are not supported by the literature, primarily because there are no studies of adequate size and duration to document such effects, and the use of metformin for these indications remains empiric.

Metformin has been associated with improvements in insulin and glucose levels in most trials of women with PCOS. Also, the Diabetes Prevention Program showed a significant reduction in the conversion to type 2 diabetes among men and women with impaired glucose tolerance [3]. Studies of glucose tolerance in American women with PCOS have shown that 35–45% have impaired glucose tolerance (≥140–199 mg/dL) or type 2 diabetes (≥200 mg/dL) by the 2 h level [5, 6].

12.3 Metformin and Ovulation Induction

In randomized controlled studies, metformin has been found to increase ovulation rates compared to placebo in women with PCOS. It has been estimated by one study to increase this about one third above the baseline ovulatory rate (most women with PCOS are oligomenorrheic and not completely amenorrheic) [7]. Additionally, it appears also to be a useful adjuvant agent increasing the ovulatory rate when used in conjunction with clomiphene citrate beyond that with either metformin or clomiphene used as single agents [8]. This finding has not been consistently replicated in all multicenter trials with these drugs, and it appears that obese women (Body mass Index (BMI ≥ 30) are more likely to benefit from combined therapy than normal or overweight women (BMI < 30) [4]. Inducing ovulation has most commonly been performed in the context of infertility treatment discussed below, but there are obvious benefits to improve ovulatory frequency in women not seeking pregnancy, such as to prevent dysfunctional bleeding and endometrial hyperplasia.

12.4 Metformin and Infertility

The best level evidence for the effects of metformin are found in recent trials that have looked at the use of metformin to treat infertility. The four trials summarized in Table 12.1 are all randomized double blind multicenter trials that used metformin and clomiphene or the combination for the treatment of infertility in women with PCOS. All trials studied participants up to six cycles, there were no adjuvant medications such as hCG to trigger ovulation, and conception was by timed intercourse without inseminations. Two of the trials were conducted by the same group in Italy and their results are disparate from the multicenter Dutch and American trials. Each trial had a unique design and endpoint.

Only one trial [4] was designed and powered to detect a difference in live birth rates between the treatment groups [9]. This and the other large Dutch trial [10], both found no

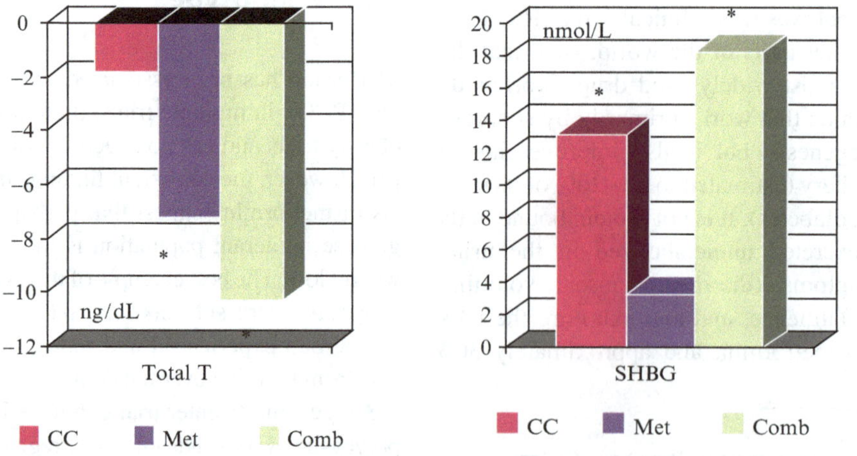

Fig. 12.1 Effect of treatment (metformin = met, cc = clomiphene, combined = metformin and clomiphene) on circulating total testosterone (T) and sex hormone binding globulin (SHBG) from baseline to end of study or last monthly visit before pregnancy in the PPCOS trial. *$P < 0.05$ compared to baseline (Adapted from [4])

Table 12.1 Summary of large randomized, blinded trials that have reported pregnancy and or live birth results

Study	N	Treatments	Cumulative 6 mos pregnancy rates	Conclusion
Palumba et al. 2005 [11]	100	Metformin/placebo vs. clomiphene/placebo	Live birth Metformin: 52% Clomiphene 18%	Metformin superior to clomiphene
Moll et al. 2006 [10]	225	Clomiphene/placebo vs. clomiphene/metformin	Ongoing pregnancy Clomiphene: 46% Metformin + Clomiphene: 40%	No benefit of combined therapy with metformin/clomiphene
Legro et al. 2007 [4]	626	Clomiphene/placebo vs. metformin/placebo vs. clomiphene/metformin	Live birth Metformin: 7% Clomiphene: 23% Metformin + Clomiphene: 28%	Clomiphene superior to metformin No benefit of combined therapy with metformin/clomiphene
Palomba et al. 2007 [12]	80	Metformin/placebo vs. clomiphene/placebo	Cumulative pregnancy rate Metformin 63% Clomiphene 49%	No benefit of metformin over clomiphene

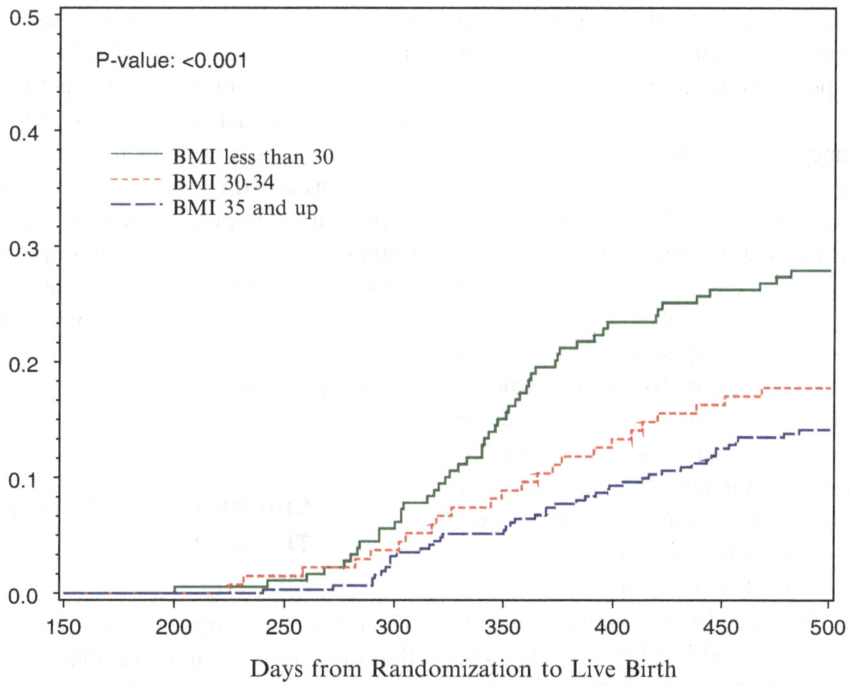

Fig. 12.2 Kaplan Meier Curve of live births by BMI group independent of treatment in the PPCOS trial (Adapted from [4])

benefit on the combination of metformin and clomiphene on live birth. The trials most at odds with one another, are the trials of Palomba et al. [11, 12], which found that metformin was significantly better or equal to clomiphene in achieving live birth and the PPCOS trial [4] which found the opposite.

12.4.1 *Metformin vs. Clomiphene*

Potential differences for the discrepant results include population differences, including genetic and environmental differences, selection criteria for the trial, and possible bias in the study design. The populations varied in terms of obesity. The Dutch and Palomba trials excluded women with PCOS with a BMI >30, whereas the PPCOS trial included them. One of the key findings of this trial is the role of BMI in predicting treatment success [4] (Fig. 12.2). Increasing obesity is clearly associated with decreasing success. However, when the primary outcome, live birth, is divided by BMI group and the highest BMI group is compared to the lowest BMI group (Table 12.2), it is obvious that the trend of each medication found in the overall study group holds regardless of weight category. The combined treatment group is still better than single agent therapy, and clomiphene is significantly better than metformin (Table 12.2). This is a post

Table 12.2 Results of the Legro et al. PPCOS trial stratified by BMI group, lowest BMI group (<30) compared to the largest group (BMI≥35) (Adapted from [4])

	BMI<30, *N*=179			BMI≥35, *N*=311		
	Clomiphene *n*=57	MET *n*=57	COMB *n*=65	Clomiphene *n*=110	MET *n*=105	COMB *n*=96
Ovulation	272/538 (50.6%)	151/554 (27.3%)	334/559 (59.7%)	190/404 (47.0%)	145/465 (31.2%)	248/405 (61.2%)
Live births	21/57 (36.8%)	5/57 (8.8%)	24/65 (36.9%)	18/110 (16.4%)	4/105 (3.8%)	22/96 (22.9%)

hoc analysis and subject to the error that multiple looks at the same data set can yield, however, the size of the normal and overweight BMI group in the PPCOS trial (*N*=179) is still substantially larger than the trial of Palomba et al. (*N*=100) [11]. Perhaps, the most relevant clinical implication is that there was a trend towards increased live birth with metformin and clomiphene in combination compared to clomiphene in the most obese subgroup, suggesting the combination may be the better choice for women with PCOS and BMI >35.

One marked discrepancy between the two trials is the different time-related trend in fecundity over the course of the trial. In the trial of Palomba et al. [11, 12] the per cycle fecundity (i.e., pregnancy/ovulation) started out at close to 15–20% for both metformin and clomiphene (i.e., consistent with normal fecundity in a fertile population) but then diverged over time with metformin approaching a per cycle of fecundity of 40% or greater by the end of the trial, whereas clomiphene declined dismally to 0%. In the follow-up, smaller clinical trial (*N*=80 subjects) by the same group that looked at of metformin vs. clomiphene as first line therapy for infertility in women with PCOS, the investigators found no significant difference between the medications in ongoing pregnancy rates (63% with metformin vs. 49% with clomiphene) [11]. In contrast, the fecundity for both clomiphene and metformin were constant in the PPCOS trial over each cycle with no time-related increase or decrease in rates (Fig. 12.3).

What did emerge from the PPCOS trial that is relevant both to clinical practice and to the FDA approval of ovulation inducing agents, is that the fecundity per ovulation was twice as good for clomiphene than metformin on a cycle basis (10.2% vs. 5.1%) and even better on a per ovulated patient basis (29.9% vs. 13.0%). This may have been due to the presumed multiple follicular recruitment of clomiphene over metformin (ultrasonography was not part of the PPCOS study), or by the improved reduction in hyperandrogenism (on the basis of reduction in the free androgen index with clomiphene compared to metformin). Some have argued that meformin's benefit requires a longer period of exposure prior to ovulation, and while no time effect was noted in the metformin only arm, a time-related improvement in pregnancy rates was noted in the combination arm of metformin and clomiphene in the PPCOS trial. However, these results are relevant to any ovulation induction agent and suggest that looking at ovulation rates alone does not answer the critical question whether that ovulation led to a pregnancy.

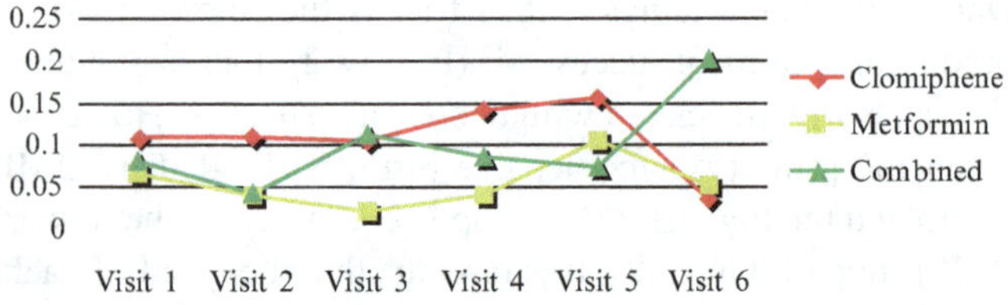

Fig. 12.3 Live birth per ovulation (as a fraction) in PPCOS trial by monthly visit. There was a significant time trend (towards improvement) in the combined arm, with constant rates noted with clomiphene and metformin alone (Adapted from [4])

12.4.2 Combination Therapy vs. Single Agent Therapy

The PPCOS trial was the only one to compare the combination of metformin and clomiphene to metformin alone and the combination was markedly more effective in achieving live birth. Both trials of Moll et al. [10] and the PPCOS, showed no benefit of combination therapy over clomiphene alone. Pregnancy rates were better in the Moll et al.trial probably because this trial also excluded obese subjects (BMI>30 kg/m). This difference in selection criteria also may explain the discrepancy in ovulation rates between the two trials. The combination of metformin and clomiphene had a significantly improved effect on the ovulation rate compared to clomiphene alone in the PPCOS trial (due to the presumed benefit of combination treatment in the more obese U.S. population), with no benefit detected in the trial of Moll et al. The women in the PPCOS trial were probably also more severely affected based on their relatively long mean period of infertility prior to participation in the trial (almost 3.5 years), and this too was likely a poor prognostic marker.

12.4.3 Metformin and Gonadotropins and Laparoscopic Ovarian Diathermy

Metformin has been used in conjunction with gonadotropins both for ovulation induction and in an IVF setting, and also as an adjunct to women who have undergone laparoscopic ovarian drilling. A recent systematic review examined the utility of metformin in this setting and concluded that there is no evidence for a positive effect of metformin on live birth when added to laparoscopic ovarian drilling (RR 1.3; 95% CI 0.39–4.0) or FSH (RR 1.6; 95% CI 0.95–2.9), or when coadministered in IVF (RR 1.5; 95% CI 0.92–2.5). In IVF, metformin led to fewer cases of ovarian hyperstimulation syndrome (OHSS) (RR 0.33; 95% CI 0.13–0.80) [13]. This latter finding, to a large extent, is based on a single well-designed, but underpowered clinical trial [14], and further, such trials are needed to establish the role of metformin in preventing OHSS.

12.5 Metformin and Multiple Pregnancy

Metformin has been recommended for use in infertility treatment partly because it is thought to be associated with monofollicular ovulation and lower multiple pregnancy rates. None of the trials was adequately powered to detect differences in multiple pregnancy rates. The multiple pregnancy rate in the clomiphene-only group was 6.4% ($N=3$, 1 triplet), 0% in the metformin-only group, and 3.3% in the combination therapy group ($N=2$) [4]. This number (~5%) is at or below what has been reported from large series of women conceiving on clomiphene citrate [15] and well below the expectations of many of an enhanced multiple pregnancy rate in response to clomiphene in women with PCOS [16]. However, given the low number of multiple pregnancies overall, there was no statistical difference in multiple pregnancy rates between treatment groups. The Dutch study reported one triplet (none survived) and one twin pregnancy on clomiphene therapy. Further research is needed, although given the relatively small multiple pregnancy rate, a very large number of pregnancies will be required to detect a significant reduction from a 5–6% multiple rate with clomiphene. The benefit of multiple pregnancy reduction must be balanced against the substantially lower pregnancy rates with metformin alone.

12.6 Metformin and Miscarriage

Metformin has been used, most commonly in women with PCOS, to prevent miscarriage. The basis for its use is primarily observational case series. There are no adequately designed and sufficiently powered randomized trials to address its risk benefit ratio in this population. The trials discussed in Table 12.1 offer some insight into early pregnancy loss, but all of them stopped study medication in study subjects upon determination of pregnancy. Therefore, they cannot address the potential risk benefit ratio of continuing medication through the first trimester or throughout pregnancy as some groups have advocated [17]. It is matter of concern that there was a non significant and unexpected trend towards an increased first trimester pregnancy loss rate in the metformin group vs. the clomiphene groups (40% in the metformin, vs. 23% in the clomiphene and 25% in the combined group) in the PPCOS trial. No similar trend in miscarriage rates was noted in the other trials, but they were significantly smaller. The Italian group in another small trial did report a significant reduction in miscarriage rates in clomiphene resistant women who conceived after metformin use, compared to laparoscopic diathermy [18]. These discrepant findings mandate further study before metformin is used routinely in women with PCOS for this indication.

12.7 Metformin for Later Pregnancy Complications

Recent data, both from a meta-analysis and from the PPCOS trial, suggests that women with PCOS are at increased risk for multiple pregnancy complications including preeclampsia, gestational diabetes, and preterm delivery [19]. The meta-analysis showed that women with PCOS demonstrated a significantly higher risk of developing gestational diabetes [odds ratio (OR) 2.94; 95% confidence interval (CI): 1.70–5.08], pregnancy-induced hypertension (OR 3.67; 95% CI 1.98–6.81), pre-eclampsia (OR 3.47; 95% CI 1.95–6.17) and preterm birth (OR 1.75; 95% CI 1.16–2.62). Their babies had a significantly higher risk of admission to a neonatal intensive care unit (OR 2.31; 95% CI 1.25–4.26) and a higher perinatal mortality (OR 3.07; 95% CI 1.03–9.21), unrelated to multiple births.

This increased risk has led to small studies using metformin throughout pregnancy to prevent these complications. Certainly, there is a rationale for using metformin to treat gestational diabetes and it is now used for this indication in many parts of the world. Theoretically, it may also be useful to prevent gestational diabetes. One randomized trial from Norway showed a remarkable reduction in pregnancy complications in women with PCOS who took metformin during pregnancy [20] , but the small sample size ($N=40$) and the clustering of unusual major pregnancy complications in the placebo arm increases the probability that this is a type 1 error (Fig. 12.4). A larger multicenter trial is now ongoing in

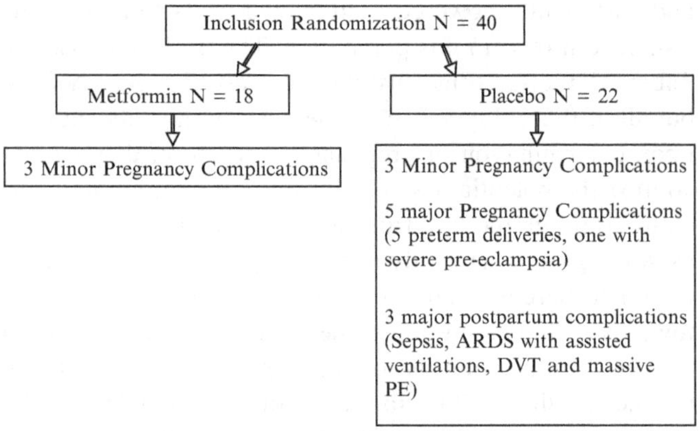

Fig. 12.4 Flow chart of randomized study of metformin or placebo throughout pregnancy in women with PCOS including outcomes of minor and major pregnancy complications (Adapted from [20])

Norway to address the benefit of metformin use during pregnancy in women with PCOS. Currently, its use must be considered experimental.

12.8 Summary: Evidence-Based Guidelines

Metformin has many potential uses in reproductive medicine, but its impact in properly designed trials has been negligible to date.

Metformin does result in modest improvements in the PCOS phenotype with reductions in circulating insulin and testosterone levels, weight loss, and improved menstrual/ovulatory frequency.

It is relatively ineffective as a solo agent to treat infertility, and further, has a relative anti-fecundity compared to clomiphene alone. Clomiphene remains the first choice for infertility therapy and the gold standard for women with PCOS.

There may be benefits of combined therapy with clomiphene and metformin on live birth rates in a very obese population.

Metformin may be useful to prevent OHSS when used in conjunction with gonadotropins.

The use of metformin to prevent pregnancy loss or to prevent pregnancy complications is still experimental and better trials are needed to guide therapy.

References

1. Fujioka K, Brazg RL, Raz I et al (2005) Efficacy, dose-response relationship and safety of once-daily extended-release metformin (Glucophage XR) in type 2 diabetic patients with inadequate glycaemic control despite prior treatment with diet and exercise: results from two double-blind, placebo-controlled studies. Diabetes Obes Metab 7(1):28–39
2. Levri KM, Slaymaker E, Last A et al (2005) Metformin as treatment for overweight and obese adults: a systematic review. Ann Fam Med 3(5):457–461
3. Knowler WC, Barrett-Connor E, Fowler SE et al (2002) Reduction in the incidence of type 2 diabetes with lifestyle intervention or metformin. N Engl J Med 346(6):393–403
4. Legro RS, Barnhart HX, Schlaff WD et al (2007) Clomiphene, metformin, or both for infertility in the polycystic ovary syndrome. N Engl J Med 356(6):551–566
5. Legro RS, Kunselman AR, Dodson WC, Dunaif A (1999) Prevalence and predictors of risk for type 2 diabetes mellitus and impaired glucose tolerance in polycystic ovary syndrome: a prospective, controlled study in 254 affected women. J Clin Endocrinol Metab 84(1):165–169
6. Ehrmann DA, Kasza K, Azziz R, Legro RS, Ghazzi MN (2005) Effects of race and family history of type 2 diabetes on metabolic status of women with polycystic ovary syndrome (PCOS). J Clin Endocrinol Metab 90(1):66–71
7. Moghetti P, Castello R, Negri C et al (2000) Metformin effects on clinical features, endocrine and metabolic profiles, and insulin sensitivity in polycystic ovary syndrome: a randomized, double-blind, placebo-controlled 6-month trial, followed by open, long-term clinical evaluation. J Clin Endocrinol Metab 85(1):139–146
8. Nestler JE, Jakubowicz DJ, Evans WS, Pasquali R (1998) Effects of metformin on spontaneous and clomiphene-induced ovulation in the polycystic ovary syndrome. N Engl J Med 338(26): 1876–1880
9. Myers ER, Silva SG, Hafley G, Kunselman AR, Nestler JE, Legro RS (2005) Estimating live birth rates after ovulation induction in polycystic ovary syndrome: sample size calculations for the pregnancy in polycystic ovary syndrome trial. Contemp Clin Trials 26(3):271–280
10. Moll E, Bossuyt PM, Korevaar JC, Lambalk CB, van der Veen F (2006) Effect of clomifene citrate plus metformin and clomifene citrate plus placebo on induction of ovulation in women with newly diagnosed polycystic ovary syndrome: randomised double blind clinical trial. BMJ 332(7556):1485
11. Palomba S, Orio F Jr, Falbo A et al (2005) Prospective parallel randomized, double-blind, double-dummy controlled clinical trial comparing clomiphene citrate and metformin as the first-line treatment for ovulation induction in nonobese anovulatory women with polycystic ovary syndrome. J Clin Endocrinol Metab 90(7): 4068–4074
12. Palomba S, Orio F Jr, Falbo A, Russo T, Tolino A, Zullo F (2007) Clomiphene citrate versus metformin as first-line approach for the treatment of anovulation in infertile patients with polycystic ovary syndrome. J Clin Endocrinol Metab 92(9):3498–3503
13. Moll E, van der Veen F, van Wely M (2007) The role of metformin in polycystic ovary syndrome: a systematic review. Hum Reprod Update 13(6):527–537
14. Tang T, Glanville J, Orsi N, Barth JH, Balen AH (2006) The use of metformin for women with PCOS undergoing IVF treatment. Hum Reprod 21(6):1416–1425
15. Asch RH, Greenblatt RB (1976) Update on the safety and efficacy of clomiphene citrate as a therapeutic agent. J Reprod Med 17(3):175–180
16. Casper RF, Mitwally MF (2006) Review: aromatase inhibitors for ovulation induction. J Clin Endocrinol Metab 91(3):760–771
17. Jakubowicz DJ, Iuorno MJ, Jakubowicz S, Roberts KA, Nestler JE (2002) Effects of metformin on early pregnancy loss in the polycystic ovary syndrome. J Clin Endocrinol Metab 87(2): 524–529

18. Palomba S, Orio F Jr, Nardo LG et al (2004) Metformin administration versus laparoscopic ovarian diathermy in clomiphene citrate-resistant women with polycystic ovary syndrome: a prospective parallel randomized double-blind placebo-controlled trial. J Clin Endocrinol Metab 89(10):4801–4809
19. Boomsma CM, Eijkemans MJ, Hughes EG, Visser GH, Fauser BC, Macklon NS (2006) A meta-analysis of pregnancy outcomes in women with polycystic ovary syndrome. Hum Reprod Update 12(6):673–683
20. Vanky E, Salvesen KA, Heimstad R, Fougner KJ, Romundstad P, Carlsen SM (2004) Metformin reduces pregnancy complications without affecting androgen levels in pregnant polycystic ovary syndrome women: results of a randomized study. Hum Reprod 19(8):1734–1740

Chapter 13
Clinical Aspects of Endometriosis

Attila Bokor, Christel Meuleman, and Thomas D'Hooghe

Abstract Endometriosis is a common, benign, estrogen-dependent, gynecological disorder associated with pelvic pain and infertility. The prevalence of this condition can reasonably be assumed to be around 10%. Endometriosis should be suspected in women with dysmenorrhea, dyspareunia, chronic pelvic pain, or subfertility; it may also be asymptomatic and can be present as a chronic disease in a subset of patients. Visual recognition during laparoscopy is required for the definitive diagnosis of endometriosis. Treatment must be individualized, taking into consideration the clinical problem in its entirety, including the impact of the disease and the effect of its treatment on quality of life. Endometriosis-associated pain can be effectively treated by surgery and by hormonal suppression. Endometriosis-associated subfertility can be effectively treated by surgery and by assisted reproduction, but not by hormonal suppression. Endometriosis can recur after treatment, and the risk increases with the severity of endometriosis and the time interval since the last surgery. However, patients with recurrent pain do not always have endometriosis and may require a multidisciplinary approach involving a pain clinic, and counseling should be considered early in the treatment plan.

Keywords Endometriosis • Infertility • Etiology • Diagnosis • Treatment • Guidelines

13.1 Pathogenesis

Endometriosis is a common, benign, estrogen-dependent, gynecological disorder associated with pelvic pain and infertility. Though endometriosis has been described for more than one hundred years, our current knowledge of its pathogenesis remains unclear.

A. Bokor, C. Meuleman, and T. D'Hooghe (✉)
Leuven University Fertility Center, UZ Gasthuisberg, K.U. Leuven, Belgium
e-mail: thomas.dhooghe@uz.kuleuven.ac.be

There are a number of theories that have been proposed to explain the pathogenesis of endometriosis:

1. Retrograde menstruation/transplantation
2. Coelomic metaplasia
3. The induction theory
4. Genetic basis
5. Altered cellular immunity
6. Environmental basis

13.1.1 The Ectopic Transplantation

The ectopic transplantation of endometrial tissue, originally proposed by Sampson in 1924, is the most widely accepted theory to explain the pathogenesis of endometriosis. It claims that the disorder originates from retrograde menstruation of endometrial tissue sloughed through patent fallopian tubes in the peritoneal cavity [1]. Retrograde menstruation occurs in 70–90% of women [2–4], and may be more common in women with endometriosis than in those without the disease [4]. The presence of endometrial cells in the peritoneal fluid, indicating retrograde menstruation, has been reported in 59–79% of women during menses or in the early follicular phase [5–7]. This hypothesis is supported by the following epidemiological data.

The development of endometriosis in the first few years after menarche has been associated with a high rate of obstructing genital tract anomalies. These include noncommunicating rudimentary uterine horns, cervical stenosis, cervical atresia, vaginal or transverse septum agenesis, or an imperforate hymen [8, 9]. As a general rule, women with a stricture at the level of the cervix have a higher incidence of endometriosis than women with a stricture lower in the genital tract. Furthermore, women with shorter intervals between menstruation and longer duration of menses are more likely to have retrograde menstruation and are at higher risk for endometriosis [2, 8, 10].

D.T. Carrell and C.M. Peterson (eds.), *Reproductive Endocrinology and Infertility: Integrating Modern Clinical and Laboratory Practice*,
DOI 10.1007/978-1-4419-1436-1_13, © Springer Science+Business Media, LLC 2010

13.1.2 The Transformation (Metaplasia) of Coelomic

The transformation (metaplasia) of coelomic epithelium into endometrial tissue has been proposed as a mechanism for the ontogenesis of endometriosis. This theory is best supported by the fact that genetic induction of ovarian endometriosis is possible in mice suggesting that ovarian endometriotic lesions may arise directly from the ovarian surface epithelium through a metaplastic differentiation process induced by activation of an onco-genic K-ras allele [11].

13.1.3 The Induction Theory

The induction theory is, in principle, an extension of the coelomic metaplasia theory. It proposes that an endogenous biochemical factor in the menstrual fluid present in the peritoneum during menstruation can induce undifferentiated peritoneal cells to develop into endometrial tissue. This theory has been somehow supported by experiments in rabbits [12, 13] but has not been substantiated in women or in primates.

13.1.4 Genetic Basis

The risk for endometriosis is seven times greater if a first-degree relative has been affected by endometriosis [14, 15]. No specific Mendelian inheritance pattern has been identified; therefore, multifactorial inheritance has been postulated. A relatíve risk for endometriosis of 7.2 has been found in mothers and sisters, and a 75% incidence has been noted in homozygotic twins of patients with endometriosis [16]. Epidemiological research in the icelandic population has shown that endometriosis occurs concordantly in monozygotic twins, that pain symptoms start at a similar age in affected nontwin sisters, and that the prevalence of endometriosis is 6 to 9 times increased among first-degree relatives of women with endometriosis when compared to the general population [16].

The induction of human-like endometriosis in mice by genetic activation of an oncogenic K-ras allele lends further support to the genetic basis of this disorder [11]. More recent studies showed aneuploidy for chromosomes 11, 16, and 17 [17], increased heterogeneity of chromosome 17 aneuploidy [18], and loss of lp and 22q (50%), 5p (33%), 6q (27%), 70 (22%), 9q (22%), and 16 (22%) of 18 selected endometriotic tissues [19].

The relationship between endometriosis and single gene polymorphisms is controversial [20]. Positive correlations have been shown for single nucleotide polymorphisms linked to cytokines and inflammation, steroid-synthesizing enzymes and detoxifying enzymes and receptors, estradiol metabolism, other enzymes and metabolic systems, and adhesion molecules and matrix enzymes. Apoptosis, cell-cycle regulation, and oncogenes seem to be negatively correlated with the disease, whereas the group of hormone receptors, growth factor systems, and especially groups of the HLA-system components show a relatively strong correlation [20].

An ongoing web project (http://www.well.ox.ac.uk/krinaz/) describes allele and genotype frequencies of SNPs in association studies and provides a useful tool for the study of genetic variants and the pathogenesis of endometriosis [20].

13.1.5 Immunologic Mechanisms

Immunologic mechanisms are believed to be involved in the pathogenesis of endometriosis. Several theories have been proposed to explain enhanced implantation and defective clearing of endometrial cells from the pelvic cavity, facilitating the development of endometriosis.

Although retrograde menstruation appears to be a common event in women, not all women who have retrograde menstruation develop endometriosis. The immune system may be altered in women with endometriosis, and it has been hypothesized that the disease may develop as a result of reduced immunologic clearance of viable endometrial cells from the pelvic cavity [21, 22]. According to this hypothesis, endometriosis can be caused by decreased clearance of peritoneal fluid endometrial cells resulting from reduced natural killer (NK) cell and macrophage activity [23]. In contrast, endometriosis can also be considered a condition of immunologic tolerance for ectopic endometrium, which essentially is self-tissue [21].

Substantial evidence suggests that endometriosis is associated with a state of subclinical peritoneal inflammation, marked by an increased peritoneal fluid volume, increased peritoneal fluid white blood cell concentration (especially macrophages with increased activation status), and increased inflammatory cytokines, growth factors, and angiogenesis-promoting substances. It has been reported in baboons that subclinical peritoneal inflammation occurs both during menstruation and after intrapelvic injection of endometrium [24, 25]. Furthermore, there are data supporting that a higher basal activation status of peritoneal macrophages in women with endometriosis may impair fertility by reducing sperm motility, increasing sperm phagocytosis, or interfering with fertilization [26, 27] possibly by increased secretion of cytokines such as tumor necrosis factor-α(TNF-α) [2, 28, 29].

Macrophages or other cells may promote the growth of endometrial cells by secretion of growth and angiogenetic factors, such as epidermal growth factor (EGF) [30], macrophage-derived growth factor (MDGF) [31], fibronectin, and adhesion molecules such as integrins [31, 32]. After attachment of endometrial cells to the peritoneum, subsequent invasion and growth appear to be regulated by matrix metalloproteinases (MMP) and their tissue inhibitors [33, 34].

Aromatase activity is absent in normal endometrium. Contrarily, aromatase is expressed aberrantly in endometriosis, which gives rise to very high levels of aromatase activity in the endometriotic tissue. Both aromatase expression and activity are stimulated by PGE2. This results in local production of estrogen, which in turn induces PGE2 formation and establishes a positive feedback cycle [35, 36].

The subclinical pelvic inflammatory status associated with endometriosis is also reflected in the systemic circulation. Increased concentrations of C-reactive protein, serum amyloid A (SAA), TNF-a, membrane cofactor protein-1, interleukin-6, interleukin-8, and chemokine (C-C motif) receptor 1 (CCR1) have been observed in peripheral blood samples of patients with endometriosis when compared with controls [2, 37].

13.1.6 Environmental Factors

The links between reproductive health, infertility, and environmental pollution are controversial. Attention has been directed to the potential role of dioxins in the pathogenesis of endometriosis, but the issue remains controversial. A recent meta-analysis concluded that currently there is insufficient evidence in women or in nonhuman primates that endometriosis is caused by dioxin exposure [38].

13.1.7 Future Research

Future research on the pathogenesis of endometriosis should focus on the early interactions between endometrial and peritoneal cells in the pelvic cavity at the time of menstruation. Proteomic and genomic approaches can detect potential differences between eutopic endometrium and myometrium in women with and without endometriosis [39].

13.2 Prevalence

Based on the few reliable data, the prevalence of the condition can reasonably be assumed to be around 10% [40]. Endometriosis is predominantly found in women of reproductive age but can also be found in adolescents and in postmenopausal women receiving hormonal replacement [40]. It is found in women of all ethnic and social groups. In women with pelvic pain or infertility, a high prevalence of endometriosis (20–90%) has been reported [41, 42]. In asymptomatic women undergoing tubal ligation, the prevalence of endometriosis ranges from 3 to 43% [2, 43].

13.3 Diagnosis

The current clinical opinion is that laparoscopy is required for definitive diagnosis of endometriosis [44]. History and physical examination can yield a number of significant findings suggestive for endometriosis including affected first degree relatives, chronic pelvic pain and dysmenorrhea, retroverted uterus, adnexal masses, cul de sac nodularity and uterosacral ligament thickening and tenderness, but none are diagnostic for endometriosis.

Well known risk factors for endometriosis include short cycle length [45], heavier menstruation, and longer flow duration [46], probably related to a higher incidence of retrograde menstruation. Patient height and weight are positively and negatively, respectively, associated with the risk of endometriosis [47]. Although a higher prevalence of endometriosis has been found among patients with coitus during menses [48], more research is needed to address the role of sexual habits in the development of endometriosis.

Endometriosis can be associated with significant gastrointestinal symptoms (pain, nausea, vomiting, early satiety, bloating and distention, altered bowel habits) as well. A characteristic motility change, along with bacterial overgrowth, has been documented the bowel system of most women with endometriosis [49].

The average delay between the onset of pain symptoms and surgically confirmed endometriosis is quite long: mean 8 years in the United Kingdom and 9 to 12 years in the United States [50]. However over the past 20 years, there has been a steady decrease in the delay in diagnosis and a decline in the prevalence of advanced endometriosis at first diagnosis [51].

13.3.1 Pain

In adult women, dysmenorrhea is especially suggestive of endometriosis if it begins after years of pain-free menses. Dysmenorrhea often starts before the onset of menstrual bleeding and continues throughout the menstrual period. In adolescents, dysmenorrhoea may be present after menarche without an interval of pain-free menses. The distribution of pain is variable but most often is bilateral [2].

Local symptoms can arise from rectal, ureteral, and bladder involvement, and lower back pain can occur. Most studies have failed to detect a correlation between the degree of pelvic pain and the severity of endometriosis [42]. Some women with extensive disease have no pain, whereas others with only minimal disease may experience severe pelvic pain. Severe pelvic pain and dyspareunia may be associated with deep infiltrating subperitoneal endometriosis [43, 52].

Possible mechanisms causing pain in patients with endometriosis include local peritoneal inflammation, deep infiltration with tissue damage, adhesion formation, fibrotic thickening, and collection of shed menstrual blood in endometriotic implants, resulting in painful traction with the physiologic movement of tissues [2, 52, 53]. In rectovaginal endometriotic nodules, a close histologic relationship has been observed between nerves and endometriotic foci and between nerves and the fibrotic component of the nodule [54].

13.3.2 Subfertility and Infertility

An association between endometriosis and subfertility is generally accepted, based on epidemiological, retrospective or cross-sectional studies in women and on nonhuman primate research [55, 56]. In women with moderate or severe endometriosis, major pelvic adhesions can impair oocyte release from the ovary or inhibit ovum pickup or transport.[2, 57]. In women with mild endometriosis, the monthly fecundity rate (MFR) is lower (5–11%) than observed in a normally fertile population (25%) [58]. The association between minimal endometriosis and infertility has been explained by numerous mechanisms (ovulatory dysfunction, luteal insufficiency, luteinized unruptured follicle syndrome, recurrent abortion, altered immunity, and intraperitoneal inflammation) [58], but remains controversial [55, 59]. It is possible that functional disorders of the endometrium may both predispose to the development of endometriosis and impair implantation mechanisms in affected women. [56]. Both the prevalence of endometriosis and the proportion of moderate to severe endometrisos are higher in infertile women (27 and 71%) than in women of proven fertility women (3 and 43%) [55].

13.3.3 Spontaneous Abortion

On the basis of on controlled prospective studies, there is no evidence that endometriosis is associated with pregnancy loss [60, 61], or that medical or surgical treatment of endometriosis reduces the spontaneous abortion rate [62, 63].

13.3.4 Endocrinologic Disorders

Endometriosis has been associated with anovulation, abnormal follicular development, reduced circulating E2 levels during the preovulatory phase, disturbed luteinizing hormone (LH) surge patterns, premenstrual spotting, the luteinized unruptured follicle syndrome, galactorrhea, and hyperprolactinemia [61]. However, there are no sufficient convincing data indicating that the prevalence of these endocrinologic abnormalities is significantly increased in women with endometriosis [2, 55, 61].

13.3.5 Clinical Examination

In many women with endometriosis, no abnormality is detected during the clinical examination. The vulva, vagina, and cervix should be inspected for any signs of endometriosis, although the occurrence of endometriosis in these areas is rare [2]. Other possible signs of endometriosis include uterosacral or cul-de-sac nodularity, lateral or cervical displacement caused by uterosacral scarring [64], painful swelling of the recto-vaginal septum, and unilateral ovarian enlargement. In more advanced disease, the uterus is often in fixed retroversion, and the mobility of the ovaries and fallopian tubes is reduced. Evidence of deeply infiltrative endometriosis (deeper than 5 mm under the peritoneum) in the rectovaginal septum with cul-de-sac obliteration or cystic ovarian endometriosis should be suspected by clinical documentation of uterosacral nodularities during menses, especially if CA125 serum levels are higher than 35 IU/mL [65, 66].

Extrapelvic endometriosis is rare (0, 5 -2%) and may result from vascular or lymphatic dissemination of endometrial cells to many gynecologic (vulva, vagina, cervix) and non-gynecologic sites [2, 67]. Although extrapelvic endometriosis is often asymptomatic, it should be suspected when symptoms of pain or a palpable mass occur outside the pelvis in a cyclic pattern. Endometriosis involving the intestinal tract, especially colon and rectum, is the most common site of extrapelvic disease, and is associated with cyclic or chronic abdominal and back pain, abdominal distention, cyclic rectal bleeding, constipation, and obstruction. Ureteral involvement can lead to obstruction and result in cyclic higher back pain, dysuria, and hematuria. Pulmonary endometriosis can manifest as pneumothorax, hemothorax, or hemoptysis during menses. Umbilical endometriosis should be suspected when a patient has a palpable mass and cyclic pain in the umbilical area [67].

Although clinical examination is a useful tool in the detection of endometriosis, the diagnosis of endometriosis should be confirmed by biopsy of suspicious lesions that are obtained laparoscopically.

13.3.6 Imaging and Endometriosis

Gynecologic transvaginal [68] or transrectal ultrasonography [69] is an important diagnostic tool [70] in the assessment of ovarian endometriotic cysts and of rectovaginal endometriosis (sensitivity, 97%; specificity, 96%). The presence of filling defects detected by hysterosalpingography has also been reported to have a significant positive correlation with endometriosis. The positive predictive value of this finding is 84% and the negatíve predictive value is 75% [71]. Other imaging techniques, including computed tomography (CT) and MRI, can be used to provide additional and confirmatory information, but they cannot be used for primary diagnosis [44].

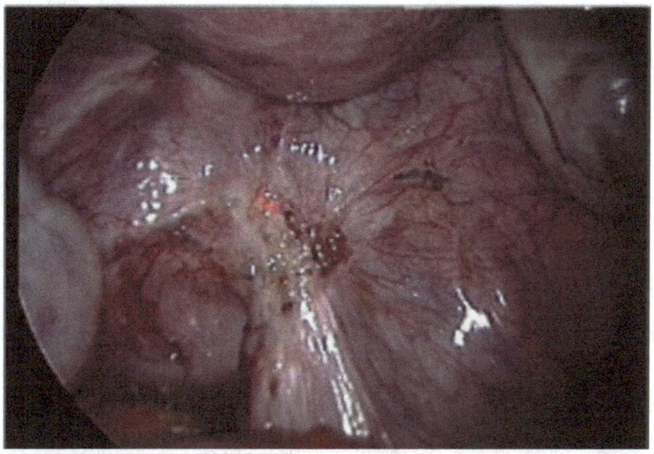

Fig. 13.1 Black peritoneal laesion, gunshot laesions, hypervascularisation (typical endometriosis)

13.3.7 Laboratory Tests

There is no blood test available for the diagnosis of endometriosis. Levels of CA125, a coelomic epithelium marker common to most nonmucinous epithelial ovarian carcinomas, have been found to be significantly higher in women with moderate or severe endometriosis, but not in women with minimal or mild disease, when compared to women with a normal pelvis [72]. Serum CA 125 levels are reported to increase during menstruation according to some [73, 74] but not all [75] investigators, and this phenomenon may be limited to patients with moderate to severe endometriosis [76]. Compared with laparoscopy, measurement of serum CA125 levels has no value as a diagnostic tool [44], but serial CA125 determinations may be useful to predict the recurrence of endometriosis after therapy [77].

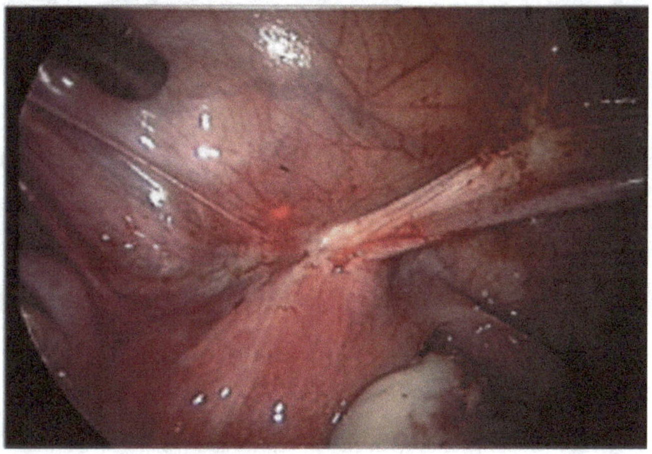

Fig. 13.2 Vesicular peritoneal endometriosis, filmy adhaesions and white plaques (atypical appearence of endometriosis)

13.3.7.1 Laparoscopic Findings and Classification

Unless disease is visible in the vagina or elsewhere, most guidelines state that laparoscopic visualization of suspicious lesions is the gold standard for the definitive diagnosis of endometriosis [44, 56]. During diagnostic laparoscopy, the pelvic and abdominal cavity should be systematically investigated for the presence of endometriosis. The type, location, and extent of all lesions and adhesions should be documented in the operative notes ideally, should be recorded [44]. Characteristic findings include typical ("powder-burn" or "gunshot") lesions on the serosal surfaces of the peritoneum. These lesions are black, dark brown, or bluish nodules or small cysts containing old hemorrhage surrounded by a variable degree of fibrosis (Fig. 13.1). Endometriosis can also appear as subtle lesions also called "atypical," including red implants (petechial, vesicular, polypoid, hemorrhagic, red flamelike), serous or clear vesicles and sometimes white plaques or scarring, yellow-brown discoloration of the peritoneum, and tubo-ovarian adhesions (Fig. 13.2) [2, 78]. Histologic confirmation of the laparoscopic impression is essential for the diagnosis of endometriosis, not only for subtle lesions but also for typical lesions reported to be histologically negative in 24% of cases [79], and should be considered as ideal practice [44]. In the presence of ovarian endometrioma (greater than 3 cm in diameter) and deeply infiltrating disease, histology should be obtained to identify endometriosis and to exclude rare instances of malignancy [78].

Deeply invasive endometriosis is associated with reduced depth and volume of the pouch of Douglas (Fig. 13.3) suggesting that this phenotype of endometriosis does not develop in the recto-vaginal septum but is the consequence of intraperitoneally buried anterior rectal wall adhesions [80].

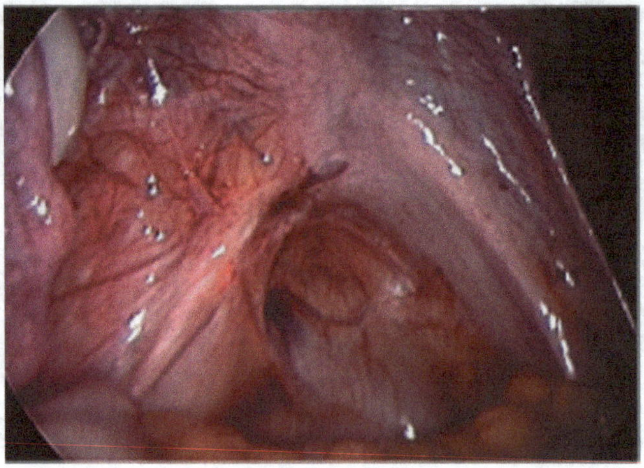

Fig. 13.3 Deeply infiltrating endometriosis nodule

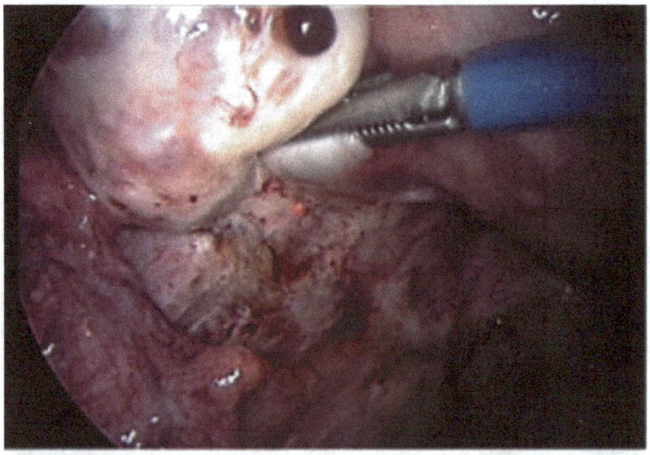

Fig. 13.4 Superficial ovarian endometriosis and typical gunshot laesions in cul de sac

Superficial ovarian endometriosis can present as both typical and subtle lesions (Fig. 13.4). Ovarian endometriotic cysts are usually located on the anterior surface of the ovary and are associated with retraction, pigmentation, and adhesions to the posterior peritoneum (Fig. 13.5). These ovarian endometriotic cysts often contain a thick, viscous dark brown fluid (chocolate fluid) composed of hemosiderin derived from previous intraovarian hemorrhage. Since such fluid may also be found in other conditions, such as in hemorrhagic corpus luteum cysts or neoplastic cysts, biopsy and preferably removal of the ovarian cyst for histologic examination is desirable [2, 81].

The current classification system of endometriosis is Revised American Fertility Society Classification (Fig. 13.7), which has been revised without major changes [57]. The classification is based on the appearance, size, and depth of peritoneal and ovarian implants; the degree of cul-de-sac obliteration and the presence, extent, and type of adnexal adhesions. In the new classification system, the morphologic aspect of the lesions is additionally categorized as red (red, red-pink, and clear lesions), white (white, yellow-brown, and peritoneal defects), and black (black and blue lesions)[2, 57]. Despite of the criticism of several authors, the revised classification of endometriosis is the only internationally accepted system, and appears to be the best available tool to describe objectively the extent of endometriosis [2].

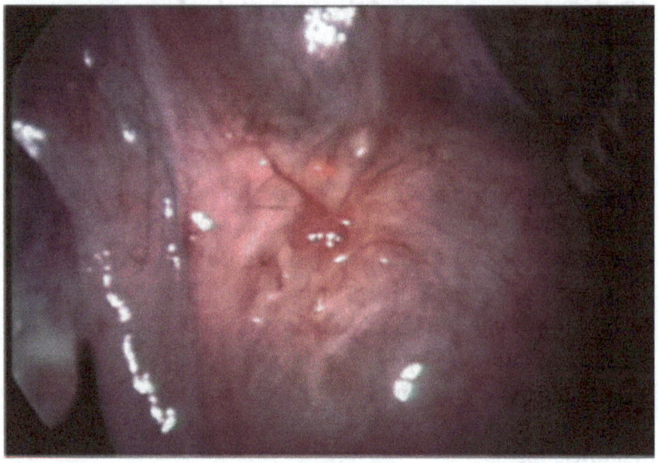

Fig. 13.5 Ovarian endometrioma

13.3.7.2 Histologic Confirmation

Histologic confirmation is essential in the diagnosis of endometriosis. In a study of 44 patients with chronic pelvic pain, endometriosis was laparoscopically diagnosed in 36%, but histologic confirmation was obtained in only 18%. This approach resulted in a low diagnostic accuracy of laparoscopic inspection with a positive predictive value of only 45%, explained by a specificity of only 77% [2, 82]. Microscopically, endometriotic implants consist of endometrial glands and stroma, with or without hemosiderin-laden macrophages (Fig. 13.6). Endometrioid stroma may be more characteristic of endometriosis than endometrioid glands [83]. Vascularization, mitotic activity, and the three-dimensional structure of endometriosis lesions are the key factors [84].

13.4 Spontaneous Evolution During Pregnancy

The characteristics of endometriosis are variable during pregnancy, and lesions tend to enlarge during the first trimester but regress thereafter [85]. Studies in baboons have

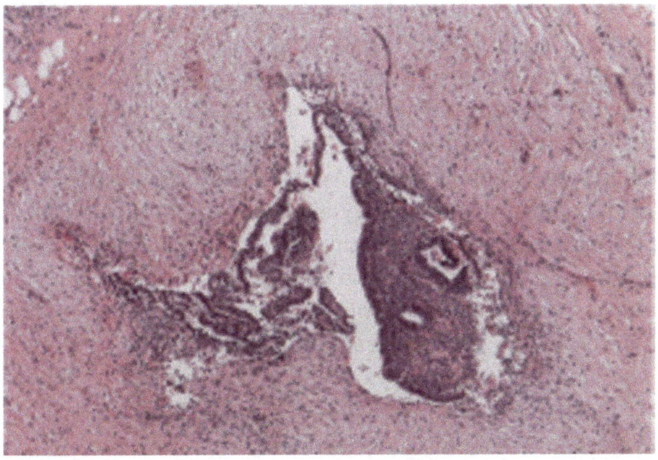

Fig. 13.6 Hystological aspect of endometriosis Photographs kindly donated by Christel Meuleman MD, Leuven University Fertility Centre, Leuven, Belgium

revealed no change in the number or surface area of endometriosis lesions during the first two trimesters of pregnancy [86]. These results do not exclude a beneficial effect that potentially may occur during the third trimester or in the immediate postpartum period.

13.5 Prevention

There are no successful strategies to prevent endometriosis. Although a reduced incidence of endometriosis has been reported in women who engaged in aerobic activity from an early age, the possible protective effect of exercise has not been investigated thoroughly [2]. There is insufficient evidence that oral contraceptive use offers protection against the development of endometriosis. In contrast, a recent report showed an increased risk for endometriosis in a selected population of women taking oral contraception [87].

13.6 Therapy

Treatment must be individualized, taking into consideration the clinical problem in its entirety, including the impact of the disease and the effect of its treatment on quality of life [44]. Complaints may persist despite adequate medical or surgical treatment of the disease. In such circumstances, a multidisciplinary approach involving a pain clinic and counseling should be considered early in the treatment plan [44].

13.6.1 Surgical Therapy

Regardless of the clinical profile, treatment of endometriosis may be justified because endometriosis appears to progress in 30–60% of patients within a year of diagnosis and because it is not possible to predict in which patients it will progress [88]. Unfortunately, elimination of the endometriotic implants by surgical or medical treatment often provides only temporary relief. In most women with endometriosis, preservation of reproductive function is desirable. Therefore, the least invasive approach that is effective should be used. Depending on the severity of disease, diagnosis and removal of endometriosis should be performed simultaneously at the time of surgery provided preoperative consent has been obtained [44, 87, 89–91]. The goal of surgery is to excise all visible endometriotic lesions and associated adhesions and to restore normal anatomy. In most women, laparoscopy can be used. This technique decreases cost, morbidity, and the possibility of recurrence of adhesions postoperatively [89, 90]. Laparotomy should be reserved for patients with advanced-stage disease, who cannot undergo a laparoscopic procedure and for those in whom fertility conservation is not necessary [2].

13.6.1.1 Peritoneal Endometriosis

Endometriosis lesions can be removed during laparoscopy by surgical excision with scissors, bipolar coagulation, or laser methods (CO2 laser, potassium-titanyl-phosphate laser, or argon laser). Although some surgeons claim that the CO_2 laser is superior because it causes only minimal thermal damage, no evidence is available to show the superiority of one technique over another [92].

13.6.1.2 Ovarian Endometriosis

Superficial ovarian lesions can be vaporized [44]. Ovarian endometrioma should be aspirated, followed by incision and removal of the cyst wall from the ovarian cortex, to prevent recurrence [2, 44]. In a recent study, coagulation or laser vaporization of endometriomas without excision of the pseudocapsule was associated with a significantly increased risk of cyst recurrence [93]. In addition, laparoscopic cystectomy for ovarian endometriomas greater than 4 cm diameter improves fertility compared with drainage and coagulation [44, 94]. Therefore, based on the current evidence, ovarian cystectomy appears to be the method of choice.

13.6.1.3 Adhesiolysis

The removal of endometriosis-related adhesions should be performed. Routine use of pharmacologic or liquid agents to prevent postoperative adhesions after fertility surgery cannot be recommended based on the evidence from randomized controlled trials [95].

13.6.1.4 Deep Rectovaginal Endometriosis

The surgical excision of deep rectovaginal and rectosigmoidal endometriosis is difficult and can be associated with major complications. Postoperative bowel perforations with peritonitis have been reported in 2–3% of cases [96].

Preoperative investigations, including gynecologic ultrasonography, intravenous pyelography, and colon contrast radiography, are essential, and MRI may be useful in specific cases. Preoperative laxatives, starch-free diet, and full bowel preparation are needed to allow perioperative bowel suturing, if needed. To allow complete excision of rectovaginal endometriosis, it is often necessary to perform discoid excision, bowel wall resection, and partial resection of the posterior vaginal fornix, and resection reanastomosis may be needed in selected cases. In the case of sigmoid bowel endometriosis, segmental resection anastomosis is ofen needed and can be performed by laparotomy, laparoscopy with intracorporeal suturing, or by laparoscopically assisted vaginal techniques [2, 96, 97].

Ureter stents may be required before excision of peritoneal endometriosis surrounding the ureter [2]. A multidisciplinary approach involving gynecologic and gastroenterologic surgeons and urologists is desirable. Radical procedures such as bilateral salpingo-oophorectomy (BSO) or total hysterectomy are indicated only in severe situations and can be performed either laparoscopically or by laparotomy. If a hysterectomy is performed, bilateral salpingo-oophorectomy should be considered as well [44, 98], and all visible endometriotic tissue should be removed at the same time [99].

13.7 Preoperative and Postoperative Hormonal Treatment

Hormonal therapy before surgery improves endometriosis scores, but there is insufficient evidence that it has any effect on pain relief after the operation [100]. In addition, a recent randomized study comparing 3 months of preoperative treatment with GnRH and no treatment in 75 women with moderate to severe endometriosis failed to show a significant difference in ease of surgery between the two groups [101].

Postoperative hormone therapy with estrogen is required after bilateral oophorectomy, but should be withheld until 3 months after surgery, as there is a negligible risk for renewed growth of residual endometriosis [102]. The addition of progestins to this regimen protects the endometrium. According to a recent Cochrane review and the ESHRE Guidelines [44, 100], compared with surgery alone or surgery plus placebo, postoperative hormonal treatment does not reduce pain recurrence at 12 or 24 months and has no effect on disease recurrence. Postoperative use of the levonorgestrel intrauterine device reduces the recurrence of painful periods in women who have had surgery for endometriosis, but there is a need for further well-designed RCTs of this approach [103].

13.8 Results of Surgical Treatment

13.8.1 Pain

Although several reports have reported pain relief with CO2-laser- laparoscopy in 60–80% of patients with very low morbidity, none was prospective or controlled [2, 104–106]. In patients with pain, the endometriosis stage was not related to pain symptoms in several studies [107]. However, more recent studies reported a positive correlation between endometriosis stage and endometriosis-related dysmenorrhea or chronic pelvic pain [108]. According to the current ESHRE guidelines, ablation of endometriotic lesions and laparoscopic uterine nerve ablation (LUNA) done at the same time in minimal–moderate disease reduces endometriosis-associated pain at 6 months compared to diagnostic laparoscopy. The smallest effect of the procedure is seen in patients with minimal disease [44]. There is no evidence that laparoscopic uterine nerve ablation is a necessary part of the treatment, because LUNA by itself has no effect on dysmenorrhea associated with endometriosis [44].

13.8.2 Subfertility

Ablation of the endometriotic lesions plus adhesiolysis to improve fertility in minimal and mild endometriosis is effective compared to diagnostic laparoscopy alone according to the ESHRE recommendations [44].

A large retrospective multicenter analysis [109] reported cumulative pregnancy rates of 39, 31, 30, and 25% in patients with endometriosis stages I, II, III, and IV, respectively, 12 months after surgical treatment. Other studies have reported a significant negative correlation between endometriosis stage and pregnancy rate and decreased pregnancy rates when the revised scores exceeded 70 [110].

Surgical management of infertile women with minimal to mild endometriosis is controversial. The cumulative pregnancy rate after 5 years without therapy has been reported to be as high as 90% in women with minimal or mild endometriosis. This is comparable to the 93% rate reported in women who do not have endometriosis [111]. Two randomized controlled studies have evaluated the effect of surgical treatment of endometriosis on fertility parameters [2, 62, 63]. Taking into account the larger patient population in the Canadian multicenter study, surgical treatment of minimal to mild endometriosis appears to offer a small but significant benefit with regard to fertility outcome [44, 62].

13.8.2.1 Preoperative and Postoperative Medical Therapy

There are no data to indicate hormonal treatment prior to surgery to improve the success of surgery [44]. Postoperative medical treatment is seldomly applied because it does not work based on randomized trials, because it prevents pregnancy, and because the highest pregnancy rates occur during the first 6 to 12 months after conservative surgery [112, 113]. Following the ESHRE guideline, medical treatment with danazol or a GnRH agonist after surgery does not improve fertility compared with expectant management [44].

However, treatment with danazol or a GnRH agonist for 6 months after surgery reduces endometriosis-associated pain and delays recurrence at 12 and 24 months compared with placebo and expectant management, whereas treatment with combined oral contraceptives does not seem to be effective [44].

13.9 Medical Treatment

Medical treatment, as a general rule, is contraindicated in women desiring to become pregnant.

13.9.1 Empirical Therapy

Empirical therapy for pain presumed to be due to endometriosis in the absence of a definitive diagnosis may include counseling, analgesia, nutritional therapy, progestins, or combined oral contraceptives. If the patient desires a treatment for pain symptoms suggestive of endometriosis in the absence of a definitive diagnosis, a therapeutic trial of a hormonal medication to reduce menstrual flow is appropriate [2, 44].

13.9.2 Hormonal Medical Therapy

Because estrogen is known to stimulate the growth of endometriosis, hormonal therapy has been designed to suppress estrogen synthesis, thereby inducing atrophy of ectopic endometrial implants or interrupting the cycle of stimulation and bleeding.

Implants of endometriosis react to gonadal steroid hormones in a manner similar but not identical to eutopic endometrium. There is strong evidence that suppression of ovarian function for 6 months reduces pain associated with endometriosis [44]. Combined oral contraceptives, danazol, gestrinone, medroxyprogesterone acetate, and GnRH agonists are all equally effective, but their side-effect and cost profiles differ [44, 114–117]. A new generation of aromatase inhibitors, estrogen receptor modulators, and progesterone antagonists may offer new hormonal treatment options in the future [2].

13.9.2.1 Oral Contraceptives

The treatment of endometriosis with continuous low-dose monophasic combination contraceptives (one pill per day for 6 to 12 months) for induction of a pseudopregnancy state with combination oral contraceptive pils has been shown to be effective in reducing dysmenorrhea and pelvic pain [44, 88]. In addition, the subsequent amenorrhea induced by oral contraceptives could potentially reduce the amount of retrograde menstruation, decreasing the risk for disease progression. On the basis of a recently published data, there is no difference in outcomes between the oral contraceptive pill (OCP) and GnRH analog in treating endometriosis-associated pain [118]. Unfortunately, endometrial implants survive during induced atrophy and are reactivated after termination of treatment, in most patients. Oral contraceptives are less costly than other treatments and may be helpful in the short-term management of endometriosis with potential long-term benefits in some women [2].

There is no convincing evidence that cyclic use of combination oral contraceptives provides prophylaxis against either the development or recurrence of endometriosis [2, 118].

13.9.2.2 Progestins

Progestins may can be considered as the first choice for the treatment of endometriosis because they are as effective as danazol or GnRH analogs and have a lower cost and a lower incidence of side effects than these agents [117, 119]. They exert an antiendometriotic effect by causing initial decidualization of endometrial tissue followed by atrophy.

There is no evidence that any single agent or any particular dose is preferable to another [117].

Medroxyprogesterone acetate (MPA) (150 mg) administered intramuscularly every 3 months is also effective for the treatment of pain associated with endometriosis, but it is not indicated in infertile women because it induces profound amenorrhea and anovulation [119]. However, a recent randomized placebo-controlled study reported a significant reduction in stages and scores of endometriosis in both the placebo group and the group treated with MPA, 50 mg/day, at laparoscopy within 3 months after cessation of therapy [2, 120]. These findings raise questions about the need for medical therapy.

13.9.2.3 Intrauterine Progesterone Treatment

Local progesterone treatment of endometriosis-associated dysmenorrhea with a levonorgestrel-releasing intrauterine system (LNR-IUS) for 12 months has resulted in a significant reduction in dysmenorrhea, pelvic pain, and dyspareunia. In addition, a high degree of patient satisfaction and a significant reduction in the volume of rectovaginal endometriotic nodules was found [120, 152].

13.9.2.4 Gestrinone

Gestrinone is a 19-nortestosterone derivative with androgenic, antiprogestagenic, antiestrogenic, and antigonadotropic effect. Gestrinone causes cellular inactivation and degeneration of endometriotic implants but not their disappearance [2, 121]. Amenorrhea occurs in 50–100% of women and is dose dependent.

The clinical side effects of gestrinone are dose dependent and similar to but less intense than those caused by danazol. They include nausea, muscle cramps, and androgenic effects such as weight gain, acne, seborrhea, and oily hair and skin [121]. In a multicenter, randomized, double-blind study, gestrinone was as effective as GnRH for the treatment of pelvic pain associated with endometriosis [122]. Pregnancy is contraindicated while taking gestrinone because of the risk for masculinization of the fetus.

13.9.2.5 Danazol

Recognized pharmacologic properties of danazol include suppression of GnRH or gonadotropin secretion, direct inhibition of steroidogenesis, increased metabolic clearance of estradiol and progesterone, direct antagonistic and agonistic interaction with endometrial androgen and progesterone receptors, and immunologic attenuation of potentially adverse reproductive effects [2, 123]. A practical strategy for the use of danazol is to start treatment with 400 mg daily (200 mg twice a day) and increase the dose, if necessary, to achieve amenorrhea and relieve symptoms [2].

The significant adverse side effects of danazol are related to its androgenic and hypoestrogenic properties. Deepening of the voice is another potential side effect that is nonreversible. The use of danazol is contraindicated in pregnancy because of its androgenic effects on the fetus. Because the many side effects of oral danazol limit its use, alternative routes (e.g., vaginal danazol ring) of administration have been studied. This treatment did not cause the classic danazol side effects and may allow ovulation and conception [2, 124].

13.9.2.6 Gonadotropin-Releasing Hormone Agonists

Gonadotropin-releasing hormone agonists bind to pituitary GnRH receptors and stimulate LH and FSH synthesis and release. However, the agonists have a much longer biologic half-life (3–8 h) than endogenous GnRH (3.5 min), resulting in the continuous exposure of GnRH receptors to GnRH agonist activity [2]. This exposure causes a loss of pituitary receptors and downregulation of GnRH activity, resulting in low FSH and LH levels. Thus, ovarian steroid production is suppressed, providing a medically induced and reversible state of pseudomenopause. A direct effect of GnRH agonists on ectopic endometrium is also possible because expression of the GnRH receptor gene has been documented in ectopic endometrium [125].

Several GnRH agonists are available including leuprolide, buserelin, nafarelin, histrelin, goserelin, deslorelin, and tritorelin. These drugs are inactive orally and must be administered intramuscularly, subcutaneously, or by intranasal absorption. The best therapeutic effect is often associated with an estradiol dose of 20–40 pg/mL. These depot formulations are beneficial because of the reduced frequency of administration and because nasal administration can be complicated by variations in absorption rates and problems with patient compliance [126]. Their side effects are caused by hypoestrogenism and include hot flashes, vaginal dryness, reduced libido, and osteoporosis. Reversibility of bone loss is equivocal and, therefore, of concern [2, 126], especially because treatment periods of longer than 6 months may be required. The goal is to suppress endometriosis and maintain serum estrogen levels of 30–45 pg/mL.

The dose of daily GnRH agonist can be regulated by monitoring estradiol levels, by the addition of low-dose progestin or estrogen-progestin in an add-back regimen, or by draw-back therapy. The goal of add-back therapy is to treat endometriosis and endometriosis-associated pain effectively while preventing vasomotor symptoms and bone loss related to the hypoestrogenic state induced by GnRH analogs.

According to ESHRE guidelines treatment for 3 months with a GnRH agonist may be as effective as 6 months in terms of pain relief. Treatment for up to 2 years with combined estrogen progestagen "add-back" appears to be effective and safe in terms of pain relief and bonedensity protection [44]. Add-back therapy can be achieved by administering progestins only, including norethisterone, 1.2 mg, and norethindrone acetate, 5 mg and also with tibolone, 2.5 mg/day or by an estrogen-progestin combination [2, 127, 128]. However, in one report, bone mineral density reduction occurred during long-term GnRH agonist use and was not fully recovered up to 6 years after treatment [2, 129]. Use of add-back therapy (2 mg estradiol and 1 mg norethisterone acetate) did not affect this process [129]. Therefore, GnRH agonists should not be prescribed to girls who have not yet attained their maximal bone density [151].

Draw-back therapy has been suggested as an alternative in a study showing that 6 months of intake of 400 μg/day of nafarelin was as effective as a draw-back regimen consisting of 1 month of intake of 400 μg/day of nafarelin followed by 5 months of 200 μg/day of nafarelin, with similar estradiol levels (30 pg/mL) but less loss of bone mineral density [2, 130].

13.9.3 Aromatase Inhibitors

Aromatase inhibitors like anastrozole and letrozole combined with an ovarian suppressant represent promising and novel treatments of postmenopusal and premenopausal endometriosis [2, 131]. The requirement for calcium, vitamin D, or bisphosphonate supplementation in premenopausal women needs further evaluation.

13.9.4 Nonhormonal Medical Therapy

13.9.4.1 Dysmenorrhea

Women suffering from dysmenorrhea are treated with analgetics. In a recent systematic Cochrane review evaluating the use of nonsteroidal anti-inflammatory drugs (NSAIDs) for primary dysmenorrhea, it was concluded that NSAIDs, except niflumic acid, were more effective than placebo for pain relief [132], but there was insufficient evidence to suggest whether any individual NSAID was more effective than another.

13.9.4.2 Pelvic Pain

Considering that endometriosis is a chronic inflammatory disease, anti-inflammatory drugs would appear to be effective for treatment. Nonsteroidal anti-inflammatory drugs may be effective in reducing endometriosis associated pain [2, 44]; however, they have significant side effects, including gastric ulceration and possible inhibition of ovulation. Women who wish to become pregnant should not take NSAIDs at the time of ovulation, because inhibition of prostaglandins may inhibit follicular rupture at ovulation [133].

13.9.4.3 Evolving Drugs

Progesterone antagonists and progesterone receptor modulators may suppress endometriosis based on their antiproliferative effects on the endometrium, without the risk for hypoestrogenism or bone loss that occurs with GnRH treatment. [2, 134]. In animal models, raloxifene therapy resulted in regression of endometriosis [135]. A recent prospective randomized placebo- and drug-controlled study in baboons showed that recombinant human TNF-a-binding protein effectively inhibits the development of endometriosis and endometriosis-related adhesions and is effective in the treatment of spontaneous endometriosis in baboons [136].

In humans, a randomized placebo-controlled trial of oral pentoxifylline, 800 mg/day for 12 months, reported after life-table analysis a similar overall pregnancy rate in treated patients (31%) and in controls (18.5%) [2, 137].

Immunomodulatory drugs inhibiting pelvic inflammation, angiogenesis or metalloproteinase activity associated with endometriosis may offer new approaches to medical treatment in the future.

13.9.5 Efficacy of Medical Treatment

Medical treatment with progestins, danazol, gestrinone, or GnRH agonists is effective in treating pain associated with endometriosis, as shown in several prospective, randomized, placebo-controlled double-blind studies [44, 138, 139]. Disadvantages of medical therapy over surgical therapy include the high cost of hormone preparations, the high prevalence of side effects, and the higher recurrence rate of endometriosis [2, 100, 139].

Conception is either impossible or contraindicated during medical treatment of endometriosis. There is no evidence that medical treatment of minimal to mild endometriosis leads to better chances of pregnancy than expectant management [44, 100].

13.10 Adolescent Endometriosis

The incidental finding of minimal to mild endometriosis in a young woman without immediate interest in pregnancy is a common clinical problem. Seventy percent of girls with chronic pelvic pain unresponsive to oral contraceptives or NSAIDs are affected by endometriosis [2, 140]. Mild disease can be treated by surgical removal of implants at the time of diagnosis, followed by continuous administration of low-dose combination oral contraceptives to prevent recurrence. More advanced disease can be treated medically for 6 months, followed by continuous oral contraceptives to prevent progression of disease [140].

13.11 Recurrence

Endometriosis tends to recur unless definitive surgery is performed. The recurrence rate is about 5–20% per year, reaching a cumulative rate of 40% after 5 years. In women treated with GnRH agonists or danazol for endometriosis associated with pelvic pain, the recurrence rates of endometriosis were similar, and associated pain symptoms usually returned after cessation of therapy [2, 141].

The rate of recurrence increases with the stage of disease, the duration of follow-up, and the occurrence of previous surgery [141, 142]. The likelihood of recurrence appears to be lower when endometriosis is located only on the right side of the pelvis than when the left side is involved [143].

13.12 Assisted Reproduction for Treatment of Endometriosis

The treatment of endometriosis-related infertility with an assisted reproduction technique is dependent on the age of the woman, the duration of infertility, the stage of endometriosis, the involvement of ovaries, tubes, or both in the endometriosis process, previous therapy, associated pain symptoms, and the priorities of the patient, taking into account her attitude toward the disease, the cost of treatment, her financial means, and the expected results [2].

13.12.1 Intrauterine Insemination

Minimal-mild endometriosis-associated infertility can be successfully treated with intrauterine insemination, proven positive outcomes were reported only in combination with superovulation therapy (SO/IUI) [44, 153].

13.12.2 In Vitro Fertilization (IVF)

According to ESHRE guidelines, IVF is an appropriate treatment especially if tubal function is compromised, if there is also male factor infertility, and/or other treatments have failed [44]. However, based on several retrospective studies [144–146], investigators have suggested that the pregnancy rate after IVF may be lower in women with endometriosis than in women without the disease. According to a recently published meta-analysis [147], IVF pregnancy rates are lower in patients with endometriosis than in those with tubal infertility [44]. This can probably be explained by reduced egg/embryo quality, since uterine implantation appears to be normal in women with endometriosis stage III or IV treated with donor egg IVF[146]. Current evidence also suggests that patients with endometriosis have a poorer ovarian response and need a higher dose of gonadotropin therapy in IVF or ICSI programs, but endometrial implantation is not reduced. Prolonged treatment with a GnRH agonist before IVF should be considered in women with moderate–severe endometriosis and discussed with patients because this therapy may result in improved pregnancy rates [44].

13.12.3 Intracytoplasmic Sperm Injection (ICSI)

A recent study in patients undergoing intracytoplasmic sperm injection (ICSI) reported a reduced number of oocytes recovered after ovarian aspiration but a normal fertilization rate, implantation rate, and pregnancy rate in women with endometriosis when compared with controls [148].

13.12.4 Gamete Intrafallopian Transfer

Gamete intrafallopian transfer has been reported to result in a higher pregnancy rate (25%) than IVF (14%). This difference may be related to selection bias, because women with less severe forms of endometriosis are more likely to be treated with gamete intrafallopian transfer than with IVF [149].

13.13 Coping with Disease

Evidence from two systematic reviews suggests that high frequency transcutaneous electrical nerve stimulation (TENS), acupuncture, vitamin B, and magnesium may help to relieve dysmenorrhea [44, 150]. Whether such treatments are effective in endometriosis-associated dysmenorrhea is unknown. Many women with endometriosis report that nutritional and complementary therapies such as reflexology, traditional Chinese medicine, herbal treatments, and homeopathy improve pain symptoms [2]. Furthermore, patient self-help groups can provide invaluable counseling, support, and advice.

13.14 Summary-Treatment/Evaluation Algorithm

Endometriosis should be suspected in women with dysmenorrhea, dyspareunia, chronic pelvic pain, or subfertility. Endometriosis may be also asymptomatic and should be perceived as a chronic disease.

Risk factors:

- Affected first degree relatives
- Short cycle length, heavier menstruation, and longer flow duration
- Height and weight are positively and negatively associated

Clinical signs:

- Signs of endometriosis on vulva, vagina, and cervix
- Uterosacral or cul-de-sac nodularity, lateral or cervical displacement, painful swelling of the recto-vaginal septum, unilateral ovarian enlargement
- Uterus in fixed retroversion, mobility reduced of the ovaries and fallopian tubes-in more advanced cases

Extrapelvic endometriosis:

- Colorectal involvement – abdominal and back pain, abdominal distention, cyclic rectal bleeding, constipation, obstruction
- Ureteral and/or bladder– obstruction resulting in cyclic pain, dysuria, and hematuria
- Pulmonary – pneumothorax, hemothorax, or hemoptysis during menses
- Umbilical – palpable mass and cyclic pain in the umbilical area

Diagnosis: visual inspection of the pelvis during laparoscopy, ideally with histological confirmation.

Imaging techniques:

- Gynecologic transvaginal or transrectal ultrasonography, MRI
- Intravenous pyelography and colon contrast radiography if needed

Treatment: must be individualized, taking the clinical problem in its entirety into account, including the impact of the disease and the effect of its treatment on quality of life.

Endometriosis-associated pain:

- Systems currently available for the classification of endometriosis are subjective and correlate poorly with pain symptoms.
- Pain symptoms suggestive of the disease can be treated without a definitive diagnosis using a therapeutic trial of a hormonal drug to reduce menstrual flow.
- Suppression of ovarian function for 6 months reduces pain. Hormonal drugs are equally effective.
- Ablation of endometriotic lesions reduces pain and the smallest effect is seen in patients with minimal(stage I) disease.
- There is no evidence that LUNA is a necessary component of treatment.
- In cases of ovarian endometrioma (>3 cm in diameter), and in deeply infiltrating disease, histology should be obtained to identify endometriosis and to exclude rare instances of malignancy.
- Severe or deeply infiltrating endometriosis should be managed in a facility with the necessary expertise to provide treatment in a multidisciplinary context, including advanced laparoscopic surgery and laparotomy.

Endometriosis-associated infertility:

- Ablation of endometriotic lesions plus adhesiolysis in minimal-to-mild endometriosis is more effective than diagnostic laparoscopy alone in improving fertility. Suppression of ovarian function is not effective in improving fertility.
- In women with stage I/II endometriosis-associated infertility, expectant management or SO/IUI after laparoscopy can be considered for younger patients. Women 35 years of age or older should be treated with SO/IUI or IVF-ET.
- IVF pregnancy rates are lower in women with endometriosis than in those with tubal infertility.
- There is insufficient evidence available to determine whether surgical excision of moderate–severe endometriosis enhances pregnancy rates.
- For women with stage III/IV endometriosis who fail to conceive following conservative surgery or because of advancing reproductive age, IVF-ET is an effective alternative.

For updated ESHRE guidlines see http://www.endometriosis.org/guidelines.html

References

1. Sampson JA (1927) Peritoneal endometriosis due to menstrual dissemination of endometrial tissue into the pelvic cavity. Am J Obstet Gynecol 14:422–469
2. D'Hooghe TM, Hill JA (2006) Chapter 29. Endometriosis. In: Williams and Wilkins, Berek JS (eds) Novak's gynecology, 14th edn. Philadelphia, USA, pp 1137–1184
3. Halme J, Becker S, Hammond MG et al (1984) Retrograde menstruation in healthy women and in patients with endometriosis. Obstet Gynecol 64:151–154
4. Liu DTY, Hitchcock A (1986) Endometriosis: its association with retrograde menstruation, dysmenorrhoea and tubal pathology. BJOG 93:859–862
5. Koninckx PR, De Moor P, Brosens IA (1980) Diagnosis of the luteinized unruptured follicle syndrome by steroid hormone assays in peritoneal fluid. BJOG 87:929–934

6. Kruitwagen RFPM, Poels LG, Willemsen WNP et al (1991) Endometrial epithelial cells in peritoneal fluid during the early follicular phase. Fertil Steril 55:297–303
7. D'Hooghe TM, Bambra CS, Isahakia M et al (1995) Intrapelvic injection of menstrual endometrium causes endometriosis in baboons (Papio cynocephalus, Papio anubis). Am J Obstet Gynecol 173:125–134
8. Olive DL, Henderson DY (1987) Endometriosis and müllerian anomalies. Obstet Gynecol 69:412–415
9. Pinsonneault O, Goldstein DP (1985) Obstructing malformations of the uterus and vagina. Fertil Steril 44:241–247
10. D'Hooghe TM, Bambra CS, Suleman MA et al (1994) Development of a model of retrograde menstruation in baboons (Papio anubis). Fertil Steril 62:635–638
11. Dinulescu DM, Ince TA, Quade BJ et al (2005) Role of K-ras and Vten in the development of mouse models of endometriosis and endometrioid ovarian cancer. Nat Med 11:63–70
12. Levander G, Normann P (1955) The pathogenesis of endometriosis: an experimentál study. Acta Obstet Gynecol Scand 34:366–398
13. Merrill JA (1966) Endometrial induction of endometriosis across millipore filters. Am J Obstet Gynecol 94:780–789
14. Kennedy SH (2004) Genetics of endometriosis. In: Tulandi T, Redwine D (eds) Endometriosis: advances and controversies. Marcel Dekker Publishing, New York, NY, pp 55–68
15. Simpson JL, Elias S, Malinak LR et al (1980) Heritable aspects of endometriosis. I. Genetics studies. Am J Obstet Gynecol 137:327–331
16. Moen MH, Magnus P (1993) The familial risk of endometriosis. Acta Obstet Gynecol Scand 72:560–564
17. Shin JC, Ross HL, Elias S et al (1997) Detection of chromosomal aneuploidy in endometriosis by multicolor in situ hybridization. Hum Genet 100:401–406
18. Kosugi Y, Elias S, Malinak LR et al (1999) Increased heterogeneity of chromosome 17 aneuploidy in endometriosis. Am J Obstet Gynecol 180:792–797
19. Gogusev J, Bouquet de Joliniere J, Telvi L et al (1999) Detection of DNA copy number changes in human endometriosis by comparative genomic hybridisation. Hum Genet 105:444–451
20. Falconer H, D'Hooghe T, Fried G (2007) Endometriosis and genetic polymorphisms. Obstet Gynecol Surv 62(9):616–628
21. D'Hooghe TM, Hill JA (1996) Immunobiology of endometriosis. In: Bronston R, Anderson DJ (eds) Immunology of reproduction. Blackwell Scientific, Cambridge, MA, pp 322–356
22. Dmowski WP, Steele RN, Baker GF (1981) Deficient cellular immunity in endometriosis. Am J Obstet Gynecol 141:377–383
23. Oosterlynck D, Cornillie FJ, Waer M et al (1991) Women with endometriosis show a defect in natural killer cell activity resulting in a decreased cytotoxicity to autologous endometrium. Fertil Steril 56:45–51
24. D'Hooghe TM, Scheerlinck JP, Koninckx PR et al (1995) Anti-endometrial lymphocytotoxicity and natural killer activity in baboons with endometriosis. Hum Repród 10:558–562
25. Hill JA (1992) Immunology and endometriosis. Fertil Steril 58:262–264
26. Zeller JM, Henig I, Radwanska E et al (1987) Enhancement of humán monocyte and peritoneal macrophage chemiluminescence activities in women with endometriosis. Am J Reprod Immunol Microbiol 13:78–82
27. Halme J, Becker S, Haskill S (1987) Altered maturation and function of peritoneal macrophages: possible role in pathogenesis of endometriosis. Am J Obstet Gynecol 156:783–789
28. D'Hooghe TM, Nugent N, Cuneo S, et al (2001) Recombinant human TNF binding protein (r-hTBP-1) inhibits the development of endometriosis in baboons: a prospective, randomized, placebo- and drug-controlled study. Paper presented at Annual Meeting of the American Society for Reproductive Medicine, Orlando, Florida, 22–24 Oct 2001
29. Hill JA, Cohen J, Anderson DJ (1989) The effects of lymphokines and monokines on human sperm fertilizing ability in the zona-free hamster egg penetration test. Am J Obstet Gynecol 160:1154–1159
30. Zhang R, Wild RA, Ojago JM (1993) Effect of tumor necrosis factor-alpha on adhesion of human endometrial stromal cells to peritoneal mesothelial cells: an in vitro system. Fertil Steril 59:1196–1201
31. Halme J, White C, Kauma S et al (1988) Peritoneal macrophages from patients with endometriosis release growth factor activity in vitro. J Clin Endocrinol Metab 66:1044–1049
32. Kauma S, Clark MR, White C et al (1988) Production of fibronectin by peritoneal macrophages and concen-tration of fibronectin in peritoneal fluid from patients with or without endometriosis. Obstet Gynecol 72:13–18
33. Sharpe-Timms KL, Keisler LW, Mclntush EW et al (1998) Tissue inhibitor of metailoproteinase-1 concentra-tions are attenuated in peritoneal fluid and sera of women with endometriosis and restored in sera by gonadotropin-releasing hormone agonist therapy. Fertil Steril 69:1128–1134
34. Kokorine I, Nisolle M, Donnez J et al (1997) Expression of interstitial collagenase (MMP-1) is related to the activity of human endometriotic lesions. Fertil Steril 68:246–251
35. Bulun SE, Yang S, Fang Z, Gurates B, Tamura M, Sebastian S (2002) Estrogen production and metabolism in endometriosis. Ann N Y Acad Sci 955:75–85; discussion 86–88, 396–406
36. Bulun SE, Zeitoun K, Takayama K et al (2000) Molecular basis for treating endometriosis with aromatase inhibitors. Hum Reprod Update 6:413–418
37. Agic A, Xu H, Finas D et al (2006) Is endometriosis associated with systemic subclinical inflammation? Gynecol Obstet Invest 62(3):139–147
38. Guo SW (2004) The link between exposure to dioxin and endometriosis: a critical reappraisal of primate data. Gynecol Obstet Invest 57:157–173
39. D'Hooghe TM, Debrock S (2003) Future directions in endometriosis research. Obstet Gynecol Clin North Am 30:221–244
40. Giudice LC, Kao LC (2004) Endometriosis. Lancet 364(9447):1789–1799
41. Koninckx PR, Meuleman C, Demeyere S et al (1991) Suggestive evidence that pelvic endometriosis is a progressive disease, whereas deeply infiltrating endometriosis is associated with pelvic pain. Fertil Steril 55:759–765
42. Mahmood TA, Templeton A (1991) Prevalence and genesis of endometriosis. Hum Reprod 6:544–549
43. Moen MH (1987) Endometriosis in women at interval sterilization. Acta Obstet Gynecol Scand 66:451–454
44. Kennedy S, Bergqvist A, Chapron C, on behalf of the ESHRE Special Interest Group for Endometriosis and Endometrium Guideline Development Group et al (2005) ESHRE guideline for the diagnosis and treatment of endometriosis. Hum Reprod 20(10):2698–2704
45. Arumugam K, Lim JMH (1997) Menstrual characteristics associated with endometriosis. BJOG 104:948–950
46. Vercellini P, De Giorgi O, Aimi G et al (1997) Menstrual characteristics in women with and without endometriosis. Obstet Gynecol 90:264–268
47. Matalliotakis IM, Cakmak H, Fragouli YG, Goumenou AG, Mahutte NG, Arici A (2008) Epidemiological characteristics in women with and without endometriosis in the Yale series. Arch Gynecol Obstet 277(5):389–393
48. Filer RB, Wu CH (1989) Coitus during menses. Its effect on endometriosis and pelvic inflammatory disease. J Reprod Med 34(11):887–890

49. Mathias JR, Franklin R, Quast DC et al (1998) Relation of endometriosis and neuromuscular disease of the gastrointestinal tract: new insights. Fertil Steril 70:81–88
50. Hadfield RM, Mardon H, Barlow D et al (1996) Delay in the diagnosis of endometriosis: a survey of women from the USA and the UK. Hum Reprod 11:878–880
51. Dmowski WP, Lesniewicz R, Rana N et al (1997) Changing trends in the diagnosis of endometriosis: a comparative study of women with endometriosis presenting with chronic pain or infertility. Fertil Steril 67:238–243
52. Chapron C, Fauconnier A, Dubuisson JB et al (2003) Deep infiltrating endometriosis: relation between severity of dysmenorrhoea and extent of disease. Hum Reprod 18:760–766
53. Barlow DH, Glynn CJ (1993) Endometriosis and pelvic pain. Baillieres Clin Obstet Gynaecol 7:775–790
54. Anaf V, Simon Ph, El Nakadi I et al (2000) Relationship between endometriotic foci and nerves in rectovaginal endometriotic nodules. Hum Reprod 15:1744–1750
55. D'Hooghe TM, Debrock S, Hill JA et al (2003) Endometriosis and subfertility: is the relationship resolved? Sem Reprod Med 21:243–254
56. Practice Committee of American Society for Reproductive Medicine. Treatment of pelvic pain associated with endometriosis. (2008) Fertil Steril. Nov;90(5 Suppl):S260–S269. Review
57. American Fertility Society (1985) Revised American Fertility Society classification of endometriosis. Fertil Steril 43:351–352
58. Haney AF (1993) Endometriosis-associated infertility. Baillieres Clin Obstet Gynaecol 7:791–812
59. D'Hooghe TM, Bambra CS, Raeymaekers BM et al (1996) Serial laparoscopies over 30 months show that endometriosis is a progressive disease in captive baboons (Papio anubis, Papio cynocephalus). Fertil Steril 65:645–649
60. Vercammen E, D'Hooghe TM, Hill JA (2000) Endometriosis and recurrent miscarriage. Semin Reprod Med 18:363–368
61. Cahill DJ, Hull MGR (2000) Pituitary-ovarian dysfunction and endometriosis. Hum Reprod Update 6:56–66
62. Marcoux S, Maheux R, Bérubé S (1997) The Canadian Collaborative Group on Endometriosis. Laparoscopic surgery in infertile women with minimal or mild endometriosis. N Engl J Med 337:217–222
63. Gruppo Italiano per lo Studio deli' Endometriosi (1999) Ablation of lesions or no treatment in minimal-mild endometriosis in infertile women: a randomized trial. Hum Reprod 14:1332–1334
64. Propst AM, Storti K, Barbieri RL (1998) Lateral cervical displacement is associated with endometriosis. Fertil Steril 70:568–570
65. Koninckx PR, Oosterlynck D, D'Hooghe TM et al (1994) Deeply infiltrating endometriosis is a disease whereas mild endometriosis could be considered a non-disease. Ann N Y Acad Sci 734:333–341
66. Koninckx PR, Meuleman C, Oosterlynck D et al (1996) Diagnosis of deep endometriosis by clinical examina-tion during menstruation and plasma CA 125 concentration. Fertil Steril 65:280–287
67. Rock JA, Markham SM (1987) Extra pelvic endometriosis. In: Wilson EA (ed) Endometriosis. AR liss, New York, NY, pp 185–206
68. Guerriero S, Paoletti AM, Mais V et al (1996) Transvaginal ultrasonography combined with CA125 plasma levels in the diagnosis of endometrioma. Fertil Steril 65:293–298
69. Fedele L, Bianchi S, Portuese A et al (1998) Transrectal ultrasonography in the assessment of rectovaginal endometriosis. Obstet Gynecol 91:444–448
70. Moore J, Copley S, Morris J et al (2002) A systematic review of the accuracy of ultrasound in the diagnosis of endometriosis. Ultrasound Obstet Gynecol 20:630–634
71. McBean JH, Gibson M, Brumsted JR (1996) The association of intrauterine filling defects on HSG with endometriosis. Fertil Steril 66:522–526
72. Bast RC, Klug TL, St. John E et al (1983) A radio-immunoassay using a monoclonal antibody to monitor the course of epithelial ovarian cancer. N Engl J Med 309:883–887
73. Pittaway DE, Fayez JA (1986) The use of CA125 in the diagnosis and management of endometriosis. Fertil Steril 46:790–795
74. Pittaway DE, Fayez JA (1987) Serum CA125 levels increase during menses. Am J Obstet Gynecol 156:75–76
75. Moloney MD, Thornton JG, Cooper EH (1989) Serum CA125 antigen levels and disease severity in patients with endometriosis. Obstet Gynecol 73:767–769
76. O'Shaughnessy A, Check JH, Nowroozi K et al (1993) CA125 levels measured in different phases of the menstrual cycle in screening for endometriosis. Obstet Gynecol 81:99–103
77. Pittaway DE (1990) The use of serial CA125 concentrations to monitor endometriosis in infertile women. Am J Obstet Gynecol 163:1032–1037
78. Nisolle M, Paindaveine B, Bourdin A et al (1990) Histological study of peritoneal endometriosis in infertile women. Fertil Steril 53:984–988
79. Moen MH, Halvorsen TB (1992) Histologic confirmation of endometriosis in different peritoneal lesions. Acta Obstet Gynecol Scand 71:337–342
80. Vercellini P, Aimi G, Panazza S et al (2000) Deep endometriosis conundrum: evidence in favor of a peritoneal origin. Fertil Steril 73:1043–1046
81. Redwine DB (1999) Ovarian endometriosis: a marker for more extensive pelvic and intestinal disease. Fertil Steril 72:310–315
82. Walter AJ, Hentz JG, Magtibay PM et al (2001) Endometriosis: correlation between histologic and visual findings at laparoscopy. Am J Obstet Gynecol 184:1407–1413
83. Czernobilsky B (1987) Endometriosis. In: Fox H (ed) Obstetrical and gynecological pathology. Churchill Livingstone, New York, NY, pp 763–777
84. Donnez J, Nisolle M, Casanas-Roux F (1992) Three-dimensional architectures of peritoneal endometriosis. Fertil Steril 57:980–983
85. McArthur JW, Ulfelder H (1965) The effect of pregnancy upon endometriosis. Obstet Gynecol Surv 20:709–733
86. D'Hooghe TM, Bambra CS, De Jonge I et al (1997) Pregnancy does not affect endometriosis in baboons (Papio anubis, Papio cynocephalus). Arch Gynecol Obstet 261:15–19
87. Italian Endometriosis Study Group (1999) Oral contraceptive use and risk of endometriosis. BJOG 106:695–699
88. Mahmood TA, Templeton A (1990) The impact of treatment on the natural history of endometriosis. Hum Reprod 5:965–970
89. Abbott JA, Hawe J, Clayton RD et al (2003) The effects and effectiveness of laparoscopic excision of endometriosis: a prospective study with 2–5 year follow-up. Hum Reprod 18:1922–1927
90. Chapron C, Fauconnier A, Vieira M et al (2003) Anatomical distribution of deeply infiltrating endometriosis: surgical implications and proposition for a classification. Hum Reprod 18:157–161
91. Fedele L, Bianchi S, Zanconato G et al (2004) Long-term follow-up after conservative surgery for rectovaginal endometriosis. Am J Obstet Gynecol 190:1020–1024
92. Redwine DB, Wright JT (2001) Laparoscopic treatment of complete obliteration of the cul-de-sac associated with endometriosis: long-term follow-up of en bloc resection. Fertil Steril 76:358–365
93. Tulandi T, Al Took S (1998) Reproductive outcome after treatment of mild endometriosis with laparoscopic excision and electrocoagulation. Fertil Steril 69:229–231
94. Vercellini P, Aimi G, Busacca M et al (2003) Laparoscopic uterosacral ligament resection for dysmenorrhea associated with endometriosis: results of a randomized, controlled trial. Fertil Steril 80(2):310–319
95. Chapron C, Vercellini P, Barakat H et al (2002) Management of ovarian endometriomas. Hum Reprod Update 8:6–7

96. Watson A, Vandekerckhove P, Lilford R (2000) Liquid and fluid agents for preventing adhesions after surgery for subfertility. Cochrane Database Syst Rev 3:CD001298
97. Koninckx PR, Timmermans B, Meuleman C et al (1996) Complications of CO-2 laser endoscopic excision of deep endometriosis. Hum Reprod 11:2263–2268
98. Redwine DB, Koning M, Sharpe DR (1996) Laparoscopically assisted transvaginal segmental resection of the rectosigmoid colon for endometriosis. Fertil Steril 65:193–197
99. Namnoum AB, Hickman TN, Goodman SB et al (1995) Incidence of symptom recurrence after hysterectomy for endometriosis. Fertil Steril 64:898–902
100. Lefebvre G, Allaire C, Jeffrey J et al (2002) SOGC clinical guidelines: hysterectomy. J Obstet Gynaecol Can 24:37–61
101. Yap C, Furness S, Farquhar C (2004) Pre and post operatíve medical therapy for endometriosis surgery. Cochrane Database Syst Rev 3:CD003678
102. Audebert A, Descampes P, Marret H et al (1998) Pre or post operatíve medical treatment with nafarelin in stage III–IV endometriosis: a French multicentered study. Eur J Obstet Gynecol Reprod Biol 79:145–148
103. Matorras R, Elorriaga MA, Pijoan JI et al (2002) Recurrence of endometriosis in women with bilateral adnexectomy (with or without total hysterectomy) who received hormone replacement therapy. Fertil Steril 77:303–308
104. Abou-Setta AM, Al-Inany HG, Farquhar CM (2006) Levonorgestrel-releasing intrauterine device (LNG-IUD) for symptomatic endometriosis following surgery. Cochrane Database Syst Rev 4:CD005072
105. Feste JR (1985) Laser laparoscopy: a new modality. J Reprod Med 30:413–417
106. Nezhat C, Winer W, Crowgey S et al (1989) Videolaparoscopy for the treatment of endometriosis associated with infertility. Fertil Steril 51:237–240
107. Sutton CJG, Hill D (1990) Laser laparoscopy in the treatment of endometriosis: a 5 year study. BJOG 97:181–185
108. Vercellini P, Cortesi I, Trespidi L et al (1996) Endometriosis and pelvic pain: relation to disease stage and localization. Fertil Steril 65:299–304
109. Guzick DS, Canis M, Silliman NP et al (1997) Prediction of pregnancy in infertile women based on the ASRM's revised classification for endometriosis. Fertil Steril 67:822–836
110. Attar E, Bulun SE (2006) Aromatase inhibitors: the next generation of therapeutics for endometriosis? Fertil Steril 85(5):1307–1318
111. Canis M, Pouly JL, Wattiez A et al (1992) Incidence of bilateral adnexal disease in severe endometriosis (revised American Fertility Society [AFS] stage IV): should a stage V be included in the AFS classification? Fertil Steril 57:691–692
112. Badawy SZA, El Bakry MM, Samuel D et al (1988) Cumulative pregnancy rates in infertile women with endometriosis. J Reprod Med 33:757–760
113. Vercellini P, Crosignani PG, Fadini R et al (1999) A gonadotropin-releasing hormone agonist compared with expectant management after conservative surgery for symptomatic endometriosis. BJOG 106:672–677
114. Parazzini F, Fedele L, Busacca M et al (1994) Postsurgical treatment of advanced endometriosis: results of a randomized clinical trial. Am J Obstet Gynecol 171:1205–1207
115. Kyama CM, Mihályi A, Mwenda JM et al (2005) The role of immunologic factors in the development of endometriosis: indications for treatment strategies. Therapy 4:623–639
116. Davis L, Kennedy SS, Moore J, Prentice A. (2007) Modern combined oral contraceptives for pain associated with endometriosis. Cochrane Database Syst Rev. 18;(3):CD001019
117. Prentice A, Deary AJ, Goldbeck WS, et al (2004) Gonadotrophin-releasing hormone analogues for pain associated with endometriosis. In: The Cochrane Library, Issue 3. John Wiley & Sons, Ltd, Chichester, UK
118. Prentice A, Deary AJ, Bland E (2004) Progestagens and anti-progestagens for pain associated with endometriosis. In: The Cochrane Library, Issue 3. John Wiley & Sons, Ltd, Chichester, UK
119. Davis L, Kennedy SS, Moore J, Prentice A (2007) Modern combined oral contraceptives for pain associated with endometriosis. Cochrane Database Syst Rev 18(3):CD001019
120. Harcison RF, Barry-Kinsella C (2000) Efficacy of medroxyprogesterone treatment in infertile women with endometriosis: a prospective, randomized, placebo-controlled study. Fertil Steril 74:24–30
121. Brosens IA, Verleyen A, Cornillie FJ (1987) The morphologic effect of short-term medical therapy of endometriosis. Am J Obstet Gynecol 157:1215–1221
122. Gestrinone Italian Study Group (1996) Gestrinone versus a GnRHa for the treatment of pelvic pain associated with endometriosis: a multicenter, randomized, double-blind study. Fertil Steril 66:911–919
123. Barbieri RL, Ryan KJ (1981) Danazol: endocrine pharmacology and therapeutic applications. Am J Obstet Gynecol 141:453–463
124. Igarashi M, Iizuka M, Abe Y et al (1998) Novel vaginal danazol ring therapy for pelvic endometriosis, in particular deeply infiltrating endometriosis. Hum Reprod 13:1952–1956
125. Borroni R, Di Blasio AM, Gaffuri B et al (2000) Expression of GnRH receptor gene in human ectopic endometrial cells and inhibition of their proliferation by leuprolide acetate. Mol Cell Endocrinol 159:37–43
126. Wingfíeld M, Healy DL (1993) Endometriosis: medical therapy. Baillieres Clin Obstet Gynecol 7:813–838
127. Hornstein MD, Surrey ES, Weisberg GW et al (1998) Leuprolide acetate depot and hormonal add-back in endometriosis: a 12-month study. Obstet Gynecol 91:16–24
128. Riis BJ, Christiansen C, Johansen JS et al (1990) Is it possible to prevent boné loss in young women treated with luteinizing hormone-releasing agonists? J Clin Endocrinol Metab 70:920–924
129. Pierce SJ, Gazvani MR, Farquharson RG (2000) Long-term use of gonadotropin-releasing hormoné analogs and hormone replacement therapy in the management of endometriosis: a randomized trial with a 6-year follow-up. Fertil Steril 74:964–968
130. Tahara M, Matsuoka T, Yokoi T et al (2000) Treatment of endometriosis with a decreasing dosage of gonadotropin-releasing hormoné agonist (nafarelin): a pilot study with low-dose agonist therapy ("draw-back" therapy). Fertil Steril 73:799–804
131. Stovall DW, Bowser LM, Archer DF et al (1997) Endometriosis-associated pain: evidence for an association between the stage of disease and a history of chronic pelvic pain. Fertil Steril 68:13–18
132. Marjoribanks J, Proctor ML, Farquhar C (2003) Nonsteroidal anti-inflammatory drugs for primary dysmen-orrhoea. Cochrane Database Syst Rev 4:CD001751
133. Duffy DM, Stouffer RL (2002) Follicular administration of a cyclooxygenase inhibitor can prevent oocyte release without alteration of normál luteal function in rhesus monkeys. Hum Reprod 17:2825–2831
134. Murphy AA, Zhou MH, Malkapuram S et al (2000) RU486-induced growth inhibition of human endometrial cells. Fertil Steril 74:1014–1019
135. Buelke SJ, Bryant HU, Francis PC (1998) The selective estrogen receptor modulátor, raloxifene: an overview of nonclinical pharmacology and reproductive and developmental testing. Reprod Toxicol 12:217–221
136. D'Hooghe TM, Nugent N, Cuneo S, et al (2001) Recombinant human TNF binding protein (r-hTBP-1) inhibits the development

of endometriosis in baboons: a prospective, randomized, placebo- and drug-controlled study. Paper presented at Annual Meeting of the American Society for Reproductive Medicine, Orlando, Florida, 22–24 October 2001
137. Balasch J, Creus M, Fabregues F et al (1997) Pentoxifylline versus placebo in the treatment of infertility associated with minimal or mild endometriosis: a pilot randomized clinical trial. Hum Reprod 12:2046–2050
138. Evers JLH (1989) The pregnancy rate of the no-treatment group in randomized clinical trials of endometriosis therapy. Fertil Steril 52:906–909
139. Bayer SR, Seibel MM, Saffan DS et al (1988) Efficacy of danazol treatment for minimai endometriosis in infertile women: a prospective randomized study. J Reprod Med 33:179–183
140. Propst AM, Laufer M (1999) Endometriosis in adolescents: incidence, diagnosis and treatment. J Reprod Med 44:751–758
141. Vercellini P, Trespidi L, Colombo A et al (1993) A gonadotropin-releasing hormone agonist versus a low-dose oral contraceptive for pelvic pain associated with endometriosis. Fertil Steril 60:75–79
142. Fedele L, Bianchi S, Di Nola G et al (1994) The recurrence of endometriosis. Ann N Y Acad Sci 734:358–364
143. Ghezzi F, Beretta P, Franchi M et al (2001) Recurrence of endometriosis and anatomical location of the primary lesion. Fertil Steril 75:136–140
144. Simon C, Guttierez A, Vidal A et al (1994) Outcome of patients with endometriosis in assisted reproduction: results from in-vitro fertilization and oocyte donation. Hum Reprod 9:725–729
145. Arici A, Oral E, Bukulmez O et al (1996) The effect of endometriosis on implantation: results from the Yale University in vitro fertilization and embryo transfer program. Fertil Steril 65:603–607
146. Diaz I, Navarro J, Blasco L et al (2000) Impact of stage III–IV endometriosis on recipients of sibling oocytes: matched case-control study. Fertil Steril 74:31–34
147. Barnhart K, Dunsmoor-Su R, Coutifaris C (2002) Effect of endometriosis on in vitro fertilization. Fertil Steril 77(6):1148–1155
148. Bukulmez O, Yarali H, Gurgan T (2001) The presence and extent of endometriosis do not effect clinical pregnancy rate and implantation rates in patients undergoing ICSI. Eur J Obstet Gynecol Reprd Biol 96:102–107
149. Rosen GE (1992) Treatment of endometriosis-associated infertility. Infert Reprod Med Clin North Am 3:721–730
150. Proctor ML, Smith CA, Farquhar CM, et al (2004) Transcutaneous electrical nerve stimulation and acupuncture for primary dysmenorrhoea (Cochrane Review). In: The Cochrane Library, Issue 3. John Wiley & Sons, Ltd, Chichester, UK
151. Ulrich U, Murano R, Skinner MA et al (1998) Women of reproductive age with endometriosis are not osteopenic. Fertil Steril 69:821–825
152. Vercellini P, Aimi G, Panazza S et al (1999) A levonorgestrel-releasing intrauterine system for the treatment of dysmenorrhea associated with endometriosis: a pilot study. Fertil Steril 72:505–508
153. Tummon IS, Asher LS, Martin JRB et al (1997) Randomized controlled trial of superovulation and insemination for infertility associated with minimai or mild endometriosis. Fertil Steril 68:8–12

Chapter 14
Common Endocrinopathies in Reproductive Endocrinology

Shawn Gurtcheff and C. Matthew Peterson

Abstract This chapter reviews two of the most common endocrinopathies in reproductive medicine and highlights the unique associations with reproductive outcomes that should be appreciated by the reproductive endocrine clinic.

Keywords Thyroid • Thyroid disorders • Iodide • Iodine • Autoimmune thyroid disease • Hashimoto's thyroiditis • Graves disease • Iodine-131 • Thyroid-stimulating receptor antibody • Antithyroid drugs • Thyroid storm • Hyperthyroidism • Gestational trophoblastic disease • Hyperemesis gravidarum • Postpartum thyroid dysfunction • Thyroid nodules • Gonadal dysgenesis • Down syndrome • Prolactin • Hyperprolactinemia • Pituitary disorder • Hypothalamic disorder • Microadenoma • Macroadenoma • MRI • Estrogen • Reproduction

14.1 Thyroid Disorders

Thyroid disorders comprise the second most common endocrinopathy in woman after polycystic ovary syndrome. Thyroid disorders are tenfold more common in women than in men [1]. Approximately 1% of the female population of the United States will develop overt hypothyroidism. Even prior to the discovery of long-acting thyroid stimulator (LATS) in women with Graves' disease in 1956, many investigators suggested a potential link between autoimmune thyroid disorders and reproductive dysfunction [2].

14.1.1 Thyroid Hormones

Iodide is the key component of the class of hormones known as thyronines, of which tri-tetraiodiothryonine (T_3) and thyroxine (T_4) are the most important. Their production is depicted in Fig. 14.1.

Iodide obtained from dietary sources is actively transported into the thyroid follicular cell for synthesis of these hormones. The sodium-iodide symporter (NIS) is key to thyroid function. It facilitates the transport of iodide from the circulation into the thyrocyte against an electrochemical gradient. The energy required by NIS is supplied by Na-K ATPase. TSH stimulates iodide uptake. The enzyme thyroid peroxidase (TPO) then oxidizes iodide near the cell-colloid surface and incorporates it into tyrosyl residues within the thyroglobulin molecule, resulting in the formation of monoiodotyrosine (MIT) and diiodotyrosine (DIT). TPO also catalyzes the secondary coupling of MIT and DIT to formTriiodothyronine (T_3) and thyroxine (T_4). TPO is a membrane-bound, heme-containing oligomer found in the rough endoplasmic reticulum, Golgi vesicles, lateral and apical vesicles, and on the follicular cell surface. Thyroglobulin, the major protein of the thyroid gland, has an iodine content of 0.1–1.1% by weight. About 33% of the iodine found in thyroglobulin is in the form of T_3 and T_4, and the remainder is MIT, DIT, or unbound iodine. Thyroglobulin is a reservoir capable of maintaining a euthyroid state for nearly two months without the formation of new thyroid hormones. The thyroid "antimicrosomal" antibodies found in patients with autoimmune thyroid disease are directed against the TPO enzyme [3, 4].

Thyroid-stimulating hormone regulates thyroid iodine metabolism by the activation of adenylate cyclase. This facilitates iodide uptake, digestion of thyroglobulin-containing colloid, and the release of thyroid hormones T_4, T_3, and reverse T_3. T_4 is released from the thyroid at 40–100 times the concentration of T_3. The concentration of reverse T_3, which has no intrinsic thyroid activity, is 30–50% of T_3 and 1% of the T_4 concentrations, respectively. Of the active and inactive thyroid hormones released, 70% are bound by circulating thyroid binding globulin (TBG). T_4 is present in the circulating storage pool in the highest concentration, however, it has a slow turnover rate (about 7 days). In contrast, the concentration of T_3 is lower but has a higher turnover rate. Approximately 30% of T_4 is converted to T_3 in the periphery. Reverse T_3cooperates in the modulation of the conversion of T_4 to T_3. T_3 is the primary physiologically functional thyroid hormone. T3 binds the nuclear receptor with 10 times the

S. Gurtcheff and C.M. Peterson (✉)
Utah Center for Reproductive Medicine, Department of Obstetrics and Gynecology, University of Utah School of Medicine, Salt Lake City, UT, 84132, USA
e-mail: c.matthew.peterson@hsc.utah.edu

D.T. Carrell and C.M. Peterson (eds.), *Reproductive Endocrinology and Infertility: Integrating Modern Clinical and Laboratory Practice*,
DOI 10.1007/978-1-4419-1436-1_14, © Springer Science+Business Media, LLC 2010

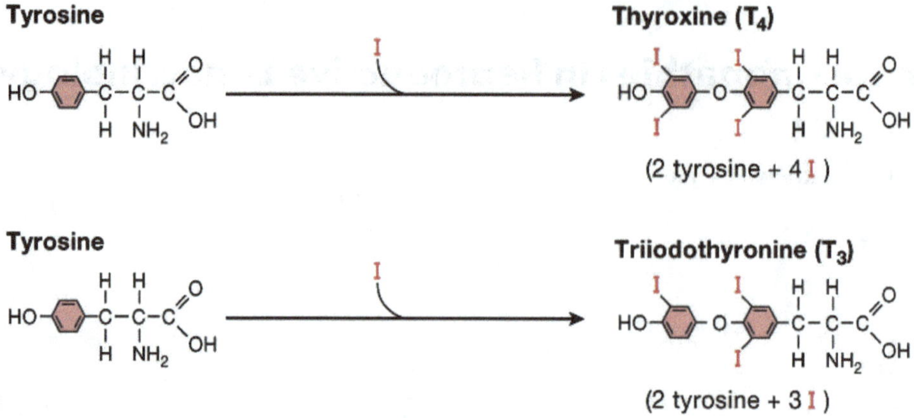

Fig. 14.1 Iodide and thyroid metabolism in the production of the thyronines: triiodothyronine (T_3) and thyroxine (T_4). Dietary iodide is actively transported into the thyroid follicular cell for synthesis of thyroid hormones. Sodium-iodide symporter (NIS) is key to thyroid function. It facilitates iodide transport from the circulation into the thyrocyte against an electrochemical gradient. The energy required by NIS is supplied by Na-K ATPase. TSH stimulates iodide uptake. The enzyme, thyroid peroxidase (TPO) then oxidizes iodide near the cell-colloid surface and incorporates it into tyrosyl residues within the thyroglobulin molecule, resulting in the formation of monoiodotyrosine (MIT) and diiodotyrosine (DIT). TPO also catalyzes the secondary coupling of MIT and DIT to form triiodothyronine (T_3) and thyroxine (T_4)

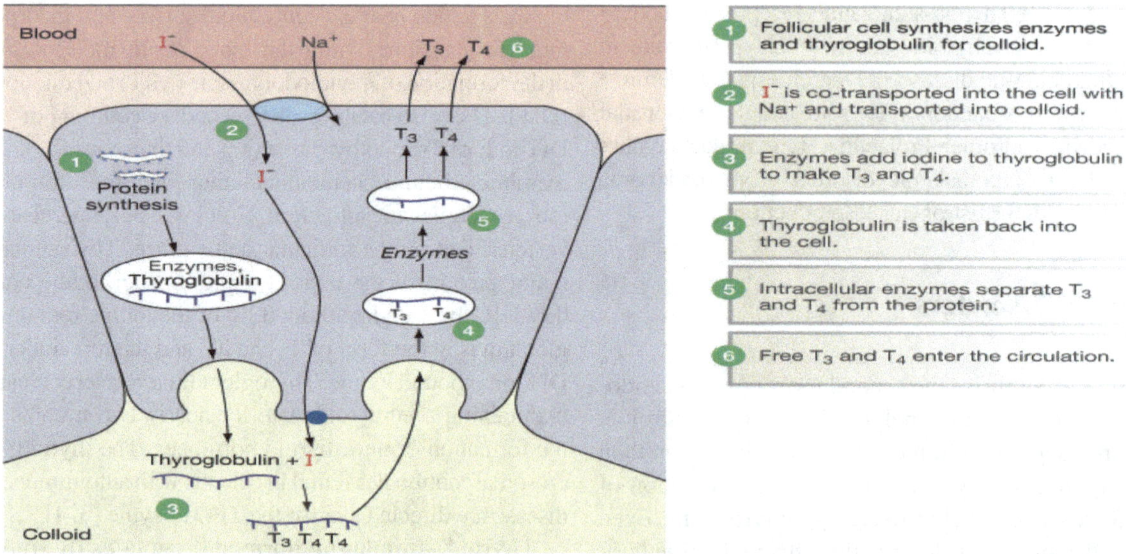

Fig. 14.2 The production and delivery of thyroid hormones. First, thyroid follicular cells synthesize enzymes and thyroglobulin for colloid production. Second, I^- is co-transported into the cell with Na^+ and transported into the colloid. Third, thyroid peroxidase (TPO) enzyme adds iodine to thyroglobulin in order to produce T_3 and T_4. Fourth, thyroglobulin is taken back into the cell. Fifth, intracellular enzymes separate T_3 and T_4 from the protein. Lastly, free T_3 and T_4 enter the circulation

affinity of T_4. Thyroid hormone causes increased oxygen consumption, heat production, and metabolism of fats, proteins, and carbohydrates. Systemically, thyroid hormone activity controls the basal metabolic rate. The production and delivery of the thyronines are outlined in Fig. 14.2.

14.1.2 Iodide Metabolism

Normal function of the thyroid gland is dependent on iodine. The recommended daily allowance by the U.S. National Research Council is 150–300 mg/day. Present daily consumption in the United States averages 200–600 mg/day due to supplements in common foodstuffs. Iodine intake is most commonly in the form of iodized salt (100 mg of potassium iodine/kg of salt) [5]. Women of childbearing age should have an average iodine intake of 150 μg/d. During pregnancy and breastfeeding, women should increase iodine intake to 250 μg/d and total intake should not exceed 500 μg/d. Iodine deficiency is the most common cause of hypothyroidism worldwide. As many as 40% of pregnant women have iodine deficiency in the UK [6].

The thyroid gland requires iodine for synthesis of thyroid hormones. In locations where dietary iodine is insufficient, goitrous hypothyroidism among adults and the consequences of inadequate fetal thyroxine are common (endemic goiter and endemic cretinism). Characterizing the narrow safety threshold for dietary iodide intake, iodine intake adequacy appears to be associated with the development of autoimmune thyroid disorders [7, 8] and decreased remission rates in patients treated for Graves' disease [9]. It appears that iodine stimulates immunoglobulin production by B lymphocytes, activates macrophages, and increases the immunogenic potential of thyroglobulin because of the higher iodide content [10–13].

14.1.3 Factors Affecting Risk for Autoimmune Thyroid Disorders

Environmental factors associated with the occurrence of autoimmune thyroid diseases include pollutants (plasticizers, polychlorinated biphenyls, and coal-processing pollutants) [14, 15] and antibodies to *Yersinia enterocolitica* [16]. The female hormonal milieu and its effects on immune surveillance appear to play a role in the tenfold increased risk in women to develop autoimmune thyroid disease. The polyclonal immunoglobulins produced against the thyroid and the multiple combinations of various antibodies present (stimulating versus blocking, complement fixing, and noncytotoxic) combine to create the clinical spectrum of autoimmune thyroid diseases (Fig. 14.3).

Stimulation of blockade of hormone receptors leads to hyperfunction or hypofunction or growth, depending on the types of immunoglobulins acting on the target cell. (TBII, TSH-binding inhibitor immunoglobulin; TGI, thyroid growth–promoting immunoglobulin; TSAb, thyroid-stimulating antibodies; TSH, thyroid-stimulating hormone.)

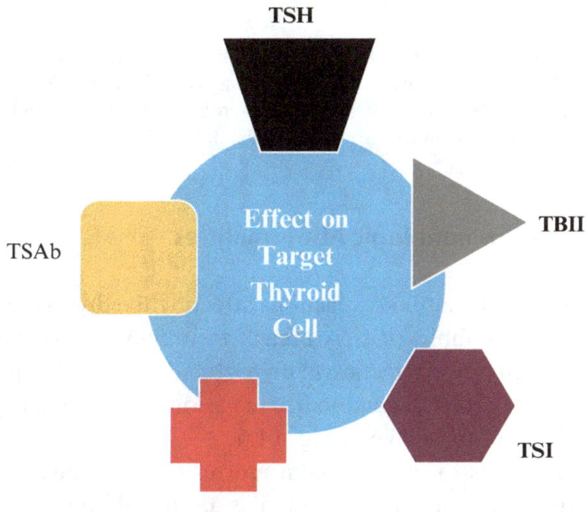

Fig. 14.3 Effects of autoimmune injury found in Hashimoto's thyroiditis depend on the algebraic sum of the activities of the various activities of the immunologic agents

14.1.4 Evaluation

14.1.4.1 Thyroid Function

Total serum T_4 is measured by radioimmunoassay and includes both freeT_4 and that bound to thyroid binding globulin (TBG). TBG levels are variable and many conditions elevate the level of TBG including: estrogen replacement, hepatitis, and genetic abnormalities of TBG, OC use, and pregnancy. Thus, an indirect estimation of the unbound ("free") T4 or its direct measurement is required for clinical evaluation. While not commonly utilized, the T_3 resin uptake can be instructive in some of the conditions noted earlier. The T_3 resin uptake determines the binding of radiolabeled T_3 to a resin that competes with TBG for T_3 binding within a serum sample. The binding capacity of TBG in the sample is inversely proportional to the amount of labeled T_3 bound to the artificial resin. Therefore, a low T_3 resin uptake indicates high TBG T_3 receptor site availability, and implies high circulating TBG levels and conversely a high T_3 resin uptake denotes low TBG T_3 receptor site availability and hence low circulating TBG levels.

The free T_4 index (FTI) is obtained by multiplying the serum T_4 concentration by the T_3 resin uptake percentage, yielding an indirect estimate of the levels of free T_4:

$$T_3RU\% \text{ x } T_4 \text{ total} = \text{free } T_4 \text{ index}$$

A high T_3RU indicates reduced TBG receptor site availability and high free T_4 index and thus hyperthyroidism, whereas a low T_3RU is a result of increased TBG receptor site binding and thus hypothyroidism. Equilibrium dialysis and ultrafiltration techniques may be used to directly determine the free T_4. Free T_4 and T_3 may also be determined by radioimmunoassay and are commonly used to evaluate thyroid function.

Because levels of TSH are sensitive to high or low levels of circulating thyroid hormone, TSH levels are commonly used to screen for primary hyper- and hypo-thyroidism. The present TSH sandwich immunoassays are extremely sensitive and are capable of differentiating low-normal from pathologic or iatrogenically subnormal values and elevations. Thus, TSH measurements provide the best single screen for thyroid dysfunction [17] and accurately predict thyroid hormone dysfunction in about 80% of cases.

During pregnancy, significant and reversible changes in thyroid physiology occur. First, there is a physiologic enlargement of the gland during pregnancy, which may prompt testing of the TSH level. Second, there is an estrogen-mediated increase in circulating levels of thyroid-binding globulin. Third, a suppressive effect caused by the thyrotropic activities of human chorionic gonadotropin (hCG) which routinely suppresses TSH values near the end of the first trimester, but not exclusively during this period (Fig. 14.4) [18].

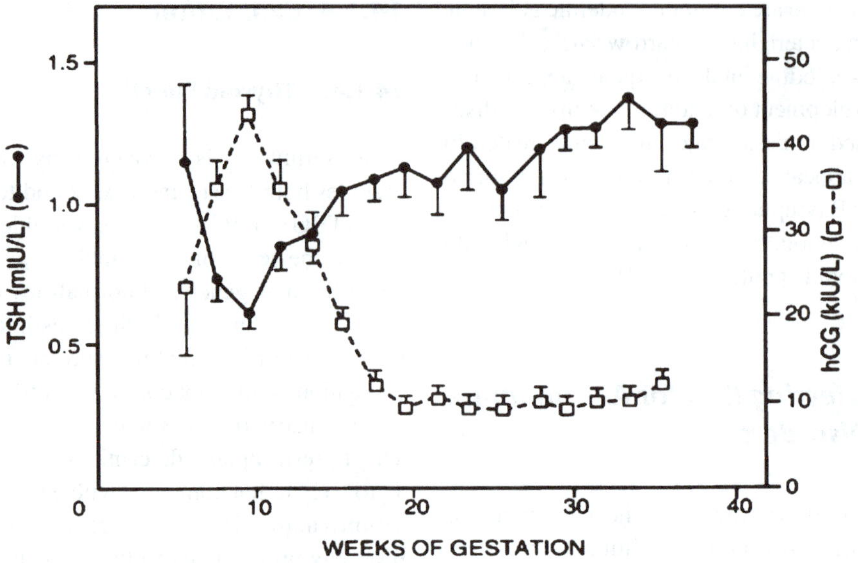

Fig. 14.4 The suppressive effect on TSH caused by the thyrotropic activities of human chorionic gonadotropin (hCG) which routinely suppresses TSH values near the end of the first trimester, but not exclusively in this period. (Reprinted with permission from Glinoer D, Denayer P, Bourdoux P, et al Regulation of maternal thyroid during pregnancy. J Clin Endocrinol Mertab 1990; 71:276–87)

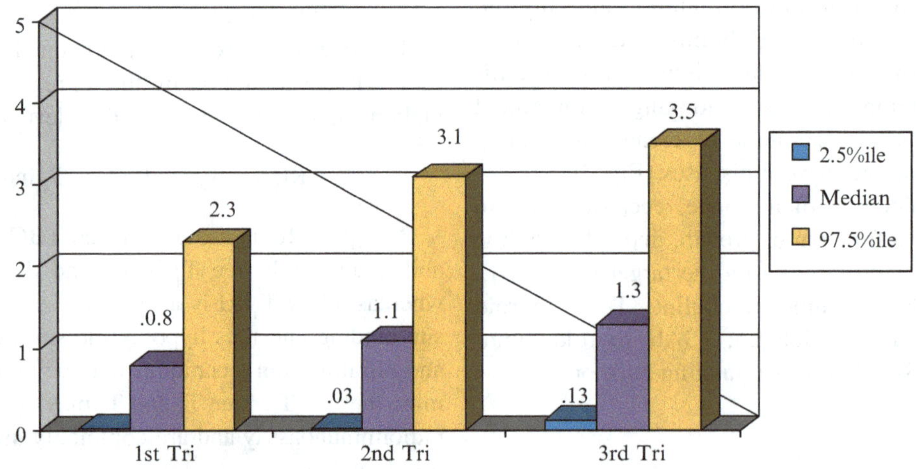

Fig. 14.5 Median and 95% confidence intervals for TSH during pregnancy (Hong Kong). The blue bar shows the 2.5th percentile and the yellow bar the 97.5th percentile in each of the trimesters of pregnancy. The purple bar is the median TSH level during the three trimesters of pregnancy. The specific values for each bar are printed above their respective bar. (Reprinted with permission from Panesar NS, Li CY, Rogers MS. Reference intervals for thyroid hormones in pregnant Chinese women. Ann Clin Biochem 2001; 38:329–332)

Fourth, there is a decline in the availability of iodide which is related to increased renal clearance and losses to the fetus and placenta. Fifth, until 10–12 weeks gestation, when the fetus acquires the ability to concentrate iodine and synthesize thyroid hormones, all thyroid hormones are supplied by the mother. Thus, the normative range for TSH during pregnancy has been defined as <2.5, <3.1 and <3.5 mIU/ml in the first, second and third trimesters, respectively, to account for these physiologic changes (Fig. 14.5) [19]. This creates new standards for normal TSH ranges – the pregnant (<2.5, 3.1 and 3.5 mIU/ml for each trimester, respectively) and nonpregnant state (<4.5 mIU/ml).

14.1.4.2 Immunologic Abnormalities

Many antigen–antibody reactions affecting the thyroid gland are listed in Table 14.1. A breach in immune surveillance allows antibody production to thyroglobulin [7, 8]. The prevalence of thyroid autoantibodies in various autoimmune thyroid disorders is shown in Fig. 14.6.

Antibodies to thyroglobulin are restricted to one minor and two major epitopes. Antibodies are mainly noncomplement-fixing immunoglobulin G (IgG) polyclonal antibodies [9]. Antithyroglobulin antibodies are found in patients with Hashimoto's thyroiditis, Graves' disease, acute thyroiditis, nontoxic goiter, and thyroid cancer. They also appear in normal women.

Antithyroid peroxidase antibodies (anti-TPO antibodies) previously referred to as anti-microsomal antibodies are directed against TPO and are found in Hashimoto's thyroiditis, Graves' disease, and postpartum thyroiditis. The antibodies produced are characteristically cytotoxic, complement-fixing IgG antibodies. Anti-TPO antibodies correlate with the histologic appearance of lymphocytic thyroiditis [20, 21]. These cytotoxic antibodies are directed against thyroid follicular cells ultimately leading to death, atrophy and hypothyroidis. These antibodies can cause artifacts in the measurement of thyroid hormone levels.

Another group of antibodies important in autoimmune thyroid disease binds the TSH receptor. These antibodies often create the signs and symptoms that lead to an evaluation. TSH receptor antibodies (TSHR-Ab or TRAb) are pathogenic and capable of activating or blocking TSH receptor functions. TSHR-Ab are detected using two approaches – competitive and functional assays. The competition between antibody and TSH for binding to the TSH receptor is the basis for the measurement of TSH-binding inhibitory immunoglobulin (TBII). The functional assay approach is on the basis of the status of the receptor induced by the antibody-receptor interaction. This functional assay measures the production and accumulation of cyclic AMP, thyroid hormone or thyroglobulin secretion, or iodide uptake in thyroid epithelial cells or Chinese hamster ovary cells transfected with the human TSH receptor. While the competitive assay does not indicate any functional activity of the antibody, the functional assay identifies whether the antibody is agonistic (thyroid-stimulating antibody [TSAb] or antagonistic TSH stimulation–blocking antibody [TSBAb or TSHBAb]). Both types of antibodies may be present in the same patient, and the effect is the algebraic sum of the two levels of activity (agonistic and antagonistic) (Fig. 14.3).

Table 14.1 Origin and function of thyroid autoantigens

Antigen	Location	Function
Thyroglobulin (Tg)	Thyroid	Thyroid hormone storage
Thyroid peroxidase (TPO) (microsomal antigen)	Thyroid	Transduction of signal from TSH
TSH receptor (TSHR)	Thyroid, lymphocytes, fibroblasts, adipocytes (including retroorbital)	Transduction of signal from TSH
Na^+/I^- symporter (NIS)	Thyroid, breast, salivary or lacrimal gland, gastric or colonic mucosa, thymus, pancreas	ATP-driven uptake of I^- along with Na^+

TSH thyroid-stimulating hormone, *ATP* adenosine triphosphate

TSAb or thyroid-stimulating immunoglobulin (TSI) activates the TSH receptor. Long-acting thyroid stimulators are monoclonal or limited polyclonal TSAb, which mimic TSH action. They are quantified by their ability to stimulate human thyroid cell cultures to produce cyclic adenosine monophosphate or to release T_3.

TBII is detectable in two varieties, those that block TSH binding and those that block both pre- and postreceptor processes. Several investigators have detected such blocking antibodies in patients with primary hypothyroidism who have atrophic thyroid glands [12, 13, 22]. The nomenclature and detection assay of TSH receptor antibodies are listed in Table 14.2.

The existence of thyroid growth-promoting immunoglobulins (TGI) thought to stimulate growth but not hormone release, have been questioned [21, 23–31]. Their immunologic antagonists would be the TGI, have been questioned blocking antibodies that are capable of inhibiting TSH-mediated

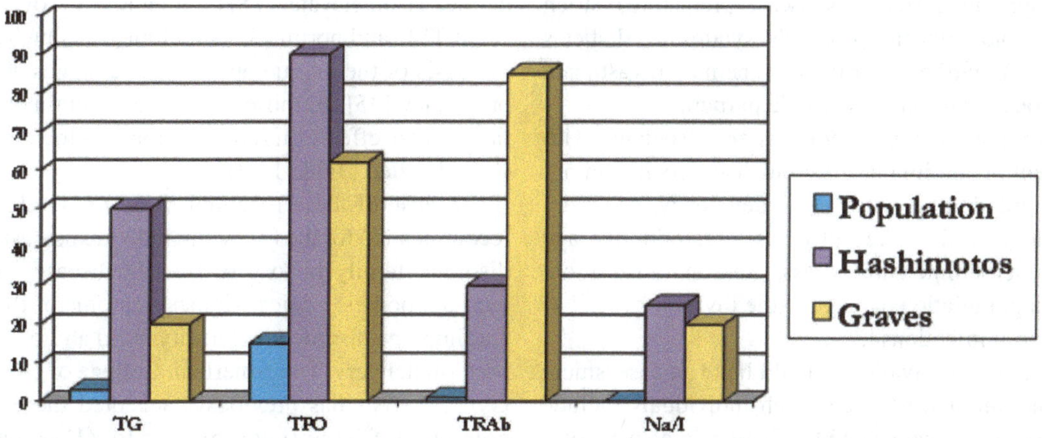

Fig. 14.6 Prevalence of thyroid autoantibodies in the most common thyroid disorders. The vertical axis represents the percentage of each group with autoantibodies (general population, Hashimoto's thyroiditis, Graves disease. The horizontal axis lists the specific target of the autoantibodies: *TG* Thyroglobulin, *TPO* Thyroid peroxidase or microsomal antibody, *TRAb* Thyroid stimulating hormone receptor antibody, NA/I Sodium–Iodide symporter

Table 14.2 Anti-TSH receptor antibody properties

Abbreviation	Term	Assay used	Refers to
TBII	TSH-binding inhibitory immunoglobulin	Competitive binding assays with TSH	Antibodies that are able to compete with TSH for TSH receptor binding, whether biologically active or not
LATS	Long-acting thyroid stimulator	In vivo assay of stimulation of mouse thyroid	Original description of the serum molecule capable of stimulation of mouse thyroid cells; no longer relevant
TSAb	Thyroid-stimulating antibodies	Bioassays of TSH receptor activation	TSH receptor- stimulating antibodies
TSBAb, TSHBAb	TSH stimulation-blocking antibodies	Competition with TSH in bioassays of TSH receptor activation	Antibodies that block activation of the TSH receptor by TSH
TSHR-Ab, TRAb	TSH receptor antibodies	Multiple	All antibodies that recognize the TSH receptor, blocking, stimulatory or biologically inactive
TSI	Thyroid-stimulating immunoglobulins	As TSAb	Identical to TSAb

TSH thyroid-stimulating hormone

growth responses in patients who may have had thyroid damage by immune destruction.

Antibodies to the NIS are prevalent in a number of thyroid conditions. Increased expression of NIS protein and NIS mRNA is found in patients with autonomous thyroid adenomas and in Graves' disease. They are decreased in Hashimoto's thyroiditis, cold nodules, and thyroid carcinoma.

14.1.4.3 Autoimmune Thyroid Disease

Autoimmune thyroid disorders commonly found in women, represent the combined effects of the multiple antibodies produced (Fig. 14.3) [32]. The various antigen–antibody reactions result in the wide clinical spectrum of these disorders. Transplacental transmission of some of these immunoglobulins may also affect thyroid function in the fetus. The presence of autoimmune thyroid disorders, particularly Graves' disease, is associated with other autoimmune conditions including: Hashimoto's thyroiditis, Addison's disease, premature ovarian failure, rheumatoid arthritis, Sjögren's syndrome, diabetes mellitus (type I), vitiligo, pernicious anemia, myasthenia gravis, and idiopathic thrombocytopenic purpura.

Furthermore, a number of conditions are associated with the development of autoimmune thyroid disorders including: low birth weight, iodine excess and deficiency, selenium deficiency, parity, oral contraceptive use, reproductive age span, fetal microchimerism, stress, seasonal variation, allergy, smoking, radiation damage to the thyroid, as well as viral and bacterial infections [33].

Certain groups of individuals should have an assessment of thyroid function at least once. Such individuals include infertile and pregnant women [34]. Testing is also recommended for women with atrial fibrillation, hyperemesis gravidarum, and hyperlipidemia. Periodic assessment of thyroid function is indicated in patients who receive amiodarone and lithium. Epidemiologists recommend that all women with diabetes be annually screened for thyroid dysfunction. Women with type 1 diabetes are three times more likely to experience postpartum thyroid dysfunction, and it is recommended that all women with diabetes be screened with a TSH evaluation in their first trimester. Any woman with a history of postpartum thyroiditis should also be offered annual surveillance of thyroid function. Because there is a high prevalence of hypothyroidism in women with Turner and Down syndrome, an annual check of thyroid function is recommended. Periodic TSH screening in mature women is advisable.

Special Considerations in Pregnancy and Postpartum

Recently, the Endocrine Society published clinical practice guidelines regarding the management of thyroid dysfunction during pregnancy and postpartum. Hypothyroidism was defined as an elevated TSH with a low T_4 (overt) and an elevated TSH and normal T_4 (subclinical) using TSH ranges on the basis of the unique physiologic changes associated with pregnancy [35]. In those guidelines, a number of the potential adverse effects on reproduction and the developing fetus were detailed (Table 14.3).

Because of these potential risks, *targeted screening* was recommended for the following individuals: history of thyroid disorder, family history of thyroid disease, goiter, thyroid auto-antibodies, clinical signs/symptoms of thyroid disease, autoimmune disorders, infertility, head and/or neck radiation, preterm delivery. The American College of Obstetricians and Gynecologists has previously accepted these conditions as criteria for TSH testing [36]. Due to: (1) potentially significant adverse effects on the neurologic development of the fetus and other adverse pregnancy events; (2) the physiologic rise in TBG and the TSH-like activity of hCG in pregnancy,

Table 14.3 Adverse and documented effects of hypothyroidism on reproduction

- Subfertility (Abalovich M. Thyroid 2002; 12:63–8)
- Miscarriage in TPO Ab+ (Negro R. JCEM 2006; 91:2587–91)
- Anemia (Davis LE. Obstet Gynecol 1988; 72:108–12)
- Gestational hypertension (Leung AS. Obstet Gynecol 1993; 81:349–53
- Abruption (Davis LE. Obstet Gynecol 1988; 72:108–12)
- Postpartum hemorrhage (Davis LE. Obstet Gynecol 1988; 72:108–12)
- Preterm delivery (Negro R. JCEM 2006; 91:2587–91)
- Impaired neuropsychological development
  - Lower IQ by 7 pts in untreated hypothyroid (Haddow JE. NEJM 1999; 341:549–55)
  - Mild reduction in global intelligence inversely correlated with 3rd trimester TSH (Rovet JF. Thyroid 14:710)
  - Iodine deficiency and deficit in IQ, ADHD (Vermiglio F. JCEM 2004; 89:6054–60)

and: (3) the potential for the above groups to have overt or subclinical hypothyroidism defined by the a reference range for pregnancy (TSH < 2.5, 3.1 and 3.5 mIU/ml for the first, second and third trimesters, respectively), targeted maternal testing for hypothyroidism was encouraged (Fig. 14.5). The *targeted screening* regimen currently recommended, allows that 30% of subclinical hypothyroidism cases may be missed. Universal screening in pregnancy is not recommended at the present time. According to these recommendations, preconceptionally diagnosed hypothyroid women (overt or subclinical) should have their T_4 dose adjusted such that the TSH value is <2.5 μU/ml before pregnancy. The T_4 dosage in women on replacement will routinely require a dose escalation at four to 6 weeks gestation in order to maintain a TSH value < 2.5 μU/ml. This adjustment may require a 30–50% increase in dosage. Pregnant women with overt hypothyroidism should be normalized as rapidly as possible to maintain TSH at less than 2.5 and 3 μU/ml in the first and second/third trimesters, respectively. The TSH value may be reevaluated every 30–40 days after dosage adjustments. Euthyroid women with thyroid autoantibodies are at risk of hypothyroidism and should also have TSH screening in each trimester. After delivery, hypothyroid women need a reduction in T_4 dosage used during pregnancy. Because subclinical hypothyroidism has been shown to be associated with adverse outcomes for mother as well and fetus, T_4 replacement is recommended.

14.1.4.4 Hashimoto's Thyroiditis

Hashimoto's thyroiditis or chronic lymphocytic thyroiditis, first described in 1912, can manifest as hyperthyroidism, hypothyroidism, euthyroid goiter, or diffuse goiter. High levels of antimicrosomal and antithyroglobulin antibody are usually present. Typically, glandular hypertrophy is found, but atrophic forms are also present. The composition of various antibodies (i.e., TBII, causing the atrophic form and congenital hypothyroidism in some neonates, and TGI, causing the goitrous variety) results in varied physical findings.

Three classic types of autoimmune injury are found in Hashimoto's thyroiditis, (a) complement-mediated cytotoxicity, (b) antibody-dependent cell-mediated cytotoxicity, and (c) stimulation or blockade of hormone receptors, which results in hypo- or hyperfunction or growth (Fig. 14.3). The clinical presentation depends on the sum and superiority of action of various antibodies possessing TSH stimulating or blocking properties.

Histologically, Hashimoto's thyroiditis demonstrates cellular hyperplasia, disruption of follicular cells, and infiltration of the gland by lymphocytes, monocytes, and plasma cells. Cervical lymphadenopathy may also be noted. Some epithelial cells are enlarged and demonstrate oxyphilic changes in the cytoplasm (Askanazy cells or Hürthle cells, which are not specific to this disorder). Interstitial cells show fibrosis and lymphocytic infiltration. Graves' disease and Hashimoto's thyroiditis may cause very similar histologic findings manifested by a similar mechanism of action. Most patients with Hashimoto's thyroiditis and about two-thirds of patients with Graves' disease have sera demonstrating antibody-dependent cell-mediated cytotoxicity. Thyroid antibody positivity is detected in 16.8% of the white U.S. female population and in 10.2% of men [37]. Within the classification of hypothyroidism, overt hypothyroidism, defined by an elevated TSH and low T_4, is found in 0.3–0.5% of the population. Subclinical hypothyroidism, defined by an elevated TSH and normal T_4 is found in 2–3% of the population. It should be remembered that women with a diagnosis of Hashimoto's thyroiditis who presently are or who are seeking pregnancy should have their thyroxine dose adjusted to keep the TSH < 2.5 μU/ml.

Clinical Characteristics and Diagnosis of Hashimoto's Thyroiditis

Most patients with Hashimoto's thyroiditis are relatively asymptomatic with painless goiter and hypothyroidism. The goiter may involve the pyramidal lobe. As the condition evolves from thyroiditis to cell death and atrophy, hypothyroidism can be found without a goiter. Notable manifestations of hypothyroidism include cold intolerance, constipation, carotene deposition in the periorbital region, carpal tunnel syndrome, dry skin, fatigue, hair loss, lethargy, and weight gain. Hashitoxicosis, the early hyperthyroid manifestation of Hashimoto's thyroiditis, may represent a variant of Graves' disease. This form is estimated to occur in 4–8% of patients with Hashimoto's thyroiditis. These patients often become hypothyroid.

Table 14.4 Etiologies of hypothyroidism

Primary
Congenital absence of thyroid gland
External thyroid gland irradiation
Familial disorders and thyroxine synthesis
Hashimoto's thyroiditis
Iodine-131 ablation for Graves' disease
Ingestion of antithyroid drugs
Iodine deficiency
Idiopathic myxedema (autoimmune)
Surgical removal of thyroid gland
Secondary
Hypothalamic thyrotropin-releasing hormone deficiency
Pituitary or hypothalamic tumors or disease

In many cases, an elevated serum level of TSH is noted during routine screening. Elevated serum antithyroglobulin and antimicrosomal antibody elevation confirm the diagnosis. The sedimentation rate may be elevated, depending on the time of recognition. Other causes of hypothyroidism should be considered as listed in Table 14.4.

Women with an elevated serum TSH and positive thyroid antibody tests have a 5% annual risk for overt hypothyroidism [32]. If the serum TSH alone is elevated, without positive thyroid antibody titers, the annual risk for hypothyroidism drops to less than 3% per year. In those seeking pregnancy, the recent guidelines encourage treatment to maintain the TSH level <2.5 mIU/ml.

Treatment

Thyroxine replacement is initiated in patients with symptomatic hypothyroidism, patients who have a goiter that is cosmetically or physically bothersome and are subclinically hypothyroid, and patients who are subclinically or overtly hypothyroid and attempting pregnancy. Regression of gland size usually does not occur, but treatment prevents further hypertrophy. All pregnant patients with an elevated TSH level should be treated with *levothyroxine*. Treatment does not slow progression of the disease. Replacement therapy is monitored by TSH determinations approximately six weeks after a change in dose. *Aluminum hydroxide* (antacids), *cholestyramine*, iron, and *sucralfate* may interfere with absorption. The half-life of *levothyroxine* is nearly 7 days; therefore, nearly six weeks of treatment are necessary before the effects of a dose change can be evaluated.

Hypothyroidism appears to be associated with decreased fertility resulting from ovulatory difficulties and possibly with spontaneous abortion [38–41]. A meta-analysis of case-control and longitudinal studies performed since 1990 reveals a possible association between miscarriage and thyroid antibodies with an odds ratio of 2.73 (2.20–3.40, 95% confidence interval). This association may be explained by a heightened autoimmune state affecting the fetal allograft, or, alternatively, a slightly higher age of women with antibodies when compared with those without (0.7 ± 1 year, $p<0.001$) [33]. Studies also suggest that early subclinical hypothyroidism may be associated with menorrhagia [42].

Severe primary hypothyroidism is associated with amenorrhea or anovulation [43, 44]. Enhanced sensitivity of the prolactin-secreting cells to thyrotropin-releasing hormone (TRH) and defective dopamine turnover resulting in hyperprolactinemia associated with a deficiency of thyroid hormone are the apparent explanations for the hyperprolactinemia [45–48]. Hyperprolactinemia-induced luteal phase defects also are associated with less severe forms of hypothyroidism [49, 50]. Replacement therapy appears to reverse hyperprolactinemia and correct ovulatory defects [51, 52].

Combined thyroxine and triiodothyronine therapy is not better than thyroxine therapy alone [53]. In patients with Hashimotos' thyroiditis and subclinical hypothyroidism, a daily dose of 0.025–0.075 mg of levothyroxine will usually normalize TSH values.

Treatment is recommended in light of the potential adverse effects on reproduction (Table 14.3). To avoid maternal hypothyroidism, *targeted screening* should be employed, recognizing that in using this strategy 30% of cases of subclinical hypothyroidism will be missed. Targeted screening should occur in individuals with:

- Autoimmune disorders
- Clinical signs/symptoms of thyroid disease
- Family history of thyroid disease
- Goiter
- Head and Neck radiation
- History of thyroid disorder
- Infertility
- Thyroid autoantibodies
- Preterm Delivery

14.1.4.5 Graves' Disease

Graves' disease, identified in 1835 is characterized by exophthalmos, goiter, and hyperthyroidism. A heritable defect in immunosurveillance by suppressor T lymphocytes is believed to result in the development of a helper T-cell population that reacts to multiple epitopes of the thyrotropin receptor and induces a B-cell–mediated response, resulting in the features of Graves' disease. The generic thyroid stimulating antibodies (TSHR-Ab) bind to conformational epitopes in the extracellular domain of the thyrotropin receptor and are detected in the serum of 90% of patients with Graves' disease (Fig. 14.6). The epitopes make up discontinuous areas that overlap the thyrotropin binding site. Human leukocyte antigen (HLA) class II antigens DR, DP, DQ, and DS can present antigens to T cells and are expressed on thyroid epithelial cells. Antibodies to the TSH receptor (TSHR-Ab) are produced when the immunogen, TSH receptor, is presented to helper T lymphocytes with the D locus antigens [54].

The class II antigens remain a focus of the genetic susceptibility to autoimmune thyroiditis [55]. The clinical use of *interferon-α* has been associated with the development of autoimmune thyroid disease [56]. Graves' disease is a complex autoimmune disorder in which several genetic susceptibility loci and environmental factors seem to play a role in the development of the disease. HLA and the CTLA-4 gene region have been established as susceptibility loci; however, the magnitude of their contributions seems to vary among patient populations and study groups. Additional loci are likely to be identified by a combination of genome-wide linkage analyses and allelic association analyses of candidate genes. The rate of concordance for Graves' disease is only 20% in monozygotic twins and even lower in dizygotic twins suggestive of a multifactorial inheritance pattern that is influenced by enviromental factors. Graves' disease is associated with polymorphisms of the cytotoxic T-lymphocyte antigen 4 (CTLA-4) gene in several populations. Linkage analysis has identified loci on chromosomes 14q31, 20q11.2, and Xq21 that are associated with susceptibility to Graves' disease [11].

Clinical Characteristics and Diagnosis

The patient with the classic diagnostic triad of exophthalmos, goiter, and hyperthyroidism in Graves' Disease confirms many of the symptoms of hyperthyroidism when asked: frequent bowel movements, heat intolerance, irritability, nervousness, palpitations or tachycardia, tremor, weight loss, and lower extremity swelling. Additional physical findings include lid lag, nontender thyroid enlargement (2–4-times normal), onycholysis, palmar erythema, proptosis, staring gaze, and thick skin. A cervical venous bruit and tachycardia are usually noted. A diagnostic clue includes a tachycardia does not respond to increased vagal tone produced with a Valsalva maneuver. Severe cases may demonstrate acropachy, chemosis, clubbing, dermopathy, exophthalmos with ophthalmoplegia, follicular conjunctivitis, pretibial myxedema, and vision loss.

Approximately 40% of patients with new onset of Graves' disease and many of those who have received treatment have elevated free T_3 and normal T_4 levels. Therefore, assessment of free T_4, free T_3, and TSH values is required. The TSH levels are suppressed, and levels may remain undetectable even for some time even after the initiation of treatment. TSH measurements are useful in evaluating medical treatment, prognosis, and anticipating fetal complications such as neonatal thyrotoxicosis. Autonomously functioning, benign thyroid neoplasias that exhibit a similar clinical picture include toxic adenomas and toxic multinodular goiter. Very rare conditions causing thyrotoxicosis include hCG-secreting choriocarcinoma, TSH-secreting pituitary adenomas, and struma ovarii. Factitious ingestion of thyroxine or desiccated thyroid must be considered in patients with eating disorders. Other potential causes of hyperthyroidism are listed in Table 14.5. Smoking appears to be an independent risk factor for relapse after medical therapy and this should be considered when planning treatment.

Table 14.5 Etiologies of hyperthyroidism

Factitious hyperthyroidism
Graves' disease
Metastatic follicular cancer
Pituitary hyperthyroidism
Postpartum thyroiditis
Silent hyperthyroidism (low radioiodine uptake)
Struma ovarii
Subacute thyroiditis
Toxic multinodular goiter
Toxic nodule
Tumors secreting human chorionic gonadotropin (molar pregnancy, choriocarcinoma)

Treatment

Iodine-131 Ablation

Treatment of women with hyperthyroidism of an autoimmune origin presents unique challenges to the physician who must consider the patient's needs and her reproductive plans. Because the drugs used to treat this disorder have potentially harmful effects on the fetus, special attention must be given to the use of contraception and the potential for pregnancy.

A single dose of radioactive iodine-131 (^{131}I) is an effective cure in about 80% of cases and is the most commonly used definitive treatment in nonpregnant women. Any woman of childbearing age should be tested for pregnancy before undergoing diagnostic or therapeutic administration of ^{131}I. Ablation of a second-trimester fetal thyroid gland and congenital hypothyroidism (cretinism) from treatment during the first trimester have been reported [57, 58]. Nuclear medicine professionals provide expertise in the administration of the radioactive isotope, and the endocrinologist continues to provide suppressive medical treatment for six to 12 weeks after administration of ^{131}I. Postablative hypothyroidism develops in 50% of patients within the first year after ^{131}I therapy and in more than 2% of patients per year thereafter.

Higher rates of miscarriage have been noted in women who received ^{131}I therapy in the year preceeding pregnancy but no reported increased rate in stillbirths, preterm birth, low birth weight, congenital malformation or death after therapy [59]. Many thyroidologists and nuclear medicine specialists ascribe the higher rates of miscarriage to unrecognized post ^{131}I induced hypothyroidism and are now more willing to allow pregnancy earlier than 1 year after therapy if patients are appropriately replaced with levothyroxine. ^{131}I therapy contraindicated while breastfeeding.

Thyroid-stimulating Receptor Antibody in Graves' Disease-Treatment Correlates

The level of TSHR-Ab (TBII) parallels the degree of hyperthyroidism as assessed by the serum levels of thyroid hormones and total thyroid volume. Studies suggest that the combination of a small goiter volume (<40 ml) and a low TBII level (<30 units/L) results in a 45% chance of remission during the 5 years after completion of a 12–24-month course of antithyroid drug therapy [57]. In contrast, the overall rate of relapse exceeds 70% in patients with a large goiter volume (>70 ml) and a higher TBII level (>30 units/L). Thus, the subgroup of patients with larger goiters and higher TBII levels had less than a 10% chance to remain in remission in the 5 years after treatment. Therefore, although it is not necessary for the diagnosis of Graves' disease, except in some cases of multinodular goiter, a TSHR-Ab measurement may be a useful marker of disease severity and, in combination with other clinical factors, may contribute to the initial decisions regarding treatment. See Table 14.2 to review the nomenclature and assay methods for TSHR-Ab.

TSHR-Ab measurements (TBII) during treatment with antithyroid drugs also are predictive of subsequent outcome. In one series, 73% of TBII-negative patients had remission when compared with only 28% of TBII-positive patients who had achieved remission after 12 months of antithyroid drug therapy [58]. Furthermore, the duration of a course of antithyroid drug therapy can be modified according to the TSHR-Ab status. In patients whose TSHR-Ab status became negative and antithyroid drug therapy was discontinued, the relapse rate was 41% when compared with a rate of 92% for those patients who remained TSHR-Ab positive [60]. Regardless of the rapidity of the disappearance of TSHR-Ab, it does seem that antithyroid drug therapy should be maintained for nine to 12 months to minimize the risk of relapse. TSHR-Ab status also appears to determine in an inverse relationship the reduction in thyroid volume after radioactive iodine therapy.

Recently, a second generation assay has been developed for assessment of TSHR-Ab using recombinant human TSH receptor [61]. This new assay has nearly 100% sensitivity and specificity in the diagnosis of Graves' disease. Its utility in monitoring treatment is being evaluated. Many patients with Graves' disease have or will develop antineutrophil cytoplasmic antibodies (ANCA), but the significance of this finding is still under study.

Antithyroid Drugs

Antithyroid drugs of the thioamide class include *propylthiouracil* (*PTU*) and *methimazole.* Low doses of either agent blocks the secondary coupling reactions that form T_3 and T_4 from MIT and DIT. At higher doses, they also block iodination of tyrosyl residues in thyroglobulin. PTU additionally blocks the peripheral coversion of T_4 to T3. Approximately one-third of patients treated by this modality alone go into remission and become euthyroid [57].

PTU causes a reduction of hyperthyroid symptoms at a dose of 100 mg taken every 8 h over 1 month. Adequate control of thyrotoxic symptoms may require considerably higher doses. PTU blocks the intrathyroid synthesis of T_3 and the peripheral conversion of T_4 to T_3 but does not cross the placenta as easily as *methimazole*, and therefore is the drug of choice during pregnancy. Drug efficacy is monitored weekly by evaluation of pulse, appetite, emotional liability, insomnia, and tremor. A general rule is to lower the dosage by 50% when thyroid function returns to normal, which frequently correlates with the return to a normal heart rate and, subsequently, normalization of TSH levels. Thyroxine is usually the first value to become normal.

Pruritus affects 3–5% of treated patients. Serious adverse reactions include agranulocytosis (occurring one to 2 months after therapy in 0.02%) and a generalized drug eruption accompanied by arthralgia, fever, and sore throat. A complete blood count determination is performed if the patient develops an upper respiratory tract infection. If adverse reactions occur, methimazole may be used.

Methimazole (10 mg) is given every eight to 24 h. Its dosage is reduced, as with *PTU*. It is not the drug of choice in pregnant women because it does not block peripheral conversion and crosses the placenta more readily than *PTU*. Its use in pregnancy is associated in some instances with the development of characteristic skin lesions in the fetus, aplasia cutis congenita. It does, however, have fewer adverse reactions, a longer dosing interval, and a lower cost than *PTU*; therefore, it is most often prescribed in nonpregnant women.

Other medical therapies include *iodide* and *lithium*, both of which reduce thyroid hormone release and inhibit the organification of iodine. *Iodide* also leads to the secondary coupling of T_3 and T_4. These medications are rarely used in women of reproductive age because of their risks to the fetal thyroid and to fetal development (*iodine* causes congenital goiter; *lithium* is associated with Ebstein's anomaly).

Surgery

A subtotal thyroidectomy is less commonly used primarily but is used routinely if medical treatment fails or if a patient is hypersensitive to medical therapy. Surgery is the most rapid and consistent method of achieving a euthyroid state in Graves' disease and avoids the possible long-term risks of radioactive iodine. Children, young women, pregnant women, and patients with coexistent thyroid nodules are potential candidates for thyroidectomy. It is felt to be the treatment of choice for a patient with significant Graves' ophthalmology. Patients should be rendered euthyroid before a thyroidectomy. The risks of surgery include postoperative hypoparathyroidism, recurrent laryngeal nerve paralysis, routine anesthetic and surgical risks, hypothyroidism, and failure to relieve thyrotoxicosis.

β-Blockers

Propranolol is occasionally used prior to surgery in patients who prove to be hypersensitive to other medical therapy and to provide symptomatic relief while awaiting a reduction in T_4 caused by *PTU* or *methimazole*.

14.1.4.6 Thyroid Storm

In severe hyperthyroidism, physiologic stress, including childbirth, systemic infection, or surgery may provoke a life threatening spectrum of symptoms. These include diarrhea, vomiting, and fever, with associated dehydration, as well as altered mental status that may proceed to coma. Patients with poorly controlled hyperthyroidism are most susceptible. Beta blockers, glucorticoids, PTU (the action of which includes inhibition T4-T3 conversion), and iodides are key elements of therapy for this life-threatening state.

14.1.4.7 Hyperthyroidism in Gestational Trophoblastic Disease and Hyperemesis Gravidarum

Because of the weak TSH-like activity of hCG, conditions with high levels of hCG such as molar pregnancy may be associated with biochemical, and clinical hyperthyroidism. Symptoms regress with removal of the abnormal trophoblastic tissue and resolution of the elevated levels of hCG. In a similar fashion, when hyperemesis gravidarum is associated with high levels of hCG, mild biochemical and clinical features of hyperthyroidism may be seen [62, 63].

14.1.4.8 Thyroid Function in Pregnancy

High levels of hCG at the end of the first trimester are sufficient to contribute to the thyrotropic effects of TSH and TSH levels show transient depression because of this phenomenon resulting in the recent guidelines from the Endocrine Society. Thyroid hormone requirements in pregnancy increase moderately. Patients depending on replacement thyroid hormone require monitoring for often needed increases in thyroid hormone replacement (estimated at 30–50%) in pregnancy commencing in the first weeks of pregnancy. Evidence suggests that optimal fetal and infant neurodevelopmental outcomes require careful titration of replacement thyroxine that addresses the frequently increased requirements of pregnancy [64, 65].

14.1.4.9 Reproductive Effects of Hyperthyroidism

High levels of TSHR-Ab in women with Graves' disease have been associated with fetal-neonatal hyperthyroidism [66, 67]. Despite both the inhibition and elevation of gonadotropins seen in thyrotoxicosis [68], most women remain ovulatory and fertile [69]. Severe thyrotoxicosis can result in weight loss, menstrual cycle irregularities, and amenorrhea. An increased risk of spontaneous abortion is noted in women with thyrotoxicosis. In the offspring of women treated with methimazole, an increased incidence of congenital anomalies, particularly apalsia cutis is noted in their offspring [70].

Autoimmune hyperthyroid Graves' disease may improve spontaneously, in which case antithyroid drug therapy may be reduced or stopped. Nevertheless, TSHR-Ab production may persist for several years after radical radioactive iodine therapy or surgical treatment for hyperthyroid Graves' disease. Thus, there is a risk of exposing a fetus to TSHR-Ab in all patients who have ever carried this diagnosis. Fetal-neonatal hyperthyroidism is observed in 2–10% of pregnancies occurring in mothers with a current or previous diagnosis of Graves' disease, secondary to the transplacental passage of maternal TSHR-Ab. This is a serious condition with a 16% neonatal mortality rate as well as a risk of intrauterine fetal death, stillbirth, and skeletal developmental abnormalities such as craniosynostosis. Caution against overtreatment with antithyroid medication is also warranted as these may cross the placenta in sufficient quantities to induce fetal goiter. Guidelines for TSHR-Ab testing during pregnancy in women with previously treated Graves' disease are found in Table 14.6.

Fetal goiters and the associated fetal hypo- or hyperthyroid status have been diagnosed accurately in mother's with Graves' disease using a combination of fetal ultrasound of the thyroid with Doppler assessing for goiter, fetal heart rate and cardiac function, bone maturation, and maternal TSHR-Ab and antithyroid drug status [71]. A number of pregnancy complications have been reported in Graves' disease including preeclampsia [11, 72, 73], intrauterine growth retatardation and low birth weight [74], and preterm delivery [72].

Postpartum Thyroid Dysfunction

This clinical entity is more common than recognized; its symptoms appear one to eight months postpartum and are often confused with postpartum depression and difficulties

Table 14.6 Guidelines for TSHR-Ab testing during pregnancy with previously treated Graves' disease

1. Women with previous Graves' disease treated with ATD and maintaining remission, have a minimal risk for fetal-neonatal hyperthyroidism, and some feel systematic measurement of TSHR-Ab is not necessary. Thyroid function should be evaluated during pregnancy to detect a possible recurrence. If noted, TSHR-Ab testing is mandatory.
2. Women with antecedent Graves' disease previously treated with radioiodine or thyroidectomy, regardless of their present thyroid status (euthyroidism with or without thyroxine substitution), should have TSHR-Ab measurement to evaluate the risk for fetal hyperthyroidism. If the TSHR-Ab level is high, careful monitoring of the fetus is mandatory for the early detection of signs of thyroid overstimulation (tachycardia, impaired growth rate, oligohydramnios, goiter). Cardiac echography and measurement of circulatory velocity may confirm fetal hyperthyroidism. Ultrasonographic size measurements of the fetal thyroid are defined from 20 weeks gestational age. Color Doppler ultrasonography is helpful in evaluating thyroid hypervascularity. Because of the risk of fetal-neonatal hyperthyroid cardiac insufficiency and the inability to measure the degree of thyroid stimulation in the mother due to previous thyroid ablation, cordocentesis can be considered . This procedure, at 25–27 weeks gestation, has less than a 1% adverse events rate (fetal bleeding, bradycardia, infection, spontaneous abortion, in utero death). Maternal ATD administration is effective in treating fetal hyperthyroidism.
3. Women with concurrent hyperthyroid Graves' disease, regardless of whether it has preceded the onset of pregnancy, should have ATD treatment monitored and adjusted to keep the free T_4 in the high-normal range. This prevents fetal hypothyroidism. TSHR-Ab should be measured in each trimester, especially if the required ATD dosage is high. If the TSHR-Ab assay is negative or the level low, fetal-neonatal hyperthyroidism is rare. If antibody levels are high (TBII ≥ 40 U/L or TSAb ≥ 300%), fetal ultrasound to detect hyperthyroidism is required. In this situation, there is usually a good correlation between maternal and fetal thyroid function such that monitoring the ATD dosage based on the mother's thyroid status is appropriate. In cases where a high dose of ATD (>300 mg/d of propylthiouracil [PTU] or >20 mg/d of methimazole) is necessary, there is a risk of goitrous hypothyroidism in the fetus which could be indistinguishable from goitrous Graves' disease. The correct diagnosis relies on the assay of fetal thyroid hormones and TSH by cordocentesis.
4. In any woman who has previously given birth to a newborn with hyperthyroidism, a TSHR-Ab assay should be performed early in the course of pregnancy and in each trimester.

ATD autoimmune thyroid disease, *TSHR-Ab* thyroid-stimulating hormone receptor antibodies, *TBII* TSH-binding inhibitory immunoglobulin, *TSAb* thyroid-stimulating antibody, T_4 thyroxine

adjusting to the demands of the neonate and infant. Following are criteria for the diagnosis of postpartum thyroiditis: (a) no history of thyroid hormonal abnormalities either before or during pregnancy, (b) documented abnormal TSH level (either depressed or elevated) during the first year postpartum, and (c) absence of a positive TSH-receptor antibody titer (Graves' disease) or a toxic nodule. Amino and others, who alerted clinicians to this condition, documented an incidence of approximately 5% in their population [75]. A number of studies now describe clinical and biochemical evidence of postpartum thyroid dysfunction in 5–10% of new mothers [76]. These women have a 25–30% chance of becoming permanently hypothyroid.

Histologically, lymphocytic infiltration and inflammation are found. Antimicrosomal antibodies are also found in this disorder [77, 78]. Women who are at greatest risk of developing this disorder are those with a personal or family history of the disorder, those with an autoimmune thyroid disorder, or those with an autoimmune disease.

Clinical Characteristics and Diagnosis

Postpartum thyroiditis begins with a transient hyperthyroid phase between 6 weeks and 6 months postpartum followed by a hypothyroid phase in nearly one quarter of the cases, while one-third have either hyperthyroidism or hypothyroidism alone. Individuals with type 1 diabetes are three times more likely to develop postpartum thyroiditis. Women with a history of postpartum thyroiditis in a previous pregnancy have nearly a 70% chance of recurrence in a subsequent pregnancy. Numerous case reports demonstrate a possible association between postpartum thyroiditis and other autoimmune disorders. The rebounding immune system in the postpartum state with the presence of thyroid autoantibodies may explain the timing of the onset. Postpartum thyroid dysfunction should be considered in all women with postpartum psychosis. The thyrotoxic phase may be subclinical and overlooked in iodine insufficient areas [79]. Those with the hyperthyroidism due to postpartum thyroiditis have a low level of radioactive isotope uptake, in contrast to those with Graves disease. The absence of thyroid tenderness, pain, fever, elevated sedimentation rate, and leukocytosis helps to rule out subacute thyroiditis (de Quervain thyroiditis).

Treatment

Most patients are diagnosed during the hypothyroid phase and require 6–12 months of T_4 replacement. Nearly 30% of women develop permanent hypothyroidism, TSH should be evaluated following discontinuation of replacement therapy. Rarely, patients are diagnosed during the hyperthyroid phase [80]. Antithyroid medications are not routinely used for these women. Propranolol may be used for symptomatic relief. Approximately two-thirds of these patients return to a euthyroid state, and one-third remain hypothyroid.

14.1.4.10 Antithyroid Antibodies and Disorders of Reproduction

Women who have antithyroid autoantibodies before and after conception appear to be at an increased risk for spontaneous abortion [81, 82]. Nonorgan-specific antibody production and pregnancy loss are documented in cases of antiphospholipid abnormalities [83]. The co-occurrence of organ-specific thyroid antibodies and nonorgan-specific autoantibody production is recognized [83–85], and in the case of recurrent pregnancy loss, thyroid autoantibodies may serve as peripheral markers of abnormal T-cell function and a potential cause of reproductive failure [86].

14.1.4.11 Thyroid Nodules

Thyroid nodules are occasionally noted on physical examination and are demonstrated by ultrasonography in more than 50% of patients [87]. Clinical and laboratory evaluations should be applied to distinguish functional from nonfunctional nodules, which are occasionally malignant. For nonfunctional "cold" nodules, fine-needle biopsy and aspiration are required to rule out malignancy. In the case of indeterminate aspirates, 2–20% are malignant; therefore, surgical biopsy is often indicated [88].

14.1.4.12 Gonadal Dysgenesis and Down Syndrome

Patients with gonadal dysgenesis (Turner syndrome, and other forms of hypergonadotropic hypogonadism associated with abnormalities of the second sex chromosome) exhibit a high prevalence of autoimmune thyroid disorders. Around 50% of adult patients with Turner syndrome have antithyroid peroxidase (anti-TPO) and antithyroglobulin (anti-TG) autoantibodies. Nearly 30% of antithyroid antibody positive, Turner patients will develop subclinical or clinical hypothyroidism. The disorder is indistinguishable from Hashimoto's thyroiditis. A susceptibility locus for Graves' disease is also noted on chromosome X [89].

Down syndrome, caused by an extra chromosome 21, is characterized by an atypical body habitus, mental retardation, cardiac malformations, an increased risk for leukemia, and a reduced life expectancy. The extra chromosome is almost always of maternal origin. Autoimmune thyroid disorders are more common in patients with Down syndrome than in the general population. The gene for autoimmune polyglandular syndrome I (APECED) has been mapped to chromosome 21 and is thought to be a transcription factor involved in immune regulation (AIRE) and may play a role in the development of autoimmune thyroid disease in these patients [90]. Hashimoto's thyroiditis is the most common abnormality in Down syndrome. Hypothyroidism develops in as many as 50% of patients over age 40 with Down syndrome. These clinical syndromes and other evidence suggest part of the genetic susceptibility to Hashimoto's thyroiditis may reside on chromosomes X and 21.

14.2 Prolactin Disorders

Prolactin was first identified as a product of the anterior pituitary in 1933 [91] and later as a hormone in 1971. The activities attributed to human prolactin (hPRL) were defined by the separation of its activity from growth hormone [92] and subsequently by the development of radioimmunoassays [93, 94]. Although the initiation and maintenance of lactation is the most visible function of prolactin, many studies have documented roles for prolactin activity both within and beyond the reproductive system.

14.2.1 Prolactin Secretion

Human prolactin has 199 amino acids, with a molecular weight (MW) of 23,000 daltons. While human growth hormone and placental lactogen have significant lactogenic activity, there is only 16% and 13% amino acid sequence homology with prolactin, respectively. A single gene on chromosome 6 encodes prolactin. The prolactin gene (10 kb) has five exons and four introns and its transcription is regulated in the pituitary by a proximal promotor region and in extrapituitary locations by a more upstream promotor [95].

Humans release three forms of prolactin, a monomer, a dimer, and a multimeric species, called *little, big, and big-big prolactin*, respectively [96–98]. Big and Big-big prolactin are degraded to the monomeric form by reducing disulfide bonds [99]. The heterogeneity of secreted forms vary with physiologic, pathologic, and hormonal stimulation [99–102]. Little prolactin (MW 23,000 daltons) represents greater than 50% of all prolactin production and is the most responsive to extrapituitary stimulation or suppression [99, 101, 102]. Clinical assays for prolactin measure the "little" prolactin. Prolactin, growth hormone, placental lactogen, gonadotropins and TSH do not require glycosylation for their primary activities. Glycosylated forms are secreted, and glycosylation does affect the bioactivity and immunoreactivity of little prolactin [103–106]. The glycosylated form is the predominant species secreted, while the most potent is the 23,000-dalton nonglycosylated form of prolactin [105]. Prolactin has over 300 known biological activities. Prolactin's activities include those associated with repoduction: lactation, luteal function, reproductive behavior; and homeostasis: immune responsivity, osomoregulation, and agiogenesis [107]. Despite these many activities, the only known disorder associated with a deficiency of prolactin secretion is inability to lactate.

Contrary to other anterior pituitary hormones, which are controlled by hypothalamic-releasing factors, prolactin secretion is primarily under inhibitory control mediated by dopamine. Dopamine, a product of tuberoinfundibular dopaminergic neurons tranmitted to portal hypophyseal vessels, is the primary prolactin-inhibiting factor. Dopamine receptors are present on pituitary lactotrophs [108], and treatment with dopamine or dopamine agonists suppress prolactin secretion [109–114]. The dopamine antagonist metaoclopramide abolishes the pulsatility of prolactin release and subsequently increases serum prolactin levels [110, 111, 115–119]. Pituitary mass lesions, or blockade of the dopamine receptor with antipsychotic, and other medications, increases serum prolactin levels. Excess thyrotropin releasing hormone (TRH) causes prolactin release, but does not appear to play an important modulatory role in the normal physiologic regulation of prolactin secretion. γ-Aminobutyric acid (GABA) and other neurohormones and neurotransmitters also may function as prolactin-inhibiting factors (Table 14.7). Numerous hypothalamic polypeptides that modulate prolactin-releasing activity are listed in Table 14.7. Dopamine and TRH are considered primary neurohormones while others (neuropeptide Y, galanin and enkephalin) acts as modulators.

Table 14.7 Factors that modulate prolactin release as well as conditions and medications that result in hyperprolactinemia

Inhibitory factors
γ-Aminobutyric acid
Dopamine
Histidyl-proline diketopiperazine
Pyroglutamic acid
Somatostatin
Stimulatory factors
β-Endorphin
Enkephalins
17β-Estradiol
Gonadotropin-releasing hormone (GnRH)
Histamine
Serotonin
Substance P
Thyrotropin-releasing hormone (TRH)
Vasoactive intestinal peptide (VIP)
Physiologic conditions
Anesthesia
Empty sella syndrome
Idiopathic
Intercourse
Newborns
Nipple stimulation
Pregnancy
Postpartum (nonnursing: days 1–7; nursing: with suckling)
Sleep
Stress (including physical examination)
Surgery on and disorders of the chest wall (burns, herpes, chest percussion)
Postpartum
Hypothalamic conditions
Arachnoid cyst
Craniopharyngioma
Cystic glioma
Cysticercosis
Dermoid cyst
Epidermoid cyst
Histiocytosis
Neurotuberculosis
Pineal tumors
Pseudotumor cerebri
Sarcoidosis
Suprasellar cysts
Tuberculosis
Pituitary conditions
Acromegaly
Addison's disease
Craniopharyngioma
Cushing's syndrome
Hypothyroidism
Histiocytosis
Lymphoid hypophysitis
Metastatic tumors from the lungs and breasts and others
Multiple endocrine neoplasia (MEN)
Nelson's syndrome
Pituitary adenomas both microadenoma and macroadenomas
Post-oral contraception
Sarcoidosis
Thyrotropin-releasing hormone administration
Trauma to pituitary stalk
Tuberculosis
Metabolic dysfunction
Ectopic production (bronchogenic sarcoma, fibroid, hypernephroma)
Hepatic cirrhosis
Renal failure
Starvation refeeding
Medications resulting in hyperprolactinemia
α Methyldopa
Antidepressants (amoxapine, imipramine, amitriptyline)
Cimetidine
Dopamine antagonists (phenothiazines, thioxanthenes, butyrophenone, diphenylbutylpiperidine, dibenzoxazepine, dihydroindolone, procainamide, metaclopramide)
Estrogen therapy
Opiates
Reserpine
Sulpiride
Verapamil

The prolactin receptor is a class 1 cytokine receptor superfamily member and is encoded by a gene on chomosome 5 [120]. Transcriptional regulation of the prolactin receptor is accomplished through three tissue specific promoter regions; promoter I for the gonads, promoter II for the liver, and III, a generic promoter which includes the mammary gland [121].

14.2.2 Hyperprolactinemia

Physiologic disturbances, pharmacologic agents or markedly compromised renal function may cause elevations in prolactin levels and transient elevations occur with acute stress or painful stimuli. Patients using antipsychotic medications, and patients using agents with antidopaminergic properties may exhibit moderately elevated prolactin levels. Drug-related and physiologic conditions resulting in hyperprolactinemia do not always require interventions to normalize prolactin levels.

14.2.2.1 Evaluation

Plasma levels of immunoreactive prolactin are 5–27 ng/ml during the normal menstrual cycle. Prolactin levels may be elevated early in the morning and after procedures. Prolactin is secreted in a pulsatile fashion with a pulse frequency ranging from about 9 to14 pulses per 24 h in the late luteal and follicular phases, respectively. Prolactin levels rise 1 h after the onset of sleep and continue to rise until peak values are reached between 5:00 and 7:00 A.M. [122, 123]. The pulse amplitude of prolactin appears to increase from early to late follicular and luteal phases [124–126].

Any single elevation of prolactin level should prompt a repeat evaluation. This sample should be drawn midmorning and not after stress, breast stimulation, physical examination, or venipuncture, all of which may increase prolactin levels.

When prolactin levels are found to be elevated, hypothyroidism and medications should first be ruled out as a cause. Prolactin and TSH determinations are basic evaluations in infertile women and hypogonadal males. Prolactin levels should be measured in the evaluation of amenorrhea, galactorrhea, amenorrhea with galactorrhea, hirsutism with amenorrhea, anovulatory bleeding, and delayed puberty. The workup of hyperprolactinemia is outlined in Fig. 14.7.

14.2.2.2 Physical Signs

Hyperprolactinemia may cause galactorrhea, anovulation causing amenorrhea, their combination, or no symptoms. Hyperprolactinemia causes amenorrhea without galactorrhea in approximately 15% of women [127, 128]. Hyperprolactinemia may cause anovulatory amenorrhea via inhibition of hypothalamic GnRH pulsatile release [109, 129–139]. In addition to the hyperprolactinemia induced hypogonadotropic state, prolactin may also impair the mechanisms of ovulation by reducing granulosa cell number and FSH binding [140], inhibition of granulosa cell 17β-estradiol production by interfering with FSH action [140–142], and by causing inadequate luteinization and progesterone secretion [143–145]. In isolated galactorrhea, prolactin levels are within the normal range in nearly 50% of such patients [146–148] (Fig. 14.7). In these cases, stimulus of the breast to produce galactorrhea may have been caused by a transient hyperprolactinemiaor other unknown factors. This situation is akin to that observed in nursing mothers in whom milk secretion, once established, continues and even increases despite a normalizedprolactin level. About one-third of women with galactorrhea have normal menses. Conversely, hyperprolactinemia commonly occurs in the absence of galactorrhea (66%), which may result from inadequate estrogenic or progestational priming of the breast.

Patients with galactorrhea and amenorrhea (including the syndromes described and named by Forbes, Henneman, Griswold, and Albright in 1951, Argonz and del Castilla in 1953, and Chiari and Frommel in 1985), demonstrate hyperprolactinemia two-thirds of the time; and in that group, about one-third will have a pituitary adenoma [149]. Anovulatory women, diagnosed with polycystic ovary disease have coexistent, and usually modest hyperprolactinemia in 3–10% [150, 151] (Fig. 14.7).

Prolactin and TSH levels should be measured in all patients with delayed puberty. In cases of delayed puberty with low basal gonadotropin levels, pituitary abnormalities, such as craniopharyngiomas and adenomas, must be considered regardless of the prolactin levels.

In the presence of prolactin secreting pituitary adenomasand delayed puberty, multiple endocrine neoplasia type 1 (MEN-1) syndrome (gastrinomas, insulinoma, parathyroid hyperplasia, and pituitary neoplasia) should be considered. It should be noted that symptoms of pituitary adenoma are rarely the presenting symptom in MEN-1. Patients with pituitary adenomas and a family history of multiple adenomas deserve particular scrutiny [152]. Prolactinomas are noted in approximately 20% of patients with MEN-1. The *MEN-1* gene is localized to chromosome 11q13 and acts as a constitutive tumor suppressor gene. Inactivating mutations result in development of the tumors. Prolactin secreting pituitary adenomas that occur in patients with MEN-1 may be more aggressive than sporadic cases [153].

Pituitary hyperprolactinemia is most often due to a microadenoma or associated with normal imaging findings. These patients should be reassured of the generally benign course of their condition. Patients with macroadenomas or

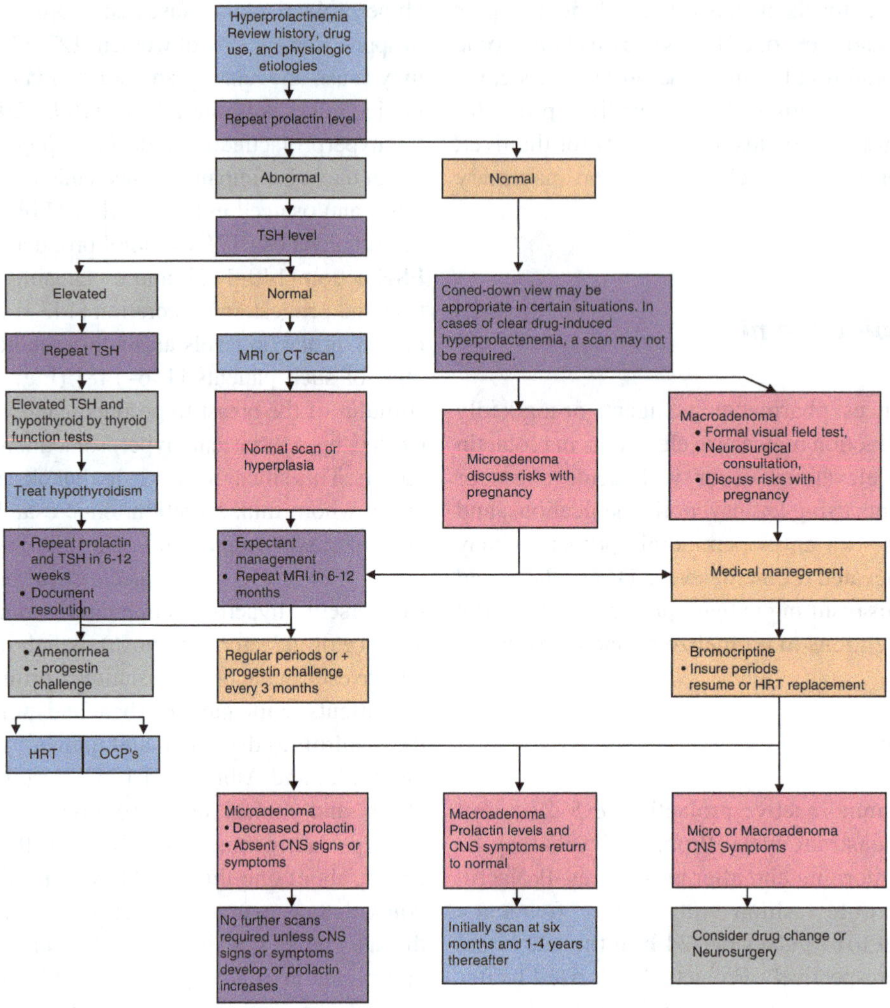

Fig. 14.7 Workup for hyperprolactinemia

juxtasellar lesions require more complex evaluations and treatment algorithms. Some will require surgical management. All patients with hyperprolactinemia should have a TSH measurement (Fig. 14.7)

14.2.2.3 Imaging Techniques

Larger microadenomas and macroadenomas result in prolactin levels that are usually higher than 100 ng/ml. However, levels lower than 100 ng/ml may be associated with smaller microadenomas, macroadenomas that produce a "stalk section" effect, and suprasellar tumors that may be missed on a "coned-down" view of the sella turcica. Because modest elevations of prolactin can be associated with microadenomas, macroadenomas, nonlactotroph pituitary tumors, and other central nervous system abnormalities, imaging of the pituitary gland must be considered for unexplained and persistent prolactin elevations (Table 14.8).

In patients with identifiable drug-induced or physiologic hyperprolactinemia, imaging is not routinely necessary unless it is accompanied by symptoms that suggest a mass lesion (headache, visual field deficits). MRI imaging of the sella and pituitary gland with gadolinium enhancement provides the best anatomic detail [154] (Fig. 14.8). It also represents the safest imaging modality because the cumulative radiation dose from multiple CT scans may cause cataracts, and the "coned-down" views or tomograms of the sella are very insensitive. For patients with hyperprolactinemia who desire future fertility, MRI is used to differentiate a pituitary microadenoma from a macroadenoma as well as to identify other potential sellar-suprasellar masses. Although rare, when pregnancy-related complications of a pituitary adenoma occur, they occur more frequently in the presence of macroadenomas.

Table 14.8 Sellar and suprasellar tumors and conditions that may result in hyperprolactinemia

Abscess
Aneurysm
Arachnoid cyst
Cephalocele
Chloroma (granulocytic sarcoma)
Colloid cyst
Craniopharyngioma
Dermoid
Ectopic neurohypophysis
"Empty" sella
Epidermoid tumor
Germinoma
Hamartoma (tuber cinereum/hypothalmus)
Histiocytosis
Hyperplasia
Hypophysitis
Lipoma
Lymphoma
Meningioma
Meningitis (bacterial, fungal, granulomatous)
Metastasis
Mucocele
Nasopharyngeal carcinoma
Opticochiasmatic-hypothalamic glioma
Osteocartilaginous tumor
Paracytic cyst
Pars intermedia cysts
Pituitary adenoma
Rathke's cleft cyst
Sarcoidosis

In over 90% of untreated women, microadenomas do not enlarge over a 4–6 year period. The rationale for medical therapy as a mechanism to prevent a microadenoma from growing is false. Additionally, while prolactin levels correlate with tumor size, both elevations and reductions in prolactin levels may occur without any change in tumor size. If during follow-up a prolactin level rises significantly or central nervous system symptoms (headache, visual changes) are noted, repeat imaging may be indicated.

14.2.2.4 Hypothalamic Disorders

Dopamine is a product of the arcuate nucleus. Dopamine-releasing neurons innervate the external zone of the median eminence. When released into the hypophyseal portal system, dopamine inhibits prolactin release in the anterior pituitary. Lesions that disrupt dopamine release can result in hyperprolactinemia. Lesions that disrupt dopamine release may arise from the suprasellar area, pituitary gland, and infundibular stalk, as well as from adjacent bone, brain, cranial nerves, dura, leptomeninges, nasopharynx, and vessels. Many pathologic entities and physiologic conditions in the hypothalamic-pituitary region can disrupt dopamine release and cause hyperprolactinemia (Table 14.7).

14.2.2.5 Pituitary Disorders

Microadenomas

More than one-third of women with hyperprolactinemia, have a radiologic abnormality consistent with a microadenoma (<1 cm). Release of pituitary stem cell growth inhibition via activation or loss-of-function mutations results in cell cycle dysregulation resulting in autonomous anterior pituitary hormone production, secretion, and cell proliferation. These mutations are critical to the development of pituitary microadenomas and macroadenomas. Microadenomas and macroadenomas are monoclonal in origin. Additional anatomic factors that contribute to adenoma formation include reduced dopamine concentrations in the hypophyseal portal system and vascular isolation of the tumor or both. Recently, the heparin-binding secretory transforming (HST) gene has been noted in a variety of cancers as well as in prolactinomas [155]. Patients with microadenomas can generally be reassured of a benign course and many of these lesions exhibit gradual spontaneous regression or perivascular fibrosis and regression after treatment with ergot alkaloids [156, 157].

Pituitary prolactinomas or lactotrope adenomas are sparsely or densely granulated histologically. The sparsely granulated lactotrope adenomas have trabecular, papillary, or solid patterns. Calcification of these tumors may take the form of a psammoma body or a pituitary stone. Densely granulated lactotrope adenomas are strongly acidophilic tumors and appear to be more aggressive than sparsely granulated lactotrope adenomas. Unusual acidophil stem cell adenomas can be associated with hyperprolactinemia with some clinical or biochemical evidence of growth hormone excess.

Microadenomas rarely progress to macroadenomas. Six large series of patients with microadenomas reveal that, with no treatment, the risk of progression for microadenoma to a macroadenoma is only 7% [158]. Treatments include expectant, medical or, rarely, surgical therapy. Affected women should be advised to notify their physicians of chronic headaches, visual disturbances (particularly tunnel vision consistent with bitemporal hemianopsia), and extraocular muscle palsies. Formal visual field testing is rarely helpful unless imaging suggests compression of the optic nerves or in monitoring symptomatic macroadenomas in pregnancy.

Autopsy series reveals that 25% of the U.S. population harbors microadenomas, and approximately 40% stains positively for prolactin. Clinically significant pituitary tumors requiring some type of intervention affect only 14 per 100,000 individuals [159].

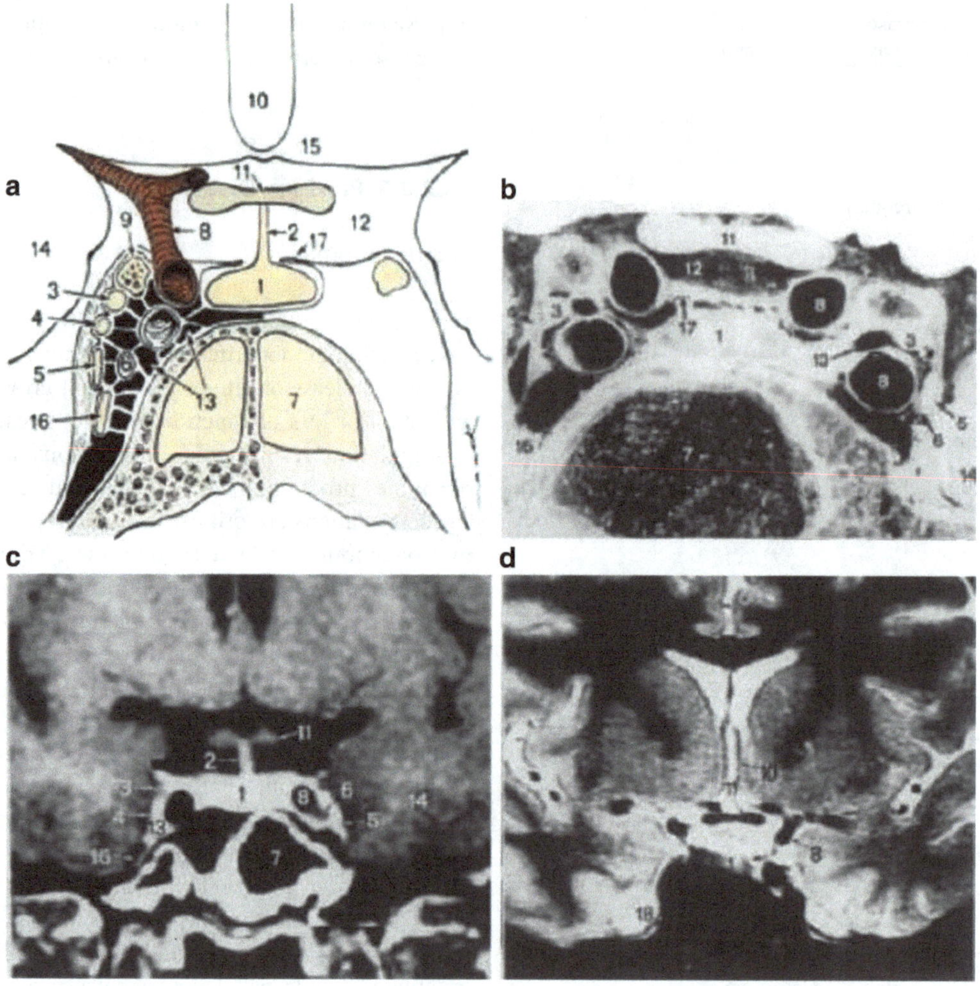

Fig. 14.8 Anatomy of the intrasellar region and cavernous sinus by: (A) anatomic diagram, (B) coronal cytomicrosome section, (C) coronal postcontrast T1-weighted MRI, and (D) coronal postcontrast T2-weighted MRI. (1, pituitary gland; 2, infundibular stalk; 3, cranial nerve (CN) III; 4, CN IV; 5, CN VI; 6, CN VI; 7, sphenoid sinus; 8, internal carotid artery; 9, anterior clinoid process; 10, third ventricle; 11, optic chiasm; 12, suprasellar cistern; 13, venous spaces of cavernous sinus; 14, temporal lobe; 15, hypothalamus; 16, CN V_2; 17, diaphragma sellae; 18, Meckel's cave.)

Expectant Management

Expectant management can be used for both microadenomas and hyperprolactinemia without an adenoma if menstrual function remains intact and fertility is not desired. Hyperprolactinemia-induced estrogen deficiency is the cause of osteopenia and osteoporosis [160]. Estrogen replacement with typical hormone replacement regimens or hormonal contraceptives is indicated for patients with amenorrhea or irregular menses. Patients with drug-induced hyperprolactinemia can also be managed expectantly with attention to the risks of osteoporosis. In the absence of symptoms of pituitary enlargement and prolactin levels remain normal, a repeat MRI may not be required after 12 months at the discretion of the practitioner.

Medical Treatment

Ergot alkaloids are the mainstay of therapy. In 1985, bromocriptine was approved for use in the United States to treat hyperprolactinemia caused by a pituitary adenoma.

These agents are dopamine agonists and cause decreasing prolactin levels. Effects on prolactin levels occur quickly (within hours) and lesion size may decrease in volume within one or two weeks. *Bromocriptine* decreases prolactin synthesis, DNA synthesis, cell multiplication, and the overall size of prolactinomas. Bromocriptine treatment results in normal prolactin blood levels or the return of ovulatory menses in 80–90% of patients.

Because ergot alkaloids, like *bromocriptine*, are excreted via the biliary tree, caution is required in patients with liver disease. Major adverse effects of bromocriptine include nausea, headaches, hypotension, dizziness, fatigue and drowsiness, vomiting, headaches, nasal congestion, and constipation. Many patients tolerate bromocriptine when the dose is increased gradually, by 1.25 mg (½ tablet) per day each week until normalization of prolactin levels is seen or until a dosage of 2.5 mg twice per day is reached. (Regimen: one-half tablet every evening (1.25 mg) for one week, one-half tablet morning and evening (1.25 mg twice daily) during the second week, one-half tablet in the morning (1.25 mg) and a full tablet every evening (2.5 mg) during the third week, and one tablet every morning and early evening during the fourth week and thereafter (2.5 mg twice per day). The lowest dose that maintains the prolactin level in the normal range is continued (1.25 mg twice daily often is sufficient to normalize prolactin levels in individuals with levels less than 100 ng/ml). Pharmacokinetic studies show peak serum levels occur 3 h after an oral dose with a trough at 7 h. There is little detectable bromocriptine in the serum by 11–14 h. Therefore, administration is required twice a day. Prolactin levels can be checked 6–24 h after the last dose.

A psychotic reaction is a rare, but notable, adverse effect of *bromocriptine*. Symptoms include auditory hallucinations, delusional ideas, and changes in mood that resolve after discontinuation of the drug [161].

Many investigators report no difference in fibrosis, calcification, prolactin immunoreactivity, or the surgical success in patients pretreated with *bromocriptine* when compared with those not receiving *bromocriptine* [158].

An alternative to oral administration is the vaginal administration of *bromocriptine* tablets. This route is well tolerated, and actually results in improved pharmacokinetic measures [162]. *Cabergoline*, another ergot alkaloid, has a very long half-life and can be given orally twice per week. Its long duration of action is attributable to slow elimination by pituitary tumor tissue, high affinity binding to pituitary dopamine receptors, and extensive enterohepatic recirculation.

Cabergoline, which is as effective as *bromocriptine* in lowering prolactin levels and in reducing tumor size, has substantially fewer adverse effects than bromocriptine. Rarely, if patients experience nausea and vomiting or dizziness with cabergoline, they may be treated with intravaginal *cabergoline* just as with *bromocriptine*. Although cabergoline appears to be safe to use during pregnancy, more extensive data regarding the use of *bromocriptine* in pregnancy are available; therefore, *bromocriptine* is preferred for pregnant patients. A gradually increasing dosage helps avoid the side effects of nausea, vomiting, and dizziness. Cabergoline at 0.25 mg twice per week is usually adequate for hyperprolactinemia with values less than 100 ng/ml. If required to normalize prolactin levels, the dosage can be increased by 0.25 mg per dose on a weekly basis to a maximum of 1 mg twice weekly.

When *bromocriptine* or *cabergoline* cannot be used, other medications such as *pergolide* or *methergoline* may be used. In patients with a microadenoma who are receiving *bromocriptine* therapy, a repeat MRI scan may be performed 6–12 months after prolactin levels are normalized, if indicated, to document tumor response. Most practitioners use normalization of prolactin as an indicator of response. While normalization of prolactin levels and resumption of menses are strong indicators, they cannot be considered an absolute proof of tumor response, thus, clinical discretion is advised. MRI scans should be performed if new symptoms appear.

Discontinuation of *bromocriptine* therapy after 2–3 years may be attempted in patients who have maintained normoprolactinemia while on therapy [163, 164]. Discontinuation of cabergoline therapy has also been successful in patients treated for 3–4 years who have maintained normoprolactinemia [165]. In general, recurrence rates are higher for macroadenomas (as compared to microadenomas or hyperprolactinemia without adenoma) after cessation of either bromocriptine or cabergoline, warranting close follow-up with serum prolactin and MRI after cessation of therapy. In patients with macroadenomas, withdrawal of therapy should proceed with caution, as rapid tumor re-expansion may occur.

Macroadenomas

Macroadenomas are pituitary tumors that are larger than 1 cm in size. *Bromocriptine* is the best initial and potentially long-term treatment option. Transsphenoidal surgery occasionally is required. Evaluation for pituitary hormone deficiencies may be indicated. Symptoms of macroadenoma enlargement include severe headaches, visual field changes and, rarely, diabetes insipidus and blindness. After prolactin has normalized following ergot alkaloid treatment, a repeat MRI is indicated within 6–12 months to document shrinkage or stabilization of the size of the macroadenoma. This examination may be performed earlier if new symptoms develop or if there is no improvement in previously documented symptoms. Normalized prolactin levels or resumption of menses cannot not be taken as absolute proof of tumor response to treatment, particularly in patients with a macroadenoma.

Medical Treatment

Macroadenomas treated with *bromocriptine* routinely show a reduction in prolactin levels and size; nearly one-half shows a 50% reduction in size, and another one-fourth show a 33% reduction after 6 months of therapy. Tumor regrowth occurs in over 60% of cases after discontinuation of *bromocriptine* therapy, therefore, long-term therapy is usually required.

After stabilization of tumor size, 6–12 months after initiating therapy, is documented, the MRI scan is only repeated as indicated by symptoms. Serum prolactin levels are measured every six months. Because tumors may enlarge despite normalized prolactin values, a reevaluation of symptoms at regular intervals (6 months) is prudent.

Long-term therapy (over 3–5 years) with dopamine agonists occasionally leads to perivascular fibrosis with cytocidal activity within the adenoma. One can consider dopamine agonist withdrawal in a microadenoma if, after ceasing dopamine agonist therapy, the prolaction level remains normal. Periodic prolactin assays and evaluation of symptoms and physical examination in the first year will detect regrowth of the microadenoma. In the case of macroadenoma, if the MRI documents: tumor resolution or >50% reduction; greater than 5 mm distance from the optic chiasm; and no cavernous sinus invasion; one could initiate a stepwise, tapered or an abrupt withdrawal of the dopamine agonist and monitor prolaction levels, symptoms, and and the physical exam every 3 months. In 30–64% of such cases, there is no tumor re-growth [165, 166].

Surgical Intervention

Tumors that are unresponsive to *bromocriptine* or that cause persistent visual field loss require surgical intervention. Some neurosurgeons have noted that a short (2–6 week) preoperative course of bromocriptine increases the efficacy of surgery in patients with larger adenomas [162]. Unfortunately, after surgical resection, recurrence of hyperprolactinemia and tumor growth is common. Complications of surgery include cerebral carotid artery injury, diabetes insipidus, meningitis, nasal septal perforation, partial or panhypopituitarism, spinal fluid rhinorrhea, and third nerve palsy. Periodic MRI scanning after surgery is indicated, particularly in patients with recurrent hyperprolactinemia.

14.2.2.6 Metabolic Dysfunction and Hyperprolactinemia

Patients with hypothyroidism may exhibit hyperprolactinemia with remarkable pituitary enlargement caused by thyrotroph hyperplasia. Thyroid replacement results in a reduction in pituitary enlargement and normalization of prolactin levels [167].

Hyperprolactinemia occurs in 20–75% of women with chronic renal failure. Prolactin levels do not normalize with hemodialysis but normalize after transplantation [168, 169]. Occasionally, women with hyperandrogenemia may have hyperprolactinemia. Elevated prolactin levels may alter adrenal function by enhancing the release of adrenal androgens such as DHEAS [129].

14.2.2.7 Drug-induced Hyperprolactinemia

Numerous drugs interfere with dopamine secretion and can therefore be responsible for hyperprolactinemia. (Table 14.7) If medication can be discontinued, prolactin levels return to normal rapidly. If the medications cannot be discontinued, management includes estrogen replacement or oral contraceptive agentsto avoid osteopenia/porosis. Treatment with dopamine agonists may be utilized if ovulation is desired and the drug inducing hyperprolactinemia cannot be discontinued.

14.2.2.8 Use of Estrogen in Hyperprolactinemia

In rodents, pituitary prolactin-secreting adenomas occur with high-dose estrogen administration [170]. Elevated levels of estrogen, such as those found in pregnancy, are responsible for hypertrophy and hyperplasia of lactotrophic cells, and account for the progressive increase in prolactin levels in normal pregnancy. However, the prolactin elevations found in pregnancy is physiologic, and reversible, and adenomas are not fostered by the hyperestrogemia of pregnancy. Indeed, pregnancy may have a favorable influence on preexisting prolactinomas [171, 172]. Studies [173–175] and autopsy surveys [176] indicate that estrogen administration is not associated with clinical, biochemical, or radiologic evidence of growth of pituitary microadenomas or the progression of idiopathic hyperprolactinemia to adenoma status. For these reasons, estrogen replacement or OC use is appropriate for hypoestrogenic patients with hyperprolactinemia secondary to microadenoma or hyperplasia.

14.2.2.9 Monitoring Pituitary Adenomas During Pregnancy

Prolactin-secreting microadenomas rarely cause complications during pregnancy. However, monitoring of patients with serial gross visual field examinations and funduscopic examination is recommended. If persistent headaches, visual field deficits, or visual or funduscopic changes occur, MRI scanning is advisable. Because serum prolactin levels progressively rise throughout pregnancy, prolactin measurements are rarely of any value.

For those women who become pregnant while taking bromocriptine due to return of spontaneous ovulations, it is recommended that bromocriptine be discontinued. Discontinuation does not preclude the subsequent use of bromocriptine during pregnancy to treat symptoms (visual field defects, headaches) that might arise from the rare enlargement of the adenoma [177, 178]. There is a physiologic increase in pituitary size in pregnancy separate from adenoma changes that rarely causes symptoms despite the adenoma. Bromocriptine has not exhibited teratogenecity in animals, and observational data in humans is reassuring.

Pregnant women with previous transsphenoidal surgery for microadenomas or macroadenomas may be monitored additionally with monthly Goldman perimetry visual field testing. Periodic MRI scanning may be necessary in women with symptoms or visual changes. Breast feeding is not contraindicated in the presence of microadenomas or macroadenomas [177, 178]. The use of bromocriptine and other dopaminergic agents classified as ergot alkaloids to inhibit postpartum lactation may cause blood pressure elevations during the postpartum period, and are contraindicated [179–183].

14.3 Conclusion: Evidence-Based Case Studies

Case 1. A 25 year old woman presents for infertility workup. A TSH evaluation yields a value of 10.68 mIU/ML. What is the work- up and treatment recommendation?

Because of a number of adverse effects on reproduction associated with hypothyroidism (Table 14.3) includingsubfertility, miscarriage, anemia, gestational hypertension, abruption, postpartum hemorrhage, preterm delivery, impaired neuropsychological development system in the fetus, a TSH evaluation is part of the standard workup for infertility. Furthermore, the currently recommended *targeted screening* guidelines designed to avoid maternal hypothyroidism in pregnancy suggest testing in individuals with autoimmune disorders, clinical signs/symptoms of thyroid disease, family history of thyroid disease, goiter, head and neck radiation, history of thyroid disorder, infertility, thyroid auto-antibodies, and preterm delivery. Thus, for the reproductive endocrinologist, nearly all patients require a TSH evaluation and treatment when elevated. Despite the widespread TSH screening associated with reproductive medicine,universal TSH screening in pregnancy is not recommended at the present time.

After confirming the elevated TSH, autoantibodies to thyroglobin and thyroid peroxidase are obtained to confirm the diagnosis of Hashimotos' thryoiditis (Table 14.1). Levothyroxine, 50 μg, is initiated with a half life of 7 days; therefore, a repeat TSH is drawn in six weeks later to assess treatment efficacy. Treatment guidelines, in this woman seeking pregnancy and others like her, recognize: (1) the potentially significant adverse effects on the neurologic development of the fetus and other adverse pregnancy events (Table 14.3); (2) the physiologic rise in TBG and the TSH-like activity of hCG in pregnancy (Fig. 14.4), and: (3) that this patient, and others like her, may have overt or subclinical hypothyroidism defined by the a reference range for pregnancy (TSH < 2.5, 3.1 and 3.5 mIU /ml for the first, second and third trimesters, respectively) (Fig. 14.5). According to these recommendations, this preconceptionally diagnosed hypothyroid woman (overt or subclinical) should have her T_4 dose adjusted such that her TSH value is < 2.5 μU/ml before pregnancy. The T_4 replacement dosage will routinely require a dose escalation at 4–6 weeks gestation in order to maintain the TSH value < 2.5 μU/ml. This adjustment may require a 30–50% increase in dosage (levothyroxine, increased from 50 μg to 75 μg). Pregnant women with overt hypothyroidism should be normalized as rapidly as possible to maintain TSH at less than 2.5 and 3 μU/ml in the first and second/third trimesters, respectively. For this patient, and others like her, it should be remembered that euthyroid women on no levothyroxine, with thyroid autoantibodies are at risk of hypothyroidism and should also have TSH screening in each trimester [35].

Case 2. A 25 year old woman with a macroadenoma treated with bromocriptine achieves pregnancy after the normalization of her prolactin level and the resumption of regular ovulation. What is the recommendation for treatment?

Macroadenomas treated with *bromocriptine* respond by decreased prolactin levels and volume; nearly one-half shows a 50% reduction in size, and another one-fourth shows a 33% reduction after six months of therapy. Tumor regrowth occurs in over 60% of cases after discontinuation of *bromocriptine* therapy, but treatment with bromocriptine during pregnancy is not necessarily required, despite the additional physiologic increase in pituitary size. Most recommend discontinuation of the bromocriptine. MRI repeat scans are only repeated as indicated by symptoms. Because serum prolactin levels progressively rise throughout pregnancy, prolactin measurements are rarely of any value. Discontinuation of bromocriptine does not exclude its later use during pregnancy to treat symptoms (visual field defects, headaches) arising from the rare enlargement of the adenoma. Bromocriptine has not exhibited teratogenecity in animals, and observational data in humans is reassuring.

This patient with a macroadenoma, and others with previous transsphenoidal surgery for macroadenomas, may be monitored additionally with monthly Goldman perimetry visual field testing. Bromocriptine would be reinitiated if deficits were noted. Breast feeding is not contraindicated in the presence of microadenomas or macroadenomas. The use of bromocriptine and other dopaminergic agents classified as ergot alkaloids to inhibit postpartum lactation may cause blood pressure elevations during the postpartum period, and are contraindicated. Thus, if bromocritine is used intrapartum, some would recommend discontinuation of bromocriptine after delivery.

After treatment for a period of time with bromocriptine, many micro and macroadenomas undergo perivascular fibrosis, cell death and regression. Discontinuation after 3–5 years of use may be indicated if MRI documents regression in size. One can consider dopamine agonist withdrawal in a microadenoma if, after ceasing dopamine agonist therapy, the prolaction level remains normal. Periodic prolactin assays and evaluation of symptoms and physical examination in the first year will detect regrowth of the microadenoma. In the case of macroadenoma, if the MRI documents: tumor resolution or >50% reduction; greater than 5 mm distance from the optic chiasm; and no cavernous sinus invasion; one could initiate a stepwise, tapered or an abrupt withdrawal of the dopamine agonist and monitor prolaction levels, symptoms, and and the physical exam every three months. In 30–64% of such cases, there is no tumor regrowth [165, 166].

References

1. Tunbridge WM, Evered DC, Hall R et al (1977) The spectrum of thyroid disease in a community: the Whickham survey. Clin Endocrinol (Oxf) 7(6):481–493
2. Whartona T (1659) Adenographoa: sive glandularum totius corporis descripto
3. Portmann L, Hamada N, Heinrich G, DeGroot LJ (1985) Anti-thyroid peroxidase antibody in patients with autoimmune thyroid disease: possible identity with anti-microsomal antibody. J Clin Endocrinol Metab 61(5):1001–1003
4. Czarnocka B, Ruf J, Ferrand M, Carayon P, Lissitzky S (1985) Purification of the human thyroid peroxidase and its identification as the microsomal antigen involved in autoimmune thyroid diseases. FEBS Lett 190(1):147–152
5. Norman AW, Litwack G (1987) Thyroid hormones. In: Norman AW, Litwack G (eds) Hormones. Academic, San Diego, p 221
6. Kibirige MS, Hutchison S, Owen CJ, Delves HT (2004) Prevalence of maternal dietary iodine insufficiency in the north east of England: implications for the fetus. Arch Dis Child Fetal Neonatal Ed 89(5):F436–F439
7. Asamer H, Riccabona G, Holthaus N, Gabl F (1968) Immunohistologic findings in thyroid disease in an endemic goiter area. Arch Klin Med 215(3):270–284
8. Boukis MA, Koutras DA, Souvatzoglou A, Evangelopoulou A, Vrontakis M, Moulopoulos SD (1983) Thyroid hormone and immunological studies in endemic goiter. J Clin Endocrinol Metab 57(4):859–862
9. Greer MA (1980) Antithyroid drugs in the treatment of thyrotoxicosis. Thyroid Today 3
10. McGregor MA, Weetman AP, Ratanchaiyavong S et al (1985) Iodide: as influence on the development of autoimune thyroid disease. In: Hall R, Kobberling J (eds) Thyroid disorders associated with iodine deficiency and excess. Raven, New York, pp 209–216
11. Weetman AP (2000) Graves' disease. N Engl J Med 343(17): 1236–1248
12. Allen EM, Appel MC, Braverman LE (1986) The effect of iodide ingestion on the development of spontaneous lymphocytic thyroiditis in the diabetes-prone BB/W rat. Endocrinology 118(5):1977–1981
13. Sundick RS, Herdegen D, Brown TR (1986) Thyroiditis induced by dietary iodine may be due to the increased immunogenicity of highly iodinated thyroglobulin. In: Dexhage HA, Wiersinga WM (eds) The thyroid and autoimmunity. Elsevier Science, Amsterdam, New York, p 213
14. Bahn AK, Mills JL, Snyder PJ et al (1980) Hypothyroidism in workers exposed to polybrominated biphenyls. N Engl J Med 302(1):31–33
15. Gaitan E, Cooksey RC, Legan J (1985) Simple goiter and autoimmune thyroiditis: environmental and genetic factors. Clin Ecol (3):158–162
16. Wenzel BE, Heesemann J (1987) Antigenic homologies between plasmid encoded proteins from enteropathogenic Yersinia and thyroid autoantigen. Horm Metab Res Suppl 17:77–78
17. Caldwell G, Kellett HA, Gow SM et al (1985) A new strategy for thyroid function testing. Lancet 1(8438):1117–1119
18. Glinoer D, de Nayer P, Bourdoux P et al (1990) Regulation of maternal thyroid during pregnancy. J Clin Endocrinol Metab 71(2):276–287
19. Panesar NS, Li CY, Rogers MS (2001) Reference intervals for thyroid hormones in pregnant Chinese women. Ann Clin Biochem 38(Pt 4):329–332
20. Mehdi SR, Vasenwala SM, Zaheer MS, Vasenwala AM (2003) Role of FNAC and antithyroid antibodies in the diagnosis of thyroid disorders. Indian J Pathol Microbiol 46(2):184–190
21. Pandit AA, Vijay Warde M, Menon PS (2003) Correlation of number of intrathyroid lymphocytes with antimicrosomal antibody titer in Hashimoto's thyroiditis. Diagn Cytopathol 28(2):63–65
22. Okamura K, Sato K, Yoshinari M, Ikenoue H, Kuroda T, Nakagawa M, Tsuji H, Washio M, Fujishima M (1990) Recovery of the thyroid function in patients with atrophic hypothyroidism and blocking type TSH binding inhibitor immunoglobulin. Acta Endocrinol (Copenh) 122(1): 107–114
23. Tang T, Wang YG, Tsuboi K, Irie M, Ma T, Ingbar SH (1991) Blocking type immunoglobulins in patients with nongoitrous primary hypothyroidism in area of iodine deficiency. Endocrinol Jpn 38(6):661–665
24. Valente WA, Vitti P, Rotella CM, Vaughan MM, Aloj SM, Grollman EF, Ambesi-Impiombato FS, Kohn LD (1983) Antibodies that promote thyroid growth. A distinct population of thyroid-stimulating autoantibodies. N Engl J Med 309(17):1028–1034
25. Zakarija M, Jin S, McKenzie JM (1988) Evidence supporting the identity in Graves' disease of thyroid-stimulating antibody and thyroid growth-promoting immunoglobulin G as assayed in FRTL5 cells. J Clin Invest. 81(3):879–884
26. Brezinschek HP, Wilders-Truschnig M, Leb G, Eber O, Dohr G, Lanzer G, Krejs GJ (1990) Thyroid growth promoting serum-IgG in endemic goiter. Acta Med Austriaca 17 Suppl 1:26–77
27. Zakarija M, McKenzie JM (1990) Do thyroid growth-promoting immunoglobulins exist?J Clin Endocrinol Metab 70(2):308–310
28. Gupta MK (1992) Thyrotropin receptor antibodies: advances and importance of detection techniques in thyroid diseases. Clin Biochem 25(3):193–199
29. Vitti P, Chiovato L, Tonacchera M, Bendinelli G, Mammoli C, Capaccioli A, Fiore E, Pretell E, Pinchera A (1994) Failure to detect thyroid growth-promoting activity in immunoglobulin G of patients with endemic goiter. J Clin Endocrinol Metab 78(5): 1020–1025
30. Wilders-Truschnig MM, Warnkross H, Leb G, Langsteger W, Eber O, Tiran A, Dobnig H, Passath A, Lanzer G, Drexhage HA (1993) The effect of treatment with levothyroxine or iodine on thyroid size and thyroid growth stimulating immunoglobulins in endemic goitre patients. Clin Endocrinol (Oxf) 39(3):281–286
31. Davies R, Lawry J, Bhatia V, Weetman AP (1995) Growth stimulating antibodies in endemic goitre: a reappraisal. Clin Endocrinol (Oxf) 43(2):189–195
32. Vanderpump MPJ, Tunbridge WMG (1996) The thyroid: a fundamental and clinical text. In, 7th edn. Lippincott-Raven, Philadelphia, pp 474–482
33. Prummel MF, Wiersinga WM (2004) Thyroid autoimmunity and miscarriage. Eur J Endocrinol 150(6):751–755
34. Haddow JE, Palomaki GE, Allan WC et al (1999) Maternal thyroid deficiency during pregnancy and subsequent neuropsychological development of the child. N Engl J Med 341(8):549–555
35. Abalovich M, Amino N, Barbour LA et al (2007) Management of thyroid dysfunction during pregnancy and postpartum: an Endocrine Society Clinical Practice Guideline. J Clin Endocrinol Metab 92(8 Suppl):S1–S47
36. American College of Obstetrics and Gynecology (2002) ACOG practice bulletin. Thyroid disease in pregnancy. Number 37, August 2002. Int J Gynaecol Obstet 79(2):171–180
37. Kabadi UM (1993) 'Subclinical hypothyroidism'. Natural course of the syndrome during a prolonged follow-up study. Arch Intern Med 153(8):957–961
38. Grodstein F, Goldman MB, Ryan L, Cramer DW (1993) Self-reported use of pharmaceuticals and primary ovulatory infertility. Epidemiology 4(2):151–156
39. Morimoto C, Reinherz EL, Schlossman SF, Schur PH, Mills JA, Steinberg AD (1980) Alterations in immunoregulatory T cell subsets in active systemic lupus erythematosus. J Clin Invest 66(5):1171–1174

40. Lao TT, Chin RK, Panesar NS, Swaminathan R (1988) Observations on thyroid hormones in hyperemesis gravidarum. Asia Oceania J Obstet Gynaecol 14(4):449–452
41. Albright F (1938) Metropathia hemorrhagica. Main MJ (29):235–238
42. Wilansky DL, Greisman B (1989) Early hypothyroidism in patients with menorrhagia. Am J Obstet Gynecol 160(3):673–677
43. Yamada T, Tsukui T, Ikejiri K, Yukimura Y, Kotani M (1976) Volume of sella turcica in normal subjects and in patients with primary hypothyroidism and hyperthyroidism. J Clin Endocrinol Metab 42(5):817–822
44. Honbo KS, van Herle AJ, Kellett KA (1978) Serum prolactin levels in untreated primary hypothyroidism. Am J Med 64(5):782–787
45. Thomas R, Reid RL (1987) Thyroid disease and reproductive dysfunction. Obstet Gynecol (70):789–798
46. Scanlon MF, Chan V, Heath M et al (1981) Dopaminergic control of thyrotropin, alpha-subunit, thyrotropin beta-subunit, and prolactin in euthyroidism and hypothyroidism: dissociated responses to dopamine receptor blockade with metoclopramide in hypothyroid subjects. J Clin Endocrinol Metab 53(2):360–365
47. Kramer MS, Kauschansky A, Genel M (1979) Adolescent secondary amenorrhea: association with hypothalamic hypothyroidism. J Pediatr 94(2):300–303
48. Feek CM, Sawers JS, Brown NS, Seth J, Irvine WJ, Toft AD (1980) Influence of thyroid status on dopaminergic inhibition of thyrotropin and prolactin secretion: evidence for an additional feedback mechanism in the control of thyroid hormone secretion. J Clin Endocrinol Metab 51(3):585–589
49. Keye WR, Yuen BH, Knopf RF, Jaffe RB (1976) Amenorrhea, hyperprolactinemia and pituitary enlargement secondary to primary hypothyroidism. Successful treatment with thyroid replacement. Obstet Gynecol 48(6):697–702
50. del Pozo E, Wyss H, Tollis G, Alcaniz J, Campana A, Naftolin F (1979) Prolactin and deficient luteal function. Obstet Gynecol 53(3):282–286
51. Bohnet HG, Fiedler K, Leidenberger FA (1981) Subclinical hypothyroidism and infertility. Lancet 2(8258):1278
52. Warfel W (1992) Thyroid regulation pathways and its effect on human luteal function. Gynakol Geburtshilfliche Rundsch (32):145–150
53. Walsh JP, Shiels L, Lim EM et al (2003) Combined thyroxine/liothyronine treatment does not improve well-being, quality of life, or cognitive function compared to thyroxine alone: a randomized controlled trial in patients with primary hypothyroidism. J Clin Endocrinol Metab 88(10):4543–4550
54. Davies TF, Roman SH, Mackenzie WA, Goldsmith N, Dower SM, Piccinini LA (1987) Thyroid cell MHC class II antigens: a perspective on the aetiology of autoimmune thyroid disease. Acta Endocrinol Suppl (Copenh) 281:13–20
55. Kong YC, Flynn JC, Wan Q, David CS (2003) HLA and H2 class II transgenic mouse models to study susceptibility and protection in autoimmune thyroid disease. Autoimmunity 36(6–7):397–404
56. Tomer Y, Blackard JT, Akeno N (2007) Interferon alpha treatment and thyroid dysfunction. Endocrinol Metab Clin North Am 36(4):1051–1066 x–xi
57. Vitti P, Rago T, Chiovato L et al (1997) Clinical features of patients with Graves' disease undergoing remission after antithyroid drug treatment. Thyroid 7(3):369–375
58. Michelangeli V, Poon C, Taft J, Newnham H, Topliss D, Colman P (1998) The prognostic value of thyrotropin receptor antibody measurement in the early stages of treatment of Graves' disease with antithyroid drugs. Thyroid 8(2):119–124
59. Schlumberger M, De Vathaire F, Ceccarelli C et al (1996) Exposure to radioactive iodine-131 for scintigraphy or therapy does not preclude pregnancy in thyroid cancer patients. J Nucl Med 37(4):606–612
60. Edan G, Massart C, Hody B et al (1989) Optimum duration of antithyroid drug treatment determined by assay of thyroid stimulating antibody in patients with Graves' disease. BMJ 298(6670):359–361
61. Iwatani Y (2004) Current topics on immunological laboratory tests-thyroid diseases. Rinsho Byori 52(9):751–758
62. Padmanabhan LD, Mhaskar R, Mhaskar A, Vallikad E (2003) Trophoblastic hyperthyroidism. J Assoc Physicians India 51:1011–1013
63. Yoshimura M, Hershman JM (1995) Thyrotropic action of human chorionic gonadotropin. Thyroid 5(5):425–434
64. Klein RZ, Sargent JD, Larsen PR, Waisbren SE, Haddow JE, Mitchell ML (2001) Relation of severity of maternal hypothyroidism to cognitive development of offspring. J Med Screen 8(1):18–20
65. Alexander EK, Marqusee E, Lawrence J, Jarolim P, Fischer GA, Larsen PR (2004) Timing and magnitude of increases in levothyroxine requirements during pregnancy in women with hypothyroidism. N Engl J Med 351(3):241–249
66. Zakarija M, McKenzie JM (1983) Thyroid-stimulating antibody (TSAb) of Graves' disease. Life Sci 32(1–2):31–44
67. Zakarija M, Garcia A, McKenzie JM (1985) Studies on multiple thyroid cell membrane-directed antibodies in Graves' disease. J Clin Invest 76(5):1885–1891
68. Tanaka T, Tamai H, Kuma K, Matsuzuka F, Hidaka H (1981) Gonadotropin response to luteinizing hormone releasing hormone in hyperthyroid patients with menstrual disturbances. Metabolism 30(4):323–326
69. Thomas R, Reid RL (1987) Thyroid disease and reproductive dysfunction: a review. Obstet Gynecol 70(5):789–798
70. Bournaud C, Orgiazzi J (2003) Antithyroid agents and embryopathies. Ann Endocrinol (Paris) 64(5 Pt 1):366–369
71. Polak M, Le Gac I, Vuillard E et al (2004) Fetal and neonatal thyroid function in relation to maternal Graves' disease. Best Pract Res Clin Endocrinol Metab 18(2):289–302
72. Millar LK, Wing DA, Leung AS, Koonings PP, Montoro MN, Mestman JH (1994) Low birth weight and preeclampsia in pregnancies complicated by hyperthyroidism. Obstet Gynecol 84(6):946–949
73. Mestman JH (2004) Hyperthyroidism in pregnancy. Best Pract Res Clin Endocrinol Metab 18(2):267–288
74. Davis LE, Lucas MJ, Hankins GD, Roark ML, Cunningham FG (1989) Thyrotoxicosis complicating pregnancy. Am J Obstet Gynecol 160(1):63–70
75. Amino N, Mori H, Iwatani Y et al (1982) High prevalence of transient post-partum thyrotoxicosis and hypothyroidism. N Engl J Med 306(14):849–852
76. Hayslip CC, Fein HG, O'Donnell VM, Friedman DS, Klein TA, Smallridge RC (1988) The value of serum antimicrosomal antibody testing in screening for symptomatic postpartum thyroid dysfunction. Am J Obstet Gynecol 159(1):203–209
77. Iwatani Y, Amino N, Tamaki H et al (1988) Increase in peripheral large granular lymphocytes in postpartum autoimmune thyroiditis. Endocrinol Jpn 35(3):447–453
78. Vargas MT, Briones-Urbina R, Gladman D, Papsin FR, Walfish PG (1988) Antithyroid microsomal autoantibodies and HLA-DR5 are associated with postpartum thyroid dysfunction: evidence supporting an autoimmune pathogenesis. J Clin Endocrinol Metab 67(2):327–333
79. Jansson R, Karlson A (1986) Autoimmune thyroid disease in pregnancy and the postpartum period. In: McGregory AM (ed) Immunology of endocrine disease. MTP Press, Lancaster, UK, pp 181–188
80. Walfish PG, Chan JY (1985) Post-partum hyperthyroidism. Clin Endocrinol Metab 14(2):417–447
81. Glinoer D, Soto MF, Bourdoux P et al (1991) Pregnancy in patients with mild thyroid abnormalities: maternal and neonatal repercussions. J Clin Endocrinol Metab 73(2):421–427

82. Stagnaro-Green A, Roman SH, Cobin RH, el-Harazy E, Alvarez-Marfany M, Davies TF (1990) Detection of at-risk pregnancy by means of highly sensitive assays for thyroid autoantibodies. JAMA 264(11):1422–1425
83. Maier DB, Parke A (1989) Subclinical autoimmunity in recurrent aborters. Fertil Steril 51(2):280–285
84. Magaro M, Zoli A, Altomonte L et al (1992) The association of silent thyroiditis with active systemic lupus erythematosus. Clin Exp Rheumatol 10(1):67–70
85. LaBarbera A, Miller MM, Ober C et al (1988) Autoimmunit etiology in premature ovarian failure. Am J Reprod Immunol (16):114–118
86. Peterson CM (1994) Thyroid disease and fertility. In Autoimmunity in Reproduction, Gleicher N (ed), Immunology and Allergy Clinics of North America WB Saunders, Philadelphia, Pa. 14:725–738.
87. Ezzat S, Sarti DA, Cain DR, Braunstein GD (1994) Thyroid incidentalomas. Prevalence by palpation and ultrasonography. Arch Intern Med 154(16):1838–1840
88. McHenry CR, Walfish PG, Rosen IB (1993) Non-diagnostic fine needle aspiration biopsy: a dilemma in management of nodular thyroid disease. Am Surgeon (59):415–419
89. Barbesino G, Tomer Y, Concepcion E, Davies TF, Greenberg DA (1998) Linkage analysis of candidate genes in autoimmune thyroid disease: 1. Selected immunoregulatory genes. International Consortium for the Genetics of Autoimmune Thyroid Disease. J Clin Endocrinol Metab 83(5):1580–1584
90. Aaltonen J, Bjorses P, Sandkuijl L, Perheentupa J, Peltonen L (1994) An autosomal locus causing autoimmune disease: autoimmune polyglandular disease type I assigned to chromosome 21. Nat Genet 8(1):83–87
91. Riddle O, Bates RW, Dykshorn S (1933) The preparation, identification and assay of prolactin. A hormone of the anterior pituitary. Am J Physiol (105):191–196
92. Frantz AG, Kleinberg DL (1970) Prolactin: evidence that it is separate from growth hormone in human blood. Science 170(959):745–747
93. Lewis UJ, Singh RN, Sinha YN, VanderLaan WP (1971) Electrophoretic evidence for human prolactin. J Clin Endocrinol Metab 33(1):153–156
94. Hwang P, Guyda H, Friesen H (1972) Purification of human prolactin. J Biol Chem 247(7):1955–1958
95. Freeman ME, Kanyicska B, Lerant A, Nagy G (2000) Prolactin: structure, function, and regulation of secretion. Physiol Rev 80(4):1523–1631
96. Suh HK, Frantz AG (1974) Size heterogeneity of human prolactin in plasma and pituitary extracts. J Clin Endocrinol Metab 39(5):928–935
97. Guyda JH (1975) Heterogeneity of human growth hormone and prolactin secreted in vitro: Immunoassay and radioreceptor assay correlations. J Clin Endocrinol Metab 41(5):953–967
98. Farkouh NH, Packer MG, Frantz AG (1979) Large molecular size prolactin with reduced receptor activity in human serum: high proportion in basal state and reduction after thyrotropin-releasing hormone. J Clin Endocrinol Metab 48(6):1026–1032
99. Benveniste R, Helman JD, Orth DN, McKenna TJ, Nicholson WE, Rabinowitz D (1979) Circulating big human prolactin: conversion to small human prolactin by reduction of disulfide bonds. J Clin Endocrinol Metab 48(5):883–886
100. Jackson RD, Wortsman J, Malarkey WB (1985) Characterization of a large molecular weight prolactin in women with idiopathic hyperprolactinemia and normal menses. J Clin Endocrinol Metab 61(2):258–264
101. Fraser IS, Lun ZG, Zhou JP et al (1989) Detailed assessment of big big prolactin in women with hyperprolactinemia and normal ovarian function. J Clin Endocrinol Metab 69(3):585–592
102. Larrea F, Escorza A, Valero A, Hernandez L, Cravioto MC, Diaz-Sanchez V (1989) Heterogeneity of serum prolactin throughout the menstrual cycle and pregnancy in hyperprolactinemic women with normal ovarian function. J Clin Endocrinol Metab 68(5): 982–987
103. Lewis UJ, Singh RN, Sinha YN, Vanderlaan WP (1985) Glycosylated human prolactin. Endocrinology 116(1):359–363
104. Markoff E, Lee DW (1985) Glycosylated prolactin is a major circulating variant in human serum. J Clin Endocrinol Metab (65):1102–1106
105. Markoff E, Lee DW, Hollingsworth DR (1988) Glycosated and nonglycosated prolactin in serum druring pregnancy. J Clin Endocrinol Metab (67):519–523
106. Pellegrini I, Gunz G, Ronin C et al (1988) Polymorphism of prolactin secreted by human prolactinoma cells: immunological, receptor binding, and biological properties of the glycosylated and nonglycosylated forms. Endocrinology 122(6):2667–2674
107. Bole-Feysot C, Goffin V, Edery M, Binart N, Kelly PA (1998) Prolactin (PRL) and its receptor: actions, signal transduction pathways and phenotypes observed in PRL receptor knockout mice. Endocr Rev 19(3):225–268
108. Goldsmith PC, Cronin MJ, Weiner RI (1979) Dopamine receptor sites in the anterior pituitary. J Histochem Cytochem 27(8):1205–1207
109. Quigley ME, Judd SJ, Gilliland GB, Yen SS (1979) Effects of a dopamine antagonist on the release of gonadotropin and prolactin in normal women and women with hyperprolactinemic anovulation. J Clin Endocrinol Metab 48(4):718–720
110. Quigley ME, Judd SJ, Gilliland GB, Yen SS (1980) Functional studies of dopamine control of prolactin secretion in normal women and women with hyperprolactinemic pituitary microadenoma. J Clin Endocrinol Metab 50(6):994–998
111. De Leo V, Petraglia F, Bruno MG, Lanzetta D, Inaudi P, D'Antona N (1989) Different dopaminergic control of plasma luteinizing hormone, follicle-stimulating hormone and prolactin in ovulatory and postmenopausal women: effect of ovariectomy. Gynecol Obstet Invest 27(2):94–98
112. Lachelin GC, Leblanc H, Yen SS (1977) The inhibitory effect of dopamine agonists on LH release in women. J Clin Endocrinol Metab 44(4):728–732
113. Hill MK, Macleod RM, Orcutt P (1976) Dibutyryl cyclic AMP, adenosine and guanosine blockade of the dopamine, ergocryptine and apomorphine inhibition of prolactin release in vitro. Endocrinology 99(6):1612–1617
114. Lemberger L, Crabtree RE (1979) Pharmacologic effects in man of a potent, long-acting dopamine receptor agonist. Science 205(4411):1151–1153
115. Braund W, Roeger DC, Judd SJ (1984) Synchronous secretion of luteinizing hormone and prolactin in the human luteal phase: neuroendocrine mechanisms. J Clin Endocrinol Metab 58(2): 293–297
116. Grossman A, Delitala G, Yeo T, Besser GM (1981) GABA and muscimol inhibit the release of prolactin from dispersed rat anterior pituitary cells. Neuroendocrinology 32(3):145–149
117. Gudelsky GA, Apud JA, Masotto C et al (1983) Ethanolamine-O-sulfate enhances gamma-aminobutyric acid secretion into hypophysial portal blood and lowers serum prolactin concentrations. Neuroendocrinology 37(5):397–399
118. Melis GB, Paoletti AM, Mais V et al (1982) The effects of the gabaergic drug, sodium valproate, on prolactin secretion in normal and hyperprolactinemic subjects. J Clin Endocrinol Metab 54(3):485–489
119. Melis GB, Fruzzetti F, Paoletti AM et al (1984) Pharmacological activation of gamma-aminobutyric acid-system blunts prolactin response to mechanical breast stimulation in puerperal women. J Clin Endocrinol Metab 58(1):201–205
120. Bazan JF (1990) Structural design and molecular evolution of a cytokine receptor superfamily. Proc Natl Acad Sci USA 87(18):6934–6938

121. Hu ZZ, Zhuang L, Meng J, Dufau ML (1998) Transcriptional regulation of the generic promoter III of the rat prolactin receptor gene by C/EBPbeta and Sp1. J Biol Chem 273(40):26225–26235
122. Sassin JF, Frantz AG, Weitzman ED, Kapen S (1972) Human prolactin: 24-hour pattern with increased release during sleep. Science 177(55):1205–1207
123. Sassin JF, Frantz AG, Kapen S, Weitzman ED (1973) The nocturnal rise of human prolactin is dependent on sleep. J Clin Endocrinol Metab 37(3):436–440
124. Carandente F, Angeli A, Candiani GB et al (1989) Rhythms in the ovulatory cycle. 1st: Prolactin. Chronobiological Research Group on Synthetic Peptides in Medicine. Chronobiologia 16(1):35–44
125. Pansini F, Bergamini CM, Cavallini AR et al (1987) Prolactinemia during the menstrual cycle. A possible role for prolactin in the regulation of ovarian function. Gynecol Obstet Invest 23(3):172–176
126. Pansini F, Bianchi A, Zito V et al (1983) Blood prolactin levels: influence of age, menstrual cycle and oral contraceptives. Contraception 28(3):201–207
127. Franks S, Gharani N, Waterworth D et al (1997) The genetic basis of polycystic ovary syndrome. Hum Reprod 12(12):2641–2648
128. Jacobs HS, Hull MG, Murray MA, Franks S (1975) Therapy-orientated diagnosis of secondary amenorrhoea. Horm Res 6(4):268–287
129. Bohnet HG, Dahlen HG, Wuttke W, Schneider HP (1976) Hyperprolactinemic anovulatory syndrome. J Clin Endocrinol Metab 42(1):132–143
130. Franks S, Murray MA, Jequier AM, Steele SJ, Nabarro JD, Jacobs HS (1975) Incidence and significance of hyperprolactinaemia in women with amenorrhea. Clin Endocrinol (Oxf) 4(6):597–607
131. Boyar RM, Kapen S, Finkelstein JW et al (1974) Hypothalamic-pituitary function in diverse hyperprolactinemic states. J Clin Invest 53(6):1588–1598
132. Moult PJ, Rees LH, Besser GM (1982) Pulsatile gonadotrophin secretion in hyperprolactinaemic amenorrhoea an the response to bromocriptine therapy. Clin Endocrinol (Oxf) 16(2):153–162
133. Buckman MT, Peake GT, Srivastava L (1981) Patterns of spontaneous LH release in normo- and hyperprolactinaemic women. Acta Endocrinol (Copenh) 97(3):305–310
134. Aono T, Miyake A, Yasuda TS, Koike K, Kurachi K (1979) Restoration of oestrogen positive feedback effect on LH release by bromocriptine in hyperprolactinaemic patients with galactorrhoea-amenorrhoea. Acta Endocrinol (Copenh) 91(4):591–600
135. Travaglini P, Ambrosi B, Beck-Peccoz P et al (1978) Hypothalamic-pituitary-ovarian function in hyperprolactinemic women. J Endocrinol Invest 1(1):39–45
136. Glass MR, Shaw RW, Butt WR, Edwards RL, London DR (1975) An abnormality of oestrogen feedback in amenorrhoea-galactorrhoea. Br Med J 3(5978):274–275
137. Koike J, Aono T, Tsutsumi H, Miyake A, Kurachi K (1982) Restoration of oestrogen-positive feedback effect on LH release in women with prolactinoma by transsphenoidal surgery. Acta Endocrinol (Copenh) 100(4):492–498
138. Rakoff J, VandenBerg G, Siler TM, Yen SS (1974) An integrated direct functional test of the adenohypophysis. Am J Obstet Gynecol 119(3):358–368
139. Zarate A, Jacobs LS, Canales ES et al (1973) Functional evaluation of pituitary reserve in patients with the amenorrhea-galactorrhea syndrome utilizing luteinizing hormone-releasing hormone (LH-RH), L-dopa and chlorpromazine. J Clin Endocrinol Metab 37(6):855–859
140. McNatty KP (1979) Relationship between plasma prolactin and the endocrine microenvironment of the developing human antral follicle. Fertil Steril 32(4):433–438
141. Dorrington J, Gore-Langton RE (1981) Prolactin inhibits oestrogen synthesis in the ovary. Nature 290(5807):600–602
142. Cutie E, Andino NA (1988) Prolactin inhibits the steroidogenesis in midfollicular phase human granulosa cells cultured in a chemically defined medium. Fertil Steril 49(4):632–637
143. Adashi EY, Resnick CE (1987) Prolactin as an inhibitor of granulosa cell luteinization: implications for hyperprolactinemia-associated luteal phase dysfunction. Fertil Steril 48(1):131–139
144. Soto EA, Tureck RW, Strauss JF 3rd (1985) Effects of prolactin on progestin secretion by human granulosa cells in culture. Biol Reprod 32(3):541–545
145. Demura R, Ono M, Demura H et al (1985) Prolactin directly inhibits basal as well as gonadotropin-stimulated secretion of progesterone and 17β-estradol in the human ovary. J Clin Endocrinol Metab (54):1246–1250
146. Kleinberg DL, Noel GL, Frantz AG (1977) Galactorrhea: a study of 235 cases, including 48 with pituitary tumors. N Engl J Med 296(11):589–600
147. Tolis G, Somma M, Van Campenhout J, Friesen H (1974) Prolactin secretion in sixty-five patients with galactorrhea. Am J Obstet Gynecol 118(1):91–101
148. Boyd AE III, Reichlin S, Turksoy RN (1977) Galactorrhea-amenorrhea syndrome: diagnosis and therapy. Ann Intern Med 87(2):165–175
149. Schlechte J, Sherman B, Halmi N et al (1980) Prolactin-secreting pituitary tumors in amenorrheic women: a comprehensive study. Endocr Rev 1(3):295–308
150. Minakami H, Abe N, Oka N, Kimura K, Tamura T, Tamada T (1988) Prolactin release in polycystic ovarian syndrome. Endocrinol Jpn 35(2):303–310
151. Murdoch AP, Dunlop W, Kendall-Taylor P (1986) Studies of prolactin secretion in polycystic ovary syndrome. Clin Endocrinol (Oxf) 24(2):165–175
152. Lythgoe K, Dotson R, Peterson CM (1995) Multiple endocrine neoplasia presenting as primary amenorrhea: a case report. Obstet Gynecol 86(4 Pt 2):683–686
153. Burgess JR, Shepherd JJ, Parameswaran B et al (1996) Spectrum of pituritary disease in multiple endocrine neoplasia type 1 (MEN-1): clinical, bichemical, and radiologic features of pituitary disease in a large MEN-1 kindred. J Clin Endocrinol Metab (81):2642–2646
154. Bohler HC Jr, Jones EE, Brines ML (1994) Marginally elevated prolactin levels require magnetic resonance imaging and evaluation for acromegaly. Fertil Steril 61(6):1168–1170
155. Gonsky R, Herman V, Melmed S, Fagin J (1991) Transforming DNA sequences present in human prolactin-secreting pituitary tumors. Mol Endocrinol 5(11):1687–1695
156. Sisam DA, Sheehan JP, Sheeler LR (1987) The natural history of untreated microprolactinomas. Fertil Steril 48(1):67–71
157. Schlechte J, Dolan K, Sherman B, Chapler F, Luciano A (1989) The natural history of untreated hyperprolactinemia: a prospective analysis. J Clin Endocrinol Metab 68(2):412–418
158. Weiss MH, Wycoff RR, Yadley R, Gott P, Feldon S (1983) Bromocriptine treatment of prolactin-secreting tumors: surgical implications. Neurosurgery 12(6):640–642
159. NIH Publication 02–3924. 2002
160. Klibanski A, Biller BM, Rosenthal DI, Schoenfeld DA, Saxe V (1988) Effects of prolactin and estrogen deficiency in amenorrheic bone loss. J Clin Endocrinol Metab 67(1):124–130
161. Turner TH, Cookson JC, Wass JA, Drury PL, Price PA, Besser GM (1984) Psychotic reactions during treatment of pituitary tumours with dopamine agonists. Br Med J (Clin Res Ed) 289(6452): 1101–1103
162. Katz E, Weiss BE, Hassell A, Schran HF, Adashi EY (1991) Increased circulating levels of bromocriptine after vaginal compared with oral administration. Fertil Steril 55(5):882–884
163. Jeffcoate WJ, Pound N, Sturrock ND, Lambourne J (1996) Long-term follow-up of patients with hyperprolactinaemia. Clin Endocrinol (Oxf) 45(3):299–303

164. Passos VQ, Souza JJ, Musolino NR, Bronstein MD (2002) Long-term follow-up of prolactinomas: normoprolactinemia after bromocriptine withdrawal. J Clin Endocrinol Metab 87(8): 3578–3582
165. Colao A, Di Sarno A, Cappabianca P, Di Somma C, Pivonello R, Lombardi G (2003) Withdrawal of long-term cabergoline therapy for tumoral and nontumoral hyperprolactinemia. N Engl J Med 349(21):2023–2033
166. Biswas M, Smith J, Jadon D et al (2005) Long-term remission following withdrawal of dopamine agonist therapy in subjects with microprolactinomas. Clin Endocrinol (Oxf) 63(1):26–31
167. Abram M, Brue T, Morange I, Girard N, Guibout M, Jaquet P (1992) Pituitary tumor syndrome and hyperprolactinemia in peripheral hypothyroidism. Ann Endocrinol (Paris) 53(5–6): 215–223
168. Nagel TC, Freinkel N, Bell RH, Friesen H, Wilber JF, Metzger BE (1973) Gynecomastia, prolactin, and other peptide hormones in patients undergoing chronic hemodialysis. J Clin Endocrinol Metab 36(3):428–432
169. Chirito E, Bonda A, Friesen HG (1972) Prolactin in renal failure. Clin Res (20):423
170. Lloyd RV (1983) Estrogen-induced hyperplasia and neoplasia in the rat anterior pituitary gland. An immunohistochemical study. Am J Pathol 113(2): p. 198–206
171. Scheithauer BW et al. (1990) The pituitary gland in pregnancy: a clinicopathologic and immunohistochemical study of 69 cases. Mayo Clin Proc 65(4):461–474
172. Weil C (1986) The safety of bromocriptine in hyperprolactinaemic female infertility: a literature review. Curr Med Res Opin 10(3): 172–195
173. Shy KK et al (1983) Oral contraceptive use and the occurrence of pituitary prolactinoma. JAMA 249(16):2204–2207
174. Corenblum B and Taylor PJ (1988) Idiopathic hyperprolactinemia may include a distinct entity with a natural history different from that of prolactin adenomas. Fertil Steril 49(3):544–546
175. Corenblum B and Donovan L (1993) The safety of physiological estrogen plus progestin replacement therapy and with oral contraceptive therapy in women with pathological hyperprolactinemia. Fertil Steril 59(3):671–673
176. Scheithauer BW et al (1989) Effects of estrogen on the human pituitary: a clinicopathologic study. Mayo Clin Proc 64(9):1077–1084
177. Ruiz-Velasco V, Tolis G (1984) Pregnancy in hyperprolactinemic women. Fertil Steril 41(6):793–805
178. Turkalj I, Braun P, Krupp P (1982) Surveillance of bromocriptine in pregnancy. JAMA 247(11):1589–1591
179. Kirsch C, Iffy L, Zito GE, McArdle JJ (2001) The role of hypertension in bromocriptine-related puerperal intracranial hemorrhage. Neuroradiology 43(4):302–304
180. Iffy L, Lindenthal J, McArdle JJ, Ganesh V (1996) Severe cerebral accidents postpartum in patients taking bromocriptine for milk suppression. Isr J Med Sci 32(5):309–312
181. Iffy L, McArdle JJ, Ganesh V (1996) Intracerebral hemorrhage in normotensive mothers using bromocriptine postpartum. Zentralbl Gynakol 118(7):392–395
182. Gittelman DK (1991) Bromocriptine associated with postpartum hypertension, seizures, and pituitary hemorrhage. Gen Hosp Psychiatry 13(4):278–280
183. Katz M, Kroll D, Pak I, Osimoni A, Hirsch M (1985) Puerperal hypertension, stroke, and seizures after suppression of lactation with bromocriptine. Obstet Gynecol 66(6):822–824

Chapter 15
Acquired Uterine Factors and Infertility

Harry H. Hatasaka

Abstract Uterine factor subfertility is defined as a structural or functional disorder of the uterus that results in reduced fertility. Between one and two percent of in vitro fertilization (IVF) procedures are recorded as being done for uterine factor in the United States as reported by Wright et al. (MMWR Surveill Summ 57:1–23, 2008). Live birth rates for isolated uterine factor are below average compared to other diagnoses for couples undergoing IVF. For example, among women <35 years of age undergoing IVF using their own fresh eggs for embryo transfer, uterine factor has the lowest live birth rate among diagnoses at 35.9% per transfer, which is even below the live birth rate for diminished ovarian reserve (40.3%) as reported by Wright et al. (MMWR Surveill Summ 57:1–23, 2008).

Although the proportion of cases of uterine factor that proceed to IVF is small, the resources spent evaluating for and treating uterine factors are disproportionately high. Uterine factors encompass a number of specific pathological entities in an endless variety of presentations and combinations which are not specified by the CDC database. Therefore, counseling couples regarding the contribution of uterine factors to their infertility is challenging. Given these considerations, the best clinical strategy is to screen for the most common uterine factors early during an infertility evaluation. When uterine pathology is encountered, general concepts and statistics for outcomes based upon the specific uterine factors, along with their locations and extent must be accounted for in relation to other infertility factors for a given couple with infertility. This chapter focuses on the evidence for an association of individual acquired uterine factors (endometrial polyps, leiomyomata, adenomyosis, and Asherman syndrome) with infertility. The clinical characterization, pathophysiology, and therapeutic principles for these commonly acquired uterine infertility factors are also reviewed.

H.H. Hatasaka (✉)
Utah Center for Reproductive Medicine, Department of Obstetrics & Gynecology, University of Utah School of Medicine, Salt Lake City, UT, USA

Keywords Acquired uterine factor subfertility • Adenomyosis • Endometrial polyps • Uterine leiomyomata • Fibroids • Asherman syndrome

15.1 Endometrial Polyps and Infertility

Polyps are endometrial tissue growths containing glands, blood vessels, and stroma. The central core consists of endometrium of the basal type covered by functionalis endometrium that can range from inactive to weakly secretory. This explains why a proportion of polyps can become cystic. The stroma is usually fibrous but can be typical endometrial stroma as well. A cluster of thick-walled vessels found in the base of the stalk tends to feed a solitary vessel in the stalk that can generally be appreciated with color flow Doppler.

A study of 215 infertile women with polyps undergoing insemination revealed that the polyps at presentation had a mean diameter of 1.6 cm (range 0.3–2.4 cm) [2]. In a different study population (243 women with abnormal uterine bleeding), the size range was from 0.5 to 5 cm with a mean diameter of 3.4 ± 0.9 cm [3]. They were solitary in 71.6%. About two-thirds of polyps are pedunculated, with the remainder being sessile [4].

Compared to the surrounding endometrium, polyps appear to have higher expression of estrogen and progesterone receptors in the glandular epithelium, but similar to slightly reduced expression in the stroma [5, 6]. The glandular epithelial component tends to be out of synchronization with the surrounding endometrium. This abnormal configuration of receptor expression may help determine the altered functional activity of polyps and help explain why polyps tend to be less sensitive to cyclic hormonal variation than eutopic endometrium [5]. However, it remains to be determined whether the high induced estrogen milieu associated with ovulation induction accelerates polyp formation.

D.T. Carrell and C.M. Peterson (eds.), *Reproductive Endocrinology and Infertility: Integrating Modern Clinical and Laboratory Practice*,
DOI 10.1007/978-1-4419-1436-1_15,

15.1.1 Diagnosis

Measurement bias is an important consideration among studies of polyps. Polyps are easily missed by endometrial biopsy and even transvaginal ultrasonography (TVUS). Transvaginal ultrasound is less sensitive than sonohysterography in identifying polyps, while sonohysterography is as accurate as hysteroscopy for detecting polyps [7]. In a comparative study, HSG had a sensitivity of approximately 50% and a PPV of 28.6% for polyp detection, whereas TVUS had a sensitivity of 75%, specificity of 97%, and a PPV of 75%. Sonohysterography and hysteroscopy were equivalent, with 100% sensitivity and 100% PPV in this particular study, although this research standard is unlikely to be realized in clinical practice by less experienced practitioners [7].

When TVUS or sonohysterography is used to diagnose polyps, rounded intrauterine filling defects often cause uncertainty as to whether they may be polyps, leiomyomata, or blood clots. There are some observations to help make the distinction, although histologic confirmation remains the gold standard. Pedunculated leiomyomata demonstrate continuity with the myometrium with echogenic endometrium overlying them. Polyps can be visualized completely within the endometrial cavity. They tend to cross the midline, pushing the endometrial stripe off center.

Color flow Doppler can sometimes also provide a clue because leiomyomata generally have no distinct feeding vessel. The vascularity of fibroids is diffuse and exhibits peripheral flow surrounding their pseudocapsules. Polyps generally have single feeding vessels, whereas cancerous masses may have multiple feeding vessels. If any flow is visualized within an intrauterine mass, it is unlikely to be a fibroid and more likely to be a polyp. Doppler flow also excludes the presence of an inanimate mass such as a blood clot.

If hysteroscopy is chosen to diagnose polyps, differences in hysteroscopic technique itself introduce more variability. In a study comparing polyp detection rates, the use of dextran 70 as a distention media identified polyps in 12% of 992 women compared to 0.6% of a similar group of 335 women using CO_2 hysteroscopy [8]. Hysteroscopy using saline as the distention medium has not been rigorously compared to the other techniques for the detection of polyps.

The inaccuracy of the hysteroscopic diagnosis of polyps compared to histologic confirmation adds yet another degree of uncertainty to reported prevalence rates. In a study of over 4,000 women with abnormal uterine bleeding, the prevalence of polyps by hysteroscopic diagnosis was 33.9%, while histology confirmed polyps in only 27.5% of the cohort [9].

15.1.2 Potential Subfertility Mechanisms Associated with Polyps

Potential mechanisms whereby endometrial polyps could diminish fecundity have been similar to those proposed for submucus fibroids including mechanical disruption of implantation, focal vascular alterations, alterations of sperm migration [4], chronic bleeding, and endometrial inflammation. One study added credence to the possibility that inflammation may play a role by noting a strong correlation between the presence of endometritis and the presence of micropolyps of the endometrium defined as polyps less than 1 mm [10].

Another intriguing mechanistic possibility is the enhanced production of the glycoprotein, glycodelin in women with polyps. It is the major secretory phase product of endometrial epithelial cells that normally appears to be stimulated by ovarian progesterone secretion and thought to facilitate implantation. Glycodelin is found in the uterine cavity in rising concentrations six days after the LH surge and peaks during the implantation interval. It has been hypothesized to suppress natural killer cell destruction of intracavitary embryos. Normally, glycodelin is found in minimal concentrations during the proliferative phase. However, in a pilot study, glycodelin concentrations from uterine flushings and in serum during the proliferative phase were found to be elevated in women with uterine polyps compared to controls [11]. Serum glyodelin is also increased in women with leiomyomata. The presence of glyodelin in the endometrium prematurely during the proliferative phase may alter endometrial receptivity during the secretory phase. Also, because glyodelin has also been shown to inhibit human sperm binding to the zona pelucida, its abnormal presence systemically during ovulation and fertilization may further contribute to subfecundity. Yet another study reported an increased level of an endometrial immunoglobulin, human decidua-associated protein 200 (hDP 200) in the endometrial cavities of women with polyps and fibroids compared to controls and also hypothesized a consequent implantation defect [12].

15.1.3 Evidence of an Association Between Endometrial Polyps and Infertility

Statistically, patients with endometrial polyps are more likely to concurrently have fibroids, adenomyosis, endometriosis, and endometrial cancer [13–15]. Estrogen is involved in the growth and maintenance of all of these lesions. Obesity is another related risk factor for the occurrence of uterine polyps [9]. This is anticipated given the excess estrogen generated from androgens via aromatase within adipocytes.

Because fibroids, obesity, and endometriosis are all independently associated with infertility, there is likely to be a statistical association between polyps and infertility as well, based solely on the frequent coexistence between polyps and the aforementioned lesions. However, whether uterine polyps directly contribute to subfertility is difficult to tease out, but concerted attempts have been made as will be reviewed below.

Routine uterine cavity assessment during evaluation for infertility frequently reveals uterine polyps. When 1,000 unselected women planning IVF underwent diagnostic office hysteroscopy, endometrial polyps were the most frequent abnormality visualized (32% of the cohort), while 0.9% had "polypoid" endometrium [16]. Only 3% had submucus fibroids and another 3% had intrauterine adhesions. A 15.6% (35/235) prevalence of polyps was found in a cohort of eumenorrheic infertile women by hysteroscopy [4]. In another study of 574 unselected patients undergoing IVF, preprocedure hysteroscopy revealed a prevalence of polyps of 26.4% [17]. The prevalence rates of polyps in infertile women planning IVF may underestimate the actual prevalence. Most women requiring IVF are likely to have previously undergone uterine cavity assessment and polypectomy. The prevalence of endometrial polyps in infertile women therefore appears to be high, but the important questions are whether they contribute to infertility and whether polypectomy improves fecundity. A number of studies have tried to answer these questions, but the study designs are generally weak. Here, the data are examined systematically, starting with the lowest quality study design first, which is comparing the prevalence of polyps in infertile populations to fertile controls.

If polyps contribute to infertility, it would be expected that infertile patients with otherwise unexplained infertility would have a higher prevalence of uterine polyps. It has not been possible to make this determination with confidence due to enormous heterogeneity between studies. Prevalence rates vary depending on the populations studied. Some factors that contribute to the variability between populations include age, obesity, abnormal uterine bleeding and menopausal status [13, 18, 19].

Despite the concerns surrounding the accurate measurement of prevalence rates, it appears that reported polyp prevalence rates in asymptomatic premenopausal women tend to be less than in infertile populations. A study of 100 asymptomatic premenopausal women found polyps in 10% by sonohysterography [13]. In studies of women undergoing preoperative evaluation for tubal reanastomosis, 15% of 99 subjects were found to have polyps hysteroscopically [20] and one of 31 (3%) in another [4]. While suggestive of a link between polyps and infertility, such uncontrolled observational studies of polyp prevalence among varied populations only help establish that polyps are frequently encountered among women with infertility.

Other studies have attempted to shed light on whether polyps contribute to infertility by calculating crude cumulative pregnancy rates before and after polypectomy. An uncontrolled study from Poland of hysteroscopic polypectomy in a group of 25 women with infertility noted a 76% clinical pregnancy rate within 12 months of polypectomy [21]. Another retrospective study divided women into those with polyps ≤1 cm ($n=31$) and those with either polyps >1 cm or multiple polyps ($n=52$). All subjects had infertility as well as abnormal uterine bleeding. After polypectomy with histological documentation, cumulative delivery rates were not significantly different (61.4% for the ≤1 cm polyp group and 54.2% for those who had polyps >1 cm) [22]. A similar uncontrolled study of 15 eumenorrheic infertile women found to have only polyps as a presumptive infertility diagnosis after thorough evaluation (including routine hysteroscopy and laparoscopy) underwent polypectomy. Of the 12 evaluable subjects after 12 months of follow-up, six conceived (50%) after polypectomy [4]. Another small study over a span of 21 years used the same design but added a comparison group [23]. The same surgeon performed 23 polypectomies for infertile women and their cumulative pregnancy rate was compared to that of 19 infertile women with normal cavities at hysteroscopy. Similar to the Polish study, 18 of 23 (78.3%) of the infertile polypectomy group became pregnant compared to eight of 19 (42.1%) of the normal cavity group. This was a significant difference in pregnancy rates, while the miscarriage rates were not significantly different.

Four non-randomized studies of IVF have looked at the reproductive outcomes of subjects with polyps who did not undergo polypectomy compared to a group who did [24, 25]. Mastrominas was the first to designate a study group where polyps were diagnosed either by hysteroscopy or sonohysterography, but who then underwent IVF without polypectomy ($n=24$) [24]. These women had polyps less than 2 cm in diameter. The treatment group had up to three polyps, all less than 2 cm in diameter and underwent polypectomy ($n=65$) prior to IVF. The polypectomy group had a 28% cumulative pregnancy rate compared to a 35% rate for those with the polyps left in situ. For the subset with polyps over 2 cm in diameter who underwent polypectomy, the pregnancy rate was 40%. The authors concluded that for women undergoing IVF, polyps less than 2 cm do not affect pregnancy rates and do not need to be removed. This study implied that polyps > 2 cm might lower IVF delivery rates (since their removal yielded the highest pregnancy rates), but this hypothesis was not directly tested by the study design. Unfortunately, the other causes for infertility were not controlled, leaving the conclusions of this study in doubt.

Another study conducted at Bourn Hall Clinic, using an untreated control group [25] was also an IVF study that only enrolled women whose polyps were less than 2 cm in diameter.

In this retrospective study, all subjects ($n=83$) were incidentally found to have polyps by transvaginal ultrasound after their IVF cycles had been initiated. In 49 subjects, the IVF cycle was completed, but in the other 34, the clinicians and patients together opted to freeze all appropriate embryos before transfer and perform hysteroscopic polypectomy immediately after the egg retrieval. Transfers were then performed several months later. Pregnancy rates could not be directly compared due to the cryopreservation step in the second group, and therefore the pregnancy and miscarriage rates of each group were compared to the historical fresh and frozen embryos transfer rates during the same time period. None of the rates were statistically different so that they concluded that polyps less than 2 cm in diameter have no effect on IVF conception rates and should not alter the planned IVF. However, the miscarriage rates of the fresh transfer conceptions with polyps left in place was nearly three times the contemporaneous clinic rate (27.3 vs. 10.3%) ($p=0.08$). Of the 34 women who decided to freeze their embryos after the diagnosis of polyps, the immediate hysteroscopy after egg retrieval only revealed polyps in 24 (58.3%). And among these 24, histology confirmed polyps in only 14. So overall, the conversion to a cryopreservation cycle did more harm than good with only 14 of 32 (44%) of the discontinued IVF cycles having histologically confirmed polyps.

A third study of women undergoing IVF also found no differences in miscarriage and pregnancy rates between 33 women with polyps and 54 controls without polyps [26]. The polyps were diagnosed by ultrasound and were all less than 1.5 cm (mean 8.3 mm, range 5–12 mm) but the ultrasound false positive rate was not reported.

A more recent study of IVF+ICSI cycles came to the same conclusion [27]. Three groups were studied retrospectively. Group 1 ($n=15$) was a group found to have polyps during the ovarian stimulation; group 2 ($n=40$) had polypectomy prior to IVF+ICSI; group 3 consisted of 956 women undergoing IVF+ICSI without polyps. Clinical pregnancy and miscarriage rates did not differ among any of the groups leading to the conclusion that polyps < 1.5 cm do not alter reproductive outcome in women undergoing IVF+ICSI.

Another small study took the aggressive approach of performing polypectomy during an IVF cycle before egg retrieval after polyps <2 cm were incidentally diagnosed between cycle days 7 and 9. Three of six such subjects conceived, but the small sample size does not yet allow recommendation of this approach [28].

Most studies of infertile women with polyps have not found an association between polyp size and implantation rates [2, 21, 22]. The exception was the uncontrolled study cited above, finding indirect evidence that polyps >2 cm may adversely affect IVF pregnancy rates [24]. Although the bulk of the evidence does not support IVF cycle cancellation or interruption due to the finding during the procedure of polyps <2 cm, this is a special circumstance that cannot be generalized to the presence of polyps in the infertile population at large. It is possible that false positive polypoid structures seen on transvaginal ultrasonography during follicular monitoring may result from hyperplastic foci of rapidly growing endometrium under the high estrogen milieu generated by ovarian FSH stimulation. Experience from the Bourne Hall study suggests caution in this setting because in those cycles converted to cryopreservation cycles due to the discovery of polyps, less than half turned out to have polyps after all. Although some small polyps detected by sonohysterography are known to spontaneously resolve given long-term untreated follow-up [29], the high rate of TVUS false positive polyp diagnoses during ovarian stimulation cycles appears to be a special situation.

To date, only one randomized trial of polypectomy with pregnancy rates as the outcome measure has been performed representing the highest quality evidence available. Women < 40 years of age, with at least 2 years of infertility, were determined to be adequate IUI candidates after a complete infertility evaluation then randomized to polypectomy or no polypectomy [2]. Up to four cycles of superovulation with FSH injections were planned starting at least three cycles after hysteroscopy (with or without polypectomy). Data were reported for 204 randomized women. In the polypectomy group, 65% of those who conceived did so before the first IUI was performed implying a strong effect from the polypectomies. Clinical pregnancy rates were subjected to survival analysis indicating a doubling of the pregnancy rate in the polypectomy group (RR 2.1 with 95% CI 1.5–2.9). The polyps in both cases and controls ranged from 3 to 24 mm (mean 16 mm). When analyzed by the size of the polyps removed, there was no difference in pregnancy rates.

15.1.4 Clinical Considerations

The incidence of new polyp formation compared to their prevalence has been little studied. This has practical significance because knowledge of the incidence would help clinicians judge how often the uterine cavity should be imaged during ongoing infertility treatment. In a prospective study observing the natural history of polyps and other uterine masses, 64 asymptomatic, premenopausal women underwent a baseline sonohysterogram (SHG) and a repeat SHG 2.6 years later on average [19]. None had interval pregnancies. Seven of 64 (11%) had polyps at baseline. Polyps persisted two and a half years later in only three of the seven women. In the remaining 57 women, seven developed new polyps over 2.6 years (for a cumulative incidence of 12% or roughly 5% annually). The polyps that regressed were of smaller diameter on average at baseline (0.7 cm, range 0.4–1.1 cm) compared to those that persisted (1.3 cm, range 0.8–1.8 cm). Of the three that persisted, their mean diameters remained the same over 2.6 years. Of the seven women with polyps at baseline, five had solitary polyps and the other two women had two polyps each.

A longitudinal study of 190 premenopausal women was performed with up to 9 years of follow-up using transvaginal ultrasound monitoring every 6 months post polypectomy. Only 1.8% had recurrence of polyps when the size was ≤2.5 cm at the initial polypectomy and 3.5% recurred with the size was >2.5 cm (difference nonsignificant) [3].

Two other factors that help in the decision of how often to perform uterine imaging are the patient's BMI and age. A BMI ≥ 30 was associated with a 52% prevalence of polyps compared to 15% in women with a BMI < 30 among 223 patients with either PCOS or unexplained infertility, undergoing pre-IVF hysteroscopy [18]. In a study of asymptomatic premenopausal women, 97% of the polyps identified using sonohysterography were in women aged 35 and older [13]. Therefore it is reasonable to consider repeating investigation of the uterine cavity more frequently for obese infertile women ≥ 35 when they are enduring prolonged conception attempts than for younger women of normal BMI. New onset of menometrorrhagia should also prompt consideration of repeat uterine cavity evaluation because women with abnormal uterine bleeding have a higher prevalence of uterine polyps than eumenorrheic women (28–30% vs. 10%) [9, 13].

At this time, while being far from definitive, there are enough data to recommend pursuing polypectomy in infertile women. The morbidity of polypectomy is low, and given the high costs (both monetary and emotional) of infertility, prophylactic polypectomy appears to be justified. Although small polyps discovered incidentally while an IVF cycle is already in progress do not appear to require cycle cancellation, the most prudent measure is to investigate the uterine cavity prior to any ART procedure at a frequency commensurate with the risk factors that an individual has.

Another reason proposed to consider hysteroscopic resection of polyps prior to conception attempts is the risk of malignancy within the polyps [30]. However, the bulk of the evidence would suggest that the risk of adenocarcinoma within polyps in premenopausal, eumenorrheic, infertile women with polyps discovered by sonohysterography is highly unlikely [31, 32].

Studies of prevalence rates of polyps in populations of women with recurrent pregnancy loss have been surprisingly low at 0.6% [33] and 5% [34]. While studies have not been performed regarding outcomes in recurrent pregnancy loss patients following polypectomy, it seems reasonable to consider polypectomy in this circumstance as well given the low complication rate of the procedure [8, 35].

15.2 Leiomyomata

Uterine leiomyomata ("fibroids," "myomas") represent a frequent dilemma in reproductive medicine with a prevalence rate as high as 40% in women of reproductive age [36–38]. The cumulative incidence of leiomyomata increases with advancing age reaching 70–80% by age 50 [39]; this contributes to the increasing cumulative reproductive hazard associated with aging. An ultrasound study identified fibroids in almost 70% of Caucasian and >80% of African American women from a randomly selected population of 35–49-year-old women regardless of whether they had symptoms attributable to fibroids [40]. Approximately 12.6% of women undergoing IVF have fibroids [41]. The impact of leiomyomata on fecundity is difficult to assess largely due to varying individual presentations that complicate the implementation of controlled trials. Furthermore, the field is muddied by the lack of functional definitions, varied fibroid detection methods, and properly designed studies [39].

Indeed, uterine fibroid classification schemes are descriptive only. They do not adequately account for fibroid size, number, contiguity, biological behavior, and spatial orientation (such as cervical, fundal, peri-ostial, etc.). Because fibroids and even a single fibroid can be located in any or all of the traditionally defined locations (subserosal, intramural, or submucosal) simultaneously, they are not readily classifiable into clinically distinct entities.

15.2.1 Diagnosis

Although most fibroids are asymptomatic, symptoms can suggest the location of the fibroids. Menorrhagia (the most common symptom associated with fibroids) is more typically associated with a submucosal fibroid location [42]. In contrast, subserosal and intramural fibroids are generally associated with pain, and when large they may compromise bowel and bladder function and lead to a pressure sensation within the pelvis [43].

During an infertility evaluation, when not palpable on pelvic exam, leiomyomata are typically discovered during pelvic ultrasonography or when there is distortion of the uterine cavity noted by hysterosalpingography. In the presence of a normal cavity by hysterosalpingography the diagnosis of uterine leiomyomata is not further enhanced by hysteroscopy [44].

Ultrasonography and in particular sonohysterography represents the most versatile and clinically useful imaging modality for localization of the fibroids and treatment planning [45]. For example, hysteroscopy, which generally offers excellent direct visualization of submucosal fibroids, cannot establish the diameter or myometrial depth of sessile submucosal fibroids. Ultrasound without saline has low precision in localizing submucosal fibroids and often overestimates their sizes. The addition of saline infusion allows an accurate assessment of fibroid impingement into the cavity. Thus, there is rarely a practical need for adjunctive MRI, CT, or hysteroscopy when planning myomectomy if sonohysterography has been successfully performed.

15.2.2 Leiomyomata and Fecundity

Although there is not yet a predictive formula regarding the impact of uterine leiomyomata on reproduction that accounts for all of the above variables, other lines of evidence have recently been systematically analyzed recently in a thoughtful and rigorous manner [46]. The evidence was summarized by first noting that case series have been used to estimate the proportion of infertility attributable to leiomyomata (approximately 2–3%). However, published case series are limited by selection and detection biases leaving the true contribution of fibroids on fecundity debatable from these studies.

A more reliable estimate of the effect could be derived from cross-sectional studies of unselected women using the most sensitive modern diagnostic technique (transvaginal ultrasonography) with pregnancy as the endpoint. But as the authors point out, such studies have not yet been performed. Despite the high prevalence of fibroids in women of reproductive age, the low estimated association of fibroids with infertility makes it challenging to ascertain the specific risk factors involved.

The next best study designs to begin to assess causation, include cohort and case-control studies. Systematic review of these study designs has convincingly revealed that parous women have a lower prevalence of fibroids than their nulliparous counterparts, and that the relative risk decreases with increasing parity [46]. The four largest such studies had relative risks of fibroids in multiparous women ranging from only 0.7 to 0.8 with none of the confidence intervals crossing one [47–50]. These studies unfortunately cannot discern whether multiparity is protective against the development of leiomyomata or whether leimomyomata may contribute to subfecundity and therefore be overrepresented in nulliparous women.

A better study design would be an analysis of infertility with or without the documented presence of fibroids. Unfortunately, only two cohort studies [49, 50] and two case-control studies [51–53] involving a total of 6,224 subjects have reported specifically on the association between infertility (albeit uncharacterized infertility) in conjunction with the presence of fibroids. Interestingly none of the four studies could statistically identify an association between fibroids and infertility.

Causation also cannot be revealed by the pregnancy outcomes of uncontrolled studies of myomectomy. Numerous such studies have been published but most have reported on series of women undergoing myomectomy without documenting whether subjects were infertile before the surgery. Only a crude estimate of pregnancy rates following myomectomy can be gleaned from the many studies and are in the range of 40–60%. Specific predictive factors for pregnancy success following myomectomy cannot be elucidated from this form of study. Taken together, these various approaches to studying the influence of fibroids on reproductive capacity have failed to identify an association.

Unfortunately, there have been no randomized trials of subfertile women undergoing myomectomy compared to expectant management using fertility outcomes as the endpoint [54]. In the absence of randomized trials, the most productive method of study regarding the impact of fibroids on reproduction has been the use of IVF. By controlling for many infertility variables, the IVF model helps to isolate the effect of fibroids on implantation and miscarriage outcomes in infertile populations. Somigliana et al. [46] reviewed 17 studies of fibroids and IVF and found inconsistent outcomes while acknowledging the limitations of the data. The IVF studies are unable to offer useful conclusions regarding the effects of larger-sized (>4 cm) fibroids that may be clinically significant due to the low numbers of large fibroids reported among the 17 studies. The study designs, methods of fibroid ascertainment, and exclusion and inclusion criteria all differed making analysis difficult. However, meta-analyses of the IVF and fibroid data have begun to reveal some important information regarding the effect of location of the fibroids on fecundity.

Whereas tubal occlusion caused by mechanical compression by fibroids is an obvious potential source of infertility, from the five meta-analyses currently available, it appears that myomas impinging into the uterine cavity increase the risk of infertility [46, 55–58]. A recent review, while acknowledging the limitations of current studies, noted trends in all major reproductive outcomes indicating that implantation in women with submucosal fibroids decreased from 11.5% to 3.0%, miscarriage rates increased over controls from 22% to 47%, and ongoing pregnancy rates demonstrated a decrease from 30% to 14% [41].

The latest two meta-analyses conclude that intramural leiomyomata may also negatively impact fecundity, although it remains uncertain whether myomectomy of intramural fibroids confers a benefit for fecundity [46, 55]. Pritts et al. also reported that subserosal fibroids do not impact fertility potential and importantly, that removal of submucosal fibroids appears to be beneficial [55]. These findings suggest that adequate implantation is compromised. Mechanistic hypotheses include endometrial thinning overlying submucosal leiomyomata, vascular alterations induced by the presence of the neoplasms, and inflammatory effects and mechanical disruption of implantation similar to the mechanisms proposed for intrauterine device contraception.

The evidence that indicates that myomectomy of submucosal fibroids prior to IVF may be beneficial is largely indirect. Three IVF studies used women without fibroids as controls compared to women who had undergone myomectomy [59–61]. The two most recent studies focused on women who had undergone myomectomy of submucus fibroids only. None of the three studies identified a difference in the pregnancy rates from those of controls. Therefore, given the evidence that submucosal fibroids diminish fecundity, their removal appears to restore fecundity back to expected levels. Direct benefit for myomectomy in IVF patients was found in one additional non-randomized study comparing myomectomy of intramural/submucosal fibroids (with at least one being >5 cm) to expectant management. The surgery group enjoyed a 25% cumulative delivery rate compared to 12% for the control group ($p=0.01$) [62].

Whereas the IVF data indicates that a submucus location of fibroids is a negative predictor of successful implantation, the impact of the number and size of leiomyomata remains to be determined. To date, the evidence suggests that the volume and number of fibroids are less important variables than their location regarding fecundity [55].

15.2.3 Treatment Options

Although estrogen is known to promote the growth of leiomyomata, exposure to and interaction with other growth factors and hormones is complex and not adequately characterized. Leiomyomata contain increased levels of estrogen and progesterone receptors as well as elevated aromatase levels compared to normal myometrium [63]. Progesterone, for some myomas, may actually be more anabolic than estrogen. Underlying the unpredictable biological behavior of fibroids is a nonrandom genetic heterogeneity, as evidenced by observations that only 60% of leiomyoma cells are cytogenetically normal. While it has been commonly believed that pregnancy is a major risk factor for the growth of leiomyomata, the hormonal milieu of pregnancy on average typically leads to the reduction in volume during the course of gestation [64].

Medical therapies meant to alter hormonal growth or maintenance of fibroids (GnRH agonists and antagonists, aromatase inhibitors, progestational agents including the levonorgestrel containing IUD, progesterone antagonists, and receptor modulators, androgenic agents, and selective estrogen modulators) currently have limited long-term utility for the treatment of infertility associated with fibroids. Although some are highly promising as adjuncts (none are curative), they are either contraceptive or not studied adequately to document therapeutic benefit for fibroid-associated infertility [65, 66].

Other surgical and non-surgical alternatives to myomectomy have been devised in an attempt to control the detrimental effects of fibroids including laparoscopic myolysis [67], uterine artery embolization (UAE) [68], and MRI-guided focused ultrasound [69].

Promising reductions in fibroid size and control of symptoms have been reported with these techniques; however, there are inadequate data regarding fertility outcomes to recommend any of these techniques at present for infertile women with leiomyomata [63, 65, 70–72]. Most of the available data regarding reproductive outcomes has been for UAE. However, most of this information comes from registries and other small series, whereas larger prospective experience will be needed to define the fecundity and pregnancy outcomes among women undergoing UAE [71, 73, 74].

A study of 51 women who underwent UAE found a high proportion (66%) of the previously normal cycling women to have abnormal hysteroscopic findings after UAE such as adhesions, protruding fibroids, and a yellow discoloration to the endometrium [75]. This raises concern for normal reproductive capability. The miscarriage rate was significantly higher following UAE in 38 women compared to laparoscopic uterine artery occlusion performed in 20 women in one prospective study [76]. Higher pregnancy complication rates and a lower fecundity rate from historically expected rates were also found in a retrospective study of 103 women attempting to conceive after UAE [63]. Only 31% of the women desiring pregnancy conceived and there were high rates of cesarean section (72.7%), postpartum hemorrhage (18.2%), prematurity (18%), spontaneous abortion (30%), and in addition there were two stillbirths and one ectopic pregnancy among the 56 pregnancies that resulted from the 33 women who conceived [63]. And in the only randomized trial of UAE and myomectomy, 121 women with at least one fibroid greater than 4 cm in diameter undergoing UAE had a lower conception rate and higher SAB rate compared to the myomectomy group [77].

Of further concern are reports of premature ovarian failure (POF) following unintended ovarian artery compromise by UAE. As many as 15% of women experience amenorrhea following UAE. Amenorrhea may remain permanently in up to approximately 7% due to either POF or endometrial compromise [78, 79]. The risk of premature ovarian failure appears to be higher with advancing age. A Doppler study of ovarian arterial perfusion after UAE noted that 54% of patients lost perfusion to the ovaries completely and another 35% demonstrated diminished perfusion [78]. It has been estimated that approximately 3% of young women undergoing UAE will develop amenorrhea as a sign of impaired ovarian function [80]. However, even without overt amenorrhea or documented premature ovarian failure, it is possible that ovarian reserve and endometrial function may be harmed by UAE. This possibility is supported by a study of 88 premenopausal women undergoing UAE for menorrhagia. Basal FSH and anti-Mullerian hormone (AMH) levels were drawn and followed for 24 months after UAE. Mean basal FSH levels increased, and AMH levels decreased compared to the expected changes due to ovarian ageing over the 2 years of follow up [81].

In contrast to the experience with UAE, expected pregnancy and miscarriage rates appear to be similar for women who undergo myomectomy prior to IVF compared to age-matched women without fibroids [59–61]. Given the data to date regarding UAE, it remains prudent to dissuade the procedure in women who desire to conceive [80, 82].

15.2.4 Planning Myomectomy

Because no medical therapies can eliminate leiomyomata, and ablative methods pose other potential reproductive hazards, surgical management remains the cornerstone of therapy when the goal is preservation and optimization of reproductive function [37]. Yet, there are no randomized trials of expectant management compared to myomectomy when fibroids are the sole detectable infertility factor. This paucity of quality literature regarding therapeutic options for uterine leiomyomata, prompting one group after having performed an extensive literature review to comment that "The current state of the literature does not permit definitive conclusions about benefit, harm, or relative costs to help guide women's choices" [39].

Even so, decisions must be made based upon the cumulative evidence to date. In an often cited review article almost 30 years old, Buttram and Reiter (1981) [36] offered some practical advice. Women with fibroids should be allowed a 6–12-month trial of conception attempts before considering myomectomy unless symptoms or rapid growth prompt quicker intervention. Since that time there are new information and new technology that have now shaped a different approach to the dilemma of fibroids in women who desire to conceive. Parker suggests that for women with fibroids desiring fertility, uterine cavity evaluation is the preliminary step to guide management. If there is no deformation of the cavity by fibroids, then pregnancy can be attempted without intervention [65]. The American Society for Reproductive Medicine's Practice Committee advises a comprehensive infertility evaluation for both partners before making an operative decision for a myomectomy [82]. In addition, before deciding on myomectomy, Somigliana et al. recommend individualized counseling including consideration of such important factors as the age of the woman, the location, number and sizes of fibroids involved, and an assessment of other symptoms related to the effect of fibroids on the quality of life of the patient [46]. Also factored into the discussion with patients should be careful review of the potential reproductive outcomes including surgical and pregnancy complications. Therefore, the pros and cons of each situation must be carefully weighed and discussed with women faced with the decision of whether to undergo myomectomy. Some of the important considerations follow.

15.2.5 Considerations Favoring Myomectomy

The perception of many gynecologists has been that myomectomy is a far riskier procedure than hysterectomy so that some recommend hysterectomy for women with symptomatic fibroids despite their desire for continued childbearing potential. There is now evidence that in the hands of properly trained gynecologic surgeons, the surgical risks of myomectomy are no higher than those of hysterectomy and may in fact be lower [83, 84]. The risk of emergency hysterectomy after initiating myomectomy appears to be less than 1% [80].

The usual common denominator for considering myomectomy as opposed to medical or interventional radiologic therapies for fibroids is the patient's desire to experience future pregnancies. Gestational surrogacy following hysterectomy for fibroids remains an option but its legal, financial, and emotional burdens make it an unpopular if not impossible option for most women.

The data from the IVF literature indicate that submucosal fibroids, and to a far lesser extent intramural fibroids, have a deleterious effect on fecundity and that successful myomectomy of submucus fibroids appears to restore fecundity to the age-expected potential. Therefore, when submucosal and/or intramural fibroids are present in an infertile but otherwise asymptomatic woman, the decision to pursue myomectomy should be carefully balanced with a number of other factors including the relative potential contribution of the fibroids to the woman's infertility after any other infertility factors have been ascertained. The decision to pursue myomectomy is often made easier when factoring in fibroid-associated symptoms such as pelvic pain or pressure, compression of the bladder causing urinary frequency, compression of the rectum leading to difficulty with defecation, and anemia and/or abnormal uterine bleeding. Cosmetic disfigurement is sometimes another factor leading some infertile women with myomas to consider myomectomy.

When leiomyomata are present, there are at least two circumstances in which direct surgical intervention is indicated as compared to hysterectomy and its alternatives. The first is the finding of hydronephrosis in the face of fibroids impinging in the vicinity of the corresponding ureter. If on the initial clinical diagnosis of leiomyomata, immobile masses emanating from the uterus are noted to fill the pelvis, it is prudent to rule out hydronephrosis by ultrasound or IVP.

The second reason for direct surgery is when cancers of the uterus including uterine sarcoma are suspected and a tissue diagnosis and staging are required. Rapid fibroid enlargement does not usually predict the presence of leiomyosarcoma (Parker, 1994) However, when associated with pelvic pain, abnormal bleeding, or a mass prolapsing through the cervix, uterine enlargement should prompt a preoperative evaluation for sarcoma that includes lactate dehydrogenase and its isoenzymes along with a pelvic MRI with gadolinium [85]. These tests in combination are highly sensitive for the diagnosis of leiomyosarcoma.

The decision of whether to pursue myomectomy for asymptomatic submucosal fibroids detected in a woman who has not yet attempted to conceive is problematic. The argument that all fibroids will eventually grow to the point of intervention cannot be substantiated. Fibroid growth cannot be predicted [39]. However, there is some risk that waiting to intervene could compromise reproductive potential by damaging tubes and/or endometrium or by making future surgery more difficult and risky. Aside from this future unpredictable risk of infertility when myomas are encountered, there are other compelling reasons to consider myomectomy in the face of submucosal fibroids. One is the probable decreased risk of spontaneous abortion following myomectomy. Mechanisms postulated to cause the increased spontaneous abortion rate associated with fibroids include fibroid degeneration, uterine vascular alterations, enhanced contractility of the myometrium, and direct impingement upon the conception site. Cohort studies have yielded mixed results but at least one well-done cohort study of pregnant women noted a significantly ($p<0.05$) higher rate of spontaneous abortion in a group of 143 women with fibroids (14.0%) compared to a control group without fibroids (7.6%) [86]. Miscarriage rates were highest in women with multiple fibroids. Furthermore, the majority of uncontrolled observational studies after myomectomy demonstrate a convincing decrease in spontaneous abortions from a presurgical rate of approximately 41% to 73%, down to the 13% to 26% range [4, 36, 41, 87].

Another logical reason to consider myomectomy is the possibility that removal of fibroids may reduce some of the risks of pregnancy complications associated with leiomyomata. A number of serious pregnancy complications, although relatively uncommon, appear to be increased in women with fibroids based on sizeable cohort studies. One of the most frequently encountered fibroid-associated symptoms is pelvic pain and pressure encountered in approximately 15% of pregnant women with fibroids [80, 88]. Fibroid-associated pregnancy complications are not restricted to the antepartum period but also include complications of labor, delivery, and the postpartum period. Increased risks have been reported for antenatal bleeding, cesarean section, preterm delivery, fetal malpresentation, obstructed labor, intrauterine growth restriction, premature rupture of membranes, placental abruption, placenta previa, and postpartum hemorrhage in association with leiomyomata [46, 80–90]. Most of these associations suffer from ascertainment bias, publication bias, and low study power so that the conclusions must be interpreted with caution. Also, increased cesarean section rates, mainly due to malpresentation, appear to be supported by the literature, whereas the bulk of the literature does not demonstrate increased rates of intrauterine growth restriction or preterm premature rupture of membranes [41].

The high estrogen and progesterone concentrations during pregnancy have been proposed as a predisposing environment for rapid fibroid growth that can outpace the fibroid blood supply leading to subsequent fibroid degeneration. Although a known entity, fortunately clinically significant fibroid degeneration requiring admission for pain control and fetal surveillance is an uncommon complication of pregnancy [64].

15.2.6 Disadvantages of Myomectomy

There is a small but real chance that myomectomy results in the loss of reproductive potential should there be surgical complications resulting in injury to the fallopian tubes, endometrium, ovaries, or even complications leading to hysterectomy. Fortunately, such serious complications are uncommon, but naturally, the risk increases with increased uterine volume and distortion of the normal anatomy due to multiple fibroids [91]. Complications common to all major abdominal surgeries remain pertinent, including pain, serious hemorrhage leading to transfusions and/or hysterectomy, damage to surrounding structures (especially the ureter and bladder when the anatomy is distorted), periadnexal and bowel adhesion formation, complications of anesthesia, infection, and thromboembolic complications. However, several residual risks are specific to myomectomy and deserve discussion with patients preoperatively. Uterine rupture is probably more likely during labor if the myometrium has been breached during myomectomy thereby obligating the recommendation for future cesarean sections following most myomectomies done to preserve fertility. Case reports of Asherman syndrome following myomectomy highlight the possibility of its occurrence but the incidence has not been estimated in large series.

Another problem is the frequent inability to adequately resect some fibroids. This may be due to difficulties with access or the inability to detect some fibroids within an enlarged and distorted uterus. It is impractical to determine clinically whether fibroids detected after initial myomectomy are persistent or newly formed. The cumulative risk for the detection of fibroids after an initial myomectomy detectable by ultrasound rises steadily to approximately 50% by 5 years postoperatively [92]. In an older study, when myomectomy of multiple fibroids was performed, 59% had recurrence and 26% of that needed either myomectomy or hysterectomy thereafter [93]. Fortunately, a more contemporary study demonstrated that 5 years after myomectomy, only approximately 5% of women will have clinically relevant fibroids from either persistent or newly formed fibroids [94].

A multicentered retrospective cohort study of 512 women analyzed the variables most predictive of fibroid recurrence following laparoscopic myomectomy [95]. The lowest recurrence rate was predicted when women at the time of surgery had only a solitary fibroid, were less than 35.5 years old, had a uterus less than 13 weeks gestational size, and had low blood loss and operative time. Achieving a pregnancy after the original myomectomy was also predictive of a low chance of recurrence [92, 95]. Interpretation of this finding remains unclear. It is possible that the hormonal milieu of pregnancy helps prevent fibroid recurrence but also possible that those women with recrudescent fibroids suffered more infertility and therefore were selected out from the group who achieved pregnancies.

When considering myomectomy, the potential gain must outweigh the possible morbidity of the procedure. When there are only intramural and/or subserosal fibroids, the modest improvement in reproductive outcomes, if any, may not justify the performance of myomectomy.

15.2.7 Myomectomy

When the decision to perform myomectomy has been made, the initial approach should include consideration of whether additional specific evaluation should be pursued for hydronephrosis and/or leiomyosarcoma. A preliminary determination of the hematocrit is also a wise precaution because women with fibroids are sometimes anemic but asymptomatic having compensated clinically because of the chronic nature of their menorrhagia. If chronic abnormal bleeding exists, then a precautionary office endometrial biopsy is necessary. Adequate pre-procedural imaging generally with sonohysterography that is best performed by the surgeon, will help to define the spatial relationships, locations, and dimensions of the fibroids so that a logical surgical approach can be planned. If there are submucus leiomyomata embedded <50% into the myometrium in an otherwise asymptomatic woman with fibroids, then hysteroscopic myomectomy will be the least invasive approach. Large transmural fibroids or intramural fibroids with a substantial submucus component are generally best removed by abdominal myomectomy, although skilled laparoscopic surgeons capable of performing multilayered myometrial closures including the important endometrial layer, may choose to consider a laparoscopic approach [65].

Once preoperative evaluation is complete, one of the first questions to address is whether a GnRH agonist (GnRH-a) or antagonist is an appropriate adjunct to facilitate the myomectomy. GnRH-agonists, mostly by lowering estrogen and progesterone exposure to fibroids (which contain receptors to both of these sex steroids), can substantially decrease fibroid size [96]. In one study, the average reduction of volume of fibroids was 30%, whereas non-fibroid uterine volume also diminished such that the total uterine volume decreased an average of 35% following 6 months of GnRH-a [98]. Despite the impressive temporary decrease in fibroid and uterine size (mostly within the first 3 months of GnRH-a use) fibroid volume returns to pretreatment size almost as quickly as it was reduced. The use of a preoperative GnRH-a has not been shown to decrease the transfusion rate with myomectomy and many gynecologists have the perception that the use of GnRH-a leads to more fibrosis of the fibroid pseudocapsule making dissection and repair of the uterus more technically difficult. One other problem with the use of GnRH agonists is the diminution in size of myomas such that they are not detectable at the time of myomectomy, only to regrow postoperatively to clinically troublesome sizes. This persistence of fibroids following the use of GnRH-a was demonstrated in a small randomized study of 24 women. In the group randomized to the use of GnRH-a for 3 months prior to myomectomy, there was a 64% rate of detection of fibroids at least 1.5 cm in diameter by ultrasound 3 months postoperatively. In the control group who did not use GnRH-a, persistent fibroids could only be detected in 13% [92].

Therefore, for a woman with fibroids desiring pregnancy, GnRH-a generally is not indicated but may be appropriate when there is anemia or when it is important for the patient to attempt to shrink the fibroids down to a point where myomectomy may be performed through a low transverse incision rather than using a less cosmetic vertical incision [96]. Likewise, a GnRH-a can potentially facilitate a laparoscopic myomectomy with its subsequent quicker recovery time [65]. When there is anemia due to fibroid-associated menorrhagia, GnRH agonists can be highly effective in reversing the anemia preoperatively [96]. A safe and effective alternative is the use of subcutaneous human recombinant erythropoietin beginning several weeks prior to the scheduled surgery [99]. Without reported side effects, erythropoietin promises to be a better tolerated therapy than GnRH agonists for the restoration of normal hemoglobin levels.

15.2.8 Minimizing Blood Loss During Myomectomy

Blood loss during myomectomy represents a major potential morbidity. Preoperative preparation can help minimize the risk. The blood loss associated with myomectomy can result from loss of control of a major vessel such as an inadvertently divided and retracted uterine artery especially when there is extreme distortion of the anatomy caused by myomas. More commonly, serious blood loss is due to deceptively slow oozing because fibroids do not have a solitary feeding vessel, rather a plexus of vessels that encircles each fibroid [100]. Along with assuring a maximal hematocrit preoperatively, the surgeon is well served to have blood typed and screened or even cross matched prior to initiating the surgery. There should be periodic communication with the anesthesiologists throughout the case regarding estimated blood loss.

Formerly, it was routine in many centers to arrange autologous blood banking prior to myomectomy. Several advances have shifted the risk–benefit ratio away from routine autologous blood banking. Cell saver technology can minimize the need for transfusions and should be available prior to myomectomies. One retrospective study of 91 abdominal myomectomies performed by one surgeon for uterine size ≥16 weeks, reported a mean estimated blood loss of 794 mL and a liberal use of the cell saver in over 75% of the cases [91]. With the use of the cell saver, homologous transfusion was limited to 8% of the patients. Intraoperative irrigation with heparinized saline (5,000 IU per liter of normal saline) allows the use of the cell saver.

Another important tool to remember when hemorrhage is life-threatening, is the use of recombinant factor VIIa. This factor promotes the terminal functions of the extrinsic clotting pathway, thereby bypassing the initial stages. After administration of 50–100 mcg/kg IV, bleeding cessation is anticipated within 40 min and can be seen as quickly as 10 min after dosing. A second dose can be used 2 h after the first when needed. Although expensive, the treatment can be life saving.

Preoperative imaging can help estimate the sizes and locations of fibroids; however optimal planning of uterine incisions when multiple fibroids are encountered awaits visualization and palpation of the uterus during abdominal myomectomy. Several principles apply when planning the number and location of uterine incisions. When possible, anterior incisions are preferable because posterior incisions are associated with more adhesion formation and exposure is more difficult to obtain [101]. The arcuate vessels in the uterus run transversely across the uterine fundus [102]. Therefore transverse incisions stand to minimize blood loss by limiting the number of arcuate arterioles that are compromised [91]. A balance must be reached between minimizing the number and length of incisions on one hand, while limiting the amount of tunneling through myometrium to reach deep fibroids, on the other. Tunneling promotes hematoma formation and diminishes exposure. In general, it is best to fastidiously close dead space in multiple hemostatic layers before making the next required myometrial incision in order to minimize blood loss and possibly reduce the probability of uterine rupture during pregnancy [101].

When the incision locations have been selected, it has become common prior to first incision to inject the synthetic vasopressin, pitressin for its vasoconstrictive effects in order to minimize blood loss. Some surgeons inject pitressin directly into the fibroids but myoma tissue itself is not well vascularized. Most bleeding appears to emanate from the vascular plexus that encircles the myoma and the surrounding vascular myometrium. Therefore, vasopressin (20U in 20 mL of normal saline) is injected directly into the myometrium and serosa surrounding fibroids. This technique has been shown to be as effective as the use of mechanical tourniquets in controlling blood loss in a randomized trial [103]. Not only does the vasoconstriction limit blood loss, but pitressin has also been postulated to stimulate myometrial contractions, thereby effecting a cleavage plane between the fibroid and its surrounding myometrium [104]. An alternate route of administration of pitressin is injection of very dilute (4 U in 80 mL of normal saline) into the cervical stroma prior to the start of myomectomy. This is done in the same manner as a paracervical block using 10 mL of the diluted pitressin into each of the four and eight o'clock positions. This technique in a randomized placebo-controlled study of 106 women undergoing operative hysteroscopy, demonstrated a significantly reduced blood loss in the pitressin group [105]. The benefit may occur from less generalized blood flow to the uterus or to a preferential decrease in bleeding from submucosal myoma sites. The technique can be used in conjunction with localized myometrial injection of pitressin.

From the first incision into the myometrium, the myomectomy should proceed expeditiously. Slow bleeding can give a false sense of security, whereas the cumulative blood loss from slow bleeding can lead to profound anemia if neglected. Also, the effective half-life of pitressin is approximately 30 min. Therefore, the majority of the myomectomy should be completed by that time. If more time and more pitressin are required, skin closure should be delayed until at least 30 min after the last pitressin was administered to help assure adequate hemostasis. Side effects of pitressin include hypertension and pulmonary edema from its antidiuretic properties. For safety, one technique has been to use dilute concentrations as low as 10 U of pitressin in 60 mL of normal saline given in 5 mL increments while monitoring for hypertension [91].

Keeping the mean arterial pressure (MAP) at approximately 60 mm of Hg will also help to minimize blood loss during myomectomy. The MAP should be raised following myomectomy and the incision sites observed for bleeding prior to skin closure.

It is prudent to be prepared to use tourniquets in the event of excessive hemorrhage during myomectomy that is resistant to the use of pitressin. Prior to first incision, survey the anatomy to plan placement of fenestrations through the broad ligaments in order to place a tourniquet around the lower uterine segment. This helps stanch the pulse pressure of the ascending uterine arteries. When needed, more tourniquets can be positioned around the ovarian artery blood supply bilaterally between the ovaries and the uterus.

If oozing continues to occur from the myometrial incision sites and that bleeding responds to pressure, another practical adjunctive technique that can be used to help secure hemostasis is placement of a B-Lynch stitch. Originally devised to control post-cesarean section bleeding from atony [106], the stitch can add another option along with pelvic artery ligations, intrauterine balloon tamponade, and interventional radiologic embolization before resorting to hysterectomy in the persistently bleeding post myomectomy patient.

Another helpful measure while performing myomectomy is the routine placement of a balloon catheter into the uterine cavity during vaginal preparation. A number 18 Foley can be used with the tip above the balloon removed. This accomplishes several tasks. First, when there is uterine distortion by fibroids the position of the uterine cavity can be deceptive. Palpation of the balloon through the myometrium can sometimes help to establish the position of the cavity. Second, indigo carmine can be passed through the catheter so that entry into the cavity can be readily appreciated. Third, the critical repair of the endometrium is facilitated by the presence of the balloon both as a stent and to ascertain when adequate reapproximation of the endometrium is accomplished by observing any leakage of indigo carmine. An intrauterine balloon can also be helpful when there is diffuse bleeding following myomectomy by applying internal pressure to endometrial sites of hemorrhage. Finally, the balloon can be left in place for 10 days following myomectomy when the endometrial cavity has been breached in an attempt to minimize intrauterine synechiae formation.

A final surgical question is whether the use of barrier products can reduce adhesion formation. To date, there are no data regarding the use of such agents in enhancing future pregnancy rates following myomectomy. However, a Cochrane review found evidence that Interceed (Ethicon, Cincinnati, OH) does reduce adhesion formation after gynecologic surgery [107]. A prospective nonrandomized study of adhesion-prevention agents following laparoscopic myomectomy confirmed the utility of Interceed and also found benefit with the use of Seprafilm (Genzyme, Cambridge, MA) and fibrin-glue [108].

15.3 Adenomyosis and Infertility

Adenomyosis uteri is a histopathological diagnosis characterized by the finding of heterotopic endometrial glands and stroma within the myometrium with surrounding smooth muscle hyperplasia. It can be suspected clinically by symptoms of uterine pain, and menorrhagia, by uterine imaging techniques and by gross inspection, but its confirmation requires microscopic examination. It was first described by Rokitansky in 1860. The diagnosis is generally made only when endometrial glands are identified >2.5 mm from the junction of the endometrium and myometrium [109].

15.3.1 The Etiology

A prevailing belief is that adenomyosis begins from eutopic endometrium that infiltrates into the myometrium [110]. The downward growth of the endometrial glands and stroma has been termed "inverted polyps." Though confirmation of this hypothesis is lacking, the frequent surgical finding of adenomyomas that are contiguous with the endometrium lend credence to the hypothesis.

An opposing hypothesis promotes the possibility that metaplasia or neoplasia of stromal cells under the influence of autocrine and/or paracrine factors, which are the intermediaries of genetic, immunologic, and endocrine influences can lead to the development of adenomyosis in situ [111–113]. Similarly, others have suggested that abnormal myometrial development is present first, and that then allows adenomyosis to develop in situ [114, 115]. In a variation of this hypothesis, the inner subendometrial layer of myometrium (called the junctional zone), which is often distinct from the outer layer of myometrium by MRI, is the proposed abnormal layer of the myometrium [116]. Indeed, the inner and outer myometrial layers originate from different embryological origins. The junctional zone and the endometrium are derived from the paramesonephric ducts, whereas the origin of the outer myometrium is nonparamesonephric [109, 117]. The inner junctional zone is approximately 5 mm thick, whereas the outer myometrium averages 10 mm in the fundal regions. Interestingly an association has been reported between trauma to the endometrial myometrial junction by surgical procedures and the presence of adenomyosis [118]. Also, the very fact that adenomyosis tends to be more common in parous women suggests that vascular/trophoblastic infiltration of the endometrial and junctional zone may be involved in the pathogenesis of adenomyosis.

A mechanistic hypothesis presents evidence that abnormal myometrial hyperperistalsis and in particular, abnormal contractility of the junctional zone may promote the dislocation and down growth of the basal endometrium into the myometrium [114, 115, 119]. The etiology of adenomyosis will require further clarification.

15.3.2 Patient Characteristics

Predisposing characteristics of patients with adenomyosis appear to include multiparity and age in the 30s and 40s [110] with the majority being over 50 [120], although rare case reports have noted that adenomyosis can occur in nulliparous juveniles as well [121]. Adenomyosis appears to become more prevalent with age [122]. A study of adenomyosis diagnosed by MRI criteria found evidence of infiltration of adenomyosis into the myometrium, beginning early in the third decade, especially in women who have concurrent endometriosis. After age 34, the presence of adenomyosis appears to accelerate in women with or without endometriosis [123]. Spontaneous abortion and dilation and curettage may be risk factors for developing adenomyosis [51, 124]. Other factors associated with adenomyosis include early menarche (≤10 years of age), short menstrual cycles (≤24 days), increasing parity and obesity, all of which are associated with greater-than-average exposure to estrogen [120].

15.3.3 Manifestations

The uterus is generally enlarged with a "boggy" feel on bimanual examination due to the spongy glandular tissue within the myometrium and the surrounding hyperplastic myocytes. Adenomyosis tends to be sporadically located throughout the myometrium, although it is more commonly observed in the posterior wall than in the anterior wall. It has occasionally been noted to extend from endometrium through to the serosa. Generally adenomyosis is not found as exophytic lesions extending submucosal or subserosal. However, ectopic locations of adenomyosis have been reported such as in the rectovaginal septum [125].

Symptoms and signs including abnormal uterine bleeding, dysmenorrhea, chronic pelvic pain, dyspareunia, and dyschezia have traditionally been ascribed to adenomyosis. However, some authors feel that adenomyosis is not the source of pathologic symptoms rather a normal variant found incidentally [126].

15.3.4 Prevalence

Reported prevalence rates for adenomyosis vary depending on the populations studied. Women undergoing hysterectomy for benign disorders have been reported to have adenomyosis ranging from 20 to 36% [117, 127]. However, it is uncertain what proportion of women of reproductive age in general have adenomyosis. An MRI study of 67 women without endometriosis found a prevalence of 9% while a corresponding group of 160 women with endometriosis detected a very high 79% prevalence of adenomyosis [122].

A higher prevalence of adenomyosis among women with unexplained infertility would imply that adenomyosis is involved in infertility, but a prevalence study of this cohort has not been done. However, a report of 26 infertile women with dysmenorrhea and/or menorrhagia and either primary or secondary infertility identified adenomyosis in over half of them (53.8%) [17]. The diagnoses were made using MRI criteria and were not confirmed histologically.

15.3.5 Diagnosis

Diagnosis requires histologic confirmation of adenomyosis. Therefore an invasive procedure to sample the uterine myometrium is required to make a definitive diagnosis. Laparoscopic and transvaginal needle biopsies are impractical not only for their invasiveness but also because adenomyosis loci tend to be scattered throughout the myometrium and not apparent on the uterine serosal surface.

An important gap in our knowledge base is the lack of correlative histologic data of women suspected of having adenomyosis only by signs and symptoms. Some clinical studies have used only clinical suspicion as their diagnostic criteria for adenomyosis. There is recent evidence from histologic examination of hysterectomy specimens that the clinical severity of adenomyosis in terms of the presence of anemia, dysmenorrhea, and menometrorrhagia correlates with the depth of infiltration of adenomyotic foci [128]. However, the study did not publish the test characteristics of clinical symptoms correlating with histologic evidence of adenomyosis.

Non invasive imaging techniques with high sensitivity and specificity are required to diagnose, treat, and follow the course of adenomyosis. The best studies of diagnostic imaging techniques have relied upon histologic confirmation of adenomyosis.

The techniques that have proven to have reasonable test characteristic for adenomyosis include transvaginal sonography and MRI. Computed tomography has poor test characteristics for adenomyosis because the foci are difficult to differentiate from myometrium [129].

Due to the large variation and presentation of adenomyosis, the use of transvaginal ultrasonography (TVUS) remains a challenging prospect for even experienced radiologists. Areas of adenomyosis scattered through the myometrium have been called the diffuse variety, whereas the less common localization of adenomyosis has been termed an adenomyoma which is frequently confused with a fibroid sonographically. Sonography may be best perfomed during the luteal phase when the glands are most active thereby enhancing the chance of detection of adenomyosis. A number of criteria have been established that correlate with the histology of adenomyosis. Most commonly, adenomyosis contains heterogeneous hyper and hypoechoic areas by ultrasound [130]. Half of the cases of adenomyosis contain cysts within the myometrium measuring up to 6 mm in diameter [131]. The borders are indistinct in comparison with leiomyomata and the network of vessels that characteristically surround myomas are absent from the borders of focal adenomyomas.

When ultrasound is correlated to histology, the areas of decreased echogenicity correlate with hypertrophic myometrium, whereas the hyperechoic areas represent islands of endometrial glands [132]. Other proposed ultrasound features of adenomyosis include subendometrial myometrial cysts, subendometrial echogenic nodules, diffuse abnormal echotexture of the myometrium, subendometrial linear striations, a nodular endometrial–myometrial junction, a poorly defined endometrial-myometrial juncture, asymmetric myometrium, and a globular configuration of the uterus.

Two experienced reviewers were blinded to the clinical presentations and histology of 102 hysterectomy cases (32 of which had histologically verified adenomyosis) then reviewed videotaped sonography of the uterine specimens. The ultrasound characteristics contributing most to the positive predictive value for adenomyosis proved to be the observation of subendometrial echogenic nodules and linear striations and asymmetric myometrial thickness [132]. The mean sensitivity, specificity, negative and positive predictive values, and accuracy of the two sonographers for the diagnosis of adenomyosis were 81%, 71%, 90%, 54%, and 74%, respectively. Along with the systematic evaluation of the ultrasound criteria, the accuracy of diagnosis is enhanced by the use of real-time imaging compared to static images [114]. Realistically, the clinically useful diagnosis of adenomyosis by ultrasonography is confined to sonographers with a special interest and experience in pursuing the diagnosis.

15.3.6 Magnetic Resonance Imaging of Adenomyosis

MRI has sensitivities and specificities comparable to those of TVUS in the hands of experienced sonographers for the diagnosis of adenomyosis [130]. T2-weighted images of adenomyosis generally demonstrate a low signal intensity of the lesions and a junctional zone thicker than the normal upper limit of 10–12 mm [122]. This thickening can be either focal or diffuse [130]. Other MRI criteria for the diagnosis of adenomyosis are similar to those for TVUS and include high signal intensity linear striations radiating from endometrium into the myometrium, high signal intensity foci situated within areas of low signal intensity, and poorly defined borders of the junctional zone [133]. The secondary criteria are used when the thickness of the junctional zone (also called the archimyometrium and stratum subvasculare) is in the gray zone of 8–12 mm [130]. The thickness depends in part on whether the uterus is contracting when the MRI images are captured, introducing some inconsistency into the interpretation of the static images.

Transvaginal ultrasound represents the most economical screen for adenomyosis in the presence of an experienced sonographer. However, if the findings are inconclusive, the addition of MRI may be of benefit in helping to make the diagnosis [134].

15.3.7 Postulated Mechanisms of Adenomyosis in Infertility

Preceding confirmation of whether adenomyosis even contributes to infertility, several potential mechanisms have been proposed for the possibility. The argument has been made that sperm transport directed to the fallopian tubes is dependent not only on normal sperm motility, but also on a properly functioning contraction pattern of the myometrium [122, 136, 135]. An observation was made that women with endometriosis have impaired sperm transportation [129]. Because there is a strong association between endometriosis and the presence of adenomyosis, it has been postulated that adenomyosis, by infiltration of the myometrial architecture, may disrupt myometrial contraction patterns and therefore contribute to infertility associated with endometriosis and adenomyosis [122].

Abnormal implantation due to disordered junctional zone structure and function has also been a proposed mechanism for infertility associated with adenomyosis. Another mechanism could be an abnormality of the inflammatory response of both the ectopic myometrial and eutopic endometrial tissue of women with adenomyosis [137]. If either of these hypotheses were correct, it would be expected that higher SAB rates and recurrent pregnancy loss would also be present, but these pregnancy complications in excess of baseline have not been confirmed consistently in association with adenomyosis.

15.3.8 Possible Involvement in Infertility

The very fact that adenomyosis is found more frequently in parous women clouds any association that the acquired condition may have with infertility. Few clinical studies have examined whether there is an association between adenomyosis and infertility. Therefore, causation cannot be ascribed currently. Indeed, the frequent coexistence of adenomyosis with endometriosis, endometrial polyps, and leiomyomata confound the ability to determine whether adenomyosis contributes to subfecundity [122]. Another major confounder is the correlation between advancing age and the increasing incidence of adenomyosis. Because advancing age correlates strongly with diminishing ovarian reserve, the possible contribution of adenomyosis to infertility becomes diluted without well-controlled studies. Currently no such studies exist. Unlike leiomyomata, there are no analyses regarding the volume and uterine location of adenomyosis contributing to implantation impairment.

The accuracy of detection of adenomyosis is clearly important and immediately poses the threat of introducing detection bias into clinical investigations. The infertility sub-populations studied also promise wide variation that can only be addressed with randomization of infertile cohorts. With these limitations in mind, an abstract from China leaves the impression that adenomyosis may indeed be associated with infertility. From a cohort of 22 married women with dysmenorrhea, hypermenorrhea, and adenomyosis documented histologically at the time of conservative surgery, seven (31.8%) also proved to have primary infertility and another 10 (45.5%) had secondary infertility and an additional three (13.6%) had recurrent pregnancy losses [138]. Overall 20 of the 22 women were affected by reproductive difficulties.

Another study of adenomyosis among an unselected group of women undergoing hysterectomy found that among 103 women histologically shown to have adenomyosis, their reproductive span was longer than for the 195 women who did not have adenomyosis [127]. This implies that the length of time between deliveries in the adenomyosis group took longer. Also, the adenomyosis group had significantly higher prevalence of nulliparous women.

15.3.9 Studies of Adenomyosis Therapy and Subsequent Fertility

Another indirect method to assess whether adenomyosis interferes with fecundity is to treat adenomyosis and observe whether there is a benefit for subsequent pregnancy rates. Fertility-sparing interventions that can be used for adenomyosis include conservative focal removal of adenomyomas and uterine artery embolization (UAE) procedures [139]. Only one report is available among women desiring continued fertility with histologically proven adenomyosis who underwent conservative surgery for adenomyosis [138] (Liu, 1998). Five of seven women with adenomyomas subsequently conceived but only one of 14 women with diffuse adenomyosis had a term delivery following conservative surgery. The study was not controlled but importantly a high proportion of these women (approximately 90%) had infertility or recurrent pregnancy loss prior to their surgery. Nonetheless, the attributable effects of adenomyosis compared to the surgery on the pregnancy rates cannot be deduced.

Likewise, no pregnancies that can be attributed to the treatment of adenomyosis have been reported from small series of UAE [140–142]. The studies have been confounded by the presence of concomitant fibroids prior to UAE. The studies were not focused on infertile cohorts but at least have generally demonstrated efficacy in reducing uterine and junctional zone size as well as a reduction in symptoms. The only such study that did examine pregnancy outcomes following UAE found that five of six women desiring fertility did conceive, but again the attributable effect of adenomyosis on fertility could not be ascertained, as the main indication for UAE was fibroids [143].

For UAE to be successful for the treatment of adenomyosis and the preservation of fertility, it would have to differentially eradicate or repress adenomyosis tissue compared to normal eutopic endometrium. This remains to be demonstrated. MRI follow-up of UAE showed some thinning of the junctional zone and areas of devascularization in areas of adenomyosis [144]. However, a study examining adenomyosis tissue histologically after UAE could identify no effect on the adenomyosis [145].

Analogous to the treatment of endometriosis, medical suppressive therapies assume that adenomyosis is treatable by estrogen deprivation. There are at least five reports involving seven infertile women in total with adenomyosis conceiving after treatment with GnRH agonist therapy and/or danazol. However, cause and effect relationships are not possible to analyze. The risk of publication bias is high with only successes being reported. Also, some of the diagnoses of adenomyosis were presumptive from imaging or symptoms alone, and in the other cases with histologic confirmation of adenomyosis, the authors also surgically treated endometriosis, fibroids, and adenomyomas prior to the medical suppressive therapy [146–150].

Risks of a combined medical and surgical approach to treating adenomyomas are likely the same as similar treatment for leiomyomata including the obstetrical risks of prematurity, uterine rupture with uterine contractions, miscarriage, and intrauterine synechiae. An epidemiologic study of gravid women who had adenomyosis diagnosed preconceptionally by either MRI or TVUS criteria, demonstrated nearly a twofold adjusted odd ratio (1.96, 95% CI 1.23–4.47) of delivering preterm [151]. For diffuse adenomyosis where a surgical approach is not practical, a rapid return of adenomyosis after medical suppressive therapy has been noted [147].

Given the high correlation between endometriosis and adenomyosis along with the uncertain mechanisms and contributions of each to infertility, it will be difficult to identify cohorts to study the reproductive effects of pure adenomyosis [152].

For infertile woman suspected of having adenomyomas by symptoms and imaging, after all other infertility causes have been addressed, it may be reasonable to consider pretreating with a GnRH agonist prior to adenomyomectomy taking all of the precautions used for performing myomectomy. When diffuse adenomyosis is diagnosed in the circumstance of otherwise unexplained infertility, the only proposed therapeutic option currently is medical suppressive therapy followed by immediate pregnancy attempts. Based upon the lack of experimental confirmation of the efficacy of this approach, it should be considered empiric therapy. This same approach has not proven effective for endometriosis-associated infertility and it is only supported by several case reports for adenomyosis. IVF is an effective therapy for endometriosis associated infertility but IVF has not been tested as a therapeutic option for adenomyosis.

15.4 Asherman Syndrome and Infertility

The diagnosis, classification, and treatment of the Asherman syndrome have been closely linked to the evolution of diagnostic technologies. Although synechiae following intrauterine trauma was first described by Fritsch in 1894 [153], the syndrome assumed its name after Joseph Asherman's series of papers starting in 1948 culminating in a 1950 paper that clinically characterized the condition and incorporated hysterosalpingography as a method of detection [154]. His observations of pregnancy-related traumatic intrauterine synechiae antedated the development of hysteroscopy.

15.4.1 Definition

The term "Asherman syndrome" has persisted and in common use has come to define a broad spectrum of physical consequences of traumatic damage to the endometrium that result in abnormal clinical manifestations, both menstrual and reproductive. The term also implies the presence of synechiae within the intrauterine cavity as opposed to only fibrotic scarring of the endometrium. Even then, inconsequential asymptomatic adhesions within the uterine cavity should not be termed Asherman syndrome [155]. Most articles on the topic have not defined Asherman syndrome in functional terms rather they simply report the presence of intrauterine adhesions (IUA) or intrauterine synechiae. All of these terms have been used interchangeably but it should be understood that Asherman syndrome when accurately defined is a functionally-designated subset of IUA.

15.4.2 Clinical Presentation

A classic review by Schenker and Margalioth has provided a basis for describing the clinical manifestations of Asherman syndrome [156]. The worldwide literature was collated up to 1982 and a total of 2,981 cases of IUA were clinically characterized. The most common manifestation of intrauterine synechiae was infertility in 43%. Amenorrhea was noted in 37% and hypomenorrhea in another 31%. Recurrent pregnancy loss represented 14% of the total. In some circumstances, Asherman syndrome may lead to amenorrhea or hypomenorrhea simply due to relative obstruction of the outflow track without intracavitary adhesions.

15.4.3 Pathophysiology

The most common predisposing history for the development of intrauterine synechiae is curettage of a gravid or postpartum uterus (over 90%) [156]. Observations indicate that there is a "critical interval" comprising the second through fourth postpartum weeks during which curettage is most likely to result in IUA compared to the first week or anytime after the fourth part partum weeks [157, 158]. The reason for this curious timing has commonly been ascribed to the low concentrations of endometrial growth-promoting estrogen in the circulation after the first postpartum week.

The importance of trauma to the gravid uterus as another predisposing factor for IUA development was emphasized in a trial of 82 women with spontaneous abortions. Subjects were randomized to medical, surgical, or expectant management and then a follow-up hysteroscopy was performed 6 months thereafter. Filmy IUA were found in 7.7% of the surgically managed group but none were observed in the expectant and medically managed groups [159]. Other traumatic antecedents resulting in Asherman syndrome have included cesarean section, uterine infections such as tuberculous endometritis, and gynecologic surgeries such as polypectomy and especially myomectomy [156].

Although there is a common belief that overly aggressive curettage and surgical trauma underlie Asherman syndrome, the seemingly innocuous nature of some procedures causing intrauterine damage suggest that other predisposing factors may be just as important [160]. Nevertheless, avoidance of the use of sharp curettage whenever possible is sensible as the incidence of IUA following suction curettage appears to be less than when sharp curettage is employed [161].

Along with a low estrogen environment hampering endometrial growth, a recently gravid uterus and uterine infection have also been implicated as predisposing factors [156]. However, each of these possible factors lacks strong experimental confirmation. Indeed some observational data revealed no correlation between serum estrogen concentrations on the day of surgical evacuation following spontaneous abortion and the development of IUA [161].

If the pregnancy state predisposes to intrauterine synechiae formation, a high degree of risk would be expected in areas where manual extraction of the placenta is practiced, but this has not been observed. Indeed just the opposite has been reported. One practitioner routinely explored the uterine cavity for retained products and swept the walls using a surgical sponge over gloved fingertips [162]. He reported not one known case of IUA in 15,000 deliveries.

Women who have used intrauterine devices where part of the contraceptive mechanism is thought to be an endometrial inflammatory reaction, have not been shown to suffer higher rates of intrauterine synechiae in the absence of perforation or overt infection upon insertion. Moreover, uterine infection alone does not appear to routinely cause IUA. A group of women suffering severe clinical endometritis prior to undergoing cesarean section was compared to a control group who had no signs of infection while undergoing cesarean section and no difference in the incidence of IUA was found between the groups [163].

A genetic predisposition may be another factor, much like some individuals appear to have a genetic predisposition toward cutaneous keloid formation. Combinations of a genetic predisposition, hypoestrogenic environment, endometrial inflammation, and trauma may be required to induce the condition.

Histological observations of the endometrium following curettage are informative regarding the pathogenesis of IUA. No endometrial activity is noted for the first 48 h, but by the third day the curetted surface becomes coated with flattened cells. Serosanguinous exudates and increased PMNs are observed in the basalis layer that ordinarily disappear within seven to nine days. However, associated with some curettage procedures, inflammatory aggregates, primarily composed of eosinophils, are seen to infiltrate into the perivascular spaces between muscle bundles within the myometrium [164]. In the case of Asherman syndrome, sections of the endometrial stroma become fibrosed and any remaining glandular tissue becomes an inactive monolayer that is generally unresponsive to hormonal stimulation [165]. Histologically, the basalis and functionalis become indistinguishable. In fact, histologic sections taken through the entire myometrium from women with Asherman syndrome demonstrated fibrous tissue three to five times that of the control proportions, occupying up to 80% of the uterine wall [166]. Another common histologic finding when there is an abnormal endometrial/myometrial interface (junctional zone) in women with IUA is an increased presence of adenomyosis [167].

The fibrous bands that connect opposing uterine walls are usually avascular. Often, the generous amount of endometrial surface area sometimes visualized at hysteroscopy does not accurately reflect the low amount of menstrual bleeding that the patient reports. This appears to represent a curious phenomenon observed by Asherman [168] wherein the endometrium becomes atretic in the presence of IUA especially when the internal ostium is occluded. The physiology of this effect is not yet known.

A clue to the development of endometrial traumatic damage has been the introduction of endometrial ablation techniques. We know from global endometrial ablation procedures that the endometrium is difficult to ablate entirely with an amenorrhea rate of less than 60% [169]. With the use of the resectoscope, endometrial resection must include the basalis (regenerative) layer to effectively prevent regrowth. It therefore gives some hope that inadvertent IUA may not necessarily preclude implantation and/or normal gestation.

The most understandable potential reasons for infertility associated with IUA include cervical, uterine, and tubal occlusion as well as reduced normal endometrial surface area for implantation. A dysfunctional endometrial/myometrial interface in areas affected by IUA and a constricted cavity with reduced vascularity and contractility may also contribute to lowered fecundity as well as the obstetrical complications of prematurity and placentation abnormalities. It is easy to imagine how in the Asherman syndrome, the functional integrity of Nitabuch's layer can be lost leading to placentation abnormalities observed in a proportion of those who conceive.

15.4.4 Classification

The Asherman syndrome historically has been a term that has been used to encompass a heterogeneous group of uterine cavity synechiae. This ranged from isolated cervical stenosis to filmy adhesions to complete obliteration of the uterine cavity. Because the definition of the syndrome involves dysfunction of menses and/or reproductive capability, classification systems must now incorporate these elements. The simple classification of the severity of Asherman syndrome by the amount of cavitary adhesions offers some correlation with the ability to conceive, but does not help predict pregnancy complications. Likely this is due to our inability to assess the damage and consequent function of the critical endometrial/myometrial junction, or to assess for the persistence of residual basalis. Unfortunately, no clinical markers have yet been described that will reliably predict the extent to which regrowth of normally functioning endometrium may occur over areas of endometrial scarring. So, whereas classification systems can classify clinical and physical findings, they still fall short of the ideal in not being able to accurately predict reproductive outcomes [155, 170].

A commonly used classification comes from the American Fertility Society (AFS, now the American Society for Reproductive Medicine) in 1988 [171]. Developed when HSG and hysteroscopy were available, the AFS classification antedated the widespread use of the newer imaging techniques that do not require instrumentation of the uterine cavity such as CT, MRI, ultrasound, and three-dimensional ultrasonography.

An advantage of the later techniques is the ability to image areas of intrauterine cavitation where contrast or hysteroscopy may be obstructed by adhesions. Among the non-instrumented techniques, only ultrasound provides a helpful, non invasive adjunct to the characterization and treatment of intracavitary adhesions. It appears that sonohysterography can be used to classify intrauterine adhesions [172], but tubal patency cannot consistently be assessed with this technique. The AFS descriptive classification attempts to combine scores regarding the extent of cavity involvement, the density of the visualized adhesions, and the concomitant menstrual pattern into mild, moderate, and severe categories. Two practical deficiencies of the classification scheme include the lack of accounting of tubal patency at the cornua, and importantly, the presence and extent of endometrial fibrosis.

The classification from the European Society of Gynecological Endoscopy accounts for all of these variables and defines seven levels of increasing severity [173]. Yet another effort to increase the prognostic value of a classification system for the Asherman syndrome has since been developed attempting to integrate the best of previous classification schemes [173].

The lack of outcome studies using any of the classification systems has not allowed reproductive prognosis to be established and has hampered the utility of classifications systems in counseling patients. Only generalizations can be used during counseling to estimate a woman's relative chance to deliver safely in the face of Asherman syndrome.

15.4.5 Prevalence

The true prevalence of the Asherman syndrome remains uncertain due to the many detection and measurement variables such as the varied populations studied, the awareness and aggressiveness of pursuing the diagnosis, definitions, and methods used to diagnose the condition. For example, the highest rates have been reported in the clinical situation of retained products of conception treated by curettage procedures where one such study reported a 40% resultant rate of Asherman syndrome [175]. Another group at high risk for intrauterine synechiae is women with recurrent pregnancy loss (RPL) where the syndrome has been variably reported in 5–39% [176–178]. This makes sense because the RPL population would tend to have more intracavitary procedures. Indeed, hysteroscopy performed after D&C procedures done for miscarriages have noted alarmingly high rates of IUA between 7 and 30% with the higher rates being associated with the use of sharp curettes [159, 161, 179]. Therefore, all ob/gyns will likely perform D&C procedures resulting in Asherman syndrome multiple times during their careers. Overall, Al-Inany has estimated the prevalence of IUA to be 1.5% in the general population [180]. Indeed, IUA would stand to be even lower for the infertile population due to fewer pregnancies and therefore fewer intrauterine interventions. In fact, one study using sonohysterography for infertility evaluation in 600 women identified IUA in only 0.3% of the cohort [181]. However, using the more sensitive detection method of hysteroscopy to screen women undergoing IVF, higher prevalence rates of IUA have been found from 3% to 22% [3, 16, 17].

15.4.6 Diagnosing Asherman syndrome

While the Asherman syndrome can be suspected by identifying a history of previous uterine cavity manipulation, especially postpartum, with a subsequent change in menstrual cycles, the diagnosis relies upon imaging or direct visualization of IUA.

Hysterosalpingography became a part of the infertility evaluation in the 1940s. It often has the advantage of outlining discreet areas of synechiae within the uterine cavity, which can assist resection attempts. One disadvantage of the HSG for IUA is if there is cervical canal or lower uterine segment occlusion, then the upper cavity cannot be imaged [3]. Another disadvantage compared to hysteroscopy is that the nature of fibrosis of the endometrium and the adhesions themselves cannot be ascertained. The test statistics for HSG, compared to hysteroscopy as the gold standard for diagnosing all visible abnormalities in an infertile population in one study included a sensitivity of 98.0%, specificity of 34.9%, positive predictive value of 69.9%, negative predictive value of 92.0%, and an accuracy rate of 73.2%, with false-positive and false-negative rates of 30.1% and 8.0%, respectively [3, 182].

When TVUS subsequently became available, it demonstrated the advantage of being able to document fluid pockets and areas of endometrium within the endometrial cavity even when the cervix is occluded. These pockets can serve as landmarks to help guide resection [183]. A stimulation test of areas of responsive endometrium can be done when there is Asherman syndrome with the help of TVUS. Estradiol (4–6 mg po daily) for a 4-week cycle can be administered, then a follow-up TVUS can identify areas of endometrial growth compared to baseline. If endometrium proliferates, this may be a helpful prognostic sign and also serve to guide resection. However, if no endometrium responds to estrogen, it may be due to the suppressive effect that IUA have on the growth of endometrium (especially when the cervical canal is occluded) such that an attempt at resection may still be worthwhile.

Overall, sensitivity, specificity, and predictive values for TVUS fall below suitable levels for the diagnosis of Asherman syndrome [7, 172, 184]. The use of three-dimensional ultrasonography is insufficiently studied for IUA to date [166]. Likewise, magnetic resonance imaging currently only has an adjunctive role in the management of the Asherman syndrome, and rarely will add more information than less expensive imaging modalities [185].

Sonohysterography (SHG) has better test characteristics than transvaginal ultrasonography for the diagnosis of Asherman syndrome on par with hysterosalpingography [184, 186]. Even when an ostium is accessible to saline, the demonstration of tubal architecture and patency by SHG is unreliable. It does not appear to add value to HSG findings for IUA, but does have better test characteristics compared to ultrasound alone.

Widely considered the gold standard for diagnosis and treatment of Asherman syndrome is hysteroscopy, with its capability of offering direct visualization of the intracavitary structures. Perhaps the most important feature that can be distinguished by no other imaging modality is the ability of hysteroscopic visualization of synechiae to correlate with histologic findings [180]. For example, fibrosis of the endometrium appears as glassy avascular patches [187]. Synechiae themselves can be composed of fibrous tissue, endometrium, and myometrium in any combination. A helpful distinguishing maneuver is to instill methylene blue into the cavity, then observe for staining, using the hysteroscope. The stain is taken up by the endometrium whereas fibrotic tissue does not stain well [188]. Another characteristic of endometrial tissue is the visible presence of surface gland ostia. But even hysteroscopic assessment of apparently adequate areas of endometrium cannot predict reproductive outcome with accuracy since overlying endometrium can mask underlying fibrosis at the level of the myometrial-endometrial junction [155].

15.4.7 Therapy

Unfortunately, therapeutic measures for Asherman syndrome are limited to attempts to restore the anatomy to a normal cavity configuration and to try to prevent reformation of the adhesions. Functional integrity can only be achieved if there is sufficient basalis to allow for adequate implantation, or if the endometrial basalis can repopulate by lateral growth over the endometrial-myometrial layer from which adhesions have been removed. Currently, there are no known growth factors, nanomolecules, or adjuncts that can reliably re-establish normal endometrial architecture to areas where the basalis has been denuded.

15.4.8 Surgical Procedures

Most reports of the surgical treatment of Asherman syndrome consist of uncontrolled case series using a number of technologies. Prior to the availability of hysteroscopy, treatment of Asherman syndrome was limited to the use of blind D&C to break up adhesions, and do hysterotomy. The experience with hysterotomy, although invasive, demonstrated at a minimum that pregnancies after hysterotomy for complete cavity obliteration were still possible. Approximately half of 31 cases conceived and one-quarter delivered at term [156]. Because these hysterotomy outcomes were subjectively better than those achieved by blind dissection of the IUA, it provided hope that precise division and removal of adhesions by hysteroscopy would be the optimum approach.

Valle and Sciarra first documented efficacy by a hysteroscopic approach, using scissors to resect IUA [188]. The rapid development of a number of techniques, including the use of hysteroscopic scissors, unipolar resectoscopes, laser energy, and more recently, intracavitary bipolar devices, has extended the menu of choices, yet randomized trials between resection techniques for Asherman syndrome have not been reported.

Although not well supported by quality data, some generalities based upon theoretic concerns are worthy of consideration. First, hemostasis should be a goal so as not to promote recurrence of adhesions. For bleeding sites within the uterine cavity, only pressure and coagulation are possible methods of hemostasis. The use of thermal energy and its potential for further collateral damage to the endometrium must be traded off with the benefit of precise hemostasis. A study could not find a difference in outcomes, including the development of IUA between use of the resectoscope, compared to hysteroscopic scissors for resection of uterine septums [189]. Another study compared outcomes between the use of a resectoscope, compared to a Versapoint bipolar electrosurgical system (Versapoint Electro-Surgical System; Gynecare Inc., Menlo Park, CA) that does not risk thermal spread into the myometrium [190]. No difference in cumulative delivery rates were observed.

A second generalization is that rather than simply dividing thick adhesions, they should be resected as close to the surface of the cavity as possible to minimize the presence of "foreign body" adhesion remnants within the cavity. Another principle is to establish patency of the cervical canal. Asherman himself described the not infrequent situation where there is stenosis of the cervix, generally at the level of the internal ostium. The interesting observation in this circumstance is that rather than the universal development of hematometra, the endometrium is quite often atretic upon curettage and visualization even when there are no intracavitary adhesions [191]. Asherman termed this circumstance, "amenorrhea traumatica atretica," and noted that most often menses return after simply re-establishing patency to the cervical canal [168]. This phenomenon implies that the presence of menstrual effluvium mediated by cytokine or growth factor signaling may shut down the cyclic development of endometrium despite the exposure to normal circulating reproductive hormones. This phenomenon itself may explain successful re-establishment of menses and reproductive potential after surgical approaches to some cases of Asherman syndrome, whereas the intracavitary adhesions may be more incidental than causative.

Whichever technique is selected, the risks of perforation and inadequate resection can be minimized by the use of adjunctive guidance. This is most helpful when there is complete obliteration of the cavity when the junction between the myometrium and endometrium is completely obscured and the entry from the cervix is obscured, risking the creation of false passages. Cervical preparation with laminaria or the use of misoprostol "cervical ripening" can be helpful to gain access to the cavity, starting 12–24 h to the procedure by using 25–50 micrograms vaginally every four–six h. We have found better success with the laminaria because the misoprostol does not soften adhesions as well as cervical tissue. Thereafter, laparoscopic guidance using the transillumination of the hysteroscopic light source helps guide resection. Alternatively, transabdominal ultrasound guidance can be a very helpful and practical adjunctive measure, using a filled bladder as the optimum ultrasound transmission window [192].

A technique we favor when complete obliteration of the cavity is encountered, was reported on the basis of six patients [193]. A 13F Pratt cervical dilator or curved uterine sound is gently worked along the lateral edge of the cavity until the tip is determined to be in the cornual region, based on the movement of the tip of the instrument under laparoscopic guidance. The basis for this maneuver is that the myometrial wall in the non-gravid uterus is more firm than the adhesions that fill the cavity. Thus, one can use the lateral wall as a tactile guide while advancing the dilator toward the cornua. The endometrium in the apex of the cornua and the tubal ostium is usually spared of adhesions in Asherman syndrome. This tunneling maneuver is done bilaterally which effectively creates a broad-based septum configuration. The intervening adhesions are then resected under continued laparoscopic guidance. The original report of six cases yielded five pregnancies and four deliveries.

In the circumstance where there are dense adhesions constricting the cavity of the uterus, a technique of scoring the uterine wall with a resectoscopic knife with six to eight longitudinal incisions into the myometrium, extending from the uterine fundus to the isthmus has been described in a series of seven patients [194]. A Collins knife electrode, set at 100 Watts of cutting power, was used with 1.5% glycine solution as the distention media. The knife makes 4 mm-deep incisions. Cervical dilation concluded the procedures in an attempt to prevent stenosis. All seven patients had subsequent increases in their menstrual flow, including two who started with amenorrhea. Two had IUDs placed and all were treated with oral estrogens postoperatively. Uterine cavity sizes returned to normal in five of the seven at hysteroscopy 2 months post operatively, but four required repeat scoring procedures. Three women conceived four pregnancies after a mean follow-up period of 12 months, however, the reproductive outcomes were guarded. One woman suffered a tubal abortion, another had an ongoing pregnancy, and a third had a first trimester missed abortion and then subsequently conceived again and delivered at 36 weeks after premature rupture of membranes. It was encouraging to learn from this series that even incisions into the myometrium could presumably yield regrowth of overlying endometrium with enough function to host an implantation to 36 weeks.

The following year, a French group reported a larger series of 31 cases of severe Asherman syndrome using a similar technique, including the 4 mm monopolar knife (Karl Storz GmbH, Tuttlingen, Germany). Prior to their procedures, all patients demonstrated at hysteroscopy, extensive firm adhesions, with agglutination of the uterine walls and both tubal ostial areas were occluded [195]. Along with longitudinal incisions, several transverse incisions were also made along the fundus. Multiple repeat scoring procedures were required until the surgeons were satisfied that adequate anatomy was achieved. Sixteen of the patients returned for one repeat procedure, seven for two repeats, seven for three repeated scoring procedures, and one woman required four repeated procedures. All had increased menstrual flow. Of the 28 patients who were followed up, 32% had live births from among the 43% who initially conceived. Of the nine live births, two had serious obstetrical complications. Both had placenta acreta, requiring hypogastric artery ligation in one and cesarean hysterectomy in the other.

As an alternative procedure for "end stage" severe Asherman syndrome with complete cavity occlusion, laparotomy with hysterotomy was reintroduced in a series of three women with severe Asherman syndrome [196]. Whereas menses were restored, none of the three conceived.

Although neither the scoring, the tunneling, or the hysterotomy techniques for obliterated cavities have sufficient published outcome information, it would seem that laparotomy is best avoided, given the outpatient alternatives and the need to recommend cesarean section when hysterotomies are made. Nonetheless, women considering any of the hysteroscopic techniques should be counseled regarding the known morbidities and the frequent need for multiple surgeries.

15.4.9 Prevention of Adhesion Reformation

In severe cases, adhesions reform in approximately half of hysteroscopic resection cases [178]. Even when IUA are not severe, adhesions reform in up to one quarter of patients [188]. Four basic strategies have been employed in an attempt to diminish adhesion reformation.

15.4.9.1 Pharmacologic

Pharmacologic adjunct used to minimize adhesion formation have included antibiotics, sex-steroids, antioxidants, anticoagulants, and anti-inflammatory agents [156, 197, 198]. Randomized clinical trials have not been published to support the theoretical values of any of these pharmacologic adjuncts. Nonetheless, in common use are supplemental doses of estrogen in an attempt to hasten the reepithelialization of the damaged endometrial surface after resection [199]. The use of estrogen clearly enhances growth of endometrium [200]. However, evidence for a beneficial reduction of adhesion reformation is not available. Various regimens have been commonly employed postoperatively. One common protocol is to prescribe oral estrogen daily for a month with or without progestational agents for the last one or 2 weeks of the course. Dosing has been empiric, with some centers using conjugated estrogen doses as high as 2.5 mg bid for anywhere from 3 to 8 weeks. Given the nausea that is frequently induced by such high doses, much lower doses such as estradiol 2 mg daily or conjugated estrogens 1.25 mg daily are probably adequate, given their proven ability to induce endometrial growth in egg donor recipients, while suppressed on GnRH analogues.

15.4.9.2 Mechanical Separation

A second early measure was the introduction of mechanical barriers into the cavity in an attempt to separate the endometrial surfaces until healing can occur. Intrauterine devices (IUDs) were tried [201, 202]. In theory, T-shaped IUDs, compared to broader IUDs, may not provide the necessary surface area to effectively combat adhesion reformation [203]. Copper containing IUDs may induce excessive inflammation that could exacerbate adhesion formation [203].

Unfortunately only T-shaped IUDs are currently available in the United States, and one of them is copper containing. For these reasons, along with the high cost, IUDs are not good choices to prevent the reformation of adhesions.

A helpful clinical study has directed clinical practice away from IUD use toward the use of 5 mL Foley catheter balloons [204]. In a comparative study from Nigeria where hysteroscopy was not available at the time, IUA were diagnosed by HSG, then treated with blind adhesiolysis. All patients in the study had IUA as their only infertility diagnosis after complete evaluation. For 4 consecutive years, from 1991 to 1995, size D Lippes loop IUDs were placed into the uterine cavity for three consecutive withdrawal bleeds in 51 patients. In the ensuing 4 years, also after blind adhesiolysis, a size 8 pediatric Foley balloon was placed into the cavity in 59 patients. The Foley stem was strapped to the inner thigh and left in place for 10 days. Patients in both groups were treated for 10 days with antibiotics and with 28 days of estrogen, followed by five days of norethisterone acetate 10 mg TID. After three withdrawal bleeds, an HSG was repeated in all subjects.

Restoration of normal menses occurred in 81.4% of the Foley group, but only 62.7% of the IUD group ($p<0.5$). Conceptions occurred in 33.9% of the Foley, compared to 22.5% of the IUD groups. No patient within the Foley group suffered perforation or infection, compared to 4% for each complication reported in the IUD group. Repeated procedures were done for 13.6% of the Foley group and 43.1% of the IUD cohort. Overall, use of the Foley was quicker, less expensive, had fewer complications, and was more efficacious.

Another non randomized study compared the use of a 3.5 mL 10F Foley balloon, left in place for 1 week ($n=32$), to using nothing ($n=18$) following operative hysteroscopy for various reasons [205]. Hysteroscopy was performed 6–8 weeks postoperatively and identified IUA in 50% of the no balloon compared to 21.9% of the Foley group ($p<0.05$). They further analyzed balloon placement after hysteroscopic resection of IUA in 12 subjects, compared to eight who did not receive a balloon. There was a non significant trend in this low-powered study toward less adhesion reformation (33.3%) in the Foley compared to the no-Foley (62.5%) group.

Some disadvantages of the Foley catheters remain. They are unpopular with patients due to the inconvenience of the length of catheter that is left protruding from the vagina postoperatively. The catheters are prone to dislodge, especially with inadvertent traction on the protruding catheter. Furthermore, the round balloon shape only separates the central uterine walls leaving the important lateral regions susceptible to agglutination. Also, the concentrated pressure that a filled balloon places on the endometrium it comes in contact with, could lead to devascularization of the affected endometrium. Some of these concerns have been addressed by the development of a triangular-shaped uterine stent (Cook; Spencer, Indiana) that comes in two sizes. The stent fits the shape of the endometrial cavity better than a Foley balloon or a Malecot catheter. It has a basic flat contour that keeps the anterior and posterior walls separated and distributes the pressure more evenly against the endometrium when filled with saline. Even when the properly placed stent is partially deflated, it still effects separation of the walls without applying excessive pressure to them. The stem that is used to inflate and deflate the stent can be rolled up and tucked into the vagina for convenience. Anecdotally, we have not yet had a stent dislodge or become infected (even without ongoing antibiotic use) from among several dozen applications. Although there are no efficacy trials using the device, it is likely that it has similar efficacy to the use of Foley balloons.

15.4.9.3 Adhesion Barriers

A third strategy to discourage IUA reformation has been the use of adhesion prevention materials placed into the uterine cavity. One such material is Seprafilm™ (Genzyme Corporation, Cambridge, MA). It is a bioresorbable membrane made up of chemically modified hyaluronic acid and carboxymethylcellulose. It is nontoxic, nonimmunogenic, and hydrates within two days into a gel that serves as a temporary mechanical barrier. When used in the abdomen, the gel resorbs within five to seven days. A randomized clinical trial of its use was performed in women undergoing suction evacuation procedures and curettage for spontaneous abortions [164]. In this population, 20–50% were expected to develop IUA. Fifty women received the Seprafilm™ and 100 controls had nothing inserted into the uterus postoperatively. The film sheets were cut in half, rolled into cylinders, and the first inserted into the cavity under aseptic conditions. The second cylinder was placed into the cervical canal such that both the internal and external ostia were covered.

In patients who had never had surgical procedures for IUA previously, all 32 who were randomized to Seprafilm™ conceived within 8 months, while only 54% of the control group conceived. In patients who had previously undergone one or more D&Cs, only 33% of the Seprafilm™ group conceived compared to 22.7% of the control group (N.S.). Of those women not conceiving, 10 Seprafilm™ and 14 controls agreed to undergo a subsequent HSG wherein one (10%) of the Seprafilm™ group and seven (50%) of the controls proved to have IUA. Importantly, no adverse reactions were observed in the Seprafilm™ group.

A different formulation of hyaluronic acid, auto-cross-linked hyaluronic acid (ACP) gel has also shown promise in diminishing adhesion reformation within the uterine in a randomized clinical trial of 92 women with IUA undergoing hysteroscopic resection [206]. The cross-linked ACP renders hyaluronic acid viscous, allowing for easier instillation into the uterus compared to film sheets. A hook-shaped monopolar electrode was used to resect adhesions hysteroscopically. Those randomized to ACP gel (Hyalobarrier gel; Baxter, Pisa, Italy) received 10 mL under hysteroscopic guidance until the entire cavity from the tubal ostia to the internal cervical ostium appeared to be filled with gel. Ultrasound was used for three consecutive days thereafter to confirm that the gel continued to separate the uterine walls. Antibiotics were administered for three days also and diagnostic hysteroscopy was performed 3 months postoperatively. While conception data were not available from this report, of the 84 subjects who completed the study, six of 43 patients given gel compared to 13 of 41 women reformed adhesions ($p < 0.05$). Also, the mean AFS adhesions scores were also significantly reduced for the ACP gel group.

A small observational study of 25 subjects reported the use of amnion grafts inserted into the endometrial cavity, draped over Foley balloons for up to 2 weeks [207]. Amnion has been successfully used to assist in the healing of other epithelial sites such as eye, abdominal wall, and vaginal wall. All subjects were undergoing hysteroscopic lysis of IUA, graded as moderate-to-severe. By a second hysteroscopy, 48% of the subjects had reformed IUA (all from the severe group of 13 subjects) but in 11 of these, the adhesions were graded as only minimal, except two, who had genital tuberculosis as the source of their IUA. Overall, five of the subjects failed to re-establish normal menstrual patterns. Both infectious and immunologic sequelae are possible from an allograft, and with the lack of fertility outcome data, this technique should be regarded as experimental. To date, there have been no trials of autologous skin, peritoneal grafts, or growth substances for use in the treatment of resected Asherman syndrome.

15.4.9.4 Serial Adhesiolysis

A fourth strategy to minimize adhesions after initial sharp hysteroscopic resection is to serially reduce filmy reformed IUA, using only a flexible hysteroscope starting 2 weeks postoperatively, and then every one to 3weeks. The intent is to intercede before the adhesions have the opportunity to become vascularized and dense. Twenty-four patients, symptomatic with Asherman syndrome, underwent this quick office technique an average of three times (range, one to nine) until no further reformation of adhesions could be observed [208]. The resulting rates for the restoration of normal menses and for clinical pregnancies compared favorably, in this small study, to other techniques. However, larger randomized studies will be needed to learn whether this strategy will have a role in optimizing reproductive outcomes in women with Asherman syndrome.

None of the four basic strategies for minimizing adhesion formation are mutually exclusive. Therefore, the best approach(es) must await systematic study. In the meantime, clinicians must individualize their approach with emphasis on minimizing risk, expense, and discomfort for women undergoing treatment for Asherman syndrome.

15.4.10 Therapeutic Outcomes

Controlled trials of therapy for Asherman syndrome should have a no-treatment arm because the spontaneous pregnancy rate appears to be relatively high, as reported by Schenker and Margalioth who observed that of 292 women with untreated Asherman syndrome, 45.5% went on to conceive spontaneously [156]. (Table 15.1) If there are adequate areas of normal endometrium remaining that are accessible to implanting embryos, then the prognosis for conception should be proportional to the available normal endometrial surface area.

As it stands, few randomized treatment trials have been performed using proper classifications, standardized techniques, and similar populations. Therefore, counseling regarding prognosis for patients must be couched in generalizations. Yu and colleagues have recently published a comprehensive review of Asherman syndrome that extends and updates the current understanding over 26 years since the review by Schenker and Margalioth [155]. This review includes a compilation of published outcome data with the use of hysteroscopic adhesiolysis, which was just becoming popular at the time the Schenker and Margolioth paper was published. Five studies of hysteroscopic resection of Asherman syndrome of all grades, including a total of 625 patients reported on the outcome of menstrual cycle resumption [188, 195, 209–212]. Normal menstrual patterns were achieved in 84.5% after hysteroscopic resection. Contrast this 84.5% to the near 100% resumption of normal menses from 10 studies (449 of 450 patients) using blind adhesiolysis and IUD placement postoperatively, as summarized by Schenker and Margalioth in 1982 [156].

Fourteen studies have reported reproductive outcomes following hysteroscopic adhesiolysis [188, 190, 193–195, 209–217]. Seven of the studies listed the proportion of treated women achieving a subsequent pregnancy [188, 210–213, 216, 217]. Overall, 468 of 632 conceived (74%). Nine studies reported spontaneous abortion rates, which totaled 84 of 477 reported pregnancies (17.6%) [188, 193–195, 209, 210, 214–216]. Another 13 studies, totaling 666 subjects who conceived following hysteroscopic adhesiolysis, reported that an impressive 79.4% delivered live born children [188, 193–195, 209–217]. However, of the four studies that listed premature deliveries, a worrisome 47% (17 of 31) delivered preterm [190, 193–195]. Abnormal placentation was reported in 23 cases from seven different studies with a total of 374 conceptions for an average incidence of 6.2% [188, 190, 193, 195, 210, 214, 215].

Table 15.1 Reproductive outcomes of published management techniques for asherman syndrome

	No treatment[a]	Hysterotomy[b]	Primary[c] IUD treatment	D&C, IUD, estrogen[d]	Vaginal adhesiolysis[e]	Hysteroscopic adhesiolysis[f]
Subjects Available[g]	$N=292$	$N=34$	$N=405$	$N=75$	$N=756$	$N=814$
Conception %[h]	46%	52%	56%	80%	48%	74%
Term Deliveries %	30%	24%	60%	77%	54%	79%
SAB %	40%	NR	27%	23%	25%	18%
Preterm %	23%	NR	7%	8%	9%	47%
Placentation Abnormalities %	13%	3%	6%	1%	6%	6.2%

NR not reported

[a]Source: Schenker and Margolioth, 1982

[b]Sources: Schenker and Margolioth, 1982; Reddy and Rock, 1997; and Protopapas et al., 1998.

[c]Source: Schenker and Margolioth, 1982. Placement of the IUD alone served as treatment of IUA without blunt or sharp adhesiolysis

[d]Source: Schenker and Margolioth, 1982. Adhesiolysis technique proposed by Schenker and Margolioth. Only cases of intrauterine adhesiolysis are reported here

[e]Source: Schenker and Margolioth, 1982. Data from studies reporting blind vaginal lysis of adhesions while removing data from Sugimoto et al. where hysteroscopic adhesiolysis was done

[f]Source: Yu et al., 2008. Reproductive outcomes abstracted from subsets of patients treated by hysteroscopic lysis of adhesions from 14 studies

[g]Proportions of pregnancy outcomes may not sum to 100% because not all outcomes were reported for all subjects

[h]Conception % refers to the % of patients who conceived

Bear in mind that among the fourteen studies, the diagnosis of infertility was not necessarily confined to isolated Asherman syndrome. In two of the studies, IVF was used for all patients. Therefore, the overall live birth rate cannot be attributed to the hysteroscopic adhesiolysis alone. Moreover, the studies represent a mixture of various techniques, disease severity, and study populations reported over a 25-year time span. Patients who desire to conceive in the face of Asherman syndrome should be informed of the imprecise nature of the reported outcome information and that serious risks of prematurity and placentation abnormalities must be carefully considered before hysteroscopic adhesiolysis is undertaken.

Table 15.1 displays data abstracted from the 1982 Schenker and Margolioth review that only includes non hysteroscopic intrauterine adhesiolysis techniques and compares their reproductive outcomes with hysteroscopic adhesiolysis from among the 14 studies reviewed by Yu et al. Caution must be used in interpreting these data due to the different populations studied, differing fertility problems and treatments, variable follow-up durations, and the few data available for some of the reproductive outcomes, notably preterm deliveries. However, both hysteroscopic and non hysteroscopic studies shared the same variety of adjunctive treatment methods, mostly composed of postoperative estrogen and Foley balloon catheter use. Overall, the hysteroscopic techniques appear to have an advantage over blind intrauterine adhesiolysis regarding conception and live birth rates. Complication rates were similar between the two techniques with the striking exception of a 47% preterm delivery rate when the hysteroscopic approach was used. However, this high preterm rate came from only four studies of hysteroscopic adhesiolysis, involving only 17 patients with preterm deliveries, out of which ten patients were contributed by a single study. Interestingly, the combined reproductive outcomes of the 14 hysteroscopic adhesiolysis studies closely mirrored the outcomes of a subset of the women undergoing vaginal adhesioysis. These were the 75 women with IUA treated using the Schenker and Margolioth protocol that included D&C, IUD, and estrogen.

15.4.11 Prevention of Intrauterine Adhesions

Because effective treatment of IUA remains only modest and obstetrical risk remains serious and frequent in the face of IUA, the obvious best management of IUA is to prevent their formation. Most cases of Asherman syndrome occur due to traumatic intervention during the postpartum period. This, therefore, is the logical place to focus on preventative measures. Perhaps one of the biggest technological advances toward reducing (but not eliminating) IUA has been the widespread use of suction curettage apparatuses for both spontaneous and elective abortions.

Because the riskiest postpartum interval for the traumatic induction of IUA is the second through fourth weeks, and for missed abortions at any time, maximal attempts to avoid the need for curettage should be made, especially during these high-risk situations. Prevention of IUA begins with sound obstetrical care in the immediate postpartum period by ensuring complete evacuation of products of conception from the uterus. This obstetrical task has been made easier with the availability of ultrasound to identify retained products and the judicious use of culture and antibiotics to minimize uterine infections after deliveries at high risk for postpartum infection. Careful labor management and the use of uterotonics when needed also stand to diminish postpartum hemorrhage, and therefore, the need for curettage. The increased use of mifepristone with prostaglandins as medical therapy for miscarriage can further reduce the risk of requiring curettage. But when curettage becomes necessary, hysteroscopy using a resectoscopic loop as a blunt curette can be directed specifically to loosely attached products of conception, and therefore in theory, stands to reduce the risk of subsequent IUA [218].

Although awaiting a cost-effectiveness analysis, there is some evidence to recommend the prophylactic use of mechanical uterine wall separation devices (stents, Foley balloons) following curettage for miscarriage [219]. Similarly, the use of these devices makes sense for scenarios presenting an elevated risk for developing IUA, such as hysteroscopic submucosal myomectomy, entrance into the uterine cavity during abdominal myomectomy, uterine perforation, and septum resections. The concomitant use of supplemental estrogen to facilitate endometrial growth, although lacking strong experimental validation, should also be considered in these situations.

15.5 Conclusions

Uterine factor infertility comprises only a small proportion of couples undergoing IVF [1]. Yet, it is a serious diagnosis because when it is recorded as the sole indication for IVF, it is accompanied by lower-than-average live birth rates [211]. Few randomized trials of infertility therapies have been done for uterine factors. Properly designed trials for treatment of acquired uterine lesions are hampered by differing study populations, detection methods, and presentations. The tendency for endometrial polyps, leiomyomata, and adenomyosis to coexist, further confounds the ability to isolate the individual effects of the lesions on fecundity, and of the effects of treatment on reproductive outcome. Nonetheless, when other infertility factors have been excluded, the balance of the evidence favors surgical removal of endometrial polyps as well as submucosal leiomyomata for infertile women. While isolated adenomyosis has been suspected of contributing to reduced fertility, there is currently no conclusive evidence to support this contention. Therefore, when all other detectable infertility factors have been excluded, surgical and medical therapies for adenomyosis remain empiric. Prevention remains the best strategy for Asherman syndrome. However, when the Asherman syndrome occurs, the optimal current surgical approach appears to be resection under hysteroscopic guidance, with the adjunctive use of estrogen and postoperative mechanical separation of the endometrial surfaces. When Asherman syndrome is severe, reproductive outcomes despite optimal treatment are guarded. Considerable risks of infertility, miscarriage, preterm delivery, and placentation abnormalities remain following the treatment of Asherman syndrome. When Asherman syndrome is less severe and the uterine cavity is not completely occluded by adhesions, hysteroscopic resection is associated with a more favorable outcome. Approximately three out of four women will conceive in these circumstances, and approximately 79% of those who conceive will deliver at term.

References

1. Wright VC, Chang J, Jeng G, Macaluso M (2008) Assisted reproductive technology surveillance – United States, 2005. MMWR Surveill Summ 57(5):1–23
2. Perez-Medina T, Bajo-Arenas J, Salazar F et al (2005) Endometrial polyps and their implication in the pregnancy rates of patients undergoing intrauterine insemination: a prospective, randomized study. Hum Reprod 20(6):1632–1635
3. Preutthipan S, Herabutya Y (2005) Hysteroscopic polypectomy in 240 premenopausal and postmenopausal women. Fertil Steril 83(3):705–709
4. Shokeir TA, Shalan HM, El-Shafei MM (2004) Significance of endometrial polyps detected hysteroscopically in eumenorrheic infertile women. J Obstet Gynaecol Res 30(2):84–89
5. Mittal K, Schwartz L, Goswami S, Demopoulos R (1996) Estrogen and progesterone receptor expression in endometrial polyps. Int J Gynecol Pathol 15(4):345–348
6. Lopes RG, Baracat EC, de Albuquerque Neto LC et al (2007) Analysis of estrogen- and progesterone-receptor expression in endometrial polyps. J Minim Invasive Gynecol 14(3):300–303
7. Soares SR, Barbosa dos Reis MM, Camargos AF (2000) Diagnostic accuracy of sonohysterography, transvaginal sonography, and hysterosalpingography in patients with uterine cavity diseases. Fertil Steril 73(2):406–411
8. Taylor E, Gomel V (2008) The uterus and fertility. Fertil Steril 89(1):1–16
9. Lasmar RB, Dias R, Barrozo PR, Oliveira MA, Coutinho Eda S, da Rosa DB (2008) Prevalence of hysteroscopic findings and histologic diagnoses in patients with abnormal uterine bleeding. Fertil Steril 89(6):1803–1807
10. Cicinelli E, Resta L, Nicoletti R et al (2005) Detection of chronic endometritis at fluid hysteroscopy. J Minim Invasive Gynecol 12(6):514–518
11. Richlin S, Ramachandran S, Shanthi A, Murphy AA, Parthasarathy S (2002) Glycodelin levels in uterine flushings and in plasma of patients with leiomyomas and polyps: implications and implantation. Hum Reprod 17(10):2742–2747
12. Golan A, Halperin R, Herman A et al (1994) Human decidua-associated protein 200 levels in uterine fluid at hysteroscopy. Gynecol Obstet Invest 38(4):217–219
13. Clevenger-Hoeft M, Syrop CH, Stovall DW, Van Voorhis BJ (1999) Sonohysterography in premenopausal women with and without abnormal bleeding. Obstet Gynecol 94(4):516–520
14. Koshiyama M, Okamoto T, Ueta M (2004) The relationship between endometrial carcinoma and coexistent adenomyosis uteri, endometriosis externa and myoma uteri. Cancer Detect Prev 28(2):94–98
15. Kim MR, Kim YA, Jo MY, Hwang KJ, Ryu HS (2003) High frequency of endometrial polyps in endometriosis. J Am Assoc Gynecol Laparosc 10(1):46–48
16. Hinckley MD, Milki AA (2004) 1000 office-based hysteroscopies prior to in vitro fertilization: feasibility and findings. JSLS 8(2):103–107
17. de Sa Rosa e de Silva AC, Rosa e Silva JC, Candido dos Reis FJ, Nogueira AA, Ferriani RA (2005) Routine office hysteroscopy in the investigation of infertile couples before assisted reproduction. J Reprod Med 50(7):501–506
18. Onalan R, Onalan G, Tonguc E, Ozdener T, Dogan M, Mollamahmutoglu L (2008) Body mass index is an independent risk factor for the development of endometrial polyps in patients undergoing in vitro fertilization. Fertil Steril 91:1056–1060
19. DeWaay DJ, Syrop CH, Nygaard IE, Davis WA, Van Voorhis BJ (2002) Natural history of uterine polyps and leiomyomata. Obstet Gynecol 100(1):3–7
20. Goerzen JL, Leader A, Taylor PJ (1983) Hysteroscopic findings in 100 women requesting reversal of a previously performed voluntary tubal sterilization. Fertil Steril 39(1):103–104
21. Spiewankiewicz B, Stelmachow J, Sawicki W, Cendrowski K, Wypych P, Swiderska K (2003) The effectiveness of hysteroscopic polypectomy in cases of female infertility. Clin Exp Obstet Gynecol 30(1):23–25
22. Stamatellos I, Apostolides A, Stamatopoulos P, Bontis J (2008) Pregnancy rates after hysteroscopic polypectomy depending on the size or number of the polyps. Arch Gynecol Obstet 277(5):395–399
23. Varasteh NN, Neuwirth RS, Levin B, Keltz MD (1999) Pregnancy rates after hysteroscopic polypectomy and myomectomy in infertile women. Obstet Gynecol 94(2):168–171
24. Mastrominas M, Pistofidis GA, Dimitropoulos K (1996) Fertility outcome after outpatient hysteroscopic removal of endometrial polyps and submucous fibroids. J Am Assoc Gynecol Laparoscs 3:S29
25. Lass A, Williams G, Abusheikha N, Brinsden P (1999) The effect of endometrial polyps on outcomes of in vitro fertilization (IVF) cycles. J Assist Reprod Genet 16(8):410–415
26. Hereter L, Carreras O, Pascual M (1998) Repercusion de la presencia de polipos endometriales en un ciclo de FIV. Prog Obstet Ginecol 41:5–7
27. Isikoglu M, Berkkanoglu M, Senturk Z, Coetzee K, Ozgur K (2006) Endometrial polyps smaller than 1.5 cm do not affect ICSI outcome. Reprod Biomed Online 12(2):199–204
28. Batioglu S, Kaymak O (2005) Does hysteroscopic polypectomy without cycle cancellation affect IVF? Reprod Biomed Online 10(6):767–769
29. DeWaay DJ, Syrop CH, Nygaard IE, Davis WA, Van Voorhis BJ (2002) Natural history of uterine polyps and leiomyomata. Obstet Gynecol 100(1):3–7
30. Lieng M, Qvigstad E, Sandvik L, Jorgensen H, Langebrekke A, Istre O (2007) Hysteroscopic resection of symptomatic and asymptomatic endometrial polyps. J Minim Invasive gynecol 14(2):189–194
31. Silberstein T, Saphier O, van Voorhis BJ, Plosker SM (2006) Endometrial polyps in reproductive-age fertile and infertile women. Isr Med Assoc J 8(3):192–195
32. Ryan GL, Syrop CH, Van Voorhis BJ (2005) Role, epidemiology, and natural history of benign uterine mass lesions. Clin Obstet Gynecol 48(2):312–324

33. Valli E, Zupi E, Marconi D et al (2001) Hysteroscopic findings in 344 women with recurrent spontaneous abortion. J Am Assoc Gynecol Laparosc 8(3):398–401
34. Guimaraes Filho HA, Mattar R, Pires CR, Araujo Junior E, Moron AF, Nardozza LM (2006) Comparison of hysterosalpingography, hysterosonography and hysteroscopy in evaluation of the uterine cavity in patients with recurrent pregnancy losses. Arch Gynecol Obstet 274(5):284–288
35. Devi Wold AS, Pham N, Arici A (2006) Anatomic factors in recurrent pregnancy loss. Semin Reprod Med 24(1):25–32
36. Buttram VC Jr, Reiter RC (1981) Uterine leiomyomata: etiology, symptomatology, and management. Fertil Steril 36(4):433–445
37. Stewart EA (2001) Uterine fibroids. Lancet 357(9252):293–298
38. Wallach EE, Vlahos NF (2004) Uterine myomas: an overview of development, clinical features, and management. Obstet Gynecol 104(2):393–406
39. Viswanathan M, Hartmann K, McKoy N et al (2007) Management of uterine fibroids: an update of the evidence. Evidence Report/Technology Assessment 154:1–122
40. Day Baird D, Dunson DB, Hill MC, Cousins D, Schectman JM (2003) High cumulative incidence of uterine leiomyoma in black and white women: ultrasound evidence. Am J Obstet Gynecol 188(1):100–107
41. Klatsky PC, Tran ND, Caughey AB, Fujimoto VY (2008) Fibroids and reproductive outcomes: a systematic literature review from conception to delivery. Am J Obstet Gynecol 198(4):357–366
42. Marino JL, Eskenazi B, Warner M et al (2004) Uterine leiomyoma and menstrual cycle characteristics in a population-based cohort study. Hum Reprod 19(10):2350–2355
43. Hart R (2003) Unexplained infertility, endometriosis, and fibroids. BMJ 327(7417):721–724
44. Fayez JA, Mutie G, Schneider PJ (1987) The diagnostic value of hysterosalpingography and hysteroscopy in infertility investigation. Am J Obstet Gynecol 156(3):558–560
45. Cicinelli E, Romano F, Anastasio PS, Blasi N, Parisi C, Galantino P (1995) Transabdominal sonohysterography, transvaginal sonography, and hysteroscopy in the evaluation of submucous myomas. Obstet Gynecol 85(1):42–47
46. Somigliana E, Vercellini P, Daguati R, Pasin R, De Giorgi O, Crosignani PG (2007) Fibroids and female reproduction: a critical analysis of the evidence. Hum Reprod Update 13(5):465–476
47. Lumbiganon P, Rugpao S, Phandhu-fung S, Laopaiboon M, Vudhikamraksa N, Werawatakul Y (1996) Protective effect of depot-medroxyprogesterone acetate on surgically treated uterine leiomyomas: a multicentre case–control study. Br J Obstet Gynaecol 103(9):909–914
48. Parazzini F, Chiaffarino F, Polverino G, Chiantera V, Surace M, La Vecchia C (2004) Uterine fibroids risk and history of selected medical conditions linked with female hormones. Eur J Epidemiol 19(3):249–253
49. Wise LA, Palmer JR, Harlow BL et al (2004) Risk of uterine leiomyomata in relation to tobacco, alcohol and caffeine consumption in the Black Women's Health Study. Hum Reprod 19(8):1746–1754
50. Marshall LM, Spiegelman D, Goldman MB et al (1998) A prospective study of reproductive factors and oral contraceptive use in relation to the risk of uterine leiomyomata. Fertil Steril 70(3):432–439
51. Parazzini F, Vercellini P, Panazza S, Chatenoud L, Oldani S, Crosignani PG (1997) Risk factors for adenomyosis. Hum Reprod 12(6):1275–1279
52. Parazzini F, Negri E, La Vecchia C, Chatenoud L, Ricci E, Guarnerio P (1996) Reproductive factors and risk of uterine fibroids. Epidemiology 7(4):440–442
53. Faerstein E, Szklo M, Rosenshein NB (2001) Risk factors for uterine leiomyoma: a practice-based case-control study. II. Atherogenic risk factors and potential sources of uterine irritation. Am J Epidemiol 153(1):11–19
54. Griffiths A, D' Angelo A, Amso N (2006) Surgical treatment of fibroids for subfertility. Cochrane database of systematic reviews (Online) 2006(19):3
55. Pritts EA, Parker WH, Olive DL (2009) Fibroids and infertility: an updated systematic review of the evidence. Fertil Steril 91: 1215–1223
56. Hart R, Khalaf Y, Yeong CT, Seed P, Taylor A, Braude P (2001) A prospective controlled study of the effect of intramural uterine fibroids on the outcome of assisted conception. Hum Reprod 16(11):2411–2417
57. Eldar-Geva T, Meagher S, Healy DL, MacLachlan V, Breheny S, Wood C (1998) Effect of intramural, subserosal, and submucosal uterine fibroids on the outcome of assisted reproductive technology treatment. Fertil Steril 70(4):687–691
58. Farhi J, Ashkenazi J, Feldberg D, Dicker D, Orvieto R, Ben Rafael Z (1995) Effect of uterine leiomyomata on the results of in-vitro fertilization treatment. Hum Reprod 10(10):2576–2578
59. Surrey ES, Minjarez DA, Stevens JM, Schoolcraft WB (2005) Effect of myomectomy on the outcome of assisted reproductive technologies. Fertil Steril 83(5):1473–1479
60. Narayan R, Rajat GK (1994) Treatment of submucous fibroids, and outcome of assisted conception. J Am Assoc Gynecol Laparosc 1(4 Pt 1):307–311
61. Seoud MA, Patterson R, Muasher SJ, Coddington CC 3rd (1992) Effects of myomas or prior myomectomy on in vitro fertilization (IVF) performance. J Assist Reprod Genet 9(3):217–221
62. Bulletti C, DEZ D, Levi Setti P, Cicinelli E, Polli V, Stefanetti M (2004) Myomas, pregnancy outcome, and in vitro fertilization. Ann N Y Acad Sci 1034:84–92
63. Walker WJ, McDowell SJ (2006) Pregnancy after uterine artery embolization for leiomyomata: a series of 56 completed pregnancies. Am J Obstet Gynecol 195(5):1266–1271
64. Hammoud AO, Asaad R, Berman J, Treadwell MC, Blackwell S, Diamond MP (2006) Volume change of uterine myomas during pregnancy: do myomas really grow? J Minim Invasive Gynecol 13(5):386–390
65. Parker WH (2007) Uterine myomas: management. Fertil Steril 88(2):255–271
66. Sankaran S, Manyonda IT (2008) Medical management of fibroids. Best Pract Res 22(4):655–676
67. Donnez J, Squifflet J, Polet R, Nisolle M (2000) Laparoscopic myolysis. Hum Reprod Update 6(6):609–613
68. Pron G, Mocarski E, Bennett J, Vilos G, Common A, Vanderburgh L (2005) Pregnancy after uterine artery embolization for leiomyomata: the Ontario multicenter trial. Obstet Gynecol 105(1):67–76
69. Stewart EA, Rabinovici J, Tempany CM et al (2006) Clinical outcomes of focused ultrasound surgery for the treatment of uterine fibroids. Fertil Steril 85(1):22–29
70. Tropeano G, Amoroso S, Scambia G (2008) Non-surgical management of uterine fibroids. Hum Reprod Update 14(3):259–274
71. Gupta JK, Sinha AS, Lumsden MA, Hickey M (2006) Uterine artery embolization for symptomatic uterine fibroids. Cochrane database of systematic reviews (Online) (1):CD005073.
72. Olive DL, Lindheim SR, Pritts EA (2004) Non-surgical management of leiomyoma: impact on fertility. Curr Opin Obstet Gynecol 16(3):239–243
73. Goodwin SC, Spies JB, Worthington-Kirsch R et al (2008) Uterine artery embolization for treatment of leiomyomata: long-term outcomes from the FIBROID Registry. Obstet Gynecol 111(1):22–33
74. Pabon IP, Magret JP, Unzurrunzaga EA, Garcia IM, Catalan IB, Cano Vieco ML (2008) Pregnancy after uterine fibroid embolization: follow-up of 100 patients embolized using tris-acryl gelatin microspheres. Fertil Steril 90:2356–2360
75. Mara M, Fucikova Z, Kuzel D, Maskova J, Dundr P, Zizka Z (2007) Hysteroscopy after uterine fibroid embolization in women of fertile age. J Obstet Gynaecol Res 33(3):316–324

76. Holub Z, Mara M, Kuzel D, Jabor A, Maskova J, Eim J (2008) Pregnancy outcomes after uterine artery occlusion: prospective multicentric study. Fertil Steril 90:1886–1891
77. Mara M, Maskova J, Fucikova Z, Kuzel D, Belsan T, Sosna O (2008) Midterm clinical and first reproductive results of a randomized controlled trial comparing uterine fibroid embolization and myomectomy. Cardiovasc Intervent Radiol 31(1):73–85
78. Tropeano G, Litwicka K, Di Stasi C, Romano D, Mancuso S (2003) Permanent amenorrhea associated with endometrial atrophy after uterine artery embolization for symptomatic uterine fibroids. Fertil Steril 79(1):132–135
79. Walker WJ, Pelage JP (2002) Uterine artery embolisation for symptomatic fibroids: clinical results in 400 women with imaging follow up. BJOG 109(11):1262–1272
80. ACOG practice bulletin (2008) Alternatives to hysterectomy in the management of leiomyomas. Obstet Gynecol 112(2 Pt 1):387–400
81. Hehenkamp WJ, Volkers NA, Broekmans FJ et al (2007) Loss of ovarian reserve after uterine artery embolization: a randomized comparison with hysterectomy. Hum Reprod 22(7):1996–2005
82. ACOG Committee Opinion (2004) Uterine artery embolization. Obstet Gynecol 103(2):403–404
83. Sawin SW, Pilevsky ND, Berlin JA, Barnhart KT (2000) Comparability of perioperative morbidity between abdominal myomectomy and hysterectomy for women with uterine leiomyomas. Am J Obstet Gynecol 183(6):1448–1455
84. Iverson RE Jr, Chelmow D, Strohbehn K, Waldman L, Evantash EG (1996) Relative morbidity of abdominal hysterectomy and myomectomy for management of uterine leiomyomas. Obstet Gynecol 88(3):415–419
85. Goto A, Takeuchi S, Sugimura K, Maruo T (2002) Usefulness of Gd-DTPA contrast-enhanced dynamic MRI and serum determination of LDH and its isozymes in the differential diagnosis of leiomyosarcoma from degenerated leiomyoma of the uterus. Int J Gynecol Cancer 12(4):354–361
86. Benson CB, Chow JS, Chang-Lee W, Hill JA 3rd, Doubilet PM (2001) Outcome of pregnancies in women with uterine leiomyomas identified by sonography in the first trimester. J Clin Ultrasound 29(5):261–264
87. Vercellini P, Oldani S, Yaylayan L, Zaina B, De Giorgi O, Crosignani PG (1999) Randomized comparison of vaporizing electrode and cutting loop for endometrial ablation. Obstet Gynecol 94(4):521–527
88. Rice JP, Kay HH, Mahony BS (1989) The clinical significance of uterine leiomyomas in pregnancy. Am J Obstet Gynecol 160(5 Pt 1):1212–1216
89. Coronado GD, Marshall LM, Schwartz SM (2000) Complications in pregnancy, labor, and delivery with uterine leiomyomas: a population-based study. Obstet Gynecol 95(5):764–769
90. Winer-Muram HT, Muram D, Gillieson MS (1984) Uterine myomas in pregnancy. J Can Assoc Radiol 35(2):168–170
91. West S, Ruiz R, Parker WH (2006) Abdominal myomectomy in women with very large uterine size. Fertil Steril 85(1):36–39
92. Fedele L, Parazzini F, Luchini L, Mezzopane R, Tozzi L, Villa L (1995) Recurrence of fibroids after myomectomy: a transvaginal ultrasonographic study. Hum Reprod 10(7):1795–1796
93. Malone LJ (1969) Myomectomy: recurrence after removal of solitary and multiple myomas. Obstet Gynecol 34(2):200–203
94. Fauconnier A, Chapron C, Babaki-Fard K, Dubuisson JB (2000) Recurrence of leiomyomata after myomectomy. Hum Reprod Update 6(6):595–602
95. Yoo EH, Lee PI, Huh CY et al (2007) Predictors of leiomyoma recurrence after laparoscopic myomectomy. J Minim Invasive Gynecol 14(6):690–697
96. Lethaby A, Vollenhoven B, Sowter M (2002) Efficacy of pre-operative gonadotrophin hormone releasing analogues for women with uterine fibroids undergoing hysterectomy or myomectomy: a systematic review. BJOG 109(10):1097–1108
97. Schlaff WD, Zerhouni EA, Huth JA, Chen J, Damewood MD, Rock JA (1989) A placebo-controlled trial of a depot gonadotropin-releasing hormone analogue (leuprolide) in the treatment of uterine leiomyomata. Obstet Gynecol 74(6):856–862
98. Friedman AJ, Hoffman DI, Comite F, Browneller RW, Miller JD (1991) Treatment of leiomyomata uteri with leuprolide acetate depot: a double-blind, placebo-controlled, multicenter study. The Leuprolide Study Group. Obstet Gynecol 77(5):720–725
99. Wurnig C, Schatz K, Noske H et al (2001) Subcutaneous low-dose epoetin beta for the avoidance of transfusion in patients scheduled for elective surgery not eligible for autologous blood donation. Eur Surg Res 33(5–6):303–310
100. Walocha JA, Litwin JA, Miodonski AJ (2003) Vascular system of intramural leiomyomata revealed by corrosion casting and scanning electron microscopy. Hum Reprod 18(5):1088–1093
101. Hurst BS, Matthews ML, Marshburn PB (2005) Laparoscopic myomectomy for symptomatic uterine myomas. Fertil Steril 83(1):1–23
102. Saeki M, Kotaki S (1974) Vasculature of uterine myoma for myomectomy. Acta Obstet Gynecol Jpn 26:335–342
103. Ginsburg ES, Benson CB, Garfield JM, Gleason RE, Friedman AJ (1993) The effect of operative technique and uterine size on blood loss during myomectomy: a prospective randomized study. Fertil Steril 60(6):956–962
104. Beyth Y, Pinkert M (2005) Local control of blood loss. Fertil Steril 84(2):548–549 author reply 9–50
105. Phillips DR, Nathanson H, Milim SJ, Haselkorn JS (1996) The effect of dilute vasopressin solution on blood loss during operative hysteroscopy. J Am Assoc Gynecol Laparosc 3(4, Supplement):S38
106. B-Lynch C, Coker A, Lawal AH, Abu J, Cowen MJ (1997) The B-Lynch surgical technique for the control of massive postpartum haemorrhage: an alternative to hysterectomy? Five cases reported. Br J Obstet Gynaecol 104(3):372–375
107. Ahmad G, Duffy JM, Farquhar C, et al. Barrier agents for adhesion prevention after gynaecological surgery. Cochrane database of systematic reviews (Online) 2008(2):CD000475.
108. Takeuchi H, Kitade M, Kikuchi I, Shimanuki H, Kumakiri J, Takeda S (2008) Influencing factors of adhesion development and the efficacy of adhesion-preventing agents in patients undergoing laparoscopic myomectomy as evaluated by a second-look laparoscopy. Fertil Steril 89(5):1247–1253
109. Uduwela AS, Perera MA, Aiqing L, Fraser IS (2000) Endometrial-myometrial interface: relationship to adenomyosis and changes in pregnancy. Obstet Gynecol Surv 55(6):390–400
110. Ferenczy A (1998) Pathophysiology of adenomyosis. Hum Reprod Update 4(4):312–322
111. Parrott E, Butterworth M, Green A, White IN, Greaves P (2001) Adenomyosis–a result of disordered stromal differentiation. Am J Pathol 159(2):623–630
112. Ota H, Igarashi S, Hatazawa J, Tanaka T (1998) Is adenomyosis an immune disease? Hum Reprod Update 4(4):360–367
113. Mai KT, Yazdi HM, Perkins DG, Parks W (1997) Pathogenetic role of the stromal cells in endometriosis and adenomyosis. Histopathology 30(5):430–442
114. Kunz G, Beil D, Huppert P, Leyendecker G (2000) Structural abnormalities of the uterine wall in women with endometriosis and infertility visualized by vaginal sonography and magnetic resonance imaging. Hum Reprod 15(1):76–82
115. Brosens JJ, Barker FG, de Souza NM (1998) Myometrial zonal differentiation and uterine junctional zone hyperplasia in the non-pregnant uterus. Hum Reprod update 4(5):496–502
116. Brosens JJ, de Souza NM, Barker FG (1995) Uterine junctional zone: function and disease. Lancet 346(8974):558–560
117. Noe M, Kunz G. Herbertz M, Mall G, Leyendecker G (1999) The cyclic pattern of the immunocytochemical expression of Oestrogen and Progesterone receptors in human myometerial

and endometerial layers: characterization of the endometerial-subendometrial unit. Hum Reprod 14(1):190–197
118. Azziz R (1989) Adenomyosis: current perspectives. Obstet Gynecol Clin North Am 16(1):221–235
119. Leyendecker G, Herbertz M, Kunz G, Mall G (2002) Endometriosis results from the dislocation of basal endometrium. Hum Reprod 17(10):2725–2736
120. Templeman C, Marshall SF, Ursin G et al (2008) Adenomyosis and endometriosis in the California teachers study. Fertil Steril 90(2):415–424
121. Dogan E, Gode F, Saatli B, Secil M (2008) Juvenile cystic adenomyosis mimicking uterine malformation: a case report. Arch Gynecol Obstet 278:593–595
122. Kunz G, Beil D, Huppert P, Noe M, Kissler S, Leyendecker G (2005) Adenomyosis in endometriosis–prevalence and impact on fertility. Evidence from magnetic resonance imaging. Hum Reprod 20(8):2309–2316
123. Kunz G, Herbertz M, Beil D, Huppert P, Leyendecker G (2007) Adenomyosis as a disorder of the early and late human reproductive period. Reprod Biomed Online 15(6):681–685
124. Curtis KM, Hillis SD, Marchbanks PA, Peterson HB (2002) Disruption of the endometrial-myometrial border during pregnancy as a risk factor for adenomyosis. Am J Obstet Gynecol 187(3):543–544
125. Domez J, Nirolle M, Casanas-Roux F, Barsil S, Anaf V (1995) Rectovaginal septum, endometriosis or adenomyosis: laparoscopic management in a series of 231 patients. Hum Reprod 10(3): 630–635
126. Weiss G, Maseelall P, Schott LL, Brockwell SE, Schocken M, Johnston JM (2009) Adenomyosis a variant, not a disease? Evidence from hysterectomized menopausal women in the study of Women's Health Across the Nation (SWAN). Fertil Steril Jan, 91(1):201–206. Epub 2008 Feb 20
127. Yeniel O, Cirpan T, Ulukus M et al (2007) Adenomyosis: prevalence, risk factors, symptoms and clinical findings. Clin Experiment Obstet Gynecol 34(3):163–167
128. Cirpan T, Yeniel O, Ulukus M et al (2008) Clinical symptoms and histopathological findings in subjects with adenomyosis uteri. Clin Experiment Obstet Gynecol 35(1):48–53
129. Levgur M (2007) Diagnosis of adenomyosis: a review. J Reprod Med 52(3):177–193
130. Reinhold C, Tafazoli F, Mehio A et al (1999) Uterine adenomyosis: endovaginal US and MR imaging features with histopathologic correlation. Radiographics 19:S147–S160
131. Reinhold C, Tafozoli F, Wang L (1998) Imaging features of adenomyosis. Hum Reprod Update 4(4):337–349
132. Atri M, Reinhold C, Mehio AR, Chapman WB, Bret PM (2000) Adenomyosis: US features with histologic correlation in an in-vitro study. Radiology 215(3):783–790
133. Devlieger R, D'Hooghe T, Timmerman D (2003) Uterine adenomyosis in the infertility clinic. Hum Reprod update 9(2):139–147
134. Dueholm M, Lundorf E (2007) Transvaginal ultrasound or MRI for diagnosis of adenomyosis. Curr Opin Obstet Gynecol 19(6): 505–512
135. Leyendecker G, Kunz G, Wildt L, Beil D, Deininger H (1996) Uterine hyperperistalsis and dysperistalsis as dysfunctions of the mechanism of rapid sperm transport in patients with endometriosis and infertility. Hum Reprod 11(7):1542–1551
136. Kissler S, Hamscho N, Zangos S et al (2006) Uterotubal transport disorder in adenomyosis and endometriosis–a cause for infertility. BJOG 113(8):902–908
137. Wang F, Li H, Yang Z, Du X, Cui M, Wen Z (2008) Expression of interleukin-10 in patients with adenomyosis. Fertil Steril 91: 1681–1685
138. Liu X, Huang H, Huang R, Lian L, Lang J (1998) Clinical observation of conservative surgery for adenomyosis. Zhongguo yi xue ke xue yuan xue bao 20(6):440–444
139. Levgur M (2007) Therapeutic options for adenomyosis: a review. Arch Gynecol Obstet 276(1):1–15
140. Lohle PN, De Vries J, Klazen CA et al (2007) Uterine artery embolization for symptomatic adenomyosis with or without uterine leiomyomas with the use of calibrated tris-acryl gelatin microspheres: midterm clinical and MR imaging follow-up. J Vasc Interv Radiol 18(7):835–841
141. Kim MD, Kim S, Kim NK et al (2007) Long-term results of uterine artery embolization for symptomatic adenomyosis. AJR Am J Roentgenol 188(1):176–181
142. Siskin GP, Tublin ME, Stainken BF, Dowling K, Dolen EG (2001) Uterine artery embolization for the treatment of adenomyosis: clinical response and evaluation with MR imaging. AJR Am J Roentgenol 177(2):297–302
143. Kim MD, Kim NK, Kim HJ, Lee MH (2005) Pregnancy following uterine artery embolization with polyvinyl alcohol particles for patients with uterine fibroid or adenomyosis. Cardiovasc Intervent Radiol 28(5):611–615
144. Kitamura Y, Allison SJ, Jha RC, Spies JB, Flick PA, Ascher SM (2006) MRI of adenomyosis: changes with uterine artery embolization. AJR Am J Roentgenol 186(3):855–864
145. Dundr P, Mara M, Maskova J, Fucikova Z, Povysil C, Tvrdik D (2006) Pathological findings of uterine leiomyomas and adenomyosis following uterine artery embolization. Pathol Res Pract 202(10):721–729
146. Lin J, Sun C, Zheng H (2000) Gonadotropin-releasing hormone agonists and laparoscopy in the treatment of adenomyosis with infertility. Chin Med J 113(5):442–445
147. Huang FJ, Kung FT, Chang SY, Hsu TY (1999) Effects of short-course buserelin therapy on adenomyosis. A report of two cases. J Reprod Med 44(8):741–744
148. Ozaki T, Takahashi K, Okada M, Kurioka H, Miyazaki K (1999) Live birth after conservative surgery for severe adenomyosis following magnetic resonance imaging and gonadotropin-releasing hormone agonist therapy. Int J Fertil Women's Med 44(5): 260–264
149. Silva PD, Perkins HE, Schauberger CW (1994) Live birth after treatment of severe adenomyosis with a gonadotropin-releasing hormone agonist. Fertil Steril 61(1):171–172
150. Hirata JD, Moghissi KS, Ginsburg KA (1993) Pregnancy after medical therapy of adenomyosis with a gonadotropin-releasing hormone agonist. Fertil Steril 59(2):444–445
151. Juang CM, Chou P, Yen MS, Twu NF, Horng HC, Hsu WL (2007) Adenomyosis and risk of preterm delivery. BJOG 114(2):165–169
152. Leyendecker G, Kunz G, Kissler S, Wildt L (2006) Adenomyosis and reproduction. Best Prac Res 20(4):523–546
153. Fritsch H (1894) Ein Fall von volligen Schwund der Gebaumutterhohle nach Auskratzung. Zentralbl gynaekol 18:1337–1342
154. Asherman J (1950) Traumatic intra-uterine adhesions. J Obstet Gynaecol Br Emp 57:892–896
155. Yu D, Wong YM, Cheong Y, Xia E, Li TC (2008) Asherman syndrome–one century later. Fertil Steril 89(4):759–779
156. Schenker JG, Margalioth EJ (1982) Intrauterine adhesions: an updated appraisal. Fertil Steril 37(5):593–610
157. Ericksen J, Kaestel C (1960) The incidence of uterine atresia after post-partum c urettage: a follow-up examination of 141 patients. Dan Med Bull 7:50–51
158. Jensen PA, Stromme WB (1972) Amenorrhea secondary to puerperal curettage (Asherman's syndrome). Am J Obstet Gynecol 113(2):150–157
159. Tam WH, Lau WC, Cheung LP, Yuen PM, Chung TK (2002) Intrauterine adhesions after conservative and surgical management of spontaneous abortion. J Am Assoc Gynecol Laparosc 9(2): 182–185
160. Klein SM, Garcia CR (1973) Asherman's syndrome: a critique and current review. Fertil Steril 24(9):722–735

161. Friedler S, Margalioth E, Kafka I, Vaffe H (1993) Incidence of post-abortion intrauterine adhesions evaluated by hysteroscopy – a prospective study. Hum Reprod 8:442–444
162. Hofmeister F (1972) Discussion. Am J Obstet Gynecol 113:150
163. Polishuk WZ, Anteby SO, Weinstein D (1975) Puerperal endometritis and intrauterine adhesions. Int Surg 60(8):418–420
164. Tsapanos VS, Stathopoulou LP, Papathanassopoulou VS, Tzingounis VA (2002) The role of Seprafilm bioresorbable membrane in the prevention and therapy of endometrial synechiae. J Biomed Mater Res 63(1):10–14
165. Buckley C (2002) Normal endometrium and non-proliferative conditions of the endometrium. In: Fox H, Wells M (eds) Obstetrical and gynaecological pathology, 5th edn. Churchill Livingstone, London, pp 391–442
166. Yaffe H, Ron M, Polishuk WZ (1978) Amenorrhea, hypomenorrhea, and uterine fibrosis. Am J Obstet Gynecol 130(5):599–601
167. Bergman P (1961) Traumatic intra-uterine lesions. Acta Obstet Gynecol Scan 40(Suppl 4):1–39
168. Asherman J (1948) Amenorrhoea traumatica (atretica). J Obstet Gynaecol Br Emp 55:23–30
169. Zarek S, Sharp HT (2008) Global endometrial ablation devices. Clin Obstet Gynecol 51(1):167–175
170. Robinson JK, Colimon LM, Isaacson KB (2008) Postoperative adhesiolysis therapy for intrauterine adhesions (Asherman's syndrome). Fertil Steril 90(2):409–414
171. (1988) The American Fertility Society classifications of adnexal adhesions, distal tubal occlusion, tubal occlusion secondary to tubal ligation, tubal pregnancies, mullerian anomalies and intrauterine adhesions. Fertil Steril 49(6):944–55
172. Sylvestre C, Child TJ, Tulandi T, Tan SL (2003) A prospective study to evaluate the efficacy of two- and three-dimensional sonohysterography in women with intrauterine lesions. Fertil Steril 79(5):1222–1225
173. Wamsteker K, DeBlock S (1998) Diagnostic hysteroscopy: technique and documentation. WB Saunders, London
174. Nasr AL, Al-Inany HG, Thabet SM, Aboulghar M (2000) A clinicohysteroscopic scoring system of intrauterine adhesions. Gynecol Obstet Invest 50(3):178–181
175. Westendorp IC, Ankum WM, Mol BW, Vonk J (1998) Prevalence of Asherman's syndrome after secondary removal of placental remnants or a repeat curettage for incomplete abortion. Hum Reprod 13(12):3347–3350
176. Weiss A, Shalev E, Romano S (2005) Hysteroscopy may be justified after two miscarriages. Hum Reprod 20(9):2628–2631
177. Ventolini G, Zhang M, Gruber J (2004) Hysteroscopy in the evaluation of patients with recurrent pregnancy loss: a cohort study in a primary care population. Surg Endosc 18(12): 1782–1784
178. Raziel A, Arieli S, Bukovsky I, Caspi E, Golan A (1994) Investigation of the uterine cavity in recurrent aborters. Fertil Steril 62(5):1080–1082
179. Adoni A, Palti Z, Milwidsky A, Dolberg M (1982) The incidence of intrauterine adhesions following spontaneous abortion. Int J fertil 27(2):117–118
180. Al-Inany H (1998) Intrauterine adhesions; an update. Acta Obstet Gynecol Scan 80:986–993
181. Tur-Kaspa I, Gal M, Hartman M, Hartman J, Hartman A (2006) A prospective evaluation of uterine abnormalities by saline infusion sonohysterography in 1, 009 women with infertility or abnormal uterine bleeding. Fertil Steril 86(6):1731–1735
182. Preutthipan S, Linasmita V (2003) A prospective comparative study between hysterosalpingography and hysteroscopy in the detection of intrauterine pathology in patients with infertility. J Obstet Gynaecol Res 29(1):33–37
183. Schlaff WD, Hurst BS (1995) Preoperative sonographic measurement of endometrial pattern predicts outcome of surgical repair in patients with severe Asherman's syndrome. Fertil Steril 63(2):410–413
184. Salle B, Gaucherand P, de Saint Hilaire P, Rudigoz RC (1999) Transvaginal sonohysterographic evaluation of intrauterine adhesions. J Clin Ultrasound 27(3):131–134
185. Bacelar A (1995) The value of MRI in the assessment of traumatic intr-uterine adhesions (Asherman's syndrome). Clin Radiol 50: 80–83
186. Confino E, Friberg J, Giglia R, Gleicher N (1985) Sonographic imaging of intrauterine adhesions. Obstet Gynecol 66:596–598
187. Taylor PJ, Hamou JE (eds) (1995) Hysteroscopy in infertility and repeated pregnancy loss. Mosby-Wolfe, London
188. Valle RF, Sciarra JJ (1988) Intrauterine adhesions: hysteroscopic diagnosis, classification, treatment, and reproductive outcome. Am J Obstet Gynecol 158(6 Pt 1):1459–1470
189. Cararach M, Penella J, Ubeda A, Labastida R (1994) Hysteroscopic incision of the septuate uterus: scissors versus resectoscope. Hum Reprod 9:87–89
190. Zikopoulos KA, Kolibianakis EM, Platteau P et al (2004) Live delivery rates in subfertile women with Asherman's syndrome after hysteroscopic adhesiolysis using the resectoscope or the Versapoint system. Reprod Biomed Online 8(6):720–725
191. Toaff R, Ballas S (1978) Traumatic hypomenorrhea-amenorrhea (Asherman's syndrome). Fertil Steril 30(4):379–387
192. Coccia M, Becattini C, Bracco G, Bargelli G, Scarselli G (2000) Intraoperative ultrasound guidance for operative hysteroscopy. a prospective study. J Reprod Med 45:413–418
193. McComb PF, Wagner BL (1997) Simplified therapy for Asherman's syndrome. Fertil Steril 68(6):1047–1050
194. Protopapas A, Shushan A, Magos A (1998) Myometrial scoring: a new technique for the management of severe Asherman's syndrome. Fertil Steril 69(5):860–864
195. Capella-Allouc S, Morsad F, Rongieres-Bertrand C, Taylor S, Fernandez H (1999) Hysteroscopic treatment of severe Asherman's syndrome and subsequent fertility. Hum Reprod 14:1230–1233
196. Reddy S, Rock JA (1997) Surgical management of complete obliteration of the endometrial cavity. Fertil Steril 67(1):172–174
197. Hellebrekers BW, Trimbos-Kemper TC, Trimbos JB, Emeis JJ, Kooistra T (2000) Use of fibrinolytic agents in the prevention of postoperative adhesion formation. Fertil Steril 74(2):203–212
198. Kappas AM, Barsoum GH, Ortiz JB, Keighley MR (1992) Prevention of peritoneal adhesions in rats with verapamil, hydrocortisone sodium succinate, and phosphatidylcholine. Eur J Surg = Acta chirurgica 158(1):33–35
199. Wood J, Pena G (1964) Treatment of traumatic uterine synechias. Int J Fertil 9:405–410
200. Farhi J, Bar-Hava I, Homburg R, Dicker D, Ben-Rafael Z (1993) Induced regeneration of endometrium following curettage for abortion: a comparative study. Hum Reprod 8(7):1143–1144
201. Massouras HG (1974) The treatment of uterine adhesions with the "Massouras Duck foot". Acta Eur Fertil 5(2):137–147
202. Polishuk WZ, Adoni A, Aviad I (1969) Intrauterine device in the treatment of traumatic intrauterine adhesions. Fertil Steril 20(2): 241–249
203. March CM (1995) Intrauterine adhesions. Obstet Gynecol Clin North Am 22(3):491–505
204. Orhue AA, Aziken ME, Igbefoh JO (2003) A comparison of two adjunctive treatments for intrauterine adhesions following lysis. Int J Gynaecol Obstet 82(1):49–56
205. Amer MI, El Nadim A, Karim H (2005) The role of intrauterine balloon after operative hysteroscopy in the prevention of intrauterine adhesions: a prospective controlled study. MEFS J 10:125–129
206. Acunzo G, Guida M, Pellicano M et al (2003) Effectiveness of auto-cross-linked hyaluronic acid gel in the prevention of

intrauterine adhesions after hysteroscopic adhesiolysis: a prospective, randomized, controlled study. Hum Reprod 18(9): 1918–1921
207. Amer MI, Abd-El-Maeboud KH (2006) Amnion graft following hysteroscopic lysis of intrauterine adhesions. J Obstet Gynaecol Res 32(6):559–566
208. Robinson JK, Colimon LM, Isaacson KB (2008) Postoperative adhesions (Asherman's syndrome). Fertil Steril 90(2):409–414. Epub 2008 Jun 20
209. Fedele L, Vercellini P, Viezzoli T, Ricciardiello O, Zamberletti D (1986) Intrauterine adhesions: current diagnostic and therapeutic trends. Acta Eur Fertil 17:31–37
210. Feng Z, Yang B, Shao J, Liu S (1999) Diagnostic and therapeutic hysteroscopy for traumatic intrauterine adhesions after induced abortions: clinical analysis of 365 cases. Gynaecol Endosc 8:95–98
211. Pabuccu R, Atay V, Orhon E, Urman B, Ergun A (1997) Hysteroscopic treatment of intrauterine adhesions is safe and effective in the restoration of normal menstruation and fertility. Fertil Steril 68(6):1141–1143
212. Preutthipan S, Linasmita V (2000) Reproductive outcome following hysteroscopic lysis of intrauterine adhesions: a result of 65 cases at Ramathibodi Hospital. J Med Assoc Thai 83(1):42–46
213. Parent B, Barbot J, Dubuisson J (1988) Synechies uterine encyclopedie medico-chirurgicale. Gynecologie 140A:10
214. Friedman A, DeFazio J, DeCherney A (1986) Severe obstetric complications after aggressive treatment of Asherman syndrome. Obstet Gynecol 67(6):864–867
215. Sugimoto O (1978) Diagnostic and therapeutic hysteroscopy for traumatic intrauterine adhesions. Am J Obstet Gynecol 131(5): 539–547
216. Roge P, Cravello L, D'Ercole C, Broussse M, Boubli L, Blanc B (1997) Intrauterine adhesions and fertility: results of hysteroscopic treatment. Gynaecol Endosc 6:225–228
217. Pistofidis GA, Dimitropoulos K, Mastrominas M (1996) Comparison of operative and fertility outcome between groups of women with intrauterine adhesions after adhesiolysis. J Am Assoc Gynecol Laparosc 3(4, Supplement):S40
218. Goldenberg M, Schiff E, Achiron R, Lipitz S, Mashiach S (1997) Managing residual trophoblastic tissue. Hysteroscopy for directing curettage. J Reprod Med 42(1):26–28
219. Massouras HG (1973) Intrauterine adhesions: a syndrome of the past with the use of the Massouras duck's foot No. 2 intrauterine contraceptive device. Am J Obstet Gynecol 116(4): 576–578

Chapter 16
Müllerian (Paramesonephric) Anomalies and Associated Wolffian (Mesonephric) Duct Malformations

Jessie Dorais and C. Matthew Peterson

Abstract The Müllerian ducts (mesodermal origin) are primordial roots of the internal female reproductive organs and differentiate to form the fallopian tubes, uterus, uterine cervix, and upper one third of the vagina. The mean incidence of uterine malformations in the general population is 4.3%, while women with infertility have a 3–6% incidence of abnormality. Patients with recurrent miscarriage have an even higher incidence. This chapter reviews the embryological basis of these important abnormalities and their clinical ramifications.

Keywords Müllerian duct • Müllerian anomaly • Müllerian defect • Müllerian malformation • Genitourinary anomaly • Gynecologic malformation • Female reproductive tract • Reproductive tract abnormalities • Uterine agenesis • Vaginal agenesis • Duplicate uterus • Duplicate vagina • Uterine anomalies • Uterine abnormalities • Uterine defect • Menstrual disorder • Infertility • Obstetric complication • Agenesis • Hypoplasia • Lateral fusion defect • Vertical fusion defect • Resorption defect • Des-related abnormalities • Diethylstilbestrol-related abnormalities • Mayer–Rokitansky–Kuster–Hauser syndrome • MRKH syndrome • Vaginoplasty • Didelphys uterus • Unicornuate uterus • Wunderlich-Herlyn-Werner syndrome • Obstructed hemivagina and ipsilateral renal agenesis • Bicornuate uterus • Bicornuate unicollis uterus • Arcuate uterus • Septate uterus • Vaginal atresia • Paramesonephric (Müllerian) ducts • Mesonephric (Wolffian) ducts • Hysterosalpingography • HSG • Sonohysterography • Saline infusion sonography • SIS

16.1 Introduction

Reproductive endocrinologists are often called upon to evaluate young women presenting with amenorrhea, cyclic pelvic pain, dysmenorrhea, persistent post menstrual spotting, recurrent miscarriage, history of preterm labor, and/or obstetrical malpresentation – all potentially consistent with genitourinary anomalies. While present evaluation paradigms emphasize the Müllerian embryologic origin of the anomalies, a knowledge of the embryology of the mesonephric ducts and the urogenital sinus are critical for a thorough evaluation of each patient.

16.2 Incidence/Prevalence

Columbo reported the first documented case of uterine and vaginal agenesis in the sixteenth century [1]. Despite the frequency of evaluations for Müllerian anomlies (MA) in reproductive medicine clinics, the actual incidence (annual diagnosis rate) and prevalence rates (percentage of the population affected at any one time) of Müllerian anomalies remain vague, at best. This may be partially due to late reporting, nonuniform classification systems, discrepant diagnostic methods, the asymptomatic nature of many Müllerian "anomalies," confounding/unclassified meosnephric anomalies, and/or differing study populations. These factors make assessment of the incidence and prevalence rates for genitourinary anomalies (Müllerian or Wolffian and/or their combinations) and their potential association with environmental endocrine disrupters problematic.

Early clinical researchers reported an incidence (annual diagnosis rate) of müllerian anomalies (MA) of 0.1–3.5% [2–5]. More recently, Grimbizis and colleagues (2001) collated data from multiple studies on uterine anomalies ($n = 3{,}000$ with an anomaly) and calculated a mean incidence for uterine malformations in the general population (i.e., general and fertile population) of 4.3% [6]. In women with infertility, the calculated incidence of uterine anomalies was higher at 3–6%. Recurrent abortions are estimated to have an incidence of 5–10%, and those experiencing third-trimester miscarriages appear to be at the greatest risk [7, 8].

In women with recurrent pregnancy loss who are undergoing hysterosalpingography (HSG), the prevalence rate of Müllerian anomalies is as high as 8–10% [9, 10]. That rate contrasts with a prevalence rate of 2–3% in women undergoing hysteroscopy

J. Dorais and C.M. Peterson (✉)
Utah Center for Reproductive Medicine, Department of Obstetrics and Gynecology, University of Utah School of Medicine, 30 N. Medical Drive, 2B200, Salt Lake City, UT, 84132
e-mail: c.matthew.peterson@hsc.utah.edu

D.T. Carrell and C.M. Peterson (eds.), *Reproductive Endocrinology and Infertility: Integrating Modern Clinical and Laboratory Practice*, DOI 10.1007/978-1-4419-1436-1_16, © Springer Science+Business Media, LLC 2010

without the diagnosis of recurrent pregnancy loss [11, 12]. Byrne et al.[13] used ultrasound examinations to establish a prevalence rate for MA in girls and women who were evaluated for reasons unrelated to the presence of uterine anomalies. These 2,065 consecutive, prospective ultrasound examinations for nonobstetric indications in girls and women (aged 8–93 years) showed eight with anomalies, including bicornuate, septate, and didelphys uteri for a prevalence of 3.87 per 1,000 women (95% confidence interval, 1.67–7.62), hence approximately *1 MA in 250 women*. The range of prevalence rates in the literature is 0.16–10% and highest when the arcuate uterus is included in the diagnostic criteria. Studies in this arena will require thoughtful epidemiological consideration for appropriate interpretation.

16.3 Embryologic Origin

The Müllerian ducts (mesodermal origin) are primordial roots of the internal female reproductive organs and differentiate to form the fallopian tubes, uterus, uterine cervix, and upper one-third of the vagina. The urogenital sinus – UGS – (endodermal origin) is thought to give rise to the lower and mid-vagina. Disruption of the developing mesoderm and its contiguous somites may account for some of the axial skeletal abnormalities seen in MA. The developing kidney and urinary system (Wolffian or mesonephric ducts) are parallel mesodermal structures and closely related to the reproductive tract, thus abnormalities in the renal/urinary system are often associated with defects in the Müllerian system and must be considered during the evaluation.

16.3.1 Embryology of the Fallopian Tubes, Uterus, and Uterine Cervix (Fig. 16.1)

Both male and female embryos at 6 weeks have paired genitourinary ducts: the paramesonephric (Müllerian) ducts and the mesonephric (Wolffian) ducts [14]. Wolffian duct development antedates the development of the Müllerian ducts. The Wolffian ducts drain the contents of the primitive mesonephric kidney into the cloaca, for a short period of time [15]. Both male and female fetuses have Müllerian ducts in the embryonic period of development. In the male, the Müllerian ducts are suppressed at 8–10 weeks due to the production of anti-Müllerian hormone (AMH) by the testis. Müllerian duct regression begins cranially and progresses caudally, which is associated with a concentration gradient in AMH protein along the length of the duct. Müllerian duct regression involves progressive apoptosis and the nuclear accumulation of beta-catenin in peri-Müllerian mesenchymal cells. The absence of AMH in females allows the Müllerian ducts to continue their differentiation. However, if the testes are incapable of secreting AMH (as in complete gonadal dysgenesis or with inactivating mutations of the AMH gene) or when there is a defect in the AMH type II receptor, a phenotypic male can be born with a uterus and fallopian tubes. This is called the persistent Müllerian duct syndrome. In males with persistent Müllerian duct syndrome, the testes usually fail to descend despite normal testosterone levels. Explanations for the undescended testes include a role for AMH in testicular descent or anatomical inhibition of descent due to the persistent Müllerian ducts. AMH is thought to have additional controlling effects on Leydig cell development, and AMH type II receptor knockout mice have Leydig cell hyperplasia.

As noted, Wolffian ducts degenerate in the female in the absence of anti-Müllerian hormone (AMH) [16]. As they degenerate, the Wolffian ducts provide an anatomic scafold for the developing Müllerian ducts which develop bidirectionally on the lateral aspects of the gonads. This unique interplay between the mesonephric and paramesonephric ducts explains the relatively frequent association between renal/urinary tract malformations and Müllerian anomalies. The American Society for Reproductive Medicine (ASRM) Müllerian Anomaly Classification system (Table 16.1) emphasizes the Müllerian duct findings. Table 16.2 details the findings in each Müllerian anomaly category based on the ASRM system. However, as Pedro and Maribel Acien have pointed out for decades, a thoughtful evaluation of renal/urinary (Wolffian) anomalies should be included in order to understand the extent of the anomaly, as well as when devising treatment plans (Table 16.3) [17].

The Müllerian ducts originate as longitudinal invaginations of coelomic epithelium on the anterolateral surface of the urogenital ridge [15]. During the 9th week of gestation, they elongate and demonstrate three regions; cranial vertical, horizontal, and caudal–vertical [15, 18, 19]. The funnel-shaped cranial vertical regions open into the primitive peritoneal cavity and form the fimbriated ends of the fallopian tubes. The horizontal segments migrate to the mesonephric ducts, cross ventrally, and then extend caudomedially. They form the isthmic structure of the fallopian tubes. Each caudal–vertical region joins its contralateral partner at the median plane of the future pelvis. These paired Müllerian duct regions fuse and form a single Y-shaped tubular structure, the uterovaginal primordium (UVP) [15, 18, 19]. Combinations of failed fusion (vertical fusion) and resorption (lateral fusion) in this segment explain many of the Müllerian anomaly configurations.

Until 1994, the unidirectional theory posited that the Müllerian ducts fuse in a caudal–cranial direction. Thus, if a duplicated cervix (bicollis) was noted, the uterus would be bicornuate and result in the uterine didelphys configuration. However, the Müllerian anomaly characterized by cervical duplication, a complete uterine septum (normal external

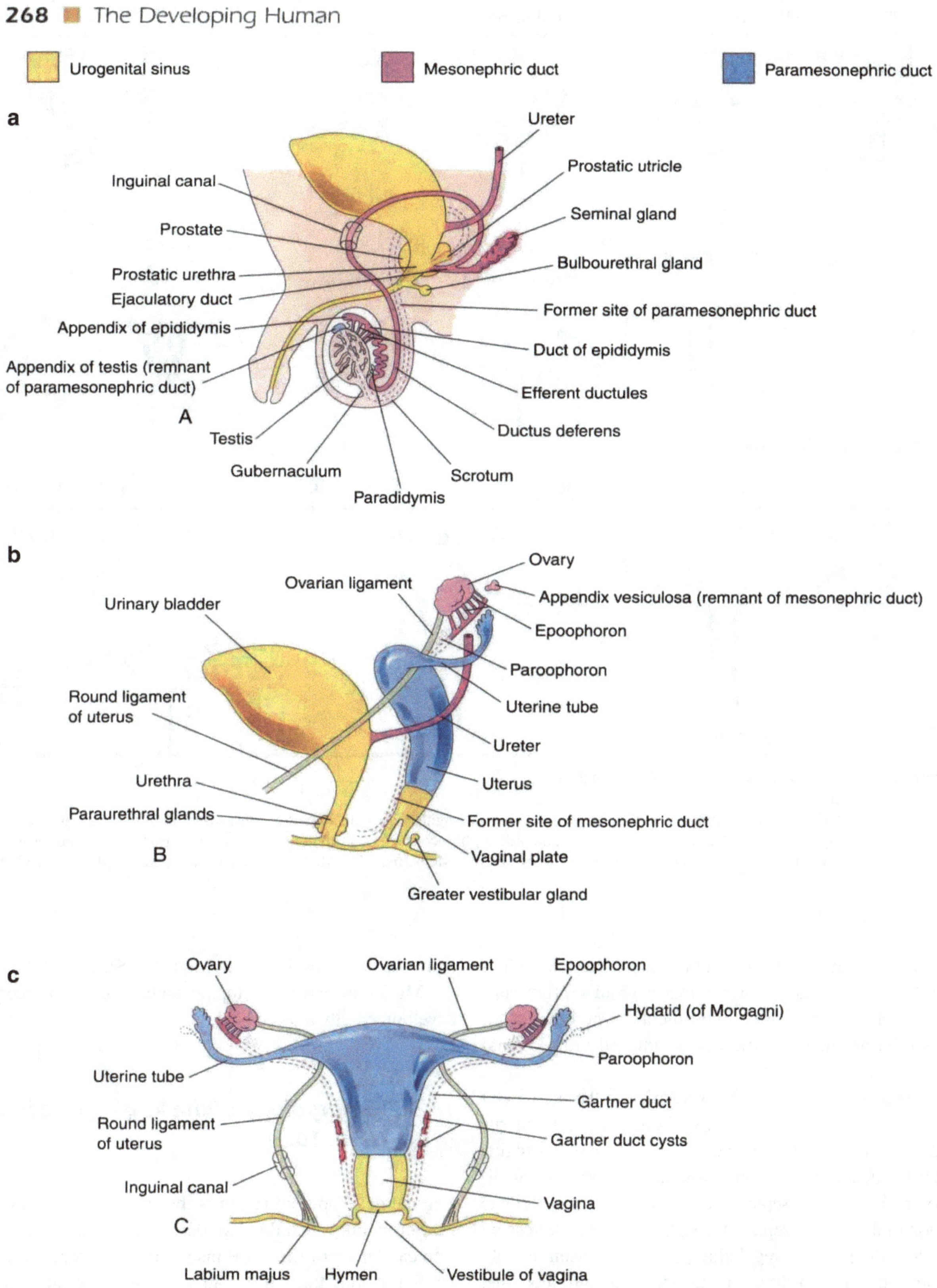

Fig. 16.1 Development of the fallopian tubes, uterus, and uterine cervix. (Reprinted with permission from Moore KL, Persaud TVN and Torchia MG, The Developing Human, Clinically Oriented Embryology, 8th Edition, Saunders/Elsevier, Philadelphia, PA, 2008; pg 268)

Table 16.1 The American Fertility Society classification of Müllerian anomalies

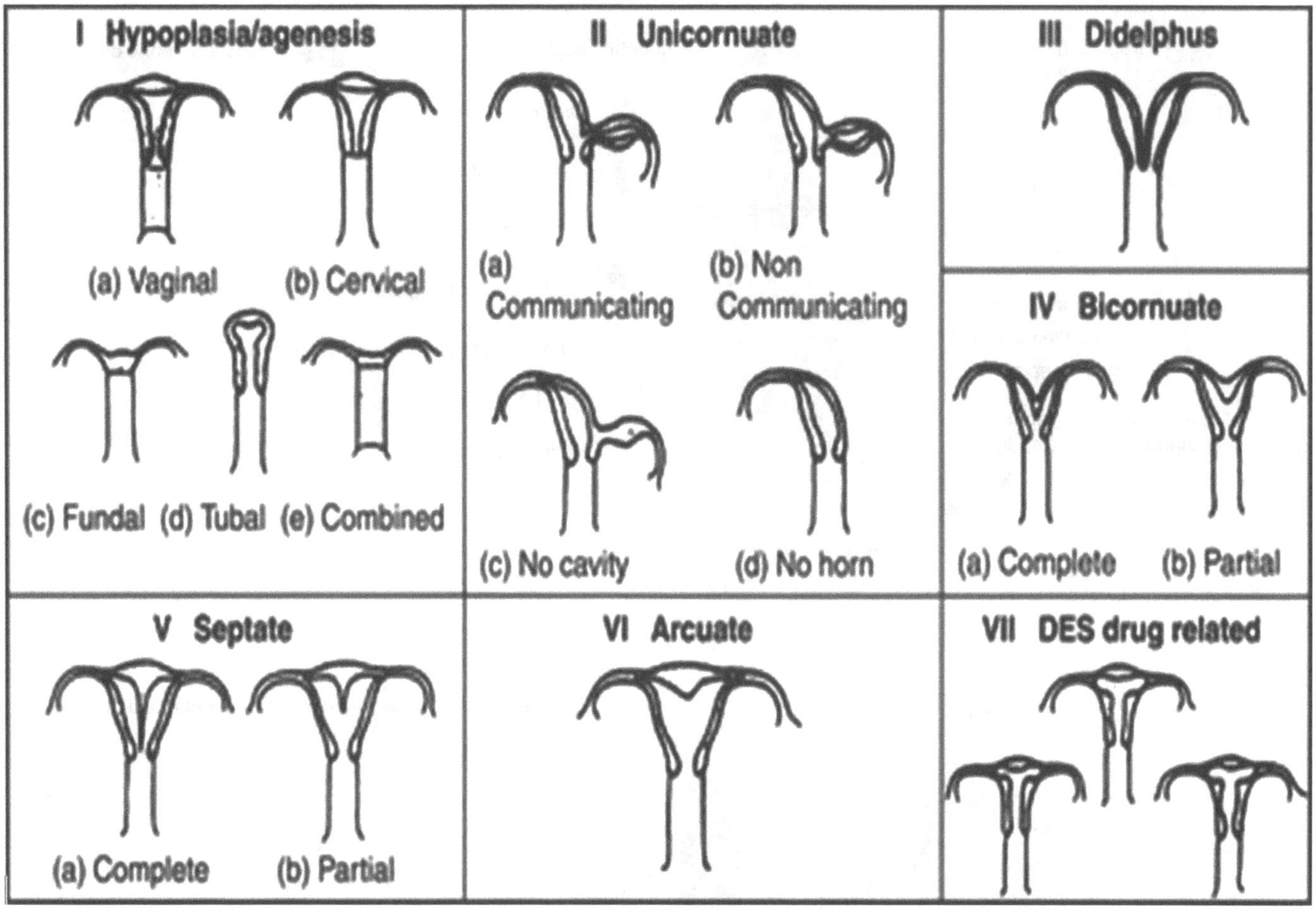

Ia the uterus may be normal or take a variety of abnormal forms
Va may have two distinct cervices

concave configuration with septate uterine cavity extending through the cervix) and a longitudinal vaginal septum supports the more recent bidirectional theory, wherein, fusion of the Müllerian ducts is both segmental and bidirectional [20, 21].

The uterine region of the UVP gives rise to the uterus and the upper third of the vagina [15, 18]. At this stage, the uterus is bicornuate, but is developmentally plastic. It continues to differentiate by means of fusion and subsequent resorption/canalization of the intervening septum. Apoptosis appears to mediate regression of the uterine septum through bcl-2 gene expression [22]. Bcl-2, an apoptosis regulating protein, has been notably absent from the septa of four septate uteri using a monoclonal antibody assay and by immunohistochemistry. At week 12, the uterus assumes its morphologic pear shape with an endometrium that is derived from the lining of the fused müllerian ducts. The endometrial stroma and myometrium originate from the adjacent mesenchyme [15, 18]. By the 22nd week, the Müllerian derived fallopian tubes, uterus, and cervix are developmentally mature [15].

16.3.2 Embryology of the Vagina and Hymen (Fig. 16.2)

Vaginal development requires the fusion of the mesodermal Müllerian ducts and the endodermal UGS (urogenital sinus). The caudal tip of the UVP inserts into the dorsal wall of the UGS forming the Müllerian or sinus tubercle. The sinus tubercle induces the formation of paired endodermal evaginations – the sinovaginal bulbs. They extend as a solid core from the UGS to the caudal aspects of the UVP, fuse, and form the vaginal plate. The vaginal plate and the sinovaginal

Table 16.2 Mullerian anomalies

Class	Major clinical finding	Descriptive	Etiology	Diagnosis/treatment
I	Segmental or complete agenesis or hypoplasia	Agenesis/hypoplasia of the mullerian ducts may involve vagina, cervix, fundus, tubes or any combination of these structures. Found in 1 in 5,000 neonates (Chen et al. 1994; ACOG 2002; Rock 2003) Complete uterovaginal agenesis Mayer–Rokitansky–Kuster–Hauser Syndrome (MRKH) is the most common variant encountered, and it is characterized by congenital absence of the vagina and the uterus in 90–95% of cases (Murray 1979). In 7–10% of women with vaginal agenesis, a normal but obstructed uterus or a rudimentary uterus with functional endometrium is present (Solomons 1956; Murray 1979; Singh and Devi 1983). The incidence of associated urologic abnormalities is 15–40%, and skeletal anomalies, such as congenital fusion or absence of vertebra, occur in approximately 12–50% of cases (Turunen and Unnerus 1967; Griffin et al. 1976). MRKH – Klippel–Feil syndrome is characterized by congenital fusion of the cervical spine, short neck, low posterior hairline, and limited range of motion in the cervical spine (Willemsen 1982). The MURCS association/ MRKH (i.e., müllerian, renal, cervicothoracic somite abnormalities) is characterized by müllerian duct aplasia, renal aplasia, and cervicothoracic somite dysplasia. (Lyons 1997).	The karyotype in müllerian agenesis is 46, XX. Familial cases occur in 4% (Cramer et al. 1987, Tiker et al. 2000). Vaginal agenesis has been associated with variants of the galactose-1-phosphate uridyltransferase enzyme (Chen et al. 1981; Cramer et al. 1987; Aughton 1993). Antimüllerian hormone or müllerian inhibitory substance (MIS) gene or receptor gene polymorphisms may play a role in its origin (Lindenman et al. 1997). De novo translocations with MRKH syndrome suggests a break point potentially involved in midmüllerian differentiation (Amesse et al. 1999). A loss-of-function mutation in the WNT4 gene identified in MRKH syndrome, with unilateral renal agenesis, androgen excess, and virilization. WNT4 gene encodes a protein that suppresses male sexual differentiation. Association between the WNT4 gene and müllerian duct differentiation may also exist in humans (Biason-Lauber et al. 2004). The absence of a uterus (without other Müllerian abnormalities) and androgen excess are pathognomonic signs of WNT4 defects, suggesting that WNT4 deficiency might be a clinical entity distinct from the typical MRKH syndrome (Biason- Lauber and Konrad 2008). Sequence analysis of coding regions of HOX candidate genes and of PBX1, a likely HOX cofactor during Müllerian duct differentiation and kidney morphogenesis, did not reveal any mutation in patients showing various forms of MRKH syndrome. This tends to show that HOX genes are not involved in MRKH syndrome. However, it does not exclude that other mechanisms leading to HOX dysfunction may account for the syndrome (Burel et al. 2006). Others feel differential ligand-specific activation of HOX genes may be a molecular mechanism by which DES signaling leads to inappropriate HOX expression and to developmental patterning distinct from that induced by estradiol in mullerian agenesis (Akbas et al. 2004).	Uterovaginal agenesis is the second most common cause of primary amenorrhea after hypergonadotrophic hypogonadism (Petrozza et al. 1997). Pelvic examination reveals a patulous urethra (Jones 1992; Amesse et al. 1999). Ultrasound or MRI shows agenesis or hypoplasia of the Mullerian duct-derived structures (Doyle 1992; Mitchell 1992; Mitchell and Outwater 1995; Imaoka et al. 2003). Nonsurgical approach to the vaginal agenesis uses graduated dilators and is routinely effective in MRKH. Surgery is also effective for complete vaginal agenesis. Surgical treatment is considered if dilator therapy fails and only when the patient will become sexually active and is motivated to use vaginal prosthesis post-operatively (Coney 1992). Psychological counseling is often helpful (David et al. 1975; Mobus et al. 1996). IVP or renal sonography is suggested (Valdes et al. 1984). Skeletal defects often can be detected on IVP. Fused cervical vertebrae (Klippel–Feil syndrome) may cause cervical rigidity and difficult intubations (Duncan et al. 1979; Willemsen 1982). Many surgical techniques have been reported in complete ueterovaginal agenesis and are commonly referred to as a McIndoe procedure (Fedele et al. 1994; Ghirardini and Popp 1994). Each technique involves developing a space between the bladder and the rectum. In many approaches, a stent or form is placed in the created space to ensure patency while graft healing occurs. Full-thickness skin grafts result in less graft contracture and stenosis compared to split-thickness grafts (Sadove and Horton 1988; Chen et al. 1994). Split-thickness skin grafts are also successful (Garcia and Jones 1977; Buttram 1983; Strickland et al. 1993). Human amnion, not stripped from the chorion, has been used as a graft for vaginoplasties (Nisolle and Donnez 1992). Motoyama et al. (2003) used absorbable adhesion barrier (Interceed; Ethicon). Bowel has also been used as neovagina (Franz 1996). Williams' vulvovaginoplasty uses full-thickness skin flaps from the labia majora to create a vaginal pouch, and fistula formation is rare (Williams 1964). The Vecchietti operation (1965) uses a designed traction device placed on abdomen. Sutures attached to the device enter and course through the abdominal cavity. Upward traction on the retrohymenal fovea by the device creates and lengthens a vaginal space over one week of traction. Laparoscopic modification is available (Brun et al. 2002). Davydov (1969) reported a laparotomy procedure using peritoneum from pouch of Douglas to create vaginal canal, and multiple modifications have been described (Soong et al. 1996; Templeman et al. 2000; Rangaswamy et al. 2001).

(continued)

Table 16.2 (continued)

Class	Major clinical finding	Descriptive	Etiology	Diagnosis/treatment
II	Unicornuate uterus with or without a rudimentary horn	Rudimentary horn may be communicating or noncommunicating. The noncommunicating horn may or may not have an endometrial cavity. The clinical significance of this classification is that the the rudimentary horn is often accompanied by ipsilateral renal agenesis (Buttram and Gibbons 1979; Acien 1992; Wagner and Woodward 1994).	Pedro and Maribel Acien have for decades made cogent arguments regarding the need to consider mesonephric anomalies as parallel and potentially causal in the evaluation of mullerian anomalies. Serious consideration should be given to consideration of Acien's Classification of genitourinary anomalies (Acien 1986, 1989, 1992, 1997, 2001, 2002; Acien et al. 1987, 1990, 1991, 2004a, 2004b, 2008) (see Table 3).	Of müllerian anomalies, 2–13% are of the unicornuate variety (Buttram and Gibbons 1979; Acien 1997; Grimbizis et al. 2001). Incidence was 0.06% in one population of over >3,000 women who desired conception (Raga et al. 1997). Unicornuate uterus is frequently associated with a rudimentary horn (Buttram and Gibbons 1979; Rock and Schlaff 1985; Heinonen 1997). Urologic anomalies are found in 44%, particularly with an obstructed horn. Urological anomalies: ipsilateral renal agenesis (67%), horseshoe kidney, and ipsilateral pelvic kidney (15%) (Rolen et al. 1966; Rock and Schlaff 1985). Noncommunicating accessory horns with endometrial cavities should be removed (Markham and Waterhouse 1992). The unicornuate uterus anomaly is at high risk for preterm labor (43%), spontaneous miscarriage (34%), ectopic pregnancy (4%), cesarean section, malpresentation, and intrauterine growth restriction (Andrews and Jones 1982; Fedele et al. 1987, 1994; Michalas 1991). Ultrasound, hysterosalpingography, and MRI are useful. The rudimentary horn may appear solid if endometrium is absent and can appear as a soft tissue mass. If endometrium is present, it may or may not communicate (Mitchell 1992; Forstner and Hricak 1994; Mitchell and Outwater 1995; Imaoka et al. 2003; Marten et al. 2003; Saleem 2003; Scarsbrook and Moore 2003). IVP or renal ultrasonography are necessary to detect ipsilateral renal agenesis, horseshoe kidney, and ipsilateral pelvic kidney (Heinonen 1997). Surgical intervention is required for functional endometrium in the accessory horn via laparoscopic hemihysterectomy (Nisolle 1996; Donnez and Nisolle 1997; Patton and Novy 1988). If significantly distended, the noncommunicating rudimentary horn can be drained with a trochar prior to removal. Ectopic pregnancies in the rudimentary horn may be treated with methotrexate and allowed to regress prior to surgical intervention (Cutner et al. 2004).

III	Didelphys uterus	Complete or partial duplication of the vagina, cervix, and uterus characterizes this anomaly.	This anomaly is characterized by the failed fusion of the paired mullerian ducts from the fundus to the cervix and upper vagina. Variations of this primary defect occur when additional mesonephric duct abnormalities are found. One variation is the Wunderlich–Herlyn–Werner (WHW) syndrome), which is caused by a developmental arrest in the ipsilateral wolffian (mesonephric) duct causing failed induction of renal structures and positioning of the ipsilateral paramesonephric (müllerian) ducts. The malpositioned müllerian duct thus cannot fuse with other hemiuteri. Familial occurrence is reported (Biedel et al. 1984; Golan et al. 1989).	Eleven percent of MA are the didelphys uterus variety (Nahum 1998). The classic form has two widely separated hemiuteri with fallopian tubes, and two endocervical canals with cervices fused at the lower uterine segment. Ovarian malposition is not uncommon (Dabirashrafi et al. 1994). The vagina commonly has a longitudinal vaginal septum which is partial or complete. (Buttram 1983; Rock and Schlaff 1985; Fedele et al. 1987). Urogenital anomalies are found in 20%, with renal agenesis the most common. (Golan et al. 1989). Other associated anomalies include: bladder exstrophy with or without vaginal hypoplasia; congenital vesicovaginal fistula with hypoplastic kidney; and cervical agenesis (Stanton 1974; Mor et al. 2002; Yang et al. 2002; Dolan et al. 2004). Obstructed hemivaginal longitudinal septum with ipsilateral renal and ureter agenesis (Wunderlich–Herlyn–Werner (WHW) syndrome), is a rare, but well-recognized anomaly within the uterine didelphys classification (Tridenti et al. 1995; Tanaka et al. 1998; Phupong et al. 2000; Burgis 2001; Pieroni et al. 2001; Mulchahey 2002; Al-Hakeem et al. 2002; Hinckley and Milki 2003; Zurawin et al. 2004).The most common presenting symptoms in WHW are early onset of dysmenorrhea soon after menarche associated with progressive pelvic pain and a unilateral pelvic mass found on the right more than the left. Additionally, there can be rectal pain, constipation or obstipation (Pieroni et al. 2001). Excision and marsupialization of the obstructed longitudinal vaginal septum can be performed via large bore needle puncture of the obstructed vagina, Kelly clamp extension of the puncture site, suction of hematometrocolpos, insertion of a small gauge foley in the obstructed hemmivagina to demonstrate the limits of the septum as it attaches to the vaginal wall, gentle cautery of the limits of the desired excision followed by cautery or Mayo scissor excision of the demarcated septum followed by suture ligation of the pedicle. Laparoscopy is often performed with the vaginal septum excision to treat commonly noted endometriosis (Stassart et al. 1992). If performed while pregnant, a large pedicle is recommended (Rock and Schlaff 1985). Hematometra and hematosalpinx may recur if the septum is inadequately excised (Tanaka et al. 1998). Biovular twins delivered over long intervals has been reported in the uterine didlphys category (Lewenthal et al. 1977; Tyagi et al. 2001; Nohara et al. 2003). Studies show the following pregnancy results: 24% ending with preterm delivery, 2% resulting in ectopic pregnancy, and 20% ending in spontaneous miscarriages (Lin 2004; Brown 1999; Nohara et al. 2003). Adverse pregnancy outcomes are attributed to decreased volume and or perfusion of hemiuteri. The most frequent complaint in uterine didelphys is difficulty with and inadequacy of tampons, and a history of breech delivery. In uterine didelphys anomalies, surgical intervention includes excision of the longitudinal vagina septum for dypareunia or persistent bleeding despite frequent tampon changes. Unification procedures for the uterine didelphys via metroplasty are not recommended and often disappointing (Rock 2003). Laparoscopic metroplasty with diagnostic hysteroscopy has been performed for the unification of the uterus (Alborizi et al. 2008). However, this anomaly can be confused with a complete uterine septum with a longitudinal vaginal septum which should be considered and is best appreciated by MRI (axial view in the plane of the uterus) or 3D ultrasound. In the case of complete longitudinal uterine septum, hysteroscopic resection may improve pregnancy outcomes. Vaginal adenosis can occur in the remnant of the excised longitudinal septum and some experts recommend serial pap smears and colposcopy (Tridenti et al. 1995). Stassart et al. (1992) reported the obstetrical outcomes in 10 pregnancies: 50% term delivery, 40% preterm delivery, and 10% early spontaneous abortion. The intercornual angle is often >105°.

(continued)

Table 16.2 (continued)

Class	Major clinical finding	Descriptive	Etiology	Diagnosis/treatment
IV	Complete or partial bicornuate uterus	The classic bicornuate uterus has two endometrial cavities separated externally in a heart-shaped configuation, with a single cervix and vagina.	A combination of failed fusion associated with various levels of failed resorption of the intervening septum between the adjacent mullerian ducts at any level from the superior fundus to the cervix results in the bicornuate uterus. In the classic bicornuate uterus, there are two endometrial cavities, a single cervix and vagina. The described classic bicornuate uterus can be considered predominately a failed fusion abnormality of the superior mullerian ducts. The length of the failed fusion and site of failed resorption determine the anatomy of the bicornuate horns and the depth of the remaining intrauterine septum and the presence or absence of a cervical or vaginal septum (Propst and Hill 2000). Uterine horn separations (by failed fusion and or resorption) extending to the internal os are known as bicornuate unicollis uteri. When the failed fusion/resoprtion abnormailities extend to the external os, the condition is called a bicornuate bicollis uterus. This latter condition represents predominantly failed fusion superiorly and failed resorption inferiorly. Bicornuate uteri are a rare component of a mild, nonlethal variant of the urorectal septum malformation (Wheeler and Weaver 2001).	A bicornuate uterus often remains unrecognized until cesarean delivery or an imaging study identifies its existence. In a study of infertile women, the incidence of bicornuate uterus was not different from that of the fertile control group, suggesting no significant fertility issues with a bicornuate uterus (Raga et al. 1997). Early observations revealed that 60% of affected can expect to deliver a viable infant, but could experience late abortion or premature labor (Rock and Jones 1977). Obstetric outcomes appear to be related to the functional uterine cavity size. In a report of women with a partial bicornuate uterus a spontaneous abortion rate of 28%, and a preterm delivery rate of 20% was noted. Higher rates of adverse reproductive outcomes are reported in complete bicornuate uterus (Heinonen et al. 1982). In rare cases, a twin pregnancy can occur in both horns (Narlawar et al. 2003). In a report on 56 bicornuate pregnancies, 14 (25%) preterm deliveries, 35 (63%) live births, 0 (0%) ectopics, and 14 (25%) spontaneous abortions were noted (Lin 2004). Overall, a bicornuate uterus rarely requires surgery and is usually associated with acceptable reproductive/obstetrical problems, while a septate uterus can be surgically corrected and has a higher association with poor reproductive outcomes. Evaluation of a suspected bicornuate uterus begins with ultrasonography during the luteal phase (hyperechoic) of the menstrual cycle (Forstner and Hricak 1994). MRI is best to differentiate a bicornuate uterus from a septate uterus. The radiologist must be reminded to take an image in the axial plane of the uterus so the external contour of the fundus can be clearly evaluated for the dimple associated with the bicornuate configuration. The intercornual distance is routinely increased to >105° in a bicornuate uterus. The myometrial tissue that separates the two horns has a signal intensity identical to that of the myometrium (Saleem 2003;2004). The external contour is outward concave in contrast to the outward convexity of normal and septate uteri (Marten et al. 2003). Laparoscopic examination of the fundal contour readily distinguishs the bicornuate from the septate uterus. In most cases, the bicornuate uterus has two distinct horns, whereas the appearance of external fundus of the septate uterus is normal. HSG is incapable of reliably distinguishing the bicornuate from the septate uterus (Carrington et al. 1990; Pellerito et al. 1992; Forstner and Hricak 1994; Mitchell and Outwater 1995). The reported accuracy of HSG in differentiating bicornuate from septate uterus is 55% (Reuter et al. 1989). In 36 women with bicornuate uterus diagnosed by HSG, 34 (94%) were subsequently identified as having septate uterus by laparoscopy/ hysteroscopy (Sheth and Sonkawde 2000). In the rare case of recurrent miscarriage or repeated second trimester births, some recommend a modified Strassmann procedure (Strassmann 1966; Rock 2003). Laparoscopic metroplasty with diagnostic hysteroscopy has been performed for the unification of the uterus (Alborizi et al. 2008). Elective cesarean sections are often recommended if a unification has been performed (Lolis et al. 2005).

V	Complete or partial septate uterus	A complete or partial midline septum is present within a single uterus.	The septate uterus is characterized by essentially complete fusion of the paired. Mullerian structures associated with varying degrees of failed resorption of the central septum, as its primary abnormality. It is the most common of all müllerian duct anomalies. The septum is composed of poorly vascularized fibromuscular tissue (Raga et al. 1996). Numerous variations include: the complete septum, which extends from the fundal area to the internal os creating two endometrial cavities; the partial septum, which does not extend to the internal os; the triad of a complete uterine septum, duplicated cervix, and vaginal septum (Giraldo et al. 2000; Hundley et al. 2001; Wai et al. 2001; Fatum et al. 2003; Chang et al. 2004 Duffy et al. 2004; Patton et al. 2004); the rare anomaly characterized by a complete septum with one noncommunicating hemiuteri (Robert 1969); and the also infrequent segmental uterine septum which allows partial communication between the endometrial cavities (Candiani et al. 1983).	Fertility is not compromised in patients with a septate uterus. However, the septate Mullerian anomaly has the poorest reproductive outcomes, overall. The septate uterus revealed: 146/1,459 (10%) preterm deliveries, 90/155 (58.1%) live births, 3/155 (1.9%) ectopics, and 1,105/1,459 (75.7%) spontaneous abortions (Lin 2004). As noted in the review, a septate uterus is not always associated with an unfavorable obstetric outcome, and thus is not a primary indication for surgical intervention. The most common presenting symptoms in the complete uterine septum anomaly are dyspareunia, pregnancy loss, and obstetrical complications. When two cervices, are noted the diagnosis of a complete uterine septum should be distinguished from that of a didelphys uterus because each has different reproductive outcomes and treatment strategies. The complete uterine septum anomaly challenged the previously held theory on Müllerian development and proved that Müllerian fusion could occur bidirectionally. Patients with a complete uterine septum with a noncommunicating hemiuterus routinely present with unilateral hematometra and dysmenorrhea (Singhal et al. 2003). MRI of the septate uterus reveals a uterine septum partially dividing the uterine cavity with intercornual angle <75°. An intercornual angle >75° but <105° could be a uterine septum or bicornuate uterus and the external fundal configuration in the axial plane of the uterus: outward convex or outward concave indicates the diagnosis, respectively. The preferred surgical intervention is the hysteroscopic metroplasty (March and Israel 1987; Litta et al. 2004). Simultaneous laparoscopy reduces the risk of perforation and offers early detection of surgical complications. Litta et al. (2008) has reported on the utility of the Verapoint in hysteroscopic resection. Uterine rupture in a subsequent pregnancy has been reported (Lobaugh et al. 1994). Uterine perforation, polyhydramnios, and/or the use of monopolar current during operative hysteroscopy increase this risk of uterine rupture in subsequent pregnancies (Sentilhes et al. 2006). Residual or reannealment of the lysed septum is found in as many as 44.1% despite the apparent success of the procedure. When residual or reannealed septa measure less than 1 cm, no adverse effects have been noted, and repeat operation is unwarranted (Fedele et al. 1996). Reproductive performance is improved after hysteroscopic surgery (Gray et al. 1984; Valle and Sciarra 1986; DeCherney et al.1986; Daly et al. 1983; Valli et al. 2004; Litta et al. 2004; Patton et al. 2004; Mollo et al. 2008; Ban-Frangez et al. 2008). Heinonen (2006) advised that lysis of a complete uterine septum with a longitudinal vaginal septum in an asymptomatic patient or before a pregnancy with an adverse outcome is not indicated. One study reported a faster procedure time with a resectoscopic excision of the vaginal portion of the complete uterine septum anomaly, but many already use electrocautery for this portion of the excision (Darwish and Elsaman 2008).

(continued)

Table 16.2 (continued)

Class	Major clinical finding	Descriptive	Etiology	Diagnosis/treatment
VI	Arcuate uterus	A small septate indentation is present at the fundus.	The arcuate uterus is a minor variant of the septate uterus category and is characterized by the near-complete resorption of the uterovaginal septum, leaving only a small intrauterine indentation less than 1 cm in depth in the mid fundus. It represents the most commonly identified uterine anomaly during HSG (Zanetti et al. 1978; Maneschi et al. 1995).	HSG reveals a single uterine cavity with a saddle-shaped fundal indentation less than 1 cm in depth from the intercornual line. MRI reveals a normal fundus with an outward convex or flat external contour. The indentation is broad and smooth. The signal intensity is myometrial in composition. A subtle indentation of arcuate vessels is sometimes detected within the fundal myometrium (Zanetti et al. 1978; Maneschi et al. 1995; Troiano, 2003). Available literature finds no evidence for primary surgical intervention. One combined review reported on 283 pregnancies: 10/195 (5.1%) had preterm deliveries, 129/195 (66.2%) had live births, 7/195 (3.6%) had ectopics, and 57/283 (20.1%) had spontaneous abortions (Lin 2004).
VII	DES-related abnormalities	The characteristic cervical findings includes a: cervical hood (vaginal fold draped over the cervix), cockscomb cervix (an abnormally shaped cervix), and adenosis (glandular cells normally located within the cervix that appear on the outside of the cervix and in the vagina). The Fallopian tubes may have abnormalities that lead to infertility. The uterus is often abnormal in size and shape. The classic sign is the T-shaped uterus.	In a mouse model DES-induced changes in the expression of genes such as Dkk2, Nkd2, and sFRP1 as well as changes in genes of the Hox, Wnt, and Eph families. These changes could be the basis for various abnormalities in reproductive tracts following exposure to this estrogenic drug (Suzuki et al. 2007). Five to ten million women were exposed between 1938 to 1971.	DES Daughters are 40 times more likely to develop CCA of the vagina and cervix than women not exposed to DES. This means that approximately one of every 1,000 women exposed to DES before birth (in the womb) will be diagnosed with CCA of the vagina and/or the cervix. Before the use of DES, CCA of the vagina and cervix only occurred in women past childbearing age. In contrast, DES Daughters have been diagnosed with CCA of the vagina and cervix at as early as age 8 and up to their late teens and early 20s. Most DES Daughters will be able to conceive and carry a healthy baby to term. However, DES Daughters are at an increased risk of reproductive problems, including complications during pregnancy and infertility. DES Daughters are at an increased risk for premature delivery (approximately 20%), ectopic pregnancy (three to five times higher risk), miscarriage (20%), and infertility (24%).

Table 16.3 Ascien's modified classification system for genitourinary anomalies

1. Agenesis or hypoplasia of a whole urogenital ridge: Unicornuate uterus with uterine, tubal, ovarian and renal agenesis on the contralateral side
2. *Mesonephric anomalies* with absence of the Wolfian duct opening to the urogenital sinus and of the urethral bud sprouting (and therefore, renal agenesis). The "inductor" function of the Wolfian duct on the Müllerian duct is also failing and there is usually:
   Utero-vaginal duplicity plus blind hemivagina ipsilateral with the renal agenesis, clinically presented as:
   (a) Large unilateral hematocolpos[a]
   (b) Gartner's pseudocyst on the anterolateral wall of the vagina[a]
   (c) Partial reabsorption of intervaginal septum, seen as a "buttonhole" on the anterolateral wall of the normal vagina which allows access to the genital organs on the renal agenesis side
   (d) Vaginal or complete cervico-vaginal unilateral agenesis, ipsilateral with the renal agenesis, and (1) with no communication, or (2) with communication between both hemiuteri (communication uteri)
3. Isolated *Müllerian anomalies*
   (a) Müllerian ducts: they are common uterine malformations as unicornuate (generally, with uterine rudimentary horn), bicornuate, septate and didelphys uterus
   (b) Müllerian tubercle: cervico-vaginal atresia and segmentary anomalies such as tranverse vaginal septum
   (c) Both, Müllerian tubercle and ducts: (uni- or bilateral) Mayer–Rokitansky–Kuster–Hauser syndrome
4. Anomalies of the urogenital sinus: cloacal anomalies and others
5. Malformative combinations: Wolfian, Müllerian and cloacal anomalies

[a]These types can associate a vaginal ectopic ureter and interseptal or interuterine communication
Reprinted with permission from Human Repro, Acien P et al. 2004; 19(10): 2377–2384 [17]

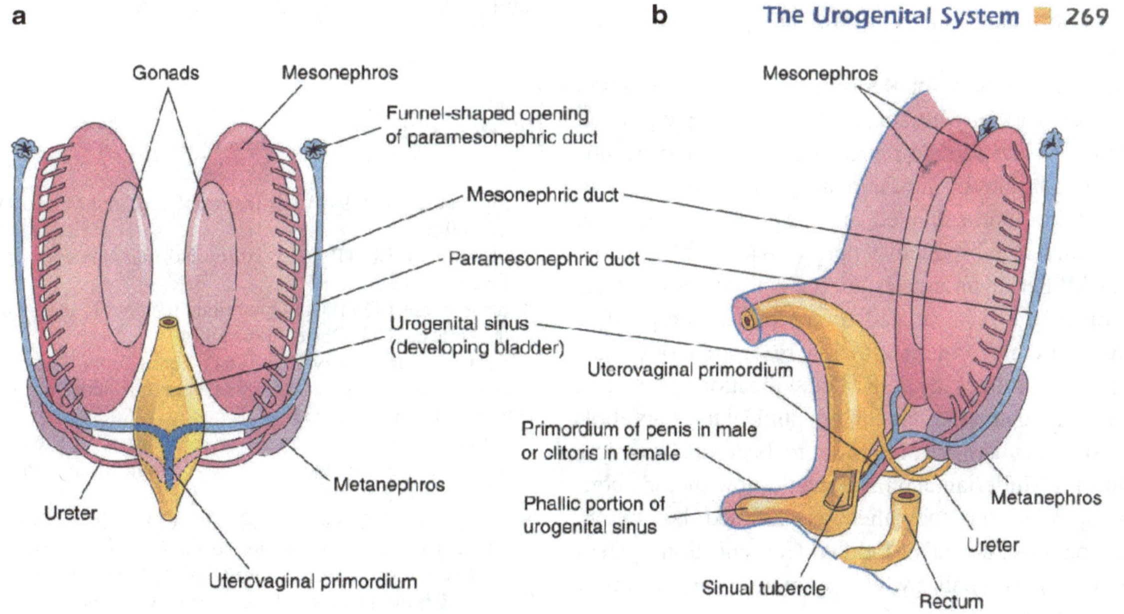

Fig. 16.2 Development of the vagina and hymen. (Reprinted with permission from Moore KL, Persaud TVN and Torchia MG, The Developing Human, Clinically Oriented Embryology, 8th Edition, Saunders/Elsevier, Philadelphia, PA, 2008; pg 269)

bulbs reform the UGS into a flat vestibule. The vaginal plate canalizes to form the vaginal canal by week 20. The vagina's fibromuscular wall comes from surrounding mesenchyme and is derived from the UVP, the UGS or a combination which remains to be determined conclusively [15].

Hart (1901) [23] and Mijsberg (1924)[24] both identified the sinovaginal bulbs as "Wolffian bulbs" and suggested they were derivatives of the caudal aspects of the Wolffian (mesonephric) and paramesonephric (Müllerian) ducts. In a mouse model, the vagina arises from the downward growth of mesonephric and paramesonephric ducts and the sinovaginal bulbs are formed by the caudal mesonephric ducts. It was also suggested that vaginal development is under negative control of androgens. Human studies of embryological development also parallel these findings by sharing a common basement membrane between the caudal Müllerian and Wolfian ducts [25]. Acien and colleagues have helped solidify the apparent union of the Wolffian and Müllerian ducts in embryological development by their extensive descriptions of MA associated with urogenital malformations. In one case report, they described a woman with complex urogenital malformations that suggested a Wolffian (mesonephric) duct and sinus tubercle origin for the vagina. The patient had a didelphys uterus, unilateral cervical–vaginal atresia, and ipsilateral renal agenesis. During hemi-hysterectomy, the atretic hemicervix opened into an atretic duct, which continued inferiorly to terminate at the existing normal vagina. Acien concluded that the histopathologic findings, suggested a role for the Wolffian ducts in vaginal formation [26]. Pedro and Maribel Acien have suggested a genitourinary classification system (Table 16.3) that includes consideration of both the Müllerian and Wolffian ducts when classifying an individual anomaly [17].

The vaginal hymen is a vestige of the endodermal membrane that differentiates into the vaginal vestibule. It separates the vaginal lumen from the UGS cavity and is formed by caudal expansion of the vagina with subsequent invagination into the posterior wall of the UGS [15]. The hymen usually ruptures perinatally and the remnants persist as a thin mucous membrane.

The American Society for Reproductive Medicine, based on the previous work of Buttram and Gibbons [27], classified the anomalies of the female reproductive tract into groups according to similarities in clinical manifestations, the degree to which normal development failed, and the possible prognoses, with treatment, for reproductive performance (Table 16.1). The various Müllerian anomalies are the consequences of the following disturbances – isolated or combined, complete or incomplete failure of: formation; fusion; resorption, or canalization. Table 16.2 utilizes the ASRM classification system and includes information on the class, major clinical findings etiology, diagnosis, and treatment of each anomaly group. Complete assessment of a Mullerian anomaly should now include consideration of Wolffian anomalies as outlined by Acien. Table 16.3 contains Ascien's Modified Classification System for Genitourinary Anomalies which we recommend as part of the evaluation exercise.

16.4 Theories for the Etiology of Reproductive Malperformance

Previous explanations for reproductive malperformance have included diminished uterine volume, cervical incompetance, muscular/connective tissue ratios of the septum, and inadequate vascularization of the uterine septum. Studies have confirmed irregular differentiation and estrogenic maturation of the endometrium covering the uterine septum [28]. This could result in a compromise of implantation and placental growth and function and result in infertility, pregnancy loss, and/or abruptio placenta. In contrast to the previously held notion of increased connective tissue in the septum, there is in fact less connective tissue and more muscle [29]. The increased muscular tissue may result in poor decidualization and placentation due to reduced connective tissue and a high degree of uncoordinated contractility due to increased muscle content. This has been confirmed both histologically and radiographically. The role of cervical incompetence in Müllerian anomalies is unclear.

16.5 Diagnostic Evaluation and Treatment

Multiple methods are available for diagnostic evaluation of suspected Müllerian anomalies, however, MRI and 3D transvaginal ultrasound are the most sensitive and specific diagnostic tools. Hysterosalpingogram or saline infusion sonogram (SIS or sonohysterography) are recommended in the initial evaluation. The evaluation, diagnosis, and treatment of MA are outlined in Tables 16.1–16.3.

References

1. Steinmetz GP (1940) Formation of artificial vagina. West J Surg 48:169-3
2. Strassmann EO (1966) Fertility and unification of double uterus. Fertil Steril 17(2):165–176
3. Strassmann EO (1961) Operations for double uterus and endometrial artesia. Clin Obstet Gynecol (4)
4. Greiss FC Jr, Mauzy CH (1961) Genital anomalies in women: an evaluation of diagnosis, incidence, and obstetric performance. Am J Obstet Gynecol 82:330–339
5. Green LK, Harris RE (1976) Uterine anomalies. Frequency of diagnosis and associated obstetric complications. Obstet Gynecol 47(4):427–429
6. Grimbizis GF, Camus M, Tarlatzis BC, Bontis JN, Devroey P (2001) Clinical implications of uterine malformations and hysteroscopic treatment results. Hum Reprod Update 7(2):161–174
7. Raga F, Bauset C, Remohi J, Bonilla-Musoles F, Simon C, Pellicer A (1997) Reproductive impact of congenital Mullerian anomalies. Hum Reprod 12(10):2277–2281
8. Acien P (1992) Embryological observations on the female genital tract. Hum Reprod 7(4):437–445
9. Stray-Pedersen B, Stray-Pedersen S (1984) Etiologic factors and subsequent reproductive performance in 195 couples with a prior history of habitual abortion. Am J Obstet Gynecol 148(2):140–146
10. Stampe Sorensen S (1988) Estimated prevalence of mullerian anomalies. Acta Obstet Gynecol Scand 67(5):441–445
11. Simon C, Martinez L, Pardo F, Tortajada M, Pellicer A (1991) Mullerian defects in women with normal reproductive outcome. Fertil Steril 56(6):1192–1193
12. Ashton D, Amin HK, Richart RM, Neuwirth RS (1988) The incidence of asymptomatic uterine anomalies in women undergoing transcervical tubal sterilization. Obstet Gynecol 72(1):28–30
13. Byrne J, Nussbaum-Blask A, Taylor WS et al (2000) Prevalence of Mullerian duct anomalies detected at ultrasound. Am J Med Genet 94(1):9–12

14. Larsen WJ (2001) Development of the urogenital system. In: Sherman LS, Potter SS, Scott WH (eds) Human Embryology, 3rd edn. Churchill Livingstone, New York, pp 277–279
15. Moore KL, Persaud TVN (2003) The urogenital system: the developmental of the genital system. In: The developing human: clinically oriented embryology, 7th edn. WB Saunders, Philadelphia
16. Lindenman E, Shepard MK, Pescovitz OH (1997) Mullerian agenesis: an update. Obstet Gynecol 90(2):307–312
17. Acien P, Acien M, Sanchez-Ferrer M (2004) Complex malformations of the female genital tract. New types and revision of classification. Hum Reprod 19(10):2377–2384
18. Shulman LP (1988) Developmental abnormalities of the female reproductive tract: pathogenesis and nosology. Acta Obstet Gynecol Scand 67
19. Puerta-Fonolla AJ (1998) Morphogenesis of the human genital tract. Ital J Anat Embryol 4(Suppl 1):3–15
20. Duffy DA, Nulsen J, Maier D, Schmidt D, Benadiva C (2004) Septate uterus with cervical duplication: a full-term delivery after resection of a vaginal septum. Fertil Steril 81(4):1125–1126
21. Chang AS, Siegel CL, Moley KH, Ratts VS, Odem RR (2004) Septate uterus with cervical duplication and longitudinal vaginal septum: a report of five new cases. Fertil Steril 81(4):1133–1136
22. Lee DM, Osathanondh R, Yeh J (1998) Localization of Bcl-2 in the human fetal mullerian tract. Fertil Steril 70(1):135–140
23. Hart DB (1901) Morphology of the human urinogenital tract. J Anat Physiol 35(Pt 3):330–375
24. Mijsberg WA (1924) Uber die entwicklung der vagina, des hymen und des sinus urogenitalis beim menschen. Z Anat Entwicklungsgesch 74:684–760
25. Hashimoto R (2003) Development of the human Mullerian duct in the sexually undifferentiated stage. Anat Rec A Discov Mol Cell Evol Biol 272(2):514–519
26. Acien P, Susarte F, Romero J et al (2004) Complex genital malformation: ectopic ureter ending in a supposed mesonephric duct in a woman with renal agenesis and ipsilateral blind hemivagina. Eur J Obstet Gynecol Reprod Biol 117(1):105–108
27. Buttram VC Jr, Gibbons WE (1979) Mullerian anomalies: a proposed classification. (An analysis of 144 cases). Fertil Steril 32(1):40–46
28. Candiani GB, Fedele L, Zamberletti D, De Virgiliis D, Carinelli S (1983) Endometrial patterns in malformed uteri. Acta Eur Fertil 14(5):311–318
29. Sparac V, Kupesic S, Ilijas M, Zodan T, Kurjak A (2001) Histologic architecture and vascularization of hysteroscopically excised intrauterine septa. J Am Assoc Gynecol Laparosc 8(1):111–116

References Table 2

Acien P (1986) Endometriosis and genital anomalies: some histogenetic aspects of external endometriosis. Gynecol Obstet Invest 22:102–107

Acien P (1989) Malformaciones genitales y embriología de la vagina humana. Rev Iber Fertilidad 6:427–436

Acien P (1992) Embryological observations on the female genital tract. Hum Reprod 7:437–445

Acien P (1997) Incidence of Mullerian defects in fertile and infertile women. Hum Reprod 12:1372–1376

Acien P (2001) Unicornuate uterus with two cavitated, non-communicating rudimentary horns? Hum Reprod 16:393–395

Acien P (2002) Obstructive mullerian anomalies. Am J Obstet Gynecol 186:854

Acien P, Arminana E (1986) Agenesia renal y malformaciones útero-vaginales: asociación sistemática. Revisión de la literatura y consideraciones sobre la embriología de la vagina. Acta Ginec 43:303–318

Acien P, Arminana E, Garcia-Ontiveros E (1987) Unilateral renal agenesis associated with ipsilateral blind vagina. Arch Gynecol 240:1–8

Acien P, Lloret M, Chehab H (1988) Endometriosis in a patient with Rokitansky-Kuster-Hauser syndrome. Gynecol Obstet Invest 25:70–72

Acien P, Garcia-Lopez F, Ferrando J, Chehab HE (1990) Single ectopic ureter opening into blind vagina, with renal dysplasia and associated utero-vaginal duplication. Int J Gynaecol Obstet 31:179–185

Acien P, Ruiz JA, Hernandez JF, Susarte F, Martin del Moral A (1991) Renal agenesis in association with malformation of the female genital tract. Am J Obstet Gynecol 165:1368–1370

Acien P, Brotons J, Quereda FJ (1992) Malformaciones genitales y endometriosis. Prog Obstet Ginec 35:88–95

Acien P, Acien M, Sanchez-Ferrer M (2004a) Complex malformations of the female genital tract. New types and revision of classification. Hum Reprod 19:2377–2384

Acien P, Sanchez-Ferrer M, Mayol-Belda MJ (2004b) Unilateral cervico-vaginal atresia with ipsilateral renal agenesis. Eur J Obstet Gynecol Reprod Biol 117:249–251

Acien P, Susarte F, Romero J et al. (2004c) Complex genital malformation: ectopic ureter ending in a supposed mesonephric duct in a woman with renal agenesis and ipsilateral blind hemivagina. Eur J Obstet Gynecol Reprod Biol 117:105–108

Acien P, Acien M, Fernandez S (2008) Segmentary atresias in Mullerian malformations. Eur J Obstet Gynecol Reprod Biol 141:188–189

Akbas GE, Song J, Taylor HS (2004) A HOXA10 estrogen response element (ERE) is differentially regulated by 17 beta-estradiol and diethylstilbestrol (DES). J Mol Biol 340:1013–1023

Alborzi S, Asadi N, Zolghadri J, Alborzi M (2009) Laparoscopic metroplasty in bicornuate and didelphic uteri. Fertil Steril 92:352–355

Al-Hakeem MM, Ghourab SA, Gohar MR, Khashoggi TY (2002) Uterine didelphus with obstructed hemivagina. Saudi Med J 23:1402–1404

American College of Obstetrics and Gynecology (2002) ACOG committee opinion. Nonsurgical diagnosis and management of vaginal agenesis. Number 274, July 2002. Committee on Adolescent Health Care. American College of Obstetrics and Gynecology. Int J Gynaecol Obstet 79:167–170

Amesse L, Yen FF, Weisskopf B, Hertweck SP (1999) Vaginal uterine agenesis associated with amastia in a phenotypic female with a de novo 46, XX, t(8;13)(q22.1;q32.1) translocation. Clin Genet 55:493–495

Andrews MC, Jones HW Jr (1982) Impaired reproductive performance of the unicornuate uterus: intrauterine growth retardation, infertility, and recurrent abortion in five cases. Am J Obstet Gynecol 144:173–176

Aughton DJ (1993) Mullerian duct abnormalities and galactosaemia heterozygosity: report of a family. Clin Dysmorphol 2:55–61

Ban-Frangez H, Tomazevic T, Virant-Klun I, Verdenik I, Ribic-Pucelj M, Bokal EV (2008) The outcome of singleton pregnancies after IVF/ICSI in women before and after hysteroscopic resection of a uterine septum compared to normal controls. Eur J Obstet Gynecol Reprod Biol 146:184–187

Biason-Lauber A, Konrad D, Navratil F, Schoenle EJ (2004) A WNT4 mutation associated with Mullerian-duct regression and virilization in a 46, XX woman. N Engl J Med 351:792–798

Biason-Lauber A, Konrad D (2008) WNT4 and sex development. Sex Dev 2:210–218

Biedel CW, Pagon RA, Zapata JO (1984) Mullerian anomalies and renal agenesis: autosomal dominant urogenital adysplasia. J Pediatr 104:861–864

Brown O (1999) Twin pregnancy in a uterus didelphys, with unilateral placental abruption and onset of labour. Aust N Z J Obstet Gynaecol 39:506–508

Brun JL, Belleannee G, Grafeille N, Aslan AF, Brun GH (2002) Long-term results after neovagina creation in Mayer-Rokitanski-Kuster-Hauser syndrome by Vecchietti's operation. Eur J Obstet Gynecol Reprod Biol 103:168–172

Burel A, Mouchel T, Odent S et al (2006) Role of HOXA7 to HOXA13 and PBX1 genes in various forms of MRKH syndrome (congenital absence of uterus and vagina). J Negat Results Biomed 5:4

Burgis J (2001) Obstructive Mullerian anomalies: case report, diagnosis, and management. Am J Obstet Gynecol 185:338–344

Buttram VC Jr (1983) Mullerian anomalies and their management. Fertil Steril 40:159–163

Buttram VC Jr, Gibbons WE (1979) Mullerian anomalies: a proposed classification. (An analysis of 144 cases). Fertil Steril 32:40–46

Candiani GB, Fedele L, Zamberletti D, De Virgiliis D, Carinelli S (1983) Endometrial patterns in malformed uteri. Acta Eur Fertil 14:311–318

Carrington BM, Hricak H, Nuruddin RN, Secaf E, Laros RK Jr, Hill EC (1990) Mullerian duct anomalies: MR imaging evaluation. Radiology 176:715–720

Chang AS, Siegel CL, Moley KH, Ratts VS, Odem RR (2004) Septate uterus with cervical duplication and longitudinal vaginal septum: a report of five new cases. Fertil Steril 81:1133–1136

Chen YT, Mattison DR, Feigenbaum L, Fukui H, Schulman JD (1981) Reduction in oocyte number following prenatal exposure to a diet high in galactose. Science 214:1145–1147

Chen YB, Cheng TJ, Lin HH, Yang YS (1994) Spatial W-plasty full-thickness skin graft for neovaginal reconstruction. Plast Reconstr Surg 94:727–731

Coney P (1992) Effect of vaginal agenesis on the adolescent: prognosis for normal sexual and psychological adjustment. Adolesc Pediatr Gyencol 5:8–12

Cramer DW, Ravnikar VA, Craighill M, Ng WG, Goldstein DP, Reilly R (1987) Mullerian aplasia associated with maternal deficiency of galactose-1-phosphate uridyl transferase. Fertil Steril 47:930–934

Cutner A, Saridogan E, Hart R, Pandya P, Creighton S (2004) Laparoscopic management of pregnancies occurring in non-communicating accessory uterine horns. Eur J Obstet Gynecol Reprod Biol 113:106–109

Dabirashrafi H, Mohammad K, Moghadami-Tabrizi N (1994) Ovarian malposition in women with uterine anomalies. Obstet Gynecol 83:293–294

Daly DC, Walters CA, Soto-Albors CE, Riddick DH (1983) Hysteroscopic metroplasty: surgical technique and obstetric outcome. Fertil Steril 39:623–628

Darwish AM, Elsaman AM (2008) Extended resectoscopic versus sequentional cold knife-resectoscopic excision of the unclassified complete uterocervicovaginal septum: a randomized trial. Fertil Steril

David A, Carmil D, Bar-David E, Serr DM (1975) Congenital absence of the vagina. Clinical and psychologic aspects. Obstet Gynecol 46:407–409

Davydov SN (1969) Colpopoeisis from the peritoneum of the uterorectal space. Akush Ginekol (Mosk) 45:55–57

DeCherney AH, Russell JB, Graebe RA, Polan ML (1986) Resectoscopic management of mullerian fusion defects. Fertil Steril 45:726–728

Dolan LM, Easwaran SP, Hilton P (2004) Congenital vesicovaginal fistula in association with hypoplastic kidney and uterus didelphys. Urology 63:175–177

Donnez J, Nisolle M (1997) Endoscopic laser treatment of uterine malformations. Hum Reprod 12:1381–1387

Doyle MB (1992) Magnetic resonance imaging in mullerian fusion defects. J Reprod Med 37:33–38

Duffy DA, Nulsen J, Maier D, Schmidt D, Benadiva C (2004) Septate uterus with cervical duplication: a full-term delivery after resection of a vaginal septum. Fertil Steril 81:1125–1126

Duncan PA, Shapiro LR, Stangel JJ, Klein RM, Addonizio JC (1979) The MURCS association: Mullerian duct aplasia, renal aplasia, and cervicothoracic somite dysplasia. J Pediatr 95:399–402

Fatum M, Rojansky N, Shushan A (2003) Septate uterus with cervical duplication: rethinking the development of mullerian anomalies. Gynecol Obstet Invest 55:186–188

Fedele L, Zamberletti D, Vercellini P, Dorta M, Candiani GB (1987) Reproductive performance of women with unicornuate uterus. Fertil Steril 47:416–419

Fedele L, Busacca M, Candiani M, Vignali M (1994) Laparoscopic creation of a neovagina in Mayer-Rokitansky-Kuster-Hauser syndrome by modification of Vecchietti's operation. Am J Obstet Gynecol 171:268–269

Fedele L, Bianchi S, Marchini M, Mezzopane R, Di Nola G, Tozzi L (1996) Residual uterine septum of less than 1 cm after hysteroscopic metroplasty does not impair reproductive outcome. Hum Reprod 11:727–729

Forstner R, Hricak H (1994) Congenital malformations of uterus and vagina. Radiologe 34:397–404

Franz RC (1996) Sigmoid colon vaginoplasty: a modified method. Br J Obstet Gynaecol 103:1148–1155

Garcia J, Jones HW Jr (1977) The split thickness graft technic for vaginal agenesis. Obstet Gynecol 49:328–332

Ghirardini G, Popp L (1994) New approach to the Mayer-von Rokitansky-Kuster-Hauser Syndrome. Adoles Pediatr 7:41–43

Giraldo JL, Habana A, Duleba AJ, Dokras A (2000) Septate uterus associated with cervical duplication and vaginal septum. J Am Assoc Gynecol Laparosc 7:277–279

Golan A, Langer R, Bukovsky I, Caspi E (1989) Congenital anomalies of the mullerian system. Fertil Steril 51:747–755

Gray SE, Roberts DK, Franklin RR (1984) Fertility after metroplasty of the septate uterus. J Reprod Med 29:185–188

Greiss FC Jr, Mauzy CH (1961) Genital anomalies in women: an evaluation of diagnosis, incidence, and obstetric performance. Am J Obstet Gynecol 82:330–339

Griffin JE, Edwards C, Madden JD, Harrod MJ, Wilson JD (1976) Congenital absence of the vagina. The Mayer-Rokitansky-Kuster-Hauser syndrome. Ann Intern Med 85:224–236

Grimbizis GF, Camus M, Tarlatzis BC, Bontis JN, Devroey P (2001) Clinical implications of uterine malformations and hysteroscopic treatment results. Hum Reprod Update 7:161–174

Heinonen PK (1997) Unicornuate uterus and rudimentary horn. Fertil Steril 68:224–230

Heinonen PK (2006) Complete septate uterus with longitudinal vaginal septum. Fertil Steril 85:700–705

Heinonen PK, Saarikoski S, Pystynen P (1982) Reproductive performance of women with uterine anomalies. An evaluation of 182 cases. Acta Obstet Gynecol Scand 61:157–162

Hinckley MD, Milki AA (2003) Management of uterus didelphys, obstructed hemivagina and ipsilateral renal agenesis. A case report. J Reprod Med 48:649–651

Hundley AF, Fielding JR, Hoyte L (2001) Double cervix and vagina with septate uterus: an uncommon mullerian malformation. Obstet Gynecol 98:982–985

Imaoka I, Wada A, Matsuo M, Yoshida M, Kitagaki H, Sugimura K (2003) MR imaging of disorders associated with female infertility: use in diagnosis, treatment, and management. Radiographics 23:1401–1421

Jones HW (1992) Reconstruction of congenital uterovaginal anomalies. In: Rock JA, Murphy A, Jones HW (eds) Female Reproducative Surgery. Lippincott Williams & Wilkins, Baltimore

Lewenthal H, Biale Y, Ben-Adereth N (1977) Uterus didelphys with a pregnancy in each horn. Case report. Br J Obstet Gynaecol 84:155–158

Lin PC (2004) Reproductive outcomes in women with uterine anomalies. J Womens Health (Larchmt) 13:33–39

Lindenman E, Shepard MK, Pescovitz OH (1997) Mullerian agenesis: an update. Obstet Gynecol 90:307–312
Litta P, Pozzan C, Merlin F et al (2004) Hysteroscopic metroplasty under laparoscopic guidance in infertile women with septate uteri: follow-up of reproductive outcome. J Reprod Med 49: 274–278
Litta P, Spiller E, Saccardi C, Ambrosini G, Caserta D, Cosmi E (2008) Resectoscope or Versapoint for hysteroscopic metroplasty. Int J Gynaecol Obstet 101:39–42
Lobaugh ML, Bammel BM, Duke D, Webster BW (1994) Uterine rupture during pregnancy in a patient with a history of hysteroscopic metroplasty. Obstet Gynecol 83:838–840
Lolis DE, Paschopoulos M, Makrydimas G, Zikopoulos K, Sotiriadis A, Paraskevaidis E (2005) Reproductive outcome after strassman metroplasty in women with a bicornuate uterus. J Reprod Med 50:297–301
Lyons JK (1997) MURSC association: müllerian duct, renal and cervical vertebral defects. In: Smith's recognizable patterns of human malformation, 5th edn. WB Saunders, Philadelphia
Maneschi F, Zupi E, Marconi D, Valli E, Romanini C, Mancuso S (1995) Hysteroscopically detected asymptomatic mullerian anomalies. Prevalence and reproductive implications. J Reprod Med 40:684–688
March CM, Israel R (1987) Hysteroscopic management of recurrent abortion caused by septate uterus. Am J Obstet Gynecol 156:834–842
Markham SM, Waterhouse TB (1992) Structural anomalies of the reproductive tract. Curr Opin Obstet Gynecol 4:867–873
Marten K, Vosshenrich R, Funke M, Obenauer S, Baum F, Grabbe E (2003) MRI in the evaluation of mullerian duct anomalies. Clin Imaging 27:346–350
Michalas SP (1991) Outcome of pregnancy in women with uterine malformation: evaluation of 62 cases. Int J Gynaecol Obstet 35:215–219
Mitchell DG (1992) Benign disease of the uterus and ovaries. Applications of magnetic resonance imaging. Radiol Clin North Am 30:777–787
Mitchell DG, Outwater EK (1995) Benign gynecologic disease: applications of magnetic resonance imaging. Top Magn Reson Imaging 7:26–43
Mobus VJ, Kortenhorn K, Kreienberg R, Friedberg V (1996) Long-term results after operative correction of vaginal aplasia. Am J Obstet Gynecol 175:617–624
Mollo A, De Franciscis P, Colacurci N et al (2008) Hysteroscopic resection of the septum improves the pregnancy rate of women with unexplained infertility: a prospective controlled trial. Fertil Steril 91:2628–2631
Mor E, Saadat P, Sokol RZ, Paulson RJ (2002) Spontaneous twin gestation after vaginal dilation in a woman with uterus didelphys and bladder exstrophy. Obstet Gynecol 100:1138–1141
Motoyama S, Laoag-Fernandez JB, Mochizuki S, Yamabe S, Maruo T (2003) Vaginoplasty with Interceed absorbable adhesion barrier for complete squamous epithelialization in vaginal agenesis. Am J Obstet Gynecol 188:1260–1264
Mulchahey KM (2002) Management quandary. Severe dysmenorrhea due to obstructive anomaly. J Pediatr Adolesc Gynecol 15:175–177
Murray JM, Gambrell RD Jr (1979) Complete and partial vaginal agenesis. J Reprod Med 22:101–105
Nahum GG (1998) Uterine anomalies. How common are they, and what is their distribution among subtypes? J Reprod Med 43:877–887
Narlawar RS, Chavhan GB, Bhatgadde VL, Shah JR (2003) Twin gestation in one horn of a bicornuate uterus. J Clin Ultrasound 31:167–169
Nisolle M, Donnez J (1992) Vaginoplasty using amniotic membranes in cases of vaginal agenesis or after vaginectomy. J Gynecol Surg 8:25–30
Nohara M, Nakayama M, Masamoto H, Nakazato K, Sakumoto K, Kanazawa K (2003) Twin pregnancy in each half of a uterus didelphys with a delivery interval of 66 days. BJOG 110:331–332
Patton PE, Novy MJ (1988) Reproductive potential of the anomalous uterus. Sem Reprod Endocrinol 6:217–233
Patton PE, Novy MJ, Lee DM, Hickok LR (2004) The diagnosis and reproductive outcome after surgical treatment of the complete septate uterus, duplicated cervix and vaginal septum. Am J Obstet Gynecol 190:1669–1675; discussion 75–78.
Pellerito JS, McCarthy SM, Doyle MB, Glickman MG, DeCherney AH (1992) Diagnosis of uterine anomalies: relative accuracy of MR imaging, endovaginal sonography, and hysterosalpingography. Radiology 183:795–800
Petrozza JC, Gray MR, Davis AJ, Reindollar RH (1997) Congenital absence of the uterus and vagina is not commonly transmitted as a dominant genetic trait: outcomes of surrogate pregnancies. Fertil Steril 67:387–389
Phupong V, Pruksananonda K, Taneepanichskul S, Tresukosol D, Virutamasen P (2000) Double uterus with unilaterally obstructed hemivagina and ipsilateral renal agenesis: a variety presentation and a 10-year review of the literature. J Med Assoc Thai 83:569–574
Pieroni C, Rosenfeld DL, Mokrzycki ML (2001) Uterus didelphys with obstructed hemivagina and ipsilateral renal agenesis. A case report. J Reprod Med 46:133–136
Propst AM, Hill JA 3rd (2000) Anatomic factors associated with recurrent pregnancy loss. Semin Reprod Med 18:341–350
Pui MH (2004) Imaging diagnosis of congenital uterine malformation. Comput Med Imaging Graph 28:425–433
Raga F, Bonilla-Musoles F, Blanes J, Osborne NG (1996) Congenital Mullerian anomalies: diagnostic accuracy of three-dimensional ultrasound. Fertil Steril 65:523–528
Raga F, Bauset C, Remohi J, Bonilla-Musoles F, Simon C, Pellicer A (1997) Reproductive impact of congenital Mullerian anomalies. Hum Reprod 12:2277–2281
Rangaswamy M, Machado NO, Kaur S, Machado L (2001) Laparoscopic vaginoplasty: using a sliding peritoneal flap for correction of complete vaginal agenesis. Eur J Obstet Gynecol Reprod Biol 98:244–248
Reuter KL, Daly DC, Cohen SM (1989) Septate versus bicornuate uteri: errors in imaging diagnosis. Radiology 172:749–752
Robert HG (1969) Uterus cloisonne avec cavite borgne sans hematometrie. CR Soc Fr Gyencol 39:767–775
Rock JA (2003) Surgery for anomalies of the mullerian ducts. In: Tompson JD, Rock JA (eds) TeLind's operative gynecology, 9th edn. JB Lippincott Williams &Wilkins, Philadelphia
Rock JA, Jones HW Jr (1977) The clinical management of the double uterus. Fertil Steril 28:798–806
Rock JA, Schlaff WD (1985) The obstetric consequences of uterovaginal anomalies. Fertil Steril 43:681–692
Rolen AC, Choquette AJ, Semmens JP (1966) Rudimentary uterine horn: obstetric and gynecologic implications. Obstet Gynecol 27:806–813
Sadove RC, Horton CE (1988) Utilizing full-thickness skin grafts for vaginal reconstruction. Clin Plast Surg 15:443–448
Saleem SN (2003) MR imaging diagnosis of uterovaginal anomalies: current state of the art. Radiographics 23:e13
Scarsbrook AF, Moore NR (2003) MRI appearances of mullerian duct abnormalities. Clin Radiol 58:747–754
Sentilhes L, Sergent F, Berthier A, Catala L, Descamps P, Marpeau L (2006) Uterine rupture following operative hysteroscopy. Gynecol Obstet Fertil 34:1064–1070
Sheth SS, Sonkawde R (2000) Uterine septum misdiagnosed on hysterosalpingogram. Int J Gynaecol Obstet 69:261–263
Singh J, Devi YL (1983) Pregnancy following surgical correction of nonfused mullerian bulbs and absent vagina. Obstet Gynecol 61:267–269

Singhal S, Agarwal U, Sharma D, Sirohiwal D (2003) Pregnancy in asymmetric blind hemicavity of Robert's uterus–a previously unreported phenomenon. Eur J Obstet Gynecol Reprod Biol 107:93–95
Solomons E (1956) Conception and delivery following construction of an artificial vagina; report of a case. Obstet Gynecol 7:329–331
Soong YK, Chang FH, Lai YM, Lee CL, Chou HH (1996) Results of modified laparoscopically assisted neovaginoplasty in 18 patients with congenital absence of vagina. Hum Reprod 11:200–203
Stanton SL (1974) Gynecologic complications of epispadias and bladder exstrophy. Am J Obstet Gynecol 119:749–754
Stassart JP, Nagel TC, Prem KA, Phipps WR (1992) Uterus didelphys, obstructed hemivagina, and ipsilateral renal agenesis: the University of Minnesota experience. Fertil Steril 57:756–761
Strickland JL, Cameron WJ, Frantz KE (1993) Long-term satisfaction of adults undergoing McIndoe vaginoplasty as adults. Adoles Pediatr Gynecol 6:135
Suzuki A, Urushitani H, Sato T et al (2007) Gene expression change in the Mullerian duct of the mouse fetus exposed to diethylstilbestrol in utero. Exp Biol Med (Maywood) 232:503–514
Tanaka YO, Kurosaki Y, Kobayashi T et al (1998) Uterus didelphys associated with obstructed hemivagina and ipsilateral renal agenesis: MR findings in seven cases. Abdom Imaging 23: 437–441
Templeman CL, Hertweck SP, Levine RL, Reich H (2000) Use of laparoscopically mobilized peritoneum in the creation of a neovagina. Fertil Steril 74:589–592
Tiker F, Yildirim SV, Barutcu O, Bagis T (2000) Familial mullerian agenesis. Turk J Pediatr 42:322–324
Tridenti G, Bruni V, Ghirardini G (1995) Double uterus with a blind hemivagina and ipsilateral renal agenesis: clinical variants in three adolescent women: case report and literature review. Adoles Pediatr Gynecol 8:201–207
Troiano RN (2003) Magnetic resonance imaging of mullerian duct anomalies of the uterus. Top Magn Reson Imaging 14:269–279
Turunen A, Unnerus CE (1967) Spinal changes in patients with congenital aplasia of the vagina. Acta Obstet Gynecol Scand 46:99–106
Tyagi A, Minocha B, Prateek S (2001) Delayed delivery of second twin in uterus didelphys. Int J Gynaecol Obstet 73:259–260
Valdes C, Malini S, Malinak LR (1984) Ultrasound evaluation of female genital tract anomalies: a review of 64 cases. Am J Obstet Gynecol 149:285–292
Valle RF, Sciarra JJ (1986) Hysteroscopic treatment of the septate uterus. Obstet Gynecol 67:253–257
Valli E, Vaquero E, Lazzarin N, Caserta D, Marconi D, Zupi E (2004) Hysteroscopic metroplasty improves gestational outcome in women with recurrent spontaneous abortion. J Am Assoc Gynecol Laparosc 11:240–244
Wagner BJ, Woodward PJ (1994) Magnetic resonance evaluation of congenital uterine anomalies. Semin Ultrasound CT MR 15:4–17
Wai CY, Zekam N, Sanz LE (2001) Septate uterus with double cervix and longitudinal vaginal septum. A case report. J Reprod Med 46:613–617
Wheeler PG, Weaver DD (2001) Partial urorectal septum malformation sequence: a report of 25 cases. Am J Med Genet 103:99–105
Willemsen WN (1982) Combination of the Mayer-Rokitansky-Kuster and Klippel-Feil syndrome–a case report and literature review. Eur J Obstet Gynecol Reprod Biol 13:229–235
Williams EA (1964) Congenital absence of the vagina: a simple operation for its relief. J Obstet Gynaecol Br Commonw 71:511–512
Yang CC, Tseng JY, Chen P, Wang PH (2002) Uterus didelphys with cervical agenesis associated with adenomyosis, a leiomyoma and ovarian endometriosis. A case report. J Reprod Med 47:936–938
Zanetti E, Ferrari LR, Rossi G (1978) Classification and radiographic features of uterine malformations: hysterosalpingographic study. Br J Radiol 51:161–170
Zurawin RK, Dietrich JE, Heard MJ, Edwards CL (2004) Didelphic uterus and obstructed hemivagina with renal agenesis: case report and review of the literature. J Pediatr Adolesc Gynecol 17:137–141

Chapter 17
Recurrent Miscarriage

D. Ware Branch and Cara Heuser

Abstract Recurrent miscarriage is a common pathology fond in 1% to 5% of reproductively active couples. This chapter discusses the possible causes of recurrent miscarriage, and delineates a cost effective, productive strategy for the clinical evaluation of couples with two or more miscarriages.

Keywords Recurrent miscarriage • Abortion • Uterine anomalies • Aneuploidy • Antiphospholipid antibodies • Alloimmunity • Thrombophilia

17.1 Background and Introduction

Spontaneous abortion, or miscarriage, is perhaps the most common complication of pregnancy, occurring in at least one-quarter of women attempting to reproduce. Many clinicians consider the loss of three or more consecutive pregnancies to be the definition of recurrent miscarriage, a condition that occurs in approximately 1% of reproductively active couples. Experts hold that two consecutive miscarriages is sufficient for the diagnosis of recurrent miscarriage; this occurs in about 5% of reproductively active couples [1].

Miscarriage is historically defined as pregnancy loss prior to 20 weeks of gestation. This rather arbitrary definition ignores the precepts of developmental biology, our currently available diagnostic capabilities, and the clinical realities of pregnancy loss.

17.1.1 Conceptus Development and Miscarriage

The development of the conceptus is, of course, a biologic continuum. However, largely different stages of development are identifiable and are useful in understanding and studying pregnancy loss. Experts debate the terminology and the exact beginning and end of each stage. One useful categorization is as follows:

- The preembryonic period lasts from conception through the 4th week, from the first day of the last menstrual period (3 weeks after conception). During this period, the early trophoblast differentiates from the tissue destined to become the embryo (the inner cell mass) and accomplishes implantation into the maternal endometrium (days 6–7 after fertilization). The pre-embryo develops into a bilaminar, and then trilaminar disk of cells and microscopically observable alterations of the cell disk define the cranial end central neural axis of the pre-embryo.
- The embryonic period begins around the 5th week of gestation, lasting through the 9th week of gestation. During the embryonic period, the trilaminar disk folds to become cylindrical, the head and tail regions become recognizable as cranial and caudal folds, definite segmentation is seen, and all organs form (organogenesis).
- The fetal period begins at the 10th week of gestation and extends through pregnancy until delivery. This period is characterized by relatively little organogenesis, but with substantial growth and differentiation of previously formed structures.

There are also distinct phases in the development of the placenta and the maternal–fetal circulation. Histological examination [2] and Doppler ultrasonography [3] indicate that normal pregnancies are characterized by obstruction of utero-placental arteries by invading trophoblastic cells. This process markedly limits maternal blood flow into the intervillous tissue during the first 10–12 weeks. During this time, the intervillous space is filled with acellular fluid [4], and the environment is relatively hypoxic [5]. Although there appears to be some individual variation, trophoblastic regression and dislocation of arteriolar trophoblastic plugs beginning at 10 weeks gestation allow initiation of true intervillous blood flow and a concomitant increase in the intervillous oxygen tension. Until this transpires, it is thought that oxygenation of the embryonic

D.W. Branch and C. Heuser (✉)
Department of Obstetrics and Gynecology, Division of Maternal Fetal Medicine, University of Utah School of Medicine, Salt Lake City, UT, USA
e-mail: ware.branch@hsc.utah.edu

D.T. Carrell and C.M. Peterson (eds.), *Reproductive Endocrinology and Infertility: Integrating Modern Clinical and Laboratory Practice*,
DOI 10.1007/978-1-4419-1436-1_17,

tissues occurs largely through diffusion across adjacent tissues, rather than through an organized circulatory delivery.

These current concepts in developmental biology are highly relevant to recurrent miscarriage because they underscore the different vulnerabilities of the conceptus at different periods in gestation. For example, it is well accepted that chromosome abnormalities render the conceptus susceptible to both developmental abnormalities and miscarriage, with different chromosome abnormalities likely to "cause" miscarriage at very different gestational ages. Our understanding of developmental abnormalities in euploid conceptions is, however, fairly limited. Early in the history of murine transgenic research, Andrew Copp noted how little was understood about developmental defects leading to embryonic or fetal demise [6]. In 1995, he summarized over 50 embryo-fetal lethal mutations in the mouse and was able to characterize them as affecting (1) the peri-implantation period, (2) the period of organogenesis, or (3) the fetal period. In each of these three periods, well-documented experimental genetic models of pregnancy loss, complete with relevant histopathology, were identified. On the basis of his analysis, Copp proposed the concept of "developmental bottlenecks," identifying, for example, three such bottlenecks in the peri-implantation period: blastocyst development, development of a connection between the blastocyst and the decidua, and completion of gastrulation. Examples of bottlenecks later in gestation included abnormalities in vasculogenesis linked to lethality during the period of organogenesis and abnormalities in hematopoesis linked to fetal death.

Currently, there is very little direct evidence of developmental defects in euploid conceptions as a cause of either sporadic or recurrent miscarriage. The primary reason for this is the lack of systematic morphological assessment of human miscarriages occurring before the early-to-mid second trimester. One group of investigators performing meticulous morphologic studies of abortuses found that 214 of 1,124 specimens (19%) were dysmorphic in nature, while only 30 (2.7%) had a recognized chromosome abnormality [7]. No such work exists for recurrent miscarriages, and our understanding of the remarkably complex field of developmental biology as it relates to human miscarriage remains infantile.

The foregoing underscores a critically important distinction in the field of recurrent miscarriage: recurrent *early* miscarriage (<10 weeks gestation) vs. recurrent *late* miscarriage (10 or more weeks gestation). Events in the latter category are often referred to as fetal deaths, whereas events in the former category may be termed as pre-embryonic or embryonic pregnancy losses. The distinction is important because the etiologies and recurrence rates of these two broad categories of pregnancy loss differ. In addition, recurrent early miscarriage is a far more common presentation than recurrent late miscarriage. Distinctions between these two conditions will be made in the ensuing discussion.

17.1.2 Epidemiology of Miscarriage and Recurrent Miscarriage

Studies of early pregnancies detected with sensitive β-human chorionic gonadotropin (βhCG) assays indicate that at least 30% of human pregnancies are lost, either as unrecognized pregnancy losses occurring before or with the expected next menses (about two-thirds of all losses) or as recognized pregnancy losses, traditionally referred to as miscarriages (about one-third of all losses). Several variables influence the rate of miscarriage, including age, number of prior spontaneous abortions, and parity (Fig. 17.1). Thus, the proportion of pregnancies ending in miscarriage ranges from approximately 9% in nulliparous and parous women aged 25–29 years without a history of prior miscarriage to >40% in nulliparous women and >70% in parous women aged 40–44 years with a history of three or more miscarriages [8]. The rate of spontaneous abortion above age 35 rises somewhat dramatically and is due in part to factors other than chromosomally abnormal conceptions [9]. The rate of second trimester fetal death follows a similar pattern, but the rate of rise begins to increase at the age of 30 [10]. The likelihood of miscarriage is also dependent upon past obstetric history. Women with a history of prior miscarriage have a higher risk and women with previous live births have a slightly lower risk.

When defined as the loss of two or more recognized pregnancies (American Society of Reproductive Medicine, 2008), recurrent miscarriage occurs in up to 5% women attempting more than one pregnancy [1], depending upon the population in question. About 1% of women present with three or more consecutive miscarriages, again depending upon the population. These figures are thought to define a distinct clinical entity because they are higher than would be expected if recurrent miscarriages were due to recurrent "sporadic" losses, which occur in some 10–15% of all pregnancies and would predict a population-based likelihood of about 0.34%. Some experts recognize *primary* recurrent miscarriage in women without any prior successful pregnancy, and *secondary* recurrent miscarriage in women whose repetitive losses follow a live birth. There is no specific classification for women who have multiple miscarriages interspersed with live births. It is generally agreed that a workup for possible causes of recurrent miscarriage is indicated in most patients after two or three miscarriages.

17.2 Etiologies of Recurrent Miscarriage

Recurrent miscarriage has been ascribed to a variety of causal factors, including specific genetic, uterine, endocrine, thrombotic, alloimmune, autoimmune, and infectious factors.

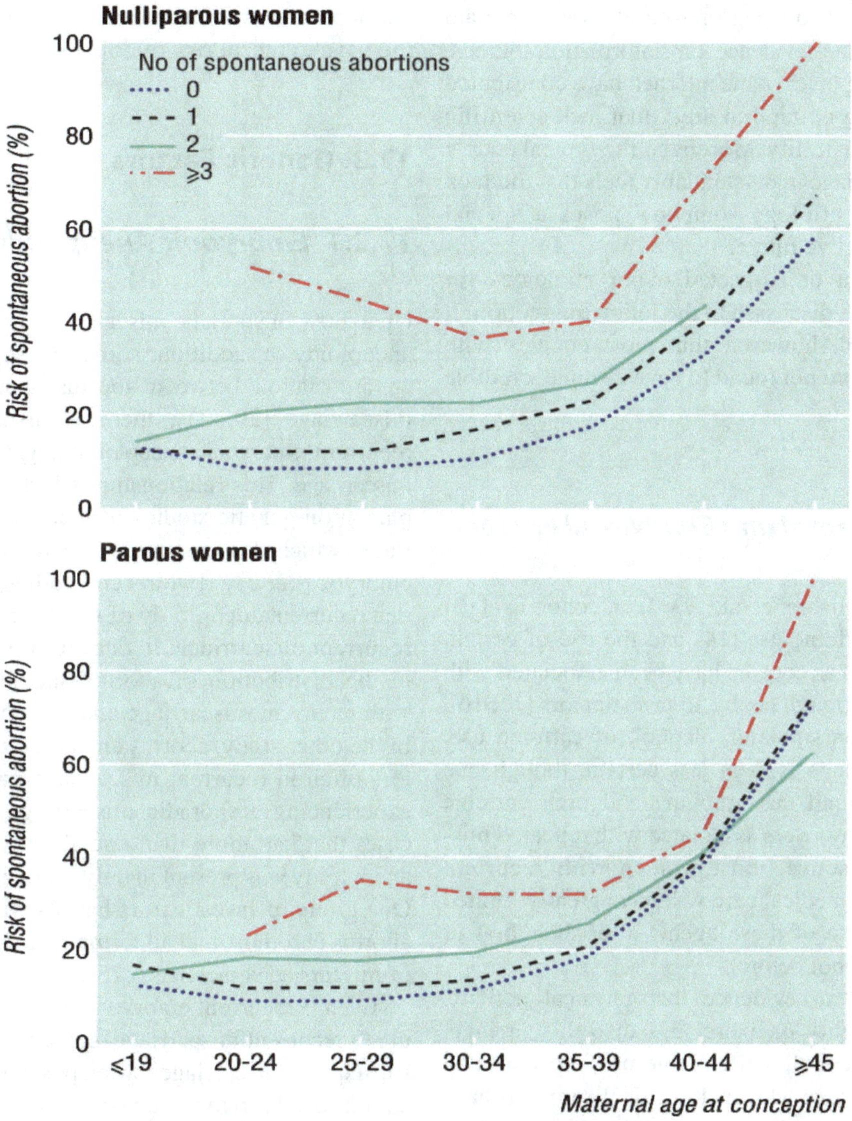

Fig. 17.1 Risk of spontaneous abortion in nulliparous and parous women according to maternal age at conception and number of spontaneous abortions in preceding 10 years [8]

However, none of these factors displays high sensitivity or specificity for recurrent miscarriage, and each may be found in couples with normal reproductive histories. Though the alleged causal factors are evaluated and managed individually in clinical practice, most couples do not have a single clear "cause." Christiansen has recently suggested that recurrent miscarriage should be seen as a "mulitfactorial" condition, much like adult arteriosclerotic heart disease [11]. Using a multifactorial paradigm, several factors would contribute to the likelihood of miscarriages, with a "threshold" effect for recurrent miscarriage being achieved by the several factors combining to elevate the likelihood of miscarriage per pregnancy attempt. In particular, maternal age and the number of prior miscarriages play important roles. Fig. 17.1 shows the miscarriage rate by maternal age at conception and number of prior miscarriages. Increasing paternal age also is independently associated with miscarriage [12], with an adjusted odds ratio of 1.6 for men over 40 years of age. One can easily see how these important variables would influence the miscarriage rate per pregnancy attempt, and thus the likelihood of having recurrent miscarriage, especially in women over 35 years of age.

Allowing that recurrent miscarriage may be best considered a multifactorial condition, most reviews of the condition discuss etiologic categories separately, a practice that is useful in clinical care and perhaps most easily understood by the average couple. While there is widespread agreement regarding a definite role for some etiologies, such as parental karyotype abnormalities, other proposed etiologies remain controversial or simply lack evidence. Lay information sources, fed by the distribution power of the internet, have contributed supposition and strong opinion to areas that lack scientific rigor and medical plausibility. Moreover, the typical couple with recurrent miscarriage understandably feels that the lack of an apparent clear etiology somehow poses a special threat to their reproductive future.

Each of the known or suspected major etiologies for recurrent miscarriage is discussed in the following section. It should be emphasized, however, that most couples with recurrent miscarriage are not found to have a single, credible etiology.

17.2.1 Environmental and Behavioral Factors

Cigarette smoking (Mishra et al. 2000), alcohol us [13] moderate-to-heavy caffeine use [14] and the use of certain recreational drugs such as cocaine have been associated with sporadic miscarriage, though not by all investigators [15, 16]. A relationship between smoking, alcohol, or caffeine use, and recurrent miscarriage is even less certain, though one case–control study found that smoking and high caffeine intake (>300 mg per day) were associated with repeated miscarriages [17]. In practice, most women with recurrent miscarriage who seek medical care will have greatly limited or discontinued the use of these agents after their first or second miscarriage, if not before.

There is virtually no evidence that physical activity, including sexual activity or exercise, cause miscarriage. As with cigarettes, alcohol, and caffeine use, most women with recurrent miscarriage who seek medical care will have greatly limited or discontinued strenuous physical activity.

Antidepressant use also might be associated with an increased rate of sporadic abortion [18], though depression itself cannot be excluded as a factor. Here again, a relationship between antidepressants and recurrent miscarriage is uncertain.

A modern-day concern is the possible association of obesity with sporadic miscarriage [19], especially with the burgeoning obesity epidemic in the U.S. Whether obesity is associated with recurrent miscarriage is uncertain, as is the role of weight reduction in subsequent pregnancy success.

17.2.1.1 Clinical Recommendations

There is no evidenced-based rationale for asking a couple with recurrent miscarriage to alter an otherwise healthy and reasonable lifestyle. It may be prudent to limit alcohol and caffeine intake, though most patients will already have done so by the time they seek medical advice. Whether or not it is similarly prudent to recommend discontinuation of antidepressants is uncertain and must be weighed against the psychological risk of doing so.

17.3 Genetic Factors

17.3.1 Embryonic Aneuploidy

Up to 60% of sporadic miscarriages are a result of embryonic aneuploidy. In addition, some investigators have suggested an association between abortus aneuploidy and recurrent miscarriage [20, 21], thereby raising the suspicion that recurrent embryonic aneuploidy might be a cause of recurrent miscarriage. This relationship is further supported by preimplantation genetic studies of women with recurrent miscarriage, which demonstrate an aneuploidy rate of 50% in all embryos [22, 23]. Two recent studies, however, did not find that recurrent aneuploidy of the conceptus was a "cause" of recurrent miscarriage. In one study, there was no difference in the distribution of abortus aneuploidy between women with recurrent miscarriage and a historic control group [20]. In the other study, abortus aneuploidy occurred significantly less often in recurrent miscarriage patients than in patients experiencing a sporadic miscarriage [24]. Furthermore, in cases that had more than one abortus karyotyped, recurrent aneuploidy was present in only a small proportion of patients. One group of investigators has shown that the likelihood of abortus chromosomal abnormalities decreases as the number of miscarriages increases [25].

Even if recurrent embryonic aneuploidy does not contribute to recurrent miscarriage, some experts favor karyotyping subsequent miscarriages when possible. Two studies indicate an improved prognosis among recurrent miscarriage patients with an aneuploid miscarriage [25, 26].

17.3.1.1 Clinical Recommendations

A modest proportion of recurrent miscarriages are chromosomally aneuploid, and couples with aneuploid recurrent miscarriages appear to have an improved prognosis for successful pregnancy compared to those with euploid recurrent miscarriages. Thus, performing karyotype analysis of a subsequent miscarriage in couples with recurrent miscarriages is of prognostic significance.

17.3.2 Parental Karyotype Abnormalities

In approximately 2–4% of couples with recurrent miscarriage, one of the reproductive partners carries a balanced structural chromosomal rearrangement, usually a balanced translocation

[27, 28]. Among these couples, the frequency of balanced translocations is twofold higher in the female partner than in the male. In such couples, it is generally held that meiotic segregation results in chromosomal duplications or deficiencies in a meaningful proportion of the gametes. In turn, chromosomal abnormalities occur in a meaningful proportion of the resulting conceptions so that spontaneous abortion is more likely and leads to recurrent miscarriage.

About 60% of balanced translocations are reciprocal (involving non-homologous translocations), while 40% are Robertsonian (involving the acrocentric chromosomes 13, 14, 15, 21, and 22). The risk of aneuploidy in the conceptus is dependent on which parent carries the translocation, as well as the chromosomes involved. In general, the risk of subsequent miscarriage is higher if the translocation is maternal in origin. Though rare, translocations involving homologous chromosomes, e.g., a 14–14 translocation, preclude the possibility of a normal live born infant.

Chromosomal *inversions* have also been linked to recurrent miscarriage, though they are less frequently found than translocations. The risk of abnormal offspring depends on the size and location of the inversion and the sex of the contributing partner. Inversions of small portions of the total chromosomal length lead to large duplications and deficiencies and are generally lethal. Paradoxically, larger inversions are more likely to be compatible with survival. The risk of abnormal offspring, and presumably recurrent miscarriage, is slightly higher if the heterozygous carrier of a *pericentric* inversion is female. *Paracentric* recombinants are universally lethal.

Parental chromosomal abnormalities do not usually preclude further attempts at pregnancy, because most couples eventually have normal offspring. For balanced translocations, the role of in-vitro fertilization with preimplantation genetic diagnosis remains controversial because of the relatively high rate of successful pregnancy with spontaneous conception [29]. For the rare homologous Robertsonian translocation that prevents genetically-normal conception, therapeutic possibilities include artificial donor insemination, in vitro fertilization with donor oocytes, and adoption.

17.3.2.1 Clinical Recommendations

Both American [30] and British [31] professional organizations recommend that the evaluation of couples with recurrent miscarriage include cytogenetic evaluation of both partners. In practice, this is often avoided initially, because it is a common practice among U.S. insurers to deny payment for this testing and because the yield is fairly low (found in only 2–4% of couples). Genetic counseling should be provided to those with parental chromosomal abnormalities in an effort to predict recurrence, and genetic amniocentesis or chorionic villus sampling should be offered in subsequent pregnancies.

17.3.3 Skewed X Inactivation

Females are mosaics for two cell populations, one with the maternal and one with the paternal X as the active chromosome. In female mammalian cells, one of the two X chromosomes is inactivated in early embryonic life, and inactivation is thought to be permanent for all descendants of a cell. Normally, there can be shown a roughly 50:50 distribution of cells with inactivated maternal X vs. paternal X chromosomes. Skewing of this normal ratio demonstrating a preferential inactivation of one X chromosome is termed as highly skewed X chromosome inactivation, or "skewed X inactivation" in short.

The finding of skewed X inactivation in a family with a high rate of miscarriage [32] led to the hypothesis that recurrent miscarriage might be due to this condition in some women [33]. One proposed mechanism by which this might occur is selective lethality of male conceptuses inheriting the deleterious X chromosome. Another proposal is that skewing and the associated mutation(s) lead to a restriction in the oocyte precursor pool and a subsequent higher miscarriage rate because of chromosomal aneuploidy. Initial excitement about a potential new cause of recurrent miscarriage has cooled, however, with the publication of several negative studies [34–36]. The fact that skewed X inactivation is associated with advancing age is potentially intriguing.

17.3.3.1 Clinical Recommendations

Testing for skewed maternal X inactivation is not clinically useful in the management or counseling of couples with recurrent miscarriage.

17.4 Structural Uterine Abnormalities

Most experts believe that structural uterine abnormalities are associated with recurrent miscarriage. The best work related to this subject comes from Jurkovic and colleagues working at King's College in London [37]. In a large, prospective case series, non-pregnant women with otherwise unexplained recurrent miscarriage were screened for uterine anomalies using two-dimensional ultrasonography. Those suspected of having a malformation were studied with three-dimensional ultrasound; anomalies were classified according to the American Fertility Society system. Controls were women referred for pelvic ultrasound for indications not related to reproductive outcomes. The investigators screened over 500 women with recurrent miscarriage and over 2,000 controls. Uterine anomalies were found in 121 (23.8%) of the recurrent miscarriage patients and 105 (5.3%) of the controls.

The most common anomalies in both groups were arcuate and subseptate uterus. The authors also found that when anomalies were present, the mean length of the uterine cavity was shorter and the mean degree of distortion of the cavity greater in the recurrent miscarriage group.

Woelfer and colleagues studied reproductive outcomes in over 1,000 women without infertility, recurrent miscarriage or fibroids deforming the uterine cavity who had been referred for pelvic ultrasound [38]. One-hundred-six women (10.7%) had uterine anomalies, including 72 arcuate, 29 subseptate, and 5 bicornuate uteri. Compared to the women with normal uteri, women with uterine anomalies were more likely to have had first trimester miscarriages (12% of all pregnancies in normal uteri; 26% of all pregnancies with arcuate or subseptate uteri). Other anomalies, particularly unicornuate uterus and hypoplastic uterus, are linked to miscarriage, though they are infrequently found anomalies.

There are several points of debate regarding the role of uterine anomalies in recurrent miscarriage. First, the frequency of these anomalies in the general population is somewhat uncertain, being reported from approximately 1.5–10.5% in relatively recent works. Thus, some studies report a frequency of anomalies in normal women that is commonly quoted as that in women with recurrent miscarriage (~10%). Second, the definition of the more subtle uterine anomalies, such as arcuate uterus, varies from study-to-study and may not be as well diagnosed with some techniques.

A third important point of debate is the mechanism of pregnancy loss in women with uterine anomalies. Diminished blood supply in malformed tissues (such as uterine septa) interfering with normal implantation and placentation has been cited as the cause of miscarriage in women with uterine anomalies. This contention has been very difficult to prove, however. Recent experimental evidence points to the endometrium in uterine malformations as the possible culprit by way of an association between structural malformations and altered uterine stroma and endometrium. For example, homeobox genes are critical in the proper structural development of the uterus, with murine mutants and human mutations associated with a variety of structural abnormalities [39]. Homeobox mutations also are associated with reduced uterine stromal tissue and decreased epidermal growth factor receptor expression [40]. Perhaps supporting a possible relationship between uterine anomalies and uterine tissue abnormalities, a hysteroscopic study of eight women with septate uterus found that the preovulatory endometrium from the septum showed alterations consistent with a decrease in the sensitivity of endometrium to preovulatory hormonal changes [41]. The implications for miscarriage are obvious, and more work in this area should prove rewarding.

A fourth area of debate is whether or not metroplasty is truly effective in women with recurrent miscarriage and uterine septum. The main point is that no well-designed studies are available. Retrospective analyses and case series, however, are nearly unanimous in claiming improved pregnancy outcomes after resection of the uterine septum [42, 43].

Uterine fibroids seem likely to impact assisted reproduction [44, 45]. The relationship between fibroids and recurrent miscarriage is less clearly established. A recent expert review concluded that fibroids, particularly multiple fibroids and intramural fibroids, were associated with an increased proportion of pregnancies ending in clinical miscarriage [46], though with an odds ratio of less than 2.0. Little can be said, however, regarding the possible benefits of myomectomy or ablation with regard to miscarriage. Given that the risks of extensive uterine surgery in subsequent pregnancy are not insubstantial, it is difficult to recommend excision of multiple fibroids as a treatment.

17.4.1 Clinical Recommendations

Women with recurrent miscarriage should undergo uterine cavity evaluation for evidence of uterine malformation or other abnormalities. Most experts would recommend hysteroscopic resection of a uterine septum if one is found. In the absence of better evidence, myomectomy or hysteroscopic resection of leiomyomas should be reserved for large fibroids that distort the uterine cavity.

17.5 Endocrinologic Factors

17.5.1 Luteal Phase Insufficiency

Luteal phase insufficiency (LPI) is a controversial condition of inadequate luteal phase preparation of the endometrium, with the most commonly hypothesized defect being in progesterone (P) preparation of the uterine lining. Though biologically plausible, the evidence linking LPI to recurrent miscarriage is far from certain. One major problem is the lack of a credible diagnostic method. Originally, LPI was diagnosed in the presence of so-called "out-of-phase" endometrial biopsies, which lagged two or more days behind the actual postovulation date, estimated by counting backward from the next menstrual period. However, the diagnostic accuracy of endometrial tissue phasing has been questioned because of considerable interobserver and intraobserver variation in pathological interpretation [47]. Also, as many as 50% of women without miscarriage can exhibit the same out-of-phase endometrial biopsies.

P levels have also been proposed as diagnostic criteria for LPI. Clearly, a single determination of P in the luteal phase of a non-pregnant cycle has little or no predictive value for subsequent pregnancy outcome in recurrent miscarriage patients [48]. Multiple determinations of P in the luteal phase also have been suggested as a requirement for the diagnosis of LPI. However, even several determinations in the same patient have inadequate predictive value for an out-of-phase endometrium. In a well-designed study of allegedly healthy, ovulatory women, some of whom were treated with P in the luteal phase, investigators found that histologic dating of the endometrium did not reflect circulating P concentrations and can not be used to assess the quality of the luteal function as indicated by immunohistochemistry for endometrial integrins, and real-time quantitative RT-PCR for putative functional makers [49].

In spite of these critical uncertainties, endometrial biopsy or luteal-phase serum P levels are widely used to make the diagnosis of LPI. In turn, many clinicians treat women with supposed LPI and recurrent miscarriage with P in a subsequent pregnancy attempt. One commonly advocated treatment is a 25–50 mg of P in suppository or gel, administered vaginally twice daily (morning and night), with treatment beginning after ovulation and continuing until either menses begin or through the first 8–12 weeks of pregnancy. Comparable doses of oral micronized P also have been used. Early studies of P supplementation reported improved pregnancy outcomes in treated women. However, the reliability of these findings has been questioned because no appropriate control groups were treated for comparison. A meta-analysis of P for women with recurrent miscarriage found no benefit in the prevention of miscarriage [50]. Results of a proposed European, placebo-controlled trial of dydrogesterone in the treatment of recurrent miscarriage may be clarifying [51].

Clomiphene and other ovulatory agents, as well as human chorionic gonadotropin (hCG), have also been tried in an attempt to improve follicular development and stimulate corpus luteum function in women with LPI with varying results. One placebo-controlled, multicentered trial with hCG found no significant improvement difference in the successful pregnancy [52].

17.5.1.1 Clinical Recommendations

An evaluation for LPI is entrenched in the field of recurrent miscarriage, and many patients will wish to have it done or insist on it. Treatment of early pregnancy with progesterone has not been shown to improve pregnancy outcome in women with recurrent miscarriage, though the treatment is widely prescribed and thought to be of minimal-to-no risk to the embryo-fetus or mother. Based on the only available trial in otherwise normal women with recurrent miscarriage, treatment with hCG is not effective.

17.5.2 Polycystic Ovarian Syndrome

A possible link between polycystic ovarian syndrome (PCOS) and recurrent miscarriage has been hypothesized. One group of investigators found ultrasonographic evidence of PCOS in 40% of recurrent miscarriage patients vs. 22% of controls [1]. It has been postulated that pregnancy loss in women with PCOS may be related to elevated serum luteinizing hormone (LH) levels, increased testosterone and androstenedione concentrations, and/or insulin resistance. However, sonographic evidence of PCOS in women with recurrent miscarriage does not predict subsequent miscarriage when compared to women with recurrent miscarriage without PCOS [1]. Also, suppression of LH in women with recurrent miscarriage and LH hypersecretion does not improve pregnancy success [53].

Some investigators have found that insulin resistance is more common in women with recurrent miscarriage compared to fertile controls regardless of whether or not they have PCOS [54]. Treatment of insulin resistance with metformin has been reported to reduce miscarriage in small studies [55]. However, well-designed trials of reasonable size are lacking. The use of metformin in pregnancy is likely safe [56], and its use in early pregnancy for women with glucose intolerance would seem reasonable.

17.5.2.1 Clinical Recommendations

Though there may be an association between recurrent miscarriage and PCOS, the diagnosis of PCOS does not alter usual care for recurrent miscarriage. Metformin may be used in pregnancy for glucose intolerance, but it is unknown as to whether or not it lessens the risk of miscarriage.

17.5.3 Glucose Intolerance and Thyroid Disease

Poorly controlled diabetes in early pregnancy has been associated with miscarriage, but well-controlled disease is not [57]. The same is true for thyroid disease [58]. Some experts, though, consider thyroid evaluation part of reasonable and comprehensive preconception care [59].

17.5.3.1 Clinical Recommendations

An otherwise healthy, non-obese woman with recurrent miscarriage does not need an evaluation for diabetes or thyroid disease as a part of her work-up. Thyroid evaluation is a reasonable part of preconception care, but subclinical thyroid disorders are not a cause of recurrent miscarriage.

17.6 Antiphospholipid Syndrome and Other Autoimmune Disorders

Antiphospholipid syndrome (APS) has been recognized as a cause of pregnancy loss in approximately 5–15% of women with recurrent miscarriage. A single prior and otherwise unexplained fetal death is also a clinical criterion for APS [60]. The diagnosis is based on the presence of either the lupus anticoagulant (LA), moderate to high levels of anticardiolipin (aCL) antibodies, or moderate-to-high levels of anti-β_2-glycoprotein I (anti-β_2-GPI) antibodies, or any combination of these. Low levels of antiphospholipid antibodies are of questionable significance and should not but used to make the diagnosis of APS. It is important to note that the diagnosis of definite APS requires positive laboratory tests (for the same antibody) on two occasions at least 12 weeks apart [60].

APS has emerged as a potentially treatable cause of recurrent miscarriage, with two studies indicating a benefit to the use of heparin in achieving successful pregnancy [61, 62]. In contrast, at least one other group of investigators found no benefit to low molecular weight heparin in women with recurrent miscarriage and APS [63].

The cause of fetal death appears to be a decidual vasculopathy that results in decidual infarction and insufficient blood flow to the placenta [64]. Intervillous thrombosis has also been described; however, these lesions are nonspecific, and the degree of pathology is not always sufficient to explain the fetal death. The mechanisms by which antiphospholipid antibodies may cause decidual vasculopathy and fetal death are unknown. A number of pathophysiologic mechanisms have been proposed, including an imbalance of local prostacyclin and thromboxane production, enhanced platelet aggregation, decreased activation of protein C, increased tissue factor, and decreased trophoblast annexin V production or availability.

Most recently, the complement system has been invoked as having a major role in APS-related pregnancy loss [65, 66]. Jane Salmon and her group at Cornell have used a murine model of APS to illustrate two critical points. First, an intact complement system is required for antiphospholipid antibody mediated pregnancy loss in the murine model. Experimental abrogation of the complement system, either by blocking C3 and C4 activation, C5 activation, or C5a-C5R interactions, salvages murine conceptuses exposed to maternally-administered antiphospholipid antibodies, even in the absence of anticoagulant treatment. Second, heparin, the widely-accepted treatment for APS to improve pregnancy outcome, likely works primarily by inhibiting complement activation rather than its anticoagulant effects. Indeed, anticoagulants that do not inhibit complement activation, such as fondaparinux and hirudin, do not block fetal loss in the murine model. Importantly, hypocomplementemia has been found in subjects with primary APS, wherein it is correlated with lupus anticoagulant activity [67].

Thus, the currently accepted mechanistic model for pregnancy complications in APS (Fig. 17.2) holds that antiphospholipid antibodies target epitopes at the maternal-fetal interface, activate complement via the classical (and perhaps lectin) pathway, cause the generation of analphylatoxins (C3a and C5a) and the mediators of effector cell actions. The local recruitment of inflammatory cells, nicely demonstrated in the murine model, is not only damaging, but also amplifies the proinflammatory cascade of events. Among other things, there is also an increase in local tissue factor production, an important pro-coagulation factor.

Maternally administered heparin, either unfractionated heparin (UF) or low molecular weight heparin (LMWH), is considered the treatment of choice for APS pregnancies, both to improve embryo-fetal outcome and protect the mother from thrombotic events (Table 17.1). Treatment regimens are usually initiated in the early first trimester after ultrasonographic demonstration of an intrauterine pregnancy. The optimal dosing regimen is debated. Some experts advocate thromboprophylactic, unadjusted, low doses of UF (e.g., 5,000–7,500 U bid.) or once daily LMWH (1 mg/kg) when treating women with APS and a history of recurrent miscarriage and other APS-related complications in the absence of prior thrombosis. However, full dose anticoagulation regimens with UF or LMWH (1 mg/kg bid.) are generally recommended for pregnant APS patients with prior thrombosis. In most case series and trials, daily low-dose aspirin is also included in the treatment regimen.

Intravenous immune globulin (IVIG) has also been used during APS pregnancy, usually in conjunction with heparin and low-dose aspirin. Two trials have demonstrated that IVIG is not beneficial with regard to pregnancy outcome in women with APS [68, 69]. Given that IVIG is expensive, requires IV administration, and appears to lack efficacy, it is not recommended by most experts [70].

Anticoagulant coverage of the postpartum period in women with APS, regardless of prior thrombosis history, is prudent. Heparin regimens may be continued or patients can be transitioned to warfarin thromboprophylaxis after delivery. In most cases, an international normalized ratio of 2.5–3.0 is desirable, and postpartum coverage should extend for 6–8 weeks after delivery. Both heparin and warfarin are safe for nursing mothers. The need for postpartum anticoagulation in women with primary APS diagnosed solely on the basis of recurrent preembryonic and embryonic losses is unclear.

Autoantibodies to thyroid antigens are associated with a modest increased rate of pregnancy loss [71] and have been

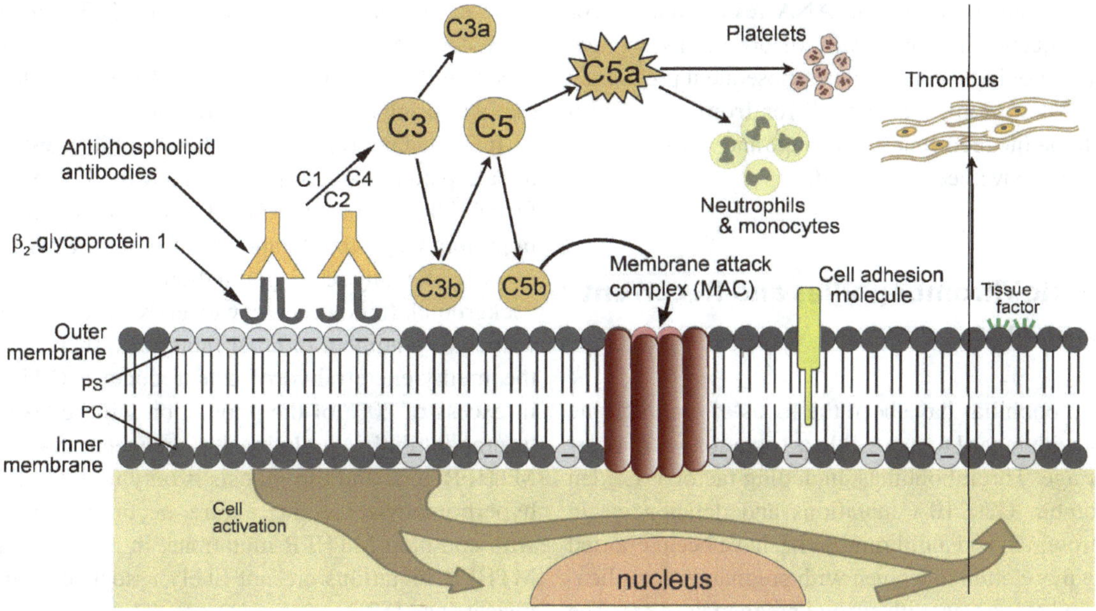

Fig. 17.2 Proposed mechanism for the pathogenic effects of antiphospholipid antibodies on tissue injury. Antiphospholipid antibodies bind to trophoblast or other cell membranes in conjunction with β2-glycoprotein I. Cell activation results in the expression of tissue factor, promoting local thombosis, and cell adhesion molecules, promoting proinflammatory interactions with the local environment. The binding of the antiphospholipid antibodies also initiates the complement cascade; C3 and subsequently, C5 are activated. C3b complexes cleave C5 into C5a and C5b. C5b complexes with C6, C7, C8, and C9 to form the membrane attack complex (MAC), which initiates cell lysis. C5a attracts and activates neutrophils, monocytes, and platelets via specific C5a receptors, and stimulates the release of inflammatory mediators, including reactive oxidants, proteolytic enzymes, chemokines, cytokines, and complement factors. This results in further influx of inflammatory cells and ultimately fetal injury. Depending on the extent of damage, either death in utero or fetal growth restriction ensues

Table 17.1 Subcutaneous heparin regimens used in the treatment of antiphospholipid syndrome during pregnancy

Prophylactic regimens
Recommended in women with no history of thrombotic events – diagnosis because of recurrent preembryonic and embryonic loss or prior fetal death or early delivery because of severe preeclampsia or severe placental insufficiency
Standard heparin
(1) 7,500–10,000 U every 12 h in the first trimester, 10,000 U every 12 h in the second and third trimesters
Low molecular weight heparin
(1) Enoxaparin 40 mg once daily or dalteparin 5,000 U once daily *or* enoxaparin 30 mg every 12 h or dalteparin 5,000 U every 12 h
Anticoagulation regimens
Recommended in women with a history of thrombotic event
Standard heparin
(1) Every 8–12 h adjusted to maintain the midinterval heparin levels[a] in the therapeutic range
Low molecular weight heparin
(1) Weight adjusted (e.g., enoxaparin 1 mg/kg every 12 h or dalteparin 200 U/kg every 12 h)

[a]Heparin levels = anti-factor Xa levels. Women without a lupus anticoagulant in whom the activated partial thromboplastin time is normal can be observed using the activated partial thromboplastin time

detected in a statistically significant proportion of women with recurrent miscarriage in some studies, but not all [72]. In one large, prospective study, pregnancy outcomes of untreated, euthyroid women with antithyroid antibodies and a history or recurrent miscarriage did not differ from those of women with recurrent miscarriage and no antithyroid antibodies [73]. Whether or not treatment improves pregnancy outcome in the euthyroid woman with antithryoid antibodies and recurrent miscarriage is uncertain because of methodological flaws in existing treatment studies [74].

A modest proportion of otherwise healthy women with recurrent miscarriage test positive for antinuclear antibodies (ANA) [75, 76]. However, subsequent pregnancy outcomes among women with a positive ANA test result are no different than those among women with a negative ANA test result. Moreover, a randomized treatment trial of women with recurrent miscarriage and a positive ANA found no benefit to treatment with prednisone and low-dose aspirin compared to treatment with placebo [76].

17.6.1 Clinical Recommendations

Women with otherwise unexplained recurrent pre-embryonic or embryonic miscarriage or one or more otherwise unexplained fetal deaths are diagnosed with APS if they have repeatedly positive antiphospholipid antibody results (at least 12 weeks apart). Such patients should be treated in subsequent pregnancies with an accepted heparin regimen (Table 17.1).

Positive thyroid autoantibody and ANA results may occur with higher frequency in women with recurrent miscarriage, but treatment is not indicated, because subsequent pregnancy outcomes in such women do not differ from those with otherwise idiopathic recurrent miscarriage and no evidenced-based treatments have been identified.

17.7 Genetic Thrombophilias and Recurrent Miscarriage

Genetic thrombophilias have been the focus of considerable recent study with regard to a possible association with recurrent miscarriage. Thrombophilias, including factor V Leiden and prothrombin G20210A mutations and deficiencies in protein C, protein S, and antithrombin III, have been reported significantly more often in women with pregnancy complications compared to women with normal pregnancies [77]. The factor V Leiden (FVL) and prothrombin G20210A mutations are the most common recognized inherited thrombophilias, present in approximately 7% and 3%, respectively, of the general Caucasian population in the United States. Some [78–80], but not all [81, 82], analyses have found an association between inherited thrombophilic disorders and recurrent early miscarriage, and the matter largely remains unsettled. A meta-analysis found a very weak, though statistically significant, odds ratios of approximately 2.0 favoring an association between recurrent miscarriage and factor V Leiden and prothrombin G20210A mutations [83]. The authors of this analysis make the cogent point that for a single gene disorder such as hemochromatosis odds ratios typically exceed 1,000! Moreover, a recent observational trial of women with inherited thrombophilias found that the presence of a thrombophilia was actually *protective* against early miscarriage in a subsequent pregnancy, likely secondary to prior adverse obstetric events and increased surveillance [84].

Though the relationship between FVL and recurrent early miscarriage is debated, some investigators have linked activated protein C resistance (APCR) to recurrent miscarriage [85, 86]. To be sure, FVL is the most common cause of APCR. However, one group has found other single nucleotide polymorphisms in the B domain of the factor V gene in a statistically significant proportion of women with non-FVL APCR and recurrent miscarriage. The investigators have hypothesized that two of these polymorphisms might be important modulators of a dysfunctional protein C anticoagulant pathway at the placental surface [87].

In contrast to recurrent early miscarriage, many authorities find the association of genetic thrombophilias with fetal loss is somewhat more compelling [88–90]; although, some controversy still exists. A recent metaanalysis found the association between late fetal death and the various genetic thrombophilias to be in the range of odds ratios of 1.5–3.5 or to have very large confidence intervals [83]. A multicenter, population-based study of fetal death after 20 weeks gestation is very likely to bring clarity to this area [91].

Informed interpretation of thombophilias testing is critical to safe patient care. Taken together, the Leiden mutation of factor V, the prothrombin G20210A mutation, and deficiencies in protein C, protein S, and antithrombin III will be found in 5–10% of many U.S. populations, depending upon racial background. If, however, one extends "thrombophilia" testing to include a number of other mutations, such as mutations in the methylenetetrahydrofolate reductase (MTHFR) gene, in excess of 20% of the population will be "positive" for a thrombophilia! A relationship between mutations in the MTHFR gene and thrombosis is only found in the setting of hyperhomocysteinemia, a rare occurrence in individuals with common MTHFR mutations. In addition, the common MTHFR mutations are not likely associated with recurrent miscarriage [82].

The high prevalence of inherited thrombophilias in women with obstetric complications has led to the use of prophylactic anticoagulation during pregnancy. One study of women with a single prior fetal death >10 weeks gestation and either FVL, prothrombin G20210A, or protein S deficiency found a benefit to treatment with low molecular weight heparin in pregnancy [92]. For the more common problem of recurrent early miscarriage, no well-designed and implemented treatment trials of anticoagulants exist.

17.7.1 Clinical Recommendations

Given the highly controversial nature of an association between recurrent early miscarriage and many genetic thrombophilias, and the complete lack of treatment trials in this population, evaluations of women with recurrent early miscarriage for genetic thrombophilias cannot be recommended. Until randomized controlled trials have been performed, prophylactic anticoagulation should be reserved for selected women with thrombophilia (e.g., those with a prior thrombotic event or with a strong family history of thrombosis) and recurrent early miscarriage after an informed discussion of the risks and limited data suggesting benefit.

17.8 Alloimmunity, Pregnancy, and Miscarriage

Few areas of medicine have generated as much controversy among experts as that of alleged alloimmune-mediated miscarriage, and a complete discussion of this area is beyond the scope of this review. The initial key concepts of reproductive (allo)immunology were (1) the embryo-fetus is a semi-allograft in so much as it bears paternal immunogenetic traits inherently foreign to the mother, (2) the semi-allogeneic fetal tissues live in intimate contact with maternal tissues, and (3) the inclination toward an adverse immunologic interaction between the conceptus and the mother must be abrogated, or at least very highly regulated, to allow for successful pregnancy. The field has undergone several major revisions and changes in focus over the last half century. Suffice it to say that normal reproductive immunology is now considered that of a unique immunologic interplay, with a partially unique cast of characters, at the maternal-fetal interface and an appropriate balance in immunoregulatory factors so as to favor, and even promote, implantation and embryo-fetal survival.

The field of reproductive alloimmunology and its possible relationship to recurrent miscarriage continues to draw interest. Some investigators propound a possible association between HLA class II alleles and unexplained recurrent miscarriage. One group has found that the frequencies of the HLA-DRB1*01 and -DRB1*03 allogenotypes are significantly increased among patients with at least four miscarriages [93]. In a prospective study of recurrent miscarriage patients, those with these allogenotypes had a higher miscarriage rate in their next pregnancy compared with other patients [94]. In addition, female relatives of recurrent miscarriage patients had a significantly higher risk of miscarriage if they had a HLA-DRB1*01 or -DRB1*03 allogenotype compared with corresponding women without these types [95]. This group has emphasized the possible role of epistatic interaction of HLA polymorphisms located in the same region, including HLA-DRB and HLA-G genes [96].

A particularly interesting set of investigations has been done by Ober and colleagues in a unique population of Hutterites in South Dakota. This population has only a small number of independent genomes represented and is one of the most genetically hemogenous populations of European origin. In studying over 1,000 Hutterites and performing high-resolution HLA haplotyping at 16 loci, these investigators found increased fetal loss rates among couples matching for the entire 16-locus haplotype and for those matching at the HLA-B locus or the flanking loci HLA-C and C4 [97]. Studies of the live born children of these couples indicate that conceptuses whose paternally inherited allele matched the mother's non-inherited allele were more likely to be miscarried. Thus, conceptuses that are HLA-genetically identical to the mother may be at a disadvantage in early pregnancy. Two critical points deserve emphasis. First, none of the Hutterite couples studied had three or more consecutive miscarriages – recurrent miscarriage is infrequent in this inbred population. Second, all of the Hutterite couples with three or more non-consecutive miscarriages also had children.

Given its likely importance in reproduction, some investigators have focused on HLA-G, a non-classical HLA gene expressed in extravillous cytotrophoblast. One study evaluated seven HLA-G polymorphisms defining 12 alleles in over 100 women with recurrent miscarriage being followed through a subsequent pregnancy [98]. The investigators found that the presence of the HLA-G *0104 or HLA-G*0105 alleles in either partner were associated with an increased risk of miscarriage in the study pregnancy. The alleles are due to polymorphisms in the a-2 domain of the HLA-G1 gene. The association between the HLA-G*0105 allele and miscarriage is confirmed in a study of German population [99]. The same group of investigators used clinical data and laboratory samples from a longitudinal study of the Hutterites to show that the presence of the −725C/G allele in both partners was associated with an increased risk of miscarriage in couples without recurrent miscarriage [100]. This allele is hypothesized to alter the binding of the transcription factor IRF-1 and the polymorphisms responsible for these alleles might downregulate HLA-G expression. However, in an immunohistochemistry study of products of conception taken from women with idiopathic recurrent miscarriage suffering another miscarriage failed to detect quantitative differences in HLA-G immunostaining when compared to women suffering trisomy 16 miscarriages or undergoing elective termination of pregnancy [101].

A Danish group first found that HLA-G alleles without a recognized 14 bp sequence (14 bp deletion) in exon 8 were prominent in the male partners of women with RM and that these women were more likely to have this same sequence present, especially as homozygotes [102]. Another group, studying Indian women with RM, found no difference in the frequency of this alleleic deletion/insertion [103], while a study of Chinese women with recurrent miscarriage found that women with recurrent miscarriage were more likely to be −14 bp/+14 bp heterozygotes [104].

Another area of interest is natural killer (NK) cells, lymphocytes of the innate immune system, which may be found in the peripheral blood and the endometrium-decidua. The populations of cells in these two environments are somewhat different, however, with the former characterized as $CD56^{dim}/CD16^{+}$ and the latter mostly $CD56^{bright}/CD16^{-}$. They are of interest in particular because the uterine NK cells are the predominant leukocyte population in the luteal phase endometrium and are particularly rich in the decidua basalis underlying the placenta. They remain present in high numbers during early pregnancy and decline after the mid-second trimester. The relationship between uterine NK cells and the population of NK cells in the peripheral circulation remains unclear.

Though their exact role in pregnancy has yet to be defined, investigators have found that the percentage, activity, or both of peripheral blood NK cells is higher among women with recurrent miscarriages or who suffer subsequent miscarriage [105–108]. However, the significance of this finding remains unclear for several reasons. First, there are potential variations and methodological flaws in the assays used, possible variations in how the samples were taken, processed or stored, and inadequate accounting for known confounding variables, including time of day and patient status with regard to activity level or recent illness. As far as the percentage of peripheral cells that should be NK cells, the threshold suggested as a meaningful cutoff by some (>12%) [106] is seemingly arbitrary and falls well within the range of normal.

A more important and truly fundamental issue is that there is no genuinely proven treatment for women with recurrent miscarriage and an "abnormal" peripheral NK cell percentage or activity level. As much as anything else, this fact renders the determination of peripheral NK cell percentages or activity meaningless. Intravenous immune globulin (IVIG), which has been proposed as a treatment in women with recurrent miscarriage and "abnormal" peripheral NK cells parameters, is not recommended outside of a research protocol by either the American College of Obstetricians and Gynecologists or the American Society of Reproductive Medicine.

Investigations into the role of uterine NK cells in normal and abnormal pregnancy may be more promising. These cells are fundamentally different than peripheral blood NK cells in that they demonstrate weak lytic activity against traditional experimental target cells and express a different cytokine profile [109]. Some [110–113], but not all [114, 115], studies of luteal phase endometrium have found either a higher proportion of $CD56^+$ or $CD16^+$ cells in women with a history of recurrent pregnancy loss. Certainly a change in uterine NK cell phenotype could be important, and two studies found a greater proportion of the cells of the $CD16^+CD56^{dim}$ phenotype in recurrent abortion patients. One group showed that oral prednisone taken in the first 21 days of the menstrual cycle reduced endometrial NK cells in women with recurrent miscarriage [116]. Such treatment has not, however, been shown to impact pregnancy outcome. In addition, a recent study that confirmed that the percentage of uterine NK cells (CD56+) was higher in women with idiopathic recurrent miscarriage also noted that the uterine NK cell numbers did not correlate with subsequent pregnancy outcome [113].

A pathologic role for alloimmunology in pregnancy failure remains confusing. The area is clearly extremely complex, and adequate human studies assessing the early pregnancy maternal-fetal interface are very difficult to perform. The area also has attracted a number of vehement "reproductive immunology" proponents who routinely advise immunologic treatments as if they were as well-accepted by mainstream medicine as immunosupression for transplantation. This practice has created something of a maelstrom of debate among miscarriage experts. In fact, properly-designed trials for most of the proposed therapies (e.g., intravenous immune globulin) are simply lacking. Existing systematic analyses also conclude that no immunomodulatory therapy is beneficial [117]. The one treatment for which adequate trials are available is leukocyte immunization. Taken together, these trials indicate either no benefit [117, 118]. Based largely on the findings of the largest and only multicenter trial [118], the U.S. Food and Drug Administration has stated that the administration of leukocyte immunotherapy may only be done as part of a clinical investigation, and then only if there is an investigational new drug application in effect.

17.8.1 Clinical Recommendations

However intriguing the immunology of HLA molecules and NK cells might be with regard to human reproduction, the field is currently confined to research because (1) existing immunologic tests are either controversial or fail to provide substantive clinical decision making distinctions, or (2) there is no "immunotherapy" known to be beneficial in promoting improved pregnancy outcome. Thus, no (allo)immunologic tests or treatments can be recommended for women with recurrent miscarriage.

17.9 Idiopathic Recurrent Miscarriage

Depending upon one's willingness to accept some "traditional" diagnoses, such as luteal phase insufficiency, at least 50% of couples with recurrent miscarriage, and perhaps more, have an idiopathic condition. As mentioned earlier, some experts have recently called for considering these cases as multifactorial in nature [11].

It should go without saying that if no definitive cause of recurrent miscarriage is found, no treatment can be recommended. It is imperative for physicians to recognize that the prognosis for idiopathic recurrent early miscarriage is by no means dismal. Numerous studies and several meta-analyses indicate that the average next pregnancy live-birth rate for placebo-treated women with idiopathic recurrent miscarriage is 60–70%. Note that these studies involved women in the early to mid 30s and with typically three to four miscarriages. Not surprisingly, the figures are less favorable for older women and for women with more miscarriages, and somewhat better for younger women and women with fewer miscarriages, e.g., only two consecutive miscarriages.

Many couples see this modestly favorable prognosis in a positive light, and it compares favorably with the prognosis for conditions, such as APS or parental karyotype abnormalities. Understanding this prognosis may allow the couple to choose against an expensive, unproven "treatment."

Importantly, the prognosis for subsequent pregnancies in women with a history of recurrent late miscarriage (fetal death) is less salutary when compared to the prognosis for women with recurrent early miscarriage. In one retrospective case series, fewer that 25% of subsequent pregnancies in women with a mean of two prior fetal losses <20 weeks gestation resulted in live birth [119].

17.9.1 Clinical Recommendations

Most couples with recurrent miscarriage will be found to have idiopathic recurrent miscarriage. Those with idiopathic recurrent early miscarriage have a relatively favorable prognosis that the practitioner should be prepared to discuss with the couple. Those couples with recurrent late miscarriage face a less favorable prognosis and should be so informed.

17.10 Recommendations for Practice in Recurrent Miscarriage

The scheme for a reasonable and cost-effective evaluation of women with RM shown in Table 17.2 is based on current guidelines published by the American College of Obstetricians and Gynecologists and the Royal College of Obstetricians and Gynaecologists. A sympathetic attitude by the physician is crucial – establishment of trust and rapport and a sincere appreciation of the distress and grief experienced by these couples permit tactful and thorough discussions with patient and partner. It is reasonable to institute an evaluation after two consecutive miscarriages in anxious women or if the patient has few reproductive years remaining or has had an infertility problem. Couples interested in an investigational protocol perhaps are best served by referral to a legitimate research center.

Table 17.2 Suggested evaluation of patients with recurrent miscarriage

History
Determine pattern and trimester of pregnancy losses and whether a live fetus was present; clues suggestive of autoimmune disease; unusual exposure to environmental toxins, drugs, infections; previous gynecologic disorders or surgery, including dilation and curettage; and previous diagnostic tests and treatments.
Physical
Abnormalities on pelvic examination, including findings suggesting abnormal cervix, diethylstilbestrol exposure, or uterine anomalies.
Tests
Lupus anticoagulant, anticardiolipin antibodies, and anti-β_2-glycoprotein I antibodies
Parental chromosome analyses (father and mother)
Uterine cavity and shape evaluation by sonohysterography, hysterosalpingography, hysteroscopy, MRI or other studies
Chromosome analysis of products of conception
Other laboratory tests if suggested by history and physical examination or personal or family history

References

1. Rai R, Regan L (2006) Recurrent miscarriage. Lancet 368(9535): 601–611
2. Hustin J, Schaaps JP (1987) Echographic [corrected] and anatomic studies of the maternotrophoblastic border during the first trimester of pregnancy. Am J Obstet Gynecol 157(1):162–168
3. Jauniaux E, Hempstock J, Greenwold N, Burton GJ (2003) Trophoblastic oxidative stress in relation to temporal and regional differences in maternal placental blood flow in normal and abnormal early pregnancies. Am J Pathol 162(1):115–125
4. Burton GJ, Watson AL, Hempstock J, Skepper JN, Jauniaux E (2002) Uterine glands provide histiotrophic nutrition for the uman fetus during the first trimester of pregnancy. J Clin Endocrinol Metab 87:2954–2959
5. Jauniaux E, Watson AL, Hempstock J, Bao YP, Skepper JN, Burton GJ (2000) Onset of maternal arterial blood flow and placental oxidative stress. A possible factor in human early pregnancy failure. Am J Pathol 157(6):2111–2122
6. Copp AJ (1995) Death before birth: clues from gene knockouts and mutations. Trends Genet 11(3):87–93
7. Shepard TH, Fantel AG, Fitzsimmons J (1989) Congenital defect rates among spontaneous abortuses: twenty years of monitoring. Teratology 39(4):325–331
8. Nybo Andersen AM, Wohlfahrt J, Christens P, Olsen J, Melbye M (2000) Maternal age and fetal loss: population based register linkage study. BMJ 320(7251):1708–1712
9. Stein Z, Kline J, Susser E (1980) Maternal age and spontaneous abortion. In: Porter I, Hook E (eds) Human embryonic and fetal death. Academic, New York
10. Harlap S, Shiono P, Ramcharan S (1980) A life table of spontaneous abortions and the effects of age, parity, and other variables. In: Porter I, Hook E (eds) Human embronic and fetal death. Academic, New York, p 145
11. Christiansen OB, Steffensen R, Nielsen HS, Varming K (2008) Multifactorial etiology of recurrent miscarriage and its scientific and clinical implications. Gynecol Obstet Invest 66(4):257–267
12. Kleinhaus K, Perrin M, Friedlander Y, Paltiel O, Malaspina D, Harlap S (2006) Paternal age and spontaneous abortion. Obstet Gynecol 108(2):369–377

12a. Mishra GD, Dobson AJ, Schofield MJ (2000) Cigarette smoking, menstrual symptoms and miscarriage among young women. Aust N Z J Public Health 24(4):413–420

13. Henriksen TB, Hjollund NH, Jensen TK et al (2004) Alcohol consumption at the time of conception and spontaneous abortion. Am J Epidemiol 160(7):661–667
14. Weng X, Odouli R (2008) Li DK (2008) Maternal caffeine consumption during pregnancy and the risk of miscarriage: a prospective cohort study. Am J Obstet Gynecol 198(3):279 e1–8
15. Maconochie N, Doyle P, Prior S, Simmons R (2007) Risk factors for first trimester miscarriage – results from a UK-population-based case–control study. BJOG 114:170–186
16. Henderson J, Gray R, Brocklehurst P (2007) Systematic review of effects of low-moderate prenatal alcohol exposure on pregnancy outcome. BJOG 114(3):243–252
17. George L, Granath F, Johansson AL, Olander B, Cnattingius S (2006) Risks of repeated miscarriage. Paediatr Perinat Epidemiol 20(2):119–126

18. Hemels ME, Einarson A, Koren G, Lanctot KL, Einarson TR (2005) Antidepressant use during pregnancy and the rates of spontaneous abortions: a meta-analysis. Ann Pharmacother 39(5): 803–809
19. The ESHRE Capri Workshop Group (2006) Nutrition and reproduction in women. Hum Reprod Update 12(3):193–207
20. Stephenson MD, Awartani KA, Robinson WP (2002) Cytogenetic analysis of miscarriages from couples with recurrent miscarriage: a case–control study. Hum Reprod 17(2):446–451
21. Stern JJ, Dorfmann AD, Gutierrez-Najar AJ, Cerrillo M, Coulam CB (1996) Frequency of abnormal karyotypes among abortuses from women with and without a history of recurrent spontaneous abortion. Fertil Steril 65(2):250–253
22. Vidal F, Gimenez C, Rubio C et al (1998) FISH preimplantation diagnosis of chromosome aneuploidy in recurrent pregnancy wastage. J Assist Reprod Genet 15(5):310–313
23. Simon C, Rubio C, Vidal F et al (1998) Increased chromosome abnormalities in human preimplantation embryos after in-vitro fertilization in patients with recurrent miscarriage. Reprod Fertil Dev 10(1):87–92
24. Sullivan AE, Silver RM, LaCoursiere DY, Porter TF, Branch DW (2004) Recurrent fetal aneuploidy and recurrent miscarriage. Obstet Gynecol 104(4):784–788
25. Ogasawara M, Aoki K, Okada S, Suzumori K (2000) Embryonic karyotype of abortuses in relation to the number of previous miscarriages. Fertil Steril 73(2):300–304
26. Carp H, Toder V, Aviram A, Daniely M, Mashiach S, Barkai G (2001) Karyotype of the abortus in recurrent miscarriage. Fertil Steril 75(4):678–682
27. De Braekeleer M, Dao TN (1990) Cytogenetic studies in couples experiencing repeated pregnancy losses. Hum Reprod 5(5):519–528
28. Clifford K, Rai R, Watson H, Regan L (1994) An informative protocol for the investigation of recurrent miscarriage: preliminary experience of 500 consecutive cases. Hum Reprod 9(7):1328–1332
29. Carp H, Feldman B, Oelsner G, Schiff E (2004) Parental karyotype and subsequent live births in recurrent miscarriage. Fertil Steril 81(5):1296–1301
30. Gynecologists ACoOa (2001) Management of recurrent early pregnancy loss. ACOG Practice Bulletin No 24
31. Gynaecologists RCoOa (2003) The investigation and treatment of women with recurrent miscarriage. TCOG Guideline No 17
32. Pegoraro E, Whitaker J, Mowery-Rushton P, Surti U, Lanasa M, Hoffman EP (1997) Familial skewed X inactivation: a molecular trait associated with high spontaneous-abortion rate maps to Xq28. Am J Hum Genet 61(1):160–170
33. Lanasa MC, Hogge WA, Kubik C, Blancato J, Hoffman EP (1999) Highly skewed X-chromosome inactivation is associated with idiopathic recurrent spontaneous abortion. Am J Hum Genet 65(1): 252–254
34. Sullivan AE, Lewis T, Stephenson M et al (2003) Pregnancy outcome in recurrent miscarriage patients with skewed X chromosome inactivation. Obstet Gynecol 101(6):1236–1242
35. Hogge WA, Prosen TL, Lanasa MC, Huber HA, Reeves MF (2007) Recurrent spontaneous abortion and skewed X-inactivation: is there an association? Am J Obstet Gynecol 196(4):384 e1–6; discussion e6–8
36. Kaare M, Painter J, Ulander V-M, Kaaja R, Aittomaoki K (2008) Sex chromosome characteristics and recurrent miscarriage. Fertil Steril 90:2328–2333
37. Salim R, Regan L, Woelfer B, Backos M, Jurkovic D (2003) A comparative study of the morphology of congenital uterine anomalies in women with and without a history of recurrent first trimester miscarriage. Hum Reprod 18(1):162–166
38. Woelfer B, Salim R, Banerjee S, Elson J, Regan L, Jurkovic D (2001) Reproductive outcomes in women with congenital uterine anomalies detected by three-dimensional ultrasound screening. Obstet Gynecol 98(6):1099–1103
39. Du H, Taylor HS (2004) Molecular regulation of mullerian development by Hox genes. Ann N Y Acad Sci 1034:152–165
40. Wong KH, Wintch HD, Capecchi MR (2004) Hoxa11 regulates stromal cell death and proliferation during neonatal uterine development. Mol Endocrinol 18(1):184–193
41. Kupesic S, Kurjak A (1998) Septate uterus: detection and prediction of obstetrical complications by different forms of ultrasonography. J Ultrasound Med 17(10):631–636
42. Heinonen PK (1997) Reproductive performance of women with uterine anomalies after abdominal or hysteroscopic metroplasty or no surgical treatment. J Am Assoc Gynecol Laparosc 4(3):311–317
43. Valli E, Vaquero E, Lazzarin N, Caserta D, Marconi D, Zupi E (2004) Hysteroscopic metroplasty improves gestational outcome in women with recurrent spontaneous abortion. J Am Assoc Gynecol Laparosc 11(2):240–244
44. Stovall DW, Parrish SB, Van Voorhis BJ, Hahn SJ, Sparks AE, Syrop CH (1998) Uterine leiomyomas reduce the efficacy of assisted reproduction cycles: results of a matched follow-up study. Hum Reprod 13(1):192–197
45. Hart R, Khalaf Y, Yeong CT, Seed P, Taylor A, Braude P (2001) A prospective controlled study of the effect of intramural uterine fibroids on the outcome of assisted conception. Hum Reprod 16(11):2411–2417
46. Klatsky PC, Tran ND, Caughey AB, Fujimoto VY (2008) Fibroids and reproductive outcomes: a systematic literature review from conception to delivery. Am J Obstet Gynecol 198(4):357–366
47. Duggan MA, Brashert P, Ostor A et al (2001) The accuracy and interobserver reproducibility of endometrial dating. Pathology 33(3):292–297
48. Ogasawara M, Kajiura S, Katano K, Aoyama T, Aoki K (1997) Are serum progesterone levels predictive of recurrent miscarriage in future pregnancies? Fertil Steril 68(5):806–809
49. Usadi RS, Groll JM, Lessey BA et al (2008) Endometrial development and function in experimentally induced luteal phase deficiency. J Clin Endocrinol Metab 93(10):4058–4064
50. Karamardian L, Grimes D (1994) Luteal phase deficiency: effect of treatment on pregnancy rates. Am J Obstet Gynecol 170:958–959
51. Walch K, Hefler L, Nagele F (2005) Oral dydrogesterone treatment during the first trimester of pregnancy: the prevention of miscarriage study (PROMIS). A double-blind, prospectively randomized, placebo-controlled, parallel group trial. J Matern Fetal Neonatal Med 18(4):265–269
52. Harrison RF (1992) Human chorionic gonadotrophin (hCG) in the management of recurrent abortion; results of a multi-centre placebo-controlled study. Eur J Obstet Gynecol Reprod Biol 47(3): 175–179
53. Clifford K, Rai R, Watson H, Franks S, Regan L (1996) Does suppressing luteinising hormone secretion reduce the miscarriage rate? Results of a randomised controlled trial. BMJ 312(7045): 1508–1511
54. Craig LB, Ke RW, Kutteh WH (2002) Increased prevalence of insulin resistance in women with a history of recurrent pregnancy loss. Fertil Steril 78(3):487–490
55. Zolghadri J, Tavana Z, Kazerooni T, Soveid M, Taghieh M (2008) Relationship between abnormal glucose tolerance test and history of previous recurrent miscarriages, and beneficial effect of metformin in these patients: a prospective clinical study. Fertil Steril 90(3):727–730
56. Rowan JA, Hague WM, Gao W, Battin MR, Moore MP (2008) Metformin versus insulin for the treatment of gestational diabetes. N Engl J Med 358(19):2003–2015
57. Mills JL, Simpson JL, Driscoll SG et al (1988) Incidence of spontaneous abortion among normal women and insulin-dependent diabetic women whose pregnancies were identified within 21 days of conception. N Engl J Med 319(25):1617–1623
58. Abalovich M, Gutierrez S, Alcaraz G, Maccallini G, Garcia A, Levalle O (2002) Overt and subclinical hypothyroidism complicating pregnancy. Thyroid 12(1):63–68

59. Christiansen OB, Nybo Andersen AM, Bosch E et al (2005) Evidence-based investigations and treatments of recurrent pregnancy loss. Fertil Steril 83(4):821–839
60. Miyakis S, Lockshin MD, Atsumi T et al (2006) International consensus statement on an update of the classification criteria for definite antiphospholipid syndrome (APS). J Thromb Haemost 4(2):295–306
61. Rai R, Cohen H, Dave M, Regan L (1997) Randomised controlled trial of aspirin and aspirin plus heparin in pregnant women with recurrent miscarriage associated with phospholipid antibodies (or antiphospholipid antibodies). BMJ 314(7076):253–257
62. Kutteh WH (1996) Antiphospholipid antibody-associated recurrent pregnancy loss: treatment with heparin and low-dose aspirin is superior to low-dose aspirin alone. Am J Obstet Gynecol 174(5): 1584–1589
63. Farquharson RG, Quenby S, Greaves M (2002) Antiphospholipid syndrome in pregnancy: a randomized, controlled trial of treatment. Obstet Gynecol 100(3):408–413
64. Branch DW, Khamashta MA (2003) Antiphospholipid syndrome: obstetric diagnosis, management, and controversies. Obstet Gynecol 101(6):1333–1344
65. Holers VM, Girardi G, Mo L et al (2002) Complement C3 activation is required for antiphospholipid antibody-induced fetal loss. J Exp Med 195(2):211–220
66. Salmon JE, Girardi G, Theodore E (2007) Woodward Award: antiphospholipid syndrome revisited: a disorder initiated by inflammation. Trans Am Clin Climatol Assoc 118:99–114
67. Oku K, Atsumi T, Bohgaki M et al (2009) Complement activation in patients with primary antiphospholipid syndrome. Ann Rheum Dis 68:1030–1035
68. Branch DW, Peaceman AM, Druzin M et al (2000) A multicenter, placebo-controlled pilot study of intravenous immune globulin treatment of antiphospholipid syndrome during pregnancy. The Pregnancy Loss Study Group. Am J Obstet Gynecol 182(1 Pt 1):122–127
69. Triolo G, Ferrante A, Ciccia F et al (2003) Randomized study of subcutaneous low molecular weight heparin plus aspirin versus intravenous immunoglobulin in the treatment of recurrent fetal loss associated with antiphospholipid antibodies. Arthritis Rheum 48(3):728–731
70. Wisloff F, Crowther M (2004) Evidence-based treatment of the antiphospholipid syndrome: I. Pregnancy failure. Thromb Res 114(2):75–81
71. Stagnaro-Green A, Roman SH, Cobin RH, el-Harazy E, Alvarez-Marfany M, Davies TF (1990) Detection of at-risk pregnancy by means of highly sensitive assays for thyroid autoantibodies. JAMA 264(11):1422–1425
72. Esplin MS, Branch DW, Silver R, Stagnaro-Green A (1998) Thyroid autoantibodies are not associated with recurrent pregnancy loss. Am J Obstet Gynecol 179(6 Pt 1):1583–1586
73. Rushworth FH, Backos M, Rai R, Chilcott IT, Baxter N, Regan L (2000) Prospective pregnancy outcome in untreated recurrent miscarriers with thyroid autoantibodies. Hum Reprod 15(7): 1637–1639
74. Abramson J, Stagnaro-Green A (2001) Thyroid antibodies and fetal loss: an evolving story. Thyroid 11(1):57–63
75. Ogasawara M, Aoki K, Katano K, Aoyama T, Kajiura S, Suzumori K (1999) Prevalence of autoantibodies in patients with recurrent miscarriages. Am J Reprod Immunol 41(1):86–90
76. Laskin CA, Bombardier C, Hannah ME et al (1997) Prednisone and aspirin in women with autoantibodies and unexplained recurrent fetal loss. N Engl J Med 337(3):148–153
77. Lockwood CJ (2002) Inherited thrombophilias in pregnant patients: detection and treatment paradigm. Obstet Gynecol 99(2):333–341
78. Brenner B, Mandel H, Lanir N et al (1997) Activated protein C resistance can be associated with recurrent fetal loss. Br J Haematol 97(3):551–554
79. Ridker PM, Miletich JP, Buring JE et al (1998) Factor V Leiden mutation as a risk factor for recurrent pregnancy loss. Ann Intern Med 128(12 Pt 1):1000–1003
80. Foka ZJ, Lambropoulos AF, Saravelos H et al (2000) Factor V leiden and prothrombin G20210A mutations, but not methylenetetrahydrofolate reductase C677T, are associated with recurrent miscarriages. Hum Reprod 15(2):458–462
81. Kutteh WH, Park VM, Deitcher SR (1999) Hypercoagulable state mutation analysis in white patients with early first-trimester recurrent pregnancy loss. Fertil Steril 71(6):1048–1053
82. Pauer HU, Neesen J, Hinney B (1998) Factor V Leiden and its relevance in patients with recurrent abortions. Am J Obstet Gynecol 178(3):629
83. Rodger MA, Paidas M, Claire M et al (2008) Inherited thrombophilia and pregnancy complications revisited. Obstet Gynecol 112(2 Pt 1):320–324
84. Roque H, Paidas MJ, Funai EF, Kuczynski E, Lockwood CJ (2004) Maternal thrombophilias are not associated with early pregnancy loss. Thromb Haemost 91(2):290–295
85. Sarig G, Younis JS, Hoffman R, Lanir N, Blumenfeld Z, Brenner B (2002) Thrombophilia is common in women with idiopathic pregnancy loss and is associated with late pregnancy wastage. Fertil Steril 77(2):342–347
86. Rai R, Shlebak A, Cohen H et al (2001) Factor V Leiden and acquired activated protein C resistance among 1000 women with recurrent miscarriage. Hum Reprod 16(5):961–965
87. Dawood F, Mountford R, Farquharson R, Quenby S (2007) Genetic polymorphisms on the factor V gene in women with recurrent miscarriage and acquired APCR. Hum Reprod 22(9):2546–2553
88. Rai R, Regan L, Hadley E, Dave M, Cohen H (1996) Second-trimester pregnancy loss is associated with activated C resistance. Br J Haematol 92(2):489–490
89. Gris JC, Quere I, Monpeyroux F et al (1999) Case–control study of the frequency of thrombophilic disorders in couples with late foetal loss and no thrombotic antecedent – the Nimes Obstetricians and Haematologists Study5 (NOHA5). Thromb Haemost 81(6): 891–899
90. Martinelli I, Taioli E, Cetin I et al (2000) Mutations in coagulation factors in women with unexplained late fetal loss. N Engl J Med 343(14):1015–1018
91. SCRN. Research on the scope and causes of stillbirth in the United States
92. Gris JC, Mercier E, Quere I et al (2004) Low-molecular-weight heparin versus low-dose aspirin in women with one fetal loss and a constitutional thrombophilic disorder. Blood 103(10): 3695–3699
93. Christiansen OB, Rasmussen KL, Jersild C, Grunnet N (1994) HLA class II alleles confer susceptibility to recurrent fetal losses in Danish women. Tissue Antigens 44(4):225–233
94. Christiansen OB, Mathiesen O, Husth M, Lauritsen JG, Jersild C, Grunnet N (1993) Prognostic significance of maternal DR histocompatibility types in Danish women with recurrent miscarriages. Hum Reprod 8(11):1843–1847
95. Christiansen OB, Andersen HH, Hojbjerre M, Kruse TA, Lauritzen SL, Grunnet N (1995) Maternal HLA class II allogenotypes are markers for the predisposition to fetal losses in families of women with unexplained recurrent fetal loss. Eur J Immunogenet 22(4):323–334
96. Hviid TV, Christiansen OB (2005) Linkage disequilibrium between human leukocyte antigen (HLA) class II and HLA-G-possible implications for human reproduction and autoimmune disease. Hum Immunol 66(6):688–699
97. Ober C (1999) Studies of HLA, fertility and mate choice in a human isolate. Hum Reprod Update 5(2):103–107
98. Aldrich CL, Stephenson MD, Karrison T et al (2001) HLA-G genotypes and pregnancy outcome in couples with unexplained recurrent miscarriage. Mol Hum Reprod 7(12):1167–1172

99. Pfeiffer KA, Fimmers R, Engels G, van der Ven H, van der Ven K (2001) The HLA-G genotype is potentially associated with idiopathic recurrent spontaneous abortion. Mol Hum Reprod 7(4):373–378
100. Ober C, Aldrich CL, Chervoneva I et al (2003) Variation in the HLA-G promoter region influences miscarriage rates. Am J Hum Genet 72(6):1425–1435
101. Patel RN, Quack KC, Hill JA, Schust DJ (2003) Expression of membrane-bound HLA-G at the maternal-fetal interface is not associated with pregnancy maintenance among patients with idiopathic recurrent pregnancy loss. Mol Hum Reprod 9(9):551–557
102. Hviid TV, Hylenius S, Hoegh AM, Kruse C, Christiansen OB (2002) HLA-G polymorphisms in couples with recurrent spontaneous abortions. Tissue Antigens 60(2):122–132
103. Tripathi P, Abbas A, Naik S, Agrawal S (2004) Role of 14-bp deletion in the HLA-G gene in the maintenance of pregnancy. Tissue Antigens 64(6):706–710
104. Xue S, Yang J, Yao F, Xu L, Fan L (2007) Recurrent spontaneous abortions patients have more -14 bp/+14 bp heterozygotes in the 3'UT region of the HLA-G gene in a Chinese Han population. Tissue Antigens 69(Suppl. 1):153–155
105. Aoki K, Kajiura S, Matsumoto Y et al (1995) Preconceptional natural-killer-cell activity as a predictor of miscarriage. Lancet 345(8961):1340–1342
106. Beer AE, Kwak JY, Ruiz JE (1996) Immunophenotypic profiles of peripheral blood lymphocytes in women with recurrent pregnancy losses and in infertile women with multiple failed in vitro fertilization cycles. Am J Reprod Immunol 35(4):376–382
107. Yamada H, Morikawa M, Kato EH, Shimada S, Kobashi G, Minakami H (2003) Pre-conceptional natural killer cell activity and percentage as predictors of biochemical pregnancy and spontaneous abortion with normal chromosome karyotype. Am J Reprod Immunol 50(4):351–354
108. Emmer PM, Nelen WL, Steegers EA, Hendriks JC, Veerhoek M, Joosten I (2000) Peripheral natural killer cytotoxicity and CD56(pos)CD16(pos) cells increase during early pregnancy in women with a history of recurrent spontaneous abortion. Hum Reprod 15(5):1163–1169
109. Dosiou C, Giudice LC (2005) Natural killer cells in pregnancy and recurrent pregnancy loss: endocrine and immunologic perspectives. Endocr Rev 26(1):44–62
110. Lachapelle MH, Miron P, Hemmings R, Roy DC (1996) Endometrial T, B, and NK cells in patients with recurrent spontaneous abortion. Altered profile and pregnancy outcome. J Immunol 156(10):4027–4034
111. Quenby S, Bates M, Doig T et al (1999) Pre-implantation endometrial leukocytes in women with recurrent miscarriage. Hum Reprod 14(9):2386–2391
112. Clifford K, Flanagan AM, Regan L (1999) Endometrial CD56+ natural killer cells in women with recurrent miscarriage: a histomorphometric study. Hum Reprod 14(11):2727–2730
113. Tuckerman E, Laird S, Prakash A, Li T (2008) Prognostic value of the measurement of uterine natural killer cells in the endometrium of women with recurrent miscarriage. Hum Reprod 22: 2208–2213
114. Michimata T, Ogasawara MS, Tsuda H et al (2002) Distributions of endometrial NK cells, B cells, T cells, and Th2/Tc2 cells fail to predict pregnancy outcome following recurrent abortion. Am J Reprod Immunol 47(4):196–202
115. Shimada S, Kato EH, Morikawa M et al (2004) No difference in natural killer or natural killer T-cell population, but aberrant T-helper cell population in the endometrium of women with repeated miscarriage. Hum Reprod 19(4):1018–1024
116. Quenby S, Kalumbi C, Bates M, Farquharson R, Vince G (2005) Prednisolone reduces preconceptual endometrial natural killer cells in women with recurrent miscarriage. Fertil Steril 84(4): 980–984
117. Porter TF, LaCoursiere Y, Scott JR (2006) Immunotherapy for recurrent miscarriage. Cochrane Database Syst Rev (2):CD000112
118. Ober C, Karrison T, Odem RR et al (1999) Mononuclear-cell immunisation in prevention of recurrent miscarriages: a randomised trial. Lancet 354(9176):365–369
119. Frias AE Jr, Luikenaar RA, Sullivan AE et al (2004) Poor obstetric outcome in subsequent pregnancies in women with prior fetal death. Obstet Gynecol 104(3):521–526

Chapter 18
Laparoscopy in the Diagnosis and Treatment of Female Infertility

Howard T. Sharp and Johnny Yi

Abstract Phillip Bozzini is credited with the first description of endoscopy in 1805, as he attempted to view the urethral mucosa with a simple tube and candlelight. Pantaleoni used a cystoscope to identify uterine polyps in 1869, thus accomplishing the first hysteroscopy. Jacobaeus of Sweden performed the first laparoscopy in 1910, when he placed a Neitze cystoscope and used a candle to illuminate a hollow tube placed into the peritoneal cavity. Eventually, Semm of Germany reported advanced operative laparoscopic procedures, such as salpingectomy, myomectomy, oophorectomy, ovarian cystectomy, and salpingostomy, in the 1970s. These pioneers of endoscopic surgery and many others have forged the way for the rest of us who now routinely perform endoscopic surgery. This chapter is to review safe and effective techniques and principles of laparoscopic surgery.

Keywords Laparoscopy • Video • Insufflations • Digital camera • Light source, camera • Fiber optic • Trocars • Optical-access trocars • Uterine manipulators • Chromotubation • Suture • Laparoscopic knots • Laparoscopic suturing • Extracorporeal knots • Intracorporeal knots • Staplers • Vascular clips • Laser • Harmonic scalpel • Electrosurgery • Monopolar • Bipolar, fulguration • Current density • Capacitative coupling • Wattage • Voltage • Nerve injury • Neuropathy • Veres needle • Hasson method • Direct trocar entry • Palmer's point • Ninth intercostal space • Inferior epigastric artery • External iliac artery • Morcellator • Adhesiolysis • Retroperitoneal space • Posterior cul de sac • Oophorectomy • Salpingo-oophorectomy • Myomectomy • Conscious sedation

H.T. Sharp (✉) and J. Yi
Division of General Gynecology, Department of Obstetrics and Gynecology, University of Utah School of Medicine, 30 N. Medical Drive, 2B200, Salt Lake City, UT, USA
e-mail: howard.sharp@hsc.utah.edu

18.1 Indications for Laparoscopy

18.1.1 Diagnostic Laparoscopy

Diagnostic laparoscopy can aid in the evaluation of patients with infertility and acute or chronic pelvic and abdominal pain including ovarian torsion, ovarian cyst rupture, ectopic pregnancy, appendicitis, pelvic inflammatory disease, pelvic adhesions, endometriosis, hernias, uterine fibroids, and adnexal masses.

18.1.2 Operative Laparoscopy

Diagnostic laparoscopy is now routinely performed in conjunction with operative laparoscopy such as adhesiolysis, treatment of endometriosis, tubal sterilation, ovarian cystectomy, oophorectomy, salpingectomy, salpingostomy, and hysterectomy. More advanced procedures include repair of pelvic organ prolapse, tubal reanastamosis, myomectomy, radical hysterectomy, and lymphadenectomy.

18.2 Equipment

Contemporary laparoscopy equipment consists of an imaging system comprised of a telescope and video camera system, an insufflation or abdominal wall lift system, and specialized surgical instruments. Robotics is an area that continues to evolve.

18.2.1 Imaging Systems

Imaging systems are designed to recreate the intrapelvic/abdominal contents onto a monitor. To make this happen, a telescope, light source, fiber optic cord, a camera unit, and monitor

D.T. Carrell and C.M. Peterson (eds.), *Reproductive Endocrinology and Infertility: Integrating Modern Clinical and Laboratory Practice*,
DOI 10.1007/978-1-4419-1436-1_18,

are used. High-definition digital cameras (1,920×1,080p) are now available that are compatible with the increased resolution capabilities of high-definition flat screen 26 in. wireless monitors. Newer minimally invasive suites have become much less cumbersome by having ceiling mounted adjustable monitors, rather than stackable monitors or rolling carts. Most new cameras allow the surgeon the ability to command the light source through programmable buttons on the camera head itself. Imaging systems are also equipped with a printer, video recorder, or DVD recorder for documentation.

Laparoscopes range from 1.8 mm to 12 cm in diameter with a distal end (objective) available in varying viewing angles. The 0° deflection angle telescope is most commonly used for gynecologic laparoscopy, and it provides a straightforward view whereas a 30° foreoblique lens allows for visualization in a large frontal view. To stay oriented with a foreoblique lens, the angle must be continuously directed to maintain field orientation.

Light sources use powerful halogen, and now more commonly 300 W xenon bulbs to introduce light through a fiber optic cable to the laparoscope. It is important that the light source have sufficient power to deliver adequate light through the fiber optic cable. The fiber optic cable transmits enough heat to burn paper drapes as well as patient's skin; therefore, caution should be taken to avoid inadvertent contact with drapes or the patient. Most cameras will allow the surgeon to place the light on stand-by mode, which will not get hot enough to cause a burn.

The camera unit consists of the camera head, cable, and camera control. The camera head attaches to the eyepiece of the laparoscope and captures images transmitted by the laparoscope. The basis of laparoscopic cameras is the solid-state silicon computer chip or charge-coupled device (CCD). This is comprised of silicon elements, which emit an electric charge when exposed to light. Each silicon element contributes one pixel unit to the image produced. The image resolution is dependent upon the number of pixels on the chip. Camera–laparoscopes complexes are now available as a combined unit, which are fully autoclavable. Three chip CCDs provide better image clarity but are more expensive as they have a separate chip for each primary color opposed to the single-chip CCD.

18.2.2 Insufflation

Insufflation systems include a Veres needle, filtered tubing, an insufflator, and gas tanks. They are designed to fill the abdominopelvic cavity with gas, usually carbon dioxide, to optimize visualization. Gas is delivered at a low rates during initial Veres needle insertion, but it must also be able to be delivered at high flow rates when gas is lost to maintain a relatively constant intraabdominal pressure during surgery. Tubing with a 0.3 micron filter is recommended to prevent intraperitoneal contamination. The Veres needle is often used to create a pneumoperitoneum. However, insufflation may be performed with other methods of abdominal wall entry such as direct trocar insertion, open laparoscopy (Hasson Method), or with optical-access trocars.

The Veres needle is available in two lengths, 120 and 150 mm, based on patient size. Reusable and disposable models are available, which contain a spring loaded tip that retracts as it pierces the abdominal wall, to avoid damaging bowel or other intraabdominal organs and allowing a blunt tip to engage on entry to the peritoneal cavity.

The most commonly used gas is carbon dioxide. It has the advantage of being the most rapidly absorbed by blood. However, it is converted to carbonic acid on moist peritoneal surface, which can cause pain. Consequently, some physicians prefer nitrous oxide or helium, especially during cases using local anesthesia or conscious sedation. Heated or hydrated gas may be used to prevent hypothermia during laparoscopy. There are alternatives to gas insufflation wherein systems comprising of a mechanical lifting arm that attaches to a fan-like retractor along the peritoneal surface of the abdominal wall. Some surgeons favor this approach in patients with cardiopulmonary risk factors.

18.2.3 Surgical Instrumentation

Laparoscopic surgical instruments are placed into the abdomen and pelvis through trocar sleeves. Trocar sleeves range from 2 to 15 mm in diameter, and are available as reusable or disposable systems. Disposable systems offer the advantage of consistent sharpness, but are more expensive. Reusable trocars are cost efficient, but must be maintained. Most trocar sleeves contain a Luer-lock port that attaches to insufflation tubing. Optical-access trocars (Optiview and Visiport) consist of a trocar/sleeve/laparoscope complex that enables the surgeon to visualize the layers of the abdominal wall during placement. Expandable trocar sheaths are available that are initially placed through the abdominal wall with a Veres needle and then expanded to accept a 5–12 mm port.

A variety of surgical instruments may be placed through secondary trocar sleeves including blunt probes, graspers (toothed and atraumatic), scissors, needle drivers, knot pushers, biopsy forceps, suction-irrigators, energy delivery tools, specimen retrieval bags, and tissue morcellators.

18.2.4 Uterine Manipulators

Uterine manipulators may be used to improve access to the uterus, fallopian tubes, ovaries, and the posterior and anterior cul-de-sacs. Reusable and disposable models are available. Some manipulators are inserted in a fixed position are allow limited uterine mobility while others are hinged and allow the uterus to be moved anteriorly, posteriorly, or laterally. Many are constructed as a catheter to allow chromotubation during the laparoscopic procedure to confirm fallopian tube patency.

18.2.5 Laparoscopic Applications of Energy

As laparoscopy has moved from diagnosis to treatment, the application of energy systems has been critical to allow surgeon to perform complex procedures with the ability to divide tissue and maintain hemostasis. Energy adapted for laparoscopic use includes electrosurgical, laser, vibrational, and mechanical systems.

18.2.6 Mechanical Energy

Endomechanical energy can be used for tissue division and hemostasis in a number of ways including suturing, stapling, and the application of vascular clips.

18.2.6.1 Suture

The laparoscopic use of suture may range from the use of pretied loops, which function as a slip knot on a push rod that is tightened around a tissue pedicle for hemostasis, to laparoscopic suturing performed with stock suture, ideally 36–48 inches in length. Laparoscopic needle drivers are available with a standard tip or with self-righting tips. Laparoscopic knots may be tied outside the laparoscopic port (extracorporeal) or within the body (intracorporeal). Extracorporeal knots are performed as sliding square knots, pushed through the trocar sleeve to the tissue by multiple passes of a knot-pusher, which serves as the surgeon's finger. Intracorporeal knots are tied within the abdomen by looping the suture material around the laparoscopic needle holders. An alternative to extracorporeal and intracorporeal knot tying is the use of the LapraTy (Ethicon). The LapraTy is used as an absorbable clip fastened taut against the tissue as it is clipped to the suture. The endostitch (US Surgical) is a device designed to obviate the use of laparoscopic needle drivers. With this device, the needle is preloaded and the suture is passed through tissue up to 2 cm thick by closing a handle and a toggle switch. The endostitch is a 10 mm instrument with jaws measuring 4 mm wide and 2 cm long.

18.2.6.2 Staplers

The endo-GIA is a stapling device for dividing tissue and laying down a staple line for hemostasis. The jaws of the instrument are closed over tissue for dividing. When the grip is fired, six staggered rows of staples 3 cm in length and 1 cm in width are placed. A knife blade simultaneously divides the tissue leaving three rows of staples on each side.

18.2.6.3 Vascular Clips

Endoscopic vascular titanium clips may be compressed over bleeding vessels or pedicles for hemostasis. These can be used near vital structures without the risk of lateral thermal damage.

18.2.6.4 Laser

Light amplification by spontaneous emission of radiation or laser was one of the early forms of laparoscopic energy. Surgical lasers available for gynecologic use include: CO_2, argon, potassium-titanyl-phosphate (KTP), and neodymium:yttrium-aluminum-garnet (Nd-YAG). They have the ability to vaporize, cut, and to varying degrees, coagulate tissue. With advances in electrosurgical energy, laser is not used with the same frequency of decades ago. If laser is to be used, most surgeons are required to undergo periodic laser safety training for each wavelength used.

18.2.6.5 Harmonic Scalpel

The harmonic scalpel (Ethicon Endosurgery) uses vibrational energy at the rate of 55,000 cycles per second to break hydrogen bonds in tissue resulting in cutting or coaptation of vessels. The harmonic scalpel is available as a 5 mm rounded "scalpel" with a blunt or hooked edge or as a 5–10 mm endoshear or harmonic ace, which can be used to grasp tissue.

18.2.6.6 Electrosurgery

Monopolar and bipolar electrosurgical instruments are frequently used in operative laparoscopy. Monopolar instruments deliver current that flows from an active electrode, through tissue, having a therapeutic effect and traveling through the patient, exiting by way of return electrode plate (usually on the patients thigh) to the electrosurgical unit. Examples of such instruments are needlepoint electrodes, L-hooks, and most endoscopic scissors. Bipolar instruments work in a very different manner, delivering current that flows from an active electrode, through tissue having a therapeutic effect, and then returning through a return electrode within the same instrument to the electrosurgical unit. Because current does not travel through the patient, a return electrode plate is not needed. The Kleppinger forceps often used in fallopian tube fulguration is an example of a bipolar instrument. Bipolar instruments have evolved significantly in recent years into devices that provide bipolar energy, which sense tissue impedance to perform controlled energy delivery. These devices, such as LigaSure (Covidien, Boulder CO), PlasmaKinetic (Gyrus ACMI, Maple Grove, MN), and EnSeal (SurgRx, Inc, Palo Alto, CA), use pressure and pulsed current to seal vessels with minimal lateral thermal spread. They use smart generator technology that integrates impedance (tissue resistance) feedback from a surgical device delivery. These devices can seal vessels up to 7 mm in diameter.

Current density refers to the amount of current flow per cross-sectional area and has several direct applications to electrosurgical energy in laparoscopy. This principle is used to safely return current from the patient to the electrosurgical unit (ESU). Applying energy per meters squared to a small area of bleeding or to a bleeding tissue pedicle will result in a measured thermal effect, inversely related to the electrode size. A needlepoint electrode will have a high current density compared to a much larger spatula tip, resulting in greater energy applied to a small surface. The current density principle also applies to current as it exits the body. Because it exits through the relatively large surface area of the return electrode, it does not cause an exit site burn due to low current density. Exit site burns have typically occurred when part of the return electrode has peeled away from the patient, resulting in a smaller area of surface contact, thus creating high current density at the exit site.

18.2.7 Basic Electrosurgical Principles

To safely use common household electricity during surgery, it must be transformed from a frequency of 60 Hz to a radiofrequency range, between 500,000 and 4,000,000 Hz. This is necessary because nerve and muscle tissue can be stimulated at frequencies below 10,000 Hz. To accomplish this, a transformer is used. The basic waveform of radiofrequency current is called continuous, cutting, or undamped if it is not altered. Cutting waveform utilizes low voltage current. Cutting current causes cells to vaporize at their boiling point (100°C) without elevating tissue temperatures to high levels, thus minimizing lateral thermal spread. This waveform can be altered by interrupting or dampening it to varying degrees. These alterations are called to blend 1 (80% on, 20% off), blend 2 (60% on, 40% off), blend 3 (50% on, 50% off), and coagulation (6% on, 94% off). As a result of current interruption (coagulation), bursts of energy with higher voltage (5,000 V) and lower current, given a constant wattage (Watts = Voltage × Current), will occur, resulting in hemostasis through denaturation and charring (fulguration).

Fulguration (coagulation mode) is best used when there is surface oozing to achieve enough superficial lateral thermal spread to cause hemostasis. Cutting current is best used in the case of a bleeding vessel or pedicle that can be desiccated by applying pressure with a tissue grasper and allowing the fibrous bonding of the dehydrated endothelium cells without significant lateral thermal spread. When the coagulation waveform is used in this scenario, rather than achieving bonding inside the vessel, superficial lateral thermal spread is more likely and eschar formation may occur on the tissue surface resulting in subsequent bleeding.

18.2.8 Glossary of Electrosurgical Terms

Ampere (A) – the rate at which current flows

Voltage (V) – electric potential expressed in volts

Ohm (Ω) – tissue resistance to current

Watt (W) – the amount of work produced or work done at a rate of one joule per second

Current (I) – electron flow measured in coulombs per second or the steady current produced by one volt applied across the resistance of one ohm

Power (P) – work per unit time

Hertz (Hz) – a unit of frequency in cycles per second

Cautery – searing through the application of a heated element

Cutting Current – (continuous or undamped current) – continuous high-frequency, low-voltage flow of current from one peak of polarity to the opposite peak without pausing at the zero polarity

Coagulating Current – (interrupted or damped current) – bursts of rapidly increasing current interrupted at intervals such that peak polarity alternated with zero polarity

Fulguration – coagulation of surface bleeding through spraying long electrical sparks

Vaporization – exploding cells at their boiling point (100°C) as a result of applied energy

Desiccation – coagulation of targeted vessels through the process of dehydration

Radiofrequency – a term given to the current frequency of electrosurgery because it is found within the AM radio frequency range (500,000–4,00,000 Hz)

Unipolar system (also monopolar) – current that flows from an active electrode, through tissue having a cutting or coagulating effect, and traveling through the patient, exiting by way of return electrode plate, usually on the patient's thigh, to the electrosurgical unit

Bipolar System – current that flows from an active electrode, through tissue having a cutting or coagulating effect, and returning through a return electrode within the same instrument directly back to the electrosurgical unit, without the need for a return electrode plate on the patient

Capacitive Coupling – transference of electrical energy from an insulated active electrode to nearby conductive material

Current Density – the amount of current flow per cross-sectional area normal to the direction of current flow described in amps per meters squared

Formulae

Energy = Wattage × Time

Watts = Voltage × Current

18.3 Patient Positioning

The proper positioning of the patient is an important aspect of successful for two reasons: access and safety. To optimize access, the patient should be placed on the operating table in the low lithotomy position with the buttocks at or slightly over the table's edge to allow placement and use of an intrauterine manipulator and to have access to the perineum during surgery. The patient's thighs should be in the same plane as the abdomen to allow freedom of motion for laparoscopic instrumentation, particularly if any work is needed to be performed in the upper abdomen. Stirrups should have adequate padding to support the lower leg without creating pressure points.

Most nerve injuries occurring during laparoscopic surgery due to stretching or compression resolve within six weeks. Femoral neuropathy occurring during laparoscopy can be associated with excessive hip flexion, abduction, or long operating times [1]. When lithotomy positioning is used in patients undergoing vaginal or laparoscopic surgery, the thigh should be flexed no greater than 90° and abducted no greater than 45°. If a patient's position is changed intraoperatively from low lithotomy to high lithotomy, these relationships should be maintained.

Sciatic neuropathy during laparoscopic surgery can be caused by nerve stretching. Injury to the sciatic nerve has been reported in procedures lasting as short as 35 min in free-hanging (candy cane) stirrups [2]. Patients at increased risk of sustaining sciatic nerve injury are long-legged, obese, or short in stature. In hanging-type stirrups, long-legged or obese patients have a tendency for external hip rotation and shorter patients have less flexion at the knee. In such patients, Allen-type stirrups that support the ankle and calf may be more appropriate.

18.4 Entering the Abdominal Cavity

Laparoscopic abdominal entry has inherent risk. In most cases, it is performed safely and routinely. The most common site of initial entry is the umbilicus. Initial entry may be performed with a Veres needle, wherein a pneumoperitoneum is created for subsequent trocar placement, by direct trocar placement, or by using the Hasson method (open trocar method) where the layers of the abdominal wall and ultimately the parietal peritoneum are entered with scissors under direct visualization. Optical-access trocars are also available that may allow the surgeon to visualize the layers of the abdominal wall laparoscopically as the trocar/laparoscope complex is being inserted. Optical-access trocars can be used after insufflation with a Veres needle or may be placed directly without pneumoperitoneum. Alternative sites to umbilical entry include the left upper quadrant (Palmer's point and 9th intercostal space), the posterior vaginal fornix, and the transuterine approach, all of which may be used primarily or may be used selectively in difficult cases.

18.4.1 Umbilical Site Veres Needle Technique

To perform the Veres needle umbilical technique, a scalpel is initially used to make a small umbilical skin incision depending on the size of trocar to be used. The umbilicus should be elevated to avoid incidentally lacerating the great vessels, which lie in close proximity to the umbilicus, particularly in thin patients. Naso-gastric suctioning will decrease the risk of inserting the Veres needle or trocar into an over-distended stomach. The patient's abdomen should be relaxed phamacologically by neural blockade if general anesthesia is being used. This allows adequate elevation of the abdominal wall for Veres needle and trocar insertion. The patient should be lying in a flat or neutral position on the operating table. Trendelenburg positioning is not recommended as it may cause the angle of the Veres needle or trocar to be closer to the great vessels rather than the pelvic cavity. In the thin patient, the Veres needle or trocar should be directed toward the hollow of the sacrum to avoid the great vessels, whereas in the obese patient, the aorta is typically above the level of the umbilicus and therefore, the Veres needle or trocar may be inserted vertically (90° to the long axis of the patient). The use of towel clamps deep in the umbilicus, or Kocher clamps on the rectus fascia may aid in properly placing the Veres needle. Separate clicks can be heard or felt as the needle traverses the rectus fascia and then peritoneum.

Correct Veres needle placement within the abdominal cavity can be assessed by several methods. The hanging drop technique is performed by placing a small amount of sterile saline in the top of the Veres needle to verify a negative intraabdominal pressure as it decends into the abdominal cavity. The syringe barrel test is performed by watching the column of saline decend the barrel of a syringe attached to the Veres needle. Low-flow insufflation should be performed at a flow rate of approximately 1–2 l/min, until further signs of intraabdominal needle placement are confirmed such as low intra-abdominal pressure (<10 mmHg) or loss of dullness to percussion over the right upper quadrant. A prospective observational study of four tests in 345 women showed that high insufflation pressures were the most sensitive for preperitoneal insufflation [3]. During insufflation, intraabdominal pressures should not exceed 20–25 mmHg to avoid interfering with diaphragmatic excursion and central venous return from caval compression. After an adequate pneumoperitoneum has been established, which may range from 1 to 5 l depending on body habitus, a trocar is inserted at the umbilicus paying attention to the angle of insertion based upon body habitus.

18.4.2 Open Laparoscopy

Hasson described the technique of open laparoscopy in 1971 as a way of avoiding blind trocar placement. A small incision is made at the umbilicus, and Allis clamps are used to grasp the rectus fascia, which is then incised. The peritoneum is tented and entered directly. A Hasson-type cannula is anchored by sutures to the rectus fascia. In a review of over 5,000 cases over nearly three decades, this technique has been shown to be associated with a low complication rate [4].

18.4.3 Direct Trocar Insertion

Direct trocar placement has also been described by placing the trocar through the umbilicus initially rather than using the Veres needle. A review of 51 pulications comparing open laparoscopy (Hasson method) and closed methods pointed out that deaths were only reported in the needle/trocar group rather than the open group [5]. However, the rarity of the outcome meant that the statistical risk could not be compared meaningfully. The meta-analysis was underpowered to adequately compare all techniques. Therefore, the question of which technique for initial port placement is safest has not been definitively answered to date.

18.4.4 Left Upper Quadrant Entry

There are two commonly used methods for gaining laparoscopic access at the left upper quadrant: Palmer's point, and the ninth intercostal space. In 1974, Raoul Palmer, a French gynecologist, described using a point located 3 cm below the left costal margin in the mid-clavicular line for laparoscopic access [6]. This is referred to as "Palmer's Point" by many surgeons. The advantage of this site for initial abdominal wall entry is the relative unlikelihood of encountering adhesions. The organs closest to this insertion site are the left lobe of the liver, spleen, transverse colon, and the stomach. Therefore, ascites, hepatomegaly, and splenomegaly are considered relative contraindications to using this technique.

To use Palmer's point for initial abdominal wall entry, the stomach should be emptied by suction and the LUQ should be palpated to exclude splenomegaly. While tenting the abdominal skin, the Veres needle is placed into the peritoneal cavity at a point 3 cm below the costal margin at the mid-clavicular line, aiming at a 45° angle from horizontal. Typically three pops are heard or felt to indicate intraperitoneal placement. Insufflation pressures of less than 10 mmHg indicate correct intraperitoneal placement. After insufflation, a 5 mm trocar is placed in a similar fashion. Alternatively, a 5 mm trocar can be placed directly, and insufflation may be carried out after intraperitoneal placement is confirmed visually.

The ninth intercostal space is often used when considering the left upper quadrant for Veres placement. With this technique, the anterior axillary line is used for reference. The Veres needle is inserted close to the upper margin of the 10th rib to avoid the neurovascular bundle that travels at the inferior margin of the 9th rib. The Veres needle is inserted at a right angle to the skin, or 45° to the horizontal between the ninth and tenth ribs. Once insufflation is complete, a 5 mm trocar is placed at Palmer's point.

18.4.5 Vaginal Approaches to Insufflation

The posterior cul-de-sac of Douglas has long been accessed through the posterior vaginal fornix for diagnostic and therapeutic purposes when culdocentesis and culdotomy were performed regularly. With ultrasound imaging, diagnostic culdocentesis has become less common, and many physicians today may not be familiar with this approach. To perform this technique, a tenaculum is placed on the cervix to gain access and to create a taut posterior fornix. The Veres needle is inserted at the posterior fornix, approximately 1.75 cm from the cervico-vaginal junction, through to the posterior cul-de-sac of Douglas, taking care to stay in the midline. Typically, a 150 mm Veres needle is used. The needle should not be advanced more than approximately 3 cm to avoid vascular injury. Once a pneumoperitneum is created, a standard umbilical trocar is placed through the abdominal wall. Fixed uterine retroversion and prior posterior fornix surgery are considered relative contraindications to using the posterior vaginal fornix approach. This should be confirmed by history and physical examination.

The transuterine approach to insufflation may be advantageous in obese patients and in patients with extreme abdominal wall laxity. Contraindications to this procedure include: suspected bowel adhesions to the uterus, previous myomectomy, and pelvic inflammatory disease. This technique is performed by placing the patient in moderate Trendelenburg positioning to allow the bowel to fall away from the uterus. A tenaculum is placed on the anterior lip of the cervix for traction and to straighten uterine flexion. Prior to placing the Veres needle, the uterus is sounded to determine a cavity length and to confirm uterine position. Originally, anteverting the uterus with the Veres needle was described so that the Veres needle tip is directed away from the sacral curve, rectosigmoid colon, and great vessels. The Veres needle tip is advanced through the myometrium and the snap of the spring loaded Veres needle mechanism prompts the operator that the needle has entered the peritoneal cavity. A 10 mmHg pressure reading should indicate peritoneal placement. Once a pneumoperitneum is created, a standard umbilical trocar is placed.

18.5 Secondary Trocar Placement

Two secondary ports are usually adequate for most laparoscopic procedures with more complicated surgeries requiring additional ports. Secondary trocars are typically placed lateral to the inferior epigastric artery or in the midline above the bladder. A 2 to 5 mm trocar may be used for diagnostic laparoscopy to maneuver pelvic organs for adequate visualization. Most instruments for tissue manipulation will fit through a 5 mm port. Some energy delivery systems and tissue retrieval systems require the use of larger ports (8–15 mm).

Lateral trocar placement can be associated with injury to the inferior epigastric artery. This vessel is a branch of the external iliac artery and can usually be seen along the anterior abdominal wall. To better visualize the relationship of the entry point to the inferior epigastric artery, a 22 gauge needle can be inserted through the anterior abdominal wall at the intended trocar site. If the vessel cannot be seen, a safe location can usually be found by measuring 5 cm superior to the pubic symphysis and 8 cm lateral [7]. Secondary trocars should be inserted in a controlled fashion, under direct vision. Placement of suprapubic secondary trocars should be placed well above the bladder. Two finger breadths measured above the pubic symphysis has been standard terminology for midline trocar placement. Due to the significant differences in finger widths, and considering the increased risk of bladder injury using the suprapubic location, particularly if the patient has had prior abdominal surgery, it may be worth placing a 22 gauge needle through the anterior abdominal wall in the midline to ensure the port is well above the bladder.

The iliohypogastic and ilioinguinal nerves can be injured from lateral trocar incisions with subsequent suture ligature and fibrotic entrapment. Care should be taken to avoid extreme lateral trocar placement; however, there is considerable anatomic variation in the course of these nerves, and injury cannot always be avoided.

In a retrospective review of over 3,500 laparoscopies in 1993, the frequency of incisional hernias was reported to be 0.17% [8]. It is recommended that fascia be closed in trocar , which are 10 mm and larger. Though there are case reports of hernia occurring at 5 mm trocar sites, closing 5 mm trocar sites would usually require enlarging the skin incision or using laparoscopic fascial closure devices, which may not be warranted in this rare possibility. Closing the fascia may not entirely prevent hernia formation. A survey of over 3,200 gynecologists noted that 18% of hernias occurred despite fascial closure and appeared to be related to the number of laparoscopies performed rather than the length of the surgeon's career [9].

18.6 Tissue Removal

Small tissue specimens such as peritoneal biopsies are simple to remove through 5 mm trocar sleeves. Larger ports (10–15 mm) are required to remove ovarian cysts or morcellated tissue. Plastic specimen removal bags are ideal to remove larger cystic structures such as ovarian cysts or medium sized singular solid structures (Endocatch, US Surgical Corp., Endopouch, Ethicon Inc.). Alternatively, posterior colpotomy can be performed for specimen removal. Colpotomy may be performed vaginally as one would when performing vaginal hysterectomy or it may be performed laparoscopically. Laparoscopic colpotomy is performed by first inserting a lubricated sponge stick in the posterior fornix for cul-de-sac elevation. An incision is made between the uterosacral ligaments into the vagina on top of the sponge by using laser, unipolar scissors, or harmonic scalpel. A wet lap pad placed in the vagina will minimize loss of pneumoperitoneum.

Morcellation is preferred for larger tissue specimens and is much simpler to perform with an electromechanical morcellator. Most morcellators require a larger post size of 15 mm. A tissue graper (tenaculum or claw) is placed through the operating port of the morcellator and the tissue is grasped carefully to avoid surrounding normal tissue. The specimen is then drawn up into the morcellator rather than pushing the morcellator into the specimen. For safety reasons, it is important that the tip of the morcellator be in view at all times. Keeping the cutting tip elevated adds to visualization and decreases the risk of inadvertently injuring bowel and other vital structures. Severe injuries have been reported including injury to the pancreas.

18.7 Operative Laparoscopy

18.7.1 Mechanical Adhesiolysis

Ideally, adhesiolysis should be used with microsurgical technique, gentle tissue handling, and meticulous hemostasis with minimal tissue fulguration. Adhesiolysis can be performed by a number of techniques including blunt and sharp dissection, electrodissection, aquadissection, and laser dissection.

Blunt dissection is the most rudimentary form of adhesiolysis. This technique is sometimes used in treating thin, avascular adhesions. Virtually, any type of laparoscopic instrument can be used to place traction on an adhesion to cause separation. If bleeding or significant resistance is encountered, this technique should be abandoned, and sharp or electrical dissection should be used.

Sharp dissection is preferred in cases of thicker avascular adhesions. The advantage of sharp dissection over electrodissection is the decreased risk of inadvertent electrosurgical injury. Similarly to laparotomy, the adhesion is held on tension with an atraumatic grasper, and laparoscopic scissors are used for dissection. Turning the tip of the scissors toward the optical viewing angle will aid in visualization to avoid inadvertent injury.

Aqua dissection can be used to free adhesions from the pelvic sidewall when operating close to the ureter or to the great vessels. It is also a useful technique in removing endometriotic nodules. With this technique, the peritoneum is grasped and a small incision is made such that the tip of a powered suction-irrigation device can be inserted. An irrigator is used to force fluid under the peritoneum, causing it to balloon out from deeper tissues. The tissue sample can then be dissected free as it is freed from its base.

18.7.2 Adhesiolysis Using Energy

Unipolar energy is frequently used to treat thicker vascular adhesions, using to avoid injury to bowel. As well-visualized areas are freed from adhesions, less well-visualized areas become recognizable. Unipolar instruments such as scissors, needle point electrodes, and L-hooks are ideal for adhesiolysis. Bipolar instruments such as Kleppinger forceps, bipolar scissors, or newer tissue-controlled bipolar energy instruments, which seal vessels, can also be used.

Laser dissection has been used in laparoscopy with great success due to minimal lateral thermal spread. The small spot size of laser makes this a useful tool for precision adhesiolysis. The CO_2 laser has a depth of penetration of 0.1 mm and is excellent for cutting.

The Harmonic scalpel is used with a technique similar to both bipolar dissection (laparosonic coagulating shears and harmonic ace) and unipolar dissection (scalpel tip) depending on which tip is used, although it does not use electrosurgery. These devices have the advantage of minimal lateral thermal spread, even compared to the newer bipolar electrosurgical instruments [10]. When using the harmonic ace, it works best if the tissue is not on tension. This allows the tissue to be treated before it is cut, reducing bleeding.

18.7.3 Sidewall and Retroperitoneal Space Dissection

When performing dissection of the sidewall or retroperitoneum surgery, which is often the case with endometriosis surgery, the course of the ureter is identified, along with the iliac vessels. If the ureter is able to be identified at the pelvic brim, but then is obscured by adhesions, endometriosis, or an ovarian mass along its caudad course, the peritoneum overlying the sidewall can be grasped and opened with scissors. A Maryland dissector can be used to gently spread the peritoneum to view the ureter. If the anatomy is distorted, it may be necessary to start the dissection high at the pelvic brim or by opening the round ligament. If the round ligament is to be opened, it should be divided with an energy source as lateral as possible. A blunt grasper can be used to dissect the avascular retroperitoneal space, while expecting the ureter to be located on the medial leaf of the broad ligament. Developing the pararectal space will also help to define anatomic landmarks to avoid inadvertent vascular or ureteral injury. Once the ureter, great vessels, and uterine artery are located, adhesions can be divided confidently with an energy system of choice.

18.7.4 Posterior Cul-de-sac Dissection

Cul-de-sac obliteration secondary to endometriosis often involves deep fibrotic endometriosis that may involve the rectum, rectovaginal septum, or uterosacral ligaments. Dissection of the posterior cul-de-sac may be necessary when partial or complete cul-de-sac obliteration has occurred and the patient has a surgical indication for treatment such as pain, mass, and in selected cases, infertility. Skilled surgeons can perform it laparoscopically.

Ideally, this condition is known or suspected preoperatively allowing for thorough bowel prep prior to surgery. A uterine manipulator is useful to antevert the uterus. A rectal probe may be placed in the rectum to help delineate and retract the rectum posteriorly. Placing a sponge stick in the vagina can further help delineate the rectum from the vagina.

The rectum is dissected from the posterior aspect of the uterus or vagina. Aqua dissection may also be useful. Dissection should continue until the loose areolar tissue of the rectovaginal space is reached. If a ureter is near the site of dissection, the position of the ureter should be confirmed before any dissection takes place. In some cases, ureteral stenting is helpful for ureteral identification. Fibrotic endometriosis can then be excised from the posterior vagina or uterosacral ligaments. If endometriosis extends to the vaginal mucosa, this is also excised.

18.7.5 Oophorectomy and Salpingo-oophorectomy

Before starting oophorectomy, the ureter should be identified. It can be identified by transperitoneal visualization of peristalsis or by dissection as described above. To gain access to the infundibulopelvic ligament, the ovary is grasped and held medial and toward the abdominal wall for optimal visualization. It is coagulated or sealed with bipolar energy or ultrasonic energy and transected. Alternately, a laparoscopic stapling device or suturing may be used. It may be suture ligated by creating an avascular window underneath the infundibulopelvic ligament and passing a ligature similar to laparotomy. The suture is tied with an extracorporeal knot pusher. The loose avascular tissue between the infundibulopelvic tissue and utero-ovarian tissue, as well as the utero-ovarian tissue is divided next with an energy device or with suture ligatures. Pedicles should be examined for hemostasis and the ovary is removed by one of the described methods of tissue removal. If the fallopian tube is to be removed with the ovary, the proximal fallopian tube and utero-ovarian ligament are coagulated or sealed before transection.

18.8 Laparoscopic Myomectomy

Laparoscopic myomectomy can be a simple procedure in the case of the pedunculated myoma, and range to one of the more difficult laparoscopic surgeries, requiring expert laparoscopic suturing skills. Two case–control studies comparing open to laparoscopic myomectomy, have both demonstrated significantly longer mean operating room time with the laparoscopic approach, but with significantly shorter hospital stays in the laparoscopic group [11, 12]. The use of a preoperative gonadotropin-releasing hormone agonist may be considered in patients who are anemic. A prospective randomized study using leuprolide acetate in patients undergoing laparoscopic myomectomy also demonstrated significantly lower blood loss and operative times in the treatment group [13]. Other studies have shown longer operative times and a higher conversion to laparotomy rate associated with the use of GnRH agonists in laparoscopic myomectomy because of difficult cleavage planes.

Pedunculated myomas can be resected by coagulating and transecting the base and then morcellated, or removed by posterior colpotomy. The small serosal defect is not typically sutured. It is best to avoid losing myoma pieces that become detached, as there have been reports of specimens becoming infected or continuing to grow at the trocar incision site and elsewhere in the pelvic cavity. Small lost myoma fragments are not necessarily an indication for laparotomy.

Intramural and subserosal fibroids require an incision to be made with scissors, laser, needle electrode, or harmonic scalpel. Prior to incising the uterine serosa, it is possible to inject hemostatic agents into the serosa and myoma. A dilute vasopressin solution or bupivacaine plus epinephrine may be injected transabdominally into the myometrium through a spinal needle or through a laparoscopic needle instrument. As the serosa is incised along the length of the myoma and the whorled white appearance of the myoma is seen, the edges of the uterine serosa may be held open with atraumatic graspers. A corkscrew retractor can be screwed into the myoma or a laparoscopic tenaculaum may be used for myoma traction. With upward traction, the myoma is peeled away from the uterine corpus. The myomas are removed by tissue morcellation, as described earlier. Hemostasis is achieved with electrosurgery or harmonic scalpel. The defect is sutured closed in two or three layers, depending on the depth of the defect using a delayed absorbable suture using intracorporeal or extracorporial suturing. Another option is to perform uterine closure through a minilaparotomy if the fundus or area to be sutured can be delivered through a small incision.

Uterine rupture has been reported in patients undergoing laparoscopic myomectomy and pregnancy should be monitored with the same caution given to patients who have undergone abdominal myomectomy. It is not known whether laparoscopic repairs are equivalent to repair by laparotomy.

18.9 Laparoscopy Using Local Anesthsia or Conscious Sedation

Laparoscopy is sometimes performed under conscious sedation or local anesthesia in the operating room or in a nonhospital environment such as physician's office with or without the assistance of an anesthesiologist. Local anesthesia and conscious sedation has long been used to perform tubal ligation, and more recently in performing pain mapping in selected patients with chronic pelvic pain [14]. Proper patient selection is important, as patients must be able to withstand lifting the abdomen at the umbilicus for Veres needle and trocar insertion and tolerate local infiltration at the umbilicus. If conscious sedation is to be performed in the office without the presence of an anesthesiologist, it is important to follow state guidelines for conscious sedation. The American College of Surgeons has developed guidelines that have been endorsed by The American College of Obstetricians and Gynecologists that detail requirements for resuscitation and an optimally safe environment.

The umbilicus is infiltrated at the skin and then down through the fascia with a 25-gauge needle, while elevating the umbilicus, using approximately 10 ml of 1% lidocaine or 0.25% bupivacaine. If conscious sedation is used, a short acting narcotic such as remifentanyl is ideal if pain mapping is to be performed such that the patient is awake and able to respond to nociceptive stimuli. If tubal sterilization is to be performed, an anxiolytic drug such as midazolam is useful.

18.10 Conclusion

Laparoscopy has become a common form of gynecologic surgery. Over the past few decades, it has become increasingly safe with improved technology. Due to this rapidly evolving technology, continued education and research are important. The main benefits of laparoscopic surgery are shorter hospitalization, improved cosmesis, and in some cases improved safety and cost.

References

1. Hershlag A, Loy RA, Lavy G, DeCherney AH (1990) Femoral neuropathy after laparoscopy. A case report. J Reprod Med 35(5): 575–576
2. Batres F, Barclay DL (1983) Sciatic nerve injury during gynecologic procedures using the lithotomy position. Obstet Gynecol 62(Suppl 3): 92s–94s
3. Teoh B, Sen R, Abbott J (2005) An evaluation of four tests used to ascertain Veres needle placement at closed laparoscopy. J Minim Invasive Gynecol 12(2):153–158
4. Hasson HM, Rotman C, Rana N, Kumari NA (2000) Open laparoscopy: 29-year experience. Obstet Gynecol 96(5 Pt 1):763–766
5. Malloy D, Kalloo P, Cooper M, Nguyen T (2002) Laparoscopic entry: a literature review and analysis of techniques and complications of primary port entry. Austrailian NZ J Obstet Gynecol 42(3):246–254
6. Palmer R (1974) Safety in laparoscopy. J Reprod Med 13(1):1–5
7. Hurd WW, Bude RO, DeLancey JO, Newman JS (1994) The location of abdominal wall blood vessels in relationship to abdominal landmarks apparent at laparoscopy. Am J Obstet Gynecol 171(3):642–646
8. Kadar N, Reich H, Liu CY, Manko GF, Gimpelson R (1993) Incisional hernias after major laparoscopic gynecologic procedures. Am J Obstet Gynecol 168(5):1493–1495
9. Montz FJ, Holschneider CH, Munro MG (1994) Incisional hernia following laparoscopy: a survey of the American Association of Gynecologic Laparoscopists. Obstet Gynecol 84(5):881–884
10. Lamberton GR, Hsi RS, Jin DH, Lindler TU, Jellison FC, Baldwin DD (2008) Prospective comparison of four laparoscopic vessel ligation devices. J Endourol 22(10):2307–2312
11. Stringer NH, Walker JC, Meyer PM (1997) Comparison of 49 laparoscopic myomectomies with 49 open myomectomies. J Am Assoc Gynecol Laparosc 4(4):457–464
12. Silva BA, Falcone T, Bradley L et al (2000) Case-control study of laparoscopic versus abdominal myomectomy. J Laparoendosc Adv Surg Tech 10(4):191–197
13. Zullo F, Pellicano M, De Stefano R, Zupi E, Mastrantonio P (1998) A prospective randomized study to evaluate leuprolide acetate treatment before laparoscopic myomectomy: efficacy and ultrasonographic predictors. Am J Obstet Gynecol 178(1 Pt 1):108–112
14. Palter SF, Olive DL (1996) Office microlaparoscopy under local anesthesia for chronic pelvic pain. J Am Assoc Gynecol Laparosc 3(3):359–364

Chapter 19
Turner Syndrome

Carolyn A. Bondy

Abstract Turner syndrome (TS) or monosomy X, is the most common cause of hypergonadotropic hypogonadism in girls and young women. This chapter reviews the prevalence and different presentations of the syndrome and explains its chromosomal origins. The interpretation of chromosomal studies in diagnosis of and prognosis for TS, including prenatal testing, is reviewed. The most recent data on the TS phenotypic spectrum indicate ~95% have short stature and ~95% have primary ovarian failure, most presenting with primary amenorrhea but a significant number is present with 2° amenorrhea. Recent studies indicate that dysmorphic features are less common than previously described but complex cardiovascular defects and metabolic problems including osteoporosis, thyroid dysfunction, diabetes, and dyslipidemia are more common than previously appreciated. A significant proportion of young girls may have viable ovarian follicles with 15–20% experiencing spontaneous puberty, and 3–5% may achieve natural pregnancy. Spontaneous and assisted pregnancies with donated oocytes are associated with serious maternal complications, including eclampsia, diabetes, and catastrophic aortic dissections in women with TS. Thus, all TS women contemplating pregnancy need thorough medical and especially cardiologic evaluations and counseling as to the risks involved. Protocols for the physiologic induction of puberty and for the maintenance of feminization and prevention of osteoporosis in adults are described. The experience of premature ovarian failure and infertility leads to impaired psychosocial and sexual functioning in many women with TS. More attention focused on the psychological aspects of premature ovarian failure may help them cope with the diagnosis in a more positive manner.

Keywords X chromosome • Ovarian failure • Primary amenorrhea • Pubertal induction • Hormone replacement therapy • Osteoporosis

C.A. Bondy (✉)
NIH, CRC 1-3330, 10 Center Drive, Bethesda, MD 20892, USA
e-mail: bondyc@mail.nih.govqa

19.1 Introduction

Turner syndrome (TS) is caused by the absence of all or significant parts of one sex chromosome in all or most somatic cells. It is the most common genetic disease of females, affecting ~1/2,000 live-born girls, as revealed by karyotypic screening of nearly 50,000 newborns. However, the number of clinically diagnosed cases is only about half that expected from these birth data [1]. Moreover, most individuals are not diagnosed until teenage years or later (Fig. 19.1). Under diagnosis is a serious problem because cardiac and metabolic defects associated with the syndrome cause morbidity and premature mortality if not properly treated. Moreover, effective hormonal treatment and psychosocial adjustment made possible with timely diagnoses greatly improve the quality of life for girls and women with TS. Until very recently, TS was viewed primarily as a pediatric disorder with medical attention focused mainly on the use of recombinant human growth hormone (GH) to increase adult height. National health registries in Great Britain and European countries provide quality epidemiological data and the ongoing National Institutes of Health (NIH) prospective genotype-phenotype study provides high quality data on genetic, physical, physiological, and psychological aspects of TS. A recent consensus conference reviewed all published and registry data to formulate updated guidelines for diagnosis, medical screening, and treatment of girls and women with TS [2]. The present chapter is based upon these sources. While young girls with TS are getting excellent care from the pediatric endocrine specialists, they seem to fall off the radar when they "graduate" from pediatric clinic. The care of adults with TS is currently far from optimal [3]. Not only do they not get the recommended medical care, but also some general practitioners have advised these young women to stop their estrogen treatment because of the publicity surrounding the Women's Health Initiative studies [4]. It would probably be best if these women receive primary care from the reproductive endocrinologist. They present a host of medically interesting problems and are generally a well informed, cooperative and rewarding group of patients.

D.T. Carrell and C.M. Peterson (eds.), *Reproductive Endocrinology and Infertility: Integrating Modern Clinical and Laboratory Practice*,
DOI 10.1007/978-1-4419-1436-1_19, © Springer Science+Business Media, LLC 2010

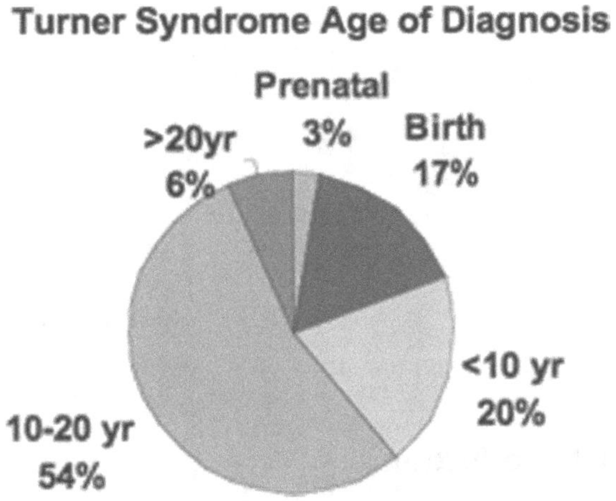

Fig. 19.1 Age at TS diagnosis for 290 girls and women aged 7–67 participating in the NIH study between 2001 and 2007. The large number diagnosed at birth was detected mainly because of persistent lymphedema or neck webbing, in some cases associated with clinically obvious congenital heart disease. Girls diagnosed in childhood up to age ten were mainly on the basis of short stature. Note that 60% were diagnosed as teens or adults, mainly because of amenorrhea

19.2 Diagnosis

19.2.1 Diagnostic Criteria

The diagnosis of TS requires both sex chromosomal abnormalities and physical features of TS, most commonly short stature and/or premature ovarian failure, in a phenotypic female [2]. The current standard for chromosomal diagnosis is the metaphase karyotype analysis of at least 30 peripheral lymphocytes. This is a time-consuming, labor intensive, and expensive test that requires cells that can divide in vitro and is limited therefore mainly to fresh lymphocytes. Comparative genomic hybridization using chromosome microarrays is likely to preempt karyotype analyses in screening for sex chromosome anomalies [5], with the karyotype reserved for confirmatory testing (Fig. 19.2). While most patients with TS have >50% abnormal cells on their karyotype, there is no specific percentage of cells that must be abnormal for the diagnosis, because a full-blown phenotype with short stature and ovarian failure may be found in a patient with less than 50% of abnormal cells on a 30-cell peripheral karyotype. This may occur because of tissue mosaicism, in which some tissues may be predominantly 45,X cells while the lymphocyte karyotype representing only a single cell lineage, may not reflect other tissues (Fig. 19.3). However, normal aging is associated with sex chromosome loss in lymphocytes [6], so normal women in their 40s may have a couple of 45,X cells on a peripheral blood karyotype without having TS. The converse situation may occur when a female presents with many typical features of TS but has a normal peripheral blood karyotype. If she has primary ovarian failure, then repeat karyotype on 50 lymphocytes and/or biopsy and analysis of genomic DNA from other tissues such as skin and buccal epithelium may reveal sex chromosome loss consistent with the diagnosis of TS. If these studies are normal, and especially if ovarian function is normal, she likely has Noonan syndrome, an autosomal dominant disorder which affects both sexes with short stature, neck webbing, and congenital heart defects with normal karyotype.

By original description [7, 8] and current consensus [2], the diagnosis of TS includes only phenotypic females. There are rare cases of phenotypic males with short stature, hypogonadism and possibly some other features of TS, and a 46,XdelY or 45,X/46,XY karyotype [9]. The underlying pathology seems to be the same as in females with TS, except that there were cells with sufficient Y-chromosome material in the developing gonadal ridge to permit the development and survival of testis long enough to induce a male phenotype. It is actually more common, however, for a male with TS features to have Noonan syndrome. Because gender identity and sexuality are major issues for individuals with these disorders, it is not appropriate to label the rare phenotypic male with TS features and Y chromosome deletions as "male TS."

19.2.2 Gonadal Dysgenesis

"Gonadal dysgenesis" means "defective development of the gonads" and was first used to refer to TS in the 1950s. This term was expanded to include unrelated disorders sharing the common feature of congenital primary hypogonadism. As distinctions between different disorders of sexual development became apparent, the terminology became increasingly cumbersome and confusing, i.e., "pure" 46,XX gonadal dysgenesis, "pure" 46,XY gonadal dysgenesis, mixed gonadal dysgenesis. These historic terms do not reflect current knowledge about the genetic etiology, molecular pathogenesis or phenotypic variation in these disorders. Moreover, the term 'gonadal dysgenesis' is not precisely accurate for TS in that the ovaries appear to develop normally but undergo accelerated atresia [10–12]. With rapid depletion of primordial follicles, the immature 45,X ovary with little stromal interstitial component, recedes into a connective tissue "streak." However, at least 15% of females with TS have sufficient follicular function to undergo spontaneous puberty [13] and ~3% have spontaneous pregnancies [14]. Thus, the historic and nonspecific "gonadal dysgenesis" terminology needs to be discarded, because it is inaccurate with respect to the TS ovary, and because it "lumps" TS with unrelated disorders. Moreover, it is more sensitive to the feelings of girls and women with TS to refer to premature ovarian failure, since this term recognizes that they have or at least at one point had

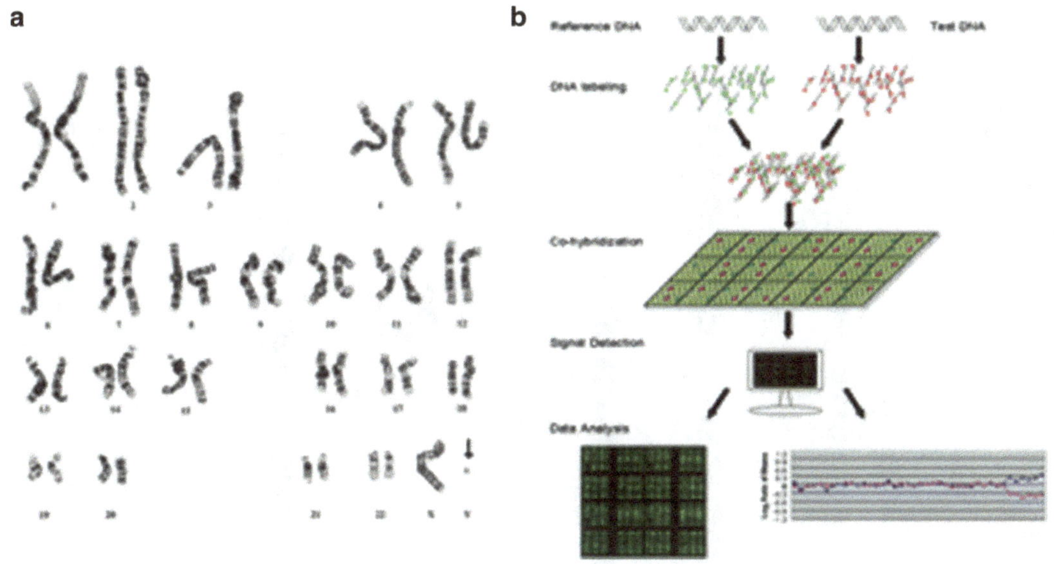

Fig. 19.2 Detection of sex chromosome anomalies. (**a**) For karyotype analysis, fresh blood cells are purified by centrifugation to enrich lymphocytes and monocytes. The mononuclear cells are cultured for 3–4 days in the presence of a mitogen like phytohemagglutinin. When there is a large population of dividing cells, the culture is treated with a drug such as Colcemid to block the cells in metaphase. After fixation, cells are plated onto microscope slides, dried and Giemsa-stained to show lightly and darkly stained bands – facilitating chromosome identification. "Good chromosome spreads" (i.e. the chromosomes are not too long or too compact and are not overlapping), are photographed or made into digital images, and the chromosomes cut out, paired up and aligned as shown in panel A. Note there is a small "marker" chromosome that represents a Y fragment (*arrow*). (**b**) Comparative genomic hybridization (CGH) using chromosomal microarrays (CMA). Whole genomic DNA from a control or reference (*left*) and from a patient (*right*) are labeled with two different fluorophores. The two genomic DNA samples are competitively cohybridized with chromosomal sequence "targets" tiled onto the microarray (*middle*). Computer imaging programs assess the relative fluorescence levels of each DNA for each target on the array (*lower left*). The ratio between control and test DNA for each clone can be linearly plotted using data analysis software to visualize dosage variations (*lower right*), indicated by a deviation from the normal log2 ratio of zero. This technology is investigational at present, but has great promise for adaptation to high throughput application that will be fast, relatively inexpensive and require simple DNA samples rather than fresh, living cells. (Reprinted from J Mol Diagn (2006) 8: 528–533 with permission from the American Society for Investigative Pathology and the Association for Molecular Pathology)

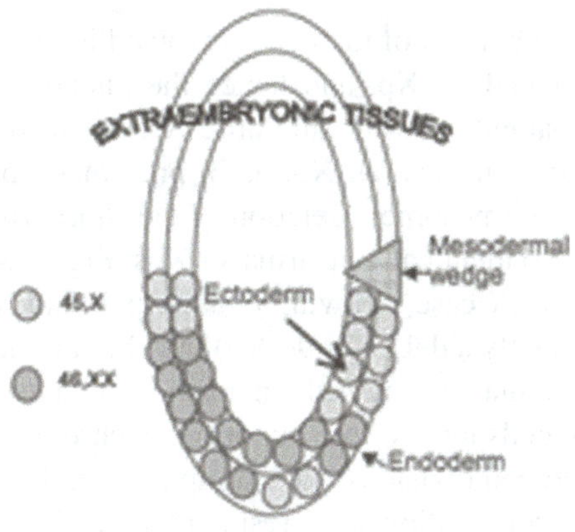

Fig. 19.3 Mosaicism for 45,X and 46,XX cell lines in an embryo at gastrulation. The 2nd X chromosome may have been lost during cell division in one or two cells during early embryo growth that give rise to clonal expansions

ovaries supporting their identification as females. Thus, the preferred nomenclature is "monosomy X (Turner syndrome)", which includes the chromosomal etiology and the familiar eponym signifying the common features of short stature and premature ovarian failure.

19.2.3 Chromosomal Origins

The X chromosome abnormalities commonly seen in TS are illustrated in Fig. 19.4 and listed in proportion to their occurrence in Table 19.1. Loss of an X or Y chromosome as a result of meiotic nondisjunction during gametogenesis will lead to a "pure" 45,X embryo if the sex chromosome null gamete joins with an opposite sex gamete that has at least one normal X chromosome. Unlike Down's syndrome, there is no association between maternal age and the risk for a TS gestation nor is there any known familial or genetic predisposition to 45,X pregnancies, and the likelihood of having a second 45,X pregnancy is not increased. The second most common group have two or three cell lines, one 45,X and the second a normal 46,XX or 46,XY karyotype, and sometimes also a third, 47,XXX cell line as well. This reflects chromosomal loss

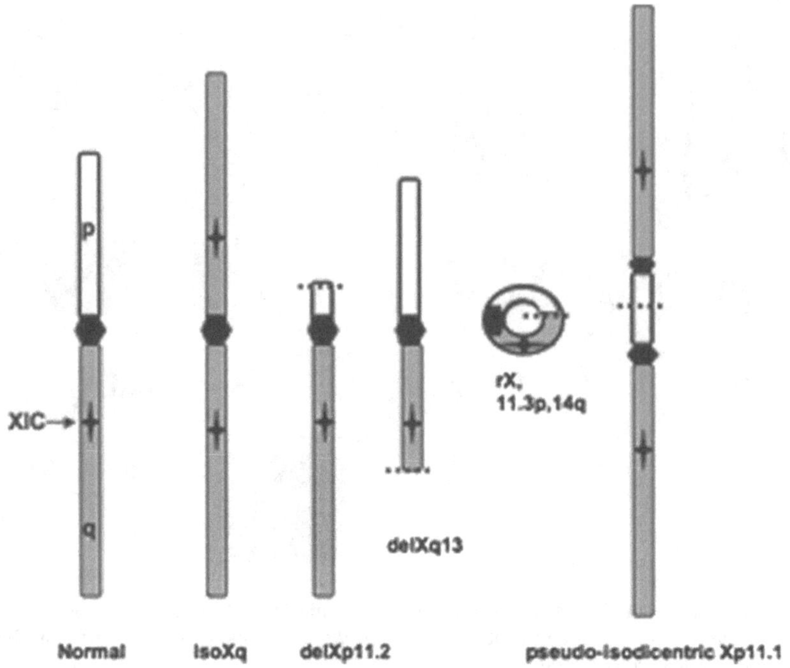

Fig. 19.4 Common X chromosome structural abnormalities found in TS. The short arm is designated "p" and the long arm "q." The XIC, or X inactivation center is located around Xq13 (the numbers refer to traditional cytogenetic staining bands) and is essential for inactivation of the 2nd (or any supernummary) X chromosomes in normal female cells. Defects involving XIC deletion are rarely seen because failure to inactivate the 2nd X chromosome is usually lethal. A common X chromosome rearrangement involves formation of an isoXq, which occurs after replication when daughter chromosomes split transversely across the centromere rather than longitudinally. Relatively proximal Xp deletions (delXp) give rise to a full TS phenotype in most cases, although ovarian function may be more sustained than in 45,X. Xq deletion may be associated with relatively mild phenotypes including normal height, since both copies of the short stature gene, SHOX, on distal X are present. Small, distal Xq deletions commonly present with isolated early menopause. A ring X (rX) chromosome forms when two breaks in an X chromosome leave "sticky" loose ends that join together. The pseudo-isodicentric Xp11.1 represents the end-to-end fusion of two copies of an Xp deleted chromosome, essentially equivalent to an isoXq

Table 19.1 Karyotype distribution in TS

Karyotype	Proportion (%)
45,X	50
45.X/46,XX & 45,X/46,XX/47,XXX	20
45,X/46,XY	3
46,XiXq & 45,X/46,XiXq	12
46,XrX & 45,X/46,XrX	6
46,XdelXp & 45,X/46,XdelXp	4
46,XdelXq & 45,X/46,XdelXq	2
46,XdelY	1
Other	2

Pooled data from the NIH study and Gravholt (2006)

(and reciprocal gain in the 47,XXX) during early embryonic mitoses (Fig. 19.5a). This mosaic individual may have a milder phenotype, if the proportion of abnormal cells present in different developing tissues is small. The other type of mosaic has an abnormal 46,XabnX cell line and a 45,X cell line. A standard 30-cell karyotype is sufficient for diagnosis in most cases and identifies a rate of 10% mosaicism with 95% confidence.

It seems that most of the genes involved in the TS phenotype are located on Xp, and hence the phenotype is quite similar in patients missing an entire X chromosome (45,X) and those missing just an Xp, as in proximal Xp deletions and Xq isochromosomes (deletion of the short arm, Xp, and joining of two identical long arms, or Xqs; Fig. 19.4). In contrast to the 45,X case, TS with an abnormal 2nd X chromosome (especially a delXq or delXp) may be familial, and the abnormal X may be passed on from mother to daughter. Embryonic cells tend to lose abnormal X chromosomes during repeated cell divisions; for example, an embryo that had a 46,XiXq constitution as a result of receiving the isoXq from one of the parents, may lose that large, unwieldy chromosome during early mitoses and thus be mosaic for 46,XiXq and 45,X cell lines (Fig. 19.5b). Both these cell lines are abnormal and monosomic for Xp, so this mosaic individual is expected to be fully affected. Females with a distal Xq deletion may be present with isolated premature ovarian failure and no other TS features; the diagnosis of TS may not be appropriate for them.

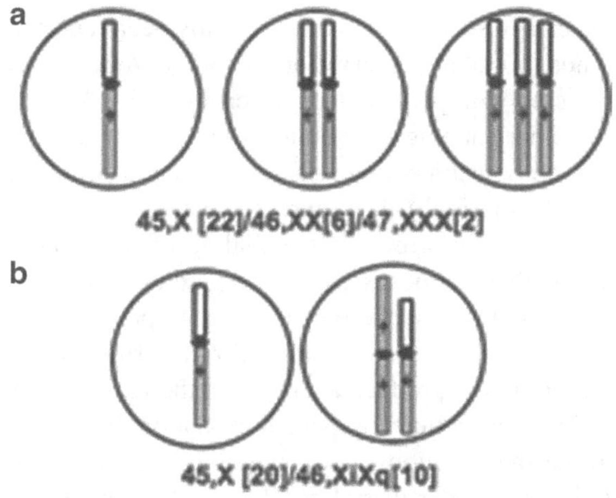

Fig. 19.5 Illustration of two types of mosaic karyotypes in TS. (**a**) From a 30-WBC karyotype, 15 cells (50%) were 45,X, 12 cells (40%) were normal 46,XX and 3 cells (10%) were 47,XXX. The standard notation reporting this karyotype is: 45,X[15]/46,XX[12]/47,XXX[3]. The triple X cell line derives from that early mitosis in which, as a result of nondisjunction, one daughter cell got only one X chromosome while the other got three. Since both 2nd and 3rd X chromosomes are (mostly) inactivated the phenotype in this patient could be relatively mild. Particularly, if there were a high proportion of 46,XX or 47,XXX in the region of gonad development, her chances for fertility may be good. (**b**) A mosaic karyotype in which both cell lines are abnormal. This cytogenetic notation tells us that 20 of the 30 cells analyzed were 45,X and the remaining third were 46,XiXq. Hence, all cells were monosomic for Xp and one expects a full TS phenotype

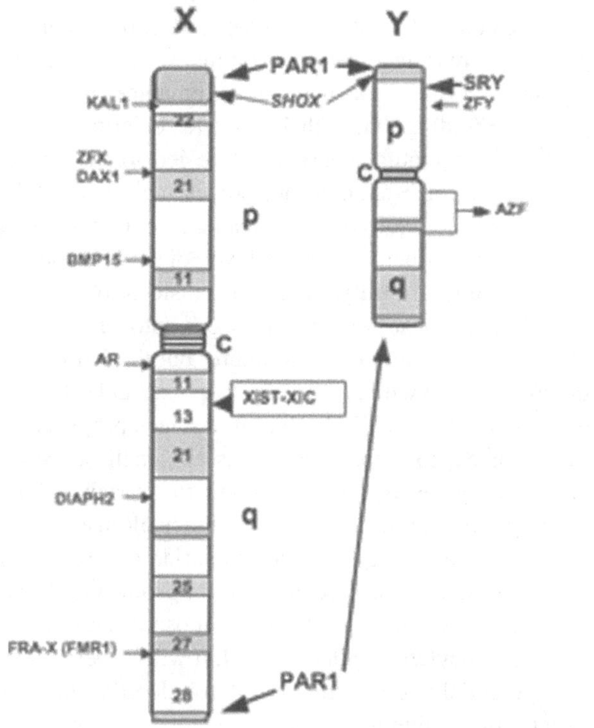

Fig. 19.6 Schematic Representation of the Sex Chromosomes. Short (p) and long (q) arms separated by the centromere (C) are indicated. The pseudo-autosomal regions (PAR1 at the p terminus and PAR2 at the q terminus) contain genes like SHOX that are expressed from both active and inactive X chromosomes in females, and from both X and Y chromosomes in males. The X-inactivation center (XIC) is a complex genomic region that transcribes XIST, a nonprotein coding RNA that coats the inactive X chromosome. The positions of several X-linked genes involved in sex determination and reproduction are shown. KAL1 – one of the genes mutation or deletion of which causes hypogonadotropic hypogonadism (IHH)/Kallmann syndrome. ZFX, BMP15, DIAPH2, and FMR have all been implicated in ovarian function. AR- androgen receptor; FRA-X – loci for the fragile X syndrome. The sex chromosomes pair only at the small terminal PAR regions, which is a weak connection and explains why loss of a sex chromosome is a common occurrence

19.2.4 Genotype and Phenotype

19.2.4.1 Short Stature

TS is the only chromosomal monosomy compatible with life. Since one sex chromosome is normally inactivated ("Lyonized") in diploid female cells, one might ask why there is any phenotype in 45,X patients. However, it turns out that a significant number of X-chromosome genes escape inactivation [15]. Some of these genes are localized in discrete "pseudoautosomal" regions of the X chromosome which have Y alleles and are normally expressed biallelically in both sexes (Fig. 19.6). The only pseudoautosomal gene implicated in the TS phenotype to date is SHOX, which encodes a homeobox transcription factor involved in skeletogenesis [16, 17]. Haploinsufficiency for SHOX, as in TS and Leri–Weill syndrome results in short stature and various skeletal anomalies [18]. Interestingly, additional X or Y chromosomes lead to tall stature secondary to extra doses of SHOX. It is likely that haploinsufficiency for other – as yet unknown – pseudoautosomal genes cause the impaired lymphatic and cardiovascular development and sensorineural deafness found in TS. In general, a mosaic karyotype with a high percent of normal cells may be associated with a relatively mild phenotype, but the phenotype is highly variable even among those females with 100% abnormal cells (e.g., see cases 1 and 2).

19.2.4.2 Premature Ovarian Failure

As noted above, the ovaries seem to develop normally in the presence of just one normal X chromosome [12]. Normal ovaries are populated with millions of germ cells early in gestation, most of which do not survive – so that at birth the typical human ovary has ~500,000 oocytes. This normal process of attrition is magnified in TS so that most girls lose all oocytes and are born with streak ovaries [19], suggesting that haploinsufficiency for unknown X-linked genes drastically impairs oocyte survival. The relation between X chromosome genes and premature ovarian failure has proven to be a complicated and frustrating subject. X chromosome breakpoints and rearrangements, involving multiple sites on both Xp and Xq are associated with premature ovarian failure [12]. The finding that both Xp and Xq deletions are associated with premature ovarian failure led to the speculation that missing or broken chromosomes may cause defects in meiotic homologous pairing leading to oocyte apoptosis [20]. To add further to the complexity of the X chromosome's influence upon fertility, balanced translocations of the long arm of the X chromosome and various autosomes are associated with premature ovarian failure, but the Xq breakpoints do not coincide with any candidate genes, and often occur in gene-poor "deserts" [21]. Thus, it has been proposed that the fusion of Xq to autosomes causes epigenetic alterations in autosomal gene expression leading to ovarian failure – an entirely different mechanism from the haploinsufficiency for X chromosome genes that causes ovarian failure in X monosomy. Thus, it seems that one X chromosome is sufficient for ovariogenesis, but that both X chromosomes are required to maintain oocyte/follicular survival. It will be very interesting and potentially clinically useful to identify the X-linked gene(s) promoting fertility in women.

19.2.5 Y Chromosome and Gonadoblastoma

This is a subject where there is much controversy and very little high quality evidence. One fact is 100% certain – any patient with TS and signs of virilization need workup for gonadal, adrenal or midline tumor, as well as further investigation of karyotype looking for Y chromosome material. The presence of Y chromosome material in patients with TS is associated with the development of gonadoblastoma in about 12%, according to a recent survey of the medical literature [22]. The risk is several fold greater in individuals with 46,XY "pure gonadal dysgenesis" or Swyer syndrome. The gonadoblastoma is a benign in situ tumor, usually microscopic in size and diagnosed histologically on ovaries removed prophylactically. Gonadoblastomas have the potential to transform into malignant germ cell neoplasms, but the frequency with which this occurs in TS is unknown. Unfortunately, there is little evidence to guide decision making on this issue. Epidemiological studies on sources of morbidity and mortality in TS do not report gonadal tumors; indeed cancer seems relatively reduced in this syndrome [23–25]. However, it is unknown whether serial ultrasound or other imaging could detect emergence of malignancy in a timely manner, and some patients may be lost to follow-up. Hence, the standard recommendation is for laparoscopic gonadectomy in these patients [22]. It was previously assumed that gonads in patients with TS and Y chromosome mosaicism have no reproductive potential, but spontaneous pregnancies in such women have recently been reported [26, 27]. Thus, possible preservation of follicles/oocytes should be discussed with patients facing gonadectomy. Many families and older patients react quite strongly to the information about Y chromosome, potential tumor, and need for gonadectomy ("castration"). Therefore, the patient and/or her parents should be informed of the finding of Y chromosome material with the utmost sensitivity regarding gender identity issues to minimize psychological harm. If a pelvic ultrasound shows no mass and there is no virilization (the majority of advancing tumors produce androgens), the family should be allowed time for adjusting to the information, further discussion or second opinions and if possible, and counseling by specialists in gender disorders. Routine testing for SRY or the presence of Y chromosome material in 45,X individuals without masculinization and without a "marker" chromosome (Fig. 19.2) is not clinically warranted at present [2] because the yield is very low and is actually in the range of test error.

19.2.6 Prenatal Diagnoses

Prenatal cytogenetic testing using chorionic villous or amniotic tissue is becoming ever more common. With the approaching wide availability of less expensive, high throughput microarray technology, chromosome screening will likely be universal. Sex chromosome anomalies are actually the most common abnormal findings from such testing. This poses a serious challenge for the clinician who asked to interpret the likely outcome of such gestations. The finding of 45,X or 45,X/46,XX or XY mosaic karyotypes in routine screening (i.e., not prompted by fetal or maternal abnormalities) creates a difficult counseling dilemma, because the outcome of such pregnancies range from fetal demise to the birth of a normal child with a normal postnatal karyotype [28–31]. If a high resolution fetal ultrasound is normal, a live birth is more likely and the child could have TS without major cardiac or lymphatic defects or could even be normal. A repeat karyotype after birth is necessary, since cytogenetic results from prenatal testing are not always confirmed in the liveborn child. The situation is less optimistic if the fetal ultrasound is abnormal in the context of a TS karyotype. The presence of cystic hygroma, heart defects or hydrops, is associated with high risk for fetal demise. Some of these fetuses survive, however, and may have an excellent outcome (See clinical case 1).

Physicians involved in counseling need to be aware that the clinical spectrum of TS is much broader and often less severe than that described in many textbooks. In particular, incidental prenatal diagnoses are associated with a mild phenotype [31, 32]. Prospective parents need to be informed about the variability of features, the likelihood of short stature and ovarian failure, and the currently available treatments. It should be emphasized that most individuals with TS have normal intelligence, and that most adults with TS function well and independently. This point is stressed because the lay person may confuse Turner with Down's syndrome.

19.2.7 Physical Diagnosis in TS

The most constant physical feature of TS is short stature (Table 19.2). Untreated adult height is about 20 cm (~8″) shorter than expected based on familial height. Thus, it is important to ask about the height of parents and sibs. Girls treated with GH for 5 years or more may reach 60–64″. Approximately 50% have skeletal malformations, including scoliosis, cubitus valgus, or a wide carrying angle and brachymetacarpia, particularly a foreshortened 4th metacarpal (Fig. 19.7), but radial bowing or Madelung deformity is actually rare. About two thirds of girls and women with TS have a high arched palate and ~25% have multiple pigmented nevi usually apparent on the head and chest. Evidence of fetal lymphedema is found in the presence of neck webbing (pterygium colli; ~30%), malrotated low set ears (~35%), and a low posterior hairline (~50%) (Fig. 19.7). Neck webbing is defined as redundant cervical skin folds arcing out from mastoid to acromium. The webbed neck has a trapezoidal shape and is always associated with a very low posterior hairline and usually with low set malrotated ears and downsloping or hooded appearing eyes. All these features are caused by the stretching of developing fetal skin and scalp over the cystic hygromata. In contrast, the common short neck in most TS patients is attributed to impaired longitudinal growth of vertebral bodies related to SHOX deficiency. It is important to identify neck webbing because these patients have nearly twice the prevalence of congenital cardiovascular defects (~50%) vs. those without the webbed neck [33, 34]. The present observations gathered from large numbers of patients examined in the 21st century show that the "classic" phenotype of dysmorphic external features (Fig. 19.7) represent only about one third of cases while, aside from short stature, most have rather subtle physical signs (Fig. 19.8). Moreover, the height deficit may not be obvious if the patients comes from a tall family (Fig. 19.8).

Table 19.2 Physical features of TS

Short stature	95%
Low post hairline	55%
High arched palate	60%
Multiple nevi	25%
Cubitus valgus	45%
Scoliosis	50%
Webbed neck	30%

Based on prospective examination of 300 participants in the NIH TS protocol 2001–2007

19.2.8 Congenital Cardiovascular and Renal Defects in TS

Congenital cardiovascular defects are the most medically significant and life-threatening consequences of monosomy for the X chromosome. Indeed, the great majority of 45,X gestations end in fetal demise due to circulatory failure. About 10% of live-born girls with TS come to medical attention early because of major cardiovascular defects, including left heart hypoplasia, aortic valve disease, and aortic coarctation. Screening of asymptomatic women with TS using cardiac magnetic resonance angiography (CMRA) reveals that ~50% have abnormalities of the aortic valve, aortic arch and/or major vessels [35]. An example of a CMRA study in a 45-year-old woman with TS and intractable hypertension, who had previous "normal" cardiac echos, is shown in Fig. 19.9. In addition to bicuspid aortic valve, aortic root dilatation and aortic coarctation, many women have very abnormal-appearing elongation of the transverse aortic arch often associated with dilatation of the aortic root [35]. Cardiac MR is invaluable in screening for congenital cardiovascular anomalies and has revolutionized our view of the spectrum of defects in TS and other disorders. CMR visualizes the aortic valve in motion and the entire configuration of the aortic arch. Unlike cardiac echo, CMR is not impeded by obesity or chest wall dimensions in obtaining accurate cardiovascular images, and all patients with TS need to have at least one comprehensive CMR evaluation.

The pathophysiology of the cardiovascular defects in TS is unknown, but there appears to be a generalized vasculopathy [36] affecting major arteries and veins. The prospective, evidence-based information available at present as well as a wealth of anecdotal reports [37, 38] indicate that women with TS are at greatly increased risk for aortic dissection or rupture even at aortic diameters that are in the normal range for normal size adults [39, 40]. Unfortunately, few ER staff members think of aortic dissection when a young woman complains of chest or back pain, and most cases go undiagnosed until it is too late. A very small percentage of individuals with TS should have proportionately small aortic diameters, and evaluation for aortic dilatation needs adjustment for body surface area. Bicuspid aortic valve, dilated aortic root, and hypertension are the major risk factors for aortic complications in TS as in the general population. Hypertension is found in ~40–50% of patients

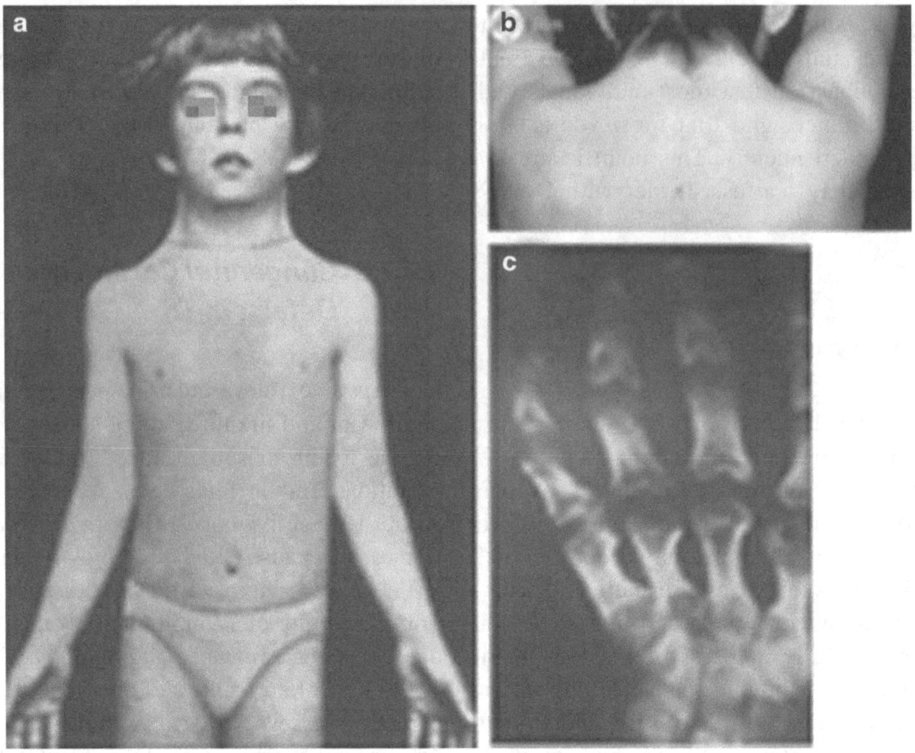

Fig. 19.7 "Classic" Stigmata of TS. These photos are from the first report in 1930 of what later came to be called TS by a German physician, Otto Ullrich (with permission from Ref. [106]). Henry Turner, an academic physician from Oklahoma published a series of 7 similar cases in 1937 and was the first to treat TS females with estrogen [8]. The patient seen in this figure has neck webbing associated with low set ears, downsloping or hooded appearing eyes (**a**) and a low posterior hairline (**b**). These features are all secondary to stretching of the head and neck skin over cystic hygroma during fetal development, and tend to make the patient look dull, or unintelligent, which is not usually true. This patient, for example, obtained a PhD in biochemistry. She also demonstrates the elbow anomaly known as cubitus valgus, or "wide carrying angle," in which she cannot hold the arms straight at her sides. In addition, she has a typical short 4th metacarpal (**c**)

with TS and is usually independent of renal or cardiovascular anomalies [41]. The high blood pressure may be part of a dysautonomia and is also characterized by resting tachycardia, already detected in utero [42, 43] and reduced heart rate variability [44]. Perhaps related to sympathetic overactivity, the renin-angiotensin system (RAS) is hyperactive in TS. Patients usually respond well to beta-adrenergic blockade and RAS inhibition. Given the risk of aortic dissection, it is highly critical to maintain good BP control.

Renal malformations are found in 20–30% of patients with TS. Horseshoe kidney, renal agenesis, and duplex collecting systems are most common abnormalities [45, 46]. In the absence of obstruction of the collecting system, the renal anomalies are usually clinically insignificant. Chronic urinary infections in a patient with TS mandate close investigation of the urologic anatomy. The prevalence of various medical problems among adults with TS is summarized in Table 19.3.

19.3 Care for Girls and Women with TS

19.3.1 Pubertal Induction

As noted above, 15–20% of girls with TS will undergo some spontaneous pubertal development [13, 47], but eventually ~95% of the individuals with TS will have premature ovarian failure. FSH level can be measured at age 11 to help predict the likelihood of spontaneous development and prepare the parents and child psychologically for initiating estrogen treatment if necessary. If there is no sign of spontaneous pubertal development and FSH is elevated by age 11–12, estrogen therapy should begin. Unfortunately, there have been and most likely never will be controlled clinical trials aimed at optimizing the pharmacological protocol for pubertal induction in TS or in any girls with primary ovarian failure. The expert consensus in the pediatric endocrine community at present is that, pubertal induction should be as physiological

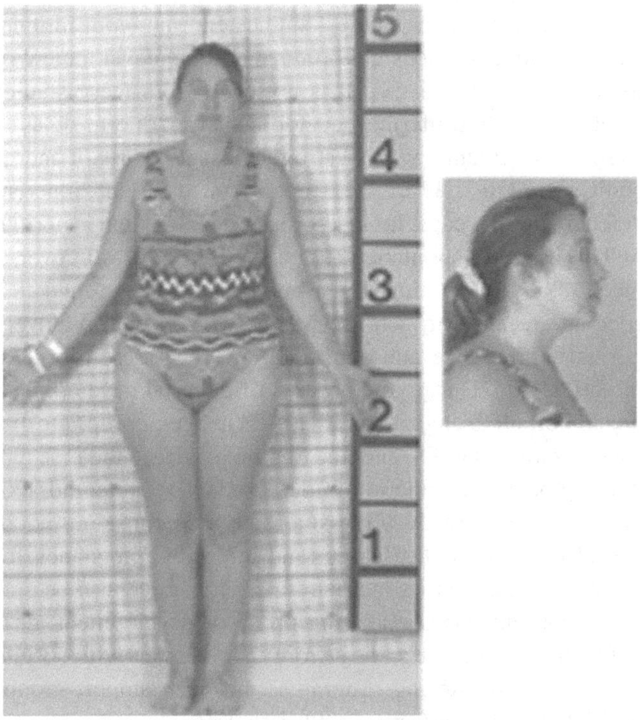

Fig. 19.8 TS Diagnosed With 2° Amenorrhea At Age 27. This figure shows a woman who had normal pubertal development, including menarche (Case 2). She went on oral contraceptives and continued them until her late mid 20s when she married and wanted to start a family. No menses occurred after discontinuation of the oral contraceptives. Her parents and sibs were tall and at ~5′1″ she is about 6 in. shorter than expected. Her karyotype is 45,X/46,XrX

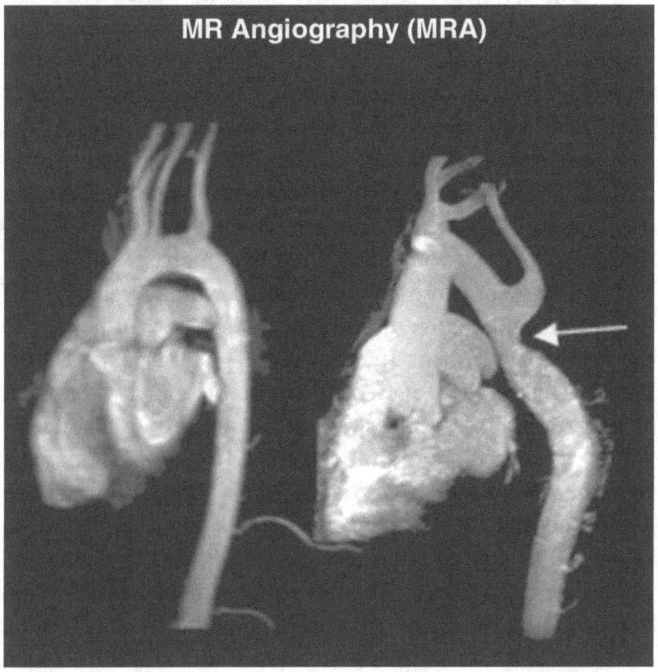

Fig. 19.9 Magnetic Resonance Angiography Reveals Aortic Coarctation. The panel on the left shows a normal, smooth, "candy cane" shaped aortic arch. On the right, there is a focal narrowing just after the origin of the left subclavian a (which is abnormally dilated). The contrast agent was gadolinium

Table 19.3 Medical problems in TS

Primary ovarian failure	97%
1° amenorrhea	85%
2° amenorrhea	12%
Congenital heart	50%
Aortic coarctation	12%
Aortic valve disease	30%
Aortic root dilatation	22%
Autoimmune thyroid	60%
Hypothyroid	56%
Hyperthyroid	4%
Hearing loss	55%
Hypertension	42%
Liver disease	60%
Mild elevation LFT	33%
Fatty liver	31%
Gastrointestinal	
IBD	5%
Celiac	5%
Intestinal telangiectasia	5%

Data from the NIH study for 200 adults (>17 years)

as possible because by trying to mimic natural puberty we are likely to do more good than harm [2]. Pubertal induction in girls with TS should begin with very small doses of (bioidentical) 17-beta estradiol (E2) at 12 years of age. Delaying estrogen therapy until 15 years of age to optimize height promotion by GH is not recommended. To quote from the recent guidelines, "This emphasis on stature tends to undervalue the psychosocial importance of age-appropriate pubertal maturation and may be deleterious to bone and other aspects of the child's health [48–50]." Moreover, we now know that very low dose of estradiol does not interfere with GH's positive effect on final adult height, so GH use may be continued for the first year on E2 [48, 51–53].

Parenteral forms of E2 are now considered to be more physiologic alternatives than traditional oral formulations [48, 52–54]. Low dose E2 patches that deliver 14 mcg/d are appropriate to begin with and more choices will likely arrive in the future. Depending on the starting age and individual tolerance and responsiveness, the dose may be doubled every 6–12 months over a period of 2–4 years until full adult dosage is achieved (e.g., 14–25–50–75–100 mcg patches). Maximizing the time between the introduction of estrogen and starting progesterone is thought to enhance breast development, thus it is advised to delay the addition of progesterone for 2 years after starting estrogen or until breakthrough bleeding occurs [2]. By the same token, the common practice of starting a low-dose combined oral contraceptive in this circumstance may not offer the best outcome of breast or uterine development. Ideally, a parenteral form of natural progesterone should be used to induce regular menses during teenage years, as this will parallel the experience of teenage peers. As a practical matter, we now use oral progesterone to induce cycles. After high school, many young women prefer

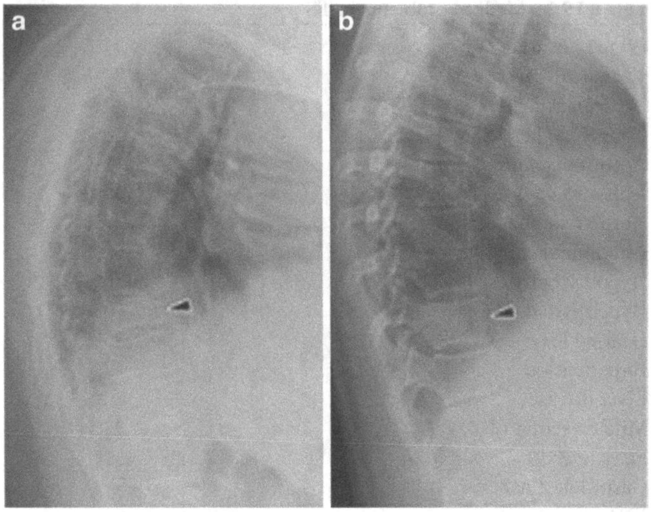

Fig. 19.10 X-rays from two 30-year-old women with TS. Both have 45,X karyotypes, both had primary amenorrhea and started on estrogen at age 12. The woman whose X-ray is seen on the left discontinued estrogen during college and the one on the right continued estrogen use to the present day. The one on the left lost 2 in. in height and has vertebral wedging and dorsal kyphosis (dowager's hump). Her vertebral BMD T-score was –4

convenience regimens that eliminate or reduce frequency of menses, and such alternatives are preferable to noncompliance. However, the use of conventional birth control pill with a "pill-free" week is not advisable. The pill-free week amounts to 3 months of estrogen deficiency each year, which is associated with bone loss. Perhaps the 3-month cycle birth control regimen is preferable. The hormone regimen should be based on the individual preferences of each patient and usually involves a trial and error approach through the wide variety of products available.

It is important to educate each patient about the importance of continued estrogen replacement therapy until the time of normal menopause to maintain feminization and prevent osteoporosis [50]. Failure to counsel the patient on the importance of compliance with estrogen treatment during adult years may have disastrous consequences, illustrated in Fig. 19.10. The patient needs to understand that clinically significant osteoporosis with fragility fractures, back pain, and height loss affects almost 50% of women who discontinue estrogen treatment prematurely [55]. To help insure adequate bone mineral accrual, teenage girls with TS should have a calcium intake of 1,200–1,500 mg per day. Vitamin D deficiency is now a major concern, so a daily multivitamin that contains at least 400IU Vitamin D is recommended for girls and young women who do not go out in the sun on a regular basis. In addition to a healthy diet, daily exercise is to be encouraged. If the girl has congenital heart disease, her exercise regimen needs to be approved by her cardiologist.

A few European studies suggested that conventional pubertal induction does not produce optimal development of the uterus in TS [56–59]. It is not clear from these studies whether impaired uterine development was due to delayed estrogen treatment, too low estrogen dosage, or use of androgenic progestins. There does not seem to be any inherent defect in uterine capacity in TS, since development is normal in TS girls with spontaneous puberty [56, 60]. Moreover, a recent study examining TS women in the U.S. found that adequate recent estrogen use was associated with relatively normal uterine size and configuration, regardless of age at initiation [61]. During the process of pubertal development, it is important to engage girls with TS in age-appropriate discussions on how TS and its treatment affect their sexual development and function and reproductive potential. For girls who seem ready for sexual activity, counseling about sexually transmitted diseases (and unwanted pregnancy for those with endogenous ovarian function) should also be provided. During this challenging phase of development, girls with TS may benefit greatly from involvement with special teen camps, mentoring programs, and peer support groups (info at https://www.turnersyndrome.org/.

19.3.2 Ovarian Hormone Replacement in Adults

Unfortunately, negative publicity about unwanted effects of hormone replacement in older postmenopausal woman has confused some practitioners and patients and many women with TS have discontinued ovarian hormone replacement (4). Our current ad hoc approach to this subject stresses the very low risk, high benefit ratio for the use of estrogen in young patients with ovarian failure with at least a 50% risk of clinically significant osteoporosis in those who discontinue estrogen at a young age. [55]. We emphasize the excellent safety record of many millions of woman-years use of oral contraceptive, the importance of estrogen for bone, and the need for estrogen effect upon the genitourinary system for adequate sexual function. We promote the physiological aspects of transdermal estradiol and its proposed relative safety in regard to thrombosis risk [62], which may be increased in TS [63–65]. We aim to parallel the normal life cycle patterns of estrogen exposure, using a higher dose (e.g., 100 mcg patch) during young adulthood, and decreasing to 50 mcg patches by 35–40 years with further reduction and cessation by age 45–50 years for most women. Of note, the use of estrogen to treat premature ovarian failure is much more liberal in Europe, where use of 4 mg oral E2 is not uncommon. Given the current preference for "natural" products, we recommend progesterone rather than any derivative, with cycling on a monthly or tri-monthly basis. These recommendations are not based on controlled clinical studies, but represent our best attempts to reconcile our patients' concerns, available medical data, and expert opinion [2]. The major contraindications to estrogen use in women with TS are similar to those for women in general, i.e., history of gynecological cancer, history of thrombosis or known clotting disorder, and possibly, familial breast cancer risk. Women with TS have significantly low androgen levels [66] and might benefit from the use of a low dose testosterone patch designed for women, but this has not yet been evaluated in any clinical study.

19.3.3 Psychosocial Concerns

The great majority of individuals with TS have normal intelligence although focal deficits in visual spatial cognition and organizational skills are noted [67, 68]. Many parents of girls with TS are now enthusiastic about defining specific "nonverbal learning disabilities" and attention deficit disorders in their daughters who will qualify for special education resources. This trend is despite the fact that earlier generations of TS patients have distinguished educational achievements with average years of formal education exceeding that of the general public [55, 69, 70]. Despite academic achievements, many women with TS have social difficulties [71]. Major psychiatric diagnoses are not increased in TS, except for depressive episodes, which occur with the same frequency seen in 46,XX women with infertility [72]. Women with TS express significantly higher levels of shyness and social anxiety and reduced self-esteem compared with normal female controls, but nearly identical to feelings expressed by 46,XX women with spontaneous premature ovarian failure, illustrated in Fig. 19.11 [73]. During open-ended interviews, this same group of women with TS reported that dealing with premature ovarian failure and loss of fertility was the most difficult part of having TS [74]. These observations suggest that the experience of premature ovarian failure and infertility cause symptoms of shyness, social anxiety, and poor self esteem.

Girls and women with TS, typically have a female pattern of gender identity, but make their sexual debut later than their peers and may be less likely to marry [71, 75, 76].

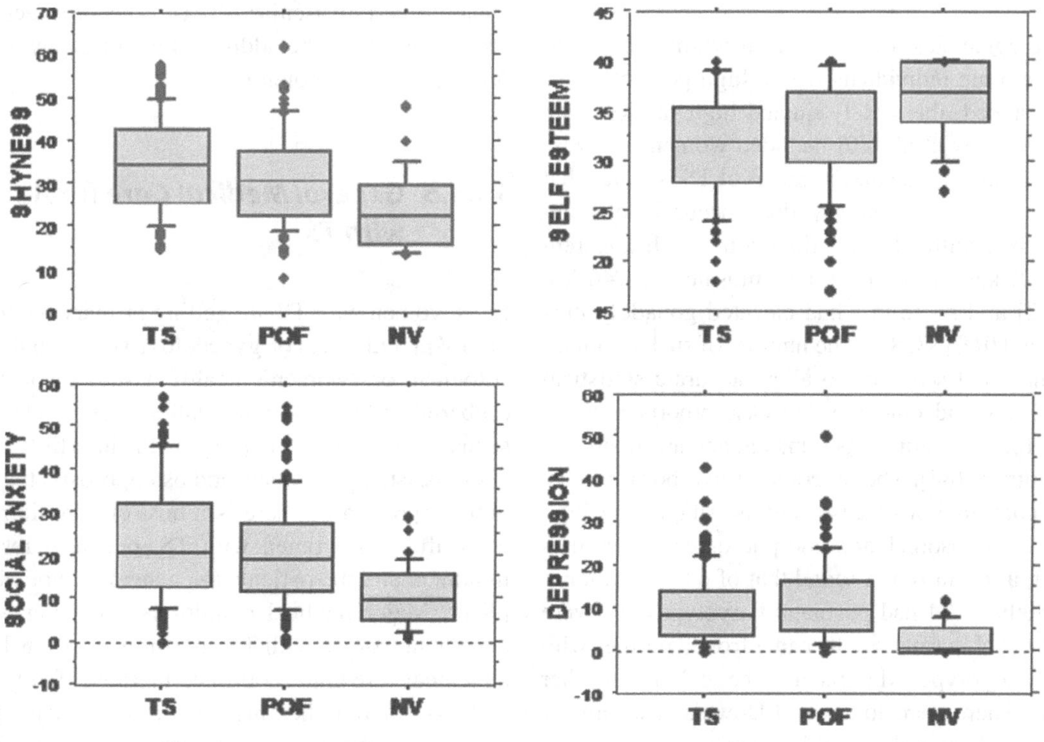

Fig. 19.11 Shyness, Social Anxiety And Impaired Self Esteem In Women With Premature Ovarian Failure. Surveys measuring these symptoms were administered to 100 women with TS, 100 women with 46,XX premature ovarian failure and 37 age-matched normal cycling female volunteers. The scores for both 45,X and 46,XX groups with premature ovarian failure show significantly greater shyness, social anxiety and depression and less self-esteem compared with control women. Adapted from [73]

The Derogatis Interview for Sexual Functioning adapted for females was administered to 100 women, average age 37 years (range 18–59), participating in the NIH TS study [77]. Sexual interest and fantasy scores were completely normal in the TS group. Sexual activity was near control levels in the partnered group (~30%), but practically nil among unmarried women [77]. Further study is needed to elucidate the nature of psychosocial impediments affecting establishment of partner relations and sexual functioning in women with TS. Several reports suggest that delayed pubertal development and miscommunications about the diagnosis and its meaning for sexual and reproductive functions, contribute to poor self esteem, social difficulties, and impaired or absent sexual functioning in TS [76, 78, 79]. Thus, it is possible that improving the management of pubertal development and providing honest and sensitive education and two-way communication about sexual aspects of the syndrome may enhance the quality of life for women with TS in the future. Psychosocial support for the individual with TS and family is critical to successful medical management, and helping them to connect with others with TS through the Turner Syndrome Society, USA. (https://www.turnersyndrome.org/) or other means is extremely important.

19.3.4 Pregnancy in TS

Spontaneous pregnancies are reported in women with TS, most often in mosaic individuals with a high percentage of normal cells. Indeed, the widely quoted high rate of ~7% reported in Birkebaek et al. [80] included women with less than 10% abnormal cells, so the diagnosis of TS is somewhat doubtful. Nevertheless, pregnancy does occur in a small number of women with TS, including some with apparent nonmosaic 45,X karyotypes [81], or a mosaic 45,X/46,XY karyotypes [82] and some that had elevated gonadotropins and had been on HRT [83, 84]. The number of such pregnancies is too small and scattered to allow accurate statistical assessment of risk and outcome, but case reports indicate increased risk for C-section, hypertension, and aortic dissection for the mothers [84]. The outcome of live-born infants, according to compilation of case reports, suggests a high incidence of chromosomal and morphological anomalies [14]. However, a recent report found that of 64 live children born to TS mothers, 24 had postnatal karyotypes; 19 were normal, and most abnormal results came from a mother with a 46,XdelXp karyotype who passed the deletion to her daughters [80]. There were no cases of Down's syndrome or other chromosomal anomalies in this series.

Although early reports suggested a poor response to embryo implantation in TS, improvement in hormonal preparation of the endometrium has apparently resulted in implantation rates equal to non-TS patients [85]. However, a recent review of women with TS participating in oocyte donation programs in the U.S. in 1997 found that of 146 women treated, 101 (69%) became pregnant; 94 of these pregnancies resulted in the birth of a live baby, for a miscarriage rate of only 6.4% [86]. While this shows a good rate of pregnancy, it was found that only ~50% of TS patients had a screening echocardiogram prior to fertility treatment. While no deaths or major complications occurred in the reviewed cases, the authors projected a mortality rate of 2.1% based on a world literature review [86]. This report was followed by a practice alert from the American Society for Reproductive Medicine [87] warning of a 100-fold increased risk for death in women with TS attempting pregnancy, and stating that TS "is a relative contraindication to pregnancy." Importantly, the warning stresses the necessity for full cardiac evaluation prior to attempting pregnancy. [87].

This is a troublesome dilemma, since the desire to experience life as a normal woman and start a family based on carrying a child to term is a very strong motivation for many young women with TS. The most intensive cardiac evaluation and current imaging technology indicate that ~50% of individuals with TS have some cardiovascular involvement. If these patients are identified at a young age, they can be counseled on alternatives to pregnancy from the early stages of pubertal development. For the ~50% of young women who have no apparent cardiovascular disease, the prospects for assisted pregnancy should be addressed on a case by case basis with full disclosure of potential risks.

19.3.5 General Medical Care for Adults with TS

Most women with TS are getting primary medical care from family practitioners or gynecologists. Given the many gynecological, or "women's health" issues involved in TS care (pubertal induction, feminization, sex education, impaired sexual functioning, coping with infertility, maintenance HRT, assisted pregnancy, and osteoporosis) the latter may be more appropriate. There is a host of chronic medical problems affecting women with TS, but most respond well to treatment and the patients are generally motivated and compliant. Major medical conditions occurring with high frequency in women with TS are summarized in Table 19.3 and a medical care plan is outlined in Table 19.4.

Sensorineural hearing loss affects many young adults with TS, worsens with age and has a significant adverse impact on quality of life [88]. Thus, regular audiological testing and aggressive promotion of hearing aid use are important for women with TS. Autoimmune thyroid disease

Table 19.4 Care plan for adult with TS

System	Baseline test(s)	Follow-up	Comments
Cardiovascular – refer to CHD specialist	Cor exam, BP in all extremities, ECG, Echocardiogram, MRA	Per cardiology	50% will have some CHD
Blood pressure	BP	Every visit	Critical if CHD
Renal	Renal ultrasound	Only if abnormal	
Thyroid	TSH	Annual	
Liver	LFTs	Annual LFTS	US if obese
Lipids	Lipid panel	Annual lipids	
Diabetes	BMI, waist, FBS	Annual waist, FBS	
Bone health	DXA BMD	At time of menopause transition or prn	
Hearing	Audiology, ENT	Audiology Q3–4 years	
Sexual health	Evaluate knowledge, activity, contraception	Annual or prn	Counseling, support groups
Psychosocial	Assess social anxiety, depression	Annual or prn	

Adapted from [2]

– usually Hashimoto's thyroiditis but occasionally Grave's disease – is greatly increased in prevalence in TS, affecting at least 50% of adults [89]. Other forms of autoimmunity that may be slightly increased in TS are celiac disease [90], inflammatory bowel disease, [91] and juvenile rheumatoid arthritis [92]. These entities are, however, very rare in the well-characterized NIH study population. About 40% of women with TS demonstrate mild to moderate elevation of hepatic transaminases TS [93]. The etiology of liver disease in TS may be heterogeneous, with some cases primarily vascular and others related to fatty infiltration [94]. Progression to clinically significant liver disease is relatively rare, at least as reported in the medical literature [94]. It is possible that the increasing prevalence of fatty liver may interact with the underlying TS liver pathology to create a more toxic condition. The abnormal liver function tests are not a contraindication to estrogen use in these patients; in fact, oral estrogens generally moderate transaminase levels in TS [93, 95].

Obesity, diabetes, and dyslipidemia are major challenges for many women with TS. It has frequently been observed that women with TS seem prone to obesity [95–97] and particularly to a central or android fat distribution [98]. Not surprisingly, there is also a high prevalence of dyslipidemia and type 2 diabetes mellitus in TS. The predisposition to metabolic problems seems to predate the onset of obesity [99], but is aggravated with excess adiposity. Women with TS, however, do not demonstrate marked insulin resistance and are actually relatively insulin sensitive for their degree of adiposity [99, 100]. Thus, diabetes in most women with TS is relatively easily controlled with diet, strictly avoiding refined carbohydrates, and by doing exercise. When diet and exercise do not suffice, usually a single agent such as metformin is effective. Lipids may benefit from diet and exercise as well, but frequently a statin is necessary to get the LDL cholesterol to a desirable level. Many women with TS have several risk factors for atherosclerotic coronary artery disease, e.g., hypertension, diabetes, and dyslipidemia, and thus the LDL cholesterol should be below 120 mg/dl.

19.3.5.1 Osteoporosis

Skeletal demineralization has been described in girls and women with TS since the first descriptions of the disorder. However, many past studies of bone mineral density (BMD) in TS were confounded by small skeletal size and variable estrogen exposure. Recent studies taking bone size into account suggest that trabecular bone mineralization, e.g., BMD at the lumbar spine and ultra distal radius, is actually normal in women who have used estrogen consistently beginning by their mid-teens [101]. Cortical bone, e.g., the radial shaft and femoral neck is, however, significantly abnormal and often in an osteoporotic range in these women [102, 103]. Appendicular fractures are increased in young women with TS, suggesting that the observed thinness of cortical bone reflects fragility as well [104]. Certainly, the fracture risk is expected to increase with age. Unfortunately, it seems that bisphosphonates and parathyroid hormone have minimal impact on cortical BMD [105]. Moreover, all safety and efficacy data for these agents apply only to older postmenopausal women. It is really unknown whether they are effective at all in TS, or whether the safety profile when used in young women will be acceptable. Thus, it seems wise to reserve the use of these potent agents for older patients who appear at great risk, or younger women who have atraumatic fractures. Further study is required to determine whether the reduction in cortical bone is an intrinsic feature of TS perhaps related to haploinsufficiency for SHOX or another X-linked gene, or due to deficient estrogen during childhood and the early teens. Current recommendations to begin low-dose estrogen treatment earlier may clarify this issue. Another untested possibility is that cortical bone deficiency in TS is related to hypoandrogenism in TS. Prophylactic treatment of low cortical BMD in young women with TS with bisphosphonates is not warranted since it is unknown if the low cortical BMD predicts fractures in young or middle-aged physically active adults, and since these agents have little if any effect on cortical bone. Evaluation of a new patient should include history of estrogen use and any other factors that pertain to bone health, history of nontraumatic fractures and/or height loss and a baseline DXA. Low scores are predictable in women less than 4′10″ tall, but can serve as the patient's baseline to measure effects of lifestyle interventions, such as weight bearing, low impact exercise programs, calcium and Vitamin D supplementation, and changes in estrogen use.

19.4 Summary: Evidence-based Guidelines

19.4.1 Diagnosis and Care for Girls and Women with TS

1. Girls/young women with hypergonadotropic hypogonadism and short stature presenting with 1° or 2° amenorrhea need sex chromosome analyses
2. All newly diagnosed patients with TS needs comprehensive medical evaluation with special focus on the cardiovascular system
   (a) Cardiology consult, echo, MRA, ECG
   (b) Renal ultrasound
   (c) Thyroid, liver function tests
   (d) Celiac screen, lipid panel
   (e) Audiology
3. Pubertal induction: Absent pubertal development, elevated FSH by age 11–12:
   (a) Begin low dose transdermal estradiol, gradually increasing over 2–3 years, adding progesterone when bleeding occurs or when adult dose E2 is reached
   (b) Attend to psychological aspects of premature ovarian failure and educate on importance of estrogen therapy
4. Transitioning from pediatric to adult care, a young woman with TS should have:
   (a) Cardiac MRA to establish adult cardiac status and aortic diameters
   (b) BP evaluation; Rx HBP with beta blocker, RAS inhibitor
   (c) DXA to establish baseline BMD
   (d) Begin annual testing of liver, thyroid, and metabolic function
   (e) Address social and sexual functioning with referral to counseling if needed.
5. Maintenance estrogen therapy for young adults 20–35 years should be at least 100 mcg/day transdermal estradiol (=1.25 mg conjugated equine estrogens, 2 mg oral estradiol, 10 mcg ethinyl estradiol) cycled with progesterone.
6. Implement bone health regimen, including low impact weight-bearing exercise, calcium and Vitamin D supplements.
7. Women with any congenital cardiovascular defects or hypertension should be counseled against attempting pregnancy. Women without apparent risk factors still need a current cardiovascular evaluation immediately prior to attempting pregnancy. If pregnancy is achieved, they should be supervised by high-risk pregnancy specialists as latent tendency for vascular compromise, hypertension, and diabetes may be expressed during pregnancy.

19.5 Clinical Cases

19.5.1 Case 1

19.5.1.1 A "Severe" Case of TS Diagnosed In Utero

A community obstetrician asks about prognosis of a mid trimester pregnancy with bilateral cystic hygromata. Amniotic karyotype done because of the abnormal fetal US was 45,X.

Figure 19.11 shows the excellent outcome of one such pregnancy. This 18-year-old college freshman was the product of a gestation complicated by bilateral cystic hygromata and oligohydraminos. The cytogenetic testing revealed a nonmosaic 45,X karyotype. At birth she had moderate webbing of the neck and mild peripheral lymphedema. The 45,X karyotype was confirmed on the infant's peripheral blood analysis. She did well, and was treated with growth hormone achieving an adult stature of 5′1 . She had premature ovarian failure with an elevated FSH, and was started on estrogen to induce pubertal development at age 12. She has had cosmetic surgery to reduce neck webbing and improve jaw line. Her social and intellectual development is normal. She has an asymptomatic bicuspid aortic valve that requires cardiology follow-up on a regular basis, but her health and QOL are excellent Fig. 19.12.

The response to the community provider should be that the risk of spontaneous fetal demise is high, probably ~90%. Live-born girls may have congenital heart defects and cosmetic issues related to the fetal lymphedema, but with modern medical and surgical management may have excellent quality of life and academic achievement.

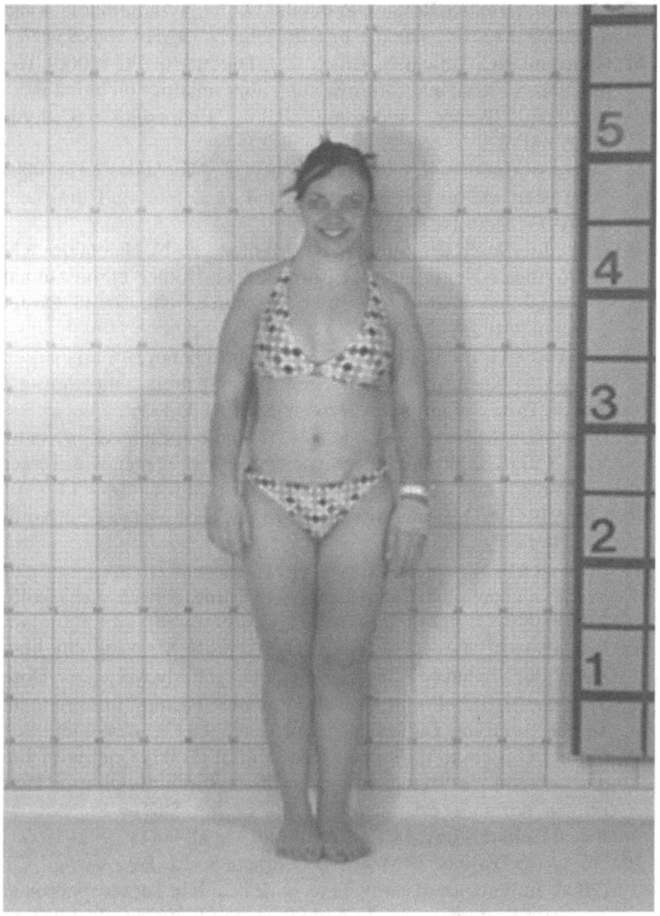

Fig. 19.12 This 17-year-old college freshman was the product of a gestation complicated by bilateral cystic hygromata and oligohydraminos (See Case 1)

19.5.2 Case 2

19.5.2.1 A "Mild" Case of TS Diagnosed at Age 27

A 27–year-old G0 P0 woman came for evaluation of infertility (Fig. 19.7). She had normal pubertal development, menarche at age 12 but menses were irregular. She went on BCP at age 16 to normalize periods and continued use until she wanted to become pregnant at age 25. She did not have a menstrual period. After 6 months, she went to a gynecologist who measured FSH of 63. Further investigation revealed that although at ~5′1″ she was not extremely short; she was a few inches shorter than her mother and ~6″ shorter than her sister. She had a high arched palate, low posterior hairline, and multiple nevi. Her karyotype was 45,X[42]/46,XrX[8].

She clearly has TS with 2° amenorrhea (masked for years by BCP). She actually has short stature for her genetic potential, and additional characteristic signs, i.e., high palate, low hairline, and multiple nevi. The karyotype is mostly 45,X with a second abnormal cell line containing a ring X chromosome. Thus, her mild phenotype is not explained by high grade mosaicism for normal cells. The relatively mild phenotype is typical of many individuals with TS, leading unfortunately to delayed diagnoses. She needs a further work up at this time, especially to examine the cardiovascular system with cardiology consultation. Additional screening tests are summarized in Table 19.3.

Acknowledgements This work was supported by the intramural research program of the NICHD, NIH.

References

1. Stochholm K, Juul S, Juel K, Naeraa RW, Gravholt CH (2006) Prevalence, incidence, diagnostic delay, and mortality in Turner syndrome. J Clin Endocrinol Metab 91(10):3897–3902
2. Bondy CA (2007) Care of girls and women with turner syndrome: A Guideline of the Turner Syndrome Study Group. J Clin Endocrinol Metab 92(1):10–25
3. Bondy C, Bakalov VK, Lange ED, Ceniceros I (2006) Deficient medical care for adults with the Turner syndrome. Ann Intern Med 145(11):866–867
4. Bondy CA, Ceniceros I, Lange E, Bakalov VK (2006) Declining estrogen use in young women with turner syndrome. Arch Intern Med 166(12):1322
5. Larrabee PB, Johnson KL, Pestova E et al (2004) Microarray analysis of cell-free fetal DNA in amniotic fluid: a prenatal molecular karyotype. Am J Hum Genet 75(3):485–491
6. Wojda A, Zietkiewicz E, Mossakowska M, Pawlowski W, Skrzypczak K, Witt M (2006) Correlation between the level of cytogenetic aberrations in cultured human lymphocytes and the age and gender of donors. J Gerontol A Biol Sci Med Sci 61(8):763–772
7. Ullrich O (1930) Über typische Kombinationsbilder multipler Abartungen. Z Kinderheilk 49:271–276
8. Turner HH (1938) A syndrome of infantilism, congenital webbed neck, and cubitus valgus. Endocrinology 23:566–574
9. Graham BH, Bacino CA (2003) Male patient with non-mosaic deleted Y-chromosome and clinical features of Turner syndrome. Am J Med Genet A 119(2):234–237
10. Ohno S (1967) Sex chomosomes and sex linked genes. Springer, Berlin
11. Opitz JM, Pallister PD (1979) Brief historical note: the concept of "gonadal dysgenesis". Am J Med Genet 4(4):333–343
12. Simpson JL, Rajkovic A (1999) Ovarian differentiation and gonadal failure. Am J Med Genet 89(4):186–200
13. Pasquino AM, Passeri F, Pucarelli I, Segni M, Municchi G (1997) Spontaneous pubertal development in turner's syndrome. J Clin Endocrinol Metab 82(6):1810–1813
14. Tarani L, Lampariello S, Raguso G et al (1998) Pregnancy in patients with Turner's syndrome: six new cases and review of literature. Gynecol Endocrinol 12(2):83–87
15. Carrel L, Willard HF (2005) X-inactivation profile reveals extensive variability in X-linked gene expression in females. Nature 434(7031):400–404
16. Rao E, Weiss B, Fukami M et al (1997) Pseudoautosomal deletions encompassing a novel homeobox gene cause growth failure in idiopathic short stature and Turner syndrome. Nat Genet 16(1):54–63
17. Ogata T (1999) SHOX: pseudoautosomal homeobox containing gene for short stature and dyschondrosteosis. Growth Horm IGF Res 9(Suppl B):53–57, discussion 7–8

18. Ross JL, Scott C Jr, Marttila P et al (2001) Phenotypes associated with SHOX deficiency. J Clin Endocrinol Metab 86(12):5674–5680
19. Reynaud K, Cortvrindt R, Verlinde F, De Schepper J, Bourgain C, Smitz J (2004) Number of ovarian follicles in human fetuses with the 45,X karyotype. Fertil Steril 81(4):1112–1119
20. Ogata T, Matsuo N (1995) Turner syndrome and female sex chromosome aberrations: deduction of the principal factors involved in the development of clinical features. Hum Genet 95(6):607–629
21. Rizzolio F, Sala C, Alboresi S et al (2007) Epigenetic control of the critical region for premature ovarian failure on autosomal genes translocated to the X chromosome: a hypothesis. Hum Genet 121(3–4):441–450
22. Cools M, Drop SLS, Wolffenbuttel KP, Oosterhuis JW, Looijenga LHJ (2006) Germ cell tumors in the intersex gonad: Old paths, new directions, moving frontiers. Endocr Rev. 2006 Aug;27(5):468–484
23. Gravholt CH, Juul S, Naeraa RW, Hansen J (1998) Morbidity in Turner syndrome. J Clin Epidemiol 51(2):147–158
24. Price WH, Clayton JF, Collyer S, De Mey R, Wilson J (1986) Mortality ratios, life expectancy, and causes of death in patients with Turner's syndrome. J Epidemiol Community Health 40(2):97–102
25. Swerdlow AJ, Hermon C, Jacobs PA et al (2001) Mortality and cancer incidence in persons with numerical sex chromosome abnormalities: a cohort study. Ann Hum Genet 65(Pt 2):177–188
26. Wei F, Cheng S, Badie N et al (2001) A man who inherited his SRY gene and Leri-Weill dyschondrosteosis from his mother and neurofibromatosis type 1 from his father. Am J Med Genet 102(4):353–358
27. Landin-Wilhelmsen K, Bryman I, Hanson C, Hanson L (2004) Spontaneous pregnancies in a Turner syndrome woman with Y-chromosome mosaicism. J Assist Reprod Genet 21(6):229–230
28. Baena N, De Vigan C, Cariati E et al (2004) Turner syndrome: evaluation of prenatal diagnosis in 19 European registries. Am J Med Genet A 129(1):16–20
29. Hamamy HA, Dahoun S (2004) Parental decisions following the prenatal diagnosis of sex chromosome abnormalities. Eur J Obstet Gynecol Reprod Biol 116(1):58–62
30. Huang B, Thangavelu M, Bhatt S, Christiansen JS, Wang S (2002) Prenatal diagnosis of 45,X and 45,X mosaicism: the need for thorough cytogenetic and clinical evaluations. Prenat Diagn 22(2):105–110
31. Koeberl DD, McGillivray B, Sybert VP (1995) Prenatal diagnosis of 45,X/46, XX mosaicism and 45,X: implications for postnatal outcome. Am J Hum Genet 57(3):661–666
32. Gunther DF, Eugster E, Zagar AJ, Bryant CG, Davenport ML, Quigley CA (2004) Ascertainment bias in turner syndrome: new insights from girls who were diagnosed incidentally in prenatal life. Pediatrics 114(3):640–644
33. Loscalzo ML, Van PL, Ho VB et al (2005) Association between fetal lymphedema and congenital cardiovascular defects in turner syndrome. Pediatrics 115(3):732–735
34. Sachdev V, Matura LA, Sidenko S, Ho VB, Arai AE, Rosing DR, Bondy CA. Aortic valve disease in Turner syndrome. J Am Coll Cardiol. 2008 May 13;51(19): 1904–1909
35. Matura LA, Ho VB, Rosing DR, Bondy CA (2007) Aortic dilatation and dissection in Turner syndrome. Circulation 116(15):1663–1670
36. Ostberg JE, Donald AE, Halcox JPJ, Storry C, McCarthy C, Conway GS (2005) Vasculopathy in turner syndrome: arterial dilatation and intimal thickening without endothelial dysfunction. J Clin Endocrinol Metab 90(9):5161–5166
37. Carlson M, Silberbach M (2007) Dissection of the Aorta in Turner Syndrome: Two new cases and review of 85 cases in the literature. In:jmg.2007.052019
38. Lin AE, Lippe B, Rosenfeld RG (1998) Further delineation of aortic dilation, dissection, and rupture in patients with Turner syndrome. Pediatrics 102(1):e12
39. Gravholt CH, Landin-Wilhelmsen K, Stochholm K et al (2006) Clinical and epidemiological description of aortic dissection in Turner's syndrome. Cardiol Young 16(5):430–436
40. Matura LA, Ho VB, Rosing DR, Bondy CA (2007) Aortic dilatation and dissection in turner syndrome. In: CIRCULATIONAHA.106.685487
41. Nathwani NC, Unwin R, Brook CG, Hindmarsh PC (2000) The influence of renal and cardiovascular abnormalities on blood pressure in Turner syndrome. Clin Endocrinol (Oxford) 52(3):371–377
42. Liao AW, Snijders R, Geerts L, Spencer K, Nicolaides KH (2000) Fetal heart rate in chromosomally abnormal fetuses. Ultrasound Obstet Gynecol 16(7):610–613
43. Hyett JA, Noble PL, Snijders RJ, Montenegro N, Nicolaides KH (1996) Fetal heart rate in trisomy 21 and other chromosomal abnormalities at 10–14 weeks of gestation. Ultrasound Obstet Gynecol 7(4):239–244
44. Gravholt CH, Hansen KW, Erlandsen M, Ebbehoj E, Christiansen JS (2006) Nocturnal hypertension and impaired sympathovagal tone in Turner syndrome. J Hypertens 24(2):353–360
45. Bondy CA, Matura LA, Wooten N, Troendle J, Zinn AR, Bakalov VK (2007) The physical phenotype of girls and women with Turner syndrome is not X-imprinted. Hum Genet 121(3–4):469–474
46. Lippe B (1991) Turner syndrome. Endocrinol Metab Clin North Am 20(1):121–152
47. Boechat MI, Westra SJ, Lippe B (1996) Normal US appearance of ovaries and uterus in four patients with Turner's syndrome and 45, X karyotype. Pediatric Radiol 26(1):37–39
48. Rosenfield RL, Devine N, Hunold JJ, Mauras N, Moshang T Jr, Root AW (2005) Salutary Effects of Combining Early Very Low-Dose Systemic Estradiol with Growth Hormone Therapy in Girls with Turner Syndrome. J Clin Endocrinol Metab 90(12):6424–6430
49. Carel J-C, Ecosse E, Bastie-Sigeac I et al (2005) Quality of life determinants in young women with Turner's Syndrome after growth hormone treatment: Results of the StaTur Population-Based Cohort Study. J Clin Endocrinol Metab 90(4):1992–1997
50. Hogler W, Briody J, Moore B, Garnett S, Lu PW, Cowell CT (2004) Importance of estrogen on bone health in Turner syndrome: A Cross-Sectional and Longitudinal Study using dual-energy X-ray absorptiometry. J Clin Endocrinol Metab 89(1):193–199
51. van Pareren YK, de Muinck Keizer-Schrama SM, Stijnen T et al (2003) Final height in girls with turner syndrome after long-term growth hormone treatment in three dosages and low dose estrogens. J Clin Endocrinol Metab 88(3):1119–1125
52. Ankarberg-Lindgren C, Elfving M, Wikland KA, Norjavaara E (2001) Nocturnal application of transdermal estradiol patches produces levels of estradiol that mimic those seen at the onset of spontaneous puberty in girls. J Clin Endocrinol Metab 86(7):3039–3044
53. Soriano-Guillen L, Coste J, Ecosse E et al (2005) Adult height and pubertal growth in Turner syndrome after treatment with recombinant growth hormone. J Clin Endocrinol Metab:jc.2005–0470
54. Piippo S, Lenko H, Kainulainen P, Sipila I (2004) Use of percutaneous estrogen gel for induction of puberty in girls with Turner Syndrome. J Clin Endocrinol Metab 89(7):3241–3247
55. Hanton L, Axelrod L, Bakalov V, Bondy CA (2003) The importance of estrogen replacement in young women with Turner syndrome. J Womens Health (Larchmt) 12(10):971–977
56. Paterson WF, Hollman AS, Donaldson MD (2002) Poor uterine development in Turner syndrome with oral oestrogen therapy. Clin Endocrinol (Oxford) 56(3):359–365
57. Snajderova M, Mardesic T, Lebl J, Gerzova H, Teslik L, Zapletalova J; The uterine length in women with turner syndrome reflects the postmenarcheal daily estrogen dose. Czech National Study Group for HRT. Optimization in Paediatric and Adolescent Endocrinology and Gynaecology. Horm Res. 2003;60(4):198–204
58. Sampaolo P, Calcaterra V, Klersy C et al (2003) Pelvic ultrasound evaluation in patients with Turner syndrome during treatment with growth hormone. Ultrasound Obstet Gynecol 22(2):172–177
59. Doerr HG, Bettendorf M, Hauffa BP et al (2005) Uterine size in women with Turner syndrome after induction of puberty with estrogens and long-term growth hormone therapy: results of

the German IGLU Follow-up Study 2001. Hum Reprod 20(5):1418–1421
60. McDonnell CM, Coleman L, Zacharin MR (2003) A 3-year prospective study to assess uterine growth in girls with Turner's syndrome by pelvic ultrasound. Clin Endocrinol 58(4):446–450
61. Bakalov VK, Shawker T, Ceniceros I, Bondy CA (2007) Uterine development in Turner syndrome. J Pediatr 151(5):528–31, 31 e1
62. Scarabin P-Y, Oger E, Plu-Bureau G (2003) Differential association of oral and transdermal oestrogen-replacement therapy with venous thromboembolism risk. The Lancet 362(9382):428–432
63. Jobe S, Donohoue P, Di Paola J (2004) Deep venous thrombosis and Turner syndrome. J Pediatr Hematol Oncol 26(4):272
64. Donal E, Coisne D, Corbi P (2000) A case report of aortic arch mobile thrombi. Heart 84(6):614
65. Pinto RB, Silveira TR, Bandinelli E, Rohsig L (2004) Portal vein thrombosis in children and adolescents: The low prevalence of hereditary thrombophilic disorders. J Pediatr Surg 39(9):1356–1361
66. Gravholt CH, Svenstrup B, Bennett P, Sandahl Christiansen J (1999) Reduced androgen levels in adult turner syndrome: influence of female sex steroids and growth hormone status. Clin Endocrinol (Oxford) 50(6):791–800
67. Rovet JF (1993) The psychoeducational characteristics of children with Turner syndrome. J Learn Disabil 26(5):333–341
68. Ross JL, Roeltgen D, Kushner H, Wei F, Zinn AR (2000) The Turner syndrome-associated neurocognitive phenotype maps to distal Xp. Am J Hum Genet 67(3):672–681
69. Verlinde F, Massa G, Lagrou K et al (2004) Health and psychosocial status of patients with turner syndrome after transition to adulthood: the Belgian experience. Horm Res 62(4):161–167
70. Okada Y (1994) The quality of life of Turner women in comparison with grown-up GH-deficient women. Endocr J 41(4):345–354
71. Boman UW, Moller A, Albertsson-Wikland K (1998) Psychological aspects of Turner syndrome. J Psychosom Obstet Gynaecol 19(1):1–18
72. Cardoso G, Daly R, Haq NA et al (2004) Current and lifetime psychiatric illness in women with Turner syndrome. Gynecol Endocrinol 19(6):313–319
73. Schmidt PJ, Cardoso GMP, Ross JL, Haq N, Rubinow DR, Bondy CA (2006) Shyness, social anxiety, and impaired self-esteem in turner syndrome and premature ovarian failure. JAMA 295(12):1374–1376
74. Sutton EJ, McInerney-Leo A, Bondy CA, Gollust SE, King D, Biesecker B (2005) Turner syndrome: four challenges across the lifespan. Am J Med Genet A 139(2):57–66
75. Pavlidis K, McCauley E, Sybert VP (1995) Psychosocial and sexual functioning in women with Turner syndrome. Clin Genet 47(2):85–89
76. Carel J-C, Elie C, Ecosse E et al (2006) Self-esteem and social adjustment in young women with Turner syndrome – influence of pubertal management and sexuality: population-based cohort study. J Clin Endocrinol Metab:jc.2005–652
77. Sheaffer A, Lange E, Bondy CA (2008) Sexual function in women with Turner syndrome. J Women's Health (Larchmt). 2008 Jan-Feb;17(1):27–33
78. Sutton E YJ, Bondy CA, Biesecker B (2006) Turner syndrome; four challenges across the lifespan. Am J Med Genet A. 2005 Dec 1;139A(2):57–66
79. Sutton EJ, Young J, McInerney-Leo A, Bondy CA, Gollust SE, Biesecker BB (2006) Truth-telling and Turner syndrome: the importance of diagnostic disclosure. J Pediatr 148(1):102–107
80. Birkebaek NH, Cruger D, Hansen J, Nielsen J, Bruun-Petersen G (2002) Fertility and pregnancy outcome in Danish women with Turner syndrome. Clin Genet 61(1):35–39
81. Cools M, Rooman RPA, Wauters J, Jacqemyn Y, Du Caju MVL (2004) A nonmosaic 45, X karyotype in a mother with Turner's syndrome and in her daughter. Fertil Steril 82(4):923–925
82. Landin-Wilhelmsen K, Bryman I, Hanson C, Hanson L (2004) Short communication: spontaneous pregnancies in a turner syndrome woman with Y-chromosome mosaicism. J Assist Reprod Genet 21(6):229–230
83. Livadas S, Xekouki P, Kafiri G, Voutetakis A, Maniati-Christidi M, Dacou-Voutetakis C (2005) Spontaneous pregnancy and birth of a normal female from a woman with Turner syndrome and elevated gonadotropins. Fertil Steril 83(3):769–772
84. Hovatta O (1999) Pregnancies in women with Turner's syndrome. Ann Med 31(2):106–110
85. Foudila T, Soderstrom-Anttila V, Hovatta O (1999) Turner's syndrome and pregnancies after oocyte donation. Hum Reprod 14(2):532–535
86. Karnis MF, Zimon AE, Lalwani SI, Timmreck LS, Klipstein S, Reindollar RH (2003) Risk of death in pregnancy achieved through oocyte donation in patients with Turner syndrome: a national survey. Fertil Steril 80(3):498–501
87. The Practice Committee of the American Society for Reproductive M (2005) Increased maternal cardiovascular mortality associated with pregnancy in women with Turner syndrome. Fertil Steril 83(4):1074–1075
88. Elsheikh M, Dunger DB, Conway GS, Wass JA (2002) Turner's syndrome in adulthood. Endocr Rev 23(1):120–140
89. Elsheikh M, Wass JAH, Conway GS (2001) Autoimmune thyroid syndrome in women with Turner's syndrome the association with karyotype. Clin Endocrinol 55(2):223–226
90. Bonamico M, Pasquino AM, Mariani P et al (2002) Prevalence and clinical picture of celiac disease in turner syndrome. J Clin Endocrinol Metab 87(12):5495–5498
91. Price WH (1979) A high incidence of chronic inflammatory bowel disease in patients with Turner's syndrome. J Med Genet 16(4):263–266
92. Zulian F, Schumacher HR, Calore A, Goldsmith DP, Athreya BH (1998) Juvenile arthritis in Turner's syndrome: a multicenter study. Clin Exp Rheumatol 16(4):489–494
93. Elsheikh M, Hodgson HJ, Wass JA, Conway GS (2001) Hormone replacement therapy may improve hepatic function in women with Turner's syndrome. Clin Endocrinol (Oxford) 55(2):227–231
94. Roulot D, Degott C, Chazouilleres O et al (2004) Vascular involvement of the liver in Turner's syndrome. Hepatology 39(1):239–247
95. Gravholt CH, Naeraa RW, Fisker S, Christiansen JS (1997) Body composition and physical fitness are major determinants of the growth hormone-insulin-like growth factor axis aberrations in adult turner's syndrome, with important modulations by treatment with 17{beta}-estradiol. J Clin Endocrinol Metab 82(8):2570–2577
96. Elsheikh M, Conway GS (1998) The impact of obesity on cardiovascular risk factors in Turner's syndrome. Clin Endocrinol (Oxford) 49(4):447–450
97. Corrigan EC, Nelson LM, Bakalov VK et al (2006) Effects of ovarian failure and X-chromosome deletion on body composition and insulin sensitivity in young women. Menopause 13(6):911–916
98. Van PL, Bakalov VK, Zinn AR, Bondy CA (2006) Maternal X chromosome, visceral adiposity, and lipid profile. JAMA 295(12):1373–1374
99. Bakalov VK, Cooley MM, Quon MJ et al (2004) Impaired insulin secretion in the Turner metabolic syndrome. J Clin Endocrinol Metab 89(7):3516–3520
100. Ostberg JE, Attar MJH, Mohamed-Ali V, Conway GS (2005) Adipokine dysregulation in turner syndrome: comparison of circulating interleukin-6 and leptin concentrations with measures of adiposity and C-reactive protein. J Clin Endocrinol Metab 90(5):2948–2953
101. Bakalov V, Chen M, Baron J et al (2003) Bone mineral density and fractures in Turner syndrome. Am J Med 115(4):257–262
102. Bakalov VK, Axelrod L, Baron J et al (2003) Selective reduction in cortical bone mineral density in turner syndrome independent

of ovarian hormone deficiency. J Clin Endocrinol Metab 88(12):5717–5722
103. Bechtold S, Rauch F, Noelle V et al (2001) Musculoskeletal analyses of the forearm in young women with Turner syndrome: a study using peripheral quantitative computed tomography. J Clin Endocrinol Metab 86(12):5819–5823
104. Gravholt CH, Vestergaard P, Hermann AP, Mosekilde L, Brixen K, Christiansen JS (2003) Increased fracture rates in Turner's syndrome: a nationwide questionnaire survey. Clin Endocrinol (Oxford) 59(1):89–96
105. Cosman F, Nieves J, Zion M, Woelfert L, Luckey M, Lindsay R (2005) Daily and cyclic parathyroid hormone in women receiving alendronate. N Engl J Med 353(6):566–575
106. Ueland T (2004) Bone metabolism in relation to alterations in systemic growth hormone. Growth Horm IGF Res 14(6):404–17

Chapter 20
Errors in Chromosome Segregation During Oogenesis and Early Embryogenesis

Maj Hultén, Edward Smith, and Joy Delhanty

Abstract Errors in chromosome segregation occurring during human oogenesis and early embryogenesis are very common. Meiotic chromosome development during oogenesis is subdivided into three distinct phases. The crucial events, including meiotic chromosome pairing and recombination, take place from around 11 weeks until birth. Oogenesis is then arrested until ovulation, when the first meiotic division takes place, with the second meiotic division not completed until after fertilization. It is generally accepted that most aneuploid fetal conditions, such as trisomy 21 Down syndrome, are due to maternal chromosome segregation errors. The underlying reasons are not yet fully understood. It is also clear that superimposed on the maternal meiotic chromosome segregation errors, there are a large number of mitotic errors taking place post-zygotically during the first few cell divisions in the embryo. In this chapter, we summarise current knowledge of errors in chromosome segregation during oogenesis and early embryogenesis, with special reference to the clinical implications for successful assisted reproduction.

Keywords Oogenesis • Embryogenesis • Chromosome segregation • Nondisjunction • Meiotic recombination • MLH1 • Crossing-over • Chiasma • Aneuploidy

M. Hultén (✉)
Warwick Medical School, University of Warwick, Coventry CV4 7AL, Coventry, England
e-mail: maj.hulten@warwick.ac.uk

E. Smith
Department of Biological Sciences, University of Warwick, Coventry, England

J. Delhanty
UCL Centre for PGD, Obstetrics & Gynecology, University College London, Gower Street, London, England

20.1 Introduction

20.1.1 Meiosis

Meiosis, derived from the Greek for diminution, means to halve. The process of meiosis halves the chromosome number of a diploid cell during gametogenesis, producing haploid gametes. This involves two cell divisions (meiosis I and meiosis II; Fig. 20.1, Table 20.1) without an intermediate DNA replication step. The first of these meiotic cell divisions is reductional, i.e., the chromosome complement of a diploid oogonial cell/primary oocyte is halved leading to haploid secondary oocytes. During the second meiotic division, chromatids separate in the same way as in mitosis, thus the chromosome number is not changed (Table 20.1). Fusion of a haploid sperm cell and a haploid oocyte at fertilization restores the somatic diploid chromosome number.

The process of meiosis is evolutionarily conserved from yeast to man, though with marked differences between sexes of the same species and between different species.

20.1.2 Differences in the Meiotic Process Between the Human Male and Female

There are drastic differences in the meiotic process between human males and females (Table 20.2). In particular, the timing of events, the numbers of gametes produced and the level of chromosome abnormalities in sperm compared to oocytes are very different.

20.1.2.1 Timing of Meiotic Events

In the human male, the testicular premeiotic spermatogonia start dividing mitotically at puberty. The meiotic process, including the reductional division at meiosis I, the equa-

D.T. Carrell and C.M. Peterson (eds.), *Reproductive Endocrinology and Infertility: Integrating Modern Clinical and Laboratory Practice*, DOI 10.1007/978-1-4419-1436-1_20, © Springer Science+Business Media, LLC 2010

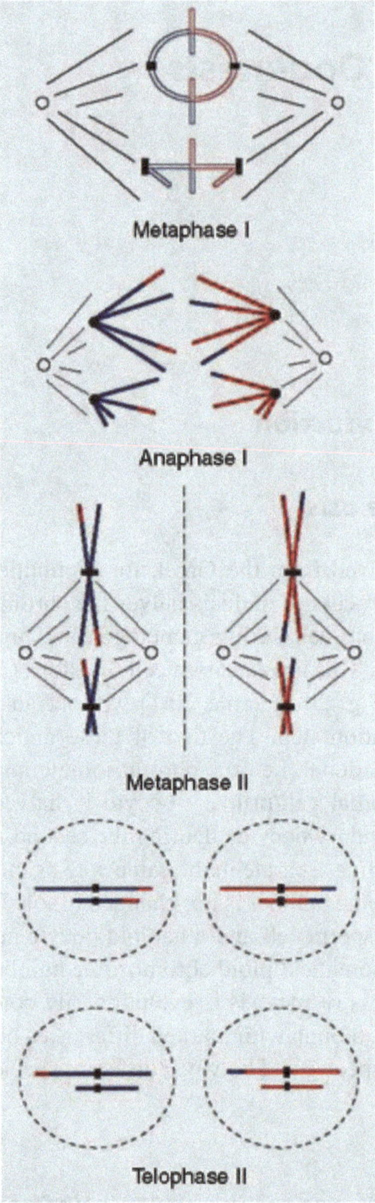

Fig. 20.1 Schematic illustration of meiosis, where following homologous chromosome synapsis, and crossing-over at the Pachytene stage of prophase I, the derivative bivalents at metaphase I progress to metaphase to anaphase I, metaphase II to anaphase II, and telophase II showing the four potential haploid gametes

tional division at meiosis II followed by maturation of spermatids to spermatozoa is ongoing in the testes throughout life. In the human female, however, meiosis is subdivided into three separate stages. The first part of meiosis I, i.e., prophase I (Table 20.1), takes place in fetal ovaries and continues until birth, at which time meiosis is arrested, and is not continued until ovulation. The second part of the reductional division of meiosis I takes place just before ovulation, and the process continues into the second meiotic division. Meiosis is then arrested again, at the metaphase II (MII) stage (Table 20.1). The anaphase and telophase stages of the second meiotic division are not completed until after the oocyte has been penetrated by the spermatozoon at fertilization.

The study of the meiotic chromosome behavior in human males is much more advanced than that in females, as the difference in timing of meiosis between the sexes means it is much easier to obtain tissue material from males. Testicular biopsies of post-pubertal men have yielded large amounts of data. However, in females, biopsies of fetal ovaries, individual oocytes at the metaphase I (MI) stage (prior to ovulation) and individual oocytes arrested at the MII stage (post-ovulation and pre-fertilization) are scarce and difficult to obtain for study. Accordingly, a large body of knowledge has accumulated over the last 40 years or so, of the meiotic chromosome behavior of normally fertile men and those with reproductive problems (see Chap. 22). The situation is very different in the human female. It is only within the last decade that technology has been developed to allow the relevant investigations of chromosome behaviour in fetal ovaries and the meiotic divisional stages occurring at ovulation and following fertilisation. Meiotic investigations of chromosome behaviour in human fetal ovaries have been performed by few research groups, while chromosome analysis of the meiosis divisional stages has primarily been undertaken as research projects within a number of Assisted Conception Units.

20.1.2.2 Frequency of Gametes Produced

With respect to availability of material for study, it should also be noted that there are incredible differences in gamete production between sexes. There are normally at least 300 million spermatozoa produced daily in post-pubertal human males, which stands in sharp contrast to the meager production of around 300–400 oocytes in the lifetime of human females.

20.1.2.3 Incidence of Meiotic Chromosome Errors

For reasons not yet fully understood, errors in meiotic chromosome behaviour giving rise to aneuploidy in offspring are more common in the human female than in the male. Remarkably, these errors are much more common in the human female than in any other species investigated to date. The reason for this species difference also remains unknown and requires further study.

Table 20.1 Features and timing of meiotic stages in oogenesis (adapted from Hultén et al. [65])

		Stage	Subdivision	Features
Fetal Development	Meiosis I	Prophase I		DNA replication of each chromosome produce sister chromatids joined at the centromere
			Leptotene	Chromosome condensation begins, formation of the lateral elements of the synaptonemal complex
			Zygotene	Chromosomes pair, completion of the synaptonemal complex
			Pachytene	Chromosomes fully paired, crossing-over completed and chiasmata fully established
			Diplotene	Initiation of separation of the synapsed chromosomes, meiosis arrested at this stage until ovulation
Adolescence ovulation		Prometaphase I	Diakinesis	Chromosomes condense and separate, except at chiasma sites
		Metaphase I		Homologous chromosomes align on the equatorial plate, the kinetochores attach to the spindles
		Anaphase I		Homologous pairs separate, sister chromatids remain together
		Telophase I		Two daughter cells form
	Meiosis II	Prophase II		Nuclear envelope dissolves, new spindle created
		Metaphase II		Chromosomes align on the spindle
Fertilization		Anaphase II		Centromeres separate, sister chromatids migrate to opposite poles
		Telophase II		Cell division results in four potential haploid gametes from each parent cell

Table 20.2 Main differences between oogenesis and spermatogenesis (adapted from Hultén et al. [65])

Oogenesis	Spermatogenesis
Can take over 40 years, few oocytes progress to the final stages, most are lost before birth	Continuous process from puberty throughout life
Two unequal cell divisions with most cytoplasm retained in the oocyte and only a minor part forming the first and second PBs. Thus only one mature egg is produced from each parent cell	All divisions are equal and each parent cell produces four gametes
Oocyte numbers appear to be limited to those present at birth, with approximately 350 ovulating between puberty and the menopause	Continual supply of gametes
Interstitial initiation of chromosome synapsis is more common	Chromosome synapsis is initiated telomerically
Poor efficiency of obligate chiasma formation	Efficient obligate chiasma formation
Higher chiasma frequency	Lower chiasma frequency
Synaptonemal complexes are relatively decondensed, associated with higher chiasma frequency	Condensed synaptonemal complexes, associated with lower chiasma frequency

20.1.3 Content of this Chapter

In this chapter, we will summarise current knowledge of errors in chromosome segregation during oogenesis and early embryogenesis, with special reference to the clinical implications for successful assisted reproduction. The main problems occurring during oogenesis are: (a) errors in meiotic chromosome pairing and recombination at the meiosis I prophase; (b) insufficient elimination of chromosomally abnormal oocytes during the meiotic chromosome pairing stage; and (c) abnormalities in segregation of chromosomes at the anaphase I (AI) and anaphase II (AII) stages. The first two of these problems may be investigated in fetal ovaries, while the segregation errors can only be analyzed on isolated oocytes at the MI stage captured at ovulation and when arrested at the following MII stage. Crucial information may also be obtained by investigation of the results of AI chromosome segregation, i.e., the secondary oocyte and the first polar body (PB). As evidenced from the analysis of chromosome constitution in early embryos, there is also a high frequency of post-zygotic mitotic chromosome segregation errors.

20.2 Investigation of Meiotic Chromosome Behaviour in Fetal Ovaries

Primordial germ cells are the gametic precursors. Around the fifth week of pregnancy, they migrate to the area of the genital ridge. Subsequently, sexual differentiation occurs and, in females, ovarian development begins. Oogonia, the precursors of oocytes, increase in number following cellular division to become oocytes. The proliferation of cells is then arrested and the oocytes begin the first stages of meiosis at around 10–11 weeks of gestation, which continues until birth (Fig. 20.2) [1]. It is at the prophase of the first meiotic cell division (Table 20.1) during this early fetal developmental stage, that the crucial events of crossing-over, chiasma for-

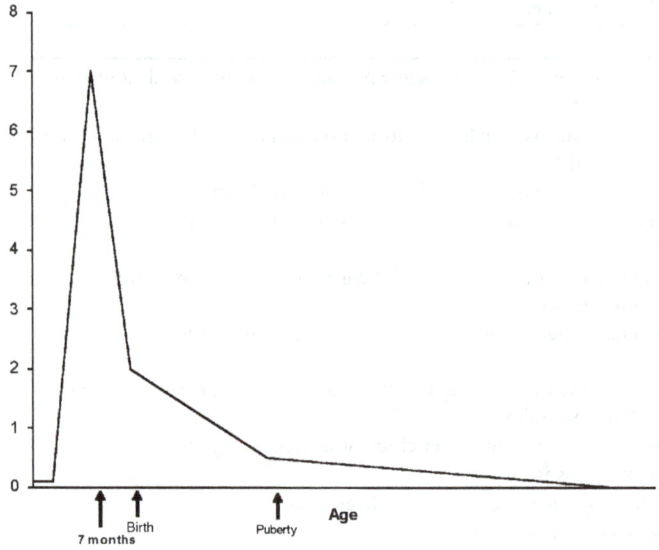

Fig. 20.2 Changes in human oocyte number (million) during prenatal and postnatal development. There is a very rapid increase in human female germ cell (oocyte) number early during fetal development with a peak at 7 months gestational age, followed by a relatively rapid decline before birth and postnatally before puberty, but a slower depletion during reproductive years until menopause

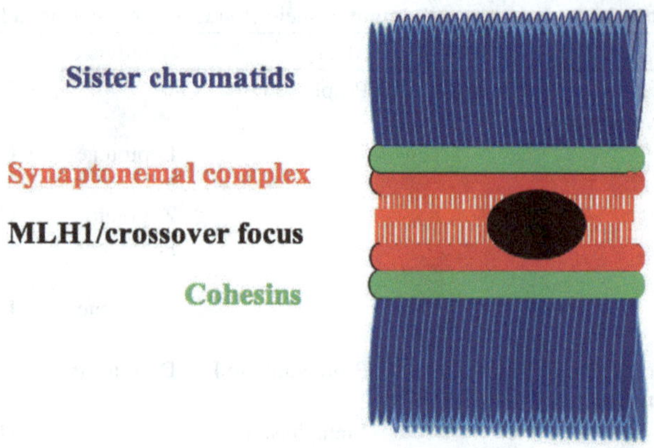

Fig. 20.3 Schematic illustration of the proteinaceous Synaptonemal Complex (SC). During meiosis I, taking place in fetal oocytes, the two homologues are paired along their entire length, held together by a number of meiosis-specific proteins (*cohesins, blue and red*). The process of crossing-over (*black dot*) takes place within the center of the SC. Note that most of the chromatin (*blue*) is not exposed within the SC

mation and recombination of parental alleles take place. As human fetal ovarian material is difficult to obtain, less knowledge is available from direct microscopy analysis of crossing-over, chiasma formation and recombination in the human female than in the male. Nevertheless, both direct investigation of fetal ovarian oocytes and indirect studies of recombination by family linkage analysis have demonstrated that meiotic recombination errors, leading to aneuploid oocytes, are common in the human female.

It is important to note that the meiotic recombination process in oocytes can be studied in three very different ways, depending on their stage of maturation. First, crossover frequency and distribution along the lengths of individual chromosomes can be identified in fetal oocytes by analysis of the meiotic chromosome pairing structure, the synaptonemal complex (SC) using immunofluorescence against recombination proteins [2–6]. Second, there is the potential to identify crossover frequency and distribution in the form of chiasmata at the MI stage [7]. Third, it is also possible to estimate crossover frequency and distribution indirectly by family linkage analysis [8–10].

20.2.1 Analysis of Meiotic Crossovers in Fetal Oocytes

Meiosis in fetal oocytes starts with pairing of the maternal and paternal homologous chromosomes along their entire length. This pairing is mediated by a meiosis-specific protein structure, the Synaptonemal Complex (SC; Fig. 20.3). Meiotic crossover points may be directly visualized by immuno-fluorescence microscopy analysis of the SC in fetal oocytes from around 12 to 24 weeks' gestational age. The visualization of the crossover/chiasma/recombination points has been made possible by the use of (commercially available) antibodies against the recombination proteins MLH1 and MLH3 (Fig. 20.4).

20.2.2 Oocyte Crossover Patterns

Meiotic crossover patterns in human fetal oocytes can vary significantly [2–6; Cheng et al 2009]. In a study of 95 oocytes from one fetus, a mean of 70.3 (range 48–102) recombination events per oocyte were detected. Chromosomes lacking a recombination focus altogether were also described [4]. A more detailed analysis indicated that fetal oocytes with defects in the formation of the SCs, such as incomplete pairing or breakage, were predisposed to recombination deficiency [4]. A study of 131 oocytes from nine cases [3] also described large variation between individual cases (range 10–107). It was concluded that if such variability persisted throughout development and into adulthood, that as many as 30% of human oocytes would be predisposed to aneuploidy, i.e., an abnormal chromosome number [3]. This is because the bivalents would lack a crossover site between the maternal and paternal homologues leading to the absence of a chiasma, which would normally hold them physically together at MI. Thus, the maternal and paternal chromosomes would not be able to orient stably at the metaphase plate in relation to

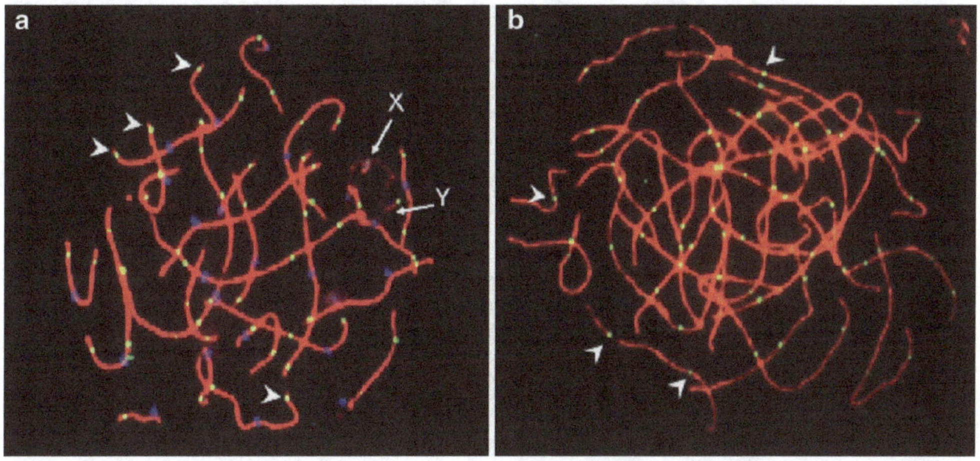

Fig. 20.4 Imaging the Synaptonemal Complex (SC) in a spermatocyte (**a**) and an oocyte (**b**) MLH1 foci are seen in yellow, the centromeres in the spermatocyte in magenta, and the SCs by SYCP3 staining in red. Note that the chromosome pairs (*bivalents*) are shorter in the spermatocyte than in the oocyte; and there are also a lower number of MLH1 foci/crossover points/chiasmata/recombination foci

the spindles, an obligatory mechanical requirement for the normal reductional chromosome segregation at AI. (Fig. 20.5a). Instead they would be expected to segregate randomly at AI (Fig. 20.5b). By chance, 50% of the two daughter cells, i.e., the secondary oocyte and the first PB would then contain both maternal and paternal chromosomes, while the remaining 50% would contain neither. Thus, if the original bivalent had been "achiasmatic" the secondary oocyte and the corresponding first PB would be expected to be aneuploid in 50% of cases. There is also the possibility that the half chromosomes (chromatids) of an unpaired chromosome (univalent) would segregate in the same way as at mitosis, leading to an extra chromatid in either the secondary oocyte or the first PB (Fig. 20.5c).

20.2.3 Natural Elimination of Abnormalities

The majority of fetal oocytes are eliminated during fetal and postnatal life, with only a small minority reaching ovulation and thus meiotic MI–AI stages (Fig. 20.2). There is evidence to suggest that natural selection against oocytes containing abnormalities in homologous chromosome pairing and crossing-over takes place during fetal development, leading to delay in their maturation or deletion by atresia and apoptosis [4]. This type of selection may also continue after birth until the onset of ovulation in adulthood. There is a paucity of data describing patterns of recombination in immature oocytes, comprising the ovarian reserve in adult women. These data could be obtained by analysis of chiasmata at the MI stage, as has been performed in spermatocytes (Fig. 20.6a). However, the scarcity of oocyte material available for study, combined with the limited clarity of chiasmata in oocytes compared to spermatocytes at this stage (Fig. 20.6b) [7] still presents challenges for obtaining this information. Chiasma analysis at the MI stage would also allow evaluation of the extent of delay and elimination by atresia and apoptosis oocytes exhibiting crossover errors during oocyte maturation from fetal life to adulthood.

20.3 Meiotic Crossover Errors Detected by Family Linkage Analysis

Meiotic crossover errors in the human female have also been investigated indirectly by linkage analysis, using DNA samples from both parents and children [8, 9]. Patterns of allelic recombination are then determined by using DNA markers along the length of individual chromosomes, including the chromosomes for which aneuploidy is common: 21 (Down syndrome), 18 (Edwards syndrome), 13 (Patau syndrome) and the sex chromosomes X and Y (e.g., Klinefelter and Turner syndromes). These studies have demonstrated that the outstanding majority of autosomal trisomies originate from recombination errors taking place during maternal oogenesis. However, errors in parental oogenesis as well as spermatogenesis give rise to the Klinefelter and XXX syndromes.

20.3.1 Linkage Analysis of Trisomy 21

It has been concluded from linkage analysis of families with a case of Down syndrome that lack of recombination during

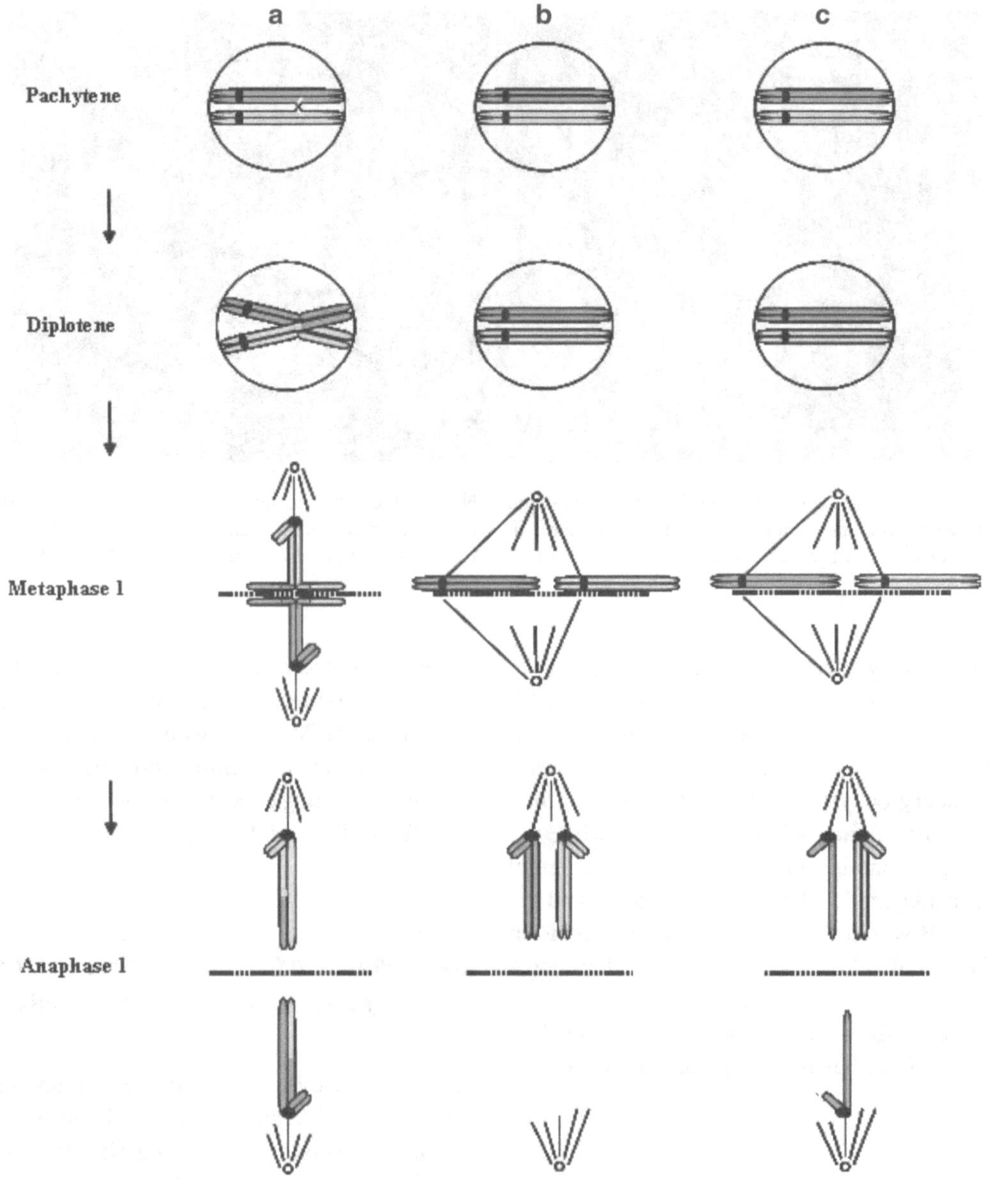

Fig. 20.5 Cartoon illustrating the different types of meiosis I segregation that may take place in a normal disomy 21 oocyte. (**a**) Normal chromosome pairing and crossing-over, attachment of the movement centers (kinetochores) at metaphase 1 and separation at anaphase 1. (**b**) Lack of crossing-over and chiasma formation may lead to primary nondisjunction at anaphase 1. (**c**) Lack of a chiasma can also lead to the same type of segregation at anaphase 1 as during mitosis (precocious meiotic disjunction). (Printed with permission from Hulten et al., Molecular Cytogenetics 2008, 1:21. doi:10.1186/1755-8166-1-21)

maternal oogenesis account for approximately half of all cases associated with chromosome nondisjunction at AI. Aberrant positioning of chiasmata (more distal or proximal than normal) on the long arm of chromosome 21 has also been detected and identified as a putative causal factor [8, 9]. Much effort has gone into explaining why such positioning would increase the risk for nondisjunction at AI [8–10]. The mechanism underlying this process remains to be elucidated; however, it should be noted that the same distal chiasma site on chromosome 21 is prevalent in human males and is not associated with a high rate of nondisjunction.

It was initially thought that the well-known maternal age effect in risk of having a child with Down syndrome (Fig. 20.7) was due to changes in patterns of maternal meiotic recombination. More recently, it has been clearly demonstrated that this is not the case, and a so-called two-hit hypothesis has been suggested to explain the maternal age affect. This postulates that bivalents with the vulnerable chiasmata positions are less readily handled by the AI machinery as women grow older. It has been suggested that one explanation could be age-related impairment of the binding of homologous grandparental chromosomes by the protein cohesin, with an

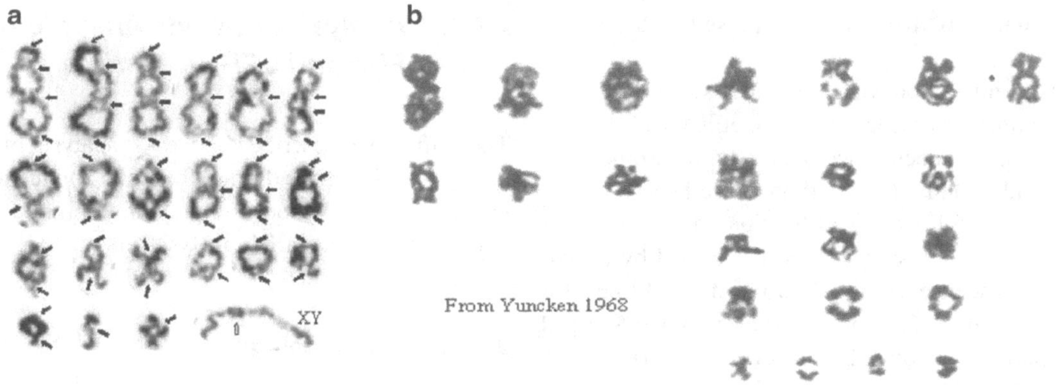

Fig. 20.6 Chromosomes at metaphase I in a spermatocyte (**a**), and an oocyte (**b**), Chiasmata can be reliably identified and counted in the spermatocyte, but this presents more difficulty in the oocyte

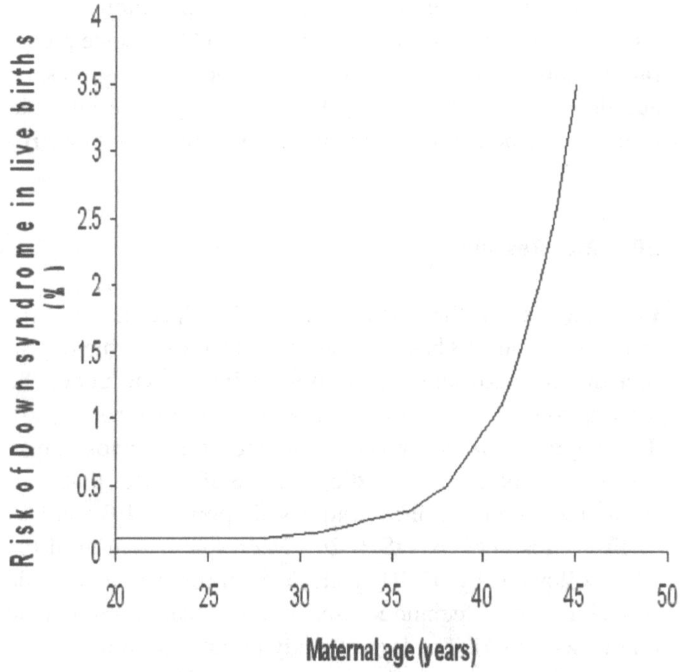

Fig. 20.7 Birth rate of T21 in relation to maternal age. The so-called maternal age effect was first recognized by Penrose in 1934, and has since been seen without much variation in different countries around the world

increased risk for primary nondisjunction of the two chromosomes 21 at AI (Fig. 20.5b, c) [10]. Most recently, it has been suggested that the maternal age effect is a multifactorial trait, and may be influenced by environmental factors [8, 9]. Another intriguing possibility is that normal women may be trisomy 21 ovarian mosaics [11–13] with the potential for oocytes containing three chromosomes 21 accumulating during maturation and when reaching MI undergoing obligatory secondary nondisjunction at AI (Hultén et al 2009).

20.3.2 Linkage Analyses of Trisomy 13 and 18

There are few data concerning trisomy 13 (Patau syndrome) and the genetic errors that can cause it. However, a recent study of 78 cases [14] indicated that over 90% of cases are due to maternal meiotic errors, with approximately one-third of these occurring at AII. This demonstrates some similarity to trisomy 18 in that a large proportion of these cases appear to arise predominantly because of errors at AII. Though, as the authors describe, the only similarity between chromosomes 13 and 18 is that they are gene poor, and any specific, potentially causative, genomic features have yet to be identified; if indeed there is a common cause of both trisomies [14].

20.4 Direct Evaluation of Oocyte Aneuploidy

To date (as far as the authors are aware), there have been no detailed studies evaluating exact oocyte aneuploidy rates in MI oocytes. However, numerous investigations have been performed on MII oocytes [15–17], obtained as immature MII oocytes or oocytes that have failed to fertilize. These studies have demonstrated that segregation errors involving both whole chromosomes and chromatids are common [18]. The material investigated consists almost exclusively of MII oocytes obtained at infertility treatment clinics, where spare oocytes, spontaneously arrested at MII, have been donated for research. However, the various stimulation regimes necessary for in vitro fertilization (IVF) do not appear to affect the chromosome constitution of the oocyte, as oocytes obtained from natural cycles show similar frequency of anomalies [19, 20]. Furthermore, the eggs that remain unfertilized after exposure to sperm are not cytogenetically different from those that are fertilized [21].

Thousands of human oocytes at the MII stage have been investigated to obtain information on the efficacy of AI segregation as well as the occurrence of structural chromosome aberrations. Traditionally, two methods have been used for analysis of oocytes, following cell fixation on a microscope slide. Chromosome analysis has been performed by karyotyping and fluorescence in situ hybridization (FISH) for selected chromosomes. Recently, however, a DNA-based method, comparative genomic hybridization (CGH) has also been used to investigate oocyte aneuploidy.

20.4.1 Analysis of Oocyte Aneuploidy by Karyotyping

20.4.1.1 Methodology

Karyotyping involves spreading and fixing a single cell on a microscope slide, followed by staining and microscopy analysis. However, use of a single cell risks the loss of one or more chromosomes, and their contracted nature does not allow for the use of conventional G-banding techniques for exact identification of individual chromosomes. Indeed, a large-scale study of unfertilized human oocytes only resulted in the successful analysis of 45.9% of samples [22].

20.4.1.2 Results

In the most recent, large-scale karyotyping study of 1,397 oocytes from 792 patients (mean age 33.7 ± 4.7 years), numerical abnormalities were detected in 20.1% of samples. The majority of these were due to extra or missing whole chromosomes or chromatids, whereas structural abnormalities (breaks, deletions, and acentric fragments) were rarer, only detected in 2.1% of cells. Numerical abnormalities caused by extra or missing chromatids were more common than aneuploidy of whole chromosomes, confirming the hypothesis that AI segregation errors of chromatids are common in human oocytes obtained through IVF studies (Fig. 20.5c) [23]. Although aneuploidy was detected in all chromosomes, the distribution was skewed toward a significantly higher frequency in the physically smallest autosomes (chromosomes 13–22); a result that has been confirmed in further studies [15, 24], irrespective of the method used.

A strong positive correlation between maternal age and rate of aneuploidy was also detected [22]. The same effect has been observed in a sample of fresh oocytes (not stimulated by hormone injections as part of IVF treatment) investigated using spectral chromosomal analysis [25].

20.4.2 Analysis of Oocyte Aneuploidy Using Fish and CGH

The difficulties described above for analysis of oocyte aneuploidy have led to the development and application of molecular cytogenetic methods: initially, multiprobe fluorescence in situ hybridization (FISH) analysis and more recently CGH.

20.4.2.1 Methodology

Similar to karyotyping, a set of FISH probes designed to hybridize to specific chromosomal regions are incubated with a cell, spread on a microscope slide. The probes are labelled, e.g., with a red or green fluorophore, and after incubation, the slides are washed and the results observed and recorded with the use of a fluorescent microscope. The application of FISH with chromosome-specific DNA probes to MII oocyte preparations allows the identification of specific chromosomes; an additional advantage of using FISH is that precise information can also be obtained from the chromatin of the first PB.

20.4.2.2 Results

FISH analysis of the first PB with probes specific for chromosomes X and 18 has been demonstrated to be able to predict the chromosome constitution of the oocyte under the assumption that the loss and gain will be reciprocal [16]. This approach has since been developed for diagnostic purposes, with the aim of avoiding the use of oocytes that have been predicted to be aneuploid based upon first PB analysis of five autosomes by FISH [26]. Micromanipulation of the PBs followed by FISH with 3–5 chromosome-specific probes is now a technique used in preimplantation genetic diagnosis (PGD). The largest study to date examined 6,733 oocytes from women above the age of 35 (average 38.5 years), and a large proportion of oocytes were aneuploid with respect to the chromosomes tested (13, 15, 18, 21 and 22) [27]. In total, 41.7% of oocytes were considered to be aneuploid because of AI malsegregation, the majority involving chromatids rather than whole chromosomes. Loss of a chromatid from the first PB was the most common anomaly scored, but it should be noted that technical FISH error could also produce this result.

Several researchers have used multiprobe FISH to analyze MII oocytes and the associated first PBs [15, 17, 28]. A number of interesting features have emerged from these studies. In agreement with karyotyping studies, anomalies were not randomly distributed between the chromosomes. The smaller chromosomes, 13, 16, 18, 21 and X were most frequently aneuploid, with no anomalies detected for chro-

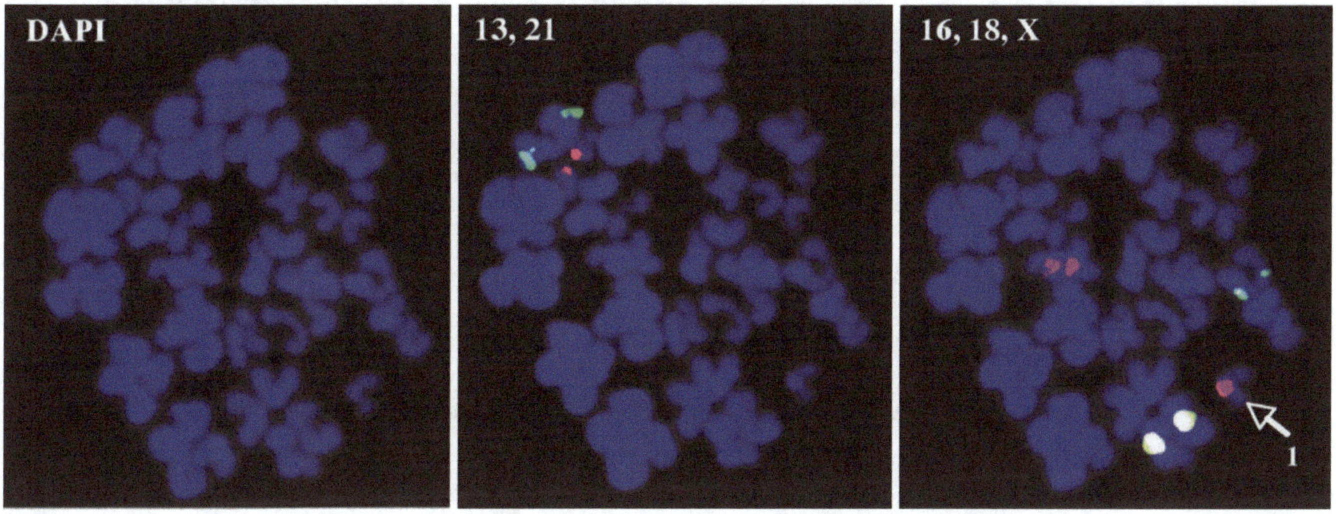

Fig. 20.8 FISH analysis of an MII oocyte to show an extra chromatid 16. Chromosomes are stained with DAPI and successively hybridized to probes for chromosomes 13 and 21, then 16, 18 and the X. (Reproduced with permission from Mahmood et al. 2000, Hum Genet 10:620–626; Copyright Springer Verlag Ltd)

mosomes 1, 9 or 12 (Fig. 20.8). In addition, analysis of an MII oocyte and its corresponding first PB revealed a previously not well-recognized mechanism leading to aneuploid gametes. In two cases, an extra chromosome was detected in the first PB with no accompanying loss in the MII oocyte; and in a third case, extra chromatids were present in both the MII oocyte and the first PB [17]. All three of these mature eggs must have been derived from cells that were trisomic for the chromosomes involved (13 and 21) when entering meiosis during fetal life. Without further investigation, it is not possible to determine whether this preexisting aneuploidy arose during the premeiotic divisions (germinal mosaicism) or if it was present in the embryonic gonad (gonadal mosaicism). The first instance of gonadal mosaicism cytogenetically proven this way was reported in a woman who had had three previous conceptions with trisomy 21 and for whom PGD was performed. FISH analysis of unfertilized MII oocytes and corresponding first PBs proved that ovarian mosaicism was the cause of the abnormal conceptions (see also Table 2 in Hultén et al. [12, 29].

20.4.3 Analysis of Oocyte Aneuploidy Using CGH

20.4.3.1 Methodology

To obtain an accurate estimate of aneuploidy in human oocytes requires a method that does not involve the spreading of chromosomes on a slide. A DNA-based method, such as CGH, is appropriate, but for single cell analysis the DNA must first be amplified from the 6–10 picograms initially present to the 200 nanograms required. DNA from a small number of cells from a chromosomally normal control source is similarly amplified, test and control DNAs are then labeled with red or green fluorochromes, respectively, and co-hybridized to prepared slides of normal male metaphase chromosomes, which act as indicators (Fig. 20.9). The two DNAs compete for hybridization sites allowing differences in the number of copies of any of the chromosomes to be detected by analysis of the green:red ratio along each indicator chromosome on the slide (Fig. 20.10). The approach of using CGH analysis to acquire data on aneuploidy in human oocytes has been validated by several recent studies [24, 30–34].

20.4.3.2 Results

As the first PB and the MII oocyte are reciprocal products of the first meiotic division, analysis of one of these cells should predict the chromosome constitution of the other, although there are exceptions as in cases of germinal or gonadal mosaicism, where there is preexisting aneuploidy in the oocyte. The first PB CGH approach has been applied in both clinical practice and research projects, providing an indirect means of assessing oocytes for aneuploidy involving any chromosome. As regards IVF treatment, the aim is the identification and transfer of embryos derived from chromosomally normal oocytes, which are likely to have the greatest chance of forming a viable pregnancy. However, the application of this technology in a clinical context to either PBs or embryonic blastomeres (i.e., Preimplantation Genetic Screening – PGS) is not without problems, one of which is the length of time

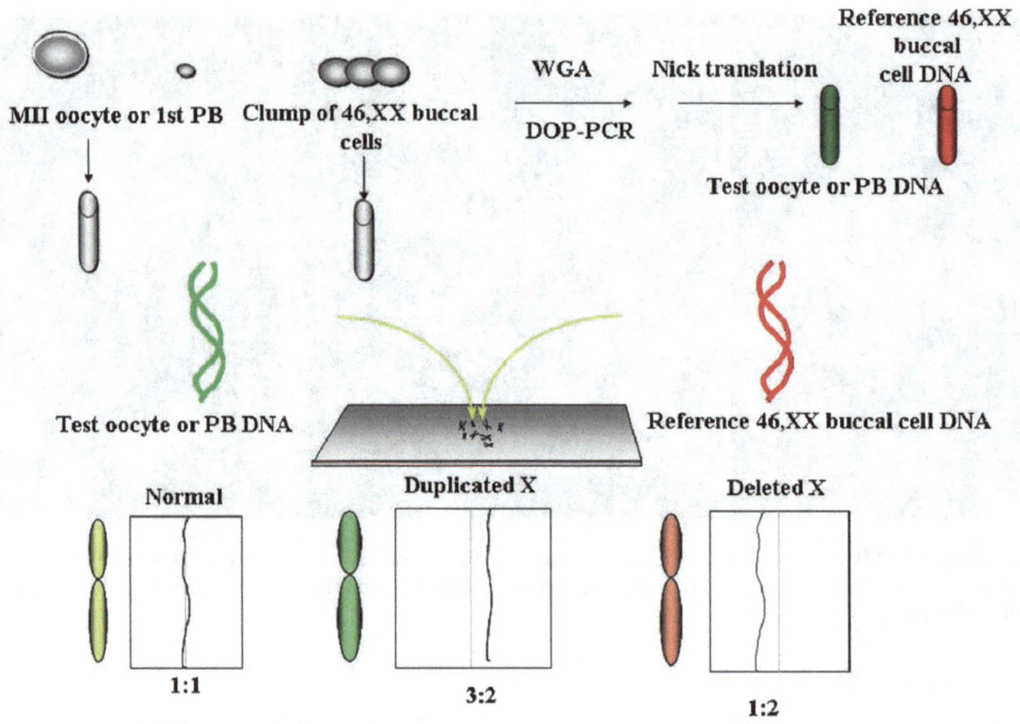

Fig. 20.9 Protocol for CGH analysis of individual MII oocyte and corresponding first PB. (Provided by Elpida Fragouli, Oxford University)

the method requires [34]. Standard CGH requires 3–4 days and the analysis is labour intensive, preventing analysis of large numbers of cells. Blastocyst transfer, usually on day-5 post-fertilization, provides sufficient time for PB CGH analysis to be completed; however, this is not appropriate for all patients undergoing IVF. An alternative is to cryopreserve the zygotes immediately after biopsy of the first and second PBs or after blastomere biopsy on day 3 of development. The success of improved freezing (vitrification) protocols in routine IVF makes this a more attractive option.

The use of lymphocyte metaphases for CGH analysis has recently been replaced by the use of genomic microarrays for pre- and postnatal genetic analysis, but for single cell analysis this approach is not yet sufficiently robust for application in clinical practice.

20.4.4 The Aneuploidy Rate in Human Oocytes

Recent karyotyping data that include chromatid anomalies and the more specific FISH analyses indicated that the overall rate of chromosome and chromatid imbalance in human oocytes is about 11% for women of maternal age 32–34 years [15, 17, 22, 35]. However, several independent studies of aneuploidy in MII oocytes and corresponding first PBs have used CGH to obtain exact information on all chromosomes. There are now data on at least 221 MII oocyte-PB complexes donated from 82 patients ([24, 30, 31] and unpublished data). The results confirm that CGH is able to detect chromatid losses and gains, as well as whole chromosome changes, and partial aneuploidies thought to be due to chromosome breakage.

Current data suggest an aneuploidy rate of 20.8% ([24, 31] and unpublished data), double the rate found by karyotyping [22]. Chromosome loss and gain occurred almost equally in the oocyte and first PB in the abnormal samples, in accordance with the theoretical expectations of the outcome of primary meiotic nondisjunction of the two homologues. These data provide no support for the frequent occurrence of anaphase lag. As evidence gained by analysis of preimplantation embryos shows that those with autosomal monosomies and with autosomal trisomies of the largest autosomes rarely progress beyond initial implantation, over half of the abnormal oocytes will lead to IVF failure. The mechanism of gonadal or germinal mosaicism involving secondary meiotic nondisjunction, leading to aneuploid oocytes was confirmed by the observation of oocytes or PBs with an additional or missing chromosome, without the reciprocal anomaly being scored in the corresponding PB or oocyte [24, 31–33].

Abnormalities affected all chromosomes except 7 and 14, but most frequently the X and then chromosomes 21, 22, followed by 8, 12 and 20 ([24, 31] and unpublished data). The mechanisms involved whole chromosome nondisjunction, chromatid imbalance due to precocious chromatid separation, chromosome breakage and, rarely, gonadal/germinal mosaicism. It is of interest that the larger autosomes,

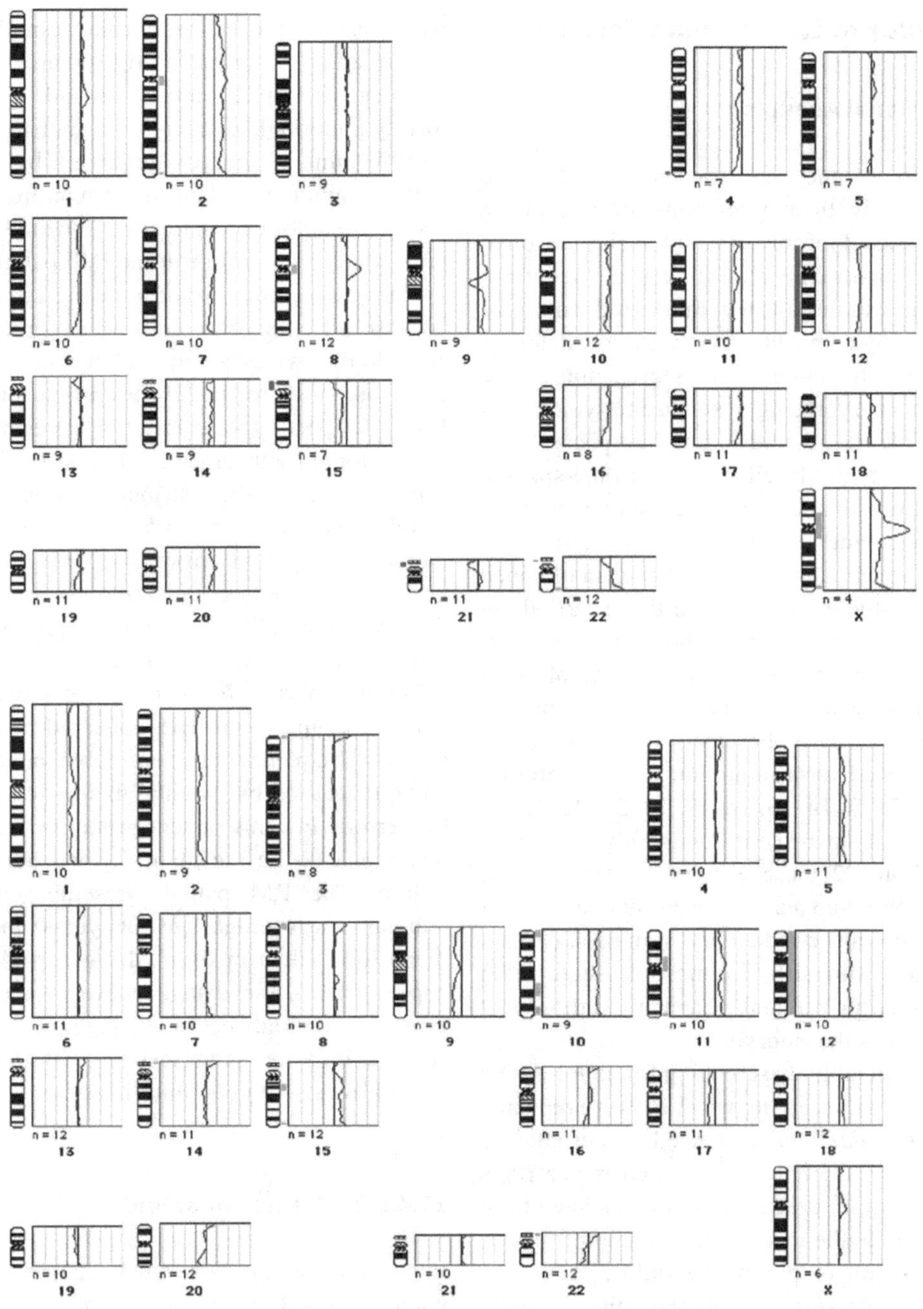

Fig. 20.10 Outcome of meiotic nondisjunction of chromosome 12 visible in an oocyte/polar body complex after CGH analysis. The oocyte has lost one chromosome 12 and the PB has gained an extra chromosome 12. Reference DNA was from a 46, XX source, labeled in red in both cases; test DNA was labeled in green. (Provided by Anna Mantzouratou, University College London Centre for PGD)

numbers 1–12, were affected solely by whole chromosome nondisjunction and unaffected by chromatid anomalies. This is thought to reflect the increased cohesion of larger bivalents as well as the role of crossing-over in holding paired homologues together, as larger chromosomes have greater numbers of chiasmata. It is further suggested that smaller chromosomes with few or no crossovers are more likely to separate early, in turn predisposing them to random disjunction as well as to chromatid anomalies. However, the X chromosome stands out as a special case, 8 of 16 X chromosome anomalies were seen in just three patients (age range 18–42). At least half of these were chromatid anomalies.

From both the X chromosome and the autosome data, it is clear that age-independent mechanisms are operating in the younger women, and there may be a causal link to their infertility. These mechanisms would include germinal or gonadal mosaicism as well as a predisposition to the production of aneuploid gametes due to reduced recombination in meiosis I.

20.4.5 Aneuploidy in Early Human Embryos

20.4.5.1 Constitutional Aneuploidy

Parental meiotic chromosome segregation errors will lead to constitutional aneuploidy, thereby affecting all cells of the embryo. Almost all recent information on the chromosomal status of the early human embryo has been derived from PGD and follow-up studies of nontransferred embryos. However, they are rarely complete enough to allow determination of parental meiotic chromosome segregation errors. Reliable conventional karyotyping of single embryonic cells is virtually impossible; but the advent of interphase FISH analysis, using fluorescently labelled chromosome-specific probes, has made it possible to determine the copy number of individual chromosomes in the nuclei of single cells obtained from preimplantation embryos. The data obtained from PGD follow-up studies, in particular those carried out for aneuploidy screening, complement those obtained from research studies on human oocytes. Munné et al. [36] reported on the diagnostic analysis of single cells from over 2,000 embryos using FISH probes for up to 14 chromosomes. Cells were tested for a minimum of four chromosomes from: 1, 4, 6, 7, 13, 14, 15, 16, 17, 18, 21, 22, X and Y. Those most frequently involved in aneuploidy were chromosomes 15, 16, 21 and 22; those least involved were 6, 14, X and Y. Because follow-up analyses were not carried out on the majority of nontransferred embryos, in most cases it was not possible to distinguish chromosome segregation errors that occurred during parental meiosis from those that arose post-zygotically in the embryo.

As a follow-up to aneuploidy screening for couples who were having difficulties conceiving via IVF due to repeated implantation failure (RIF) or advanced maternal age (AMA) or who were experiencing repeated miscarriage (RM), mainly after natural pregnancies, studies have been carried out to determine the mechanisms leading to aneuploidy and implantation or pregnancy failure. Embryos from 75 couples undergoing preimplantation genetic screening (PGS) have been investigated for abnormalities of chromosomes 13, 15, 16, 18, 21 and 22 using FISH in two rounds of hybridization ([37] and unpublished data). This included the screening of single blastomeres on day 3 and full follow-up analysis on day 5/6 of all the cells of nontransferred embryos. In total, 94 PGS cycles were included in the study, and 847 embryos biopsied, with results obtained for 91% of these. Approximately one-fifth (19%) were normal disomic for the chromosomes tested at diagnosis on day 3, while 81% showed an abnormal result. Despite the low normality rate, the pregnancy rate per cycle that progressed to embryo biopsy was 29.5%; 32.9% per cycle in which embryos were suitable to be transferred. Satisfactory follow-up was obtained from 536 embryos. All those diagnosed as chromosomally abnormal were confirmed as abnormal on follow-up, of which 94% were mosaics with mixed cell types and only 5.3% were uniformly abnormal. Although mosaicism in general is common in human embryos generated by IVF and increases with the number of days spent in culture, this almost universal aneuploid mosaicism is beyond what is normally seen in embryos from routine IVF patients [38–42].

Parental meiotic chromosome segregation errors, detected because all embryonic cells were affected with the same aneuploidy, were identified overall in only 14.8% of embryos, most frequently for chromosomes 18, 21 and 22. Errors in post-zygotic mitotic segregation were detected mostly for chromosomes 13, 15 and 16. There was a significant difference in the distribution of embryos that were uniformly abnormal ($p<0.005$) and those caused by parental meiotic segregation errors ($p<0.005$) between the referral groups. The rates for parental meiotic errors were 24% for the RM group, 20% for the AMA group and only 8.9% for RIF patients. There were similarities in the abnormalities affecting embryos from the couples with RM and AMA, whereas couples with RIF appeared to be different due to the low frequency of identifiable abnormalities in their embryos caused by parental meiotic chromosome segregation errors. For this patient group, post-zygotic abnormalities appear to be the main factor leading to implantation failure. The RM patients resemble those with AMA, although the average age (36 years) in the RM group is much lower than in the AMA group (42 years). It would appear from these data that even for the RM and AMA groups, aneuploidy caused by parental meiotic chromosome segregation errors is far less of a risk than the mosaic form caused by post-zygotic mitotic errors.

20.4.5.2 Mosaic Aneuploidy

In general, the embryos of women undergoing IVF who are younger than 37 years of age are chiefly at risk of mosaic aneuploidy caused by post-zygotic segregation errors rather than the full constitutional type with all embryo cells being aneuploid, this type originating from parental meiotic segregation errors. Interphase FISH detection of the X and Y chromosomes for the purposes of embryo sexing first indicated that mosaicism is a common feature of human preimplantation embryos [38]. Subsequent studies using autosomal probes for testing between three and nine chromosomes detected mosaic aneuploidy in more than half of the embryos investigated [39, 41, 42]. The development of single cell CGH analysis, allowing the copy number of every chromosome to be determined, and its application to analyze every cell from a total of 24 good quality 3-day-old embryos demonstrated that 62% were mosaic [43, 44]. The extent of mosaic abnormality varied between the presence of a single abnormal cell to every cell being abnormal, but with the chromosomal constitution varying randomly from cell to cell (a feature termed "chaotic"). Importantly, the CGH analysis also showed that a quarter of the embryos were totally euploid, with no chromosome imbalance by day 3 of development. Clearly, it is these euploid embryos that have the greatest potential to implant and develop normally thereafter.

20.5 Preimplantation Genetic Diagnosis for Chromosomal Disorders

Preimplantation genetic diagnosis (PGD) for chromosomal disorders involves analysis of a single cell, either the first PB or a blastomere taken on day 3 of development. As it is not possible to visualize the whole chromosome set with accuracy, PGD almost always involves FISH with chromosome-specific DNA probes. This enables the number of copies of each chromosome to be determined. The highest efficiency and accuracy is achieved by using probes for three pairs of chromosomes for each hybridization experiment. Probe mixes to detect five chromosomes are available commercially, but they involve some compromise on efficiency and accuracy.

20.5.1 Specific PGD for Carriers of Chromosomal Rearrangements

One of the most common reasons for requesting specific PGD is where one parent is a carrier of a balanced chromosomal rearrangement (such as a translocation or an inversion) and this has led to infertility or frequent miscarriage. For each couple, an individual protocol must be developed to detect embryos that have an unbalanced form of the rearrangement. A three-probe strategy has been designed for reciprocal translocations, such that two of the probes are located either side of the breakpoint on one of the involved chromosomes and the third probe maps to any position on the second involved chromosome (Fig. 20.11) [45]. The main risk for these couples is due to segregation problems of the rearranged chromosomes at the first meiotic division, leading to the production of a high proportion of unbalanced gametes [46, 47]. However, from the data gathered on the outcome of this type of specific PGD, it is apparent that the level of abnormality detected far exceeds that expected due to parental meiotic segregation errors alone. Much of the abnormality is chaotic in nature (affecting multiple chromosomes) and clearly post-zygotic in origin [46–49]. The frequency of abnormality in the embryos from these cycles approaches 75%, adding weight to the suggestion that these particular couples are afflicted by two pathologies, the increased risk of parental meiotic segregation errors, compounded by additional factors that result in above normal rates of post-zygotic anomalies. It is possibly these additional factors that lead to the couple being referred for PGD. It should be noted, however, that it is nevertheless possible for most of the parents who carry a translocation or inversion to achieve a normal pregnancy by this type of advanced specific PGD, with the option available for confirmation of a normal pregnancy by prenatal diagnosis using fetal cells obtained by chorionic villus sampling at 12–13 weeks of pregnancy or amniocentesis at around 16 weeks.

20.5.2 Preimplantation Genetic Screening for Aneuploidy

PGS was developed to improve the outcome for couples that were unable to achieve an ongoing pregnancy due to AMA, RIF or RM. In all these situations, the parents themselves have normal somatic karyotypes. The aim is to provide a general screen for the most common aneuploidies affecting implantation and spontaneous abortion. Probe sets used invariably contain those specific for chromosomes 13, 18 and 21; and frequently also include probes for chromosomes 16 and 22. The X and Y chromosomes may also be selected.

20.5.3 First Polar Body or Blastomere for the Diagnosis of Aneuploidy?

Up to 20% of embryos overall will have an error that is due to meiotic chromosome segregation errors during the production of gametes in either parent, of these, 90% will be maternal. Initially, it might seem that analysis of the first PB would be the most effective procedure for the identification of aneuploid embryos. However, as previously stated, at least 50% of embryos created by IVF are chromosomally mosaic, with a mixture of normal and abnormal cells [42, 50] and this proportion increases in couples with RIF [37, 51]. This type of aneuploidy is due to errors in post-zygotic mitotic divisions.

20.5.4 Problems with First PB Analysis

There are several problems with analysis limited to the first PB. Meiotic segregation of the primary oocyte will lead to

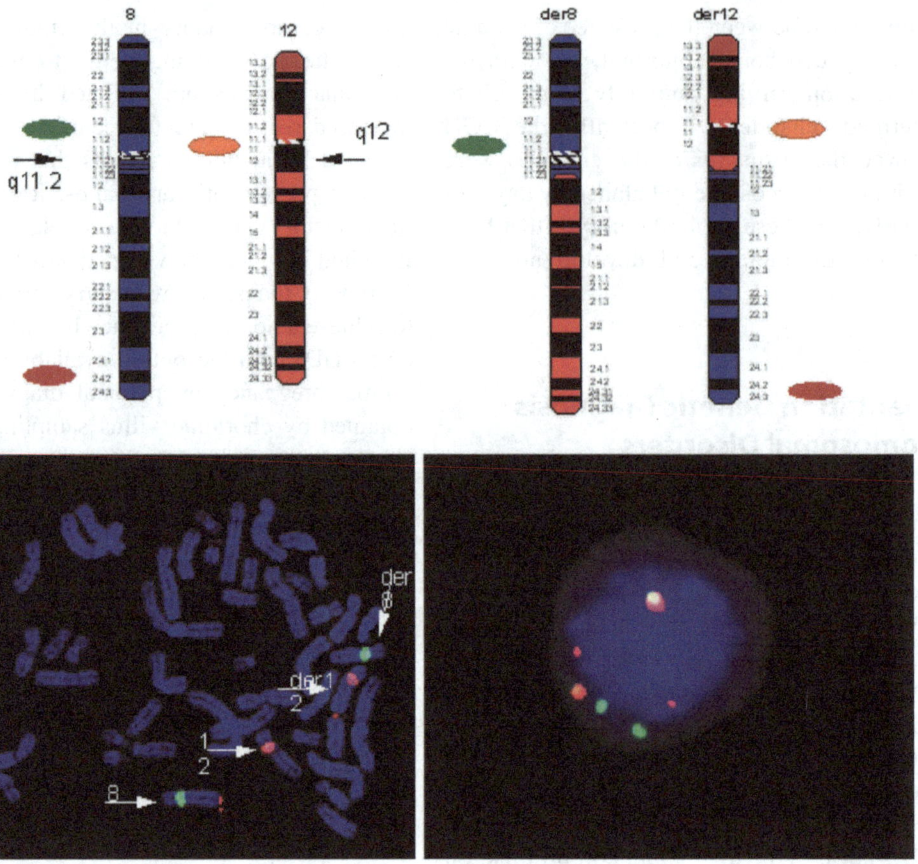

Fig. 20.11 Three-probe strategy for detection of reciprocal translocations. Probes are located on both sides of the breakpoint on one of the chromosomes involved, and the third maps to the second involved chromosome. This example illustrates the FISH probe strategy for a carrier of 46XX, t(8;12)(q11.2;q12) for use in PGD. Probes are shown hybridized to the chromosomes of carrier parent (*left*) and to an embryonic nucleus, which is balanced for the translocation. (Provided by Anna Mantzouratou, University College London Centre for PGD)

two haploid cell nuclei, each normally expected to contain 23 chromosomes. Each chromosome will then consist of two chromatids that should still be attached at the centromere. Many of the chromosome-specific probes used for FISH hybridize to the centromere region and should appear as a doublet signal, but this is not always clear. Therefore, the distinction between the presence of one or two chromatids may be difficult, especially as the first PB rapidly degenerates. Assuming the primary oocyte is normal disomic, loss of a chromosome or a chromatid from the first PB should be mirrored by a gain in the secondary oocyte, as these are the two haploid products of the first meiotic oocyte division. While an extra whole chromosome will always lead to a trisomic embryo, an extra chromatid in the secondary oocyte will lead to a trisomic embryo in 50% of cases, since it is likely to segregate randomly at A2 after fertilization. This in turn highlights a second problem with first PB analysis – namely that events at A2 will determine the eventual outcome. Ideally, therefore, both first and second PBs should be analysed where possible. If the first PB alone is analysed this will lead to the discarding of oocytes with chromatid anomalies that could lead to a chromosomally normal embryo if the additional chromosome material is passed to the second PB.

In cases of PGD for maternal carriers of chromosomal rearrangements, usually reciprocal or Robertsonian translocations, there are additional problems posed by crossingover during the prophase of meiosis I. As oogenesis progresses in the mother (occurring during fetal development), crossingover within the chromosome segment between the centromere and the breakpoint (the interstitial segment) will create a "hybrid" chromosome with one normal chromatid and the other unbalanced due to the translocation. This may be detected by the use of "chromosome paints" – collections of probes that hybridize along each chromosome arm – but once again it is not possible to predict whether the normal or the abnormal chromatid will pass to the oocyte [52]. The corresponding oocytes complementary to such first PBs can thus not be used for fertilization. In summary, unless analysis of the second PB is also possible, many of the oocytes will unfortunately have to be discarded due to the uncertainty of the outcome after AII segregation.

20.5.5 Problems with Single Blastomere Analysis

A single blastomere will provide an interphase nucleus for analysis. FISH analysis of interphase chromatin is less efficient than that of metaphase chromosomes, especially when locus-specific probes are used. Hybridization failure is one source of error. Probes that detect multiple copies of a sequence, e.g., alpha satellite DNA associated with the centromere, give larger signals and are less prone to this type of technical error. Another major problem is that of chromosomal mosaicism, the cell chosen for biopsy and analysis may not be representative of the embryo as a whole. In the case of specific PGD for chromosomal rearrangements it would be advisable to take two cells for analysis, as embryos that are a mosaic of balanced and abnormal cells occur quite frequently [49]. Unfortunately, however, the indications for PGS are such that removal of two cells is not considered advisable as this may retard embryonic development.

Embryo mosaicism is of two basic types, firstly, diploid/aneuploid mosaicism where the embryo began with a normal diploid complement and an aneuploid cell line developed during post-zygotic cleavage divisions, usually due to loss or gain of a chromosome (or similarly diploid/aneuploid mosaicism where the embryo began with an aneuploid complement and a normal cell line developed during post-zygotic cleavage divisions, due to loss of the extra chromosome); and secondly a mixture of different aneuploid cells. Clearly, it is the first type where there is a mixture of normal and abnormal cells that has the most potential to cause misdiagnosis. The outcome of diploid/aneuploid mosaicism cannot then be predicted with certainty. In cases where an aneuploid cell is detected, the chances are that many of the remaining cells are normal. Equally, when a normal cell has been biopsied, it is still possible that a large proportion of the remaining cells are aneuploid. Analysis of a single blastomere out of eight available at 3 days post-conception is not likely to detect aneuploidy that affects one or two cells only. However, such embryos do have a reasonable chance of implantation and progression to a normal pregnancy.

20.5.6 Controversies Over PGS

Given the high rates of chromosome abnormalities seen in embryos created by IVF, screening a cell from each embryo for aneuploidy should improve the outcome, especially for high risk couples. There is a large amount of evidence to indicate that PGS improves implantation and reduces miscarriage [53–57]. However, these studies were retrospective and nonrandomized. Others using randomized control trials (RCTs) were not able to demonstrate a significant difference between couples treated by PGS and a control group [18, 58] at least when there was no restriction on the number of embryos to be replaced per cycle. Most recently, an RCT demonstrated a negative effect [59]. There are crucial differences between these studies, quite apart from being randomized or not being so; the methodology used in the RCTs has been widely criticized [60]. For example, in the studies by Staessen et al. [61] and Mastenbroek et al. [59], chromosomes 15 and 22 were not tested – the latter is a particularly important omission as it is one of those most frequently involved in the production of aneuploid oocytes originating from parental meiotic segregation errors. Most striking is the poor diagnostic success rate in the Mastenbroek et al. [59] study with 20% of embryos remaining undiagnosed, far higher than in any other reported study. This fact alone suggests that the group was not experienced at carrying out PGS, and other data presented indicates that the biopsy technique used was detrimental [59]. In conclusion, evidence to date suggests that if PGS is carried out efficiently and is applied to appropriately chosen groups of patients who are at high risk of producing aneuploid embryos then it is beneficial [37]. Couples who are likely to benefit from aneuploidy screening include those where the maternal age is over 40, couples experiencing repeated miscarriage (where the parents have normal chromosomes) and couples with recurrent implantation failure. The former two groups have been shown to have an increased risk of meiotic errors and the third group to have a very high rate of post-zygotic anomalies [37, 51].

20.5.7 Screening the Whole Chromosome Complement

At the preimplantation embryonic stage, trisomy or monosomy can affect any chromosome; this has led to the development of technology which enables the whole chromosome complement to be screened for aneuploidy. The most effective method is that of CGH. This was first applied to analyse single blastomeres from cleavage stage embryos [43, 44] and provided concrete support for the findings of the interphase FISH studies. Namely that mosaicism was very common (60%) and that some of it was "chaotic" in nature, with differing abnormalities in cells from the same embryo. The most striking finding from both studies was that only 25% of embryos were normal euploid.

The problem with diagnostic CGH analysis of single blastomeres is that the time taken precludes transfer of the embryo in the same cycle, requiring it to be frozen while analysis is carried out [62]. With more efficient freezing (vitrification) protocols, there is hope that this may now be feasible. In the meantime, others have approached the problem by subjecting the first PB to CGH analysis [34].

This provides an extra 2 days for analysis, allowing embryo selection and transfer in the same cycle, albeit with a very labor-intensive protocol. As with any analysis involving the first PB, there needs to be confirmation either with the second PB or by analysis of a blastomere. Some recent reports have failed in this respect [63, 64]. However, post-conception diagnosis is banned in Italy and Germany; for those countries first PB analysis is all that is available.

When dealing with extremely high-risk patient groups, the level of embryonic aneuploidy is so high that screening the whole chromosome set is not necessary since much of the mosaicism is chaotic [37]. Additionally, certain groups of chromosomes are more likely to be affected by aneuploidy caused by parental meiotic chromosome segregation errors [24] and these are the ones chosen for PGS. Paradoxically, the net effect of these considerations is that when dealing with groups of patients at lower risk, a more thorough screen of a wider range of chromosomes is needed to demonstrate any beneficial effect.

20.6 Conclusions

Mammalian oogenesis, leading up to mature eggs having half the chromosome number in comparison to somatic cell nuclei, is a complex process. Uniquely, in human females, this process is also highly error-prone, with a high proportion of mature eggs showing an abnormal chromosome number, aneuploidy. Superimposed on the segregation errors taking place during the meiotic cell divisions at oogenesis, there is a high amount of mitotic segregation errors during early embryogenesis, so that a high proportion of embryos are aneuploidy mosaics. The underlying reasons for these problems are not yet fully understood. Much work has been devoted within Assisted Conception Units to the development of schedules for preselection of embryos that, following IVF treatment, have the optimal chance of being implanted and the successful outcome of the pregnancy. This includes analysis of chromosome copy number in the first and the second PBs as well as in individual cells, blastomeres, micromanipulated from the embryo at the eight-cell stage. Both types of investigation are labour intensive with limited success rate. Nevertheless, there are indications that these methods, if carried out efficiently and applied to appropriately chosen groups of patients, who are at high risk of producing aneuploid embryos, then they are beneficial.

References

1. Bendsen E, Byskov AG, Andersen CY, Westergaard LG (2006) Number of germ cells and somatic cells in human fetal ovaries during the first weeks after sex differentiation. Hum Reprod 21(1):30–35
2. Barlow AL, Hulten MA (1998) Crossing over analysis at pachytene in man. Eur J Hum Genet 6(4):350–358
3. Lenzi ML, Smith J, Snowden T et al (2005) Extreme heterogeneity in the molecular events leading to the establishment of chiasmata during meiosis I in human oocytes. Am J Hum Genet 76(1):112–127
4. Tease C, Hartshorne G, Hulten M (2006) Altered patterns of meiotic recombination in human fetal oocytes with asynapsis and/or synaptonemal complex fragmentation at pachytene. Reprod Biomed Online 13(1):88–95
5. Tease C, Hartshorne GM, Hulten MA (2002) Patterns of meiotic recombination in human fetal oocytes. Am J Hum Genet 70(6): 1469–1479
6. Tease C, Hulten MA (2004) Inter-sex variation in synaptonemal complex lengths largely determine the different recombination rates in male and female germ cells. Cytogenet Genome Res 107(3–4): 208–215
7. Yuncken C (1968) Meiosis in the human female. Cytogenetics 7(3):234–238
8. Hunt PA, Hassold TJ (2008) Human female meiosis: what makes a good egg go bad? Trends Genet 24(2):86–93
9. Oliver TR, Feingold E, Yu K et al (2008) New insights into human nondisjunction of chromosome 21 in oocytes. PLoS Genet 4(3):e1000033
10. Jones KT (2008) Meiosis in oocytes: predisposition to aneuploidy and its increased incidence with age. Hum Reprod Update 14(2): 143–158
11. Delhanty JD (2005) Mechanisms of aneuploidy induction in human oogenesis and early embryogenesis. Cytogenet Genome Res 111(3–4):237–244
12. Hultén MA, Patel S, Tankimanova M et al (2008) On the origin of trisomy 21 Down syndrome. Mol Cytogenet 1:21
13. Kovaleva NV (2007) Parental mosaicism for trisomy 21: problems with its detection and an approach to determining its population rate. Genet Test 11(3):341–344
14. Hall HE, Chan ER, Collins A et al (2007) The origin of trisomy 13. Am J Med Genet A 143A(19):2242–2248
15. Cupisti S, Conn CM, Fragouli E et al (2003) Sequential FISH analysis of oocytes and polar bodies reveals aneuploidy mechanisms. Prenat Diagn 23(8):663–668
16. Dyban A, Freidine M, Severova E, Cieslak J, Ivakhnenko V, Verlinsky Y (1996) Detection of aneuploidy in human oocytes and corresponding first polar bodies by fluorescent in situ hybridization. J Assist Reprod Genet 13(1):73–78
17. Mahmood R, Brierley CH, Faed MJ, Mills JA, Delhanty JD (2000) Mechanisms of maternal aneuploidy: FISH analysis of oocytes and polar bodies in patients undergoing assisted conception. Hum Genet 106(6):620–626
18. Pellestor F, Andreo B, Arnal F, Humeau C, Demaille J (2003) Maternal aging and chromosomal abnormalities: new data drawn from in vitro unfertilized human oocytes. Hum Genet 112(2):195–203
19. Gras L, McBain J, Trounson A, Kola I (1992) The incidence of chromosomal aneuploidy in stimulated and unstimulated (natural) uninseminated human oocytes. Hum Reprod 7(10):1396–1401
20. Hassold T, Hunt P (2001) To err (meiotically) is human: the genesis of human aneuploidy. Nat Rev Genet 2(4):280–291
21. Almeida PA, Bolton VN (1994) The relationship between chromosomal abnormalities in the human oocyte and fertilization in vitro. Hum Reprod 9(2):343–346
22. Pellestor F, Andreo B, Arnal F, Humeau C, Demaille J (2002) Mechanisms of non-disjunction in human female meiosis: the co-existence of two modes of malsegregation evidenced by the karyotyping of 1397 in-vitro unfertilized oocytes. Hum Reprod 17(8): 2134–2145
23. Angell R (1997) First-meiotic-division nondisjunction in human oocytes. Am J Hum Genet 61(1):23–32
24. Fragouli E, Wells D, Doshi A, Gotts S, Harper JC, Delhanty JD (2006) Complete cytogenetic investigation of oocytes from a young

cancer patient with the use of comparative genomic hybridisation reveals meiotic errors. Prenat Diagn 26(1):71–76
25. Sandalinas M, Marquez C, Munné S (2002) Spectral karyotyping of fresh, non-inseminated oocytes. Mol Hum Reprod 8(6):580–585
26. Kuliev A, Cieslak J, Verlinsky Y (2005) Frequency and distribution of chromosome abnormalities in human oocytes. Cytogenet Genome Res 111(3–4):193–198
27. Kuliev A, Cieslak J, Ilkevitch Y, Verlinsky Y (2003) Chromosomal abnormalities in a series of 6,733 human oocytes in preimplantation diagnosis for age-related aneuploidies. Reprod Biomed Online 6(1):54–59
28. Pujol A, Boiso I, Benet J et al (2003) Analysis of nine chromosome probes in first polar bodies and metaphase II oocytes for the detection of aneuploidies. Eur J Hum Genet 11(4):325–336
29. Cozzi J, Conn CM, Harper J et al (1999) A trisomic germ cell line and precocious chromatid segregation leads to recurrent trisomy 21 conception. Hum Genet 104(1):23–28
30. Fragouli E, Wells D, Thornhill A et al (2006) Comparative genomic hybridization analysis of human oocytes and polar bodies. Hum Reprod 21(9):2319–2328
31. Fragouli E, Wells D, Whalley KM, Mills JA, Faed MJ, Delhanty JD (2006) Increased susceptibility to maternal aneuploidy demonstrated by comparative genomic hybridization analysis of human MII oocytes and first polar bodies. Cytogenet Genome Res 14(1):30–38
32. Gutierrez-Mateo C, Benet J, Wells D et al (2004) Aneuploidy study of human oocytes first polar body comparative genomic hybridization and metaphase II fluorescence in situ hybridization analysis. Hum Reprod 19(12):2859–2868
33. Gutierrez-Mateo C, Wells D, Benet J et al (2004) Reliability of comparative genomic hybridization to detect chromosome abnormalities in first polar bodies and metaphase II oocytes. Hum Reprod 19(9):2118–2125
34. Wells D, Escudero T, Levy B, Hirschhorn K, Delhanty JD, Munné S (2002) First clinical application of comparative genomic hybridization and polar body testing for preimplantation genetic diagnosis of aneuploidy. Fertil Steril 78(3):543–549
35. Anahory T, Andreo B, Regnier-Vigouroux G et al (2003) Sequential multiple probe fluorescence in-situ hybridization analysis of human oocytes and polar bodies by combining centromeric labelling and whole chromosome painting. Mol Hum Reprod 9(10):577–585
36. Munné S, Bahce M, Sandalinas M et al (2004) Differences in chromosome susceptibility to aneuploidy and survival to first trimester. Reprod Biomed Online 8(1):81–90
37. Mantzouratou A, Mania A, Fragouli E et al (2007) Variable aneuploidy mechanisms in embryos from couples with poor reproductive histories undergoing preimplantation genetic screening. Hum Reprod 22(7):1844–1853
38. Delhanty JD, Griffin DK, Handyside AH et al (1993) Detection of aneuploidy and chromosomal mosaicism in human embryos during preimplantation sex determination by fluorescent in situ hybridisation, (FISH). Hum Mol Genet 2(8):1183–1185
39. Delhanty JD, Harper JC, Ao A, Handyside AH, Winston RM (1997) Multicolour FISH detects frequent chromosomal mosaicism and chaotic division in normal preimplantation embryos from fertile patients. Hum Genet 99(6):755–760
40. Evsikov S, Verlinsky Y (1998) Mosaicism in the inner cell mass of human blastocysts. Hum Reprod 13(11):3151–3155
41. Munné S, Cohen J (1998) Chromosome abnormalities in human embryos. Hum Reprod Update 4(6):842–855
42. Munné S, Lee A, Rosenwaks Z, Grifo J, Cohen J (1993) Diagnosis of major chromosome aneuploidies in human preimplantation embryos. Hum Reprod 8(12):2185–2191
43. Voullaire L, Slater H, Williamson R, Wilton L (2000) Chromosome analysis of blastomeres from human embryos by using comparative genomic hybridization. Hum Genet 106(2):210–217
44. Wells D, Delhanty JD (2000) Comprehensive chromosomal analysis of human preimplantation embryos using whole genome amplification and single cell comparative genomic hybridization. Mol Hum Reprod 6(11):1055–1062
45. Conn CM, Harper JC, Winston RM, Delhanty JD (1995) Preimplantation diagnosis for trisomies 13, 14, 18 and 21 using multicolour fluorescent in situ hybridisation. Am J Hum Genet 57(Suppl):A1611
46. Conn CM, Harper JC, Winston RM, Delhanty JD (1998) Infertile couples with Robertsonian translocations: preimplantation genetic analysis of embryos reveals chaotic cleavage divisions. Hum Genet 102(1):117–123
47. Munné S, Fung J, Cassel MJ, Marquez C, Weier HU (1998) Preimplantation genetic analysis of translocations: case-specific probes for interphase cell analysis. Hum Genet 102(6):663–674
48. Iwarsson E, Malmgren H, Inzunza J et al (2000) Highly abnormal cleavage divisions in preimplantation embryos from translocation carriers. Prenat Diagn 20(13):1038–1047
49. Simopoulou M, Harper JC, Fragouli E et al (2003) Preimplantation genetic diagnosis of chromosome abnormalities: implications from the outcome for couples with chromosomal rearrangements. Prenat Diagn 23(8):652–662
50. Delhanty JD, Handyside AH (1995) The origin of genetic defects in the human and their detection in the preimplantation embryo. Hum Reprod Update 1(3):201–215
51. Voullaire L, Wilton L, McBain J, Callaghan T, Williamson R (2002) Chromosome abnormalities identified by comparative genomic hybridization in embryos from women with repeated implantation failure. Mol Hum Reprod 8(11):1035–1041
52. Munné S, Bahce M, Schimmel T, Sadowy S, Cohen J (1998) Case report: chromatid exchange and predivision of chromatids as other sources of abnormal oocytes detected by preimplantation genetic diagnosis of translocations. Prenat Diagn 18(13):1450–1458
53. Gianaroli L, Magli MC, Ferraretti AP, Fiorentino A, Garrisi J, Munné S (1997) Preimplantation genetic diagnosis increases the implantation rate in human in vitro fertilization by avoiding the transfer of chromosomally abnormal embryos. Fertil Steril 68(6):1128–1131
54. Munné S (2005) Analysis of chromosome segregation during preimplantation genetic diagnosis in both male and female translocation heterozygotes. Cytogenet Genome Res 111(3–4):305–309
55. Munné S, Fischer J, Warner A, Chen S, Zouves C, Cohen J (2006) Preimplantation genetic diagnosis significantly reduces pregnancy loss in infertile couples: a multicenter study. Fertil Steril 85(2):326–332
56. Munné S, Magli C, Cohen J et al (1999) Positive outcome after preimplantation diagnosis of aneuploidy in human embryos. Hum Reprod 14(9):2191–2199
57. Verlinsky Y, Tur-Kaspa I, Cieslak J et al (2005) Preimplantation testing for chromosomal disorders improves reproductive outcome of poor-prognosis patients. Reprod Biomed Online 11(2): 219–225
58. Platteau P, Staessen C, Michiels A, Van Steirteghem A, Liebaers I, Devroey P (2005) Preimplantation genetic diagnosis for aneuploidy screening in women older than 37 years. Fertil Steril 84(2): 319–324
59. Mastenbroek S, Twisk M, van Echten-Arends J et al (2007) In vitro fertilization with preimplantation genetic screening. N Engl J Med 357(1):9–17
60. Cohen J, Grifo JA (2007) Multicentre trial of preimplantation genetic screening reported in the New England Journal of Medicine: an in-depth look at the findings. Reprod Biomed Online 15(4):365–366
61. Staessen C, Platteau P, Van Assche E et al (2004) Comparison of blastocyst transfer with or without preimplantation genetic diagnosis for aneuploidy screening in couples with advanced maternal

age: a prospective randomized controlled trial. Hum Reprod 19(12):2849–2858

62. Wilton L, Williamson R, McBain J, Edgar D, Voullaire L (2001) Birth of a healthy infant after preimplantation confirmation of euploidy by comparative genomic hybridization. N Engl J Med 345(21):1537–1541
63. Sher G, Keskintepe L, Keskintepe M et al (2007) Oocyte karyotyping by comparative genomic hybridization provides a highly reliable method for selecting "competent" embryos, markedly improving in vitro fertilization outcome: a multiphase study. Fertil Steril 87(5):1033–1040
64. Fragouli E, Delhanty JD, Wells D (2007) Single cell diagnosis using comparative genomic hybridization after preliminary DNA amplification still needs more tweaking: too many miscalls. Fertil Steril 88(1):247–248 author reply 8–9
65. Hultén M, Tankimanova M, Baker H (2005) Meiosis and meiotic errors. In: Jorde LB, Little PFR, Dunn MJ, Subramaniam S (eds) Encyclopedia of genetics, proteomics and bioinformatics (online edition). John Wiley and Sons Ltd, Chichester
66. Cheng EY, Hunt PA, Naluai-Cecchini TA, Fligner CL, Fujimoto VY, Pasternack TL, Schwartz JM, Steinauer JE, Woodruff TJ, Cherry SM, Hansen TA, Vallente RU, Broman KW, Hassold TJ. (2009) PLoS Genet. 5(9):e1000661. Epub 2009 Sep 18
67. Hultén M, Patel S, Jonasson J, Iwarsson E. (2009) Reproduction. [Epub ahead of print]PMID: 19755486 [PubMed - as supplied by publisher]

Part III
Male Reproductive Physiology and Medicine

Chapter 21
An Overview of Sperm Production

Louis Hermo and Bernard Robaire

Abstract With every heartbeat, men produce approximately 1,000 spermatozoa. Although the regulatory mechanisms are still only partially understood, the remarkably well-organized process needed for this consistent, high level of production of unique haploid cells has been resolved and is presented in the first section of this review. The numerous unique cellular features needed for the extraordinary sperm cell to undertake its function are then discussed.

Keywords Spermatogenesis • Stem cell renewal • Meiosis • Spermatid • Acrosome • Flagellum

21.1 Introduction

The main focus of this chapter is on male germ cells: their mode of renewal and differentiation, their ultrastructural features, their spatial arrangement within the testis, and the functional significance of their genes and proteins. Although some of the data discussed will be from animal models, whenever feasible, focus has been placed on literature related to the human testis. The primary objective of this review is to present the adult situation; it does not deal with the complex changes that take place during development or senescence. Many topics have had to be excluded. These include studies of the effects of hormones, therapeutic and nontherapeutic drugs, and environmental factors (chemicals, radiation, etc.) that regulate or can affect sperm production. A rapidly growing number of mouse models (null mutation, gene overexpression, induced random mutations) give new insight into the function of many specific genes and the large array of clinical conditions that result in abnormal sperm production.

L. Hermo
Department of Anatomy and Cell Biology, McGill University, Montreal, Quebec, Canada

B. Robaire (✉)
Department of Pharmacology and Therapeutics and Obstetrics and Gynecology, McGill University, Montreal, Quebec, Canada
e-mail: bernard.robaire@mcgill.ca

21.2 General Features of Testicular Histology

The testes of mammals are paired organs that essentially perform two functions: production of spermatozoa and hormones, mostly androgens, and also estrogens. The testicular parenchyma is composed of numerous seminiferous tubules and the intervening interstitial space [1–3]. Seminiferous tubules are coiled structures forming loops that empty at both ends into the rete testis, an anastomotic channel located at one pole of the testis and lined by a cuboidal epithelium [4]. Seminiferous tubules consist of an epithelium composed of germ cells and supporting Sertoli cells, with the latter being mitotically inactive in adults. Sertoli cells perform a multitude of functions that support and nourish germ cells and that have been extensively described [5, 6]. The interstitial space consists of the hormone-producing Leydig cells, macrophages, blood and lymphatic channels as well as nerves [1, 7, 8].

21.3 Spermatogenesis

The process of spermatogenesis has been investigated by many groups of researchers [1–3]. It is defined as the process whereby germ cells develop, differentiate, and metamorphose into spermatozoa. It is an orderly and well-defined process, occurring in seminiferous tubules of the testis and requiring an intimate communication with Sertoli cells. The temporal events whereby undifferentiated spermatogonial germ cells develop into spermatozoa over a period of several weeks require hormonal, autocrine, paracrine, and juxtacrine signaling between the different testicular compartments (germ, Sertoli, myoid, and Leydig cells, and macrophages). These signals, regulating cell growth and/or cellular differentiation, encompass gonadotropins (LH, FSH), steroids (androgens and estrogens), growth factors, and peptides [9–12].

Spermatogenesis is characterized by three specific functional phases: proliferation, meiosis, and spermiogenesis.

D.T. Carrell and C.M. Peterson (eds.), *Reproductive Endocrinology and Infertility: Integrating Modern Clinical and Laboratory Practice*,
DOI 10.1007/978-1-4419-1436-1_21,

In the proliferation phase, spermatogonia undergo several mitotic divisions to form spermatocytes that after the process of two meiotic divisions form the haploid spermatids. The latter develop into spermatozoa as a result of a complicated metamorphosis involving dramatic structural modifications of the shape of their nucleus, compaction of the nuclear chromatin, formation of an acrosome, and establishment of a flagellum permitting eventual motility. The series of modifications occurring in spermatids is referred to as spermiogenesis, a subdivision of spermatogenesis. Spermatogenesis thus constitutes undifferentiated spermatogonial renewal and proliferation, spermatogonial differentiation, meiosis of spermatocytes, and spermatid development.

21.3.1 The Cycle of the Seminiferous Epithelium

In the middle of the last century [13], it was noted that in cross sections of seminiferous tubules of the testis of rodents, germ cells were organized in concentric layers within the seminiferous epithelium with immature germ cells, spermatogonia, residing at the base of the epithelium adjacent to the limiting membrane, and more advanced germ cells (spermatocytes, early and late spermatids) occupying successive layers situated closer to the tubular lumen. In addition, several distinct generations of germ cells, each at the same step of development and developing in synchrony, were seen in any given tubular cross sectional profile; it was also noted that the various generations of germ cells in different cross sectional profiles gave rise to specific cellular associations, referred to as the stages of the cycle of the seminiferous epithelium. In the rat, 14 distinct stages occur, each with generations of germ cells at specific steps in their development; the stages were designated by roman numerals I-XIV. As a result, it was observed that four or five generations of germ cells occupied a given tubular cross section, depending on the specific stage of the cycle of the seminiferous epithelium. In fact, stages I-VIII showed five generations of germ cells, while stages IX-XIV presented four generations [2, 13].

The formation of specific stages of the cycle and their sequential appearance in a given area of tubule was found to be highly synchronous. A generation of germ cells at a specific step of their development associated with other generations of germ cells, each at their own step of development; such cellular associations were precise and constant. Since spermatozoa were periodically released from the seminiferous epithelium, the idea of a cycle of the seminiferous epithelium was proposed. The precise sequential occurrence of the 14 cellular associations that occurred over time in a given area of the tubule was defined as a cycle of the seminiferous epithelium [13]. Using a variety of techniques, the duration of each stage and hence the cycle of the seminiferous epithelium could be determined. The cycle was found to be different for different species and even varied among strains of the same species. The duration of a cycle was constant and was calculated to be about 12 days in the rat [13], 8.65 days in mouse [14], and 10–11 days in primates [15]. In the human testis, generations of germ cells also developed in synchrony; however, cross sectional tubular profiles did not display any single stage, but, rather, several different stages, thus making analysis of the human testis more complex. Also unlike rodents, there were only six stages of the cycle of the seminiferous epithelium, with a cycle lasting 16 days and spermatogenesis taking 64 days in man (Fig. 21.1) [16, 17].

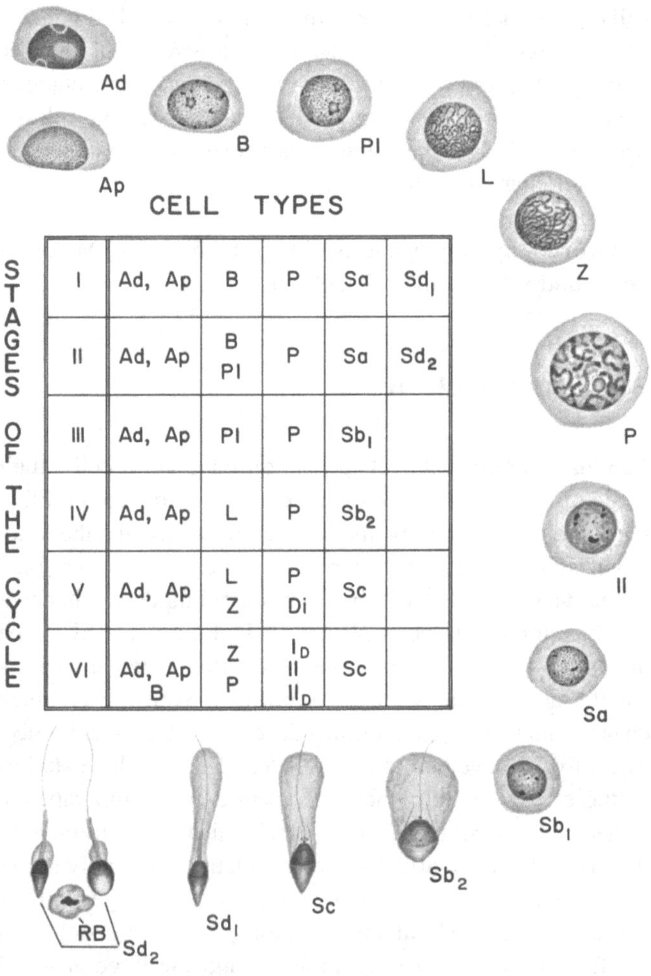

I	Ad, Ap	B	P	Sa	Sd_1
II	Ad, Ap	B Pl	P	Sa	Sd_2
III	Ad, Ap	Pl	P	Sb_1	
IV	Ad, Ap	L	P	Sb_2	
V	Ad, Ap	L Z	P Di	Sc	
VI	Ad, Ap B	Z P	I_D II II_D	Sc	

Fig. 21.1 Stages of the spermatogenic cycle in man. Starting from the upper left corner of the figure and encircling the table, drawings illustrate the steps of spermatogenesis in man. The table in the center of the figure gives the cellular composition of the six stages of the cycle of the seminiferous epithelium (Roman numerals, I–VI). *Ad* dark type A spermatogonium; *Ap* pale type A spermatogonium; *B* type B spermatogonium; *Pl* preleptotene primary spermatocyte; *L* leptotene spermatocyte; *Z* zygotene spermatocyte; *P* pachytene spermatocyte; II: secondary spermatocyte; Sa, Sb_1, Sb_2, Sc, Sd_1, Sd_2: correspond to steps of spermiogenesis; Rb: residual body; Di: diakinesis; ID and IID: first and second maturation divisions of spermatocytes. Reproduced from Clermont [16]

21.3.2 The Wave of the Seminiferous Epithelium

The wave of the seminiferous epithelium is in space what the cycle is in time. Specific stages of the cycle of the seminiferous epithelium are arranged in consecutive order throughout the length of a seminiferous tubule, and move distally from the rete testis, with the stages showing a decreasing order. Since tubules are loops with both ends emptying into the rete testis, the sequence of stages reverses in the middle of the loop to permit the formation of a descending order in both limbs of the loop. The sequential order is broken occasionally for a short distance; such breaks are coined modulations of the segmental order. The wave is defined as a series of adjacent stages that include, in the rat, the 14 possible types in addition to any stage involved in modulation [18].

21.3.3 Spermatogonial Stem Cell Renewal

Spermatozoa are continuously produced in the testis and this requires the presence of stem cells. Although the periodic renewal of type A spermatogonia was recognized early in the last century [19], the process of spermatogonia renewal is complex and is only beginning to be understood [19]. The undifferentiated stem cells produce sperm throughout adult life, thereby transmitting genetic information to future generations and simultaneously renewing themselves to maintain a constant supply. While studies have been done on several species, the majority of studies in recent years were done on the mouse and rat [20–23]. In the 1950s, Clermont and Leblond developed the initial significant concepts on stem cells that have led the way for all subsequent investigations. These investigators demonstrated that there are five classes of type A spermatogonia (A1–4 and Ao), in addition to more differentiated intermediate (In) and B spermatogonia; while the majority are actively engaged in proliferation, the Ao, now referred to as Aisolated (As), acts as reserve stem cells. Extensive analyses of these cells have been done on cross sections of seminiferous tubules and on whole mounts, where the spermatogonial cells can be seen in face view, allowing an analysis of their overall shape and topographical distribution along the tubule. Examining whole mounts of seminiferous tubules and recording mitotic and labeling indices using ^{3}H-thymidine, Clermont and associates proposed that the type A4 spermatogonia were the stem cells and that they gave rise to A1 and In spermatogonia at each cycle of the seminiferous epithelium, while the As acted as reserve stem cells to be used after assault to the testis [24–27].

In the early 1970s, an alternative model was proposed by Huckins [28]. It stated that all spermatogonia fall into three categories: stem cells (As); proliferating cells, Apair (Apr) and Aaligned (Aal); and differentiating cells (A1–A4, In, B). The As, Apr, and Aal are morphologically undifferentiated spermatogonia, while the A1–4, In, and B are differentiated cells. Huckins [29] also demonstrated that the As are located singly in the basal compartment of the seminiferous epithelium and that they divide periodically, but randomly to yield either two new daughter cells that separate to become two new As stem cells or two daughter cells (Apr) that remain connected by intercellular bridges and are committed to differentiate. Most of the As cells are in a short cell cycle (60 h), while a few As spermatogonia have a very long cell cycle, remaining in G1 phase for up to 13 days, from which they exit randomly to reenter the common stem cell pool and resume mitosis [30]. The latter were defined as cells that are highly resistant to irradiation and other noxious agents and thus constitute a population of cells that ensures the continuation of spermatogenesis over a lifetime [31].

In the rat, the production of paired daughter cells by the As spermatogonia signals a commitment to differentiation. Most of these cells undergo a variable number of synchronous divisions before beginning to differentiate, whereupon they are referred to as the Aal undifferentiated proliferating compartment. This activity increases the size of the germ cell population. Cyclically, spermatogonia in the proliferating compartment morphologically transform into differentiating spermatogonia, the type A1 spermatogonia; this occurs at stage VII–VIII of the cycle. Type B spermatogonia eventually divide to give rise to preleptotene (PL) spermatocytes. Over the past decade, this model appears to have been widely accepted by many investigators [24, 32, 33].

In the human testis, essentially three types of spermatogonia are recognized (Adark, Apale and B) in the light microscope, but other types of A spermatogonia have been suggested by electron microscopy [33–37]. Adark have been considered reserve stem cells, with Apale being active stem cells [16, 17]. However, some investigators stated that the Adark may be representative of a phase of the cell cycle since in many testicular abnormalities, the Apale usually persist [38]. Recent investigations on the human testis [39] suggest that spermatogenesis begins with the first division of a pair or quadruplet of Apale spermatogonia at stage I–II. These clones of cells split and enter a second division that leads to pairs, quadruplets, or eight-cell clones of B spermatogonia, as well as a pair or quadruplet of Apale spermatogonia to replenish the pool of Apale spermatogonia. Thus, in the human testis, more committed Apale spermatogonia may act as stem cells, with the Adark dividing only rarely [39].

Another noted feature of spermatogonia derived from early studies revealed that many of these cells undergo degeneration during their differentiation [40]. In fact, because of extensive degeneration of dividing spermatogonia (A2, A3), the theoretically expected number of preleptotene (PL) spermatocytes is considerably reduced (25%). It has been estimated that 75% of spermatogonia do not survive to become mature sperm [41]. Apoptosis is the process by which most germ cell death occurs in the seminiferous tubules. Spontaneous apoptosis occurs primarily during the very late and early stages of spermatogenesis [42, 43]. Cell death associated with exposure to toxicants increases apoptosis primarily at these same stages [43–45], whereas androgen withdrawal causes an increased rate of apoptosis primarily during the middle stages, at the time of germ cell release from the tubules. Several different signaling molecules, including the TNFα/TNFR1, Fas/FasL, TRAIL/DR5, and Bcl2 family proteins have been shown to play roles in regulating germ cell apoptosis depending on the nature of the insult, e.g., heat, drugs, and radiation [46–49].

21.3.4 Spermatocyte Development

Meiosis, involving many genes, is unique to germ cells and is a process of cell division required for the production of healthy haploid spermatids [3, 50]; it serves two important cellular activities: meiotic recombination and synapsis of homologous chromosomes. The recombination of homologous chromosomes during prophase of the first meiotic division assists in orienting chromosomes on the meiotic spindle as well as introducing genetic variability. Proliferating type B spermatogonia differentiate and enter meiosis as primary spermatocytes that undergo the first meiotic division. The latter is composed of prophase, metaphase, anaphase and telophase. Prophase is lengthy, taking up to 90% of the time required for the completion of meiosis [51, 52]. It consists of the following defined cells: preleptotene spermatocytes, the first cells to be formed, are actively engaged in DNA synthesis and are the most mature cells capable of incorporating thymidine into DNA; they are followed by leptotene spermatocytes, involved in chromosome condensation; chromosomal pairing known as synapsis occurs in zygotene spermatocytes; during pachytene, spermatocytes undergo a thickening and shortening of chromosomes and exchange of chromosomal material by the process of crossing over; diplotene is where desynapsis occurs and chromosomes partially separate; diakenesis involves shortening of chromosomes, with each one composed of two chromatids. Prophase is followed by metaphase, where attachment of paired chromatids to the equator of the spindle occurs. Anaphase involves movement of paired chromatids to opposite poles of the spindle, and telophase results in daughter cells called secondary spermatocytes. The latter have a short half life with a haploid number of chromosomes though their DNA content is diploid. They undertake the second meiotic division to form spermatids with a haploid DNA content and a haploid chromosomal number. The duration of spermatocyte maturation is of the order of 20.9 days in rats and 25.3 days in humans.

The nucleus of spermatocytes contains specialized structures such as the synaptonemal complexes and the sex vesicle (XY or sex body), described in detail by several investigators [53–55]. Synapsis of homologous chromosomes is mediated by the synaptonemal complex (SC). The relationship between abnormalities of the synaptonemal complex and male fertility in the human has been documented in several recent articles [56–58]. The temporal aspects of synaptonemal complex assembly, relationship between the synaptonemal complex and meiotic recombination, and the structural composition of the synaptonemal complex and its associated proteins have been reviewed recently [59].

There is a remarkable stage-specific gene expression in both rats [60] and humans [61]. The expression pattern of genes in germ cells throughout spermatogenesis and during development can be found at: http://mrg.genetics.washington.edu. The mechanisms for this selective turn on and off of large families of genes, such as those associated with the cell cycle, DNA repair, and embryonic neuron development, is far from resolved. In addition, many genes are expressed uniquely by germ cells once they enter meiosis; neither the need for having these genes expressed nor the mechanism regulating such expression are resolved; however, proposed mechanisms include alternative splicing, and epigenetic mechanisms, such as DNA methylation, histone modifications and piRNAs [62–66]. For example, in humans, the cytochrome c oxidase II gene is expressed in primary spermatocytes where it may serve the high energy demands of these cells as they enter the final stages of meiosis. The rescue factor-humanin gene is also expressed by these cells and may prevent germ cell death and/or apoptosis, allowing spermatogenesis to proceed [60].

21.3.5 Spermiogenesis: Associated Processes Involved in the Formation of Spermatids

During spermiogenesis, several major changes occur to spermatids as they metamorphose into spermatozoa: (1) the shape of the cell and its nucleus undergo major modifications that are species specific; (2) there is a compaction and condensation of the nuclear chromatin; (3) the acrosome develops on the surface of the nucleus; (4) the connecting piece and other components of the flagellum are formed; (5) the excess cytoplasm of the spermatid, referred to as the residual body, is eliminated; (6) the release of spermatids, known as spermiation, occurs. Many of the details of these processes have been described by others [3, 67–69]. Spermiogenesis extends over 22.7 days in rats and 21.6 days in humans.

21.4 The Spermatozoon

Over a few weeks, the transition that occurs from the somatic diploid spermatogonium to the haploid, highly specialized spermatozoon (Fig. 21.2), with a number of organelles and cellular features that are distinct from every other cell type in the body, is remarkable. Highlights of some of these cellular characteristics are described below.

21.4.1 Role of the Golgi Apparatus in Acrosome Formation

The acrosome is a membrane bound lysosomal structure that functions in sperm–egg binding; it is formed from the Golgi apparatus of early spermatids [70–72]. The acrosome is made up of three major subdivisions: apical segment, principal segment and equatorial segment. The membrane of the acrosome consists of an outer acrosomal membrane, underlying the plasma membrane of the spermatid, and the inner acrosomal membrane, facing the nucleus and being apposed to the perinuclear electron dense material, referred to as the perforatorium. The acrosome contains a variety of hydrolytic enzymes, with hyaluronidase and acrosin being most prominent; they both facilitate sperm penetration of the egg investments [73, 74]. Acrogranin and dipeptidyl peptidase II are found in the guinea pig acrosome and acrosomal antigen SP-10 in the human. It has been suggested that the acrosomal infrastructure is made up of spatially segregated distinct matrix components that may interact with and define the distribution of selected hydrolases [75].

21.4.2 Endoplasmic Reticulum

The endoplasmic reticulum (ER) undergoes extensive structural modifications during spermiogenesis [76]. In addition to being closely related to the Golgi apparatus, in steps 1–7

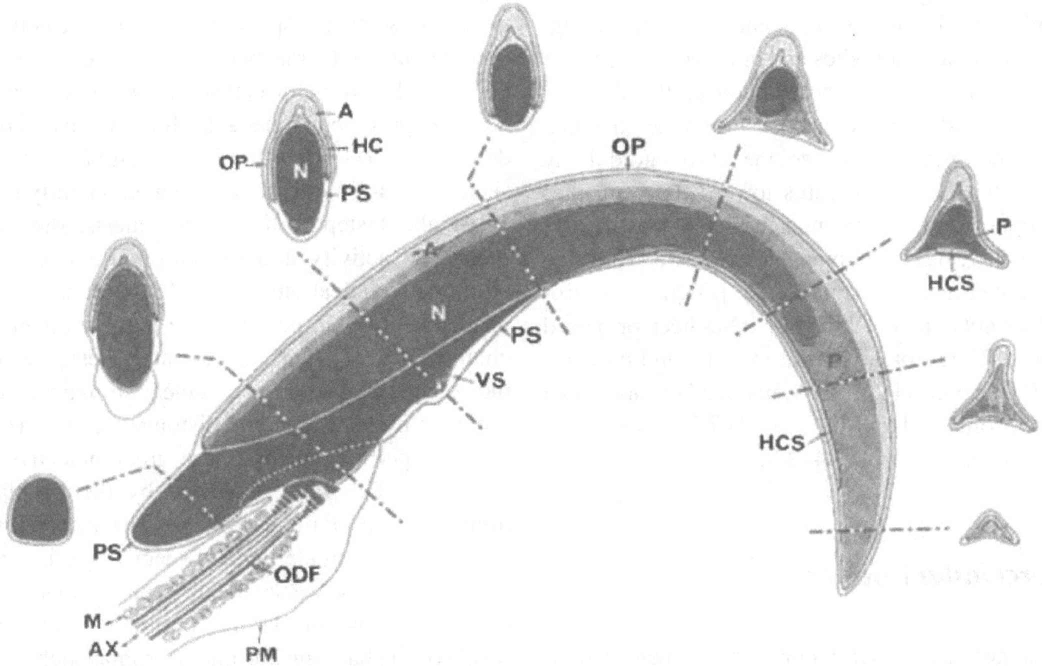

Fig. 21.2 Drawing of the head of a rat spermatozoa as seen from the side and accompanied by representative cross-sectional views. The region of the perinuclear theca delineated in smooth gray and lying between the acrosomic system (A: stippled in light gray) and the nucleus (N: dark black) represents the perforatorium (P). The region of the perinuclear theca beginning where the acrosomic system ends and lying between the nucleus and the plasmalemma is the post-acrosomal sheath (PS). The ventral spur (VS) refers to the ventral prominence of the sperm head, which is due to the ventral thickening of the postacrosomal sheath. The inner part of the ventral spur is colored in smooth gray to convey that this part of the ventral spur is similar in composition to the perforatorium. The acrosomic system is composed of the acrosome (A), head cap (HC) and separated head cap segment (HCS). The outer periacrosomic layer (OP), lying between the plasmalemma and the acrosomic system, is continuous structurally with the perforatorium and acrosomal sheath. The region of the outer periacrosomal layer adjacent to the acrosornic head cap is denoted in smooth gray to convey that this part of outer periacrosomal layer is similar in composition to the perforatorium. The dashed white line at the base of the nucleus indicates the borderline of the perifossal zone. Labels: PM, plasma membrane; *A* axoneme; *M* mitochondria; *ODF* outer dense fibers. Reproduced from Oko RI, Clermont Y (1991) Biogenesis of specialized cytoskeletal elements of rat spermatozoa. Ann N Y Acad Sci 637:203–223

(rat) the ER cisternae are dispersed in the cytoplasm where they are arranged as a 3-D network of spherical and tubular cisternae connected by small tubules that line the plasma membrane. In steps 8–14, the ER lines the microtubules of the manchette as long tubes or plates, appears along the flagellum in the form of a fenestrated sleeve, and encloses large vacuoles as fenestrated spherules. The ER is also continuous with the annulate lamellae and an aggregate of radially arranged collapsed cisternae termed the radial body. At steps 15–19, the ER regresses, fragments, and then disappears from the cytoplasm [76].

21.4.3 Chromatoid Body: Structure and Functions

The chromatoid body is a spongy-looking mass of electron dense granulofilamentous material with areas of low electron density that are associated with numerous small vesicles [77–80]. It first appears as an inter-mitochondrial dense material in pachytene spermatocytes. During early spermiogenesis, the chromatoid body is closely associated with the Golgi apparatus and multivesicular bodies and moves on the nuclear envelope, where continuities are noted between the chromatoid body material and intranuclear dense particles through nuclear pore complexes [81]. Later, the chromatoid body moves away for the Golgi apparatus toward the centrioles occupying the opposite pole of the nucleus where it associates with the annulus [77, 82]; in humans, it is transferred to the residual body at the time of spermiation [83]. While the chromatoid body does not contain DNA [84], it has been proposed to be involved in RNA storage and processing and contains snRNP, hnRNP proteins, TP2 mRNA, histone H4, ribosomal RNAs, large ribosomal subunit proteins P1/P2, and mRNA-binding proteins p48/52 [79, 80, 84–88].

21.4.4 Intercellular Bridges

During spermatogenesis, numerous mitotic and meiotic divisions occur in which cytokinesis begins, but is arrested such that daughter cells remain connected by intercellular bridges. The intercellular bridges are large (approximately 1 μm) open channels between clones of germ cells that are lined by an electron dense layer on the inner aspect of their membrane and that contain ER, mitochondria, ribosomes, filaments and microtubules [89–91]; it has been shown that, thanks to these bridges, genetically distinct spermatids can share the product of transgenes, thus making them phenotypically equivalent [92]. Hundreds or even thousands of germ cells may be connected by intercellular bridges [41, 91]. Intercellular bridges provide physical support and synchronous development for the clones of developing germ cells by facilitating the spread of regulatory substances throughout the clone [41, 90, 93]; removal of a specific protein (TEX14) prevents the formation of these bridges, blocking spermatogenesis at the first meiotic division, thus resulting in infertility [94].

21.4.5 Sperm Head and Nuclear Modifications

During spermiogenesis, the nucleus undergoes several major modifications, including a change in shape, compaction of its chromatin, protein expression and metabolic activity. In the early steps of rat spermiogenesis, the spermatid nucleus is round, occupies the center of the cytoplasm of the cell and is metabolically active. In the rat, when the acrosome is fully formed at the end of stage VIII, the spherical spermatid nucleus migrates to the periphery of the cell and becomes oriented with the acrosome intimately apposed to the overlying plasma membrane. From stage IX onward, the nucleus takes on its species-specific shape. The structure of the head components of the rat spermatid has been studied extensively [72, 95]. The transformation of the nucleus, acrosomic system, and perinuclear theca (perforatorium and postacrosomal dense lamina) during the maturation phase of spermiogenesis (steps 14–19) has been reviewed recently [96].

At about step 8 of spermiogenesis, the nucleus ceases metabolic activity and the chromatin begins to condense along with nuclear elongation. Despite the cessation of RNA synthesis at this time, the male gamete undergoes dramatic changes [68, 97]. During spermatogenesis, before and during meiosis, most of the basic nuclear somatic-type histones are replaced by testis-specific histones, such as H1t and others. During spermiogenesis, these are replaced with transition proteins (TP1, TP2), followed by their replacement with highly basic protamines [98, 99]. These proteins are involved in molecular remodeling and species specific compaction of the male genome within the differentiating spermatid nucleus [100]. The loss of H1t in spermatid nuclei appears to be involved in changing chromatin from a euchromatin to a filamentous form; the appearances of TP1 and TP2 are related to chromatin condensation [88]. This is followed by further DNA compaction induced when protamines bind to DNA, displacing the other chromatin proteins [101, 102].

Protamines are arginine-rich proteins of the testis. Two types of protamines are present, protamine 1 and 2, both are hypermethylated and evident in round spermatids. Protamine 1 is present in most mammals [103], while protamine 2 is found in a few mammals, including humans [104]. Protamine 1 has polyarginine DNA binding domains, while protamine 2 is synthesized as a precursor protein processed after binding to DNA in late spermatids. Binding of protamines to DNA condenses the DNA into a highly compact form. Protamine binding to DNA induces the coiling of DNA into donut or toroidal structures [105]. Histone to protamine exchange in spermatids is preceded by hyperacetylation of core histones resulting in decreased DNA–histone interaction. In the human testis, hyperacetylated histone H4 displays a strong signal in nuclei of elongating spermatids and spermatogonia, wherein it appears to play an important role in correct histone-to-protamine exchange [106]. In human sperm, histones remain as 15% of the nuclear proteins, whereas in rodents, the proportion of histone remaining in spermatozoa is in the range of 1% [107, 108].

The dramatic change in chromatin architecture also requires the appearance of DNA strand breaks because most of the DNA supercoiling is eliminated in the maturing sperm [109]. In the human testis, there is an increase in DNA strand breaks in the nuclei of round spermatids coincident with chromatin remodeling [110]. Chromatin in pachytene spermatocyte nuclei is loosely packed because of the poor DNA and chromatin condensing property of the testis specific linker histone H1t, which lacks a DNA condensing domain. TP1 is a DNA melting protein, while TP2 is a DNA condensing protein [101]. TP2 has two zinc finger modules and is phosphorylated by sperm specific protein kinase A. The phosphorylation and dephosphorylation cycle plays a role in the chromatin condensation process [111]. The chromatin domain containing the two human protamines and TP2 forms a DNase I-sensitive conformation in pachytene spermatocytes; this persists in mature sperm [112, 113]. In addition, this domain contains an enrichment of histones, and the distribution of histones and protamines within the sperm nucleus is nonrandom [114].

The protamine mRNAs are stored in the cytoplasm for about a week before the protamine protein is synthesized. Testis Brain RNA-binding protein (TB-RBP, translin, TSN) is present in the cytoplasm of round spermatids, functions with the cytoskeleton and facilitates both translational regulation of stored mRNAs and their transportation between cells [115]. It accumulates in the cytoplasm of spermatogonia and during meiosis enters the nuclei of pachytene spermatocytes, functioning as a DNA-binding protein for gene rearrangements. It travels from cell to cell via the intercellular bridges [116]. Given the large number of proteins that are synthesized in spermatids well after transcription stops, it is likely that there are a number of other RNA binding proteins yet to be identified in these cells.

Translationally inactive, sperm nuclei have been shown recently to contain both mRNAs and noncoding RNAs, i.e., miRNA and piRNAs [117–120]; the functional significance of these RNAs is unclear since sperm cannot synthesize proteins, and their contribution to the zygote is likely to be extensively diluted by the contribution of the oocute; however, they may play a role in selective activation of paternal genes after fertilization.

21.4.6 Structure of the Flagellum

As the acrosome grows on one pole of the nuclear surface, paired centrioles move to the opposite pole, where they initiate formation of the flagellum. The flagellum consists of a neck or connecting piece, and middle, principal and end pieces. Throughout its length, the flagellum shows specific modifications [96]. A central axoneme consists of nine microtubular doublets circularly arranged to form a cylinder around a central pair of single microtubules. In the middle piece, the axoneme is surrounded by an outer cylinder of nine outer dense fibers arranged as nine rod-like structures that run parallel to the axoneme; they play a role in protecting sperm against shearing forces, defining waveform and generating motility [121, 122]. A discontinuous helix of individual elongated mitochondria is arranged around this cylinder. In the principal piece, the mitochondrial helix is absent and a fibrous sheath composed of its own unique proteins replaces two of the outer dense fibers. The fibrous sheath may play a role in directing the sperm wave form [123]. The principal piece is 10 times the length of the middle piece and terminates in the end piece. In humans, the total length of the flagellum is 45 μm. The annulus is the site of junction between the middle and principal piece.

A-kinase-anchoring protein, or AKAP, controls cAMP-dependent protein kinase (PKA) [124] and has been localized to the flagellum, midpiece and acrosome [125–127]. WAVE1, a member of the Wiskott–Aldrich syndrome family of adaptor proteins, has been identified as an AKAP that targets actin and is localized to the Golgi apparatus of spermatocytes and round spermatids, whereas in elongating spermatids, it is localized to the mitochondrial sheath [128]. Several putative partners of WAVE1, such as the regulatory subunit II of PKA, are also localized to the flagellar mid piece. Collectively, these data suggest that a functional signaling unit is established by WAVE1 and associated proteins in maturing sperm [128].

The outer dense fiber proteins are synthesized during the latter part of spermiogenesis [129, 130], long after transcriptional activity in the haploid germ cell has ended. They are translationally regulated, with their mRNAs being stored in an electron dense amorphous granulated body which is abundant in the cytoplasm of elongated spermatids at steps 15–17, at the time of peak outer dense fiber assembly.

The fibrous sheath extends throughout the principal piece, where it lies under the plasma membrane and surrounds the outer dense fibers and axoneme [96]. It consists of two longitudinal dense columns connected by circumferential ribs. It provides form and rigor to the flagellum and determines the shape of the flagellar beat [131]; infertility is associated with sperm with defective fibrous sheaths [132]. Several proteins have been identified, with the most abundant being phosphorylated [133, 134]. Intermediate filament-like proteins also appear to be present in the fibrous sheath [123]. Interestingly, a number of glycolytic enzymes have been shown to be bound to the fibrous sheath [135], and null mutations for enzymes such as glyceraldehyde 3-phosphate dehydrogenase-S result in immotile sperm and consequent male infertility [136].

The perforatorium is the expanded subacrosomal region of the perinuclear theca [72]. The perforatorial proteins are synthesized during the meiotic prophase, reaching a peak in early spermiogenesis prior to the initiation of the condensation of the nucleus of spermatid at which time RNA synthesis stops. The perforatorial proteins are concentrated in the nuclei of pachytene spermatocytes and round spermatids until their displacement into the cytoplasm during nuclear condensation [137]. The perforatorium contains several proteins of different molecular weights [138, 139]. The major protein of the perforatorium is PERF 15, a 15-kDa protein that shares similarities with members of the family of fatty acid-binding proteins. It appears that the outer aspect of PERF 15 may play a role in development and stabilization of the acrosome and shaping the sperm [140]. The extracellular protein coat of the inner acrosomal membrane (IAM38), facing the perinuclear theca, is involved in secondary sperm–zona binding and penetration during fertilization [141].

The axoneme is essential for motility and consists of over 240 different proteins [142]. In humans, the radial spoke protein 44 gene, also termed RSP44, produces the protein designated as human meichroacidin. The latter localizes to the tails of elongating spermatids, where it appears within radial spokes of the axonemal complex and plays a role in sperm motility [143].

21.5 Conclusions

The last half of the twentieth century saw an explosion in our understanding of the process of spermatogenesis and of the remarkably complex and unique cellular elements that constitute spermatozoa. Over the last 10 years, the functions of many germ-cell specific proteins are being resolved thanks to ever-rapidly developing molecular biology tools. However, we still have a very limited understanding of the regulatory factors that control the assembly of spermatozoa, of the cell signaling mechanisms that allow for the complex communication among germ, Sertoli and Leydig cells, and of how extrinsic factors such as drugs and environments conditions modulate changes in both the quantity and quality of spermatozoa that are produced. With the rapid development of our understanding of the genetic and epigenetic mechanisms that regulate the sperm proteome and function, we can look forward to resolving the underlying causes of male infertility, to developing new therapeutic approaches for its treatment, and to identifying specific and selective approaches for male contraception.

References

1. Roosen-Runge EC (1962) The process of spermatogenesis in mammals. Biol Rev Camb Philos Soc 37:343–377
2. Clermont Y (1972) Kinetics of spermatogenesis in mammals: seminiferous epithelium cycle and spermatogonial renewal. Physiol Rev 52:198–236
3. Kerr JB, Loveland KL, O'Bryan MK, de Kretzer DM (2006) Cytology of the testis and intrinsic control mechanisms. In: Neill JD (ed) Knobil and Neill's Physiology of Reproduction, vol 1, 3rd edn. Academic Press, Amsterdam, pp 827–947
4. Huckins C, Clermont Y (1968) Evolution of gonocytes in the rat testis during late embryonic and early post-natal life. Arch Anat Histol Embryol 51(1):341–354
5. Griswold MD, McLean D (2006) The Sertoli cell. In: Neill JD (ed) Knobil and Neill's Physiology of Reproduction, vol 1, 3rd edn. Academic Press, Amsterdam, pp 949–976
6. Skinner MK, Griswold MD (2004) Sertoli cell biology, vol. 1. Academic Press, Amsterdam, 512 p
7. Setchell BP, Breed WG (2006) Anatomy, vasculature and innervation of the male reproductive tract. In: Neill JD (ed) Knobil and Neill's Physiology of Reproduction, vol 1, 3rd edn. Academic Press, Amsterdam, pp 771–825
8. Payne AH, Hardy MP (2007) The Leydig cell in health and disease. Humana Press, Totowa, Amsterdam, 476 p
9. Steinberger E (1971) Hormonal control of mammalian spermatogenesis. Physiol Rev 51:1–22
10. Skinner MK (1991) Cell–cell interactions in the testis. Endocr Rev 12(1):45–77
11. Zirkin BR, Awoniyi C, Griswold MD, Russell LD, Sharpe R (1994) Is FSH required for adult spermatogenesis? J Androl 15:273–276
12. O'Donnell L, Meachem SJ, Stanton PG, McLachlan RI (2006) Endocrine regulation of spermatogenesis. In: Neill JD (ed) Knobil and Neill's Physiology of Reproduction, vol 1, 3rd edn. Academic Press, Amsterdam, pp 1017–1070
13. Leblond CP, Clermont Y (1952) Definition of the stages of the cycle of the seminiferous epithelium in the rat. Ann N Y Acad Sci 55(4):548–573
14. Clermont Y, Trott M (1969) Duration of the cycle of the seminiferous epithelium in the mouse and hamster determined by means of 3H-thymidine and radioautography. Fertil Steril 20:805–817
15. Clermont Y, Leblond CP (1959) Differentiation and renewal of spermatogonia in the monkey, *Macacus rhesus*. Am J Anat 104:237–273
16. Clermont Y (1966) Renewal of spermatogenesis in man. Am J Anat 118:509–524
17. Heller CG, Clermont Y (1963) Spermatogenesis in man: an estimate of its duration. Science 140:184–186
18. Perey B, Clermont Y, Leblond CP (1961) The wave of the seminiferous epithelium of the rat. Am J Anat 108:47–77
19. Regaud C (1901) Etudes sur la structure des tubes séminifères et sur la spermatogenèse chez les mammifères. Arch Anat Microsc 4:101–156
20. Brinster RL (2007) Male germline stem cells: from mice to men. Science 316:404–405
21. Dym M (1994) Spermatogonial stem cells of the testis. Proc Natl Acad Sci U S A 91:11287–11289
22. Brinster RL (2002) Germline stem cell transplantation and transgenesis. Science 296:2174–2176
23. de Rooij DG (2001) Proliferation and differentiation of spermatogonial stem cells. Reproduction 121:347–354
24. Clermont Y, Bustos-Obregon E (1968) Re-examination of spermatogonial renewal in the rat by means of seminiferous tubules mounted "in toto". Am J Anat 122:237–247
25. Dym M, Clermont Y (1970) Role of spermatogonia in the repair of the seminiferous epithelium following x-irradiation of the rat testis. Am J Anat 128:265–282

26. Clermont Y, Hermo L (1975) Spermatogonial stem cells in the albino rat. Am J Anat 142:159–175
27. Bartmanska J, Clermont Y (1983) Renewal of type A spermatogonia in adult rats. Cell Tissue Kinet 16:135–143
28. Huckins C (1971) Cell cycle properties of differentiating spermatogonia in adult Sprague–Dawley rats. Cell Tissue Kinet 4:139–154
29. Huckins C (1971) The spermatogonial stem cell population in adult rats. I. Their morphology, proliferation and maturation. Anat Rec 169:533–557
30. Huckins C (1971) The spermatogonial stem cell population in adult rats. 3. Evidence for a long-cycling population. Cell Tissue Kinet 4:335–349
31. Huckins C (1971) The spermatogonial stem cell population in adult rats II. A radioautographic analysis of their cell cycle properties. Cell Tissue Kinet 4:313–334
32. de Rooij DG, Grootegoed JA (1998) Spermatogonial stem cells. Curr Opin Cell Biol 10:694–701
33. Yoshida S, Takakura A, Ohbo K, Abe K, Wakabayashi J, Yamamoto M, Suda T, Nabeshima Y (2004) Neurogenin3 delineates the earliest stages of spermatogenesis in the mouse testis. Dev Biol 269:447–458
34. Roosen-Runge EC, Barlow FD (1953) Quantitative studies on human spermatogenesis. I. Spermatogonia. Am J Anat 93(2):143–169
35. Mancini RE, Narbaitz R, Lavieri JC (1960) Origin and development of the germinative epithelium and Sertoli cells in the human testis: cytological, cytochemical, and quantitative study. Anat Rec 136:477–489
36. Rowley MJ, Berlin JD, Heller CG (1971) The ultrastructure of four types of human spermatogonia. Z Zellforsch Mikrosk Anat 112(2):139–157
37. Schulze W (1978) Light and electron microscope studies of the morphology of A spermatogonia in men with normal spermatogenesis and in patients treated with antiandrogens. Andrologia 10(4):307–320
38. Oakberg EF, Gosslee DG, Huckins C, Cummings CC (1986) Do spermatogonial stem cells have a circadian rhythm? Cell Tissue Kinet 19:367–375
39. Ehmcke J, Schlatt S (2006) A revised model for spermatogonial expansion in man: lessons from non-human primates. Reproduction 132(5):673–680
40. Clermont Y (1962) Quantitative analysis of spermatogenesis of the rat: a revised model for the renewal of spermatogonia. Am J Anat 111:111–129
41. Huckins C (1978) Spermatogonial intercellular bridges in whole-mounted seminiferous tubules from normal and irradiated rodent testes. Am J Anat 153(1):97–121
42. Blanco-Rodríguez J, Martínez-García C (1996) Spontaneous germ cell death in the testis of the adult rat takes the form of apoptosis: re-evaluation of cell types that exhibit the ability to die during spermatogenesis. Cell Prolif 29:13–31
43. Brinkworth MH, Weinbauer GF, Schlatt S, Nieschlag E (1995) Identification of male germ cells undergoing apoptosis in adult rats. J Reprod Fertil 105:25–33
44. Cai L, Hales BF, Robaire B (1997) Induction of apoptosis in the germ cells of adult male rats after exposure to cyclophosphamide. Biol Reprod 56:1490–1497
45. Blanco-Rodríguez J, Martínez-García C (1998) Apoptosis pattern elicited by several apoptogenic agents on the seminiferous epithelium of the adult rat testis. J Androl 19:487–497
46. Pentikäinen V, Erkkilä K, Suomalainen L, Otala M, Pentikäinen MO, Parvinen M, Dunkel L (2001) TNFalpha down-regulates the Fas ligand and inhibits germ cell apoptosis in the human testis. J Clin Endocrinol Metab 86:4480–4488
47. McKee CM, Ye Y, Richburg JH (2006) Testicular germ cell sensitivity to TRAIL-induced apoptosis is dependent upon p53 expression and is synergistically enhanced by DR5 agonistic antibody treatment. Apoptosis 11:2237–2250
48. Richburg JH, Johnson KJ, Schoenfeld HA, Meistrich ML, Dix DJ (2002) Defining the cellular and molecular mechanisms of toxicant action in the testis. Toxicol Lett 135:167–183
49. Sugiyama N, Obinata M, Matsui Y (2001) Bcl-2 inhibits apoptosis of spermatogonia and growth of spermatogonial stem cells in a cell-intrinsic manner. Mol Reprod Dev 58:30–38
50. Hackstein JH, Hochstenbach R, Pearson PL (2000) Towards an understanding of the genetics of human male infertility: lessons from flies. Trends Genet 16:565–572
51. Cobb J, Handel MA (1998) Dynamics of meiotic prophase I during spermatogenesis: from pairing to division. Semin Cell Dev Biol 9:445–450
52. Handel MA, Sun F (2005) Regulation of meiotic cell divisions and determination of gamete quality: impact of reproductive toxins. Semin Reprod Med 23:213–221
53. Solari AJ (1972) Ultrastructure and composition of the synaptonemal complex in spread and negatively stained spermatocytes of the golden hamster and the albino rat. Chromosoma 39: 237–263
54. Heyting C, Dietrich AJ, Moens PB, Dettmers RJ, Offenberg HH, Redeker EJ, Vink AC (1989) Synaptonemal complex proteins. Genome 31:81–87
55. Hoyer-Fender S, Costanzi C, Pehrson JR (2000) Histone macroH2A1.2 is concentrated in the XY-body by the early pachytene stage of spermatogenesis. Exp Cell Res 258:254–260
56. Liu JY, Dai XH, Zeng XL, Zhang CS, Hao S, Song YC (2005) The relationship between abnormity of synaptonemal complex and male fertility impairment in human. Yi Chuan 27:819–827
57. Sun F, Greene C, Turek PJ, Ko E, Rademaker A, Martin RH (2005) Immunofluorescent synaptonemal complex analysis in azoospermic men. Cytogenet Genome Res 111:366–370
58. Geoffroy-Siraudin C, Aknin-Seiffer I, Metzler-Guillemain C, Ghalamoun-Slaimi R, Bonzi MF, Levy R, Guichaoua MR (2007) Meiotic abnormalities in patients bearing complete AZFc deletion of Y chromosome. Hum Reprod 22(6):1567–1572
59. Vallente RU, Cheng EY, Hassold TJ (2006) The synaptonemal complex and meiotic recombination in humans: new approaches to old questions. Chromosoma 115:241–249
60. Johnston DS, Wright WW, Dicandeloro P, Wilson E, Kopf GS, Jelinsky SA (2008) Stage-specific gene expression is a fundamental characteristic of rat spermatogenic cells and Sertoli cells. Proc Natl Acad Sci U S A 105:8315–8320
61. Liang G, Zhang XD, Wang LJ, Sha YS, Zhang JC, Miao SY, Zong SD, Wang LF, Koide SS (2004) Identification of differentially expressed genes of primary spermatocyte against round spermatid isolated from human testis using the laser capture microdissection technique. Cell Res 14:507–512
62. Maclean JA 2nd, Wilkinson MF (2005) Gene regulation in spermatogenesis. Curr Top Dev Biol 71:131–197
63. Hogeveen KN, Sassone-Corsi P (2006) Regulation of gene expression in post-meiotic male germ cells: CREM-signalling pathways and male fertility. Hum Fertil (Camb) 9:73–79
64. Elliott DJ, Grellscheid SN (2006) Alternative RNA splicing regulation in the testis. Reproduction 132:811–819
65. Yin H, Lin H (2007) An epigenetic activation role of Piwi and a Piwi-associated piRNA in *Drosophila melanogaster*. Nature 450:304–308
66. Hecht NB (1990) Regulation of 'haploid expressed genes' in male germ cells. J Reprod Fertil 88:679–693
67. Clermont Y, Oko R, Hermo L (1993) Cell biology of mammalian spermatogenesis. In: Desjardins C (ed) Cell and Molecular biology of the testis. Oxford University Press, New York: pp332-376
68. Hecht NB (1995) The making of a spermatozoon: a molecular perspective. Dev Genet 16:95–103
69. Kierszenbaum AL, Rivkin E, Tres LL (2007) Molecular biology of sperm head shaping. Soc Reprod Fertil Suppl 65:33–43

70. Susi FR, Leblond CP, Clermont Y (1971) Changes in the golgi apparatus during spermiogenesis in the rat. Am J Anat 130(3):251–267
71. Mollenhauer HH, Morré DJ (1978) Polyribosomes associated with forming acrosome membranes in guinea pig spermatids. Science 200:85–86
72. Lalli M, Clermont Y (1981) Structural changes of the head components of the rat spermatid during late spermiogenesis. Am J Anat 160:419–434
73. Moreno RD, Alvarado CP (2006) The mammalian acrosome as a secretory lysosome: new and old evidence. Mol Reprod Dev 73:1430–1434
74. Salicioni AM, Platt MD, Wertheimer EV, Arcelay E, Allaire A, Sosnik J, Visconti PE (2007) Signalling pathways involved in sperm capacitation. Soc Reprod Fertil Suppl 65:245–259
75. Olson GE, Winfrey V (1991) Structure-function relationships in the sperm acrosome. Ann N Y Acad Sci 637:240–257
76. Clermont Y, Rambourg A (1978) Evolution of the endoplasmic reticulum during rat spermiogenesis. Am J Anat 151(2):191–211
77. Fawcett DW, Eddy EM, Phillips DM (1970) Observations on the fine structure and relationships of the chromatoid body in mammalian spermatogenesis. Biol Reprod 2:129–153
78. Susi FR, Clermont Y (1970) Fine structural modifications of the rat chromatoid body during spermiogenesis. Am J Anat 129:177–191
79. Parvinen M (2005) The chromatoid body in spermatogenesis. Int J Androl 28:189–201
80. Kotaja N, Sassone-Corsi P (2007) The chromatoid body: a germ-cell-specific RNA-processing centre. Nat Rev Mol Cell Biol 8:85–90
81. Söderström KO, Parvinen M (1976) Transport of material between the nucleus, the chromatoid body and the Golgi complex in the early spermatids of the rat. Cell Tissue Res 168:335–342
82. Russell L, Frank B (1978) Ultrastructural characterization of nuage in spermatocytes of the rat testis. Anat Rec 190:79–97
83. Breucker H, Schäfer E, Holstein AF (1985) Morphogenesis and fate of the residual body in human spermiogenesis. Cell Tissue Res 240:303–309
84. Biggiogera M, Fakan S, Leser G, Martin TE, Gordon J (1990) Immunoelectron microscopical visualization of ribonucleoproteins in the chromatoid body of mouse spermatids. Mol Reprod Dev 26:150–158
85. Saunders PT, Millar MR, Maguire SM, Sharpe RM (1992) Stage-specific expression of rat transition protein 2 mRNA and possible localization to the chromatoid body of step 7 spermatids by in situ hybridization using a nonradioactive riboprobe. Mol Reprod Dev 33:385–389
86. Moussa F, Oko R, Hermo L (1994) The immunolocalization of small nuclear ribonucleoprotein particles in testicular cells during the cycle of the seminiferous epithelium of the adult rat. Cell Tissue Res 278:363–378
87. Werner G, Werner K (1995) Immunocytochemical localization of histone H4 in the chromatoid body of rat spermatids. J Submicrosc Cytol Pathol 27:325–330
88. Oko R, Korley R, Murray MT, Hecht NB, Hermo L (1996) Germ cell-specific DNA and RNA binding proteins p48/52 are expressed at specific stages of male germ cell development and are present in the chromatoid body. Mol Reprod Dev 44:1–13
89. Burgos MH, Fawcett DW (1955) Studies on the fine structure of the mammalian testis. I. Differentiation of the spermatids in the cat (*Felis domestica*). J Biophys Biochem Cytol 1:287–300
90. Fawcett DW, Ito S, Slautterback D (1959) The occurrence of intercellular bridges in groups of cells exhibiting synchronous differentiation. J Biophys Biochem Cytol 5:453–460
91. Dym M, Fawcett DW (1971) Further observations on the numbers of spermatogonia, spermatocytes, and spermatids connected by intercellular bridges in the mammalian testis. Biol Reprod 4:195–215
92. Braun RE, Behringer RR, Peschon JJ, Brinster RL, Palmiter RD (1989) Genetically haploid spermatids are phenotypically diploid. Nature 337:373–376
93. Gondos B, Zemjanis R (1970) Fine structure of spermatogonia and intercellular bridges in *Macaca nemestrina*. J Morphol 131:431–446
94. Greenbaum MP, Yan W, Wu MH, Lin YN, Agno JE, Sharma M, Braun RE, Rajkovic A, Matzuk MM (2006) TEX14 is essential for intercellular bridges and fertility in male mice. Proc Natl Acad Sci U S A 103(13):4982–4987
95. Fawcett DW, Anderson WA, Phillips DM (1971) Morphogenetic factors influencing the shape of the sperm head. Dev Biol 26:220–251
96. Eddy EM (2006) The spermatozoon. In: Neill JD (ed) Knobil and Neill's Physiology of Reproduction, vol 1, 3rd edn. Academic Press, Amsterdam, pp 3–54
97. Hecht NB (1998) Molecular mechanisms of male germ cell differentiation. Bioessays 20:555–561
98. Kistler WS, Henriksén K, Mali P, Parvinen M (1996) Sequential expression of nucleoproteins during rat spermiogenesis. Exp Cell Res 225:374–381
99. Steger K, Klonisch T, Gavenis K, Drabent B, Doenecke D, Bergmann M (1998) Expression of mRNA and protein of nucleoproteins during human spermiogenesis. Mol Hum Reprod 4:939–945
100. Sassone-Corsi P (2002) Unique chromatin remodeling and transcriptional regulation in spermatogenesis. Science 296:2176–2178
101. Brewer L, Corzett M, Balhorn R (2002) Condensation of DNA by spermatid basic nuclear proteins. J Biol Chem 277:38895–38900
102. Balhorn R (2007) The protamine family of sperm nuclear proteins. Genome Biol 8:227
103. Queralt R, Adroer R, Oliva R, Winkfein RJ, Retief JD, Dixon GH (1995) Evolution of protamine P1 genes in mammals. J Mol Evol 40:601–607
104. McKay DJ, Renaux BS, Dixon GH (1986) Human sperm protamines. Amino-acid sequences of two forms of protamine P2. Eur J Biochem 156:5–8
105. Ward WS (1993) Deoxyribonucleic acid loop domain tertiary structure in mammalian spermatozoa. Biol Reprod 48:1193–1201
106. Sonnack V, Failing K, Bergmann M (2002) Steger K Expression of hyperacetylated histone H4 during normal and impaired human spermatogenesis. Andrologia 34:384–390
107. Churikov D, Zalenskaya IA, Zalensky AO (2004) Male germline-specific histones in mouse and man. Cytogenet Genome Res 105:203–214
108. Kimmins S, Sassone-Corsi P (2005) Chromatin remodelling and epigenetic features of germ cells. Nature 434:583–589
109. Laberge RM, Boissonneault G (2005) Chromatin remodeling in spermatids: a sensitive step for the genetic integrity of the male gamete. Arch Androl 51:125–133
110. Marcon L, Boissonneault G (2004) Transient DNA strand breaks during mouse and human spermiogenesis new insights in stage specificity and link to chromatin remodeling. Biol Reprod 70:910–918
111. Pradeepa MM, Rao MR (2007) Chromatin remodeling during mammalian spermatogenesis: role of testis specific histone variants and transition proteins. Soc Reprod Fertil Suppl 63:1–10
112. Choudhary SK, Wykes SM, Kramer JA, Mohamed AN, Koppitch F, Nelson JE, Krawetz SA (1995) A haploid expressed gene cluster exists as a single chromatin domain in human sperm. J Biol Chem 270:8755–8762
113. Kramer JA, McCarrey JR, Djakiew D, Krawetz SA (1998) Differentiation: the selective potentiation of chromatin domains. Development 125:4749–4755
114. Wykes SM, Krawetz SA (2003) The structural organization of sperm chromatin. J Biol Chem 278:29471–29477
115. Cho YS, Iguchi N, Yang J, Handel MA, Hecht NB (2005) Meiotic messenger RNA and noncoding RNA targets of the

RNA-binding protein Translin (TSN) in mouse testis. Biol Reprod 73:840–847
116. Morales CR, Wu XQ, Hecht NB (1998) The DNA/RNA-binding protein, TB-RBP, moves from the nucleus to the cytoplasm and through intercellular bridges in male germ cells. Dev Biol 201:113–123
117. Ostermeier GC, Dix DJ, Miller D, Khatri P, Krawetz SA (2002) Spermatozoal RNA profiles of normal fertile men. Lancet 360:772–777
118. Marcon E, Babak T, Chua G, Hughes T, Moens PB (2008) miRNA and piRNA localization in the male mammalian meiotic nucleus. Chromosome Res 16:243–260
119. Lalancette C, Miller D, Li Y, Krawetz SA (2008) Paternal contributions: new functional insights for spermatozoal RNA. J Cell Biochem 104:1570–1579
120. Gilbert I, Bissonnette N, Boissonneault G, Vallée M, Robert C (2007) A molecular analysis of the population of mRNA in bovine spermatozoa. Reproduction 133:1073–1086
121. Shao X, Tarnasky HA, Schalles U, Oko R, van der Hoorn FA (1997) Interactional cloning of the 84-kDa major outer dense fiber protein Odf84. Leucine zippers mediate associations of Odf84 and Odf27. J Biol Chem 272:6105–6113
122. O'Bryan MK, Sebire K, Meinhardt A, Edgar K, Keah HH, Hearn MT, De Kretser DM (2001) Tpx-1 is a component of the outer dense fibers and acrosome of rat spermatozoa. Mol Reprod Dev 58:116–125
123. Eddy EM, Toshimori K, O'Brien DA (2003) Fibrous sheath of mammalian spermatozoa. Microsc Res Tech 61:103–115
124. Rubin CS (1994) A kinase anchor proteins and the intracellular targeting of signals carried by cyclic AMP. Biochim Biophys Acta 1224:467–479
125. Vijayaraghavan S, Liberty GA, Mohan J, Winfrey VP, Olson GE, Carr DW (1999) Isolation and molecular characterization of AKAP110, a novel, sperm-specific protein kinase A-anchoring protein. Mol Endocrinol 13:705–717
126. Miki K, Eddy EM (1999) ingle amino acids determine specificity of binding of protein kinase A regulatory subunits by protein kinase A anchoring proteins. J Biol Chem 274:29057–29062
127. Turner RM, Eriksson RL, Gerton GL, Moss SB (1999) Relationship between sperm motility and the processing and tyrosine phosphorylation of two human sperm fibrous sheath proteins, pro-hAKAP82 and hAKAP82. Mol Hum Reprod 5:816–824
128. Rawe VY, Ramalho-Santos J, Payne C, Chemes HE, Schatten G (2004) WAVE1, an A-kinase anchoring protein, during mammalian spermatogenesis. Hum Reprod 19:2594–2604
129. Clermont Y, Oko R, Hermo L (1990) Immunocytochemical localization of proteins utilized in the formation of outer dense fibers and fibrous sheath in rat spermatids: an electron microscope study. Anat Rec 227:447–457
130. Henkel R, Stalf T, Mertens N, Miska W, Schill WB (1994) Outer dense fibres of human spermatozoa: partial characterization and possible physiological functions. Int J Androl 17:68–73
131. Phillips DM (1972) Comparative analysis of mammalian sperm motility. J Cell Biol 53:561–573
132. Baccetti B, Collodel G, Gambera L, Moretti E, Serafini F, Piomboni P (2005) Fluorescence in situ hybridization and molecular studies in infertile men with dysplasia of the fibrous sheath. Fertil Steril 84:123–129
133. El-Alfy M, Moshonas D, Morales CR, Oko R (1999) Molecular cloning and developmental expression of the major fibrous sheath protein (FS 75) of rat sperm. J Androl 20:307–318
134. Brito M, Figueroa J, Maldonado EU, Vera JC, Burzio LO (1989) The major component of the rat sperm fibrous sheath is a phosphoprotein. Gamete Res 22:205–217
135. Krisfalusi M, Miki K, Magyar PL, O'Brien DA (2006) Multiple glycolytic enzymes are tightly bound to the fibrous sheath of mouse spermatozoa. Biol Reprod 75:270–278
136. Miki K, Qu W, Goulding EH, Willis WD, Bunch DO, Strader LF, Perreault SD, Eddy EM, O'Brien DA (2004) Glyceraldehyde 3-phosphate dehydrogenase-S, a sperm-specific glycolytic enzyme, is required for sperm motility and male fertility. Proc Natl Acad Sci U S A 101:16501–16506
137. Oko R, Clermont Y (1991) Origin and distribution of perforatorial proteins during spermatogenesis of the rat: an immunocytochemical study. Anat Rec 230:489–501
138. Olson GE, Hamilton DW, Fawcett DW (1976) Isolation and characterization of the perforatorium of rat spermatozoa. J Reprod Fertil 47:293–297
139. Oko R, Clermont Y (1988) Isolation, structure and protein composition of the perforatorium of rat spermatozoa. Biol Reprod 39:673–687
140. Pouresmaeili F, Morales CR, Oko R (1997) Molecular cloning and structural analysis of the gene encoding PERF 15 protein present in the perinuclear theca of the rat spermatozoa. Biol Reprod 57:655–659
141. Yu Y, Xu W, Yi YJ, Sutovsky P, Oko R (2006) The extracellular protein coat of the inner acrosomal membrane is involved in zona pellucida binding and penetration during fertilization: characterization of its most prominent polypeptide (IAM38). Dev Biol 290:32–43
142. Ostrowski LE, Blackburn K, Radde KM, Moyer MB, Schlatzer DM, Moseley A, Boucher RC (2002) A proteomic analysis of human cilia: identification of novel components. Mol Cell Proteomics 1:451–465
143. Shetty J, Klotz KL, Wolkowicz MJ, Flickinger CJ, Herr JC (2007) Radial spoke protein 44 (human meichroacidin) is an axonemal alloantigen of sperm and cilia. Gene 396:93–107

Chapter 22
Meiotic Recombination and Errors During Spermatogenesis

Helen Ghislaine Tempest and Renee Halo Martin

Abstract It has been suggested that reduced recombination is associated with the production of paternally derived aneuploid gametes. Recent studies have shown major defects in recombination and synapsis of chromosomes in infertile men who have an increased frequency of aneuploid sperm. Given this information, the aim of this chapter is to provide a brief overview of human spermatogenesis and meiosis, and to investigate previous and current techniques used to further our understanding of chromosomal synapsis and genetic recombination. The chapter also covers the: current understanding of the timing and progression of synaptonemal complex (SC) formation, SC abnormalities, the frequency and variation of meiotic recombination in control males and azoospermic infertile males, and the clinical implications for meiotic recombination studies.

Keywords Meiosis • Spermatocytes • Recombination • Synaptonemal complex • Aneuploidy • Chromosomal synapsis • Pachytene

22.1 Introduction

Spermatogenesis in the male begins at the onset of puberty, takes approximately 70 days to complete in humans and is a continual process occurring in the seminiferous tubules within the testes. Spermatogonia (containing a diploid number ($n=46$) of chromosomes) develop from primordial germ cells that lie within the tubules, and at puberty the spermatogonia undergo mitosis. Of these progeny, some continue to divide indefinitely, while others undergo meiosis and become primary spermatocytes. These primary spermatocytes continue on to division I of meiosis, becoming secondary spermatocytes. By the end of the second meiotic division, these cells are spermatids, which then undergo a series of morphological differentiation steps in order to become spermatozoa.

22.2 Meiosis

From a genetic point of view, the two key features of spermatogenesis are the specialised form of cell division (meiosis) that takes place to halve the number of chromosomes within the gametes, and the generation of genetic variation among the population through genetic recombination. The most important meiotic stage is considered to be meiosis I prophase, during which, homologous chromosomes come together (synapsis) and an intimate physical coupling of the homologous chromosomes allows exchange of genetic material (genetic recombination) [1]. During subsequent stages of meiosis I, homologous chromosomes segregate and the cell divides into two cells. During meiosis II, sister chromatids in each of these cells separate and the cells divide again, resulting in the generation of four germ cells containing a haploid number of chromosomes ($n=23$). It is hypothesised that chromosome pairing and recombination of chromosomes is critical for the normal progression of spermatogenesis and to ensure that chromosome segregation occurs correctly. Any alteration in these vital meiotic events results in chromosomal non-disjunction (abnormal segregation of chromosomes) and sperm that have missing or extra chromosomes (aneuploidy).

Aneuploidy is the leading cause of infertility, birth defects, developmental defects and pregnancy loss in humans. Aneuploidy in humans is surprisingly prevalent, estimated to affect 0.3% of live births, 4% of stillbirths and up to 35% of spontaneous abortions [2]. Information is emerging that while meiotic recombination is essential for providing genetic variability within the population, it also appears to play a crucial role for correct chromosome segregation, ensuring the formation of haploid gametes [3]. Several studies to date have

H.G. Tempest
Department of Medical Genetics, University of Calgary, Calgary, AB, Canada
Herbert Wertheim College of Medicine, Department of Human and Molecular Genetics, Florida International University, Miami, Florida, USA, 33199

R.H. Martin (✉)
Department of Medical Genetics, University of Calgary, 3330 Hospital Drive, Calgary, AB, Canada T2N 4N1
e-mail: rhmartin@ucalgary.ca

D.T. Carrell and C.M. Peterson (eds.), *Reproductive Endocrinology and Infertility: Integrating Modern Clinical and Laboratory Practice*,
DOI 10.1007/978-1-4419-1436-1_22,

demonstrated that a reduction in genetic recombination in lower organisms is associated with increased frequencies of aneuploidy in the gametes [4]. Single sperm typing has also provided evidence of this association in human sex chromosomes – reduced recombination within the pseudoautosomal pairing region is associated with increased sex chromosome aneuploidy [5]. Reduced recombination between the sex chromosomes has also been observed in paternally derived cases of Klinefelter syndrome (47,XXY) [6, 7]. However, little is known about the patterns of meiotic recombination in human germ cells or the mechanisms through which these are controlled [8]. Our current understanding of the progression and patterns of recombination will form the basis of this review.

22.2.1 Techniques Used to Study Genetic Recombination

Genetic recombination in human spermatogenesis has been studied for several decades through genetic linkage studies, single sperm typing by PCR, the cytogenetic study of chiasmata at diplotene and diakinesis and, more recently, through immunocytogenetic studies.

Genetic linkage studies allow genetic measures of recombination to be calculated over relatively short genomic segments (typically regions of individual chromosomes) through the identification of genotype data in families [9, 10]. The use of this method to study the entire genome in individual meioses is inefficient, however [9], and few genome wide studies have been reported [11].

Microsatellite typing using PCR on single sperm cells has also been utilised to estimate the frequency of recombination between two selected markers on a given chromosome [5]. Again, while this is a useful technique, it is technically demanding and can generate information only on the region between the two microsatellite markers chosen on the chromosome of interest.

Hultén and colleagues have been at the forefront of cytogenetic studies of genetic recombination, and have conducted numerous studies on meiotic recombination in both mice and human meiocytes by studying chiasmata at diplotene and diakinesis stages of metaphase I. This technique is limited by technical difficulties, as chiasmata at the diplotene stage are difficult to distinguish from chromosome twists, while diakinesis preparations are notoriously difficult to analyse due to highly condensed chromatin and poor chromosome morphology/banding [1]. These conditions make it difficult to pinpoint chiasmata to individual chromosomes or specific chromosome regions. Some of the technical difficulties in identifying individual chromosomes can be overcome by using multi-colour fluorescence in-situ hybridisation (FISH) on diakinesis preparations, but due to the extreme condensation of the chromatin, specific chromosome regions are still indistinguishable. In addition, the amount of data that can be generated by these techniques is restricted, as the diplotene and diakinesis stages are relatively short, so only a small proportion of nuclei are found at these stages. Thus, this method is able to generate relatively crude recombination maps, but not high-resolution maps [9].

More recent immunocytogenetic techniques have proved advantageous. The identification of meiotic proteins in knockout mice has enabled researchers to study chromosome pairing and recombination in spermatogenesis using relatively simple immunocytogenetic methods. The use of immunocytogenetic studies on pachytene spermatocytes has alleviated the technical disadvantages of traditional cytogenetic methods, as there are a large number of readily accessible cells in which the synaptonemal complex can be studied. Fine mapping of individual chiasmata is possible using a combination of immunocytogenetic and FISH techniques to identify individual chromosomes [1, 8]. The major limiting factor in these studies is the difficulty in obtaining the testicular material required to undertake this type of analysis. As a result, studies to date are predominantly focused on men undergoing vasectomy reversals and infertile men with obstructive and non-obstructive azoospermia. The advantage of such studies are that they enable the total number and position of recombination events within a single nucleus to be observed, and provide an overview unavailable from linkage or sperm typing analyses [1].

22.2.2 Identification of Key Proteins Involved in Mammalian Chromosome Synapsis and Recombination

Until relatively recently, the vast majority of research in meiotic recombination has been carried out in lower eukaryotes such as *saccharomyces cerevisiae* and *drosophila.* Recently, an immunocytogenetic approach, identifying proteins at the pachytene stage of prophase I in the mammalian meiotic recombination pathway, has been used to investigate mammalian recombination [3]. Since large numbers of spermatocytes (derived from testicular tissue) are available per individual for investigation at pachytene, normal baseline values for meiotic events can be established [8, 9]. Visualisation of meiotic proteins has been possible by using antibodies to the synaptonemal complex (SC; SCP1 and SCP3), to sites of genetic recombination (MLH1) and to the centromere (CREST – calcinosis, Raynaud's phenomenon, oesophageal dysfunction, sclerodactyly, telangiectasia). The SC is a proteinaceous complex composed of axial elements (SCP3) and transverse elements (SCP1), that "zipper up" homologous chromosomes, linking them together during prophase of meiosis I [12]. During this period, the chromatin of each chromatid is organised into an array of loops [13] around the SC.

The use of anti-CREST antibodies to pinpoint the centromere aids in analysis of pachytene spreads. A mismatch repair protein, MutL homologue 1 (MLH1), was identified when it was observed that meiotic recombination was practically absent in a male knock-out mouse cancer model missing the gene for this protein [14]. In wild-type mice with functional copies of the mlh1 gene, discrete foci were observed on SCs during pachytene, and the overall number and positions of the foci corresponded to previous cytogenetic studies of chiasmata in mice. This finding suggested that in addition to its function as a mismatch repair protein, MLH1 was also involved in the process of meiotic recombination, localising at the sites where genetic exchanges take place during pachytene – and that absence of MLH1 results in a breakdown of this process. Initial data on the number and location of foci (generated to determine whether MLH1 is a suitable marker for genetic recombination) are reassuring, producing markedly consistent results when compared to both conventional genetic linkage studies and cytogenetic studies [15]. Marcon and Moens [16] provided further corroboration: using okadaic acid (a phosphatase inhibitor), they demonstrated that MLH1 foci are localised at chiasmata. Through the rapid and reliable analysis of the localisation of these proteins, it is possible to generate both chromosome-specific and genome-wide genetic maps [8, 17].

22.2.3 Timing and Progression of SC Formation

Immunocytogenetic studies have been crucial to the unravelling of molecular events during meiotic recombination, including the timing and progression of SC formation (chromosomal synapsis). It is apparent that the first components of the SC that form are those of the axial elements (SCP3), which are first visible during the leptotene phase of prophase I. By zygotene, these become full-length axial elements along the length of sister chromatids. As these sister chromatids come into close proximity, transverse elements (SCP1) form between the axial elements, and by pachytene, the homologous axial elements have been "zippered up" [12, 18]. Immunocytogenetic studies have begun to shed light on not only the timing of SC assembly, but also on the process by which homologous SCs synapse. In humans, it appears that the initiation of synapsis is tightly controlled, with few inter-individual differences [19]. In acrocentric chromosomes, initiation of synapsis occurs at the distal end of the long arm; in metacentric and sub-metacentric chromosomes, there are two initiation sites, located distally on the p- and q-arms of the chromosomes, and synapsis proceeds towards the centromere. In non-acrocentric chromosomes, the centromere itself appears to act as a barrier, and hinders synapsis: if synapsis is completed on one arm prior to the other, it does not proceed past the centromere to the other arm [19]. While the initiation of synapsis occurs preferentially at the distal ends of chromosome arms, Brown et al. [19] have provided evidence that the site of initiation is found in sub-telomeric regions rather than within the telomere itself. To date, however, it remains to be established whether synapsis start sites require specific DNA sequence(s) or whether they are found within sub-telomeric repeat regions.

22.2.4 Fidelity of Meiotic Chromosome Synapsis

Immunocytogenetic analyses, when SC formation is complete in all bivalents at pachytene, have revealed potential perturbations in chromosome synapsis [8]. In particular, the observation of discontinuities (gaps) and unpaired regions (splits) along the length of the SC is indicative of abnormal fidelity in chromosome pairing during prophase I (Fig. 22.1). These SC abnormalities are not attributable to the immunocytogenetic technique itself, as they have been previously observed using silver staining and light microscopy [20]. On average, Sun et al. [8] found gaps in 35% and splits in 7.5% of spermatocytes in 11 control males. However, a large degree of variation was found between individuals, with ranges of 20–58% and 0–37% for gaps and splits, respectively. Identification of individual SCs has revealed that gaps occur most commonly within the heterochromatin regions of chromosomes 1 and 9 [8], with 91% of events located on 9qh. Splits in the SC were primarily located on chromosomes 1 and 9, with 9qh splits accounting for 58% of events [21]. Since correct pairing and meiotic recombination are required to ensure correct chromosome disjunction, abnormalities in chromosome pairing and synapsis may lead to aneuploidy and all its resultant clinical implications.

22.2.5 Variation in Meiotic Recombination Frequencies

Physical interaction of DNA molecules through reciprocal recombination [22] enables the formation of chiasmata between homologous chromosomes [18]. It has long been recognised that the process of meiotic recombination is controlled genetically, and that there is strict regulation of both the number and distribution of these exchanges [8]. There is however, evidence of inter-species variations in the overall frequency of recombination (in flies, bacteria, fungi, plants and mammals) and sex-specific differences within the same species [23–25]. For example, in most studies, the frequency

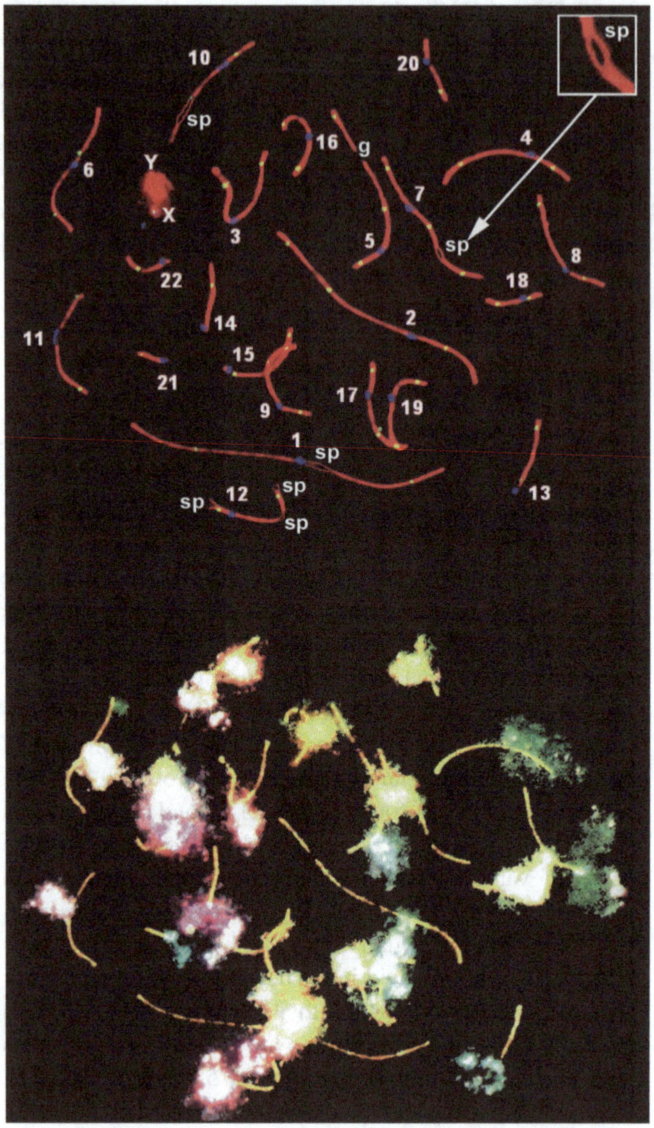

Fig. 22.1 Human pachytene spermatocyte. (*upper*) SCs are shown in *red*, centromeres in *blue* and MLH1 foci in *yellow*. Discontinuities within the SCs are indicated (SC gaps -g; SC splits -sp an enlarged example is inset *top right*). (*lower*) Subsequent cenM-FISH analysis allows identification of individual chromosomes so that recombination (MLH1) foci can be analysed for each SC. Numbers positioned by the centromeres (*upper*) correspond to individual chromosomes as identified by cenM-FISH

and distribution of meiotic recombination foci is markedly different between the sexes in humans, with a much higher frequency of recombination events in females than in males (approximately 95 MLH1 foci per oocyte, vs. 50 per spermatocyte) [1, 8, 9, 17, 26, 27]. In one of the few studies where the frequency of MLH1 foci was lower (approximately 70 per oocyte), Tease and Hultén [28] noted that SC length in oocytes is longer that that in spermatocytes, suggesting that perhaps SC length may be the determining factor for recombination focus frequency. It is clear that recombination events are not fixed, but are subject to intrinsic factors (e.g. genetic background) [29] and extrinsic factors (e.g. environmental and age effects) [30–32] that contribute to the significant intra- and inter-individual variability observed.

In normal men, there is a significant amount of variability in recombination frequencies between individuals (% difference) and among cells from the same individual (range). This variation was first shown cytologically when Laurie et al. [33] reported significant variation in chiasmata frequency between chromosome arms (especially for larger chromosomes), and was further confirmed when Laurie and Hultén [34] reported a 16% difference in the mean number of chiasmata per cell among 13 donors (range 46.3–53.7). The more recent use of immunocytogenetic methods gave similar results, with the following levels of variability observed in control donors: 23% difference among 11 donors (range 42.5–55.0) [8]; 20% among 25 donors (range 46.2–55.3) [9]; 15% among 14 donors (range 46.2–52.8) [26] and 13% in 10 donors (range 46.4–53.2) [17]. Studies have sought to identify the source of this well-reported variability in human male spermatocytes. Although SC formation is essential for the production of recombination nodules, Sun et al. [8] found no evidence of an association between reduced recombination frequencies and the number of gaps/splits per SC or per individual, so recombination frequency variability does not appear to be associated with errors in chromosome synapsis. To date, the underlying cause of this variability remains to be elucidated.

22.2.5.1 Age Effect

The question of an age effect on genetic recombination is something that has sparked a great deal of interest. The presence of an age effect in females does not seem improbable, especially given the well-established association between the elevated risk of the producing an aneuploid conceptus and increasing maternal age. Indeed, there is evidence that a decreased recombination frequency in females is correlated with advancing age in mice [35–37], hamsters [38] and in humans for the telomeric and pericentromeric regions of chromosome 21 [31]. A similar association between paternal age and decreased recombination in mammals has not been identified [8, 11, 26, 39] with the exception of two studies carried out by Sun et al. [17, 40].

22.2.5.2 Achiasmate Bivalents

Achiasmate autosomal bivalents (i.e. bivalents lacking a recombination event) are found in approximately 0.1–5% of control men [8, 17, 18, 41]. Achiasmate bivalents are clinically relevant, as these bivalents that lack recombination foci and are thus unable to orientate themselves on the metaphase plate in order to segregate to daughter cells correctly [18]. The absence or reduction of recombination can increase sperm aneuploidy frequencies, or can even arrest spermatogenesis, resulting in infertility [8, 22, 42]. No relationship between the mean numbers of autosomal MLH1 and SCs containing no MLH1 foci was found in control males, that is, individuals with low frequencies of recombination did not have an increased frequency of achiasmate bivalents. The frequency of sex bodies lacking MLH1 foci was, however, notably higher than that found in autosomes, with MLH1 foci absent in approximately 27–31% of sex bodies [17, 18, 43]. One study has provided evidence linking a reduction of recombination within the sex body to a reduction in autosomal recombination frequencies, suggesting that the presence of recombination within the sex body may be a marker for general recombination and for the continuation of the meiotic process [43].

22.2.5.3 Meiotic Recombination Maps for Individual Chromosomes

Analysis of the frequency of recombination across the genome is a useful tool, but the identification of potential chromosome-specific effects on recombination in normal men provides detailed information on recombination formation and chromosome–chromosome variation. This enables an assessment of the incidence of aneuploidy for individual chromosomes, and could ultimately provide clues to identify the source of clinically observed trisomies [40]. Although it was possible to study the progression of chromosome synapsis and recombination, recombination frequencies and errors in chromosomal synapsis using immunocytogenetic methods, this technique could not, at first, identify or study specific chromosomes. Recently, however, the number and position of recombination foci and errors in chromosome synapsis for individual chromosomes has been made possible by following immunocytogenetic techniques with centromere-specific multi-colour fluorescent in-situ hybridisation (cenM-FISH) on the same spermatocytes. After capturing and analysing immunocytogenetic images of SCs, sites of recombination and the centromeres in an individual spermatocyte and recording its exact position on a slide, cenM-FISH is performed, and the same pachytene spread is re-captured for analysis and identification of individual chromosomes [17, 40, 44, 45] (Fig. 22.1). The combination of these two strategies enables the analysis of crossover frequencies, distributions and synaptic defects in human germ cells in a precise manner, thus providing a means to determine patterns of recombination across the whole genome at a chromosomal level that is not readily available by other means [40]. The first recombination maps for individual autosomal chromosomes was published in 2004 using this method [44]. These recombination maps address questions about the position and distribution of recombination foci across chromosomes [40, 44] and the analysis of achiasmate bivalents [40]. Data obtained from these studies showed that MLH1 foci preferentially occur near medial and terminal regions of the chromosomes, with an apparent repression of foci around the centromere [40, 44]. With the exception of the short arms of the acrocentric chromosomes, where recombination rarely occurs, each chromosome bivalent typically had at least one MLH1 focus per chromosome arm. The frequency of MLHI foci per SC varies according to SC size, with up to five MLH1 foci observed on the larger chromosomes. On average, there is one MLH1 focus per SC for the smallest chromosomes and 3.9 MLH1 foci for chromosome 1, the largest chromosome [44]. There also appears to be positive interference – the presence of one recombination focus inhibits the formation of a second one in close proximity, and MLH1 foci are rarely found next to the centromere [40]. Not surprisingly, a strong association between SC length and the number of MLH1 foci has also been identified [17, 26, 44]. Analysis of MLH1 foci in 10 control men revealed that 5% of spermatocytes had one or more achiasmate autosomal SCs and that 27% of sex bodies were achiasmate [17]. In this study, MLH1 foci were always present on SCs 1–10; of the 60 spermatocytes lacking MLH1, in decreasing order of frequency, the following SCs were involved: SCs 21; 22; 14; 16; 15; 17; 18; 20; 13; 11; 12 and 19. A significantly higher frequency of achiasmate chromosomes was found for chromosomes 21, 22 and the sex chromosomes, with the highest autosomal frequency observed for chromosome 21 [17, 43]. This observation may in part be explained by the association between SC length and MLH1 focus frequency. Chromosomes 21 and 22 are the smallest in the genome, and recombination can take place only in the small pseudoautosomal region of the sex chromosomes, so typically only a single recombination event takes place in these chromosomes. These findings echo the data provided by both sperm karyotyping studies and sperm FISH analysis, demonstrating that chromosomes 21, 22, X and Y have the highest frequencies of aneuploidy within sperm [46–48].

22.2.6 Meiotic Recombination and Chromosome Synapsis in Infertile Males

Even as data on genetic recombination and chromosome synapsis in normal men (typically vasectomy reversal patients) are being generated, studies have begun to investigate infertile men with obstructive azoospermia (OA) and non-obstructive azoospermia (NOA), to determine the prevalence of errors in chromosome synapsis and recombination within these populations.

22.2.6.1 Chromosome Synapsis Errors in Infertile Men

Evidence from both light- [49, 50] and electron-microscopic analyses [51–53] and from immunocytogenetic methods indicate that synaptic errors (gaps and splits within the SC) can occur at significantly higher frequencies in material derived from infertile azoospermic men [18, 41]. Ferguson et al. [41] found a significantly increased frequency of SC gaps in men with NOA and oligoasthenoteratozoospermia (OAT) (32.7% and 38.1%, respectively, versus 26.6% in controls). In 14 NOA men, Sun et al. [18] found a significantly increased frequency of splits compared to controls (24% vs. 10%). Similarly, two NOA males had significantly increased frequencies of SC gaps compared to controls (68% and 62% vs. 37%), but in the overall cohort, there was no significant difference in the occurrence of gaps compared to controls (37% of cells in both groups). Several studies indicate that abnormal chromosome synapsis may lead to complete [54, 55] and partial meiotic arrest [56] in men with idiopathic infertility. Asynapsis in pachytene may be regarded as a cytological manifestation of a spermatocyte whose progress through gametogenesis has run into difficulties, and in which there is an increased probability of atresia [57–59]. It has been suggested that higher levels of extended asynapsis may arise from a primary meiotic defect that could be responsible for infertility [60]. This hypothesis is supported by Sun et al. [18], whose data showed a significantly higher proportion of cells in leptotene compared to controls. This suggests a delay in the formation of the SC, which could in turn lead to a partial meiotic arrest in NOA males. It has been speculated that in NOA men, the succession of meiotic prophase sub-stages does not progress normally due to high frequencies of asynapsed regions in pachytene. These asynapsed regions may trigger a checkpoint leading to partial spermatogenic arrest, and when meiotic defects are severe it may lead to complete spermatogenic arrest [18].

22.2.6.2 Recombination Frequency Errors in Infertile Men

A number of interesting observations have come from several studies investigating recombination frequencies in infertile men with OAT, OA and NOA. In a significant proportion of NOA men (45–53%), meiotic cells are absent [18, 27, 54, 61] or reduced (approximately 10%) due to partial or nearly complete meiotic arrest at the zygotene stage [54]. Pachytene is the longest of the meiotic stages, and the majority of cells (80–90%) are found at this stage in controls [18, 27, 41, 54]. However, in NOA men, there is a significantly decreased frequency of pachytene cells (approximately 62%) [18], and an increased frequency of cells at other stages [41, 54], suggesting a developmental block during prophase in these individuals. In addition to the abnormal progression of meiosis, the majority of studies have noted that NOA males have a significant reduction in the number of MLH1 foci per cell compared to controls (40–42 vs. 46–49) [18, 27, 54], although two studies did not observe such a reduction [41, 43]. Interestingly, OA males have also been shown to have a small but significant reduction in the MLH1 focus frequency compared to controls (44.8 vs. 45.9 foci per cell) [27, 54]. In a study of infertile men with NOA, OA and OAT, Ferguson et al. [41] observed a reduction in recombination in the OAT males studied (33.9 vs. 47.6 in controls). Although they reported inter-individual variation with significant reductions in recombination for some OA and NOA men, overall, they did not observe reduced recombination in these patients. In a number of reports on NOA patients [18, 27, 41, 54], the proportion of achiasmate autosomal bivalents was also found to be significantly higher in NOA males compared to controls (29% vs. 5%) [18].

Increased sperm aneuploidy in infertile men is long established, and affects the sex chromosomes in particular [48]. Overall, Sun et al. [18] found no significant increase in the frequency of sex bodies lacking MLH1 foci in NOA patients compared to controls (34.4% vs. 29.1%), although two individuals did have significantly higher frequencies (76% and 80%). Codina-Pascual et al. [43] also found no elevation in the frequency of sex bodies without MLH1 foci. Interestingly, Ferguson et al. [41] found a novel recombination deficiency in two men enrolled in their study: a complete absence of recombination between the sex chromosomes. Data from immunocytogenetic studies indicate that an increased frequency of sex bodies lacking recombination foci (i.e. abnormalities in sex chromosome recombination) may be responsible in some NOA males for the increased levels of aneuploid sperm found in these men [18, 43], and thus has the potential to give rise to offspring with a sex chromosome abnormality [62].

22.3 Conclusions

Increased aneuploidy frequencies found in the sperm of infertile men [48] have been mirrored in an increase in chromosome abnormalities in offspring conceived through intracytoplasmic sperm injection (ICSI) – a technique used to achieve pregnancies in couples faced with male factor infertility [63, 64]. The underlying mechanism for the increased production of aneuploid sperm remains unknown, but a plausible explanation lies in asynapsis and aberrant genetic recombination. Chromosomes 21, 22 and the sex chromosomes are particularly prone to non-disjunction in sperm [47, 48], and have a higher frequency of non-recombination than all other chromosomes [18, 27, 41, 43]. This may trigger a meiotic checkpoint interfering with the completion of meiosis, potentially leading to meiotic arrest and hence oligozoospermia

[17]. However, non-recombinant chromosomes may escape such checkpoints and are thus at an increased risk of producing aneuploid gametes. Paternally derived cases of liveborn aneuploid conceptuses have been associated with reduced recombination for the involved chromosomes [6, 7, 41], providing evidence that a reduced and/or absent genetic recombination is a molecular risk factor for chromosome non-disjunction in human males [17, 22].

Although the genetic basis of meiotic defects in infertile men remains largely unknown, it is clear that affected individuals have significantly increased frequencies of errors in chromosome synapsis and recombination. Indeed mutations within the murine SCP3 gene results in sterile mice that have unsynapsed chromosomes, as the SC is unable to form resulting in massive apoptotic cell death during meiotic prophase [65]. Similar mutations in genes involved in chromosome synapsis are now being identified in azoospermic men including mutations in SCP3 [66] and FKBP6 [67] genes.

Clinical applications arising from this research may also have applications for cancer and cryptochidism patients in the future. The incidence of cancer and cryptochidism in pre-pubertal boys in the Western world is on the rise, and treatment often results in infertility or sterility. Freezing and storing testicular tissue from these individuals may be the only method that will allow them to conceive later in life. Development of methods that enable pachytene spermatocyte maturation either through in-vivo or in-vitro methods will be required before sperm derived from frozen testicular tissue can be used to establish pregnancies. Immunocytogenetic studies on testicular samples are likely to provide important practical and functional information during the development of these techniques, allowing monitoring and testing of both the culture methods and the meiotic progression of the maturing spermatocytes. [68].

While the use of immunocytogenetic studies for meiotic recombination is presently only a research tool, there is clear potential for clinical applications in the future, including: the detection and interpretation of abnormal meiotic profiles; generating important risk assessments for gamete aneuploidy in infertile males; and enabling the use of reproductive technologies in boys treated for cancer or cryptorchidism. These clinical applications, in conjunction with a furthering of our understanding of the aetiology of idiopathic infertility, spermatogenic failure and human trisomies will undoubtedly greatly impact genetic counselling, and will provide expanded insights and opportunities for patients pondering their reproductive choices.

Acknowledgements The authors gratefully acknowledge Evelyn Ko for her technical expertise and assistance in the preparation of the text and figures. R.H.M holds the Canada Research Chair in Genetics, and the research was funded by the Canadian Institutes of Health Research (CIHR) grant MA7961. H.T. is a recipient of a CIHR Strategic Training Fellowship in Genetics, Child Development and Health.

References

1. Barlow AL, Hultén MA (1998) Crossing over analysis at pachytene in man. Eur J Hum Genet 6:350–358
2. Hassold T, Abruzzo M, Adkins K, Griffin D, Merrill M, Millie E, Saker D, Shen J, Zaragoza M (1996) Human aneuploidy: incidence, origin, and etiology. Environ Mol Mutagen 28:167–175
3. Hassold T, Sherman S, Hunt P (2000) Counting cross-overs: characterizing meiotic recombination in mammals. Hum Mol Genet 9:2409–2419
4. Koehler K, Hawley R, Sherman S, Hassold T (1996) Recombination and nondisjunction in humans and flies. Hum Mol Genet 5: 1495–1504
5. Shi Q, Spriggs E, Field L, Ko E, Barclay L, Martin R (2001) Single sperm typing demonstrates that reduced recombination is associated with the production of aneuploid 24, XY human sperm. Am J Med Genet 99:34–38
6. Lorda-Sanchez I, Binkert F, Maechler M, Robinson WP, Schinzel AA (1992) Reduced recombination and paternal age effect in Klinefelter syndrome. Hum Genet 89:524–530
7. MacDonald M, Hassold T, Harvey J, Wang L, Morton N, Jacobs P (1994) The origin of 47, XXY and 47, XXX aneuploidy: heterogeneous mechanisms and role of aberrant recombination. Hum Mol Genet 3:1365–1371
8. Sun F, Trpkov K, Rademaker A, Ko E, Martin RH (2005) Variation in meiotic recombination frequencies among human males. Hum Genet 116:172–178
9. Hassold T, Judis L, Chan ER, Schwartz S, Seftel A, Lynn A (2004) Cytological studies of meiotic recombination in human males. Cytogenet Genome Res 107:249–255
10. Kong A, Gudbjartsson DF, Sainz J, Jonsdottir GM, Gudjonsson SA, Richardsson B, Sigurdardottir S, Barnard J, Hallbeck B, Masson G, Shlien A, Palsson ST, Frigge ML, Thorgeirsson TE, Gulcher JR, Stefansson K (2002) A high-resolution recombination map of the human genome. Nat Genet 31:241–247
11. Broman K, Murray J, Sheffield V, White R, Weber J (1998) Comprehensive human genetic maps: individual and sex-specific variation in recombination. Am J Hum Genet 63:861–869
12. Topping D, Brown P, Hassold T (2007) The immunocytogenetics of human male meiosis: a progress report. In: Carrell DT (ed) The genetics of male infertility. Humana Press Inc, Totowa, pp 115–128
13. Kleckner N, Zickler D, Jones GH, Dekker J, Padmore R, Henle J, Hutchinson J (2004) A mechanical basis for chromosome function. Proc Natl Acad Sci U S A 101:12592–12597
14. Baker SM, Plug AW, Prolla TA, Bronner CE, Harris AC, Yao X, Christie DM, Monell C, Arnheim N, Bradley A, Ashley T, Liskay RM (1996) Involvement of mouse Mlh1 in DNA mismatch repair and meiotic crossing over. Nat Genet 13:336–342
15. Lynn A, Ashley T, Hassold T (2004) Variation in human meiotic recombination. Annu Rev Genomics Hum Genet 5:317–349
16. Marcon E, Moens P (2003) MLH1p and MLH3p localize to precociously induced chiasmata of okadaic-acid-treated mouse spermatocytes. Genetics 165:2283–2287
17. Sun F, Oliver-Bonet M, Liehr T, Starke H, Turek P, Ko E, Rademaker A, Martin RH (2006) Analysis of non-crossover bivalents in pachytene cells from 10 normal men. Hum Reprod 21:2335–2339
18. Sun F, Turek P, Greene C, Ko E, Rademaker A, Martin RH (2007) Abnormal progression through meiosis in men with nonobstructive azoospermia. Fertil Steril 87:565–571
19. Brown PW, Judis L, Chan ER, Schwartz S, Seftel A, Thomas A, Hassold TJ (2005) Meiotic synapsis proceeds from a limited number of subtelomeric sites in the human male. Am J Hum Genet 77:556–566
20. Fletcher JM (1979) Light microscope analysis of meiotic prophase chromosomes by silver staining. Chromosoma 72:241–248

21. Sun F, Oliver-Bonet M, Liehr T, Starke H, Trpkov K, Ko E, Rademaker A, Martin RH (2005) Discontinuities and unsynapsed regions in meiotic chromosomes have a cis effect on meiotic recombination patterns in normal human males. Hum Mol Genet 14:3013–3018
22. Hassold T, Hunt P (2001) To err (meiotically) is human: the genesis of human aneuploidy. Nat Rev Genet 2:280–291
23. Brooks L (1988) The evolution of recombination rates. In: Michod RE, Levin BR (eds) The evolution of sex: an examination of current ideas. Sinauer, Sunderland, MA, pp 87–105
24. Fisher-Lindahl K (1991) His and hers recombinational hotspots. Trends Genet 7:273–276
25. Robinson WP (1996) The extent, mechanism, and consequences of genetic variation, for recombination rate. Am J Hum Genet 59:1175–1183
26. Lynn A, Koehler KE, Judis L, Chan ER, Cherry JP, Schwartz S, Seftel A, Hunt P, Hassold TJ (2002) Covariation of synaptonemal complex length and mammalian meiotic exchange rates. Science 296:2222–2225
27. Sun F, Greene C, Turek PJ, Ko E, Rademaker A, Martin RH (2005) Immunofluorescent synaptonemal complex analysis in azoospermic men. Cytogenet Genome Res 111:366–370
28. Tease C, Hultén MA (2004) Inter-sex variation in synaptonemal complex lengths largely determine the different recombination rates in male and female germ cells. Cytogenet Genome Res 107:208–215
29. Koehler KE, Cherry JP, Lynn A, Hunt PA, Hassold TJ (2002) Genetic control of mammalian meiotic recombination. I. Variation in exchange frequencies among males from inbred mouse strains. Genetics 162:297–306
30. Rose A, Baillie D (1979) The effect of temperature and parental age on recombination and nondisjunction in C. elegans. Genetics 92:409–418
31. Tanzi RE, Watkins PC, Stewart GD, Wexler NS, Gusella JF, Haines JL (1992) A genetic linkage map of human chromosome 21: analysis of recombination as a function of sex and age. Am J Hum Genet 50:551–558
32. Williamson JH, Parker DR, Manchester WG (1970) X-ray-induced recombination in the fourth chromosome of Drosophila melanogaster females. I. Kinetics and brood patterns. Mutat Res 9:287–297
33. Laurie DA, Hulten M, Jones GH (1981) Chiasma frequency and distribution in a sample of human males: chromosomes 1, 2, and 9. Cytogenet Cell Genet 31:153–166
34. Laurie D, Hultén M (1985) Further studies on chiasma distribution and interference in the human male. Ann Hum Genet 49:203–214
35. Jagiello G, Fang JS (1979) Analyses of diplotene chiasma frequencies in mouse oocytes and spermatocytes in relation to ageing and sexual dimorphism. Cytogenet Cell Genet 23:53–60
36. Luthardt FW, Palmer CG, Yu P (1973) Chiasma and univalent frequencies in aging female mice. Cytogenet Cell Genet 12:68–79
37. Speed RM (1977) The effects of ageing on the meiotic chromosomes of male and female mice. Chromosoma 64:241–254
38. Sugawara S, Mikamo K (1983) Absence of correlation between univalent formation and meiotic nondisjunction in aged female Chinese hamsters. Cytogenet Cell Genet 35:34–40
39. Shi Q, Spriggs E, Field L, Rademaker A, Ko E, Barclay L, Martin R (2002) Absence of age effect on meiotic recombination between human X and Y chromosomes. Am J Hum Genet 71:254–261
40. Sun F, Oliver-Bonet M, Liehr T, Starke H, Turek P, Ko E, Rademaker A, Martin RH (2006) Variation in MLH1 distribution in recombination maps for individual chromosomes from human males. Hum Mol Genet 15:2376–2391
41. Ferguson KA, Wong EC, Chow V, Nigro M, Ma S (2007) Abnormal meiotic recombination in infertile men and its association with sperm aneuploidy. Hum Mol Genet 16:2870–2879
42. Hale D (1994) Is X-Y recombination necessary for spermatocyte survival during mammalian spermatogenesis? Cytogenet Cell Genet 65:278–282
43. Codina-Pascual M, Oliver-Bonet M, Navarro J, Campillo M, Garcia F, Egozcue S, Abad C, Egozcue J, Benet J (2005) Synapsis and meiotic recombination analyses: MLH1 focus in the XY pair as an indicator. Hum Reprod 20:2133–2139
44. Sun F, Oliver-Bonet M, Liehr T, Starke H, Ko E, Rademaker A, Navarro J, Benet J, Martin RH (2004) Human male recombination maps for individual chromosomes. Am J Hum Genet 74:521–531
45. Oliver-Bonet M, Liehr T, Nietzel A, Heller A, Starke H, Claussen U, Codina-Pascual M, Pujol A, Abad C, Egozcue J, Navarro J, Benet J (2003) Karyotyping of human synaptonemal complexes by cenM-FISH. Eur J Hum Genet 11:879–883
46. Martin RH (2006) Meiotic chromosome abnormalities in human spermatogenesis. Reprod Toxicol 22:142–147
47. Shi Q, Martin R (2000) Aneuploidy in human sperm: a review of the frequency and distribution of aneuploidy, effects of donor age and lifestyle factors. Cytogenet Cell Genet 90:219–226
48. Tempest HG, Griffin DK (2004) The relationship between male infertility and increased levels of sperm disomy. Cytogenet Genome Res 107:83–94
49. Vidal F, Navarro J, Templado C, Marina S, Egozcue J (1984) Development and behavior of synaptonemal complexes in human spermatocytes by light and electron microscopy. Hum Genet 68:142–147
50. Vidal F, Templado C, Navarro J, Brusadin S, Marina S, Egozcue J (1982) Meiotic and synaptonemal complex studies in 45 subfertile males. Hum Genet 60:301–304
51. Johannisson R, Schulze W, Holstein AF (2003) Megalospermatocytes in the human testis exhibit asynapsis of chromosomes. Andrologia 35:146–151
52. Lange R, Krause W, Engel W (1997) Analyses of meiotic chromosomes in testicular biopsies of infertile patients. Hum Reprod 12:2154–2158
53. Solari AJ, Ponzio R, Rey Valzacchi G (1991) Synaptonemal complex karyotyping in an oligospermic patient with heterochromatin duplication in chromosome n. 9. Medicina (B Aires) 51:217–221
54. Gonsalves J, Sun F, Schlegal P, Hopps C, Turek P, Greene C, Martin RH, Reijo-Pera RA (2004) Defective recombination in infertile men. Hum Mol Genet 13:2875–2883
55. Judis L, Chan ER, Schwartz S, Seftel A, Hassold T (2004) Meiosis I arrest and azoospermia in an infertile male explained by failure of formation of a component of the synaptonemal complex. Fertil Steril 81:205–209
56. Sun F, Kozak G, Scott S, Trpkov K, Ko E, Mikhaail-Philips M, Bestor TH, Moens P, Martin RH (2004) Meiotic defects in a man with non-obstructive azoospermia: case report. Hum Reprod 19:1770–1773
57. Egozcue J, Templado C, Vidal F, Navarro J, Morer-Fargas F, Marina S (1983) Meiotic studies in a series of 1100 infertile and sterile males. Hum Genet 65:185–188
58. Hultén M (1970) Meiosis in XYY men. Lancet 1:717–718
59. Mittwoch U, Mahadevaiah SK (1992) Unpaired chromosomes at meiosis: cause or effect of gametogenic insufficiency? Cytogenet Cell Genet 59:274–279
60. Guichaoua MR, Perrin J, Metzler-Guillemain C, Saias-Magnan J, Giorgi R, Grillo JM (2005) Meiotic anomalies in infertile men with severe spermatogenic defects. Hum Reprod 20:1897–1902
61. Topping D, Brown P, Judis L, Schwartz S, Seftel A, Thomas A, Hassold TJ (2006) Synaptic defects at meiosis I and non-obstructive azoospermia. Hum Reprod 21:3171–3177
62. Hassold T, Sherman S, Pettay D, Page D, Jacobs P (1991) XY chromosome nondisjunction in man is associated with diminished recombination in the pseudoautosomal region. Am J Hum Genet 49:253–260
63. Aboulghar H, Aboulghar M, Manour R, Serour G, Amin Y, Al-Inany H (2001) A prospective controlled study of karyotyping for 430 consecutive babies conceived through intracytoplasmic sperm injection. Fertil Steril 76:249–254

64. Van Steirteghem A, Bonduelle M, Devroey P, Liebaers I (2002) Follow-up of children born after ICSI. Hum Reprod Update 8:111–116
65. Yuan L, Liu JG, Zhao J, Brundell E, Daneholt B, Hoog C (2000) The murine SCP3 gene is required for synaptonemal complex assembly, chromosome synapsis, and male fertility. Mol Cell 5:73–83
66. Miyamoto T, Hasuike S, Yogev L, Maduro MR, Ishikawa M, Westphal H, Lamb DJ (2003) Azoospermia in patients heterozygous for a mutation in SYCP3. Lancet 362:1714–1719
67. Miyamato T, Sato H, Yogev L, Kleiman S, Namiki M, Koh E, Sakugawa N, Hayashi H, Ishikawa M, Lamb DJ, Sengoku K (2006) Is a genetic defect in Fkbp6 a common cause of azoospermia in humans? Cell Mol Biol Lett 11:557–569
68. Lyrakou S, Mantas D, Msaouel P, Baathalah S, Shrivastav P, Chrisostomou M, Mihalopoulos Y, Hasiakos D, Baka S (2007) Crossover analysis using immunofluorescent detection of MLH1 foci in frozen-thawed testicular tissue. Reprod Biomed Online 15:99–105

Chapter 23
Clinical Evaluation and Treatment of Male Factor Infertility

Michael A. Poch and Mark Sigman

Abstract The work up of the infertile couple should begin after 1 year of unprotected intercourse or sooner if infertility risk factors are present. A thorough history and physical examination are key components of the evaluation and should not be underestimated, as varicoceles and other causes of male factor infertility can easily be identified. The semen analysis is the only laboratory test that should be obtained in all patients. On the basis of the history, physical examination, and semen analysis, the decision to pursue further testing and the type of testing should be methodical and aimed at refining the differential diagnosis. This will allow the clinician to counsel the infertile couple about appropriate management options.

Keywords Infertility, male • Azoospermia • Oligozoospermia • Infertility, evaluation • Semen analysis

23.1 Introduction

23.1.1 Epidemiology

A male factor is commonly involved in infertility with approximately 30% of cases due to a male factor alone and 20% due to combined male and female factors. Since the total contribution of the male factor can be as high as 50%, it is imperative that both members of the infertile couple undergo proper evaluations.

23.1.2 Goals of the Evaluation

The evaluation of the infertile male should proceed with several goals in mind: (1) to identify potentially correctable causes of the male factor; (2) to identify non-correctable causes of male factor infertility in which the male partner's sperm may be utilized in the assisted reproductive techniques; (3) to identify uncorrectable causes of male infertility that are not amenable to the assisted reproductive techniques with the male partner's sperm but may best be managed by donor insemination or adoption; (4) to identify genetic and chromosomal abnormalities in order to counsel the patient about implications to himself or his potential offspring; (5) lastly to identify underlying systemic and potentially life threatening diseases including, testicular cancer, pituitary tumors, and spinal cord tumors [1–4]. Without a full evaluation, these diagnoses may go unnoticed.

23.1.3 Timing

A thorough, cost effective male evaluation should be initiated when, after 1 year of unprotected intercourse, the couple has not conceived. Evaluation may occur earlier if the female is above age 35 or if the male has a pertinent history of known infertility risk factors, such as testicular cancer or cryptorchidism [5].

23.2 History

23.2.1 Sexual and Reproductive History

The history should begin with a sexual and reproductive history. It is important to distinguish between primary and secondary infertility. Those patients who have never conceived are considered to have primary infertility, and the differential diagnosis of those patients is often larger than those whose paternity has been established.

The sexual history should initially focus on the details associated with the current attempts at conception. These include the length of time the couple has been trying to conceive,

M.A. Poch and M. Sigman (✉)
Department of Urology, Brown University, Providence, RI, USA
e-mail: MSigman@lifespan.org

D.T. Carrell and C.M. Peterson (eds.), *Reproductive Endocrinology and Infertility: Integrating Modern Clinical and Laboratory Practice*,
DOI 10.1007/978-1-4419-1436-1_23, © Springer Science+Business Media, LLC 2010

the frequency of sexual intercourse and masturbation, and the time during the female cycle at which the couple is having sexual intercourse. Patients should be educated regarding the timing of the menstrual cycle and ovulation. Couples should be advised that intercourse should occur up to 6 days prior to ovulation and 1 day after ovulation in order to optimize fertilization [6].

There are very little data to support the optimal frequency of sexual intercourse, however, most experts advise vaginal intercourse every 2 days during the time of ovulation. Increased frequency of ejaculation through masturbation or intercourse can decrease sperm concentrations. Sexual intercourse around ovulation ensures that viable sperm are potentially present during the 12–24 h, when the oocyte is in the fallopian tube and capable of being fertilized. Many commercial lubricants as well as saliva have been shown to be detrimental to sperm motility in vitro although in vivo studies are lacking [7, 8]. Substances such as peanut oil, safflower oil, vegetable oil, and raw egg white as well as a few commercial lubricants appear not to be detrimental to sperm function and should be recommended if a lubricant is needed.

23.2.2 Childhood History

Childhood history should focus on trauma to the scrotum or genital region, prior inguinal or scrotal surgery or a history of cryptorchidism. Individuals with a history of unilateral cryptorchidism have been shown to have variable sperm counts; however, their paternity rates remain similar to that of the general population [9]. In contrast, a history of bilateral cryptorchidism is associated with significantly decreased paternity rates compared to controls [10].

Testicular trauma has been associated with the production of antisperm antibodies. Some retrospective studies have shown that testicular salvage procedures may improve semen parameters compared with those that underwent orchiectomy after testicular trauma [11]. However, the variable indications for orchiectomy could have resulted in selection bias affecting the findings. There is conflicting data regarding the effects of testicular torsion on semen parameters [11, 12].

Surgery in the pelvis, retroperitoneum, and groin may affect fertility potential. Pelvic and retroperitoneal surgery can cause erectile or ejaculatory dysfunction. During inguinal surgery, structures contained within the spermatic cord are at risk. Damage to the vas deferens is more likely to be caused by ischemia or scarring rather than direct ligation. Specifically, hernia repairs with polypropylene mesh have been implicated in vasal obstruction due to a dense inflammatory reaction [13]. Damage to the testicular artery may cause testicular atrophy [2].

23.2.3 Past Medical History

Spermatogenesis, ejaculate volume, and sexual function are all complex processes that require coordination of hormonal and physiologic events. Medical conditions that disrupt these processes can thereby affect overall fertility. Obtaining a detailed medical history is paramount when determining possible factors associated with male infertility.

Diabetes has been associated with ejaculatory dysfunction as well as erectile dysfunction. Recent studies of insulin dependent diabetics have reported an increased rate of DNA fragmentation compared to controls, which may put those patients at risk for lower paternity rates [14].

Patients with spinal cord injuries often have erectile dysfunction and ejaculatory dysfunction [15]. Additionally, similar recent reports have shown increased DNA fragmentation in sperm of spinal cord patients compared to controls. The clinical implication of this remains uncertain [16]. Other neurologic diseases with ejaculatory dysfunction include multiple sclerosis and Parkinson's disease. End stage renal disease has been shown to impair fertility in a number of ways including affecting the hypothalamic-pituitary axis and decreasing ejaculate volume [17, 18].

Sexually transmitted diseases and urinary tract infections, bacterial and viral, can adversely affect fertility and should, therefore, be elicited as part of the history. Genital tract infections may impair fertility by direct cytotoxic effect to sperm and spermatogenesis. Additionally, infections can also cause local inflammatory reactions resulting in obstruction of the epididymis or ejaculatory ducts. Lastly, spermatogenesis occurs in a protected environment via the blood testis barrier, and if an inflammatory reaction is severe enough to violate this barrier, the formation of anti-sperm antibodies may theoretically follow. HIV infection has also been shown to affect semen parameters, specifically motility [19].

A history of recurrent sinopulmonary infections is common in patients with, cystic fibrosis, ciliary dyskinesia syndrome (and Kartagener Syndrome when associated with situs inversus), or Young's syndrome. Anosmia has also been associated with Kallman syndrome, which is a cause of hypogonadotropic hypogonadism.

23.2.4 Past Surgical History

As stated earlier, surgical procedures in the groin, scrotum, retroperitoneum, or pelvis during childhood or as an adult can affect fertility. Transurethral surgery may result in retrograde ejaculation or failure of antegrade ejaculation as seen with transurethral resection of the prostate (TURP), laser enucleation procedures, and transurethral microwave surgery [20, 21]. Deep pelvic surgery for rectal cancer, inflammatory bowel disease, and diverticulitis can all injure pelvic nerves resulting in erectile dysfunction.

Retroperitoneal surgery may result in ejaculatory dysfunction. RPLND for advanced testicular tumors can affect the para-aortic sympathetic chain resulting in ejaculatory dysfunction. Recent advancements in chemotherapy and changes in the template for lymphadenectomy have resulted in improvements in ejaculatory function [22]. Additionally, anterior lumbar fusions have reported complications of ejaculatory dysfunction postoperatively [23].

23.2.5 Medications

Medications have been implicated in impairing multiple aspects of fertility by affecting sperm production through a direct gonadal toxic effect, altering the hypothalamic pituitary axis, or causing disruptions in transport of sperm by impairment of erectile function, ejaculation or libido.

There is clear data linking medications to impairment in sexual function, but despite suggestive in vitro data, there is a dearth of evidence supporting the in vivo affects of most medications on fertility and ultimate paternity. Antihypertensive medications have been implicated in effecting multiple aspects of male fertility. Calcium channel blockers have been the most studied of the antihypertensive medications suspected of affecting fertilization [24, 25]. This theory, however, has been challenged by studies demonstrating similar IVF fertility rates of those who were on calcium channel blockers and those who were not [26]. The antihypertensive spironolactone has also been implicated in infertility because of its effect as an anti-androgen. Spironolactone has been found to inhibit testosterone synthesis as well as to act peripherally on androgen receptors [27]. Beta- blockers, specifically, propranolol have been found to impair erectile function [28]. Alpha-blockers have been associated with decreased ejaculatory volumes and lack of emission. Tamsulosin has been implicated in decreased contractility of seminal vesicles and vas deferens as well as acting on central nervous system theoretically affecting neurostimulation of ejaculation [29–31].

Medications that interfere with hormone regulation can have a significant effect on fertility. Exogenous testosterone supplementation may inhibit the hypothalamic pituitary axis, inducing a lack of intratesticular testosterone production, which results in decreased spermatogenesis. In addition, androgen deprivation therapy for the treatment of prostate cancer with GnRH (gonadotropin releasing hormone) agonists will lead to impairment of spermatogenesis. These affects are typically reversible if therapy is discontinued. Low doses of the 5-alpha reductase inhibitor, finasteride, utilized for the prevention of male pattern baldness have been shown not to inhibit sperm production [32]. A variety of antibiotics have been linked to adverse effects on fertility. High dose, long-term nitrofurantoin has been shown to cause maturation arrest, but the lower, shorter term doses most commonly used in clinical practice are likely safe [33]. Erythromycin, tetracycline, gentamycin, and neomycin have all been shown to adversely affect sperm in vitro, but studies of clinical use and subsequent effects on semen parameters is lacking [34, 35].

Antidepressants, specifically the serotonin reuptake inhibitors, may lead to decreased libido and anorgasmia [36, 37]. Various other medications including cimetidine, sulfasalazine, colchicine, and allopurinol can all impair fertility either by affecting spermatogenesis, semen parameters, or fertilization [38].

The online databases Reprotox and Reprotext, are comprehensive databases covering the fertility effects of specific medications and should be consulted regarding the effects of a patients current medication list. These resources are typically available through hospitals and university libraries.

23.2.6 Malignancy

A history of malignancy should be elicited. Patients with Hodgkin's disease, acute lymphocytic leukemia, a variety of solid neoplasms as well as testis cancer often demonstrate impaired spermatogenesis prior to therapy. Many chemotherapeutic regimens for these cancers are gonadotoxic [39]. The gonadal toxicity of chemotherapy depends on the agent used, timing, and dosing of therapy. Alkylating agents, platinum based agents, vinca alkaloids, and antimetabolites have all been shown to be gonadotoxic [40, 41]. For those patients who have received chemotherapy, FSH values have been shown to be a reliable marker indicative of injury to the germinal epithelium and for return of normal sperm concentrations.

Radiation therapy for malignancy may be gonadotoxic, and like chemotherapy, the damage is dose dependent. For those patients with testicular cancer who undergo radiotherapy for seminoma, permanent infertility is uncommon. However, unlike chemotherapy, FSH is a less reliable marker for return to normal sperm concentration [4]. Radioactive iodine, for the treatment of thyroid cancer, has also been shown to transiently increase FSH levels; however, it has not shown to permanently effect male fertility [42].

23.2.7 Social History

Social factors have also been implicated as etiologic causes of infertility. While controversial, cigarette smoking has been associated with adverse effects on semen parameters [43].

Use of recreational drugs including cocaine and heavy marijuana use have also been associated with worsening semen parameters [44].

Spermatogenesis is temperature dependent and optimally occurs 2–4°C below core body temperature. Exposure to occupational environments, which theoretically increase scrotal temperatures, has been associated with decreased paternity [45]. Regular use of hot tubs or saunas has been linked to adverse effects on semen parameters. However, the type of undergarments worn, boxers, or briefs has not been shown to affect the semen analysis [46].

The use of anabolic steroids by athletes has also been shown to impair fertility by inducing hypogonadotropic hypogonadism. The increased peripheral testosterone causes negative feedback on the hypothalamic pituitary axis, causing oligospermia or azoospermia. Some reports have shown that the effects of anabolic steroid use are reversible; however, there are case reports of irreversible damage [47, 48].

23.3 Physical Examination

The physical examination should be focused and thorough. General factors that affect overall health can theoretically affect sperm production and sexual function. The presence of breast development and lack of virilization should be noted. These findings may be indicative of a primary or acquired endocrinopathy. Kartagener Syndrome is associated with primary ciliary dyskinesia (immotile cilia syndrome) with situs inversus. The presence of an inguinal scar suggestive of prior surgery may be a clue to a potential injury to the vas deferens or testicular artery. The focus of the physical examination should be centered on the male genitalia. The finding of Tanner stage less than stage V should be documented and suggests impaired androgen action. The presence of penile abnormalities should be noted including the presence of chordee, penile plaques, or a hypospadiac meatus which could impair erectile function, penetration, intercourse, or vaginal deposition of the ejaculate.

The scrotal exam should focus on abnormality or absence of the normal scrotal contents including the testis, epididymis, and vas deferens. Congenital absence of the vas deferens is noted in 1.4% of infertile male population and is associated with mutations in the cystic fibrosis transmembrane regulator protein (CFTR) gene [49]. These patients should be offered genetic testing for CFTR mutations and genetic counseling.

Testis size should be measured, keeping in mind that, in the adult, a normal testis size is greater than 20 ml in Caucasian or African American males. Asians have been reported to have smaller testes. Smaller testis size is suggestive of impaired spermatogenesis. Testicular masses may be indicative of testis cancer, which is often associated with decreased sperm production.

The patient should be examined in the standing position for the presence of a varicocele. Large varicoceles (grade III) are easily discovered by inspection of the scrotum with the typical "bag of worms" appearance. A moderate (grade II) varicocele is palpable by physical examination without a Valsalva maneuver. A small (grade I) varicocele is palpable only when the patient performs a Valsalva.

23.3.1 Duplex Ultrasonography

Duplex ultrasonography is not necessary in the presence of the easily diagnosed varicocele by physical examination. The Male Infertility Best Practice Policy Committee of the AUA recommends duplex ultrasonography for the work up of the infertile male only for those patients with inconclusive physical examination. The use of ancillary testing to detect non-palpable "subclinical" varicoceles is not recommended. Varicoceles are discussed further in the chapter by Tanrikut and Schlegel.

23.4 Laboratory Assessment

23.4.1 Semen Analysis

The semen analysis is generally the initial laboratory test for evaluation of the infertile male. A minimum of two properly collected specimens should be obtained from all patients. If the two samples are very discrepant, a third specimen should be obtained. It should be noted that while the semen analysis helps guide the diagnostic evaluation, it does not provide for definitive separation between those patients who are sterile and those who are fertile, but rather may help differentiate those patients that are likely fertile from those who may be subfertile.

In order for accurate evaluation, at least two specimens should be obtained with specific collection and transportation guidelines provided by the physician or laboratory. Specimens may be collected by masturbation or by special condoms for use during intercourse and deposited in a container provided by the physician. Samples may be collected at home or at the physicians' office [50]. If collected at home, the specimen should be kept warm, typically in a shirt pocket, and brought to the office within approximately 1 h.

The semen analysis is typically divided into seven parameters: volume, sperm concentration, morphology, motility, forward progression, and pH. Sperm concentration on average is usually reported as total concentration or per ml. The WHO reference value for sperm concentration is greater than

20×10^6 per ml or 40×10^6 per ejaculate. It should be noted that the average sperm concentrations and what is described as the reference value does not mean that an individual with a sperm concentration below two standard deviations from the mean is infertile or that a man with a "normal" sperm concentration will be fertile. The seminal analysis is discussed in detail in the chapter by Bjorndahl.

Low seminal volumes can be caused by incomplete collection, obstruction, retrograde ejaculation, or congenital absence of the vas deferens. The pH is determined by a balance between the acidic prostatic secretions, which enter directly through prostatic ducts into the urethra, and the alkaline seminal vesicle fluid, which enters the ejaculatory ducts. Normal pH is approximately 7.2. Therefore, a patient with semen analysis with a low volume and low pH suggests either obstruction of the ejaculatory ducts or absence or dysfunction of the seminal vesicles as is found in patients with CBAVD. Whereas, low volume but normal pH, may suggest retrograde ejaculation or ejaculatory dysfunction.

Defects in other semen parameters may be indicative of specific causes of infertility. For example, sperm that agglutinate is suggestive of the presence of anti-sperm antibodies. Additionally, sperm morphology is an evaluation of the sperm shape. Because there is variation within the infertility literature as to what criteria are used to define normal and abnormal as well as what percentage of normal sperm are the lower limits of normal, it is important for the clinician to be familiar with the laboratory performing the examination.

Under wet mount microscopy, both immature germ cells (such as spermatocytes) and white blood cells appear similar and are termed "round cells." While there is a growing shift in laboratories to differentiate between these two cell types in the semen analysis report, many laboratories still report all round cells as white blood cells. It is therefore important for the clinician to understand the distinction that must be made if round cells are reported [51]. Special staining to differentiate germ cells from leukocytes is recommended, when the patient has greater than 10–15 round cells per high power field. The presence of greater than 1 million white blood cells per milliliter within the semen sample is termed pyospermia. While excess leukocytes does not necessarily indicate a genital tract infection, genital cultures for Mycoplasma genitalia and, Chlamydia Trachoma should be performed since these organisms have been shown to be detrimental to sperm. A morning, first voided urine may be sent for nucleic acid testing for the presence of these organisms [52].

23.4.2 Hormonal Evaluation

Endocrine causes of male infertility are present in less than 3% of patients and are extremely rare among men with normal semen parameters [53]. The results of hormonal studies may diagnose true endocrine abnormalities responsible for the infertility or may be of prognostic value for patient management. The primary indication for hormonal evaluation of sperm concentration is less than 10 million per ml. Additional indications include the presence of gynecomastia, decreased androgenization, sexual dysfunction, or decreased libido. The initial plasma tests should consist of an FSH and a morning testosterone determination. While gonadotropins are secreted in a pulsatile manner, single determinations are usually adequate with pooled blood samples reserved for situations when the results of one hormonal determination does not fit the clinical situation [54]. Since much of the plasma testosterone is protein bound, bioavailable testosterone levels are preferred since they yield more accurate determinations of true tissue available testosterone levels [55].

Most laboratories provide references ranges for "normal" FSH; however, these ranges are not from populations of men of known normal fertility. Similar to sperm concentration, FSH level should be considered a spectrum and must be interpreted in the clinical context rather than be viewed in absolutes. High "normal" FSH values are suggestive of spermatogenic impairment, while most men with normal spermatogenesis have FSH values of less than 5–7 mIU. An elevated FSH with a normal testosterone indicates a significant impairment of spermatogenesis. On the other hand, those individuals with elevated FSH and low testosterone may have primary testicular failure with a deficiency in both spermatogenesis and testosterone production.

Oligospermic or azoospermic patients with low FSH and low testosterone may have hypogonadotropic hypogonadism. This is typically caused by a failure of the pituitary gland and patients should, therefore, undergo determinations of LH, prolactin, and repeat testosterone. Normal prolactin levels in the setting of hypogonadotropic hypogonadism can be due to Kallman syndrome or other genetically inherited disorders. Elevated prolactin levels may be indicative of a prolactinoma of the pituitary. Pituitary imaging with MRI should be performed in all patients with hypogonadotropic hypogonadism, as some pituitary tumors may be non-functioning adenomas.

23.5 Development of a Differential Diagnosis

On the basis of the initial history, physical, and semen analysis with or without hormonal studies, a differential diagnosis should be developed. Additional advanced testing may be required to narrow down the diagnostic possibilities. The included diagnostic algorithms may be used to pursue the evaluation in an efficient, organized fashion. A useful initial categorization groups the potential etiologies based on the findings of the semen analyses. Common categories include low seminal volume, defects in isolated parameters, defects in multiple parameters, or all parameters normal. Defects in semen parameters can be due to intrinsic deficiency in sperm production or a defect in the transport of viable sperm to the oocyte. The algorithms will help direct an efficient evaluation (Fig. 23.1–23.4).

23.5.1 Low Seminal Volume

The absence of an antegrade ejaculate is termed ejaculatory failure or aspermia and results in a "dry ejaculate." This may be due to retrograde ejaculation in which semen travels retrograde from the prostatic urethra into the bladder or due to lack of emission, when no semen is deposited in the prostatic urethra. Ejaculatory failure is different from azoospermia, in

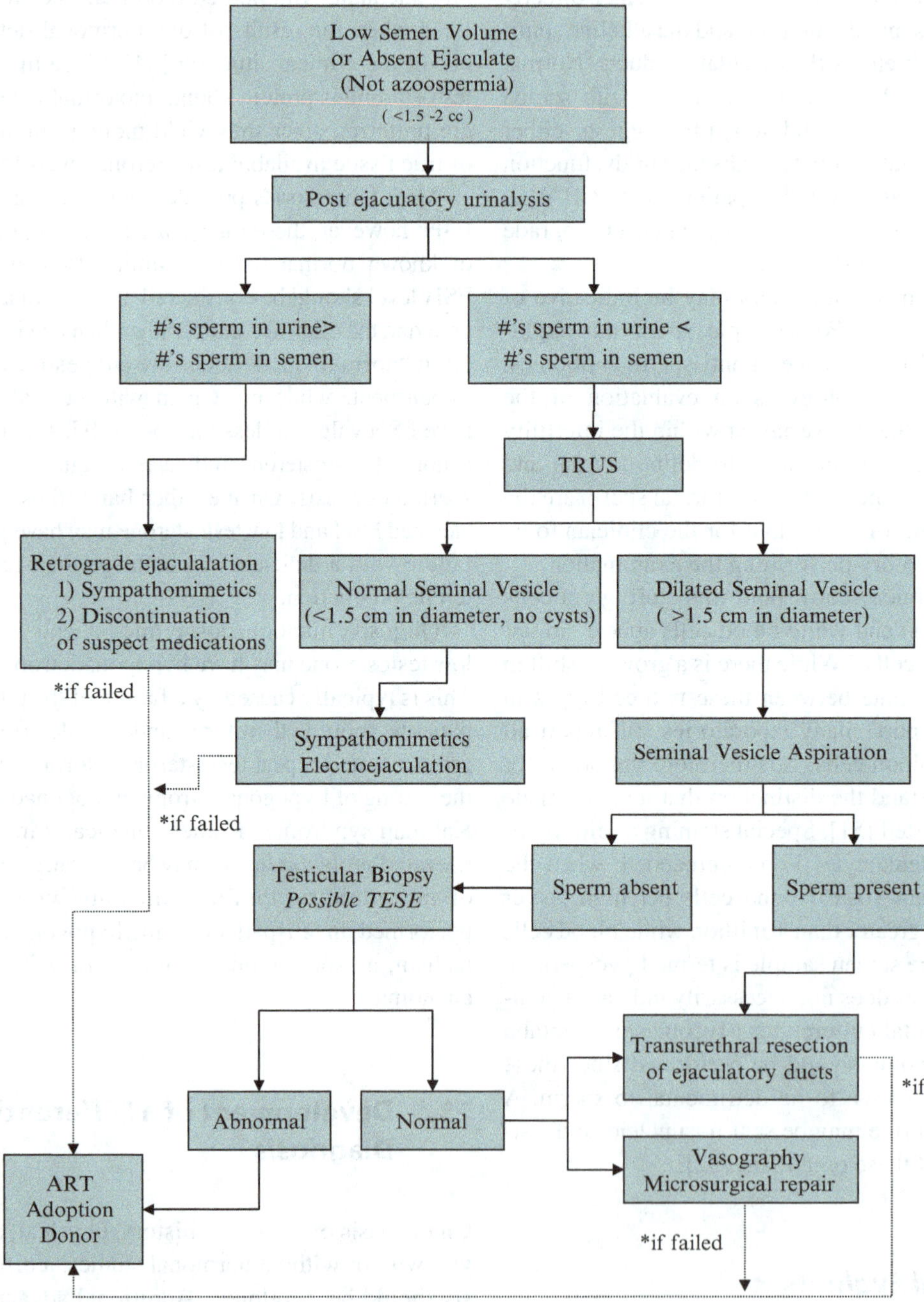

Fig 23.1 Algorithm for evaluation of low volume ejaculate. Excludes azoospermic specimens. TESE = testicular sperm extraction, ART = assisted reproductive techniques, Donor = insemination with donor sperm

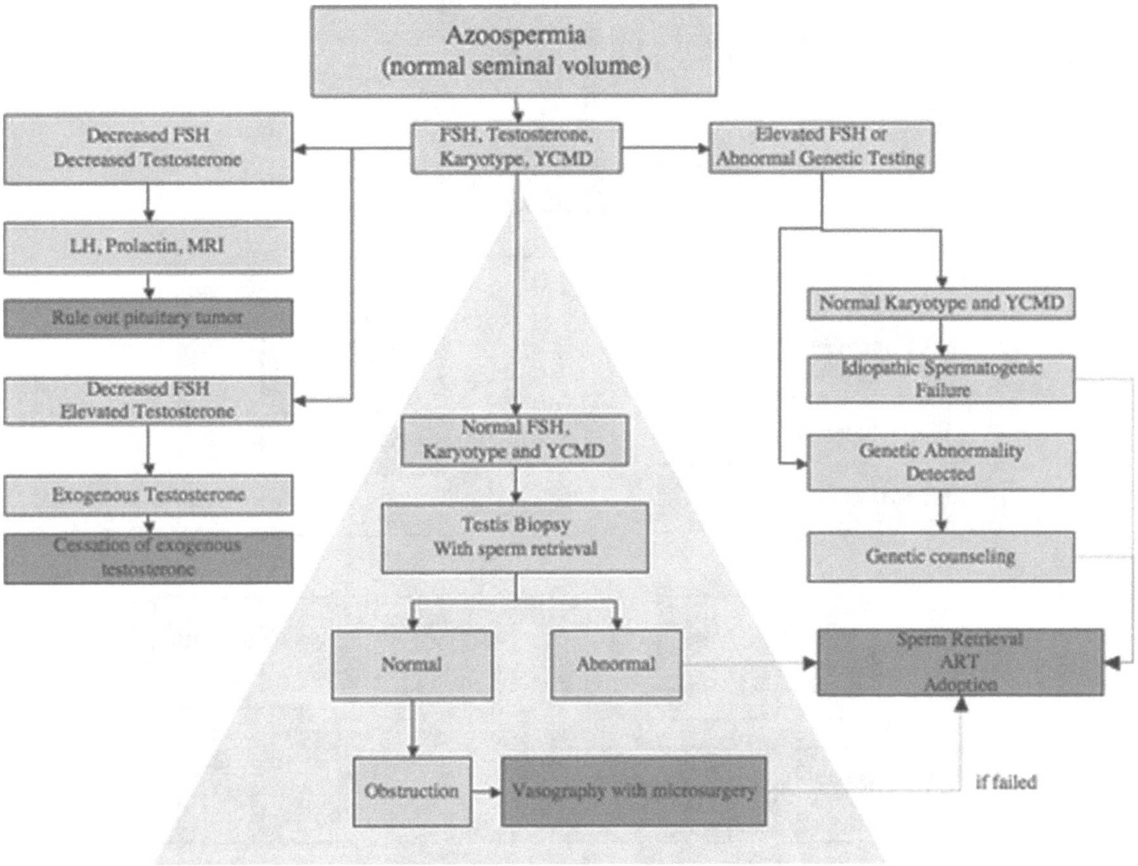

Fig 23.2 Algorithm for normal volume azoospermia. TESE = testicular sperm extraction, ART = assisted reproductive techniques

which there is an antegrade ejaculate but no sperm are present in the seminal fluid. Neurologic disorders such as spinal cord injury, multiple sclerosis, Parkinson's disease, retroperitoneal surgery, as well as diabetes, and the use of alpha blockers may cause ejaculatory failure. All patients with ejaculatory failure or low volume ejaculates should be evaluated with post-ejaculate urinalyses.

The presence of sperm in the post ejaculatory urinalysis in patients with aspermia indicates retrograde ejaculation or the passage of some sperm into the urethra. In addition, it rules out complete bilateral ductal obstruction. In patients with low volume oligospermic semen samples, the finding of greater numbers of sperm in the urine than in the semen suggests an important component of retrograde ejaculation. Low volume azoospermic specimens suggest the presence of ejaculatory duct obstruction or CBAVD. Semen from these patients will be acidic and of low volume. The physical exam will determine if CBAVD is present. Genetic testing for mutations in the CFTR gene and analysis for the 5 T polymorphism should be offered to all patients with low volume azoospermia, even if vas are palpable, since some patients who have palpable vas deferens are congenitally obstructed. In a minority of patients, CBAVD is due to an embryologic defect not related to CFTR mutations. These patients should be offered renal ultrasonography since unilateral absence of the kidney is often associated with the vasal defect.

Ejaculatory duct obstruction may be evaluated by transrectal ultrasonography (TRUS) to determine if the seminal vesicles are present and whether they are dilated. The normal width of the seminal vesicles is 0.4–1.4 cm. A measurement of 1.5 cm or greater on TRUS should raise concern for ejaculatory duct obstruction. Transrectal aspiration of dilated seminal vesicles can be done at the same time as ultrasound evaluation. The presence of sperm with the seminal vesicle is diagnostic of ejaculatory duct obstruction [56].

23.5.2 Azoospermia

All azoospermic semen samples should be centrifuged. The presence of sperm in the centrifuged pellet rules out complete

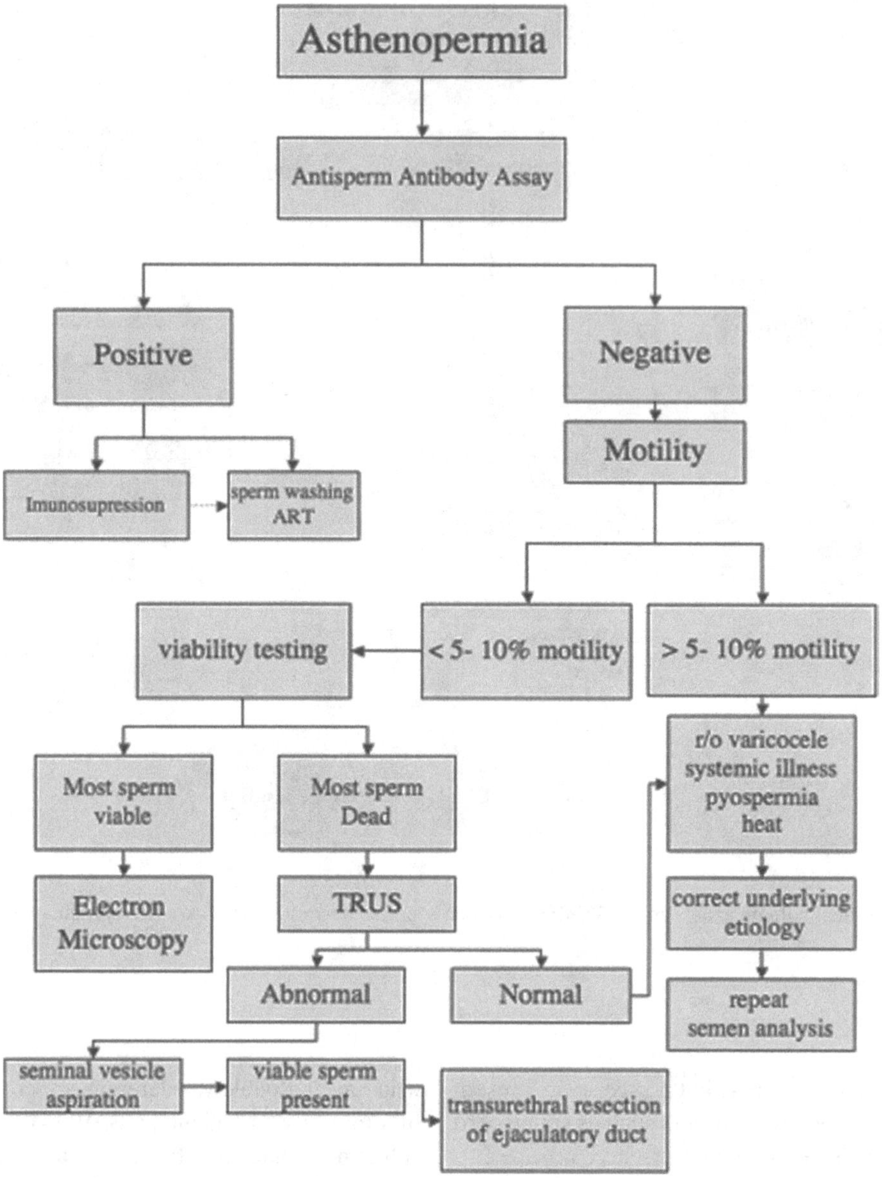

Fig 23.3 Algorithm for asthenospermia. ART = assisted reproductive techniques, TRUS = transrectal ultrasonography of prostate and seminal vesicles

bilateral ductal obstruction. The finding of atrophic testes in patients with normal volume azoospermia suggests a defect in spermatogenesis (non-obstructive azoospermia). The results of FSH and testosterone studies will determine if this is due to a primary spermatogenic defect or is secondary to a hormonal deficiency (see Table 23.1). Those azoospermic patients who are not thought to have an obstructive etiology or a hormonal deficiency should be offered genetic testing with karyotype and Y chromosome microdeletion analysis. Patients with normal volume azoospermia and normal testicular volume, FSH, and testosterone levels may have ductal obstruction. A testicular biopsy with the option of sperm cryopreservation if sperm are present should be offered. With the availability of ICSI, a purely diagnostic testicular biopsy, without an attempt at sperm retrieval is rarely indicated. The finding of normal spermatogenesis indicates obstructive azoospermia.

23.5.3 Oligospermia

All patients with sperm densities of less than 10 million sperm per milliliter should undergo hormonal evaluation

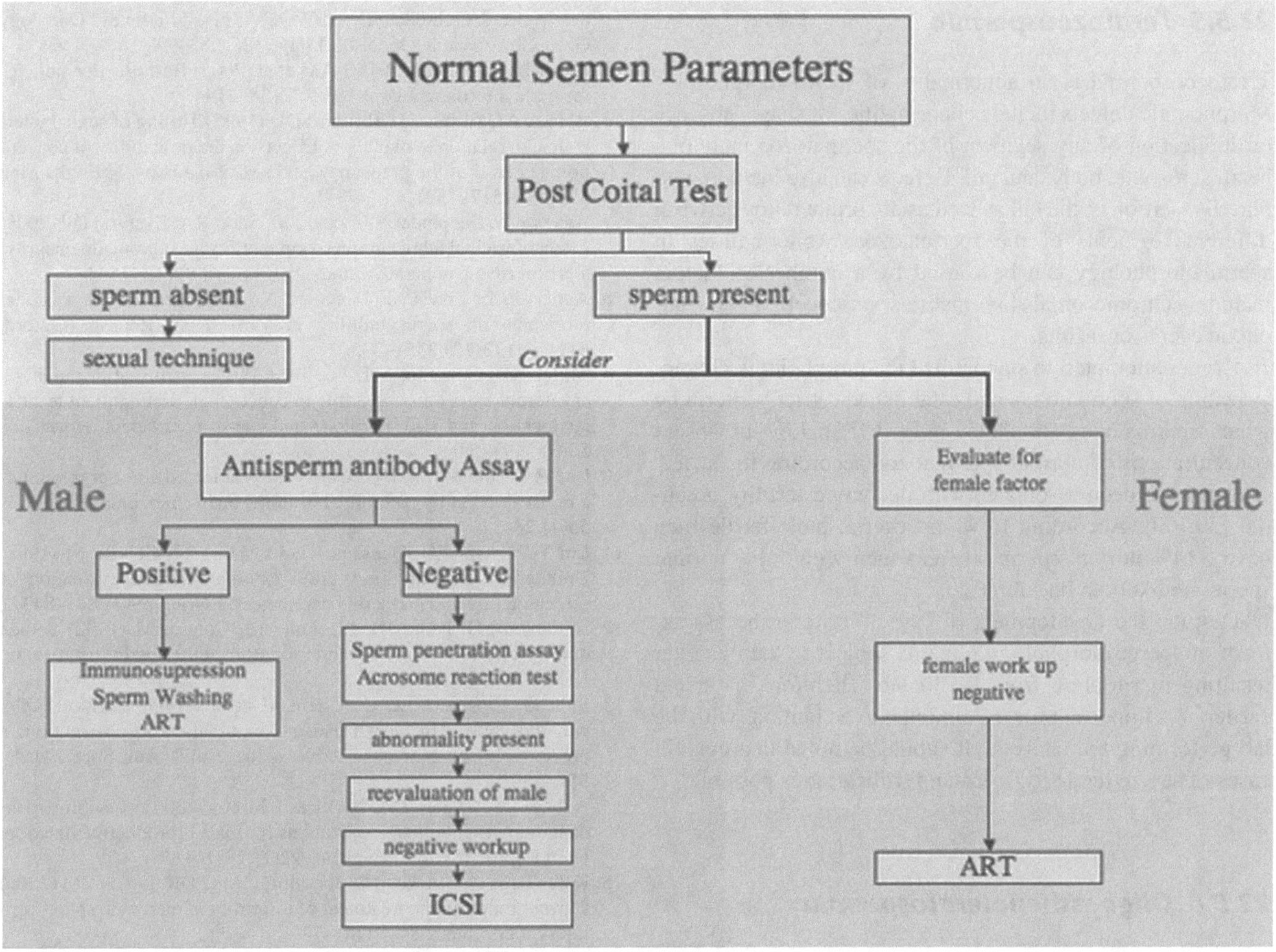

Fig 23.4 Algorithm for normal semen parameters. ART = assisted reproductive techniques, ICSI = intracytoplasmic sperm injection

Table 23.1 Hormone levels in various endocrinopathies

Condition	FSH	LH	Testosterone	Prolactin
Hypogonadotropic hypogonadism	⇓	⇓	⇓	nl
Testicular failure	⇑	⇑	⇓	nl
Spermatogenic failure	⇑	nl	nl	nl
Prolactinoma	⇓	⇓	⇓	⇑
Exogenous testosterone	⇓	⇓	⇑	nl

with an FSH and testosterone. Since the vast majority of patients with chromosomal abnormalities affecting sperm production or AZF deletions have sperm densities of less than 5 million sperm per milliliter, karyotype and YCMD studies should be reserved for this group of patients [57]. Most commonly, isolated oligospermia is idiopathic.

23.5.4 Asthenospermia

Asthenospermia is a defect in sperm motility and can be caused by a number of factors including infection with pyospermia, varicocele, antisperm antibodies, partial ductal ejaculatory duct obstruction, impaired transport of sperm through the ductal system (as may occur with diabetes), prolonged abstinence periods, and ultrastructural abnormalities such as primary ciliary dyskinesia. Ultrastructural defects are most commonly associated with motilities of less that 5–10%. These patients should undergo sperm viability testing. The finding of very low motility with high viability indicates an ultrastructural abnormality which may be further evaluated with electron microscopy of the sperm.

23.5.5 Teratozoospermia

Teratozoospermia is an abnormality of sperm morphology. Morphologic defects include abnormalities of shape, absence or duplication of any segment of the spermatozoa including head, acrosome, body, and tail. Defects can also include misplaced insertion of the tail as well as abnormal ratios between different segments of the spermatozoa. Abnormalities in sperm morphology can be caused by a number of factors including chromosomal abnormalities, varicocele, and gonadotoxic events or insults.

Kruger attempted to standardize the morphologic characterization of spermatozoa and established "strict" criteria by which spermatozoa should be judged [58]. Low or absent concentrations of normal spermatozoa according to "strict" criteria have been associated with decreased fertility potential [59, 60]. According to strict criteria, most fertile men have $>14\%$ normal sperm whereas men with $<4\%$ normal sperm are likely to be subfertile.

Despite, the development of "strict" criteria the assessment of sperm morphology remains subject to the observer resulting in variation from lab to lab. Therefore, as stated earlier, it is important for the clinician to be familiar with the lab performing the analysis. It should be noted that even in cases of severe teratozoospermia, fertilization is possible.

23.5.6 Oligoasthenoteratospermia

A defect in all semen parameters (density, motility, and morphology) is called Oligoasthenoteratospermia (OAT). The most common causes of OAT include varicocele, testicular trauma, history of cryptorchidism, environmental insults and toxins, medications, drugs, partial ejaculatory duct obstruction, idiopathic causes as well as temporary insults to spermatogenesis including recent illness. The criteria for the diagnosis of partial ejaculatory duct obstruction remain controversial. In most cases, it is not possible to differentiate partial obstruction from idiopathic causes.

References

1. American Urologic Association and the American Society of Reproductive Medicine (2001) Report on the optimal evaluation of the infertile male. American Urological Association, Baltimore, MD
2. Jarow JP (1994) Life-threatening conditions associated with male infertility. Urol Clin North Am 21(3):409–415
3. Raman JD, Nobert CF, Goldstein M (2005) Increased incidence of testicular cancer in men presenting with infertility and abnormal semen analysis. J Urol 174(5):1819–1822 discussion 1822
4. Gordon W Jr, Siegmund K, Stanisic TH et al (1997) A study of reproductive function in patients with seminoma treated with radiotherapy and orchidectomy: (SWOG-8711). Southwest Oncology Group. Int J Radiat Oncol Biol Phys 38(1):83–94
5. Jarow JP, Sharlip ID, Belker AM et al (2002) Best practice policies for male infertility. J Urol 167(5):2138–2144
6. Wilcox AJ, Weinberg CR, Baird DD (1995) Timing of sexual intercourse in relation to ovulation. Effects on the probability of conception, survival of the pregnancy, and sex of the baby. N Engl J Med 333(23):1517–1521
7. Agarwal A, Deepinder F, Cocuzza M, Short RA, Evenson DP (2008) Effect of vaginal lubricants on sperm motility and chromatin integrity: a prospective comparative study. Fertil Steril 89(2):375–379
8. Anderson L, Lewis SE, McClure N (1998) The effects of coital lubricants on sperm motility in vitro. Hum Reprod (Oxford, England) 13(12):3351–3356
9. Miller KD, Coughlin MT, Lee PA (2001) Fertility after unilateral cryptorchidism. Paternity, time to conception, pretreatment testicular location and size, hormone and sperm parameters. Horm Res 55(5):249–253
10. Lee PA, Coughlin MT (2001) Fertility after bilateral cryptorchidism. Evaluation by paternity, hormone, and semen data. Horm Res 55(1):28–32
11. Lin WW, Kim ED, Quesada ET, Lipshultz LI, Coburn M (1998) Unilateral testicular injury from external trauma: evaluation of semen quality and endocrine parameters. J Urol 159(3):841–843
12. Anderson MJ, Dunn JK, Lipshultz LI, Coburn M (1992) Semen quality and endocrine parameters after acute testicular torsion. J Urol 147(6):1545–1550
13. Shin D, Lipshultz LI, Goldstein M et al (2005) Herniorrhaphy with polypropylene mesh causing inguinal vasal obstruction: a preventable cause of obstructive azoospermia. Ann Surg 241(4): 553–558
14. Agbaje IM, Rogers DA, McVicar CM et al (2007) Insulin dependant diabetes mellitus: implications for male reproductive function. Hum Reprod (Oxford, England) 22(7):1871–1877
15. Kafetsoulis A, Brackett NL, Ibrahim E, Attia GR, Lynne CM (2006) Current trends in the treatment of infertility in men with spinal cord injury. Fertil Steril 86(4):781–789
16. Brackett NL, Ibrahim E, Grotas JA, Aballa TC, Lynne CM (2008) Higher sperm DNA damage in semen from men with spinal cord injuries compared to controls. J Androl 29(1):93–99 discussion 100–101
17. Palmer BF (1999) Sexual dysfunction in uremia. J Am Soc Nephrol 10(6):1381–1388
18. Prem AR, Punekar SV, Kalpana M, Kelkar AR, Acharya VN (1996) Male reproductive function in uraemia: efficacy of haemodialysis and renal transplantation. Br J Urol 78(4):635–638
19. Umapathy E, Simbini T, Chipata T, Mbizvo M (2001) Sperm characteristics and accessory sex gland functions in HIV-infected men. Arch Androl 46(2):153–158
20. Briganti A, Naspro R, Gallina A et al (2006) Impact on sexual function of holmium laser enucleation versus transurethral resection of the prostate: results of a prospective, 2-center, randomized trial. J Urol 175(5):1817–1821
21. Ahmed M, Bell T, Lawrence WT, Ward JP, Watson GM (1997) Transurethral microwave thermotherapy (Prostatron version 2.5) compared with transurethral resection of the prostate for the treatment of benign prostatic hyperplasia: a randomized, controlled, parallel study. Br J Urol 79(2):181–185
22. Jonker-Pool G, Van de Wiel HB, Hoekstra HJ et al (2001) Sexual functioning after treatment for testicular cancer – review and meta-analysis of 36 empirical studies between 1975–2000. Arch Sex Behav 30(1):55–74
23. Kleeman TJ, Michael Ahn U, Clutterbuck WB, Campbell CJ, Talbot-Kleeman A (2002) Laparoscopic anterior lumbar interbody fusion at L4-L5: an anatomic evaluation and approach classification. Spine 27(13):1390–1395

24. Hershlag A, Cooper GW, Benoff S (1995) Pregnancy following discontinuation of a calcium channel blocker in the male partner. Hum Reprod (Oxford, England) 10(3):599–606
25. Benoff S, Cooper GW, Hurley I et al (1994) The effect of calcium ion channel blockers on sperm fertilization potential. Fertil Steril 62(3):606–617
26. Katsoff D, Check JH (1997) A challenge to the concept that the use of calcium channel blockers causes reversible male infertility. Hum Reprod (Oxford, England) 12(7):1480–1482
27. Corvol P, Michaud A, Menard J, Freifeld M, Mahoudeau J (1975) Antiandrogenic effect of spirolactones: mechanism of action. Endocrinology 97(1):52–58
28. Rosen RC, Kostis JB, Jekelis AW (1988) Beta-blocker effects on sexual function in normal males. Arch Sex Behav 17(3):241–255
29. Giuliano FA, Clement P, Denys P, Alexandre L, Bernabe J (2006) Comparison between tamsulosin and alfuzosin on the expulsion phase of ejaculation in rats. BJU Int 98(4):876–879
30. Giuliano F, Bernabe J, Droupy S, Alexandre L, Allard J (2004) A comparison of the effects of tamsulosin and alfuzosin on neurally evoked increases in bladder neck and seminal vesicle pressure in rats. BJU Int 93(4):605–608
31. Hellstrom WJ, Sikka SC (2006) Effects of acute treatment with tamsulosin versus alfuzosin on ejaculatory function in normal volunteers. J Urol 176(4 Pt 1):1529–1533
32. Overstreet JW, Fuh VL, Gould J et al (1999) Chronic treatment with finasteride daily does not affect spermatogenesis or semen production in young men. J Urol 162(4):1295–1300
33. Albert PS, Mininberg DT, Davis JE (1974) Nitrofurans: sperm-immobilizing agents. Their tissue toxicity and clinical application. Urology 4(3):307–310
34. Schlegel PN, Chang TS, Marshall FF (1991) Antibiotics: potential hazards to male fertility. Fertil Steril 55(2):235–242
35. Hargreaves CA, Rogers S, Hills F, Rahman F, Howell RJ, Homa ST (1998) Effects of co-trimoxazole, erythromycin, amoxycillin, tetracycline and chloroquine on sperm function in vitro. Hum Reprod (Oxford, England) 13(7):1878–1886
36. Hu XH, Bull SA, Hunkeler EM et al (2004) Incidence and duration of side effects and those rated as bothersome with selective serotonin reuptake inhibitor treatment for depression: patient report versus physician estimate. J Clin Psychiatry 65(7):959–965
37. Tanrikut C, Schlegel PN (2007) Antidepressant-associated changes in semen parameters. Urology 69(1):185.e5–185.e7
38. Nudell DM, Monoski MM, Lipshultz LI (2002) Common medications and drugs: how they affect male fertility. Urol Clin North Am 29(4):965–973
39. Kreuser ED, Xiros N, Hetzel WD, Heimpel H (1987) Reproductive and endocrine gonadal capacity in patients treated with COPP chemotherapy for Hodgkin's disease. J Cancer Res Clin Oncol 113(3):260–266
40. Howell SJ, Shalet SM (2001) Testicular function following chemotherapy. Hum Reprod Update 7(4):363–369
41. Tal R, Botchan A, Hauser R, Yogev L, Paz G, Yavetz H (2000) Follow-up of sperm concentration and motility in patients with lymphoma. Hum Reprod (Oxford, England) 15(9):1985–1988
42. Hyer S, Vini L, O'Connell M, Pratt B, Harmer C (2002) Testicular dose and fertility in men following I(131) therapy for thyroid cancer. Clin Endocrinol 56(6):755–758
43. Chia SE, Lim ST, Tay SK, Lim ST (2000) Factors associated with male infertility: a case-control study of 218 infertile and 240 fertile men. BJOG 107(1):55–61
44. Bracken MB, Eskenazi B, Sachse K, McSharry JE, Hellenbrand K, Leo-Summers L (1990) Association of cocaine use with sperm concentration, motility, and morphology. Fertil Steril 53(2):315–322
45. Thonneau P, Bujan L, Multigner L, Mieusset R (1998) Occupational heat exposure and male fertility: a review. Hum Reprod (Oxford, England) 13(8):2122–2125
46. Munkelwitz R, Gilbert BR (1998) Are boxer shorts really better? A critical analysis of the role of underwear type in male subfertility. J Urol 160(4):1329–1333
47. Gazvani MR, Buckett W, Luckas MJ, Aird IA, Hipkin LJ, Lewis-Jones DI (1997) Conservative management of azoospermia following steroid abuse. Hum Reprod (Oxford, England) 12(8): 1706–1708
48. Menon DK (2003) Successful treatment of anabolic steroid-induced azoospermia with human chorionic gonadotropin and human menopausal gonadotropin. Fertil Steril 79(Suppl 3):1659–1661
49. Anguiano A, Oates RD, Amos JA et al (1992) Congenital bilateral absence of the vas deferens. A primarily genital form of cystic fibrosis. JAMA 267(13):1794–1797
50. Shetty Licht R, Handel L, Sigman M (2008) Site of semen collection and its effect on semen analysis parameters. Fertil Steril 89(2):395–397
51. Johanisson E, Campana A, Luthi R, de Agostini A (2000) Evaluation of 'round cells' in semen analysis: a comparative study. Hum Reprod Update 6(4):404–412
52. Jensen JS, Bjornelius E, Dohn B, Lidbrink P (2004) Comparison of first void urine and urogenital swab specimens for detection of Mycoplasma genitalium and Chlamydia trachomatis by polymerase chain reaction in patients attending a sexually transmitted disease clinic. Sex Transm Dis 31(8):499–507
53. Sigman M, Jarow JP (1997) Endocrine evaluation of infertile men. Urology 50(5):659–664
54. Bain J, Langevin R, D'Costa M, Sanders RM, Hucker S (1988) Serum pituitary and steroid hormone levels in the adult male: one value is as good as the mean of three. Fertil Steril 49(1):123–126
55. Ashok S, Sigman M (2007) Bioavailable testosterone should be used for the determination of androgen levels in infertile men. J Urol 177(4):1443–1446 quiz 591
56. Jarow JP (1996) Transrectal ultrasonography in the diagnosis and management of ejaculatory duct obstruction. J Androl 17(5):467–472
57. Ferlin A, Arredi B, Speltra E et al (2007) Molecular and clinical characterization of Y chromosome microdeletions in infertile men: a 10-year experience in Italy. J Clin Endocrinol Metab 92(3): 762–770
58. Kruger TF, Menkveld R, Stander FS et al (1986) Sperm morphologic features as a prognostic factor in in vitro fertilization. Fertil Steril 46(6):1118–1123
59. Coetzee K, Kruge TF, Lombard CJ (1998) Predictive value of normal sperm morphology: a structured literature review. Hum Reprod Update 4(1):73–82
60. Guzick DS, Overstreet JW, Factor-Litvak P et al (2001) Sperm morphology, motility, and concentration in fertile and infertile men. N Engl J Med 345(19):1388–1393

Chapter 24
Semen Analysis: Essentials for the Clinician

Lars Björndahl

Abstract Basic semen analysis comprises sperm number, motility, vitality, and morphology. The clinical usefulness has been under debate due to variable reliability and poor prognostic value. There are now reliable and robust methods possible to train and obtain lower interobserver variability and also to control variability with modern laboratory quality control procedures. Still, the results from semen analysis cannot alone give the clinical diagnosis for the subfertile couple; results from basic semen analysis must be combined with other clinical data in order to set a proper diagnosis. In this chapter, basic technical aspects of semen analysis are discussed to give a basis for the clinician to set appropriate demands on the local andrology service. The limitations of basic semen analysis as well as semen biochemistry, antisperm antibody testing, some sperm function tests, sperm DNA damage tests and the present status of stem cell research are also discussed in relation to the clinical usefulness of the methods.

Keywords Semen analysis • Biological variability • Technical variability • Quality control • Sequence of ejaculation • Predictive value • Prognostic value • Terminology

24.1 Introduction

Semen analysis is the starting point for the investigation of the man in the infertile couple [1–3], but the clinical value of semen analysis has been under debate for a long time [4]. The doubts of the usefulness of semen analysis must, however, be seen in relation to somewhat exaggerated expectations for what an analysis of semen parameters really can contribute. The intention of this chapter is to discuss what can be learned from semen analysis and which the limitations are. Some information on the basic technical aspects is also included to give the clinician a basis to understand which laboratories that can deliver reliable results and which are less likely to do that.

When the usefulness of semen analysis is discussed, one important aspect is to differentiate between prognostic (or predictive) capacity and correlation between analysis parameters and various fertility success parameters. A laboratory test with a good predictive ability will help the clinician in the individual investigation: the result of a test (or a combined set of test) corresponds to a high degree of likelihood that the man has a certain disorder, or that a certain treatment will solve the problem with high likelihood. This is not the case with most results from semen analysis. Although many components of semen analysis are significantly correlated to fertility, it is usually impossible to give the individual man a reliable prediction of the couple's fertility just from the semen analysis results. One factor is, of course, that semen analysis extremely seldom discloses problems in the female partner. More importantly, semen analysis results overlap between fertile and infertile men. Therefore, single semen analysis results are seldom helpful to determine the fertility potential of the man in the infertile couple while combination of several parameters can is predictive (Guzick et al 2001, Jedrzejczak et al 2008). The recommendation is, therefore, to regard semen analysis not as a predictive tool, but as all other laboratory tests: important jigsaw puzzle pieces for the clinician to evaluate together with patient history, physical examination, and blood analyses of hormone levels etc.

A probable contributing factor for this confusion of predictive and descriptive laboratory investigations is the unfortunate terminology [5] that can give the false impression that results from semen analyses can be used as prognostic tools. As in the development of all areas of medicine, the descriptive terms were developed before the discovery of causes and treatment methods. From qualitative assessments (many, few, none), quantitative measures were developed, and the quite arbitrary terms were given quantitative limits. Although semen samples with less than 20 million sperm per milliliter can be defined as oligozoospermic, there is no prognostic value in this term, and it can be questioned if 22 millions/mL is very much better than 18 millions/mL, but categorizing the patient with the latter result as "oligozoospermic" does indicate that there is relevant information in such a limit and that

L. Björndahl (✉)
Centre for Andrology and Sexual Medicine, Endocrinology Clinic Karolinska University Hospital, Huddinge and Department of Medicine, Huddinge, Karolinska Institute, Stockholm, Sweden
e-mail: Lars.Bjorndahl@ki.se

D.T. Carrell and C.M. Peterson (eds.), *Reproductive Endocrinology and Infertility: Integrating Modern Clinical and Laboratory Practice*,
DOI 10.1007/978-1-4419-1436-1_24,

semen analysis can give accurate diagnoses without other sources of information. The exaggerated use of these arbitrary limits giving the false impression of a true dichotomous outcome of semen analysis has, most likely, also influenced clinical research, where men have been sorted into male factor or not male factor categories based on such categorical limits. Thus, all studies supposedly investigating "male factor" infertility must be read with very critical eyes and interpreted with great caution. So we should, instead of regarding the semen analysis as the miracle test that will reveal all, look for what information that can be gained. In general, semen analysis gives combined information about quantitative sperm production and transport, some basic functional aspects and the overall structural appearance of sperm in the ejaculate.

Not only pathological processes affect the results of semen analysis; there is a considerable biological variability in semen analysis, and the variation between two different samples from one man can be significant, although the clinical importance has been questioned [6–8]. Furthermore, if the laboratory does not apply modern methods and quality control, the technical variability can cause significant errors resulting in couples being subjected to inadequate investigations and treatment alternatives. It is also essential to consider that the semen sample examined in the semen laboratory is not likely to be representative for what the man delivers during sexual intercourse. Under the latter circumstances, the first, sperm rich fractions with mainly prostatic fluid, are expelled onto the cervical mucus [9] and the sperm are most likely to enter the cervical mucus without any essential contact with seminal vesicular fluid from the later fractions of the ejaculate [10]. In the laboratory investigation, the entire ejaculate is collected in one container and the first fractions are trapped in the coagulum formed by proteins in the seminal vesicular fluid. Before sperm can be examined, enzymes of prostatic origin must degrade proteins forming the coagulum, causing increased osmolarity in the laboratory sample. Also pH changes during in vitro storage; sperm motility decreases by time, varying between different samples, in semen. However, presently there is no better alternative, but these basic problems with semen analysis should to be known by anyone using and interpreting semen analysis results.

24.2 Problems in Conducting the Semen Analysis

24.2.1 Biological Variability Affecting Semen Analysis

The number, or concentration, of sperm a man can produce in a semen sample does not appear to have Gaussian (normal) distribution. It is well known that testicular size [11] as well as the number of abstinence days [12, 13] influence the sperm output in semen samples, but the variation among men with regard to abstinence time is considerable [14]. Also the duration and quality of sexual stimulation appears to be important for the output of sperm in the ejaculate [15–17].

24.2.2 Causes for Technical Variability in Semen Analysis

A modern andrology laboratory should apply methods and techniques that reduce the sources of errors to a minimum. In order to allow comparisons of results from different laboratories, as well as to implementation of discoveries from other laboratories in the local laboratory, it is absolutely necessary to have implemented standardized techniques and participate in the same type of external quality control. The World Health Organization has issued a series of manuals to give a basis for global standardization [5]. On the basis of these recommendations as well as on recent developments in the field of laboratory science, detailed laboratory methods have been published [18], and a practical training course has been developed and used in several different countries in Europe, in Canada, and in South Africa [19–21].

Quality Control is a continuous process that should be implemented in any laboratory producing data used for the investigation and treatment of individuals [22]. Although robust and reliable methods are available with adequate training programs for staff members, it is only by systematic testing of the performance of the laboratory that the laboratory can ascertain that the quality of service actually is at the level defined in the quality manual of the laboratory and in accordance with any contracts with customers (patients, clinicians, other parties paying for the services).

One basic component of quality control is to make assessments in duplicate and to compare the two assessments. Only if the difference is likely to be due to random factors can the two assessments be accepted and the result is calculated on both assessments. Another basic requirement for reliable results is that sufficient numbers of sperm have been assessed. The theories of probability tell us that with few observations, random factors will have a considerable influence of the results. In general, counting 400 cells will give a variability of ±10% due to random factors, while counting only 100 cells will give a variability of around ±20% [18]. Furthermore, if only ten sperm are counted to, for example, obtain the result of sperm preparation for Assisted Reproductive Techniques (ART), the level of uncertainty (95% Confidence Interval) can be calculated to be larger than ±50%.

24.3 Components of Basic Semen Analysis

Since the patient will be responsible for preparations before and at the actual sample collection, comprehensive and understandable information that support patient compliance is absolutely essential for reliable results, no less important than adequate equipment and materials, and well trained staff using controllable technical procedures.

24.3.1 Sample Collection: Preanalytical Issues

Besides informing the patient about abstinence time (or even frequency of ejaculation), it is important to be aware that the intensity and duration of stimulation during sample collection is essential to optimize the results of semen collection [15–17]. Although it may be more comfortable for the patient to collect the semen sample at home, long transportation by car or bus/train can introduce uncontrollable factors as temperature drops at long delay before start of examination. However, the facilities provided for the patients to collect semen samples must be suitable, allowing privacy, and avoid any disturbance. A long delay before analysis will affect the sperm motility, but the variability between different samples is considerable. Thus, a sample with poor motility 2 h after ejaculation may have had completely satisfactory motility 30 min after ejaculation. The recommendation is therefore to initiate all investigations with motility assessments as close to 30 min after ejaculation as possible. Also morphological disturbances can occur as a result of long storage of sperm in semen on the lab bench.

Since it is difficult to define and correctly maintain "room temperature" during the microscopic examinations, the recommendation is that the sample should be kept at and investigated at 37°C at least until sperm motility has been assessed. The proportion and velocity of rapidly progressive sperm appears to vary a lot with different ambient temperatures, and since this parameter is considered important for fertilizing ability, it is reasonable to try to maintain a standardized temperature.

24.3.2 Semen Volume

It is important to determine the total semen volume accurately since this value is used to calculate the total sperm number in the ejaculate from the measured sperm concentration. The dominant part of semen volume is constituted by seminal vesicular fluid and prostatic fluid; the sperm concentration thus depends on the total number of sperm recruited from the epididymis and the dilution caused by the accessory sex gland secretion at ejaculation. Traditionally, semen volume has been measured in graduated centrifugations tubes, but the graduation is often too inaccurate for this purpose. Other types of volume measuring devices (cylinders, pipettes) are much more accurate, but do induce volume losses of varying magnitude [23]. The recommendation is therefore that semen volume is assessed by weighing. Taking into consideration that the density (mass/volume) of semen is sufficiently constant and around 1.0 g/mL, the volume can easily be measured with a calibrated scale.

24.3.3 Sperm Motility

A basic sperm function that is very apparent in basic semen analysis is the motility. It is quite easy to understand that with no or very poor motility, the chance for a man to cause a spontaneous pregnancy is very small. It is more difficult to establish a clear threshold under which pregnancy will not occur, or a threshold above which pregnancies are very likely to occur. There are studies clearly indicating that the rapid progressive motility is related to normal fertilization [24, 25]. Although most of the studies were based on Computer Assisted Sperm Analysis (CASA), manual methods are possible to use. Human examiners can be trained to a high degree of concordance and repeatability and to distinguish between slowly and rapidly progressive sperm [26]. Therefore, the recommendation is that sperm motility should be assessed in four categories: immotile, nonprogressive, slowly progressive, and rapidly progressive [5, 18]. To decrease the influence from random factors due to sampling errors and possible remaining heterogeneity in a well mixed sample, the analysis should be based on at least two different aliquots sampled from a well mixed semen and in each aliquot at least 200 sperm should be assessed in at least four different fields. The results from the two aliquots should be compared and found similar enough to exclude random errors in order to be accepted [18]. CASA can not accurately distinguish immotile sperm crystals and debris in the ejaculate, why this technology can not replace the manual assessment of sperm motility in semen [27, 28]. However, CASA can give much more detailed information about the motility patterns of sperm than trained laboratory staff can obtain with manual methods.

24.3.4 Sperm Vitality

In a sense, sperm motility can be said to be a sperm vitality test, since dead sperm do not swim by themselves in semen. However, when very few, or no sperm, are motile the question arises whether some or many of the immotile sperm still are alive. This can be tested by dye exclusion (live sperm with intact membranes do not take up stain) or a hypoosmotic swelling test (live sperm with intact membranes take up some water when exposed to hypoosmotic environment; dead sperm do not swell, and sperm with poor adaptive ability to adapt to osmotic stress may even burst). The recommended staining method [29] uses ordinary bright field microscopy and in contrast to the corresponding method in the 1999 WHO manual, this method does not kill a certain portion of sperm [30]. The HOS test is mainly helpful when sperm are not only investigated for diagnostic purposes; HOS-tested sperm can in principle be used for treatment purposes while those exposed to stain are not suitable for treatments [31].

24.3.5 Sperm Concentration

Sampling of an exact volume of well mixed semen for sperm concentration assessment should be done with positive displacement pipette [32]. The viscosity of semen is variable between different samples, but invariably significantly higher than water. Therefore, the most common types of pipettes – air displacement pipettes – are not suitable for semen. Furthermore, even in well mixed samples, there may still be heterogeneity at the microscopic level. Therefore, the sampling volume should not be too low, since a low volume (3–5 μL) does increase the risk for poor representativity of the sampled aliquots. The recommended standard sampling volume is therefore 50 μL. The diluted sperm suspension (where sperm are fixed, meaning that the sperm will not swim around and, therefore, will be easier to count) should be examined in a counting chamber with a well controlled chamber volume. The best accuracy is found among haemocytometers, and the type called improved Neubauer chamber is recommended since its type of pattern is easiest to utilize for sperm counting purposes. The Neubauer chamber is 100 μm deep, which means that a relatively large volume will be assessed after the immotile sperm have sedimented. Shallow chambers (20 μm) which fill by capillary forces do not distribute sperm evenly, causing counting errors [33, 34]. Other chambers with only 10 μm depth contain too low volumes to obtain accurate counts [18]. It would be advantageous with fixed 100 μm deep, disposable chambers, but it is essential that different optics in plastic material does not hinder proper sperm counting [35].

For sperm concentration assessment, duplicate counts with comparisons is essential to avoid random errors in sampling and dilution. At least 200 sperm should be counted in each of the duplicates to reduce influence of random on the final results.

24.3.6 Sperm Morphology

It is no exaggeration to say that human sperm morphology is seen as very controversial. For the interpretation of human sperm morphology assessments, it is thus essential to know the criteria used and the techniques and equipment used for assessment [36]. Although there are recommendations for standardized methods [5, 18], the variability between laboratories is considerable. There are many factors contributing to the global confusion about human sperm morphology. The first is of course the criteria used for morphology classification. In contrast to earlier definitions, where abnormalities were defined from findings in microscopic examination of semen samples, the so called strict criteria (or strict Tygerberg criteria) are based on the studies of morphology of sperm that have passed through cervical mucus, and even binding to the zona pellucida of the oocyte [37]. With the starting point from these definitions of "normal" sperm morphology, several studies have established a relation to both spontaneous pregnancies and pregnancies after ART [38–42].

Another important factor is the technique for preparation of sperm – smearing and fixation of slides, staining, mounting of cover slip – and the optics used for assessing the slides. Many different staining techniques exist, but the Papanicolaou staining adapted especially for sperm is the staining that gives the best overall staining of different sperm parts. Singular stains may be slightly better for certain details, but will then lack quality in most other details. A microscope with poor light or suboptimal optics will not allow the examiner to see details well. A stained and mounted slide with a well prepared smear should look empty to the eye, but show sperm with good contrast under 100× oil immersion bright field optics.

When human sperm morphology is assessed using strict criteria, many men will have less than 10–15% normal sperm. Therefore, information about what errors that occur is of interest.

The recommendation is that morphology abnormalities are recorded in four categories: head, neck or midpiece, tail, and abnormal cytoplasmic residue. An abnormal sperm can have abnormalities in any of these four categories. It is not uncommon with sperm with more than one abnormality. It is possible to calculate an index (Teratozoospermia index) based on these four categories of abnormalities, giving the average number of abnormalities on the abnormal sperm [18]. There are results indicating that multiple abnormalities on sperm is a negative factor for fertility [43, 44].

24.4 Other Investigations

During the last decades, a number of additional methods have been developed and tested to supplement the existing basic semen analyses. The usefulness of some methods is still controversial – both from the diagnostic or prognostic aspect, as well as from technical and practical aspects. Due to the complexity of some techniques and their demand for advanced and expensive equipment, they have not become standard methods [27]. Some other methods also lack standardization, thorough basic evaluations as well as clinical reference limits and the clinical value have therefore not been proven yet.

24.4.1 Semen Biochemistry

Analyses of biochemical markers give important information about the composition of the mixture of secretions the sperm encounters in the laboratory pot. The secretory functions of the epididymis (α-glucosidase), prostate (zinc), and seminal vesicles (fructose) [45] are important for normal sperm function and can give clues to the reasons for abnormal results in basic semen analysis. Among men with fairly normal semen analysis, some can have an abnormal sequence of ejaculation, leading to a decreased protection of the nuclear chromatin. The majority of their sperm are expelled together with mainly the zinc binding seminal vesicular fluid and have lower zinc content in the nuclear chromatin. The only way to discover this anomaly is to investigate a split ejaculate: assess sperm number, motility, and biochemistry in the different ejaculate fractions [46]. Poor sperm motility combined with decreased prostatic secretion should awaken the suspicion of subacute prostatitis and result in a full physical examination to detect any signs of prostatic affection. A semen sample without sperm, low volume, and only normal zinc level indicates lack of Wolffian ducts (epididymis, vas deference, seminal vesicles) and is related to mutation in genes involved in Cystic Fibrosis [47]. The biochemical markers can be assessed with spectrophotometric assays [48–51]. Quality control is equally important for these basically chemical assessments, and schemes for external quality control of semen biochemistry already exist.

24.4.2 White Blood Cells and Bacteria

The significance of white blood cells and bacteria in semen is controversial [52–55]. First, round blood cells in semen must be distinguished from immature germ cells. This is virtually impossible to do in the neat, wet preparation. In stained morphology smears it easier to make the distinction, and methods that more easily are concluded on the day when the sample is collected are based on immunological or biochemical identification of leukocytes or inflammatory cells. Secondly, the interpretation of leukocytes in semen is difficult. Very high presence of inflammatory cells is not so controversial, but the limit for when the concentration of leukocytes indicate a condition that should be treated is not absolute. The recommendation for when specific identification of leukocytes should be done has more or less arbitrarily been set to 1 million cells/mL [5]. However, for the best clinical use of data on suspected inflammatory cells, it is advisable to interpret these together with results from sperm motility assessment, patient history, and results from physical examination [56]. Presence of bacteria in semen is notoriously difficult to prove [57]. Semen is believed to contain factors that counteract bacterial proliferation. Best results of bacterial cultures from semen is in general obtained when (a) semen is collected in a sterile container (b) after hands and penis have been washed [58], and (c) if semen is diluted or cellular component concentrated by centrifugation [59].

24.4.3 Antisperm Antibodies

There are two main types of screening tests for antisperm antibodies on the market: a mixed antiglobulin reaction test (MAR) and an immunobead test. Tests for antibodies of IgG type are most widely used, but also IgA and IgM tests exist. Reports indicate that the presence of antisperm antibodies of IgA type should be most important to explain inability to penetrate human cervical mucus [60]. However, after the introduction of ART procedures that bypass the human cervical mucus, the importance of testing for these antisperm antibodies has been questioned [61]. There is also a problem to interpret the results of the two types of scanning test. For both tests, a possible immunological problem is said to be likely when at least half of motile sperm bind markers. However, the tests can give quite different results for the same sample [18]. One could ask if there is biologically significant binding if not all sperm are covered by antisperm antibodies – or could the test at least in part be due to more unspecific binding? Furthermore, the screening tests are dependent on motile sperm. That means that for example, cytotoxic antisperm antibodies cannot be measured properly with these tests, only those antibodies with no or only marginal effect on sperm motility.

Cytotoxic antisperm antibodies, probably together with complement reactions, cause cell death [62]. Other antisperm antibodies are supposed to cause less damage, for example, only decrease the motility or perhaps hinder proper binding of sperm to different receptors essential for sperm–oocyte interaction and fertilization. It is likely that due to an acute infection, infiltrating immuno-competent cells can settled in the reproductive tract epithelium and function as a source for continuous production of antibodies. It is believed that due to the partially different genetic composition of sperm, the immune system could be able to produce antibodies towards sperm and not only towards invading micro organisms. If such immuno-competent cells in the male reproductive tract produce antibodies that bind to sperm, this could explain also the presence of low levels of antisperm antibodies even in the absence of an acute inflammation.

24.4.4 Hyperactivation

Sperm that have undergone capacitation (changes necessary before fertilization can occur) usually exhibit a change pattern of motility: high frequency, high amplitude tail movements with poor progressive motility. The pattern of motility is best studied with CASA, provided a higher frequency of frames can be recorded than with standard video recording, and with sperm in a 50 μm deep chamber to allow free tail movement. The clinical value of hyperactivation motility has not been established. Hyperactivation is certainly of interest in the study of sperm physiology to understand more about how the sperm change to enable all events around the oocyte to enable fertilization [63].

24.4.5 Zona Binding

The binding of the sperm to the gelatinous Zona Pellucida (ZP) surrounding the oocyte is an essential step for the sperm to be able to continue to fertilization. In laboratory experiments, the zona appears to be an important species specific barrier [64] and it is therefore also likely that disorders in the sperm may impact the capacity to bind to the ZP. Among mammals, the mouse zona has for a long time been used as a model for zona structure and sperm interaction. However, it has been shown that in human, there are four main ZP proteins which opens for a sperm–zona interaction in human that is different from the binding pattern quite extensively studied in mice [65, 66].

In theory, ZP not used for IVF could be used for in vitro testing of human sperm binding to human zona pellucida. Protocols including control sperm are available, but the main obstacle is the very limited access to the biological material as well as relatively complicated immuno cytochemic fluorescence microscopy necessary to perform the test. This is probably the reason why positive small scale experiments have not been followed by full scale clinical evaluations that could have given a better ground for a clinical use of the test [27].

24.4.6 Acrosome Reaction

The acrosome reaction is an essential event for the sperm to be able to get in contact with the oocyte. Techniques based on fluorescent dyes have shown basically three types of cells: intact acrosome, initiated acrosome reaction, and full acrosome reaction with staining only at the equatorial segment. Many different physiological and pharmacological substances have been tested and found possible to interact with the reaction. However, the high costs (demand for extensive training and in general time consuming procedures) in combination with poor standardization and limited prognostic value does not presently motivate its use in clinical settings [27].

24.4.7 Sperm–Oocyte Interaction and Penetration

The testing of sperm fertilizing ability was historically developed from a research test in which zona-free hamster oocytes were used to assess human sperm function [64]. From an ethical point of view, it is reasonable only to let human sperm fertilize human oocytes as part of a treatment procedure, not as a diagnostic test. However, during IVF procedures, the lack of ability of sperm to fertilize any of the available oocytes indicate a possible sperm disorder; if donor oocytes are used in parallel treatments, differentiation between sperm and oocyte factors may be possible. Originally, the hamster egg penetration test was aimed to prognosticate total fertilization failure and thereby avoid useless treatment cycles, but in most centers, the test was too complicated and time consuming – a clinical treatment trial is usually considered much easier, less expensive, and more informative. Furthermore, by the introduction of Intracytoplasmic Sperm Injection (ICSI), the clinics obtained the possibility to by-pass also the fertilization step, which even more reduced the clinical interest in the method. There is some clinical value, but the test is not commonly used presently, not even in research [27].

24.4.8 Reactive Oxygen Species

Chemically active agents like the reactive oxygen species (ROS) are very common in semen and could be the cause of many problems occurring in sperm. Besides white blood cells in semen, also sperm can generate ROS [67]. However, prostatic fluid is rich in antioxidants [68], and sperm expelled together with this fluid and kept out of reach for the ROS rich seminal vesicular fluid ought to have a better situation than sperm stored in the laboratory together with large amounts of seminal vesicular fluid. Under these circumstances, it is likely that ROS can also affect the sperm DNA in a negative way. Also the assessment of ROS requires further laboratory resources beyond basic semen analysis:

at least spectrofluorimetric or spectrophotometric methods. This in combination with absence of clinical evaluations of prognostic value limits is usefulness in clinical practice.

24.4.9 Sperm DNA Integrity

In recent years, a large number of studies related to sperm DNA and possible DNA damages as causes for male factor infertility have been published [69, 70]. An ever increasing number of investigations showing correlations between different fertility parameters and a variety of possible markers for issues in sperm DNA integrity and protection indicate that these assays have important information that cannot be revealed by basic semen analysis. However, before becoming useful for the clinician, methods must be standardized, what is actually measured must be established, and clinically important reference limits must be established [71–73].

24.4.9.1 Sperm Chromatin Structure Assay

This technique originates from studies on the ability of acridine orange to bind to double stranded DNA (intact DNA: green fluorescence) and single stranded DNA (damaged DNA: red flourescence), respectively [74, 75]. In 1980, a study using flow cytometry demonstrated a variability of DNA in sperm from bull, mice and human sperm with regard to ability to resist heat denaturation as revealed by acridine orange [76].

24.4.9.2 Comet Assay: Single Cell DNA Electrophoresis

This assay is based on electrophoretic migration of small DNA fragments, from the experimentally decondensed sperm nucleus, into the surrounding gel. The highly compacted DNA-protamine structural organization must be changed in vitro to liberate DNA from the crystalline like structure. It is not unlikely that these in vitro modifications may induce DNA damages in sperm with poor structural organization [71].

24.4.9.3 TdT-mediated dUTP Nick-End Labelling Assay

This method was originally developed to detect DNA fragmentation as a sign of apoptosis in somatic cells with DNA associated with histones [77]. In spermatozoa, the organization of the nuclear chromatin is completely different, with DNA inactivated and condensed to 1/6 of its original volume. To use essay kits developed for somatic cells to investigate human sperm chromatin, the sperm DNA must be made accessible for the active compounds. Whether these procedures per se can affect the sperm DNA integrity has not been thoroughly elucidated. The principle of the TdT-mediated dUTP Nick-End Labelling (TUNEL) kit is enzymatic incorporation of modified nucleotides (dUTP) on DNA structures ("DNA nicks," representing DNA breaks) that should mainly be found in apoptotic human somatic cell DNA. The fluorescence of the incorporated nucleotides is further enhanced, and the final result of the test is measured as fluorescence from sperm heads [71].

24.4.10 Stem Cells

For men with genetic disorders, hindering an efficient sperm production, a theoretical remedy, could be production of gametes from somatic nuclei. This is still theory and requires substantial advances in the field of stem cell development and culture. The knowledge of how genes are reprogrammed in the fertilized oocyte to allow the development of a germ cell line is very meagre – subtle changes in culturing conditions are now known to favour the development in certain directions but the exact mechanisms are still unknown. Furthermore, essentially nothing is known about how stem cell techniques should be applied to ascertain that no new harm is introduced during the laboratory procedures. Besides these far from trivial problems, it is also essential to learn how to specifically repair the DNA damages resulting in testicular problems.

24.5 Aspects of Evaluation and Identification of Clinical Pathologies

The best use of results from semen analysis is thus to combine these observations with other information about the man and the couple. In cases where no sperm has been observed, the reason could be either a testicular failure or lack of patent communication with the testicles and the outside of the body. In the former cases, blood analysis of the hormone FSH can indicate failure of the testis to respond to gonadotrophins. In the latter case, normal blood hormone levels together with low semen volume and low semen pH indicates agenesis of the entire Wolffian duct system, including the vasa deferentia and the seminal vesicles. There are other possible causes for hinders to sperm transportation. From the middle of the epididymis to the urethra, there is only one single canal for sperm transport on each side. Thus, even minor inflammatory reactions – although bilaterally – are believed to be able to block the sperm transport, and inflammations in the accessory sex glands can also reduce sperm transportation and cause a reduced sperm motility [78].

Severe reduction of sperm number and function due to testicular problems has been reported after systemic inflammatory disease like febrile illness [79]. Due to the long time needed for sperm to develop and mature (approximately 10–12 weeks), effects of episodes of high fever and inflammation may not be revealed until months after the man has recovered. Therefore, a full patient history is essential to interpret low sperm numbers; if a period of high fever or systemic inflammatory process has occurred during the last 6 months, a sample with poor results should be repeated after another 3–6 months. It is a well established fact that high temperature in the testicles is negative for the spermatogenesis. Testicles that have not migrated to their position in the scrotum are, therefore, not expected to be able to produce sperm. Furthermore, there is a significantly increased risk for development of cancer in a non migrated testis and if it is not possible to surgically correct the position of the gonad the recommendation is to remove it before puberty [80]. There are also other possible causes for absence of sperm in the ejaculate, e.g., orchitis (e.g., occurring as a complication of mumps after puberty – quite easy caught by taking a full patient history) and also technical faults. A laboratory with poor procedures can erroneously report cases with very low sperm numbers as lacking sperm completely. A situation when even low numbers of sperm must be detected is controls after vasectomy, due to the risk for recanalization, which has been reported to occur relatively frequently [81]. Poor – or no – sperm motility could be due to genetical disorders or for instance, infections and inflammatory disorders leading to disturbed secretion from the accessory sex glands with secondary sperm motility problems. The immotile cilia syndrome, characterized by completely immotile sperm with straight and stiff tails, is a very rare condition caused by any genetic mutation that disable ciliary movements. In its originally described form, some 50% of men have also situs inversus as well as symtoms from the respiratory tract (Kartagener's syndrome) [82, 83].

An aspect of sperm motility that has not been in focus for a long time is a possible effect of abnormal ejaculation sequence. Since seminal vesicular fluid has a negative influence on sperm motility and survival, it is likely that men where most spermatozoa are expelled together with this fluid instead of prostatic secretion show decreased sperm motility and survival [9]. Calcifications and other changes occurring after chronic inflammations in the prostate are likely to cause disturbances in the normal prostatic secretion [78, 84, 85] and most probably also the sequence of ejaculation. The only way to discover if a man's sequence of ejaculation is abnormal and which portions that may have the most optimal conditions for sperm to use for ART, is to investigate a split ejaculate [9]. The structural appearance of sperm ("morphology") can be affected by genetic and other disorders expressed in the testis, but morphological abnormalities can also be due to factors affecting sperm after the formation in the testis. There are observations also on the sperm morphology indicating that inflammatory processes in the male reproductive tract can have a negative impact on the general sperm morphology [86]. Sperm morphology is usually the most distorted in cases with severe testicular dysfunction. Thus, a combination of low sperm numbers, poor motility, and poor sperm morphology indicate a serious testicular problem. On the other hand, good numbers of sperm and good progressive motility make a possibly decreased sperm morphology less likely to be a sign of seriously decreased fertility. It could even be that a relatively long abstinence time (or low frequency of ejaculation) has increased the number of senescent and possibly deteriorating sperm, all in all a subgroup of sperm less likely to participate in fertilization. Problems during the epididymal transfer and storage are believed to give rise to abnormal cytoplasmic residues in many sperm. Cytoplasmic residues can be found among many sperm after ejaculation, but during the drying procedure involved in slide preparation for morphology assessment most of them disappear – remaining cytoplasmic residues after preparation for sperm morphology is thus indicative for a physiological problem among the sperm, i.e., an inability to adjust to the rapidly changing osmotic pressure during the preparation procedures [87, 88].

Sperm senescence in the laboratory can also influence what is finally assessed in the microscope. It is well established that coiled tails are more likely to be found among sperm that have been kept in semen for several hours, than those smeared within 30 min after ejaculation [18]. Furthermore, recent studies on sperm morphology with Hoffman optics indicate that vacuoles can actually increase with time after ejaculation [89].

References

1. MacLeod J (1950) The male factor in fertility and infertility; an analysis of ejaculate volume in 800 fertile men and in 600 men in infertile marriage. Fertil Steril 1(4):347–361
2. McLachlan RI, Baker HW, Clarke GN et al (2003) Semen analysis: its place in modern reproductive medical practice. Pathology 35(1):25–33
3. Barratt CL (2007) Semen analysis is the cornerstone of investigation for male infertility. Practitioner 251(1690):2, 5–7, 8–10
4. Niederberger C (2003) Responses to semen analysis CART report. J Androl 24(3):329–331
4b. Guzick DS, Overstreet JW, Factor-Litvak P, Brazil CK, Nakajima ST, Coutifaris C, Carson SA, Cisneros P, Steinkampf MP, Hill JA, Xu D, Vogel DL (2001) National Cooperative Reproductive Medicine Network. Sperm morphology, motility, and concentration in fertile and infertile men. N Engl J Med. 345(19):1388–1393.
4c. Jedrzejczak P, Taszarek-Hauke G, Hauke J, Pawelczyk L, Duleba AJ (2008) Prediction of spontaneous conception based on semen parameters Int J Androl. 31(5):499–507
5. World Health Organization (1999) WHO laboratory manual for the examination of human semen and sperm–cervical mucus interactions, 4th edn. Cambridge University Press, Cambridge, UK

6. Francavilla F, Barbonetti A, Necozione S et al (2007) Within-subject variation of seminal parameters in men with infertile marriages. Int J Androl 30(3):174–181
7. Keel BA (2006) Within- and between-subject variation in semen parameters in infertile men and normal semen donors. Fertil Steril 85(1):128–134
8. Stokes-Riner A, Thurston SW, Brazil C et al (2007) One semen sample or 2? Insights from a study of fertile men. J Androl 28(5):638–643
9. Björndahl L, Kvist U (2003) Sequence of ejaculation affects the spermatozoon as a carrier and its message. Reprod biomed online 7(4):440–448
10. MacLeod J, Gold RZ (1951) The male factor in fertility and infertility. III. An analysis of motile activity in the spermatozoa of 1000 fertile men and 1000 men in infertile marriage. Fertil Steril 2(3):187–204
11. Pasqualotto FF, Lucon AM, de Goes PM et al (2005) Semen profile, testicular volume, and hormonal levels in infertile patients with varicoceles compared with fertile men with and without varicoceles. Fertil Steril 83(1):74–77
12. Levitas E, Lunenfeld E, Weiss N et al (2005) Relationship between the duration of sexual abstinence and semen quality: analysis of 9,489 semen samples. Fertil Steril 83(6):1680–1686
13. MacLeod J, Gold RZ (1952) The male factor in fertility and infertility. V. Effect of continence on semen quality. Fertil Steril 3(4):297–315
14. De Jonge C, LaFromboise M, Bosmans E, Ombelet W, Cox A, Nijs M (2004) Influence of the abstinence period on human sperm quality. Fertil Steril 82(1):57–65
15. Pound N, Javed MH, Ruberto C, Shaikh MA, Del Valle AP (2002) Duration of sexual arousal predicts semen parameters for masturbatory ejaculates. Physiol Behav 76(4–5):685–689
16. van Roijen JH, Slob AK, Gianotten WL et al (1996) Sexual arousal and the quality of semen produced by masturbation. Hum Reprod 11(1):147–151
17. Yamamoto Y, Sofikitis N, Mio Y, Miyagawa I (2000) Influence of sexual stimulation on sperm parameters in semen samples collected via masturbation from normozoospermic men or cryptozoospermic men participating in an assisted reproduction programme. Andrologia 32(3):131–138
18. Kvist U, Björndahl L (eds) (2002) Basic semen analysis. Oxford University Press, Oxford, UK
19. Björndahl L, Barratt CL, Fraser LR, Kvist U, Mortimer D (2002) ESHRE basic semen analysis courses 1995–1999: immediate beneficial effects of standardized training. Hum Reprod 17(5):1299–1305
20. Punjabi U, Spiessens C (1998) Basic semen analysis courses: experience in Belgium. In: Ombelet W, Bosmans E, Vandeput H, Vereecken A, Renier M, Hoomans E (eds) Modern ART in the 2000s – andrology in the nineties. The Parthenon Publishing Group, London, UK, pp 107–113
21. Vreeburg JTM, Weber RFA (1998) Basic semen analysis courses: experience in the Netherlands. In: Ombelet W, Bosmans E, Vandeput H, Vereecken A, Renier M, Hoomans E (eds) Modern ART in the 2000s – andrology in the nineties. The Parthenon Publishing Group, London, UK, pp 103–106
22. Mortimer D, Shu MA, Tan R (1986) Standardization and quality control of sperm concentration and sperm motility counts in semen analysis. Hum Reprod 1(5):299–303
23. Cooper TG, Brazil C, Swan SH, Overstreet JW (2007) Ejaculate volume is seriously underestimated when semen is pipetted or decanted into cylinders from the collection vessel. J Androl 28(1):1–4
24. Donnelly ET, Lewis SE, McNally JA, Thompson W (1998) In vitro fertilization and pregnancy rates: the influence of sperm motility and morphology on IVF outcome. Fertil Steril 70(2):305–314
25. Verheyen G, Tournaye H, Staessen C, De Vos A, Vandervorst M, Van Steirteghem A (1999) Controlled comparison of conventional in-vitro fertilization and intracytoplasmic sperm injection in patients with asthenozoospermia. Hum Reprod 14(9):2313–2319
26. Mortimer D (1994) Laboratory standards in routine clinical andrology. Reprod Med Rev 3:97–111
27. ESHRE SIGA (1996) Consensus workshop on advanced diagnostic andrology techniques. ESHRE (European Society of Human Reproduction and Embryology) Andrology Special Interest Group. Hum Reprod 11(7):1463–1479
28. Mortimer D, Aitken RJ, Mortimer ST, Pacey AA (1995) Workshop report: clinical CASA – the quest for consensus. Reprod Fertil Dev 7(4):951–959
29. Björndahl L, Söderlund I, Kvist U (2003) Evaluation of the one-step eosin-nigrosin staining technique for human sperm vitality assessment. Hum Reprod 8(4):813–816
30. Björndahl L, Söderlund I, Johansson S, Mohammadieh M, Pourian MR, Kvist U (2004) Why the WHO recommendations for eosin-nigrosin staining techniques for human sperm vitality assessment must change. J Androl 25(5):671–678
31. Verheyen G, Joris H, Crits K, Nagy Z, Tournaye H, Van Steirteghem A (1997) Comparison of different hypo-osmotic swelling solutions to select viable immotile spermatozoa for potential use in intracytoplasmic sperm injection. Hum Reprod Update 3(3):195–203
32. Mortimer D, Shu MA, Tan R, Mortimer ST (1989) A technical note on diluting semen for the haemocytometric determination of sperm concentration. Hum Reprod 4(2):166–168
33. Douglas-Hamilton DH, Smith NG, Kuster CE, Vermeiden JP, Althouse GC (2005) Capillary-loaded particle fluid dynamics: effect on estimation of sperm concentration. J Androl 26(1):115–122
34. Douglas-Hamilton DH, Smith NG, Kuster CE, Vermeiden JP, Althouse GC (2005) Particle distribution in low-volume capillary-loaded chambers. J Androl 26(1):107–114
35. Kirkman-Brown J, Björndahl L (2008) Evaluation of a disposable plastic Neubauer counting chamber for semen analysis. Fertil Steril 91(2):627–631.
36. Mortimer D, Menkveld R (2001) Sperm morphology assessment – historical perspectives and current opinions. J Androl 22(2):192–205
37. Menkveld R, Franken DR, Kruger TF, Oehninger S, Hodgen GD (1991) Sperm selection capacity of the human zona pellucida. Mol Reprod Dev 30(4):346–352
38. Eggert-Kruse W, Reimann-Andersen J, Rohr G, Pohl S, Tilgen W, Runnebaum B (1995) Clinical relevance of sperm morphology assessment using strict criteria and relationship with sperm–mucus interaction in vivo and in vitro. Fertil Steril 63(3):612–624
39. Enginsu ME, Dumoulin JC, Pieters MH, Bras M, Evers JL, Geraedts JP (1991) Evaluation of human sperm morphology using strict criteria after Diff-Quik staining: correlation of morphology with fertilization in vitro. Hum Reprod 6(6):854–858
40. Menkveld R, Kruger TF (1995) Advantages of strict (Tygerberg) criteria for evaluation of sperm morphology. Int J Androl 18(Suppl 2):36–42
41. Obara H, Shibahara H, Tsunoda H et al (2001) Prediction of unexpectedly poor fertilization and pregnancy outcome using the strict criteria for sperm morphology before and after sperm separation in IVF-ET. Int J Androl 24(2):102–108
42. Vawda AI, Gunby J, Younglai EV (1996) Semen parameters as predictors of in-vitro fertilization: the importance of strict criteria sperm morphology. Hum Reprod 11(7):1445–1450
43. Jouannet P, Ducot B, Feneux D, Spira A (1988) Male factors and the likelihood of pregnancy in infertile couples. I. Study of sperm characteristics. Int J Androl 11(5):379–394
44. Rowe PJ, Comhaire FH, Hargreave TB, Mahmoud AMA (2000) WHO manual for the standardized investigation, diagnosis and management of the infertile male. Cambridge University Press, Cambrige
45. Cooper TG, Jockenhovel F, Nieschlag E (1991) Variations in semen parameters from fathers. Hum Reprod 6(6):859–866
46. Björndahl L, Kjellberg S, Kvist U (1991) Ejaculatory sequence in men with low sperm chromatin-zinc. Int J Androl 14(3):174–178
47. von Eckardstein S, Cooper TG, Rutscha K, Meschede D, Horst J, Nieschlag E (2000) Seminal plasma characteristics as indicators of

cystic fibrosis transmembrane conductance regulator (CFTR) gene mutations in men with obstructive azoospermia. Fertil Steril 73(6):1226–1231
48. Cooper TG, Weidner W, Nieschlag E (1990) The influence of inflammation of the human male genital tract on secretion of the seminal markers alpha-glucosidase, glycerophosphocholine, carnitine, fructose and citric acid. Int J Androl 13(5):329–336
49. Cooper TG, Yeung CH, Nashan D, Jockenhovel F, Nieschlag E (1990) Improvement in the assessment of human epididymal function by the use of inhibitors in the assay of alpha-glucosidase in seminal plasma. Int J Androl 13(4):297–305
50. Karvonen MJ, Malm M (1955) Colorimetric determination of fructose with indol. Scand J Clin Lab Invest 7(4):305–307
51. Johnsen O, Eliasson R (1987) Evaluation of a commercially available kit for the colorimetric determination of zinc in human seminal plasma. Int J Androl 10(2):435–440
52. Lackner J, Schatzl G, Horvath S, Kratzik C, Marberger M (2006) Value of counting white blood cells (WBC) in semen samples to predict the presence of bacteria. Eur urol 49(1):148–152; discussion 52–53
53. Schaeffer AJ, Knauss JS, Landis JR et al (2002) Leukocyte and bacterial counts do not correlate with severity of symptoms in men with chronic prostatitis: the National Institutes of Health Chronic Prostatitis Cohort Study. J Urol 168(3):1048–1053
54. Rodin DM, Larone D, Goldstein M (2003) Relationship between semen cultures, leukospermia, and semen analysis in men undergoing fertility evaluation. Fertil Steril 79(Suppl 3):1555–1558
55. Trum JW, Mol BW, Pannekoek Y et al (1998) Value of detecting leukocytospermia in the diagnosis of genital tract infection in subfertile men. Fertil Steril 70(2):315–319
56. Esfandiari N, Saleh RA, Abdoos M, Rouzrokh A, Nazemian Z (2002) Positive bacterial culture of semen from infertile men with asymptomatic leukocytospermia. Int j fertil women's med 47(6):265–270
57. Damirayakhian M, Jeyendran RS, Land SA (2006) Significance of semen cultures for men with questionable semen quality. Arch Androl 52(4):239–242
58. Kim FY, Goldstein M (1999) Antibacterial skin preparation decreases the incidence of false-positive semen culture results. J Urol 161(3):819–821
59. Villanueva-Diaz CA, Flores-Reyes GA, Beltran-Zuniga M, Echavarria-Sanchez M, Ortiz-Ibarra FJ, Arredondo-Garcia JL (1999) Bacteriospermia and male infertility: a method for increasing the sensitivity of semen culture. Int j fertil women's med 44(4):198–203
60. Hjort T (1999) Antisperm antibodies. Antisperm antibodies and infertility: an unsolvable question? Hum Reprod 14(10):2423–2426
61. Vujisic S, Lepej SZ, Jerkovic L, Emedi I, Sokolic B (2005) Antisperm antibodies in semen, sera and follicular fluids of infertile patients: relation to reproductive outcome after in vitro fertilization. Am J Reprod Immunol 54(1):13–20
62. Francavilla F, Santucci R, Barbonetti A, Francavilla S (2007) Naturally occurring antisperm antibodies in men: interference with fertility and clinical implications. An update. Front Biosci 12:2890–2911
63. Mortimer ST (1997) A critical review of the physiological importance and analysis of sperm movement in mammals. Hum Reprod Update 3(5):403–439
64. Yanagimachi R, Yanagimachi H, Rogers BJ (1976) The use of zona-free animal ova as a test-system for the assessment of the fertilizing capacity of human spermatozoa. Biol Reprod 15(4):471–476
65. Conner SJ, Lefievre L, Hughes DC, Barratt CL (2005) Cracking the egg: increased complexity in the zona pellucida. Hum Reprod 20(5):1148–1152
66. Lefievre L, Conner SJ, Salpekar A et al (2004) Four zona pellucida glycoproteins are expressed in the human. Hum Reprod 19(7): 1580–1586
67. Ebisch IM, Thomas CM, Peters WH, Braat DD, Steegers-Theunissen RP (2007) The importance of folate, zinc and antioxidants in the pathogenesis and prevention of subfertility. Hum Reprod Update 13(2):163–174
68. Yeung CH, Cooper TG, De Geyter M et al (1998) Studies on the origin of redox enzymes in seminal plasma and their relationship with results of in-vitro fertilization. Mol Hum Reprod 4(9):835–839
69. O'Brien J, Zini A (2005) Sperm DNA integrity and male infertility. Urology 65(1):16–22
70. Sakkas D, Moffatt O, Manicardi GC, Mariethoz E, Tarozzi N, Bizzaro D (2002) Nature of DNA damage in ejaculated human spermatozoa and the possible involvement of apoptosis. Biol Reprod 66(4):1061–1067
71. Perreault SD, Aitken RJ, Baker HW et al (2003) Integrating new tests of sperm genetic integrity into semen analysis: breakout group discussion. Adv Exp Med Biol 518:253–268
72. Schlegel PN, Paduch DA (2005) Yet another test of sperm chromatin structure. Fertil Steril 84(4):854–859
73. Zini A, Libman J (2006) Sperm DNA damage: importance in the era of assisted reproduction. Curr Opin Urol 16(6):428–434
74. Gledhill BL, Gledhill MP, Rigler R Jr, Ringertz NR (1966) Atypical changes of deoxyribonucleo-protein during spermiogenesis associated with a case of infertility in the bull. J Reprod fertil 12(3): 575–578
75. Rigler R Jr (1966) Microfluorometric characterization of intracellular nucleic acids and nucleoproteins by acridine orange. Acta Physiol Scand 267:1–122
76. Evenson DP, Darzynkiewicz Z, Melamed MR (1980) Relation of mammalian sperm chromatin heterogeneity to fertility. Science (NY) 210(4474):1131–1133
77. Gorczyca W, Traganos F, Jesionowska H, Darzynkiewicz Z (1993) Presence of DNA strand breaks and increased sensitivity of DNA in situ to denaturation in abnormal human sperm cells: analogy to apoptosis of somatic cells. Exp Cell Res 207(1): 202–205
78. Dohle GR (2003) Inflammatory-associated obstructions of the male reproductive tract. Andrologia 35(5):321–324
79. Carlsen E, Andersson AM, Petersen JH, Skakkebaek NE (2003) History of febrile illness and variation in semen quality. Hum Reprod 18(10):2089–2092
80. Pettersson A, Richiardi L, Nordenskjold A, Kaijser M, Akre O (2007) Age at surgery for undescended testis and risk of testicular cancer. N Engl J Med 356(18):1835–1841
81. Labrecque M, Hays M, Chen-Mok M, Barone MA, Sokal D (2006) Frequency and patterns of early recanalization after vasectomy. BMC urol 6:25
82. Afzelius BA (1976) A human syndrome caused by immotile cilia. Science (NY) 193(4250):317–319
83. Afzelius BA, Stenram U (2006) Prevalence and genetics of immotile-cilia syndrome and left-handedness. Int J Dev Biol 50(6):571–573
84. Christiansen E, Tollefsrud A, Purvis K (1991) Sperm quality in men with chronic abacterial prostatovesiculitis verified by rectal ultrasonography. Urology 38(6):545–549
85. Leib Z, Bartoov B, Eltes F, Servadio C (1994) Reduced semen quality caused by chronic abacterial prostatitis: an enigma or reality? Fertil Steril 61(6):1109–1116
86. Menkveld R, Kruger TF (1998) Sperm morphology and male urogenital infections. Andrologia 30(Suppl 1):49–53
87. Cooper TG, Yeung CH, Fetic S, Sobhani A, Nieschlag E (2004) Cytoplasmic droplets are normal structures of human sperm but are not well preserved by routine procedures for assessing sperm morphology. Hum Reprod 19(10):2283–2288
88. Fetic S, Yeung CH, Sonntag B, Nieschlag E, Cooper TG (2006) Relationship of cytoplasmic droplets to motility, migration in mucus, and volume regulation of human spermatozoa. J Androl 27(2):294–301
89. Peer S, Eltes F, Berkovitz A, Yehuda R, Itsykson P, Bartoov B (2007) Is fine morphology of the human sperm nuclei affected by in vitro incubation at 37°C? Fertil Steril 88(6):1589–1594

Chapter 25
Sperm Capacitation, the Acrosome Reaction, and Fertilization

Peter Sutovsky

Abstract Recent advances in our understanding of fertilization are summarized, highlighting newly discovered molecules implicated in sperm interactions with the epithelia of the female reproductive system (spermadhesins, BSP-proteins), sperm–zona binding (ZP4, ZP3R, IAM38/ZPBP), sperm oolemma binding and fusion (IZUMO, CD9, CD81), oocyte activation (PLCzeta, SRC-family kinases and their activators), and pronuclear development (nucleoplasmin, oocyte-specific histones). Sperm-contributed RNAs and signaling molecules are discussed, and the mechanisms of gamete interactions and antipolyspermy defense during natural fertilization are compared with fertilization events following intracytoplasmic sperm injection (ICSI).

Keywords Sperm • Oocyte • Capacitation • Hyperactivation Sperm reservoir • Fertilization • Zona pellucida • Acrosome • Oolemma • Perinuclear theca • Oocyte activation • Pronucleus • Zygote

25.1 Introduction

25.1.1 A Zygote is an Accident that has Already Happened

To fertilize a single human oocyte, ovulated at one time, hundreds of millions of spermatozoa are initially deployed in the female reproductive system just to be filtered out by barriers such as the cervix and uterotubal junction. Other spermatozoa become prematurely capacitated and destined for death, with only a few dozen spermatozoa reaching the site of fertilization in the oviductal isthmus. These few remaining viable spermatozoa undergo an intricate series of changes (Table 25.1) induced by sperm binding to the egg coat [zona pellucida (ZP)], initiation of acrosomal exocytosis (AE), and sperm–zona penetration and sperm binding to the oocyte plasma membrane, the oolemma. The first spermatozoon to fuse with the oolemma releases signaling molecules from its perinuclear theca that awaken the oocyte cell cycle and activate the antipolyspermy defense. Even at this step, the success of embryo development is not guaranteed as the release of the sperm centriole and its conversion into an active zygotic centrosome is needed for the formation of the sperm aster (not the case in rodents), and the reversal of spermatogenetic protamine–histone exchange has to occur in the sperm nucleus before it is transformed into a male pronucleus. These last few steps also determine the success of assisted human fertilization by intracytoplasmic sperm injection (ICSI), a technique that skips the early steps of fertilization while depositing a single, intact spermatozoon directly in the ooplasm. Changes that occur in gametes during their journey to fertilization are irreversible and may only result in the death of gametes or new life of a zygote.

Given the amount of literature on fertilization and the page limits of this chapter, it is impossible to give details on all pathways involved. Consequently, the purpose of this chapter is to reference the important historical milestones in the discovery of fertilization mechanisms and to highlight the recent progress in studying each of the above steps of fertilization in the order of their natural occurrence. Without losing the focus on human fertilization, an overwhelming majority of fertilization research in mammals has been accomplished by using rodent and large animal models, as reflected by citations in this chapter. Each section is introduced by a brief summary of currently prevailing interpretation of the main event during each described step of fertilization.

25.2 Gamete Transport and Recognition

The current model of gamete transport has been proposed by Suarez [1]. In this paradigm, ejaculated spermatozoa bypass a series of hurdles in the female reproductive system, resulting

P. Sutovsky (✉)
Animal Science and Clinical Obstetrics and Gynecology, Cell and Tissue Research, University of Missouri-Columbia, Columbia, MO, USA
e-mail: sutovskyp@misouri.edu

D.T. Carrell and C.M. Peterson (eds.), *Reproductive Endocrinology and Infertility: Integrating Modern Clinical and Laboratory Practice*, 389
DOI 10.1007/978-1-4419-1436-1_25, © Springer Science+Business Media, LLC 2010

Table 25.1 Steps of mammalian fertilization and their effect on gamete structure

Step and main events	Major change in sperm	Major change in oocyte
Gamete transport		
Sperm deposition Passage through cervix Passage through uterus and uterotubal junction Formation of oviductal sperm reservoir Ovulation Oocyte pickup and descent	Acquisition of progressive motility, removal of some seminal plasma proteins from sperm surface	Ovulation, binding of oviductal glycoproteins to zona/ and/or their accumulation in perivitelline space
Gamete recognition		
Capacitation Hyperactivation Detachment from sperm reservoir Chemotaxis Cumulus penetration	Plasma membrane remodeling; cholesterol efflux; increased plasma membrane fusogenicity; hyaluronidase release	Secretion of chemoatractants (hypothetical); cumulus dispersal
Sperm–egg coat binding and penetration		
Sperm–zona pellucida binding Calcium influx Acrosomal exocytosis Sperm penetration	Acrosomal exocytosis; loss of outer acrosomal membrane and acrosomal matrix; release of acrosin and hyaluronidase	Digestion of fertilization slit; retraction and loss of the cumulus cells
Sperm oolemma fusion and oocyte activation		
Sperm oolemma binding and fusion Release of SOAF Completion of meiosis II Activation of anti-polyspermy defense Sperm incorporation	Membrane fusion, sperm demembranation; localized solubilization of perinuclear theca; excision of head from tail; release of the sperm centriole (non-rodent species only)	Formation of fertilization cone, calcium release from ER; plasma membrane depolarization; release from second meiotic metaphase arrest; cortical granule exocytosis; zona hardening, second polar body extrusion
Pronuclear development		
Reversal of histone–protamine exchange Reconstitution of nuclear envelope PN formation and apposition Minor zygotic genome activation Paternal and maternal DNA replication	Protamine removal from sperm nucleus; male PN formation; remodeling of sperm centriole into zygotic centrosome and sperm aster formation	Chromosome decondensation, female PN formation and apposition with male PN

SOAF sperm borne-oocyte activating factor; *PN* pronucleus

in the culling of spermatozoa from hundreds of millions to a few dozen that actually reach the egg. The posttesticular/postepididymal life of spermatozoa starts with the deposition in the vagina (primates, ruminants, carnivores), cervix (rodents) or uterus (sow, mare). At the time of deposition, spermatozoa acquire progressive motility allowing them to swim through the cervix (where applicable) and move through the uterine cavity. Sperm velocity is reduced at the uterotubal junction or at the isthmus, where they bind to the oviductal epithelium/oviductal sperm reservoir. Here, the capacitation, hyperactivation, and sperm release occur in waves, induced by ovulation. Concomitant to these late events, the ovulated oocyte is picked up by cilia on fimbria and moved down the ampula by oviductal cilia and contractions. Fertilization occurs at the ampullary–isthmic junction.

25.2.1 Sperm Interactions with the Vaginal Environment, Cervix, and Uterus

Sperm transport within the female reproductive system is aided by sperm motility. This activity is suppressed while the spermatozoa are stored in the epididymis by low pH and low lactate content of the epididymal fluid. Upon ejaculation, motility is induced, possibly by sex accessory gland secretions present in semen, causing sperm cAMP elevation through a soluble, sperm-borne adenylate cyclase [2, 3]. The cAMP elevation stimulates the activation of sperm flagellar protein kinase A (PKA) [3] tethered to the flagellar fibrous sheath by the A-kinase anchoring proteins (AKAPs) [4].

In vaginal depositors, such as humans/primates, ruminants, and carnivores, spermatozoa initially encounter the cervix. Spermatozoa are thought to migrate along the mucosal channels formed within the folds of the cervical wall rather than through the lumen [5]. In their subsequent travel, spermatozoa face challenges in the long uterine body and horns as well as leukocytic infiltration of the uterus (sperm phagocytosis is observed). To support sperm transport, uterine muscle contractions increase in the late follicular phase ([6], [7]), and the cervical mucus may serve as a vehicle for sperm and a filter for seminal plasma. Protease inhibitors [8], prostaglandins [9], and immuno suppressors are present in seminal plasma [10, 11]. A protective coating of immunoprotective N-glycans are present on the human sperm surface [12]. The timing of immune response to spermatozoa (leukocyte infiltration of the uterine cavity) is delayed for several hours after coitus in the rodents [13].

25.2.2 Uterotubal Junction, Oviductal Transport, and Oviductal Sperm Reservoir

Similar to the cervical canal, spermatozoa in the uterotubal junction and isthmus encounter mucosal folds filled with viscous fluid [14] that could also present a biochemical barrier to sperm transport. This obstacle is thought to remove spermatozoa with reduced motility as well as the remnants of seminal plasma, particularly in intrauterine depositors [1]. Consequently, bull spermatozoa with gross morphological defects are less likely to reach the fertilization site [15]. Sperm passage through uterotubal junction is aided by waves of contraction stimulated by coitus [16, 17]. Most boar spermatozoa are delivered to uterotubal junction in a sperm-rich fraction (SRF) followed by a postSRF containing increasing amounts of spermadhesin heterodimer PSP I/PSP II. The heterodimer acts as leukocyte chemoattractant both in vivo and in vitro, contributing to the phagocytosis of those spermatozoa not reaching the sperm reservoir [18].

Approximately 9 h is required for bull spermatozoa to reach the fertilization site after copulation, and the spermatozoa can remain sequestered in the site of the oviductal sperm reservoir for over 20 h. [19]. The timing of coitus is not synchronized with the timing of ovulation. It is thus important to extend the lifespan of spermatozoa inside the oviduct so that sufficient numbers are present at the time of ovum descent [20]. First described in the hamster [21], the oviductal sperm reservoir has been studied extensively in large animal models using in situ techniques and cultured oviductal epithelial explants. Human spermatozoa can be stored for an extended period of time in the oviduct, but it has yet to be clearly demonstrated that sperm reservoirs similar to that of the ruminants form at a discrete site within the human oviductal ampula [22]. Specific glycoproteins secreted by the epididymis and/or accessory glands coat the sperm acrosomal surface to mediate the sperm attachment to the epithelial surface of the oviductal sperm reservoir. Among those best characterized accessory gland products are bovine seminal plasma proteins BSP-A1/BSP-A2, BSP-A3, and BSP-30-kDa [23, 24] produced by accessory sex glands. Spermadhesins are another group of multifunctional proteins showing a range of ligand-binding activities implicated in sperm reservoir function [25, 26]. Spermadhesin AQN1 on the acrosomal surface is thought to contribute sperm-oviduct binding by recognizing D-mannose-containing oviductal surface ligands [27–29]. To promote the detachment from the sperm reservoir, capacitation allows the spermatozoa to release the oviductal epithelium-binding proteins by shedding or perhaps by active proteolysis. Partial removal of AQN1 from the acrosomal surface occurs within the first 30 min of capacitation [28]. Beta defensin, an immunoprotective sperm surface protein, appears to be released from the sperm surface during primate sperm detachment from the oviductal epithelial explants in vitro [30].

25.2.3 Sperm Capacitation

Both capacitation [31] and hyperactivation [32] are thought to accelerate or enable sperm detachment from the oviductal sperm reservoir [33, 34]. Spermatozoa are thought to be capacitated and released from the sperm reservoir in waves rather than all at the same time [35], thus extending the window of opportunity during which fertilization-competent spermatozoa can reach the ovulated ovum. The capacitated state is transient and lasts up to 240 min in human spermatozoa [35]. The timing of sperm release is likely controlled by the dominant ovarian follicle and synchronized with ovulation by endocrine secretion of steroids [36]. Plasma membrane remodeling during capacitation gives the spermatozoon the ability to undergo acrosomal exocytosis and to fuse with the oolemma [37]. Capacitation is an irreversible event. Once the spermatozoa commit to it, they either reach the ovum or die. Seminal plasma removal is necessary for capacitation [38]. Decapacitating factors in the seminal plasma are thought to maintain spermatozoa in the decapacitated state during early stages of sperm transport. These include spermine in the ram [39], uteroglobin and transglutaminase in humans [40], and beta1, 4-galactosyltransferase in the mouse [41]. Capaciation may start even before the spermatozoa reach the sperm reservoir, but is completed following their release from this storage pool. Progesterone present in oviductal secretions may be a female factor regulating sperm capacitation and priming of the sperm head membranes for acrosomal exocytosis [38, 42].

A complex and only partially understood network of signaling pathways regulates the sperm-plasma membrane priming during capacitation [38, 43]. The proposed sequence of events [38] starts with the removal of cholesterol causing an influx of Ca^{2+} ions and an increase in intra-acrosomal pH, which results in phospholipid redistribution within the sperm plasma membrane and activation of sperm adenyl cyclase. The resultant cAMP elevation triggers the activation of protein kinase A and a set of tyrosine kinases, leading to tyrosine phosphorylation of multiple substrates [44, 45], including but not limited to ERK1 and ERK2 [46]. Phospholipids within the noncapacitated plasma membrane are asymmetrically distributed over the lipid membrane bilayer, while sterols (including cholesterol) are diffusely distributed. The activation of cAMP-dependent protein phosphorylation leads to scrambling of the phospholipids and formation of distinct membrane microdomains, lipid rafts [43], enriched in cholesterol and saturated fatty acids [47]. Changes in plasma membrane phospholipid content and distribution [48] are followed by cholesterol efflux during capacitation that dramatically reduces cholesterol to phospholipid ratio in sperm plasma membrane [49]. Lipid binding proteins in the oviductal and follicular fluids are the likely natural acceptors of cholesterol during capaciation in vivo [50]. Serum albumin [51] or heparin [52] are commonly used for this purpose during in vitro capacitation. Sodium bicarbonate is also essential in the in vitro capacitation media [45]. Phospholipid remodeling in the plasma membrane is thought to be controlled by ATP-dependent enzymes such as aminophospholipid transporter/translocase [53, 54]. On the basis of their function and affinity to certain phopsholipids, these enzymes have been described as flippases, floppases, and scramblases [43]. Altogether, the changes in sperm plasma membrane, and possibly in the outer acrosomal membrane, result in increased fluidity and fuseability of these sperm membranes [55]. Phosphorylation of multiple plasma membrane substrates on Ser/Thr or Tyr is a prominent event accompanying sperm capacitation [56]. Capacitation induced phosphorylation and membrane remodeling are impaired in the spermatozoa of some infertile, asthenozoospermic men [57].

25.2.4 Sperm Hyperactivation

Sperm hyperactivation could be considered a late event of sperm capacitation although a disconnection between capacitation and hyperactivation is observed under certain experimental conditions in vitro [38, 58]. Hyperactivation is defined by an increased amplitude and frequency of the flagellar movement, and increased lateral displacement of the sperm head, altogether resulting in an increased sperm velocity [32]. Increased motility is thought to promote sperm detachment from the oviductal reservoir and sperm passage through egg vestments. Sperm hyperactivation is calcium-dependent [59], which is consistent with the proposed role of Ca^{2+} ions during sperm capacitation. Sperm Ca^{2+} oscillations coincide with flagellar bend oscillations in the midpiece of the hyperactivated golden hamster spermatozoa [60]. While the events of capacitation mainly affect the architecture of sperm plasma membrane, the events of hyperactivation affect the motile apparatus of the sperm flagellum. One of the Ser-phosphorylated proteins during capacitation/hyperactivation was identified as AKAP3 [61]. AKAP3/AKAP110 is a major protein kinase A-anchoring protein in the sperm tail fibrous sheath [62]. Through sequestration of PKA, AKAP3 and related AKAP-proteins likely modulate a change in sperm motility that is induced during capacitation, causing sperm hyperactivation [63]. Several infertile transgenic mouse models have been described recently, implicating the cAMP-dependent signaling in the regulation of sperm motility [64, 65]. Similarly, the knock-out of GAPDH, one of many glycolytic enzymes residing in the sperm tail fibrous sheath [66], results in the loss of motility [67]. It is not clear, however, whether this is the effect on general motility, or a specific effect on hyperactivated motility.

25.2.5 Ovulation, Oocyte Pickup, and Sperm–Egg Recognition

Ovulation is induced by the preovulatory gonadotropin surge and facilitated by the synergistic action of increased intrafollicular pressure and a timely, localized digestion of the follicular wall by ovarian metaloproteinases and other proteases [68–70]. The expulsed, expanded oocyte cumulus complex is captured by the fimbriae of the oviductal bursa, a process aided by the contractions of mesossalphinx casing, a sweeping movement of fimbria across the ovarian surface [1]. In the absence of the cumulus, the ovulated oocytes fall through without being captured by the fimbria [71]. Oocytes of multiparous animals are picked up in a large mass of oocyte–cumulus complexes, and they travel down the oviduct together ("ovulatory product"). Consequently, the diameter of oviductal lumen in the studied mammalian species matches the size of the whole ovulatory mass of oocytes, not that of a single cumulus-enclosed oocyte [72]. The ovulatory product moves down the oviduct with a back and forth movement pattern aided by smooth muscle concentrations and motility of the cilia on the apical surface of oviductal epithelium [73, 74]. Suarez [1] suggested that the back and forth movement could aid the infiltration of ovarian secretions in the cumulus extracellular matrix. As will be discussed below, the exposure of the oocyte or zona pellucida surface to oviductal secretory proteins plays an important, albeit underappreciated, role in fertilization and antipolyspermy defense.

The molecular mechanism of sperm–egg recognition is poorly understood. In the invertebrates and lower vertebrates, oocyte-secreted proteins are thought to stimulate sperm motility and chemotaxis. Examples include the sperm motility initiation factor SMIF in fish [75], and the SPERACT and RESACT peptides in sea urchin species [76, 77]. Allurin, a sperm attractant protein, has been isolated from Xenopus egg jelly [78]. The mammalian homologs of these proteins, which could be present in the ovarian follicular fluid or directly secreted by the ovulated oocyte, are yet to be identified. Importantly, olfactory receptors have been identified in human spermatozoa [79–81]. In this gamete-recognition pathway, the oocyte-produced substances are thought to stimulate the G-protein coupled cAMP signaling pathway in spermatozoa, leading to a calcium signaling response in the sperm tail midpiece that eventually spreads to the sperm head [82].

Cumulus expansion prior to ovulation produces a large mass with high content of extracellular matrix proteins that may be important for sequestration of growth factors and other molecules influencing sperm and oocyte physiology [83, 84]. The cumulus ECM is particularly rich in hyaluronan [85], a large hydrated polysaccharide capable of binding water and thus greatly increasing its volume. Reciprocally, a hyaluronidase enzymes such as PH20 and HYAL5 are present on the sperm surface, probably to support sperm penetration through cumulus matrix and dispersion of cumulus cells during fertilization [86, 87]. Capacitation appears to be a prerequisite for successful cumulus penetration [88], perhaps because proteolytic processing, unmasking, or release of the sperm hyaluronidases occurs at that time. In contrast, premature acrosomal exocytosis precludes sperm–cumulus penetration [89].

25.3 Sperm–Egg Coat Binding and Acrosomal Exocytosis

According to the prevailing view, the fertilizing mammalian spermatozoa are primed for zona binding and acrosomal exocytosis (AE) during capacitation. Upon contact with the ZP3/ZPC sperm receptor protein (or a complex of ZP3 and another ZP-protein in pigs and humans) on the zona surface, one or more receptors on the sperm plasma membrane trigger signaling pathways that mediate external calcium influx in the acrosome and mobilize the internal calcium within the acrosome. Calcium-dependent signaling then triggers the vesiculation of the outer acrosomal membrane, which remains associated with the spermatozoon in form of an acrosomal shroud or ghost. Acrosomal matrix proteins appear to be released in layers rather than being rejected at once; possibly creating a microenvironment for acrosomal enzymes to act on zona pelluicida underneath the sperm head. Acrosomal exocytosis removes some acrosomal matrix proteins while exposing other proteins on the inner acrosomal membrane (IAM). Propelled by the [altered] motility of the sperm flagellum, the sperm head progresses through ZP, leaving behind a sharply etched fertilization slit. Disagreement still exists as to whether the formation of fertilization slit is caused by proteolytic and glycolytic activities of acrosomal enzymes or by mechanical severing of the zona matrix helped by an oscillating thrust movement of the sperm head.

25.3.1 Oocyte Zona Pellucida Composition and Assembly

The mammalian egg coat, zona pellucida (ZP), has been studied most extensively in the mouse. The murine ZP is composed of three major glycoproteins, ZP1, ZP2, and ZP3 [90]. A fourth major glycoprotein, ZP4, has been reported in humans [91], and more recently in the rat [92] and bonnet monkey [93]. The nomenclature of ZP proteins (Table 25.2) may be confusing as it varies significantly among mammalian species [94–96]. In the mouse, the ZP proteins are heavily glycosylated, expressing both N- and O-linked glycans [97, 98]. Initially studies suggested that O-linked glycans were responsible for initial sperm–egg binding in this model [99]. However, more recent knockout studies confirm that the majority of murine sperm–egg binding is dependent on N-glycosylation [100]. N-linked glycans have also been implicated in initial porcine sperm–egg binding [101]. Evidence for carbohydrate mediated binding has also been presented in the human [102].

The current model of mouse zona structure proposes a parallel fiber organization of ZP2-ZP3 heterodimers cross-linked with ZP1 molecules [103, 104]. Glycosylation of ZP differs between the inner and outer layers of ZP; lectin and antiZP antibody labeling experiments reveal distinct layers and aggregates of ZP proteins with distinct patterns of lectin-binding and saccharide composition [105, 106]. Proteins other than ZP-proteins could contribute to some layers of ZP, particularly in the ovulated oocytes exposed to oviductal secretions [107, 108]. In the mouse, the ZP-proteins are translated and secreted exclusively by the oocyte [109], while ZP-protein mRNAs have been reported in the cumulus cells of other species [110], including nonhuman primates [111] and possibly humans [112]. In lower vertebrates, ZP proteins can even be produced outside of the ovary, e.g., in liver [113]. The function of ZP is believed to be oocyte protection, sperm binding, species specificity of fertilization and anti-polyspermy defense. It may also play an active role in abrogating immune responses directed against this cell type [114]. Murine ZP3 protein is believed to be the primary

Table 25.2 Protein and gene nomenclatures of major ZP components in mammals. Compiled by using information from genome sequence data and nomenclature from Hasegawa and Koyama [94]; Yonezawa et al. [101]; Harris et al. [96]

Nascent MW less glycosylation, and aminoacid residue number	*H. sapiens*	*M. musculus*	*S. scrofa*	*B. taurus*
63–65 kDa, 623 aa	ZP1 *(Zp1/ZpB1)*	ZP1 *(Zp1/ZpB)*	X	X
70–75 kDa, 713–716 aa	ZP2 *(Zp2/ZpA)*	ZP2 *(Zp2/ZpA)*	ZPA/ZP2*(ZpA)*	ZPA/ZP2 *(ZpA)*
43–45 kDa, 421 aa	ZP3[a] *(Zp3/ZpC)*	ZP3[a] *(Zp3/ZpC)*	ZPC/ZP3β[a] *(ZpC)*	ZPC/ZP3B[a] *(ZpC)*
~55 kDa, 532–540 aa	ZP4[a] *(Zp4/ZpB2)*	X	ZPB/ZP3α[a] *(ZpB)*	ZPB/ZP4 *(ZpB)*

[a]Proposed primary sperm receptor

sperm receptor [115]. In humans, both ZP3 and ZP4 proteins bind to the sperm acrosome and induce acrosomal exocytosis in recombinant form [116]. In the pig, a heterodimer complex of ZPB and ZPC proteins is thought to act as primary sperm receptor [117].

25.3.2 Sperm Acrosome Biogenesis and Structure

While often compared to a secretory lysosome because of its content of lysosomal enzymes, the acrosomal biogenesis displays unique features not observed in somatic cell secretory vesicles [118]. Some acrosomal components may already be synthesized during spermatocyte meiosis [119]. However, the acrosome as an organelle only arises during the haploid phase of spermatogenesis from the fusion of proacrosomic membrane vesicles released from the Golgi in step 1–2 round spermatids (reviewed in [120, 121]). Deletion of the gene encoding for Golgi-associated GOPC protein prevents acrosomal biogenesis and elicits a phenotype similar to human globozoospermia in the GPC –/– mice [122]. The proacrosomic vesicles are coated with perinucelar theca (PT) proteins before they reach the surface of the spermatid nucleus [123, 124]. Deletion of the gene encoding for a proacrosomic-vesicle coating membrane-fusion protein HRB/RAB disrupts acrosomal biogenesis in the mouse [125]. The proacrosomic vesicles settle on the apical spermatid nucleus and fuse into a large acrosomal granule, lay down the subacrosomal PT-layer, and start stretching distally to form the acrosomal cap (step 4–8 in mouse spermiogenesis). The subacrosomal PT and the inner acrosomal membrane become closely adjacent and the mutation of at least one IAM gene *(ZPBP2)* disrupts acrosomal biogenesis in the mouse [126]. An alternative model of acrosomal biogenesis proposes that the assembly of subacrosomal cytoskeletal plate, the acroplaxome precedes the tethering of the proacrosomic vesicles to the apex of the spermatid nucleus [127]. The fully differentiated acrosome is delimited by the inner acrosomal membrane (IAM) and outer acrosomal membrane (OAM), together concealing the acrosomal matrix. The subacrosomal PT fuses with the inner face of IAM, while the equatorial segment leaf of PT partially covers the outer distal face of OAM and may even extend proximally to separate the OAM from the overlying plasma membrane [128]. Besides acrosin, the acrosomal matrix contains a number of proteolytic enzymes, proteinases and glycohydrolases, that have been implicated in different steps of sperm passage through egg vestments [129].

25.3.3 Sperm–Zona Binding

Just like many other steps of fertilization, the sperm–zona binding step is not fully understood. Two distinct steps are recognized by some investigators during mouse sperm–zona adhesion: primary binding to ZP3 and secondary binding to ZP2 [130]. Sperm–ZP binding is thought to involve multiple sperm surface receptors [131]. It is still being debated whether the primary adhesion is an absolute requirement for fertilization since, at least in the guinea pig, the acrosome-reacted spermatozoa can adhere to ZP [132]. The majority of biochemical data obtained by using solubilized zona proteins implicate the O-linked and N-linked oligosaccharide residues of ZP3 in primary sperm binding and induction of acrosomal exocytosis [97, 99, 101, 102]. It has been estimated that 75–80% of sperm–ZP adhesion depends on sperm–ZP carbohydrate interaction and only the remaining portion is dependent on protein–protein interaction [114, 133]. The ZP2 protein has been proposed as a secondary mouse sperm receptor, destined to sustain sperm–zona adhesion after acrosomal exocytosis [130]. Genetic ablation of *Zp2* and *Zp3* genes in the mouse causes infertility due to a failure of zona assembly, and targeted mutation of the *Zp1* gene results in early embryo loss and small litter sizes [134–137]. The knock-in of human *Zp3* and *Zp2* gene in the *Zp3 –/– Zp2 –/–* double-mutant mouse restored fertility. Unexpectedly, such hybrid zonae were unable to bind human spermatozoa [138, 139]. A likely explanation is that the ZP2 and ZP3 proteins translated from the inserted human genes were glycosylated or otherwise postranslationally modified by the mouse ova in a murine-like pattern, allowing for the binding of mouse, but not of the human, spermatozoa. In fact, the hybrid zonae of the *huZp3* expressing mice and the zonae of wild type mice share a set of identical O-glycans [98]. Baculovirus expressed, but not yeast expressed, human ZPB2 and ZPC (ZP4 and ZP3, respectively) proteins were able to bind to the human sperm acrosome and induce acrosomal exocytosis [140]. Only the baculovirus expressed ZP proteins were properly glycosylated. Contrary to biochemical evidence, studies of transgenic mice deficient in certain glycosyltransferases demonstrated that female mutant mice lacking certain types of ZP3-borne glycans, such as core-1-derived O-glycans and complex and hybrid N-glycans, are fertilization-competent [141]. However, these double knockout mice display extremely low fertility. It is to be determined whether other ZP3-borne glycans compensate for the lack of the above glycans-types, or if other ZP-proteins contribute to sperm–ZP binding in the mouse. Alternatively, it is to be considered that some of the competitive inhibition studies with isolated glycans designed to mimic the ZP3-borne glycans could have caused reduced sperm–ZP interaction by binding to glycans expressed on the sperm surface that are not directly involved in sperm–zona binding. During natural fertilization, the oviductal glycoproteins picked up by zona or accumulated in the perivitelline space during oocyte descent to oviductal ampula could affect sperm–zona binding [108]. Sperm zona-interactions are thought to be responsible for species specificity of fertilization during the initial binding as well as during sperm penetration through vitelline coat, although some promiscuity may exist [142].

25.3.4 Sperm Acrosomal Proteins Implicated in Sperm–Zona Interactions

While the involvement of ZP3 (or ZPB–ZPC complex in pig) in sperm–zona binding is well supported experimentally, there is more confusion with regard to which sperm surface proteins bind to these ZP-proteins. Reviewing all of the proposed candidate ZP-receptor molecules [143, 144] is beyond the scope of this chapter, so the focus is on a few candidates who have been thoroughly examined.

SP56 (AM67/ZP3receptor/ZP3R)[145] is an acrosomal matrix protein implicated in sperm–ZP3 binding [146]. Mice immunized with recombinant SP56/ZP3R had significantly smaller litter sizes than control mice [147]. SP56/ZP3R is related to complement component 4-binding proteins, a family of surface-bound complement regulatory glycoproteins involved in cell adhesion.

β1,4-galactosyl transferase (GalT) is expressed on the sperm acrosomal surface and is believed to bind terminal galactose residues of the oligosaccharide chains of mouse ZP3 [144] . Male GalT –/– mice are fertile, but show a somewhat reduced sperm–ZP binding and acrosomal exocytosis during in vitro fertilization [148]. However, sperm from GalT –/– mice displays greatly increased binding to eggs in vitro when compared with sperm from wild type male mice. By contrast, mice overexpressing GalT on the sperm surface undergo precocious acrosomal exocytosis [149]. Recent genetic studies suggest that neither terminal galactose nor the *N*-acetylglucosamine of the O-linked zona pellucida glycoproteins are necessary for fertilization in the mouse [141], confirming that sperm GalT is not obligatory for murine fertilization. However, such knockout mice are so subfertile that it is very likely that glycosylation of the ZP is obligatory for the survival of this species.

Zonadhesin (ZAN) is a transmembrane-receptor protein carrying five von Willenbrand factor D-domains. Zonadhesin may be the only sperm protein identified so far to bind zona pellucida in a species-specific manner [150]. The evolution of the zonadhesin precursor gene, driven by positive selection, could be a tool of speciation [151]. It has been suggested that zonadhesin only becomes exposed on the acrosomal surface after acrosomal exocytosis and thus may serve to tether the acrosomal shroud to the ZP [152]. An alternative view is that zonadhesin precursor protein is processed and transferred to posterior acrosome to mediate sperm–ZP binding during initial stages of exocytosis [153].

Spermadhesins PSP-I/PSP-II, AQN1, AQN3, and AWN [154] are secreted in the seminal plasma by accessory sex glands of boar reproductive systems and become absorbed onto the acrosomal surface after ejaculation. AWN is the only known spermadhesin also expressed in the female reproductive system [154]. Isolated spermadhesins and anti-spermadhesin antibodies inhibit in vitro sperm–zona binding and penetration in the pig [155–159]. Spermadhesin AQN1 may also be involved in sperm interaction with the oviductal epithelium and in the formation of the oviductal sperm reservoir [27–29]. Spermadhesins interact with another secretory protein of seminal plasma, the sperm-associated acrosin-inhibitor (SAAI) [160, 161]. Formation of the complex between SAAI and spermadhesins was detected both by gel chromatography [162] and by Western blotting [163]. It is thought that SAAI protects the zona pellucida binding sites of spermadhesins on the sperm surface against proteolytic degradation from the moment of ejaculation, until the sperm–zona binding [161].

Arylsulfatase A (ASA) has a cumulus matrix-dispersing activity because of its affinity toward chondroitin sulfate B [164]. The ASA was not found to act on ZP-associated sulfated glycans [165], but the purified ASA inhibits sperm–zona binding and induces acrosomal exocytosis in the mouse [166], presumably through its binding to sperm surface sulfoglycolipids. The ASA-deficient transgenic male mice are fertile [167] but display delayed dispersion of cumulus oophorus during fertilization [164].

P34H: Some infertile men appear to be deficient in epididymal sperm binding protein P34H [168], which has been implicated in sperm–zona binding [169]. P34H is a member of the short chain dehydrogenase/reductase family [170]. The mechanism of P34H interaction with zona pellucida is yet to be established.

Proacrosin/acrosin is a major acrosomal protease [171, 172] with mannose-binding properties [173]. Proacrosin binds to recombinant human ZP2/ZPA with high affinity [174]. Proacrosin null mice are fertile but exhibit a delayed sperm–zona penetration [175]. A fraction of proacrosin remains associated with sperm IAM after acrosomal exocytosis [176, 177]. Proacrosin is thought to bind to zona pellucida glycoproteins through a sulfate-recognition mechanism [178].

SP38/IAM38/ZPBP1&2: Secondary sperm–ZP binding is thought to sustain the adhesion of the spermatozoa to ZP after acrosomal exocytosis. Most likely receptor proteins for this interaction would be found on the inner acrosomal membrane (IAM), which remains patent after acrosomal exocytosis [176]. Antibodies against the IAM protein SP38/IAM38 inhibit sperm ZP-binding and fertilization in the pig [179], and the protein has been shown to bind to ZP [180, 181]. Mutant mice lacking the *ZPBP2* gene, encoding one of the two ZPBP isoforms are subfertile because of their reduced ability to penetrate zona pellucida, and mice lacking the other gene, *ZPBP1,* are completely infertile because of a failure to form a normal acrosome during spermiogenesis [126].

PH20/SPAM1: The GPI-linked guinea pig sperm hyaluronidase PH20 [182] has been implicated in secondary sperm–zona binding [183]. Anti-PH20 antibodies block sperm–ZP binding. Immunization with PH20 elicited a reversible contraceptive effect in male guinea pigs [184]. However, this effect could have been due to an autoimmune disease/orchitis rather than to a specific block of sperm–zona interaction [185]. Mice immunized with PH20 protein remained fertile despite developing high specific antibody titers [186]. The PH20/SPAM1-deficient mice are fertile and exhibit sperm hyaluronidase activity [187], supporting the existence of additional sperm-borne hyaluronidases. A novel testis-specific, cell-surface anchored hyaluronidase, HYAL5, has been described recently [188].

25.3.5 Acrosomal Exocytosis (AE)

The signaling cascade of acrosomal exocytosis is triggered by sperm binding to their complementary receptor on the zona pellucida [189, 190], or it can occur spontaneously in some spermatozoa exposed to a variety of experimental conditions [108]. This event, most likely carbohydrate dependent for the most part, induces the influx of external Ca^{2+} ions in the acrosome [191], as well as the release of intracellular calcium from the intraacrosomal store [192, 193]. Calcium influx is an early event of AE. Following Ca^{2+} influx and concomitant increase in intraacrosomal pH, the first morphologically discernible step of acrosomal exocytosis (AE) is the acrosomal membrane vesiculation [194]. Acrosomal membrane vesiculation distinguishes true acrosomal exocytosis from acrosomal damage that may also result in the loss of OAM and acrosomal matrix. Formation of acrosomal vesicles could occur either by the fusion of OAM with plasma membrane, resulting in the formation of hybrid OAM-plasma membrane vesicles [108], or by the vesiculation of OAM alone [195] while the plasma membrane is still intact or removed before the OAM vesiculation. The SNARE hypothesis proteins, involved in membrane vesicle fusion in neurons, are present in the OAM [196] and may be contributing to its vesiculation during AE [197]. In either case, the rupture of acrosomal membranes exposes the acrosomal matrix to the ZP. Following acrosomal exocytosis, the vesiculated acrosomal shroud or ghost remains associated with the sperm tail or with zona pellucida near the exocytosed spermatozoon. It is possible that the shroud, surrounding the sperm head during intial stages of sperm–zona penetration, may provide an environment rich in proteases and ATP necessary for the digestion of the outer ZP-layers during sperm–zona penetration [108].

Two basic models of acrosomal exocytosis have been proposed: The analog model and the binary model [198]. The older, binary model assumes that the acrosome is either intact (ON/1) or reacted (OFF/2) and there are no intermediates. Should any intermediates exist, they would be short-lived, and the spontaneous AR is not assumed to be physiological. In this paradigm, the sperm–ZP interactions are governed by acrosomal status, and the intact acrosome is needed for sperm–ZP binding and penetration. This model is not supported by studies showing that the acrosome-reacted spermatozoa do bind to zona by their retained acrosomal shroud or acrosomal matrix proteins on the IAM [e.g., [199, 200]]. The analog concept of acrosomal exocytosis, proposed by Gerton [198], assumes the existence of transitional intermediates of AE. In this model, capacitation promotes AE, and sperm–ZP binding accelerates it. Spontaneous AE is a physiological event according to this hypothesis; it may be slower yet mechanistically similar to ZP-induced AE. Importantly, the acrosomal matrix in this scenario is not dispersed at once, but layer after layer [201, 202]. Differential release of enzymes from the acrosome was also observed during AE in the guinea pig [203].

Signaling pathways implicated in the induction of acrosomal exocytosis are too numerous to list here [129, 204]. These pathways, triggered by distinct receptors on the sperm acrosomal surface may act in concert under physiological conditions, or one pathway could prevail when the spermatozoa are stimulated experimentally to induce acrosomal exocytosis. The receptors involved in zona-binding and AE-induction could be clustered within distinct plasma membrane domains that also sequester the downstream elements of corresponding signaling pathways. As a consequence of cholesterol removal from plasma membrane during capacitation, lipid rafts form on the plasma membrane overlying the acrosome [43, 205]. Lipid rafts are unique membrane domains with a high density of membrane receptors and underlying signaling molecules, that are likely involved in cell signaling during acrosomal exocytosis [43, 206].

Some of the examined signaling pathways may contribute to acrosomal membrane priming during capacitiation rather than to the actual induction of AE during sperm–zona binding [204]. The opening of the ion channels responsible for the sustained calcium influx may be triggered by sperm receptor binding to a G-protein coupled receptor on the acrosomal surface [207] or by a plasma membrane associated phosphatidyl-inositol phosphate (PIP2) [208]. Transient receptor potential (TRP) proteins are the likely components of the ion channels transporting Ca^{2+} across the acrosomal membranes [209]. Acrosomal surface galactosyl-transferase, previously implicated in the process of sperm zona binding, activates pertussis toxin sensitive G-protein signaling cascade leading to AE [210]. Besides Ca^{2+} ions, the second messenger cAMP has been implicated in the induction of AE which is known to trigger the activation of the cAMP-dependent protein kinase PKA [211]. Tyrosine and Ser/Thr phosphorylation of several distinct substrates accompany acrosomal exocytosis [212–214]. Some studies found that tyrosine kinase inhibitors prevent the ZP-induced or progesterone-induced acrosomal exocytosis in human spermatozoa, most likely at a point downstream of calcium signaling [215]. Phospholipases (PLC) are enzymes capable of hydrolyzing phosphatidyl-inositol-4,5-bisphosphate (PIP2) into two distinct second messenger molecules, inositol 1,4,5-triphosphate (IP3) and diacylglycerol. Mutliple PLCs are present in the acrosome [216] and calcium transients/oscillations have been recorded during mammalian AE [60]. Spermatozoa of male mice deficient in phopholipase PLCdelta4 are unable to undergo AE [217]. The acrosome reaction can be triggered by progesterone [218] via progesterone receptors present on the plasma membrane [219]. At present, it is not clear which of the early mentioned pathways are physiologically relevant. A common endpoint of calcium signaling during AE may be the severing of microfilament barrier that separates OAM from the inner face of plasma membrane [220]. This event allows for the fusion of OAM with plasma membrane, resulting in acrosomal membrane vesiculation. For the sake of brevity, Fig. 25.1 shows the simplified signaling cascade during AE, as interpreted earlier [221]. The AE induced in the capacitated human spermatozoa by nascent or recombinant ZP proteins can be blocked by the inhibitors of the 26 S proteasome [222, 223], a multisubunit protease specific to ubiquitinated protein substrates. This proteasome inhibitor-sensitive step of AE occurs upstream of calcium influx, as the calcium ionophore-induced AE is not sensitive to proteasomal inhibitors [222, 223]. The occurrence of proteasomal proteolysis during AE suggests that some acrosomal proteins are postranslationally modified and proteolytically processed during AE. We are currently investigating the acrosomal proteins that could be degraded by the resident proteasomes during AE.

25.3.6 Sperm–Zona Penetration

Sperm motility shifts from progressive to nonprogressive upon sperm–zona binding, as shown by the incubation of human sperm with recombinant human ZP-proteins [224]. Both nonenzymatic egg coat lysis and proteolytic mechanism of egg coat penetration have been described in the invertebrates. In abalone, a sperm-borne vitteline envelope (VE) lysin breaks down the VERL glycoprotein (viteline envelope receptor for lysin) by outcompeting the VERL molecules for binding within the VERL fibers of VE. This mechanism is highly species-specific. [225]. Mammalian fertilization biologists remain divided over the issue of mechanical versus enzymatic egg coat penetration. There is no doubt that sperm motility is required for sperm passage through ZP [226]. Videorecordings of the fertilizing spermatozoa document a sweeping movement of the sperm head interpreted as cutting through ZP [227]. However, biophysical studies do not support the mechanical hypothesis of sperm–ZP penetration because the calculated forces generated by sperm motility were found to be insufficient to push the spermatozoon through the ZP by purely mechanical means [228, 229].

Duve first proposed that sperm–zona penetration is assisted by hydrolases released from the acrosome. Acrosin was a popular candidate for mammalian egg coat lysin until the male acrosin mutant mice proved to be fertile, albeit with somewhat delayed AE [175]. This observation revived the mechanical hypothesis of sperm–ZP penetration, inspiring reinterpretation of the earlier studies [227, 230]. Antibodies against sperm acrosomal proteins acrin 1 (MN7) and acrin 2 (MC41) inhibit early stages of sperm–ZP penetration in the mouse, without affecting sperm–ZP binding and AE [231]. Testis specific proteases TESP1, TESP2 and TESP5 are present in the mouse sperm acrosome, and at least TESP5 appears to be enriched in the acrosomal membrane lipid rafts [232, 233].

The ubiquitin proteasome pathway [234] has been implicated in various steps of fertilization, employing the ATP-dependent covalent ligation of multiubiquitin chains to proteolytic substrates followed by proteolytic degradation by a multisubunit, ubiquitin-specific protease, the 26 S proteasome

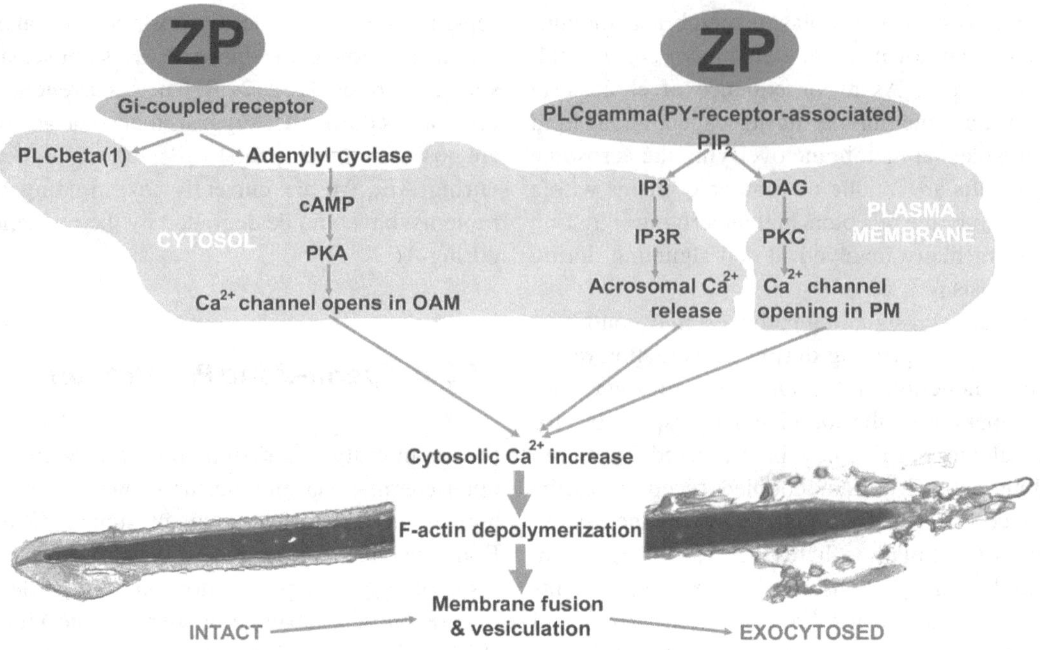

Fig. 25.1 Signaling pathways of acrosomal exocytosis, as proposed by Breitbart [221]. Gi-coupled receptor pathway: Binding of sperm plasma membrane to ZPC/ZP3 activates adenylyl cyclase which causes increased production of second messenger cyclic adenosine-monophosphate (cAMP), which activates protein kinase A (PKA), stimulating the phopshorylation and opening of Ca^{2+} channels in the outer acrosomal membrane (OAM). PLCgamma/phosphotyrosine receptor pathway: Binding of ZPC/ZP3 to a tyrosine kinase receptor (PY-receptor) activates the PY receptor-associated phospholipase C gamma (PLCgamma), which hydrolyses phopshatidyl-inositol diphosphate (PIP2) into two second messenger products: inositol-1,4,5-triphosphate (IP3) that is released in the cytosol and diacyl-glycerol (DAG) that remains associated with plasma membrane. IP3 causes acrosomal Ca^{2+} release when it binds to the intraacrosomal IP3-receptors (IP3R). DAG causes external Ca^{2+} influx when it activates protein kinase C (PKC) which causes phosphorylation and opening on Ca^{2+} channel in plasma membrane. At the same time, DAG increases the fuseability of plasma membrane. Downstream effects of cytoslic calcium release: Altogether, external Ca^{2+} influx and intracarosomal Ca^{2+} mobilization cause an increase in sperm cytosolic Ca^{2+} ion-content which stimulates microfilament severing proteins to break down filamentous actin (F-actin) barrier that separates the OAM from sperm plasma membrane. Consequently, the outer face of OAM and the inner face of the plasma membrane bind and fuse together, giving rise to acrosomal membrane vesicles. Adapted from [221]

[235, 236]. In ascidians and echinoderms, proteasomes are present in the sperm head and the sperm receptor on viteline envelope, a homologue of the mouse ZP3 protein is ubiquitinated [237–240]. Since ATP is required for some, but not all, steps of proteasome-substrate recognition, depletion of extracellular ATP from the surface of sea urchin sperm by apyrase added in the sea water surrounding the sea urchin eggs inhibits fertilization in a dose-dependent manner [241]. The ubiquitinated sperm receptor on VE, HrVC70, is the ascidian homologue of murine ZP3 [240]. Evidence from several laboratories demonstrates the presence of proteolytically active proteasomes in the mammalian and human sperm acrosome [222, 242–244], and ubiquitinated proteins have been detected in pig zona pellucida [244]. As mentioned earlier, an early step in ZP-induced human sperm AE is sensitive to proteasomal inhibitors [222, 245], suggesting that proteasomal proteolysis has multiple functions during fertilization. At low concentrations, proteasomal inhibitors and antiproteasome antibodies are permissive to sperm–ZP binding and AE, but efficiently block the sperm–ZP penetration during porcine IVF [244]. It is now being investigated whether the sperm receptors on mammalian ZP are ubiquitinated and whether they are degraded by the sperm-associated proteasomes during fertilization.

25.4 Sperm–Oolemma Binding, Sperm Incorporation and Oocyte Activation

Sperm–oolemma fusion is mediated by tetraspanins CD9 and CD81 on the oolemma and by the tetraspanin-binding IZUMO protein on sperm plasmalemma. The incorporation of the spermatozoon in the ooplasm is aided by microfilaments of the oocyte cortex and not by motility of the sperm flagellum that ceases upon sperm–oolemma fusion. Oocyte activation is induced by the sperm borne oocyte activating factor(s) (**SOAF**) amalgamated in the sperm perinulcear theca, for which the current hottest candidate is phospholipase C-zeta.

25.4.1 Sperm–Oolemma Binding and Fusion

The first serious candidate ligand-receptor duo implicated in sperm–oolemma binding was a disintegrin, ADAM disintegrin-metaloproteinase family member, fertilin beta (PH30/ADAM2) on the sperm plasmalemma, binding to integrin alpha6 beta1 on the oolemma [246, 247]. Later, cyritestin (ADAM3), a fertilin-related sperm ADAM-family protein, was added to the list [248]. Although integrins likely contribute to proper oolemma architecture conducive to fertilization, they are not indispensable for either sperm oolemma binding or fusion [249]. Spermatozoa of mutant mice lacking fertilin beta and cyritestin fail to adhere to zona pellucida and oolemma [250], possibly because the deletions have a profound effect on sperm plasma membrane composition and fusability as well as on sperm ability to migrate through the oviduct [251].

More recently, the tetraspanins CD9 and CD81 on the oolema has been found to be essential for sperm oolemma fusion in the mouse [252–255]. The CD9-CD81 double knockout mice are completely infertile [256]. It was predicted that the protein would interact with a sperm protein from the immunoglobulin superfamily. One such protein, IZUMO, named after a fertility shrine in Japan, has indeed been found to be essential for sperm–oolemma fusion [257]. *Izumo* –/– mouse males are completely infertile due to a failure to fuse with oolemma, after normal sperm–zona penetration. IZUMO is not absent from spermatozoa of infertile men, suggesting that its lack is not a contributor to human male infertility [258]. Immunization of female mice with an IZUMO-based contraceptive vaccine caused significant reduction in fertility [259].

The cysteine-rich secretory proteins (CRISP)[260], including epididymal protein DE (CRISP1) and testicular protein TXP1 (CRISP2), have been implicated in sperm–oolemma fusion [261]. Both male and female mice immunized with recombinant CRISP1 displayed reduced fertility [262]. This result could be due to an effect on sperm–oolemma fusion, but also due to the block of CRISP1-dependent tyrosine kinase signaling during sperm capacitation [263]. While CRISP family has been initially deemed to be uniquely expressed in the male reproductive system, allurin, a sperm-atracting chemoatractant protein, is expressed by the *Xenopus* egg [78].

25.4.2 Sperm Incorporation

While sperm–zona penetration requires sperm flagellar motility, the beating of the flagellum stops once the sperm head reaches the perivitelline space and binds to the oolemma [264]. Consequently, it is not thought that sperm motility is required for sperm–oolema fusion, or for sperm incorporation in the ooplasm. Acrosomal exocytosis primes the sperm plasma membrane for fusion with oolemma, by exposing/processing the receptor molecules on the equatorial segment part of the acrosome such as IZUMO or equatorin [257, 265]. Acrosome-intact spermatozoa can bind to oolema, but are incapable of fusion and incorporation [108]. Actin-microfilament rich oocyte microvilli bind to equatorial segment of the perivitelline spermatozoa prior to sperm incorporation [108, 266]. Disruption of cortical actin filaments during bovine fertilization efficiently prevents sperm incorporation without preventing the localized solubilization of the perinuclear theca in the area of contact between sperm plasmalemma and oolemma [128, 267, 268]. Consequently, such oocytes are activated but contain only the female pronucleus. The involvement of actin microfilaments in sperm incorporation is even more obvious in rodents, where a large fertilization cone is formed around the fertilizing spermatozoon composed largely of actin microfilaments [269]. The microfilament stabilizing drug, jasplakinoide, inhibits both the formation of mouse fertilization cone (if applied during fertilization) and its disassembly (if applied after fertilization) [270]. Microfilament cytoskeleton helps in the organization of various oolemma receptors and in the propagation of oolemma-dependent antipolyspermy defense [271].

25.4.3 Solubilization of Sperm Perinuclear Theca and the Release of SOAF

The perinuclear theca (PT) is an important, though often underemphasized, accessory structure of the sperm head. It is a high density coat-like structure containing amalgamated cytosolic proteins, histones, cytoskeleletal and signaling proteins [272, 273]. Molecular composition of the PT varies according to the segment of the sperm head covered, which can be divided into a subacrosomal layer (SAL), outer periacrosomal layer (OPL) overlying the equatorial segment (ES), and postacrosomal sheath (PAS) [128]. These three distinct segments of PT play differing roles during spermiogenesis. The postacrosomal sheath is the most likely player during fertilization as it harbors factors involved in oocyte activation (Fig. 25.2a–d) [128, 274, 275]. To discuss oocyte activation and the role of PT in it, this chapter adopts the acronym SOAF (sperm borne oocyte activating factor) [275, 276], which, in the author's opinion, adequately describes the properties of signaling molecules harbored in postacrosomal PT. Initial oocyte fusion between a small stretch of sperm postacrosomal sheath and oolemma transfers sufficient amount of SOAF to activate an oocyte [267]. The oocyte's capacity to reduce disulfide bonds in the sperm PT and the proteolytic activity of the ooplasm facilitate SOAF release during fertilization or after ICSI [277]. Before we discuss

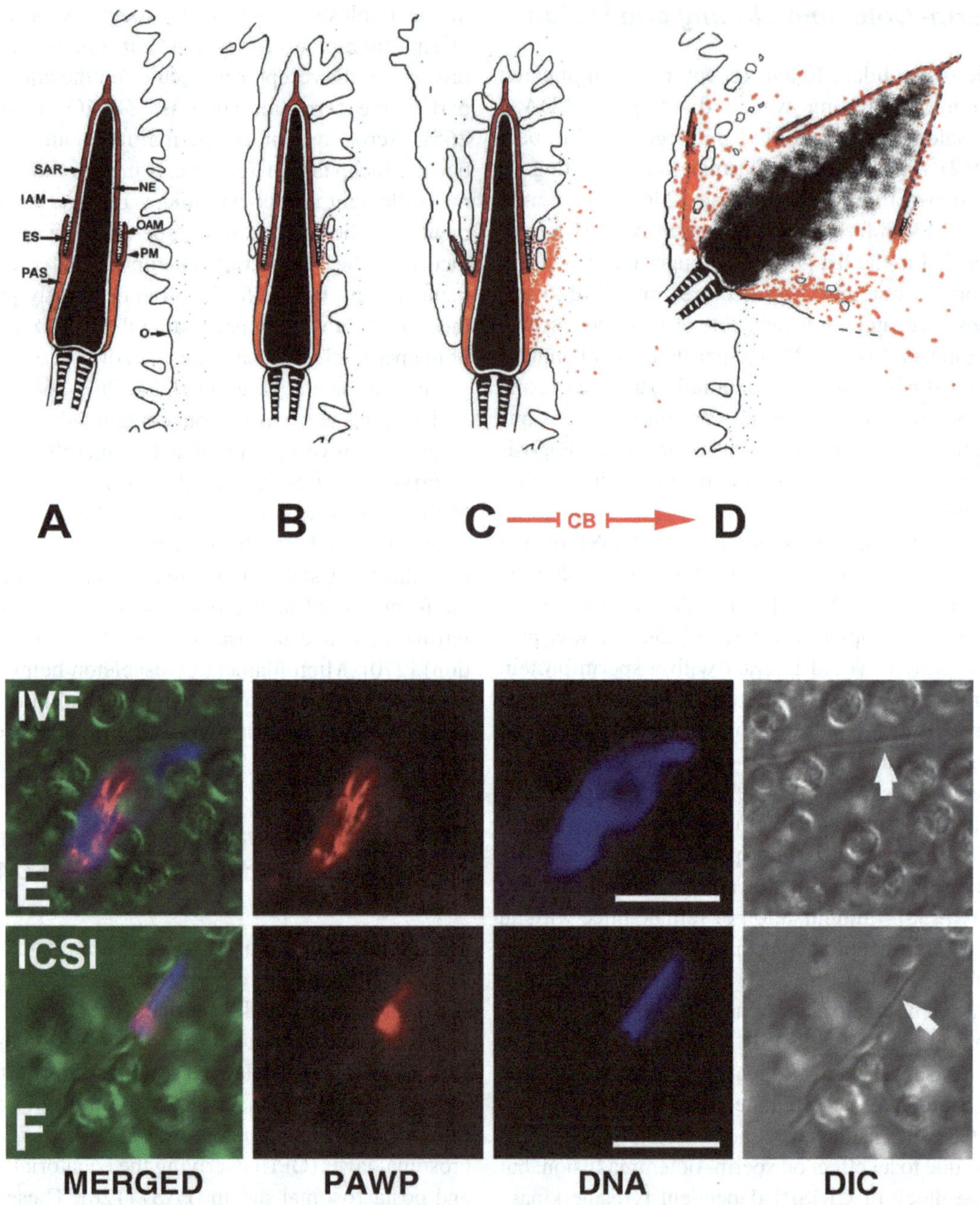

Fig. 25.2 Transmission of the sperm PT-borne, oocyte activating factors (SOAF) into ooplasm at fertilization. (**a–e**) Schematic interpretation of the release of SOAF into oocyte cytoplasm. (**a**) Acrosome reaction exposes the inner acrosomal membrane (IAM), and the subacrosomal PT layer (SAR), equatorial segment (ES), and the postacrosomal sheath (PAS) regions of the sperm head are accessible to the oocyte microvilli once the spermatozoon reaches the perivitelline space. (**b**) Oocyte microvilli fuse with the sperm plasma membrane over the equatorial segment, effectively exposing the perinuclear theca to the oocyte cytoplasm. (**c**) PT (PAS) in the regions already fused with the oolema becomes solubilized very rapidly, releasing the SOAF and possibly other factors into oocyte cytoplasm. Disulfide-bond-reducing and chromatin-remodeling factors such as glutathione and proteases, present in the oocyte cytoplasm, may facilitate the dissolution and dispersion of sperm PT at this stage. (**d**) The oocyte microvilli pull the PT and sperm nucleus into the ooplasm, and the PT starts to solubilize in the oocyte cytoplasm. The arrest of sperm-incorporation (at step **c**), induced by microfilament disruption with cytochalasin B (CB), does not prevent oocyte activation, as the oocyte microvilli retain their ability to fuse with the sperm plasma membrane, effectively exposing the sperm PT to oocyte cytoplasm. PT from those parts of the sperm head engulfed by the oocyte is then released into the oocyte cytoplasm, thus explaining the ability of spermatozoa to activate the oocytes in the absence of complete sperm incorporation after CB-treatment. *ES* equatorial segment; *IAM* inner acrosomal membrane; *NE* nuclear envelope; *OAM* outer acrosomal membrane; *PM* plasma membrane; *PAS* post-acrosomal sheath; *SAR* sub-acrosomal region. Original drawings were adapted from Yanagimachi [108], after Bedford and Cooper [266]. Panels (**a–e**) were reprinted from [128] with permission from the publishers. (**e, f**) Transmission of the PAWP protein (red) from sperm PT to ooplasm after in vitro fertilization (IVF; **e**) and intracytoplasmic sperm injection (ICSI; **f**). PAWP is a sperm-specific WW-domain binding signaling protein in the SRC-family tyrosine kinase pathway. Porcine zygotes were fixed 8 h after IVF (**e**) or 3 h after ICSI (**f**) and processed with a rabbit polyclonal antibody against sperm PT protein PAWP (red) and DNA stain DAPI (blue), and photographed under epifluorescence illumination and differential interference contrast (DIC). Anti-PAWP antibody kindly provided by Dr. Richard Oko, Queen's University, Kingston, ON. See [315] for details

proposed SOAF components, the main features of the SOAF should be outlined. The definition of SOAF properties is based on studies using the microinjection of whole spermatozoa or soluble sperm cytosol in the metaphase-II arrested mammalian, lower vertebrate, and invertebrate oocytes. A credible mammalian SOAF-candidate must satisfy many criteria: (1) Male germ cell specificity: since somatic cells extracts typically do not induce oocyte activation, the SOAF is a sperm/male germ cell specific protein [278, 279]; (2) Presence in elongated spermatids and spermatozoa only: Early haploid cells, the early step round spermatids, do not induce oocyte activation [280] when injected in the ooplasm, but the later stage, elongating spermatids do [281]. Therefore, SOAF component-encoding genes should be transcribed in late secondary spermatocytes or early spermatids, and their mRNAs should only be translated during spermatid elongation; (3) Localization in the PAS and/or OPL: Sperm PT-solubilization restricted to PAS and outer layer of the ES following sperm–oolemma fusion is sufficient to trigger oocyte activation [128, 267]; (4) Lack of species-specificity: SOAF is not species-specific although differences in oocyte calcium response to crude sperm extract injections or ICSI have been noted [282–285]. Consequently, microinjecting spermatozoa and sperm extract from one mammal can activate ova of a different mammalian species or of a lower vertebrate species; and (5) Ability to induce repetitive release of calcium (calcium oscillations in mammals) from the oocyte's internal stores [275, 278].

Besides SOAF, the fertilizing spermatozoon may contribute other molecules that could affect early embryo development. Human spermatozoa carry a transcriptome of more than 5,000 mRNAs and microRNAs; many of them could be translation-competent [286–288]. The human sperm transcriptome may reflect donor's fertility as the sperm borne transcriptomes of some cellular pathways, such as ubiquitin–proteasome pathway mRNAs, show major difference between fertile and infertile human sperm transcriptome [289]. Consequently, the interrogation of sperm transcriptome could have a diagnostic application in the male infertility field. It is not clear where and how the sperm RNAs are stored by the spermatozoa. Somatic cell type histones, ribonucleoprotein, and/or other nucleic acid binding proteins in the perinucelar theca could mediate sperm mRNA binding, explaining why spermatozoa can be used as a DNA vector for transgenic ICSI or IVF in animals [290, 291]. Thus far, the evidence does not suggest that the sperm borne mRNAs are transcribed by the oocyte, and the small sperm borne microRNAs that could cause RNA-interference do not seem to have a profound effect on the zygote [292]. Until now, it was believed that the fully differentiated spermatozoa themselves cannot translate their mRNA, a notion recently challenged by a report of mRNA translation in the sperm mitochondrial sheath [293].

25.4.4 Oocyte Activation and the Identity of SOAF

Oocyte activation is a key event of fertilization. The hallmark of oocyte activation in mammals is the cyclic release of free calcium ions from the oocyte's endoplasmic reticulum (ER), referred to as calcium oscillations [294]. The proposed cascade of activation events [295] starts with the solubilization of SOAF from sperm perinucelar theca into ooplasm, which either releases a sperm-specific phospholipase C (PLC) species or activates an ooplasmic PLC. The activated PLC hydrolyses IP3 into PIP2 and DAG (as already outlined for acrosomal exocytosis). IP3 binds to IP3 receptor on the calcium store in the ER and causes calcium release through the opening of an ion channel on the ER-membrane. The released Ca^{2+}-ions activate the Calcium–calmodulin Kinase II (CaMKII), SRC-family kinases and their downstream kinases (PKA, PKC), causing a series of phosphorylation events responsible for the cortical granule exocytosis and for the release of oocyte meiosis from metaphase-II. One of the activated kinases, PKC, is thought to act on the plasma membrane-associated transient receptor potential channels (TRP-C) to potentiate influx of external calcium in the oocyte, which then refills the ER with Ca^{2+}-ions. In presence of IP3, the cycle keeps repeating itself, resulting in an oscillatory pattern of calcium release [295]. By releasing the SOAF (see previous section) and activating CaMKII, the fertilizing spermatozoon releases the oocyte's cell cycle from metaphase-II arrest via activating the anaphase-promoting complex (APC) [296], an ubiquitin–ligase complex that causes ubiquitination and proteasomal degradation of the cyclin B1 component of the meiosis-promoting factor (MPF) [297]. Calcineurin, a calcium–calmodulin dependent protein phosphatase, plays an important role in releasing the *Xenopus* oocyte from MII-arrest [298].

Much debate has occurred on the identity of the SOAF component that triggers calcium oscillations. Readers new to the field should be aware of the literature on "oscillin," which was proposed earlier to be the SOAF [299] but later disproved experimentally [300]. More recently, the phospholipase Cζ, a sperm/male germ cell specific PLC isoforms, has become a favorite SOAF candidate [301]. Indeed, overexpression of PLCζ through cRNA or recombinant protein injection triggers calcium oscillations nearly identical to those seen during natural fertilization in the mouse and other species [302, 303]. Also, the GFP-tagged, oocyte-translated PLCζ becomes sequestered in the pronuclei after activation, which is a predicted sequestration pattern of the SOAF after fertilization [304]. Consistent with the requirement of proteolysis for SOAF release and activity, the activation inducing boar sperm extracts contain hydrolyzed, bioactive C-terminal and N-terminal fragments of PLCζ [305]. A mouse PLCζ knock-out is not yet available. Despite repeated attempts, the transmission of PLCzeta from the sperm head to ooplasm during fertilization has not been documented.

Perry et al. [277] proposed that mammalian SOAF is a multi-component factor. At least two recently proposed mammalian candidate SOAF-components other than PLCζ are signaling molecules in the SRC-family tyrosine kinase pathways. Localized activation of oocyte SRC-family kinases FYN, SRC, and YES occurs downstream of calcium release during mouse fertilization [306, 307]. Tyrosine kinase activation before or after calcium release could trigger some events of oocyte activation and zygotic development, such as pronuclear apposition and entry to mitosis [308], by activating the downstream protein kinases such as the PKC [309, 310]. The requirement for SRC-family kinase-dependent signaling of sperm-induced oocyte activation has been established in invertebrates, namely the starfish eggs, by the injection of dominant negative-inhibitory SH2 domains of SRC-family kinases SRC and FYN [311, 312]. In the mouse, similar experiments did not prevent calcium oscillations, but the injection of SH2 domain peptides did prevent embryonic development, suggesting that at least these two tyrosine kinases may act as downstream effectors of calcium signaling induced by the fertilizing spermatozoon [308]. The injection of testis/sperm specific truncated c-KIT tyrosine kinase (trKIT) into mouse ova causes the activation of ooplasmic PLCγ, calcium release from ER and oocyte activation [313, 314]. In this case, the injection of SH2-domain of FYN kinase, thought to be necessary for c-KIT activation, did inhibit mouse oocyte activation [314]. Such data keep open a possibility that a sperm-borne phospholipase species such as PLCζ may not be the only factors essential for oocyte activation. To my knowledge, there is no precedent for one PLC species activating a different PLC species, as the PLCζ studies would suggest, although indirect activation through other kinases could occur. With regard to presence of phospholipases in the sperm head, calcium oscillations have been recorded in the acrosome and postacrosomal region during hamster sperm hyperactivation [60].

Recently, we have described a male germ cell-specific, sperm PT-borne protein PAWP, which is transmitted from sperm PAS-PT to ooplasm during fertilization [315] and contains multiple repeats of the WW-binding, proline-rich PPXY motif initially implicated in the activation of SRC-family tyrosine kinases [316]. WW-motif containing SRC-kinase adaptor proteins, the potential binding partners of PAWP have also been implicated in the regulation of transcription and cell cycle progression [317], both of which have a central role during oocyte activation and zygotic development. PAWP transcription and translation coincide with the acquisition of the oocyte-activating ability by the differentiating spermatid [318], and the the competitive peptides and antibodies recognizing PAWP's WW-binding motifs block oocyte activation when coinjected with spermatozoon by ICSI [315]. The relationship between PAWP transmission to ooplasm (Fig. 25.2e, f) and calcium release at fertilization is being investigated. Of note, ungulate PLCζ also contains one PPXY domain, but its functionality or ability to bind to WW domain containing proteins has not been examined.

One of the earlier theories of oocyte activation attributed this process to ligand receptor binding events between sperm plasmalemma and oolemma. There is some justification for this "receptor mechanism" to be at least a cofactor of the SOAF-induced oocyte activation. Calcium oscillations occur normally but fail to activate an efficient antipolyspermy defense after ICSI in the mouse [319]. This finding suggests that the SOAF release alone is not sufficient to induce full antipolyspermy defense, and either a receptor-ligand binding-induced signalling or the contribution of sperm plasma membrane components to oolemma are necessary for complete oocyte activation. The interest in the "receptor hypothesis" has been renewed by the studies of interactions between sperm disintegrins (ADAM2 and ADAM3) and their oocyte receptor, integrin alpha6 beta1. While knock-out studies indicate that this pathway is not the main mechanism of sperm–oolemma fusion, studies using synthetic RGD peptides (the disintegrins' active, integrin-binding motif) showed that beads coated with such peptides can trigger oocyte activation at least in some mammalian species [320]. Peptides mimicking the RGD-motif containing extracellular receptor domain of disintegrins bind to zona free oocytes and induce their parthenogenetic activation, including some calcium release with a limited number of transients [321, 322]. A recent study showed that binding of RGD peptides induced calcium release in mouse oocytes and implicated tyrosine kinases and PKC in the downstream events of disintegrin-integrin binding [323]. Altogether, it is reasonable to conclude that the main oocyte activating signal comes in the form of sperm SOAF release while sperm–oolemma interactions may activate parallel signaling events supportive of complete oocyte activation. While some studies attribute the oscillatory pattern of calcium release in the oocyte solely to sperm-contributed PLC species, a recent paper suggests that the oocyte's resident PLCs can convey calcium oscillations [324].

25.4.5 Antipolyspermy Defense

The simplest method of antipolyspermy defense in vivo may be via regulation of the number of spermatozoa that actually reach the descending ovum [325]. The actual antipolyspermy defense in an individual mammalian ovum is achieved at two different levels; that of the zona and that of the oolemma. Different mammalian species studied can be divided based on which mechanism is thought to be primary, as shown in Table 25.3 adapted from a previous review [108] and other reports. Notwithstanding the filtering of spermatozoa by

Table 25.3 Zona pellucida and oolemma based anti-polyspermy defense in mammals

Species	Human	Pig	Mouse	Rabbit
Predominant anti-polyspermy defense site	ZP	ZP	Both ZP and oolemma	Oolemma
Supernumerary spermatozoa accumulate in perivetelline space	No/rarely	No/rarely	Yes (few)	Yes (many)
Polyspermy in vitro	Moderate	High	Low	?
Other species with this pattern of sperm accumulation	Dog, golden hamster, sheep, field vole, ferret		Rat, guinea pig, cat	Pika, mole, bat
AE induction by ZP binding	In most ZP-bound spermatozoa		In some ZP-bound spermatozoa	?
Superfluous sperm detach from ZP after IVF and ZP hardening	No	No	Yes	?
Proteasomal inhibitors block sperm–ZP binding	No	No	Yes	?
Proteasomal inhibitors block AE	Yes	Yes	Yes	?
Proteasomal inhibitors block sperm–ZP penetration	Yes	Yes	?	?
Proteasomal inhibitors block sperm–oolemma fusion	No	No	Yes	?

Proteasomal involvement in sperm–zona interactions is also reviewed. References for the data summarized in Table 25.3: [108, 222, 223, 244, 327, 435–438]

cumulus oophorus, zona pellucida is thought to be the primary antipolyspermy barrier in most mammals. The fusion of the fertilizing spermatozoon with the oolemma triggers the exocytosis of cortical granules (CG), commonly referred to as cortical reaction [326, 327]. The CG-exudate contains enzymes thought to alter zona pellucida of the newly fertilized oocyte via proteolysis, lectin binding and deglycosylation [328]. Following the cortical granule exocytosis, the oligosaccharide composition of the zona is altered [329], and the ZP2 protein is hydrolyzed into two fragments of 90 kDa and 30 kDa, respectively, in the mouse [330]. The changes to ZP caused by cortical reaction are referred to as zona hardening and are observed in all mammals except hamster [331]. In the mouse, the ZP2-cleavage alone seems to prevent the binding of spermatozoa to ZP in activated eggs. However, the cortical reaction or ZP2 cleavage alone is not sufficient to fend off polyspermy in other species such as the rabbit [332] or the pig [333]. In the pig, the antipolyspermy defense mechanism employs oviductal glycoproteins (OGP) expressed in a segment specific manner [334]. Consequently, porcine ova are highly polyspermic in vitro when they are not exposed to oviductal secretions, but less polyspermy is observed after coincubation with oviductal fluid or with oviductal fluid components such as the OGP [334] or osteopontin [335]. Pertinent to the proposed role of sperm proteasome in sperm–zona interactions, inhibitors of sperm and oocyte-borne deubiqutinating enzymes, the ubiquitin-C-terminal hydrolases, increase polyspermy during porcine fertilization in vitro [333]. Similarly, the *gad* mutant mice expressing mutant ubiquitin-C-teminal hydrolase L1 in the oocyte cortex are subfertile because of high polyspermy [336]. In lower vertebrates, the release of CG lectins is thought to desensitize the egg coat to further sperm binding after oocyte activation, and this mechanism could also be applicable to mammals [328]. At the oolemma level, membrane depolarization is thought to be the main mechanism of anti-polyspermy defense [337]. Contribution of sperm membranes may alter the composition of oolemma and cortical cytoskeletal architecture to support antipolyspermy defense, as suggested by mouse ICSI experiments in which oocyte activation by sperm injection failed to activate the oolemma-based antipolyspermy defense [319].

25.5 Zygotic/Pronuclear Development

During spermiogenesis, the removal of sperm nuclear histones and their replacement with protamines allows for the hypercondensation of sperm DNA. This histone–protamine exchange is reversed shortly after sperm incorporation in the ooplasm and removal of the sperm nuclear envelope (NE). The NE is then reformed, and oocyte-specific histones infiltrate the paternal chromatin. Simultaneouly, oocyte chromosomes complete second meiosis and start decondensing into female pronucleus (PN). An early wave of transcription is observed mainly from the male PN. The pronuclei are brought together during the process of PN-apposition guided by microtubule sperm aster, organized by the sperm-contributed centriole-turned zygotic centrosome. DNA replication and first embryo cleavage follow. While the sperm nucleus and proximal centriole are transformed into male PN and zygotic centrosome, sperm mitochondrial sheath, fibrous sheath, and flagellar axoneme are degraded by the zygote. Contrary to natural fertilization, the ICSI fails to trigger oolemma-based antipolyspermy defense and may result in the asynchronous development of male and female PN.

25.5.1 Sperm Chromatin Remodeling and Formation of Pronuclei

The crucial event of male pronuclear development is the reversal of histone–protamine exchange. During spermiogenesis, nuclear DNA packaging proteins, histones become dislodged by transitional proteins (TP1 and TP2) [338], then replaced by protamines, the arginine rich DNA-binding proteins [339], and ultimately ubiquitinated for degradation by the 26 S proteasome [340]. Male mice deficient in ubiquitin-conjugating enzyme HR6B are infertile due to a failure of spermatid chromatid remodeling [341]. Protamine binding to sperm DNA allows for hypercondensation of sperm chromatin, which is important for the protection of sperm DNA until fertilization, but not permissive to transcription [339]. Consequently, the histone–protamine exchange is reversed after fertilization, when protamines are removed and replaced first by oocyte specific histones and later by somatic cell type histones in a predetermined developmental program [342–344]. Protamine removal and male PN formation requires the disulfide-bond reducing capacity of ooplasmic peptide glutathione, produced during oocyte maturation [345]. Consequently, oocytes depleted of glutathione during maturation are capable of fertilization but not of normal PN development [346]. While protamines are removed, other sperm chromatin or nuclear matrix proteins may be retained by the male pronucleus to support pronuclear development [347]. Chromatin remodeling during pronuclear development after initial sperm nucleus decondensation is supported by nucleoplasmin-related protein NPM2, as shown by mouse knockout studies [348]. Apart from a small pool of redundant nuclear envelopes at the base of the sperm head, the NE of the fertilizing spermatozoa is deprived of nuclear pore complexes and has to be removed prior to sperm chromatin decondensation [349]. Nuclear pore complexes (NPC) are inserted in the de novo formed NE at an early stage of male and female PN development, and their saturation with NPC-binding lectins prevents pronuclear development [349]. Association of microtubule motor proteins, dynein and dynactin, with the NPC on male and female pronuclei anchors the sperm aster microtubules to pronuclear NE, thus facilitating pronuclear apposition [350].

25.5.2 Early Transcriptional Activity

Most of the stored maternal mRNA is degraded after fertilization [351, 352], and a similar fate may meet stored maternal proteins [333, 353] (Fig. 25.3). Zygotic genome transcription starts as early as one cell stage [354, 355], mainly confounded to the male PN [356, 357]. Accordingly, male pronucleus attracts hyperacetylated histones to a higher degree than female PN [356], and has a higher content of transcription factors SP1 and TBP [358]. The appearance of compact nucleolus precursor bodies (NPBs) is a hallmark of

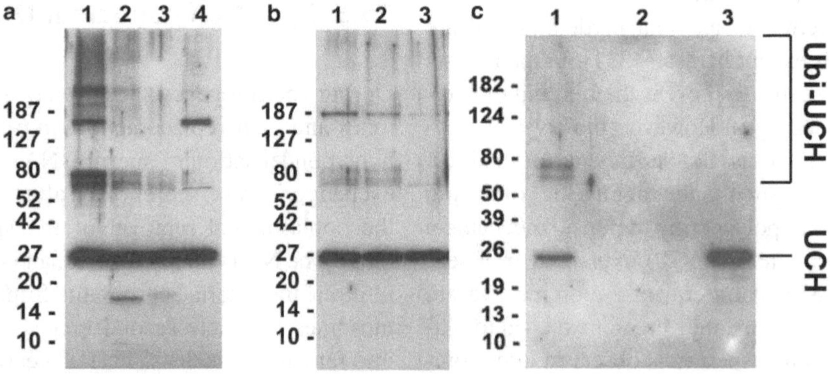

Fig. 25.3 Proteasome-dependent degradation of ubiquitin-C-terminal hydrolase UCHL1 following in vitro fertilization of porcine oocytes. Biochemical analysis of UCH-turnover after porcine oocyte-activation (**a**) and parthenogenetic activation (**b**) was conducted by western blotting of in vitro matured porcine oocytes harvested at consecutive time points after fertilization/activation. Evidence is provided that oocyte UCHL1 is postranslationally modified by ubiquitination prior to fertilization and degraded by the oocyte 26 S proteasome after fertilization/oocyte activation. (**a**) High molecular mass bands (Ubi-UCH) immunoreactive with anti-UCHL1 antiserum suggest that UCHL1 is ubiquitinated in MII oocytes. *Lane 1*: 100 MII oocytes; *lane 2*: 100 zygotes cultured for 13 h after IVF; *lane 3*: 100 parthenogenetic oocytes cultured for 13 h after parthenogenetic activation; *lane 4*: 100 MII oocytes treated with 10 μM proteasomal inhibitor MG-132 at 6 h after insemination, a proteolysis blocking treatment that prevents the degradation of ubiquitinated proteins. (**b**) Time-lapse western blot of UCHL1 in porcine zygotes at 6 (*lane 1*), 7 (*lane 2*) and 8 (*lane 3*) h after insemination. Fifty oocytes were loaded per lane. (**c**) Affinity purification of ubiquitinated UCHL1 species from porcine in vitro matured ova by using agarose-imobilized, recombinant ubiquitin-binding protein p62. *Lane 1*: anti-UCHL1 immunoreactive bands in the ubiquitinated oocyte–protein fraction purified by p62; *lane 2*: control elution of p62-agarose matrix not coincubated with oocyte proteins; *lane 3*: whole oocyte-extract (no p62-purification). Ubi-UCH=high mass, ubiquitinated UCHL1 species; UCH=nascent, 24 kDa UCHL1-band. Reprinted from [333] with permission from the publishers

PN development [359] and some limited transcription of ribosomal genes may be occurring at the periphery of NPBs in one cell embryos [360]. Eventually, the NPBs are transformed into reticulate nucleoli, the sites of ribosomal gene transcription and rRNA processing during later stages of preimplantation development. Oocytes of mutant mice lacking the mammalian homologue of *Xenopus* nucleoplasmin, the NPM2 gene product implicated in nucleolar biogenesis, fail to make normal NPBs and pronuclei [348]. It is thus not surprising that ribosomal and ribonucleoprotein-encoding genes are found in the first wave of transcription at one cell stage in the mouse. In addition, genes encoding for products involved in proton transport, ion transport, ribonucleotide triphosphate metabolism and proteasomal subunit genes are expressed by the zygote [355]. These early transcribed gene products may be rapidly translated to regulate zygotic development. Altogether, the first round of zygotic transcription is referred to as minor genome activation and is followed by major genome activation occurring at two to eight cell stage in different mammalian species [361]. Major activation of the mouse genome occurs at two-cell stage and is controlled by a mechanism known as the "zygotic clock" that schedules zygotic gene transcription and translation based on time lapsed from fertilization [362]. Alternatively, the male PN-restricted transcription at one cell stage could serve as a proofreading mechanism assuring that there is no irreparable DNA damage left after sperm chromatin decondensation and protamine removal. A number of knockouts of genes involved in DNA repair and cell cycle checkpoints are embryonic-lethal at an early stage of zygote/embryo development [363]. Chromatin remodeling after fertilization and pronuclear DNA replication and during the zygotic S-phase provides window of opportunity prior to nucleosome reformation during which the maternal transcription factors gain easy access to their bidning sites on the paternal DNA [364, 365]. The deletion of BRG1 catalytic subunit of the chromatin remodeling complex SWI/SNF causes two-cell embryonic arrest [366]. Ablation of transcription intermediary factor 1α (TIF1α) that translocates into the pronuclear transcription foci in the mouse zygote, compromises zygotic transcription and embryo development [367]. Schultz [368] speculates that transcription at one cell stage in the mouse serves to mark promoters that will be utilized at two-cell stage during the onset of major genome activation.

Similar to other cells and tissues, the gene expression in gametes and embryos is in part controlled by epigenetic modification, cytosine methylation that occurs in pairs of cytosine and guanosine found within gene promoter sequences (CpG islands)[369]. The pattern of DNA methylation is erased immediately after fertilization, likely mediating a profound epigenetic effect on the embryo. Remethylation/genome reprogramming then occurs after implantation [370]. The X-chromosome silencing or X-inactivation is an important event of preimplantation development that dependents on DNA methylation [371–373]. If the fertilizing spermatozoon carries an X-chromosome, meaning the embryo is destined to be a female with XX sex chromosome configuration, then one of the two X-chromosomes has to be silenced in order to promote gene dosage compensation by preventing redundant and potentially detrimental expression from both copies of the X-chromosome bound genes. Originally thought to occur at or shortly before blastocyst stage, X-silencing is now believed to be initiated at one-cell stage in humans and at two-cell stage of embryo development in the mouse when the X-inactivation-specific transcript *(X-ist)* gene is first transcribed [374, 375]. The *Xist* gene is expressed exclusively by the to-be-silenced copy of X-chromosome and the *Xist* RNA becomes associated with the silenced copy of X-chromosome early after fertilization [376]. The association of *Xist* noncoding RNA with the silenced X-chromosome triggers an extensive chromatin modification of the silenced X [377, 378]. Altered X-inactivation is observed in cloned mice [379], cattle [380], and in the neonatal-deceased cloned pigs [381].

25.5.3 Sperm Aster Formation and PN Apposition

The pinnacle of fertilization is the union of maternal and paternal genomes in the first mitotic metaphase plate. This integration is achieved through pronuclear apposition mediated by microtubule cytoskeleton [382, 383]. The means of PN apposition by microtubule networks are common in all mammals, but the mechanisms of microtubule organization are strikingly different between rodents and other eutherian mammals, including primates [384]. In most plant and animal cells, the organization of microtubules in the meiotic/mitotic spindle or in the interphase networks is governed by the centrosome, a microtubule organizing center (MTOC) composed of two centrioles and a halo of pericentriolar materials [385]. Uniquely, the MTOCs found at the spindle poles of mammalian oocytes are acentriolar [386] and the sperm centrosome is reduced to a single, proximal centriole devoid of pericentriolar material during spermiogenesis [387, 388]. In all mammals but rodents, the fertilizing spermatozoon contributes this single centriole to the zygote [389–391]. During fertilization, the sperm proximal centriole is released from the sperm tail connecting piece by active proteolysis [392], then duplicates while attracting maternal, ooplasmic pericentriolar material and forms an active zygotic centrosome [267, 393] (Fig. 25.4a–e). This newly formed zygotic centrosome has the ability to nucleate the polymerization of microtubules into a radial array referred to as sperm aster [269]. Sperm aster microtubules reach

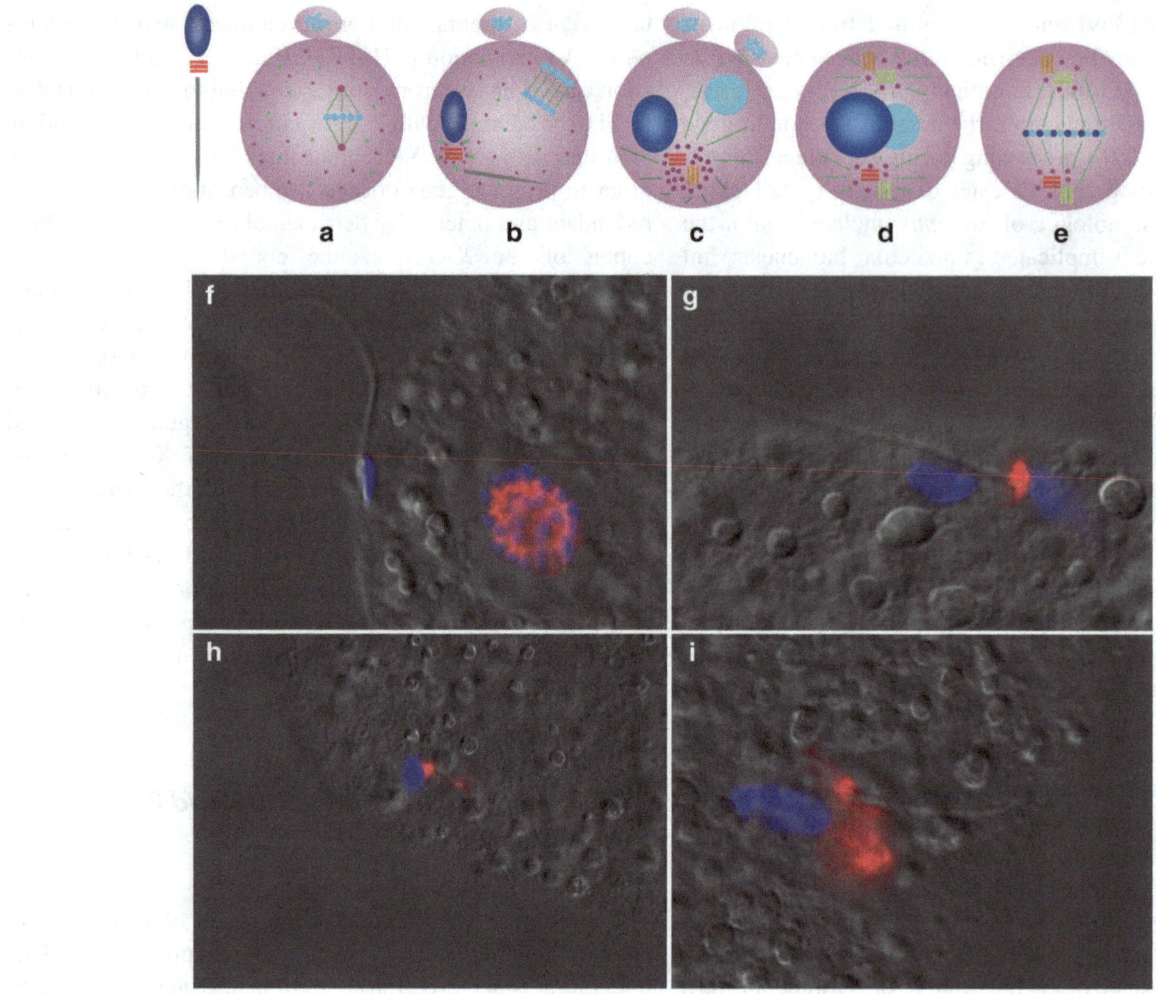

Fig. 25.4 Centrosomal inheritance following fertilization in nonrodent mammals. (**a–e**) Diagram of zygotic centrosome reconstitution. (**a**) The fertilizing spermatozoon (*left*) carries a single centriole, termed proximal centriole, embedded in the connecting piece of its flagellum. The mature, fertilization-competent oocyte carries a metaphase-II-spindle with one acentriola microtubule-organizing center (MTOC) on each of its poles. Ooplasm contains tubulin molecules and centrosomal proteins necessary for de novo synthesis of centrioles and pericentriolar material. (**b**) After sperm incorporation and head-flagellum-excision, the proximal centriole is released and starts attracting ooplasmic tubulin and pericentriolar proteins. (**c**) Tubulin nucleation and microtubule polymerization around the assembled pericentriolar material results in the formation of the sperm aster. The sperm centriole duplicates giving rise to a de novo synthesized daughter centriole (yellow centriole). (**d**) Pronuclear apposition occurs on the tracks of sperm aster microtubules, and the daughter centriole migrates to the opposite pole of the future mitotic spindle. Both sperm centriole and daughter centriole duplicate giving rise to two complete centrosomes on the opposite sides of apposed pronuclei. Each centrosome contains two centrioles. The DNA inside both pronuclei has now been replicated. Hence, two cycles of centriole duplication occurred within one cycle of DNA replication and centrosome duplication. (**e**) First mitotic spindle forms with aligned maternal and paternal chromosomes. (**f–i**) Sperm aster formation during bovine fertilization starts even before complete incorporation of the whole sperm flagellum in the ooplasm. (**f**) Sperm–oolemma fusion, no sperm aster yet; only the microtubules of the oocyte meiotic spindle are stained red. (**g, h**) Early stages of sperm tail incorporation. Sperm head and flagellar connecting piece have already been exposed to ooplasm, resulting in sperm head decondensation and nucleation of nascent sperm aster microtubules (red) around the sperm proximal centriole. (**i**) Advanced stages of sperm incorporation; sperm aster is formed to approx. 1/3 final size. All zygotes were fixed at 7.5 h after gamete mixing during IVF and processed with anti-tubulin antibody E7 (Developmental Studies Hybridoma Bank, Iowa City, IA) and DNA stain DAPI. Perfocal epifluorescence images were superimposed onto DIC background

toward the male and female pronuclei, fitted with nuclear envelope-bound microtubule motor proteins [350], and the male and female PN are brought together. Failure of sperm aster formation and pronuclear apposition has been revealed in the postfertilization-arrested human IVF and ICSI zygotes [394–397]. Injection of patients' spermatozoa into bovine ova has been introduced as a prospective test of sperm centrosomal function for infertility patients [398]. Attempts have been made to relieve centrosome disfunction-related male infertility by "centrosomal donation" of the sperm centriole from a fertile donor, coinjected during ICSI, but they failed to rescue pronuclear apposition in the injected embryos [399].

25.5.4 Degradation of Sperm Accessory Structures

Akin to a space shuttle rejecting its engines after reaching orbit, the accessory structures of the sperm flagellum become separated from the sperm head early after sperm incorporation in the ooplasm and degraded [267, 268]. This process starts with the excision of the sperm tail from the head at the implantation fossa [267, 346]. This development, instrumental in the release of the sperm borne centriole and sperm aster formation, starts even before the whole length of the sperm flagellum is incorporated in the ooplasm (see Fig. 25.4f-I). At least in bovine and rat zygotes, the earliest event of sperm tail degradation is the dissolution of the fibrous sheath enveloping the sperm tail principal piece [267, 400]. The FS serves as a flexible scaffold of the sperm flagellar apparatus affording it both structural support and movement required for flagellar motility [401, 402]. It contains A-kinase anchoring proteins and glycolytic enzymes necessary for the regulation of flagellar motility and ATP production, respectively [63]. Apart from the centriole, it is thought that the accessory, axonemal, and periaxonemal structures of the flagellum are not essential for postfertilization development. However, it should be considered whether cytosolic proteins amalgamated in the dense ribs of the FS could serve some function during early development, especially if they are released so quickly after fertilization.

The next degradation event during fertilization targets sperm mitochondria [267, 403] and is executed by ubiquitin-dependent proteasomal proteolysis [404–407]. Sperm mitochondria are thus targeted for degradation selectively without the oocyte inflicting damage to its own mitochondria [407]. Degradation of paternal mitochondria prevents the mixing of two different mitochondrial genomes (maternal and paternal) within the zygote, an anomaly referred to as heteroplasmy [408]. An additional reason for the destruction of sperm mitochondria after fertilization is the likelihood that they have been exposed to reactive oxygen species prior to fertilization and thus could carry damaged mtDNA [409, 410]. However, the recognition mechanism for the degradation of paternal mitochondria does not appear to screen for DNA mismatch between maternal and paternal mitochondrial genomes; the interspecific mouse crosses are heteroplasmic, carrying both maternal and paternal mtDNA, and viable [411]. Back-crossed interspecific mouse hybrids carrying foreign mtDNA on the background of homologous nuclear-encoded mitochondrial membrane proteins eliminate paternal mitochondria and paternal mtDNA just like wild type mice [412]. This selective depletion suggests that foreign mitochondrial membrane proteins, not the foreign mtDNA, are recognized by the zygote. Proteasomal degradation is the likely endpoint of a yet to be identified event that leads to the recognition of foreign mitochondrial membranes inside the zygote in a species-specific manner. One recently proposed candidate is the mitochondrial membrane translocator system, including proteins TOM22 and TOM40 [413]. The degradation of sperm mtDNA coincides with, but does not precede, morphological changes in sperm mitochondrial membranes inside the zygote [414]. Thus far, only one case of maternal mtDNA leakage has been reported in humans. It involved a male patient with severe mitochondrial pathology because of a deletion of NADH dehydrogenase subunit-2 gene (ND2) [415]. To date, there are no reports of human IVF or ICSI causing aberrant mtDNA transmission [416]. In contrast, the experimental ooplasm donation procedure, causing heteroplasmy by transfer of mitochondria between donor and recipient oocytes, had to be discontinued because of occurrences of miscarriage and chromosomal anomalies [417].

The motile and supporting structures of the sperm axoneme, including microtubule doublets and outer dense fibers, persist in the zygote/embryo cytoplasm for several embryonic cell cycles [267, 268, 418, 419]. Although not likely to contribute to early embryo development, these structures, if not processed in a timely manner, could interfere with embryo cleavage and development.

25.5.5 Differences Between Natural Fertilization and ICSI

During natural fertilization, the fertilizing spermatozoon is deprived of its plasma membrane during sperm–oocyte fusion, and its acrosome is lost even earlier during sperm–zona binding. Consequently, the ooplasm is brought into direct contact with sperm internal structures, allowing for their degradation or remodeling [268]. Besides direct exposure, sperm demembranation may support oocyte activation via membrane receptor binding events and contribute membrane components to the oolemma [128]. In contrast, ICSI introduces spermatozoa with more or less intact plasma membrane and acrosome directly into the ooplasm, skipping multiple steps of fertilization and omitting sperm–oolemma binding events. Essentially, the major differences between ICSI and natural fertilization are in the mechanism of oocyte activation, anti-polyspermy defense, and in the processing of sperm accessory structures by the ooplasm.

As established earlier in this review, the processing of the sperm plasma membrane, acrosome, perinuclear theca, and sperm nuclear envelope during fertilization exposes the

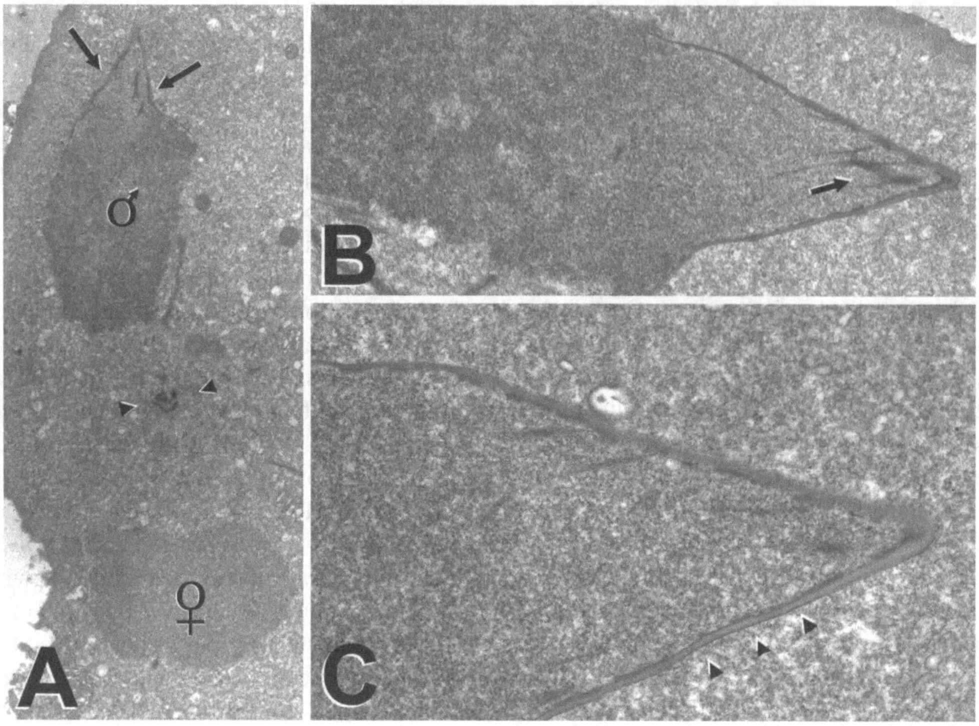

Fig. 25.5 Retention of the subacrosomal perinulear theca layer following ICSI in the rhesus monkey oocytes. (**a**) The retained PT (*arrows*) restricts the apical pole of the nascent male pronucleus (♂), causing the uneven decondensation of paternal chromatin and the aberrant formation of the female proncuelus (♀). (**b**, **c**) Detail of the apical region of injected sperm head showing cords of condensed heterochromatin (*arrow*) and an intact subacrosomal perinuclear theca layer (*arrowheads*). The phenomenon of delayed male PN development after ICSI been described in detail by [420, 421]

sperm chromatin to ooplasmic factors in charge of decondensation and male PN-formation. In rhesus monkey, the postacrosomal sheath disperses shortly after the vesiculation of the plasma membrane after ICSI, but the subacrosomal perinuclear theca layer, often with the attached inner acrosomal membrane and acrosomal matrix, can severely restrict the decondensation at the apical pole of the sperm nucleus, causing a fertilization failure [420] (Fig. 25.5). Such a delayed sperm nuclear decondensation can result in an asynchronous development of male and female pronuclei in the ICSI zygotes [420–422]. The apical pole of the sperm nucleus, sheltered by the subacrosomal PT, seems to be the preferential location of sex chromosomes. It was suggested that subacrosomal PT persistence after ICSI could contribute to a slight increase of sex chromosome anomalies seen in ICSI children [423].

Earlier ICSI experiments demonstrated that sperm–oolema binding is not necessary for oocyte activation, conveyed primarily by the release of SOAF from the sperm head perinuclear theca. While some oocytes may fail to demembranate the injected spermatozoon and solubilize its PT after ICSI (see above), oocyte activation is typically not the primary reason for post-ICSI fertilization arrest. If necessary, the lack of oocyte-activating sperm substances can be relieved by artificial activation following ICSI [424–426]. Even if not essential for triggering calcium oscillations, sperm–oolemma fusion and contribution of sperm membrane components to the oolemma may be necessary for establishing normal antipolyspermy defense at the oolemma level. Maleszewski et al. [319] demonstrated the lack of antipolyspermy defense in mouse ICSI-zygotes. Similar observations were later made in humans [427]. Recently, the anomalous remodeling of oocyte-cortical actin cytoskeleton after mouse ICSI has been suggested to be a contributing factor for the failure of post-ICSI antipolyspermy defense in the mouse [428].

Acrosomal matrix proteases transferred by ICSI could be harmful for the zygote [429] (Fig. 25.6). The removal of the acrosome by sperm membrane permeabilization [430] or by induction of acrosomal exocytosis coupled with mechanical membrane disruption [431] improves oocyte activation and PN development after ICSI in animals. Similarly, rubbing of the sperm tail midpiece seems to generate mechanical forces along the plasmalemma that cause acrosomal disruption and plasma membrane vesiculation in the postacrosomal sheath of human ICSI spermatozoa that could promote oocyte activation and PN development [432–434].

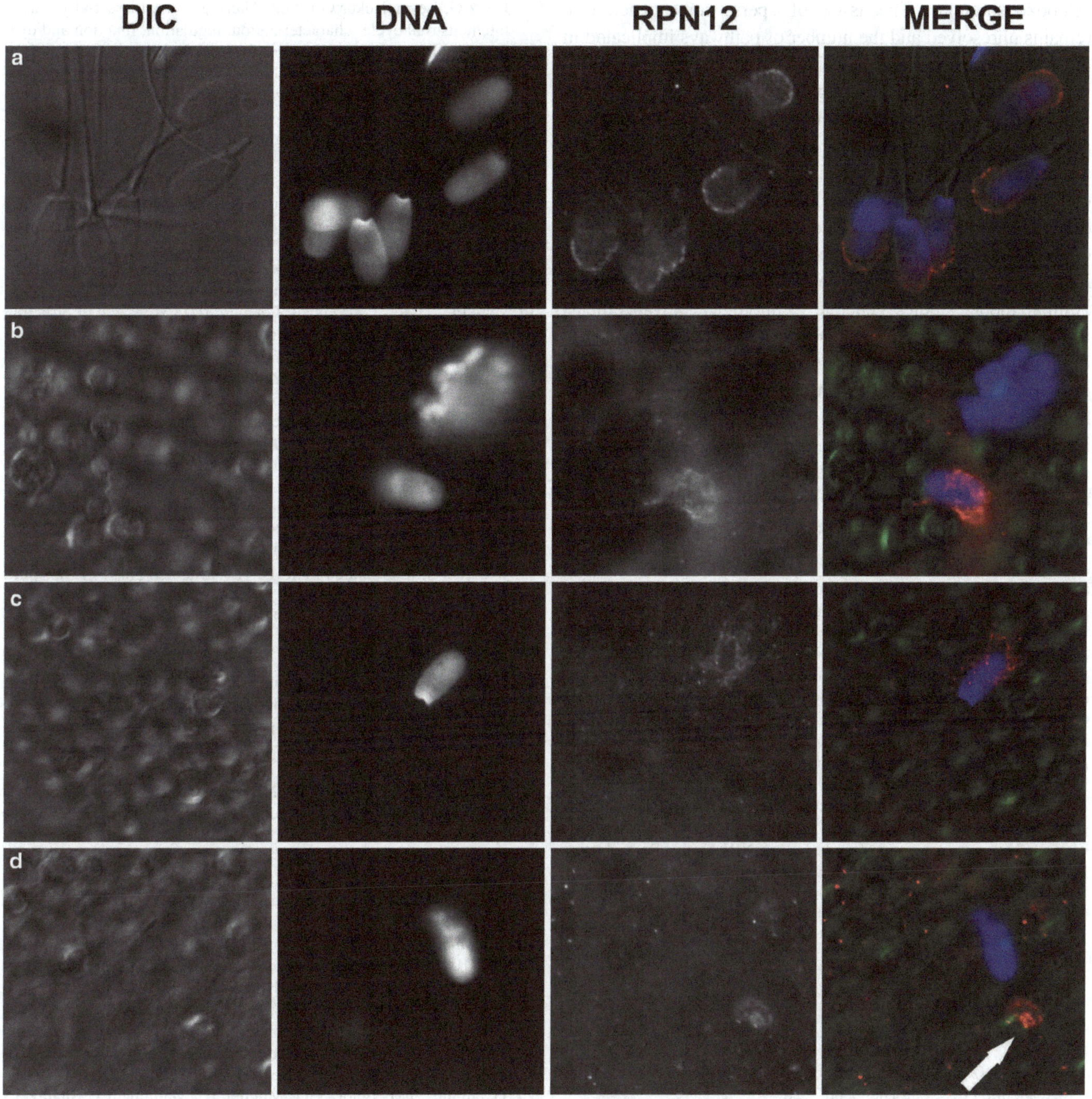

Fig. 25.6 Fate of the sperm head accessory structures following porcine ICSI. Resident proteasomes of the boar sperm acrosome were labeled red and sperm DNA blue. (**a**) Intact spermatozoa prior to ICSI. (**b**, **c**) Partial release of the acrosomal matrix from the injected spermatozoa found inside early stage ICSI zygotes. (**d**) Sperm head decondensation coincides with rejection of acrosome (*arrow*). Persistence of the redundant subacrosomal perincuelar theca (PT; *arrows*) hinders the decondensation of the apical sperm nucleus following rhesus monkey ICSI

25.6 Conclusions

Substantial progress was made in understanding human/mammalian fertilization in the last decade. There are numerous issues to be resolved. Credible candidates have been identified for mediating sperm–oolemma binding and fusion and oocyte activation though the latter in particular may require further validation. Such knowledge could be used to optimize oocyte activation procedures during human ICSI, particulary in patients with anomalous or missing sperm head skeleton (globozoospermia). The issue of sperm–zona penetration remains unresolved and the number of pathways implicated in the downstream events of capacitation and acrosomal exocytosis is tantalyzing. Advances in glycobiology of zona pellucida will have to be made to fully understand the mechanism of sperm–zona binding and antipolyspermy defense. Better understanding of acrosomal exocytosis and sperm–zona interactions could result in new gamete quality testing and selection procedures for IVF and ICSI. Many described steps of fertilization could be manipulated to induce a contraceptive effect or to increase the yield of viable embryos for embryo transfer. Animal model studies generate technological advancements for better efficiency and safeguarding of IVF and ICSI. Without diminishing the importance of mouse as a genetic model, caution should be exercised when extrapolating rodent data to human fertilization. Inter-strain differences in fertility are also important and should be accounted for when examining the results of mouse fertilization studies. Alternative models such as large animals will probably be used increasingly in future fertilization research for these reasons.

Acknowledgments I would like to acknowledge the support from my past and present associates and graduate students at the University of Missouri, including Gauri Manandhar, Young-Joo Yi, Kathleen Baska, Kyle Lovercamp, Alex Wu, Katie Fischer, Shawn Zimmerman, Jen Antelman, and Miriam Sutovsky. Clerical and editorial assistance from Kathy Craighead is much appreciated. Support from my colleagues and collaborators, Drs. Randy Prather, Jon Green, Billy N. Day and Gary Clark, and their associates are much appreciated. Special thanks to Dr. Richard Oko for sharing unpublished data from our collaborative research projects for the purpose of this chapter and to the staff of the Electron Microscopy Core Facility of UM for sample procesing. Critical reading of this manuscript by Drs. Vera Jonakova, Richard Oko and Gary Clark is gratefully acknowledged. In the last 7 years, my laboratory was/has been supported by generous grants from the USDA-NRI Animal Reproduction Program, the NIH, Canadian Institutes of Health Research, Pfizer Inc., Monsanto Inc, and seed funding from the Food for the twenty-first Century Program of the University of Missouri-Columbia.

References

1. Suarez S (2002) Gamete transport. In: Hardy D (ed) Fertilization. Academic Press, San Diego, pp 3–28
2. Garbers DL, Kopf GS (1980) The regulation of spermatozoa by calcium cyclic nucleotides. Adv Cyclic Nucleotide Res 13:251–306
3. Vijayaraghavan S, Goueli SA, Davey MP, Carr DW (1997) Protein kinase A-anchoring inhibitor peptides arrest mammalian sperm motility. J Biol Chem 272(8):4747–4752
4. Lin RY, Moss SB, Rubin CS (1995) Characterization of S-AKAP84, a novel developmentally regulated A kinase anchor protein of male germ cells. J Biol Chem 270(46):27804–27811
5. Mullins KJ, Saacke RG (1989) Study of the functional anatomy of bovine cervical mucosa with special reference to mucus secretion and sperm transport. Anat Rec 225(2):106–117
6. Kunz G, Beil D, Deininger H, Wildt L, Leyendecker G (1996) The dynamics of rapid sperm transport through the female genital tract: evidence from vaginal sonography of uterine peristalsis and hysterosalpingoscintigraphy. Hum Reprod 11(3):627–632
7. Kunz G, Leyendecker G (2002) Uterine peristaltic activity during the menstrual cycle: characterization, regulation, function and dysfunction. Reprod Biomed Online 4(Suppl 3):5–9
8. Fritz H, Schiessler H, Schleuning WD (1973) Proteinases and proteinase inhibitors in the fertilization process: new concepts of control? Adv Biosci 10:271–286
9. Samuelsson B (1963) Prostaglandins of human seminal plasma. Blue Sheet 89:34
10. Dostal J, Veselsky L, Marounek M, Zelezna B, Jonakova V (1997) Inhibition of bacterial and boar epididymal sperm immunogenicity by boar seminal immunosuppressive component in mice. J Reprod Fertil 111(1):135–141
11. Kelly RW (1995) Immunosuppressive mechanisms in semen: implications for contraception. Hum Reprod 10(7):1686–1693
12. Pang PC, Tissot B, Drobnis EZ et al (2007) Expression of bisecting type and Lewisx/Lewisy terminated N-glycans on human sperm. J Biol Chem 282(50):36593–36602
13. Austin CR (1957) Fate of spermatozoa in the uterus of the mouse and rat. J Endocrinol 14(4):335–342
14. Jansen RP (1980) Cyclic changes in the human fallopian tube isthmus and their functional importance. Am J Obstet Gynecol 136(3):292–308
15. Saacke RG, DeJarnette JM, Bame JH, Karabinus DS, Whitman SS (1998) Can spermatozoa with abnormal heads gain access to the ovum in artificially inseminated super- and single-ovulating cattle? Theriogenology 50(1):117–128
16. Overstreet JW, Cooper GW (1978) Sperm transport in the reproductive tract of the female rabbit: II. The sustained phase of transport. Biol Reprod 19(1):115–132
17. Overstreet JW, Cooper GW (1978) Sperm transport in the reproductive tract of the female rabbit: I. The rapid transit phase of transport. Biol Reprod 19(1):101–114
18. Rodriguez-Martinez H, Saravia F, Wallgren M et al (2005) Boar spermatozoa in the oviduct. Theriogenology 63(2):514–535
19. Hunter RH, Wilmut I (1984) Sperm transport in the cow: peri-ovulatory redistribution of viable cells within the oviduct. Reprod Nutr Dev 24(5A):597–608
20. Dalton JC, Nadir S, Bame JH, Noftsinger M, Nebel RL, Saacke RG (2001) Effect of time of insemination on number of accessory sperm, fertilization rate, and embryo quality in nonlactating dairy cattle. J Dairy Sci 84(11):2413–2418
21. Yanagimachi R, Chang MC (1963) Sperm ascent through the oviduct of the hamster and rabbit in relation to the time of ovulation. J Reprod Fertil 6:413–420
22. Williams M, Hill CJ, Scudamore I, Dunphy B, Cooke ID, Barratt CL (1993) Sperm numbers and distribution within the human fallopian tube around ovulation. Hum Reprod 8(12):2019–2026
23. Ignotz GG, Lo MC, Perez CL, Gwathmey TM, Suarez SS (2001) Characterization of a fucose-binding protein from bull sperm and seminal plasma that may be responsible for formation of the oviductal sperm reservoir. Biol Reprod 64(6):1806–1811
24. Gwathmey TM, Ignotz GG, Mueller JL, Manjunath P, Suarez SS (2006) Bovine seminal plasma proteins PDC-109, BSP-A3, and BSP-30-kDa share functional roles in storing sperm in the oviduct. Biol Reprod 75(4):501–507
25. Haase B, Schlotterer C, Hundrieser ME et al (2005) Evolution of the spermadhesin gene family. Gene 352:20–29
26. Topfer-Petersen E, Petrounkina AM, Ekhlasi-Hundrieser M (2000) Oocyte-sperm interactions. Anim Reprod Sci 60–61:653–662
27. Liberda J, Manaskova P, Prelovska L, Ticha M, Jonakova V (2006) Saccharide-mediated interactions of boar sperm surface proteins with components of the porcine oviduct. J Reprod Immunol 71(2):112–125
28. Ekhlasi-Hundrieser M, Gohr K, Wagner A, Tsolova M, Petrunkina A, Topfer-Petersen E (2005) Spermadhesin AQN1 is a candidate receptor molecule involved in the formation of the oviductal sperm reservoir in the pig. Biol Reprod 73(3):536–545

29. Jelinkova P, Liberda J, Manaskova P, Ryslava H, Jonakova V, Ticha M (2004) Mannan-binding proteins from boar seminal plasma. J Reprod Immunol 62(1–2):167–182
30. Tollner TL, Yudin AI, Tarantal AF, Treece CA, Overstreet JW, Cherr GN (2008) Beta-defensin 126 on the surface of macaque sperm mediates attachment of sperm to oviductal epithelia. Biol Reprod 78(3):400–412
31. Austin CR (1952) The capacitation of the mammalian sperm. Nature 170(4321):326
32. Yanagimachi R (1970) The movement of golden hamster spermatozoa before and after capacitation. J Reprod Fertil 23(1):193–196
33. Demott RP, Suarez SS (1992) Hyperactivated sperm progress in the mouse oviduct. Biol Reprod 46(5):779–785
34. Lefebvre R, Suarez SS (1996) Effect of capacitation on bull sperm binding to homologous oviductal epithelium. Biol Reprod 54(3):575–582
35. Cohen-Dayag A, Tur-Kaspa I, Dor J, Mashiach S, Eisenbach M (1995) Sperm capacitation in humans is transient and correlates with chemotactic responsiveness to follicular factors. Proc Natl Acad Sci U S A 92(24):11039–11043
36. Hunter RH (2008) Sperm release from oviduct epithelial binding is controlled hormonally by peri-ovulatory graafian follicles. Mol Reprod Dev 75(1):167–174
37. Abou-Haila A, Tulsiani DR (2003) Evidence for the capacitation-associated membrane priming of mouse spermatozoa. Histochem Cell Biol 119(3):179–187
38. Jaiswal BS, Eisenbach M (2002) Capacitation. In: Hardy DM (ed) Fertilization. Academic Press, San Diego, pp 57–117
39. Rubinstein S, Breitbart H (1991) Role of spermine in mammalian sperm capacitation and acrosome reaction. Biochem J 278(Pt 1):25–28
40. Luconi M, Muratori M, Maggi M et al (2000) Uteroglobin and transglutaminase modulate human sperm functions. J Androl 21(5):676–688
41. Rodeheffer C, Shur BD (2004) Sperm from beta1, 4-galactosyltransferase I-null mice exhibit precocious capacitation. Development 131(3):491–501
42. Roldan ER, Murase T, Shi QX (1994) Exocytosis in spermatozoa in response to progesterone and zona pellucida. Science 266(5190): 1578–1581
43. Gadella BM, Visconti PE (2006) Regulation of capacitation. In: De Jonge C, Barratt CL (eds) The sperm cell. Cambridge University Press, Cambridge, UK, pp 134–169
44. Visconti PE, Bailey JL, Moore GD, Pan D, Olds-Clarke P, Kopf GS (1995) Capacitation of mouse spermatozoa. I. Correlation between the capacitation state and protein tyrosine phosphorylation. Development 121(4):1129–1137
45. Visconti PE, Moore GD, Bailey JL et al (1995) Capacitation of mouse spermatozoa. II. Protein tyrosine phosphorylation and capacitation are regulated by a cAMP-dependent pathway. Development 121(4):1139–1150
46. Luconi M, Barni T, Vannelli GB et al (1998) Extracellular signal-regulated kinases modulate capacitation of human spermatozoa. Biol Reprod 58(6):1476–1489
47. Rajendran L, Simons K (2005) Lipid rafts and membrane dynamics. J Cell Sci 118(Pt 6):1099–1102
48. Snider DR, Clegg ED (1975) Alteration of phospholipids in porcine spermatozoa during in vivo uterus and oviduct incubation. J Anim Sci 40(2):269–274
49. Davis BK (1981) Timing of fertilization in mammals: sperm cholesterol/phospholipid ratio as a determinant of the capacitation interval. Proc Natl Acad Sci U S A 78(12):7560–7564
50. Langlais J, Kan FW, Granger L, Raymond L, Bleau G, Roberts KD (1988) Identification of sterol acceptors that stimulate cholesterol efflux from human spermatozoa during in vitro capacitation. Gamete Res 20(2):185–201
51. Jaiswal BS, Cohen-Dayag A, Tur-Kaspa I, Eisenbach M (1998) Sperm capacitation is, after all, a prerequisite for both partial and complete acrosome reaction. FEBS Lett 427(2):309–313
52. Valencia A, Wens MA, Merchant H, Reyes R, Delgado NM (1984) Capacitation of human spermatozoa by heparin. Arch Androl 12(Suppl):109–113
53. Muller K, Pomorski T, Muller P, Zachowski A, Herrmann A (1994) Protein-dependent translocation of aminophospholipids and asymmetric transbilayer distribution of phospholipids in the plasma membrane of ram sperm cells. Biochemistry 33(33): 9968–9974
54. Wang L, Beserra C, Garbers DL (2004) A novel aminophospholipid transporter exclusively expressed in spermatozoa is required for membrane lipid asymmetry and normal fertilization. Dev Biol 267(1):203–215
55. Gadella BM, Flesch FM, van Golde LM, Colenbrander B (1999) Dynamics in the membrane organization of the mammalian sperm cell and functionality in fertilization. Vet Q 21(4):142–146
56. Flesch FM, Colenbrander B, van Golde LM, Gadella BM (1999) Capacitation induces tyrosine phosphorylation of proteins in the boar sperm plasma membrane. Biochem Biophys Res Commun 262(3):787–792
57. Buffone MG, Calamera JC, Verstraeten SV, Doncel GF (2005) Capacitation-associated protein tyrosine phosphorylation and membrane fluidity changes are impaired in the spermatozoa of asthenozoospermic patients. Reproduction 129(6):697–705
58. Suarez SS (1996) Hyperactivated motility in sperm. J Androl 17(4):331–335
59. Yanagimachi R, Usui N (1974) Calcium dependence of the acrosome reaction and activation of guinea pig spermatozoa. Exp Cell Res 89(1):161–174
60. Suarez SS, Varosi SM, Dai X (1993) Intracellular calcium increases with hyperactivation in intact, moving hamster sperm and oscillates with the flagellar beat cycle. Proc Natl Acad Sci U S A 90(10): 4660–4664
61. Ficarro S, Chertihin O, Westbrook VA et al (2003) Phosphoproteome analysis of capacitated human sperm. Evidence of tyrosine phosphorylation of a kinase-anchoring protein 3 and valosin-containing protein/p97 during capacitation. J Biol Chem 278(13): 11579–11589
62. Vijayaraghavan S, Liberty GA, Mohan J, Winfrey VP, Olson GE, Carr DW (1999) Isolation and molecular characterization of AKAP110, a novel, sperm-specific protein kinase A-anchoring protein. Mol Endocrinol 13(5):705–717
63. Eddy EM, Toshimori K, O'Brien DA (2003) Fibrous sheath of mammalian spermatozoa. Microsc Res Tech 61(1):103–115
64. Esposito G, Jaiswal BS, Xie F et al (2004) Mice deficient for soluble adenylyl cyclase are infertile because of a severe sperm-motility defect. Proc Natl Acad Sci U S A 101(9):2993–2998
65. Ren D, Navarro B, Perez G et al (2001) A sperm ion channel required for sperm motility and male fertility. Nature 413(6856):603–609
66. Krisfalusi M, Miki K, Magyar PL, O'Brien DA (2006) Multiple glycolytic enzymes are tightly bound to the fibrous sheath of mouse spermatozoa. Biol Reprod 75(2):270–278
67. Miki K, Qu W, Goulding EH et al (2004) Glyceraldehyde 3-phosphate dehydrogenase-S, a sperm-specific glycolytic enzyme, is required for sperm motility and male fertility. Proc Natl Acad Sci U S A 101(47):16501–16506
68. Stouffer RL, Xu F, Duffy DM (2007) Molecular control of ovulation and luteinization in the primate follicle. Front Biosci 12:297–307
69. Curry TE Jr, Smith MF (2006) Impact of extracellular matrix remodeling on ovulation and the folliculo-luteal transition. Semin Reprod Med 24(4):228–241
70. Richards JS (2002) Delivery of the oocyte from the follicle to the oviduct: a time of vulnerability. Ernst Schering Res Found Workshop (41):43–62

71. Mahi-Brown CA, Yanagimachi R (1983) Parameters inlfuencing ovum pickup by oviductal fimbria in the golden hamster. Gamete Res 8:1–10
72. Bedford JM (1996) What marsupial gametes disclose about gamete function in eutherian mammals. Reprod Fertil Dev 8(4):569–580
73. Halbert SA, Tam PY, Adams RJ, Blandau RJ (1976) An analysis of the mechanisms of egg transport in the ampulla of the rabbit oviduct. Gynecol Invest 7(5):306–320
74. Halbert SA, Tam PY, Blandau RJ (1976) Egg transport in the rabbit oviduct: the roles of cilia and muscle. Science 191(4231): 1052–1053
75. Vines CA, Yoshida K, Griffin FJ et al (2002) Motility initiation in herring sperm is regulated by reverse sodium-calcium exchange. Proc Natl Acad Sci U S A 99(4):2026–2031
76. Suzuki N, Garbers DL (1984) Stimulation of sperm respiration rates by speract and resact at alkaline extracellular pH. Biol Reprod 30(5):1167–1174
77. Suzuki N, Shimomura H, Radany EW et al (1984) A peptide associated with eggs causes a mobility shift in a major plasma membrane protein of spermatozoa. J Biol Chem 259(23):14874–14879
78. Olson JH, Xiang X, Ziegert T et al (2001) Allurin, a 21-kDa sperm chemoattractant from Xenopus egg jelly, is related to mammalian sperm-binding proteins. Proc Natl Acad Sci U S A 98(20): 11205–11210
79. Spehr M, Schwane K, Riffell JA, Zimmer RK, Hatt H (2006) Odorant receptors and olfactory-like signaling mechanisms in mammalian sperm. Mol Cell Endocrinol 250(1–2):128–136
80. Parmentier M, Libert F, Schurmans S et al (1992) Expression of members of the putative olfactory receptor gene family in mammalian germ cells. Nature 355(6359):453–455
81. Spehr M, Gisselmann G, Poplawski A et al (2003) Identification of a testicular odorant receptor mediating human sperm chemotaxis. Science 299(5615):2054–2058
82. Spehr M, Schwane K, Riffell JA et al (2004) Particulate adenylate cyclase plays a key role in human sperm olfactory receptor-mediated chemotaxis. J Biol Chem 279(38):40194–40203
83. Elvin JA, Yan C, Matzuk MM (2000) Oocyte-expressed TGF-beta superfamily members in female fertility. Mol Cell Endocrinol 159(1–2):1–5
84. Camaioni A, Salustri A, Yanagishita M, Hascall VC (1996) Proteoglycans and proteins in the extracellular matrix of mouse cumulus cell-oocyte complexes. Arch Biochem Biophys 325(2): 190–198
85. Eppig JJ (1981) Prostaglandin E2 stimulates cumulus expansion and hyaluronic acid synthesis by cumuli oophori isolated from mice. Biol Reprod 25(1):191–195
86. Myles DG, Primakoff P (1997) Why did the sperm cross the cumulus? To get to the oocyte. Functions of the sperm surface proteins PH-20 and fertilin in arriving at, and fusing with, the egg. Biol Reprod 56(2):320–327
87. Kim E, Baba D, Kimura M, Yamashita M, Kashiwabara S, Baba T (2005) Identification of a hyaluronidase, Hyal5, involved in penetration of mouse sperm through cumulus mass. Proc Natl Acad Sci U S A 102(50):18028–18033
88. Austin CR (1960) Capacitation and the release of hyaluronidase from spermatozoa. J Reprod Fertil 3:310–311
89. Cummins JM, Yanagimachi R (1986) Development of ability to penetrate the cumulus oophorus by hmster speratozoa capaciatetd in vivo in relation to the timing of the acrosome reaction. Gamete Res 15:187–212
90. Bleil JD, Wassarman PM (1980) Structure and function of the zona pellucida: identification and characterization of the proteins of the mouse oocyte's zona pellucida. Dev Biol 76(1):185–202
91. Lefievre L, Conner SJ, Salpekar A et al (2004) Four zona pellucida glycoproteins are expressed in the human. Hum Reprod 19(7): 1580–1586
92. Boja ES, Hoodbhoy T, Garfield M, Fales HM (2005) Structural conservation of mouse and rat zona pellucida glycoproteins. Probing the native rat zona pellucida proteome by mass spectrometry. Biochemistry 44(50):16445–16460
93. Ganguly A, Sharma RK, Gupta SK (2008) Bonnet monkey (Macaca radiata) ovaries, like human oocytes, express four zona pellucida glycoproteins. Mol Reprod Dev 75(1):156–166
94. Hasegawa A, Koyama K (2007) Contribution of zona proteins to oocyte growth. Soc Reprod Fertil Suppl 63:229–235
95. Yonezawa N, Fukui N, Kuno M et al (2001) Molecular cloning of bovine zona pellucida glycoproteins ZPA and ZPB and analysis for sperm-binding component of the zona. Eur J Biochem 268(12):3587–3594
96. Harris JD, Hibler DW, Fontenot GK, Hsu KT, Yurewicz EC, Sacco AG (1994) Cloning and characterization of zona pellucida genes and cDNAs from a variety of mammalian species: the ZPA, ZPB and ZPC gene families. DNA Seq 4(6):361–393
97. Easton RL, Patankar MS, Lattanzio FA et al (2000) Structural analysis of murine zona pellucida glycans. Evidence for the expression of core 2-type O-glycans and the Sd(a) antigen. J Biol Chem 275(11):7731–7742
98. Dell A, Chalabi S, Easton RL et al (2003) Murine and human zona pellucida 3 derived from mouse eggs express identical O-glycans. Proc Natl Acad Sci U S A 100(26):15631–15636
99. Florman HM, Wassarman PM (1985) O-linked oligosaccharides of mouse egg ZP3 account for its sperm receptor activity. Cell 41(1):313–324
100. Hoodbhoy T, Joshi S, Boja ES, Williams SA, Stanley P, Dean J (2005) Human sperm do not bind to rat zonae pellucidae despite the presence of four homologous glycoproteins. J Biol Chem 280(13):12721–12731
101. Yonezawa N, Amari S, Takahashi K et al (2005) Participation of the nonreducing terminal beta-galactosyl residues of the neutral N-linked carbohydrate chains of porcine zona pellucida glycoproteins in sperm–egg binding. Mol Reprod Dev 70(2):222–227
102. Ozgur K, Patankar MS, Oehninger S, Clark GF (1998) Direct evidence for the involvement of carbohydrate sequences in human sperm–zona pellucida binding. Mol Hum Reprod 4(4):318–324
103. Wassarman PM, Mortillo S (1991) Structure of the mouse egg extracellular coat, the zona pellucida. Int Rev Cytol 130:85–110
104. Wassarman PM, Jovine L, Litscher ES (2004) Mouse zona pellucida genes and glycoproteins. Cytogenet Genome Res 105(2–4):228–234
105. El-Mestrah M, Castle PE, Borossa G, Kan FW (2002) Subcellular distribution of ZP1, ZP2, and ZP3 glycoproteins during folliculogenesis and demonstration of their topographical disposition within the zona matrix of mouse ovarian oocytes. Biol Reprod 66(4):866–876
106. Shalgi R, Maymon R, Bar-Shira B, Amihai D, Skutelsky E (1991) Distribution of lectin receptors sites in the zona pellucida of follicular and ovulated rat oocytes. Mol Reprod Dev 29(4):365–372
107. Sinowatz F, Kolle S, Topfer-Petersen E (2001) Biosynthesis and expression of zona pellucida glycoproteins in mammals. Cells Tissues Organs 168(1–2):24–35
108. Yanagimachi R (1994) Mammalian fertilization, 2nd edn. Raven Press, New York
109. Greve JM, Salzmann GS, Roller RJ, Wassarman PM (1982) Biosynthesis of the major zona pellucida glycoprotein secreted by oocytes during mammalian oogenesis. Cell 31(3 Pt 2):749–759
110. Lee VH, Dunbar BS (1993) Developmental expression of the rabbit 55-kDa zona pellucida protein and messenger RNA in ovarian follicles. Dev Biol 155(2):371–382
111. Bogner K, Hinsch KD, Nayudu P, Konrad L, Cassara C, Hinsch E (2004) Localization and synthesis of zona pellucida proteins in the marmoset monkey (*Callithrix jacchus*) ovary. Mol Hum Reprod 10(7):481–488

112. Tesarik J, Kopecny V (1986) Late preovulatory synthesis of proteoglycans by the human oocyte and cumulus cells and their secretion into the oocyte–cumulus-complex extracellular matrices. Histochemistry 85(6):523–528
113. Yamagami K, Hamazaki TS, Yasumasu S, Masuda K, Iuchi I (1992) Molecular and cellular basis of formation, hardening, and breakdown of the egg envelope in fish. Int Rev Cytol 136:51–92
114. Clark GF, Dell A (2006) Molecular models for murine sperm–egg binding. J Biol Chem 281(20):13853–13856
115. Wassarman PM (1990) Profile of a mammalian sperm receptor. Development 108(1):1–17
116. Chakravarty S, Kadunganattil S, Bansal P, Sharma RK, Gupta SK (2008) Relevance of glycosylation of human zona pellucida glycoproteins for their binding to capacitated human spermatozoa and subsequent induction of acrosomal exocytosis. Mol Reprod Dev 75(1):75–88
117. Yurewicz EC, Sacco AG, Gupta SK, Xu N, Gage DA (1998) Hetero-oligomerization-dependent binding of pig oocyte zona pellucida glycoproteins ZPB and ZPC to boar sperm membrane vesicles. J Biol Chem 273(13):7488–7494
118. Moreno RD, Alvarado CP (2006) The mammalian acrosome as a secretory lysosome: new and old evidence. Mol Reprod Dev 73(11):1430–1434
119. Anakwe OO, Gerton GL (1990) Acrosome biogenesis begins during meiosis: evidence from the synthesis and distribution of an acrosomal glycoprotein, acrogranin, during guinea pig spermatogenesis. Biol Reprod 42(2):317–328
120. Clermont Y, Oko R, Hermo L (1993) Cell and molecular biology of the testis. In: Desjardins C, Ewing L (eds) Cell biology of mammalian spermatogenesis. Oxford University Press, New York, pp 332–376
121. Barth AD, Oko RJ (1989) Abnormal morphology of bovine spermatozoa, 1st edn. Iowa State University Press, Ames, IA
122. Yao R, Ito C, Natsume Y et al (2002) Lack of acrosome formation in mice lacking a Golgi protein, GOPC. Proc Natl Acad Sci U S A 99(17):11211–11216
123. Aul RB, Oko RJ (2001) The major subacrosomal occupant of bull spermatozoa is a novel histone H2B variant associated with the forming acrosome during spermiogenesis. Dev Biol 239(2): 376–387
124. Aul RB, Oko RJ (2002) The major subacrosomal occupant of bull spermatozoa is a novel histone H2B. Dev Biol 242(2):376–387
125. Kang-Decker N, Mantchev GT, Juneja SC, McNiven MA, van Deursen JM (2001) Lack of acrosome formation in Hrb-deficient mice. Science 294(5546):1531–1533
126. Lin YN, Roy A, Yan W, Burns KH, Matzuk MM (2007) Loss of zona pellucida binding proteins in the acrosomal matrix disrupts acrosome biogenesis and sperm morphogenesis. Mol Cell Biol 27(19):6794–6805
127. Kierszenbaum AL, Rivkin E, Tres LL (2003) Acroplaxome, an F-actin-keratin-containing plate, anchors the acrosome to the nucleus during shaping of the spermatid head. Mol Biol Cell 14(11):4628–4640
128. Sutovsky P, Manandhar G, Wu A, Oko R (2003) Interactions of sperm perinuclear theca with the oocyte: implications for oocyte activation, anti-polyspermy defense, and assisted reproduction. Microsc Res Tech 61(4):362–378
129. Tulsiani DR, Abou-Haila A, Loeser CR, Pereira BM (1998) The biological and functional significance of the sperm acrosome and acrosomal enzymes in mammalian fertilization. Exp Cell Res 240(2):151–164
130. Bleil JD, Greve JM, Wassarman PM (1988) Identification of a secondary sperm receptor in the mouse egg zona pellucida: role in maintenance of binding of acrosome-reacted sperm to eggs. Dev Biol 128(2):376–385
131. Thaler CD, Cardullo RA (1996) The initial molecular interaction between mouse sperm and the zona pellucida is a complex binding event. J Biol Chem 271(38):23289–23297
132. Huang TT, Fleming AD, Yanagimachi R (1981) Only acrosome-reacted spermatozoa can bind to and penetrate zona pellucida: a study using the guinea pig. J Exp Zool 217(2):287–290
133. Litscher ES, Juntunen K, Seppo A et al (1995) Oligosaccharide constructs with defined structures that inhibit binding of mouse sperm to unferti lized eggs in vitro. Biochemistry 34(14):4662–4669
134. Wassarman PM, Liu C, Chen J, Qi H, Litscher ES (1998) Ovarian development in mice bearing homozygous or heterozygous null mutations in zona pellucida glycoprotein gene mZP3. Histol Histopathol 13(1):293–300
135. Rankin T, Familari M, Lee E et al (1996) Mice homozygous for an insertional mutation in the Zp3 gene lack a zona pellucida and are infertile. Development 122(9):2903–2910
136. Rankin TL, O'Brien M, Lee E, Wigglesworth K, Eppig J, Dean J (2001) Defective zonae pellucidae in Zp2-null mice disrupt folliculogenesis, fertility and development. Development 128(7): 1119–1126
137. Liu C, Litscher ES, Mortillo S et al (1996) Targeted disruption of the mZP3 gene results in production of eggs lacking a zona pellucida and infertility in female mice. Proc Natl Acad Sci U S A 93(11):5431–5436
138. Rankin TL, Coleman JS, Epifano O et al (2003) Fertility and taxon-specific sperm binding persist after replacement of mouse sperm receptors with human homologs. Dev Cell 5(1):33–43
139. Rankin TL, Tong ZB, Castle PE et al (1998) Human ZP3 restores fertility in Zp3 null mice without affecting order-specific sperm binding. Development 125(13):2415–2424
140. Chakravarty S, Suraj K, Gupta SK (2005) Baculovirus-expressed recombinant human zona pellucida glycoprotein-B induces acrosomal exocytosis in capacitated spermatozoa in addition to zona pellucida glycoprotein-C. Mol Hum Reprod 11(5):365–372
141. Williams SA, Xia L, Cummings RD, McEver RP, Stanley P (2007) Fertilization in mouse does not require terminal galactose or N-acetylglucosamine on the zona pellucida glycans. J Cell Sci 120(Pt 8):1341–1349
142. Evans JP (2000) Getting sperm and egg together: things conserved and things diverged. Biol Reprod 63(2):355–360
143. Evans JP, Florman HM (2002) The state of the union: the cell biology of fertilization. Nat Cell Biol 4(Suppl):s57–s63
144. Ensslin MA, Lyng R, Raymond A, Copland S, Shur BD (2007) Novel gamete receptors that facilitate sperm adhesion to the egg coat. Soc Reprod Fertil Suppl 63:367–383
145. Cheng A, Le T, Palacios M et al (1994) Sperm–egg recognition in the mouse: characterization of sp56, a sperm protein having specific affinity for ZP3. J Cell Biol 125(4):867–878
146. Foster JA, Friday BB, Maulit MT et al (1997) AM67, a secretory component of the guinea pig sperm acrosomal matrix, is related to mouse sperm protein sp56 and the complement component 4-binding proteins. J Biol Chem 272(19):12714–12722
147. Hardy CM, Mobbs KJ (1999) Expression of recombinant mouse sperm protein sp56 and assessment of its potential for use as an antigen in an immunocontraceptive vaccine. Mol Reprod Dev 52(2):216–224
148. Lu Q, Shur BD (1997) Sperm from beta 1, 4-galactosyltransferase-null mice are refractory to ZP3-induced acrosome reactions and penetrate the zona pellucida poorly. Development 124(20): 4121–4131
149. Youakim A, Hathaway HJ, Miller DJ, Gong X, Shur BD (1994) Overexpressing sperm surface beta 1, 4-galactosyltransferase in transgenic mice affects multiple aspects of sperm–egg interactions. J Cell Biol 126(6):1573–1583
150. Hardy DM, Garbers DL (1995) A sperm membrane protein that binds in a species-specific manner to the egg extracellular matrix

is homologous to von Willebrand factor. J Biol Chem 270(44):26025–26028
151. Herlyn H, Zischler H (2005) Sequence evolution, processing, and posttranslational modification of zonadhesin D domains in primates, as inferred from cDNA data. Gene 362:85–97
152. Lea IA, Sivashanmugam P, O'Rand MG (2001) Zonadhesin: characterization, localization, and zona pellucida binding. Biol Reprod 65(6):1691–1700
153. Bi M, Hickox JR, Winfrey VP, Olson GE, Hardy DM (2003) Processing, localization and binding activity of zonadhesin suggest a function in sperm adhesion to the zona pellucida during exocytosis of the acrosome. Biochem J 375(Pt 2):477–488
154. Ekhlasi-Hundrieser M, Sinowatz F, Greiser De Wilke I, Waberski D, Topfer-Petersen E (2002) Expression of spermadhesin genes in porcine male and female reproductive tracts. Mol Reprod Dev 61(1):32–41
155. Caballero I, Vazquez JM, Rodriguez-Martinez H et al (2005) Influence of seminal plasma PSP-I/PSP-II spermadhesin on pig gamete interaction. Zygote 13(1):11–16
156. Manaskova P, Liberda J, Ticha M, Jonakova V (2000) Aggregated and monomeric forms of proteins in boar seminal plasma: characterization and binding properties. Folia Biol (Praha) 46(4):143–151
157. Veselsky L, Peknicova J, Cechova D, Kraus M, Geussova G, Jonakova V (1999) Characterization of boar spermadhesins by monoclonal and polyclonal antibodies and their role in binding to oocytes. Am J Reprod Immunol 42(3):187–197
158. Calvete JJ, Carrera E, Sanz L, Topfer-Petersen E (1996) Boar spermadhesins AQN-1 and AQN-3: oligosaccharide and zona pellucida binding characteristics. Biol Chem 377(7–8):521–527
159. Veselsky L, Jonakova V, Sanz ML, Topfer-Petersen E, Cechova D (1992) Binding of a 15 kDa glycoprotein from spermatozoa of boars to surface of zona pellucida and cumulus oophorus cells. J Reprod Fertil 96(2):593–602
160. Jonakova V, Cechova D, Topfer-Petersen E, Calvete JJ, Veselsky L (1991) Variability of acrosin inhibitors in boar reproductive tract. Biomed Biochim Acta 50(4–6):691–695
161. Jonakova V, Calvete JJ, Mann K, Schafer W, Schmid ER, Topfer-Petersen E (1992) The complete primary structure of three isoforms of a boar sperm-associated acrosin inhibitor. FEBS Lett 297(1–2):147–150
162. Jelinkova P, Manaskova P, Ticha M, Jonakova V (2003) Proteinase inhibitors in aggregated forms of boar seminal plasma proteins. Int J Biol Macromol 32(3–5):99–107
163. Sanz L, Calvete JJ, Jonakova V, Topfer-Petersen E (1992) Boar spermadhesins AQN-1 and AWN are sperm-associated acrosin inhibitor acceptor proteins. FEBS Lett 300(1):63–66
164. Wu A, Anupriwan A, Iamsaard S et al (2007) Sperm surface arylsulfatase A can disperse the cumulus matrix of cumulus oocyte complexes. J Cell Physiol 213(1):201–211
165. Dudkiewicz AB (1984) Purification of boar acrosomal arylsulfatase A and possible role in the penetration of cumulus cells. Biol Reprod 30(4):1005–1014
166. Carmona E, Weerachatyanukul W, Xu H et al (2002) Binding of arylsulfatase A to mouse sperm inhibits gamete interaction and induces the acrosome reaction. Biol Reprod 66(6):1820–1827
167. Hess B, Saftig P, Hartmann D et al (1996) Phenotype of arylsulfatase A-deficient mice: relationship to human metachromatic leukodystrophy. Proc Natl Acad Sci U S A 93(25):14821–14826
168. Moskovtsev SI, Jarvi K, Legare C, Sullivan R, Mullen JB (2007) Epididymal P34H protein deficiency in men evaluated for infertility. Fertil Steril 88(5):1455–1457
169. Boue F, Berube B, De Lamirande E, Gagnon C, Sullivan R (1994) Human sperm–zona pellucida interaction is inhibited by an antiserum against a hamster sperm protein. Biol Reprod 51(4):577–587
170. Xia XY, Huang YF, Xu XF (2002) [Epididymal sperm protein P34H and male reproduction]. Zhonghua Nan Ke Xue 8(5):356–358 362
171. Meizel S, Mukerji SK (1975) Proacrosin from rabbit epididymal spermatozoa: partial purification and initial biochemical characterization. Biol Reprod 13(1):83–93
172. Barros C, Crosby JA, Moreno RD (1996) Early steps of sperm–egg interactions during mammalian fertilization. Cell Biol Int 20(1):33–39
173. Furlong LI, Veaute C, Vazquez-Levin MH (2005) Binding of recombinant human proacrosin/acrosin to zona pellucida glycoproteins. II. Participation of mannose residues in the interaction. Fertil Steril 83(6):1791–1796
174. Furlong LI, Harris JD, Vazquez-Levin MH (2005) Binding of recombinant human proacrosin/acrosin to zona pellucida (ZP) glycoproteins. I. Studies with recombinant human ZPA, ZPB, and ZPC. Fertil Steril 83(6):1780–1790
175. Baba T, Azuma S, Kashiwabara S, Toyoda Y (1994) Sperm from mice carrying a targeted mutation of the acrosin gene can penetrate the oocyte zona pellucida and effect fertilization. J Biol Chem 269(50):31845–31849
176. Huang TT Jr, Yanagimachi R (1985) Inner acrosomal membrane of mammalian spermatozoa: its properties and possible functions in fertilization. Am J Anat 174(3):249–268
177. Tesarik J, Pilka L, Drahorad J, Cechova D, Veselsky L (1988) The role of cumulus cell-secreted proteins in the development of human sperm fertilizing ability: implication in IVF. Hum Reprod 3(1):129–132
178. Moreno RD, Sepulveda MS, de Ioannes A, Barros C (1998) The polysulphate binding domain of human proacrosin/acrosin is involved in both the enzyme activation and spermatozoa–zona pellucida interaction. Zygote 6(1):75–83
179. Yu Y, Xu W, Yi YJ, Sutovsky P, Oko R (2006) The extracellular protein coat of the inner acrosomal membrane is involved in zona pellucida binding and penetration during fertilization: characterization of its most prominent polypeptide (IAM38). Dev Biol 290(1):32–43
180. Mori E, Kashiwabara S, Baba T, Inagaki Y, Mori T (1995) Amino acid sequences of porcine Sp38 and proacrosin required for binding to the zona pellucida. Dev Biol 168(2):575–583
181. Mori E, Baba T, Iwamatsu A, Mori T (1993) Purification and characterization of a 38-kDa protein, sp38, with zona pellucida-binding property from porcine epididymal sperm. Biochem Biophys Res Commun 196(1):196–202
182. Primakoff P, Hyatt H, Myles DG (1985) A role for the migrating sperm surface antigen PH-20 in guinea pig sperm binding to the egg zona pellucida. J Cell Biol 101(6):2239–2244
183. Hunnicutt GR, Primakoff P, Myles DG (1996) Sperm surface protein PH-20 is bifunctional: one activity is a hyaluronidase and a second, distinct activity is required in secondary sperm–zona binding. Biol Reprod 55(1):80–86
184. Primakoff P, Woolman-Gamer L, Tung KS, Myles DG (1997) Reversible contraceptive effect of PH-20 immunization in male guinea pigs. Biol Reprod 56(5):1142–1146
185. Tung KS, Primakoff P, Woolman-Gamer L, Myles DG (1997) Mechanism of infertility in male guinea pigs immunized with sperm PH-20. Biol Reprod 56(5):1133–1141
186. Hardy CM, Clydesdale G, Mobbs KJ et al (2004) Assessment of contraceptive vaccines based on recombinant mouse sperm protein PH20. Reproduction 127(3):325–334
187. Baba D, Kashiwabara S, Honda A et al (2002) Mouse sperm lacking cell surface hyaluronidase PH-20 can pass through the layer of cumulus cells and fertilize the egg. J Biol Chem 277(33):30310–30314
188. Reitinger S, Laschober GT, Fehrer C, Greiderer B, Lepperdinger G (2007) Mouse testicular hyaluronidase-like proteins SPAM1 and HYAL5 but not HYALP1 degrade hyaluronan. Biochem J 401(1):79–85
189. Saling PM, Sowinski J, Storey BT (1979) An ultrastructural study of epididymal mouse spermatozoa binding to zonae pellucidae

in vitro: sequential relationship to the acrosome reaction. J Exp Zool 209(2):229–238

190. Bleil JD, Wassarman PM (1983) Sperm–egg interactions in the mouse: sequence of events and induction of the acrosome reaction by a zona pellucida glycoprotein. Dev Biol 95(2):317–324
191. Yanagimachi R (1978) Calcium requirement for sperm–egg fusion in mammals. Biol Reprod 19(5):949–958
192. Meizel S, Turner KO (1993) Initiation of the human sperm acrosome reaction by thapsigargin. J Exp Zool 267(3):350–355
193. O'Toole CM, Arnoult C, Darszon A, Steinhardt RA, Florman HM (2000) Ca(2+) entry through store-operated channels in mouse sperm is initiated by egg ZP3 and drives the acrosome reaction. Mol Biol Cell 11(5):1571–1584
194. Barros C, Bedford JM, Franklin LE, Austin CR (1967) Membrane vesiculation as a feature of the mammalian acrosome reaction. J Cell Biol 34(3):C1–C5
195. Nagae T, Yanagimachi R, Srivastava PN, Yanagimachi H (1986) Acrosome reaction in human spermatozoa. Fertil Steril 45(5): 701–707
196. Ramalho-Santos J, Moreno RD, Sutovsky P et al (2000) SNAREs in mammalian sperm: possible implications for fertilization. Dev Biol 223(1):54–69
197. Tomes CN, Michaut M, De Blas G, Visconti P, Matti U, Mayorga LS (2002) SNARE complex assembly is required for human sperm acrosome reaction. Dev Biol 243(2):326–338
198. Gerton G (2002) Function of the sperm acrosome. Academic Press, San Diego
199. VandeVoort CA, Yudin AI, Overstreet JW (1997) Interaction of acrosome-reacted macaque sperm with the macaque zona pellucida. Biol Reprod 56(5):1307–1316
200. Valdivia M, Sillerico T, De Ioannes A, Barros C (1999) Proteolytic activity of rabbit perivitelline spermatozoa. Zygote 7(2):143–149
201. Kim KS, Gerton GL (2003) Differential release of soluble and matrix components: evidence for intermediate states of secretion during spontaneous acrosomal exocytosis in mouse sperm. Dev Biol 264(1):141–152
202. Kim KS, Foster JA, Gerton GL (2001) Differential release of guinea pig sperm acrosomal components during exocytosis. Biol Reprod 64(1):148–156
203. Hardy DM, Oda MN, Friend DS, Huang TT Jr (1991) A mechanism for differential release of acrosomal enzymes during the acrosome reaction. Biochem J 275(Pt 3):759–766
204. Darszon A, Espinosa F, Galindo B, Sanchez D, Beltran C (2002) Regulation of sperm ion currents. In: Hardy D (ed) Fertilization. Academic Press, San Diego
205. Travis AJ, Merdiushev T, Vargas LA et al (2001) Expression and localization of caveolin-1, and the presence of membrane rafts, in mouse and Guinea pig spermatozoa. Dev Biol 240(2):599–610
206. Tanphaichitr N, Carmona E, Bou Khalil M, Xu H, Berger T, Gerton GL (2007) New insights into sperm–zona pellucida interaction: involvement of sperm lipid rafts. Front Biosci 12:1748–1766
207. Endo Y, Lee MA, Kopf GS (1987) Evidence for the role of a guanine nucleotide-binding regulatory protein in the zona pellucida-induced mouse sperm acrosome reaction. Dev Biol 119(1):210–216
208. Tomes CN, McMaster CR, Saling PM (1996) Activation of mouse sperm phosphatidylinositol-4, 5 bisphosphate-phospholipase C by zona pellucida is modulated by tyrosine phosphorylation. Mol Reprod Dev 43(2):196–204
209. Jungnickel MK, Marrero H, Birnbaumer L, Lemos JR, Florman HM (2001) Trp2 regulates entry of Ca^{2+} into mouse sperm triggered by egg ZP3. Nat Cell Biol 3(5):499–502
210. Shi X, Amindari S, Paruchuru K et al (2001) Cell surface beta-1, 4-galactosyltransferase-I activates G protein-dependent exocytotic signaling. Development 128(5):645–654
211. De Jonge CJ, Han HL, Lawrie H, Mack SR, Zaneveld LJ (1991) Modulation of the human sperm acrosome reaction by effectors of the adenylate cyclase/cyclic AMP second-messenger pathway. J Exp Zool 258(1):113–125
212. Leyton L, Saling P (1989) 95 kd sperm proteins bind ZP3 and serve as tyrosine kinase substrates in response to zona binding. Cell 57(7):1123–1130
213. Furuya S, Endo Y, Oba M, Matsui Y, Nozawa S, Suzuki S (1992) Protein phosphorylation regulates the mouse sperm acrosome reaction induced by the zona pellucida. J Assist Reprod Genet 9(4):384–390
214. Burks DJ, Carballada R, Moore HD, Saling PM (1995) Interaction of a tyrosine kinase from human sperm with the zona pellucida at fertilization. Science 269(5220):83–86
215. Kirkman-Brown JC, Lefievre L, Bray C, Stewart PM, Barratt CL, Publicover SJ (2002) Inhibitors of receptor tyrosine kinases do not suppress progesterone-induced $[Ca^{2+}]i$ signalling in human spermatozoa. Mol Hum Reprod 8(4):326–332
216. Roldan ER, Shi QX (2007) Sperm phospholipases and acrosomal exocytosis. Front Biosci 12:89–104
217. Fukami K, Nakao K, Inoue T et al (2001) Requirement of phospholipase Cdelta4 for the zona pellucida-induced acrosome reaction. Science 292(5518):920–923
218. Osman RA, Andria ML, Jones AD, Meizel S (1989) Steroid induced exocytosis: the human sperm acrosome reaction. Biochem Biophys Res Commun 160(2):828–833
219. Blackmore PF, Neulen J, Lattanzio F, Beebe SJ (1991) Cell surface-binding sites for progesterone mediate calcium uptake in human sperm. J Biol Chem 266(28):18655–18659
220. Spungin B, Margalit I, Breitbart H (1995) Sperm exocytosis reconstructed in a cell-free system: evidence for the involvement of phospholipase C and actin filaments in membrane fusion. J Cell Sci 108(Pt 6):2525–2535
221. Breitbart H (2002) Role and regulation of intracellular calcium in acrosomal exocytosis. J Reprod Immunol 53(1–2):151–159
222. Morales P, Kong M, Pizarro E, Pasten C (2003) Participation of the sperm proteasome in human fertilization. Hum Reprod 18(5): 1010–1017
223. Chakravarty S, Bansal P, Sutovsky P, Gupta SK (2008) Role of proteasomal activity in the induction of acrosomal exocytosis by recombinant zona pellucida glycoproteins in human spermatozoa. Reprod Biomed Online 16(3):391–400
224. Caballero-Campo P, Chirinos M, Fan XJ et al (2006) Biological effects of recombinant human zona pellucida proteins on sperm function. Biol Reprod 74(4):760–768
225. Lyon JD, Vacquier VD (1999) Interspecies chimeric sperm lysins identify regions mediating species-specific recognition of the abalone egg vitelline envelope. Dev Biol 214(1):151–159
226. Olds-Clarke P (1996) How does poor motility alter sperm fertilizing ability? J Androl 17(3):183–186
227. Bedford JM (1998) Mammalian fertilization misread? Sperm penetration of the eutherian zona pellucida is unlikely to be a lytic event. Biol Reprod 59(6):1275–1287
228. Green DPL (2002) Fertilization biophysics. In: Hardy DM (ed) Fertilization. Academic Press, San Diego, pp 387–399
229. Green DP (1987) Mammalian sperm cannot penetrate the zona pellucida solely by force. Exp Cell Res 169(1):31–38
230. Olds-Clarke P (2003) Unresolved issues in mammalian fertilization. Int Rev Cytol 232:129–184
231. Saxena DK, Tanii I, Yoshinaga K, Toshimori K (1999) Role of intra-acrosomal antigenic molecules acrin 1 (MN7) and acrin 2 (MC41) in penetration of the zona pellucida in fertilization in mice. J Reprod Fertil 117(1):17–25
232. Kohno N, Yamagata K, Yamada S, Kashiwabara S, Sakai Y, Baba T (1998) Two novel testicular serine proteases, TESP1 and TESP2, are present in the mouse sperm acrosome. Biochem Biophys Res Commun 245(3):658–665
233. Honda A, Yamagata K, Sugiura S, Watanabe K, Baba T (2002) A mouse serine protease TESP5 is selectively included into lipid

rafts of sperm membrane presumably as a glycosylphosphatidylinositol-anchored protein. J Biol Chem 277(19):16976–16984
234. Wilkinson KD (2005) The discovery of ubiquitin-dependent proteolysis. Proc Natl Acad Sci U S A 102(43):15280–15282
235. Sakai N, Sawada MT, Sawada H (2004) Non-traditional roles of ubiquitin-proteasome system in fertilization and gametogenesis. Int J Biochem Cell Biol 36(5):776–784
236. Baska KM, Sutovsky P (2005) Protein modification by ubiquitination and is consequences for spermatogenesis, sperm maturation, fertilization and pre-implantation embryonic development. Research Signpost, Kerala
237. Yokota N, Sawada H (2007) Effects of proteasome inhibitors on fertilization of the sea urchin *Anthocidaris crassispina*. Biol Pharm Bull 30(7):1332–1335
238. Saitoh Y, Sawada H, Yokosawa H (1993) High-molecular-weight protease complexes (proteasomes) of sperm of the ascidian, *Halocynthia roretzi*: isolation, characterization, and physiological roles in fertilization. Dev Biol 158(1):238–244
239. Sawada H, Pinto MR, De Santis R (1998) Participation of sperm proteasome in fertilization of the phlebobranch ascidian *Ciona intestinalis*. Mol Reprod Dev 50(4):493–498
240. Sawada H, Sakai N, Abe Y et al (2002) Extracellular ubiquitination and proteasome-mediated degradation of the ascidian sperm receptor. Proc Natl Acad Sci U S A 99(3):1223–1228
241. Yokota N, Sawada H (2007) Sperm proteasomes are responsible for the acrosome reaction and sperm penetration of the vitelline envelope during fertilization of the sea urchin *Pseudocentrotus depressus*. Dev Biol 308(1):222–231
242. Bialy LP, Ziemba HT, Marianowski P, Fracki S, Bury M, Wojcik C (2001) Localization of a proteasomal antigen in human spermatozoa: immunohistochemical electron microscopic study. Folia Histochem Cytobiol 39(2):129–130
243. Pizarro E, Pasten C, Kong M, Morales P (2004) Proteasomal activity in mammalian spermatozoa. Mol Reprod Dev 69(1):87–93
244. Sutovsky P, Manandhar G, McCauley TC et al (2004) Proteasomal interference prevents zona pellucida penetration and fertilization in mammals. Biol Reprod 71(5):1625–1637
245. Chakravarty S, Pankaj Bansal P, Sutovsky P, Gupta S (2008) Role of proteasomal activity in the induction of acrosomal exocytosis by recombinant zona pellucida glycoproteins in human spermatozoa. Reprod Biomed Online 16(3):391–400
246. Blobel CP, Wolfsberg TG, Turck CW, Myles DG, Primakoff P, White JM (1992) A potential fusion peptide and an integrin ligand domain in a protein active in sperm–egg fusion. Nature 356(6366):248–252
247. Almeida EA, Huovila AP, Sutherland AE et al (1995) Mouse egg integrin alpha 6 beta 1 functions as a sperm receptor. Cell 81(7):1095–1104
248. Yuan R, Primakoff P, Myles DG (1997) A role for the disintegrin domain of cyritestin, a sperm surface protein belonging to the ADAM family, in mouse sperm–egg plasma membrane adhesion and fusion. J Cell Biol 137(1):105–112
249. He ZY, Brakebusch C, Fassler R, Kreidberg JA, Primakoff P, Myles DG (2003) None of the integrins known to be present on the mouse egg or to be ADAM receptors are essential for sperm–egg binding and fusion. Dev Biol 254(2):226–237
250. Nishimura H, Cho C, Branciforte DR, Myles DG, Primakoff P (2001) Analysis of loss of adhesive function in sperm lacking cyritestin or fertilin beta. Dev Biol 233(1):204–213
251. Cho C, Bunch DO, Faure JE et al (1998) Fertilization defects in sperm from mice lacking fertilin beta. Science 281(5384):1857–1859
252. Rubinstein E, Ziyyat A, Wolf JP, Le Naour F, Boucheix C (2006) The molecular players of sperm–egg fusion in mammals. Semin Cell Dev Biol 17(2):254–263
253. Miller BJ, Georges-Labouesse E, Primakoff P, Myles DG (2000) Normal fertilization occurs with eggs lacking the integrin alpha-6beta1 and is CD9-dependent. J Cell Biol 149(6):1289–1296
254. Le Naour F, Rubinstein E, Jasmin C, Prenant M, Boucheix C (2000) Severely reduced female fertility in CD9-deficient mice. Science 287(5451):319–321
255. Kaji K, Oda S, Miyazaki S, Kudo A (2002) Infertility of CD9-deficient mouse eggs is reversed by mouse CD9, human CD9, or mouse CD81; polyadenylated mRNA injection developed for molecular analysis of sperm–egg fusion. Dev Biol 247(2):327–334
256. Rubinstein E, Ziyyat A, Prenant M et al (2006) Reduced fertility of female mice lacking CD81. Dev Biol 290(2):351–358
257. Inoue N, Ikawa M, Isotani A, Okabe M (2005) The immunoglobulin superfamily protein Izumo is required for sperm to fuse with eggs. Nature 434(7030):234–238
258. Hayasaka S, Terada Y, Inoue N, Okabe M, Yaegashi N, Okamura K (2007) Positive expression of the immunoglobulin superfamily protein IZUMO on human sperm of severely infertile male patients. Fertil Steril 88(1):214–216
259. Naz RK (2008) Immunocontraceptive effect of Izumo and enhancement by combination vaccination. Mol Reprod Dev 75:336–344
260. Cohen DJ, Da Ros VG, Busso D et al (2007) Participation of epididymal cysteine-rich secretory proteins in sperm–egg fusion and their potential use for male fertility regulation. Asian J Androl 9(4):528–532
261. Da Ros V, Busso D, Cohen DJ, Maldera J, Goldweic N, Cuasnicu PS (2007) Molecular mechanisms involved in gamete interaction: evidence for the participation of cysteine-rich secretory proteins (CRISP) in sperm–egg fusion. Soc Reprod Fertil Suppl 65:353–356
262. Ellerman DA, Busso D, Maldera JA, Cuasnicu PS (2007) Immunocontraceptive properties of recombinant sperm protein DE: implications for the development of novel contraceptives. Fertil Steril 89(1):199–205
263. Roberts KP, Wamstad JA, Ensrud KM, Hamilton DW (2003) Inhibition of capacitation-associated tyrosine phosphorylation signaling in rat sperm by epididymal protein Crisp-1. Biol Reprod 69(2):572–581
264. Gaddum-Rosse P, Blandau RJ, Langley LB, Battaglia DE (1984) In vitro fertilization in the rat: observations on living eggs. Fertil Steril 42(2):285–292
265. Manandhar G, Toshimori K (2001) Exposure of sperm head equatorin after acrosome reaction and its fate after fertilization in mice. Biol Reprod 65(5):1425–1436
266. Bedford J, Cooper G (1978) Membrane fusion events in fertilization of vertebrate eggs. In: Poste G, Nicolson G (eds) Membrane surface reviews. Elsevier, Amsterdam, North-Holland, pp 65–125
267. Sutovsky P, Navara CS, Schatten G (1996) Fate of the sperm mitochondria, and the incorporation, conversion, and disassembly of the sperm tail structures during bovine fertilization. Biol Reprod 55(6):1195–1205
268. Sutovsky P, Schatten G (2000) Paternal contributions to the mammalian zygote: fertilization after sperm–egg fusion. Int Rev Cytol 195:1–65
269. Longo FJ (1985) Fine structure of the mammalian egg cortex. Am J Anat 174(3):303–315
270. Terada Y, Simerly C, Schatten G (2000) Microfilament stabilization by jasplakinolide arrests oocyte maturation, cortical granule exocytosis, sperm incorporation cone resorption, and cell-cycle progression, but not DNA replication, during fertilization in mice. Mol Reprod Dev 56(1):89–98
271. McAvey BA, Wortzman GB, Williams CJ, Evans JP (2002) Involvement of calcium signaling and the actin cytoskeleton in the membrane block to polyspermy in mouse eggs. Biol Reprod 67(4):1342–1352
272. Oko R, Maravei D (1994) Protein composition of the perinuclear theca of bull spermatozoa. Biol Reprod 50(5):1000–1014

273. Oko R, Aul RB, Wu A, Sutovsky P (2001) The sperm head skeleton. In: Robaire B, Chemes HE, Morales CR (eds) Andrology in the 21st century. Medimond Publishing Company, Englewood, NJ
274. Sutovsky P, Oko R, Hewitson L, Schatten G (1997) The removal of the sperm perinuclear theca and its association with the bovine oocyte surface during fertilization. Dev Biol 188(1):75–84
275. Kimura Y, Yanagimachi R, Kuretake S, Bortkiewicz H, Perry AC, Yanagimachi H (1998) Analysis of mouse oocyte activation suggests the involvement of sperm perinuclear material. Biol Reprod 58(6):1407–1415
276. Perry AC, Wakayama T, Yanagimachi R (1999) A novel trans-complementation assay suggests full mammalian oocyte activation is coordinately initiated by multiple, submembrane sperm components. Biol Reprod 60(3):747–755
277. Perry AC, Wakayama T, Cooke IM, Yanagimachi R (2000) Mammalian oocyte activation by the synergistic action of discrete sperm head components: induction of calcium transients and involvement of proteolysis. Dev Biol 217(2):386–393
278. Swann K (1990) A cytosolic sperm factor stimulates repetitive calcium increases and mimics fertilization in hamster eggs. Development 110(4):1295–1302
279. Stice SL, Robl JM (1990) Activation of mammalian oocytes by a factor obtained from rabbit sperm. Mol Reprod Dev 25(3):272–280
280. Kimura Y, Yanagimachi R (1995) Mouse oocytes injected with testicular spermatozoa or round spermatids can develop into normal offspring. Development 121(8):2397–2405
281. Yanagida K, Yazawa H, Katayose H, Kimura Y, Hayashi S, Sato A (2000) Oocyte activation induced by spermatids and the spermatozoa. Int J Androl 23(Suppl 2):63–65
282. Palermo GD, Avrech OM, Colombero LT et al (1997) Human sperm cytosolic factor triggers Ca^{2+} oscillations and overcomes activation failure of mammalian oocytes. Mol Hum Reprod 3(4):367–374
283. Malcuit C, Kurokawa M, Fissore RA (2006) Calcium oscillations and mammalian egg activation. J Cell Physiol 206(3):565–573
284. Malcuit C, Maserati M, Takahashi Y, Page R, Fissore RA (2006) Intracytoplasmic sperm injection in the bovine induces abnormal $[Ca^{2+}]i$ responses and oocyte activation. Reprod Fertil Dev 18(1–2):39–51
285. Wu H, He CL, Fissore RA (1997) Injection of a porcine sperm factor triggers calcium oscillations in mouse oocytes and bovine eggs. Mol Reprod Dev 46(2):176–189
286. Ostermeier GC, Miller D, Huntriss JD, Diamond MP, Krawetz SA (2004) Reproductive biology: delivering spermatozoan RNA to the oocyte. Nature 429(6988):154
287. Krawetz SA (2005) Paternal contribution: new insights and future challenges. Nat Rev Genet 6(8):633–642
288. Boerke A, Dieleman SJ, Gadella BM (2007) A possible role for sperm RNA in early embryo development. Theriogenology 68(Suppl 1):S147–S155
289. Platts AE, Dix DJ, Chemes HE et al (2007) Success and failure in human spermatogenesis as revealed by teratozoospermic RNAs. Hum Mol Genet 16(7):763–773
290. Lavitrano M, Busnelli M, Cerrito MG, Giovannoni R, Manzini S, Vargiolu A (2006) Sperm-mediated gene transfer. Reprod Fertil Dev 18(1–2):19–23
291. Perry AC, Wakayama T, Kishikawa H et al (1999) Mammalian transgenesis by intracytoplasmic sperm injection. Science 284(5417):1180–1183
292. Amanai M, Brahmajosyula M, Perry AC (2006) A restricted role for sperm-borne microRNAs in mammalian fertilization. Biol Reprod 75(6):877–884
293. Gur Y, Breitbart H (2007) Protein translation in mammalian sperm. Soc Reprod Fertil Suppl 65:391–397
294. Whitaker M (2006) Calcium at fertilization and in early development. Physiol Rev 86(1):25–88
295. Malcuit C, Fissore RA (2007) Activation of fertilized and nuclear transfer eggs. Adv Exp Med Biol 591:117–131
296. Nixon VL, Levasseur M, McDougall A, Jones KT (2002) Ca(2+) oscillations promote APC/C-dependent cyclin B1 degradation during metaphase arrest and completion of meiosis in fertilizing mouse eggs. Curr Biol 12(9):746–750
297. Glotzer M, Murray AW, Kirschner MW (1991) Cyclin is degraded by the ubiquitin pathway. Nature 349(6305):132–138
298. Nishiyama T, Yoshizaki N, Kishimoto T, Ohsumi K (2007) Transient activation of calcineurin is essential to initiate embryonic development in *Xenopus laevis*. Nature 449(7160):341–345
299. Parrington J, Swann K, Shevchenko VI, Sesay AK, Lai FA (1996) Calcium oscillations in mammalian eggs triggered by a soluble sperm protein. Nature 379(6563):364–368
300. Wolny YM, Fissore RA, Wu H et al (1999) Human glucosamine-6-phosphate isomerase, a homologue of hamster oscillin, does not appear to be involved in Ca2+ release in mammalian oocytes. Mol Reprod Dev 52(3):277–287
301. Saunders CM, Larman MG, Parrington J et al (2002) PLC zeta: a sperm-specific trigger of Ca(2+) oscillations in eggs and embryo development. Development 129(15):3533–3544
302. Kouchi Z, Fukami K, Shikano T et al (2004) Recombinant phospholipase Czeta has high Ca^{2+} sensitivity and induces Ca^{2+} oscillations in mouse eggs. J Biol Chem 279(11):10408–10412
303. Cox LJ, Larman MG, Saunders CM, Hashimoto K, Swann K, Lai FA (2002) Sperm phospholipase Czeta from humans and cynomolgus monkeys triggers Ca^{2+} oscillations, activation and development of mouse oocytes. Reproduction 124(5):611–623
304. Yoda A, Oda S, Shikano T et al (2004) Ca^{2+} oscillation-inducing phospholipase C zeta expressed in mouse eggs is accumulated to the pronucleus during egg activation. Dev Biol 268(2):245–257
305. Kurokawa M, Yoon SY, Alfandari D, Fukami K, Sato KI, Fissore RA (2007) Proteolytic processing of phospholipase Czeta and [Ca(2+)](i) oscillations during mammalian fertilization. Dev Biol 312(1):407–418
306. McGinnis LK, Albertini DF, Kinsey WH (2007) Localized activation of Src-family protein kinases in the mouse egg. Dev Biol 306(1):241–254
307. Talmor-Cohen A, Tomashov-Matar R, Eliyahu E, Shapiro R, Shalgi R (2004) Are Src family kinases involved in cell cycle resumption in rat eggs? Reproduction 127(4):455–463
308. Meng L, Luo J, Li C, Kinsey WH (2006) Role of Src homology 2 domain-mediated PTK signaling in mouse zygotic development. Reproduction 132(3):413–421
309. Bement WM, Capco DG (1990) Protein kinase C acts downstream of calcium at entry into the first mitotic interphase of *Xenopus laevis*. Cell Regul 1(3):315–326
310. Sun QY, Wang WH, Hosoe M, Taniguchi T, Chen DY, Shioya Y (1997) Activation of protein kinase C induces cortical granule exocytosis in a Ca(2+)-independent manner, but not the resumption of cell cycle in porcine eggs. Dev Growth Differ 39(4):523–529
311. Giusti AF, Carroll DJ, Abassi YA, Terasaki M, Foltz KR, Jaffe LA (1999) Requirement of a Src family kinase for initiating calcium release at fertilization in starfish eggs. J Biol Chem 274(41):29318–29322
312. Giusti AF, Xu W, Hinkle B, Terasaki M, Jaffe LA (2000) Evidence that fertilization activates starfish eggs by sequential activation of a Src-like kinase and phospholipase cgamma. J Biol Chem 275(22):16788–16794
313. Sette C, Bevilacqua A, Bianchini A, Mangia F, Geremia R, Rossi P (1997) Parthenogenetic activation of mouse eggs by microinjection of a truncated c-kit tyrosine kinase present in spermatozoa. Development 124(11):2267–2274

314. Sette C, Paronetto MP, Barchi M, Bevilacqua A, Geremia R, Rossi P (2002) Tr-kit-induced resumption of the cell cycle in mouse eggs requires activation of a Src-like kinase. Embo J 21(20):5386–5395
315. Wu AT, Sutovsky P, Manandhar G et al (2007) PAWP, a sperm-specific WW domain-binding protein, promotes meiotic resumption and pronuclear development during fertilization. J Biol Chem 282(16):12164–12175
316. Sudol M, Chen HI, Bougeret C, Einbond A, Bork P (1995) Characterization of a novel protein-binding module – the WW domain. FEBS Lett 369(1):67–71
317. Sudol M, Sliwa K, Russo T (2001) Functions of WW domains in the nucleus. FEBS Lett 490(3):190–195
318. Wu AT, Sutovsky P, Xu W, van der Spoel AC, Platt FM, Oko R (2007) The postacrosomal assembly of sperm head protein, PAWP, is independent of acrosome formation and dependent on microtubular manchette transport. Dev Biol 312(2):471–483
319. Maleszewski M, Kimura Y, Yanagimachi R (1996) Sperm membrane incorporation into oolemma contributes to the oolemma block to sperm penetration: evidence based on intracytoplasmic sperm injection experiments in the mouse. Mol Reprod Dev 44(2):256–259
320. Fenichel P, Durand-Clement M (1998) Role of integrins during fertilization in mammals. Hum Reprod 13(Suppl 4):31–46
321. White KL, Passipieri M, Bunch TD, Campbell KD, Pate B (2007) Effects of arginine–glycine–aspartic acid (RGD) containing snake venom peptides on parthenogenetic development and in vitro fertilization of bovine oocytes. Mol Reprod Dev 74(1):88–96
322. Campbell KD, Reed WA, White KL (2000) Ability of integrins to mediate fertilization, intracellular calcium release, and parthenogenetic development in bovine oocytes. Biol Reprod 62(6): 1702–1709
323. Yue LM, Zhang L, He YP et al (2004) Integrins mediate the increase of concentration of intracellular free calcium in mouse eggs. Sheng Li Xue Bao 56(3):347–352
324. Igarashi H, Knott JG, Schultz RM, Williams CJ (2007) Alterations of PLCbeta1 in mouse eggs change calcium oscillatory behavior following fertilization. Dev Biol 312(1):321–330
325. Hunter RH (1996) Ovarian control of very low sperm/egg ratios at the commencement of mammalian fertilisation to avoid polyspermy. Mol Reprod Dev 44(3):417–422
326. Monroy A (1953) A model for the cortical reaction of fertilization in the sea-urchin egg. Experientia 9(11):424–425
327. Sun QY (2003) Cellular and molecular mechanisms leading to cortical reaction and polyspermy block in mammalian eggs. Microsc Res Tech 61(4):342–348
328. Hedrick JL (2007) A comparative analysis of molecular mechanisms for blocking polyspermy: identification of a lectin-ligand binding reaction in mammalian eggs. Soc Reprod Fertil Suppl 63:409–419
329. Aviles M, Jaber L, Castells MT, Ballesta J, Kan FW (1997) Modifications of carbohydrate residues and ZP2 and ZP3 glycoproteins in the mouse zona pellucida after fertilization. Biol Reprod 57(5):1155–1163
330. Bleil JD, Beall CF, Wassarman PM (1981) Mammalian sperm–egg interaction: fertilization of mouse eggs triggers modification of the major zona pellucida glycoprotein, ZP2. Dev Biol 86(1):189–197
331. Drobnis EZ, Andrew JB, Katz DF (1988) Biophysical properties of the zona pellucida measured by capillary suction: is zona hardening a mechanical phenomenon? J Exp Zool 245(2):206–219
332. Gould K, Zaneveld LJ, Srivastava PN, Williams WL (1971) Biochemical changes in the zona pellucida of rabbit ova induced by fertilization and sperm enzymes. Proc Soc Exp Biol Med 136(1):6–10
333. Yi YJ, Manandhar G, Sutovsky M et al (2007) Ubiquitin C-terminal hydrolase-activity is involved in sperm acrosomal function and anti-polyspermy defense during porcine fertilization. Biol Reprod 77(5):780–793
334. McCauley TC, Buhi WC, Wu GM et al (2003) Oviduct-specific glycoprotein modulates sperm–zona binding and improves efficiency of porcine fertilization in vitro. Biol Reprod 69(3):828–834
335. Hao Y, Mathialagan N, Walters E et al (2006) Osteopontin reduces polyspermy during in vitro fertilization of porcine oocytes. Biol Reprod 75(5):726–733
336. Sekiguchi S, Kwon J, Yoshida E et al (2006) Localization of ubiquitin C-terminal hydrolase L1 in mouse ova and its function in the plasma membrane to block polyspermy. Am J Pathol 169(5): 1722–1729
337. Gwatkin RB, Rasmusson GH, Williams DT (1976) Induction of the cortical reaction in hamster eggs by membrane-active agents. J Reprod Fertil 47(2):299–303
338. Brewer L, Corzett M, Balhorn R (2002) Condensation of DNA by spermatid basic nuclear proteins. J Biol Chem 277(41):38895–38900
339. Balhorn R (2007) The protamine family of sperm nuclear proteins. Genome Biol 8(9):227
340. Chen HY, Sun JM, Zhang Y, Davie JR, Meistrich ML (1998) Ubiquitination of histone H3 in elongating spermatids of rat testes. J Biol Chem 273(21):13165–13169
341. Roest HP, van Klaveren J, de Wit J et al (1996) Inactivation of the HR6B ubiquitin-conjugating DNA repair enzyme in mice causes male sterility associated with chromatin modification. Cell 86(5):799–810
342. Gao S, Chung YG, Parseghian MH, King GJ, Adashi EY, Latham KE (2004) Rapid H1 linker histone transitions following fertilization or somatic cell nuclear transfer: evidence for a uniform developmental program in mice. Dev Biol 266(1):62–75
343. Tanaka Y, Kato S, Tanaka M, Kuji N, Yoshimura Y (2003) Structure and expression of the human oocyte-specific histone H1 gene elucidated by direct RT-nested PCR of a single oocyte. Biochem Biophys Res Commun 304(2):351–357
344. Teranishi T, Tanaka M, Kimoto S et al (2004) Rapid replacement of somatic linker histones with the oocyte-specific linker histone H1foo in nuclear transfer. Dev Biol 266(1):76–86
345. Perreault SD, Wolff RA, Zirkin BR (1984) The role of disulfide bond reduction during mammalian sperm nuclear decondensation in vivo. Dev Biol 101(1):160–167
346. Sutovsky P, Schatten G (1997) Depletion of glutathione during bovine oocyte maturation reversibly blocks the decondensation of the male pronucleus and pronuclear apposition during fertilization. Biol Reprod 56(6):1503–1512
347. Ward WS, Kishikawa H, Akutsu H, Yanagimachi H, Yanagimachi R (2000) Further evidence that sperm nuclear proteins are necessary for embryogenesis. Zygote 8(1):51–56
348. Burns KH, Viveiros MM, Ren Y et al (2003) Roles of NPM2 in chromatin and nucleolar organization in oocytes and embryos. Science 300(5619):633–636
349. Sutovsky P, Simerly C, Hewitson L, Schatten G (1998) Assembly of nuclear pore complexes and annulate lamellae promotes normal pronuclear development in fertilized mammalian oocytes. J Cell Sci 111(Pt 19):2841–2854
350. Payne C, Rawe V, Ramalho-Santos J, Simerly C, Schatten G (2003) Preferentially localized dynein and perinuclear dynactin associate with nuclear pore complex proteins to mediate genomic union during mammalian fertilization. J Cell Sci 116(Pt 23): 4727–4738
351. Alizadeh Z, Kageyama S, Aoki F (2005) Degradation of maternal mRNA in mouse embryos: selective degradation of specific mRNAs after fertilization. Mol Reprod Dev 72(3):281–290
352. Tadros W, Houston SA, Bashirullah A et al (2003) Regulation of maternal transcript destabilization during egg activation in Drosophila. Genetics 164(3):989–1001

353. DeRenzo C, Seydoux G (2004) A clean start: degradation of maternal proteins at the oocyte-to-embryo transition. Trends Cell Biol 14(8):420–426
354. Memili E, First NL (1999) Control of gene expression at the onset of bovine embryonic development. Biol Reprod 61(5):1198–1207
355. Hamatani T, Carter MG, Sharov AA, Ko MS (2004) Dynamics of global gene expression changes during mouse preimplantation development. Dev Cell 6(1):117–131
356. Adenot PG, Mercier Y, Renard JP, Thompson EM (1997) Differential H4 acetylation of paternal and maternal chromatin precedes DNA replication and differential transcriptional activity in pronuclei of 1-cell mouse embryos. Development 124(22): 4615–4625
357. Aoki F, Worrad DM, Schultz RM (1997) Regulation of transcriptional activity during the first and second cell cycles in the preimplantation mouse embryo. Dev Biol 181(2):296–307
358. Worrad DM, Ram PT, Schultz RM (1994) Regulation of gene expression in the mouse oocyte and early preimplantation embryo: developmental changes in Sp1 and TATA box-binding protein, TBP. Development 120(8):2347–2357
359. Maddox-Hyttel P, Svarcova O, Laurincik J (2007) Ribosomal RNA and nucleolar proteins from the oocyte are to some degree used for embryonic nucleolar formation in cattle and pig. Theriogenology 68(Suppl 1):S63–S70
360. Hay-Schmidt A, Viuff D, Greve T, Hyttel P (2001) Transcriptional activity in in vivo developed early cleavage stage bovine embryos. Theriogenology 56(1):167–176
361. Dieleman SJ, Hendriksen PJ, Viuff D et al (2002) Effects of in vivo prematuration and in vivo final maturation on developmental capacity and quality of pre-implantation embryos. Theriogenology 57(1):5–20
362. Schultz RM (1993) Regulation of zygotic gene activation in the mouse. Bioessays 15(8):531–538
363. Brown EJ (2004) Analysis of cell cycle progression and genomic integrity in early lethal knockouts. Methods Mol Biol 280:201–212
364. Schultz RM, Davis W Jr, Stein P, Svoboda P (1999) Reprogramming of gene expression during preimplantation development. J Exp Zool 285(3):276–282
365. Morgan HD, Santos F, Green K, Dean W, Reik W (2005) Epigenetic reprogramming in mammals. Hum Mol Genet 14(Spec No 1):R47–R58
366. Bultman SJ, Gebuhr TC, Pan H, Svoboda P, Schultz RM, Magnuson T (2006) Maternal BRG1 regulates zygotic genome activation in the mouse. Genes Dev 20(13):1744–1754
367. Torres-Padilla ME, Zernicka-Goetz M (2006) Role of TIF1alpha as a modulator of embryonic transcription in the mouse zygote. J Cell Biol 174(3):329–338
368. Schultz RM (2002) The molecular foundations of the maternal to zygotic transition in the preimplantation embryo. Hum Reprod Update 8(4):323–331
369. Bird A (2002) DNA methylation patterns and epigenetic memory. Genes Dev 16(1):6–21
370. Dean W, Lucifero D, Santos F (2005) DNA methylation in mammalian development and disease. Birth Defects Res C Embryo Today 75(2):98–111
371. Hamerton JL, Giannelli F, Collins F et al (1969) Non-random x-inactivation in the female mule. Nature 222(5200):1277–1278
372. Mohandas T, Sparkes RS, Shapiro LJ (1981) Reactivation of an inactive human X chromosome: evidence for X inactivation by DNA methylation. Science 211(4480):393–396
373. Lyon MF (1961) Gene action in the X-chromosome of the mouse (Mus musculus L.). Nature 190:372–373
374. Daniels R, Zuccotti M, Kinis T, Serhal P, Monk M (1997) XIST expression in human oocytes and preimplantation embryos. Am J Hum Genet 61(1):33–39
375. Zuccotti M, Boiani M, Ponce R et al (2002) Mouse Xist expression begins at zygotic genome activation and is timed by a zygotic clock. Mol Reprod Dev 61(1):14–20
376. Brown CJ, Ballabio A, Rupert JL et al (1991) A gene from the region of the human X inactivation centre is expressed exclusively from the inactive X chromosome. Nature 349(6304):38–44
377. Plath K, Mlynarczyk-Evans S, Nusinow DA, Panning B (2002) Xist RNA and the mechanism of X chromosome inactivation. Annu Rev Genet 36:233–278
378. Masui O, Heard E (2006) RNA and protein actors in X-chromosome inactivation. Cold Spring Harb Symp Quant Biol 71:419–428
379. Senda S, Wakayama T, Yamazaki Y et al (2004) Skewed X-inactivation in cloned mice. Biochem Biophys Res Commun 321(1):38–44
380. Xue F, Tian XC, Du F et al (2002) Aberrant patterns of X chromosome inactivation in bovine clones. Nat Genet 31(2):216–220
381. Jiang L, Lai L, Samuel M, Prather RS, Yang X, Tian XC (2008) Expression of X-linked genes in deceased neonates and surviving cloned female piglets. Mol Reprod Dev 75(2):265–273
382. Longo FJ (1976) Sperm aster in rabbit zygotes: its structure and function. J Cell Biol 69(3):539–547
383. Schatten H, Schatten G (1986) Motility and centrosomal organization during sea urchin and mouse fertilization. Cell Motil Cytoskeleton 6(2):163–175
384. Manandhar G, Schatten H, Sutovsky P (2005) Centrosome reduction during gametogenesis and its significance. Biol Reprod 72(1):2–13
385. Azimzadeh J, Bornens M (2007) Structure and duplication of the centrosome. J Cell Sci 120(Pt 13):2139–2142
386. Szollosi D, Ozil JP (1991) De novo formation of centrioles in parthenogenetically activated, diploidized rabbit embryos. Biol Cell 72(1–2):61–66
387. Manandhar G, Simerly C, Schatten G (2000) Highly degenerated distal centrioles in rhesus and human spermatozoa. Hum Reprod 15(2):256–263
388. Manandhar G, Sutovsky P, Joshi HC, Stearns T, Schatten G (1998) Centrosome reduction during mouse spermiogenesis. Dev Biol 203(2):424–434
389. Le Guen P, Crozet N (1989) Microtubule and centrosome distribution during sheep fertilization. Eur J Cell Biol 48(2):239–249
390. Szollosi D, Szollosi MS, Czolowska R, Tarkowski AK (1990) Sperm penetration into immature mouse oocytes and nuclear changes during maturation: an EM study. Biol Cell 69(1):53–64
391. Sathananthan AH, Kola I, Osborne J et al (1991) Centrioles in the beginning of human development. Proc Natl Acad Sci U S A 88(11):4806–4810
392. Rawe VY, Díaz ES, Abdelmassih R et al (2008) The role of sperm proteasomes during sperm aster formation and early zygote development: Implications for fertilization failure in humans. Hum Reprod 23(3):573–580
393. Navara CS, First NL, Schatten G (1994) Microtubule organization in the cow during fertilization, polyspermy, parthenogenesis, and nuclear transfer: the role of the sperm aster. Dev Biol 162(1):29–40
394. Asch R, Simerly C, Ord T, Ord VA, Schatten G (1995) The stages at which human fertilization arrests: microtubule and chromosome configurations in inseminated oocytes which failed to complete fertilization and development in humans. Hum Reprod 10(7): 1897–1906
395. Obasaju M, Kadam A, Sultan K, Fateh M, Munne S (1999) Sperm quality may adversely affect the chromosome constitution of embryos that result from intracytoplasmic sperm injection. Fertil Steril 72(6):1113–1115
396. Kovacic B, Vlaisavljevic V (2000) Configuration of maternal and paternal chromatin and pertaining microtubules in human oocytes

failing to fertilize after intracytoplasmic sperm injection. Mol Reprod Dev 55(2):197–204
397. Palermo GD, Colombero LT, Rosenwaks Z (1997) The human sperm centrosome is responsible for normal syngamy and early embryonic development. Rev Reprod 2(1):19–27
398. Terada Y, Simerly CR, Hewitson L, Schatten G (2000) Sperm aster formation and pronuclear decondensation during rabbit fertilization and development of a functional assay for human sperm. Biol Reprod 62(3):557–563
399. Van Blerkom J, Davis P (1995) Evolution of the sperm aster after microinjection of isolated human sperm centrosomes into meiotically mature human oocytes. Hum Reprod 10(8):2179–2182
400. Shalgi R, Magnus A, Jones R, Phillips DM (1994) Fate of sperm organelles during early embryogenesis in the rat. Mol Reprod Dev 37(3):264–271
401. Escalier D (2006) Knockout mouse models of sperm flagellum anomalies. Hum Reprod Update 12(4):449–461
402. Fawcett DW (1975) The mammalian spermatozoon. Dev Biol 44(2):394–436
403. Ankel-Simons F, Cummins JM (1996) Misconceptions about mitochondria and mammalian fertilization: implications for theories on human evolution. Proc Natl Acad Sci U S A 93(24): 13859–13863
404. Sutovsky P (2003) Ubiquitin-dependent proteolysis in mammalian spermatogenesis, fertilization, and sperm quality control: killing three birds with one stone. Microsc Res Tech 61(1):88–102
405. Sutovsky P, Moreno RD, Ramalho-Santos J, Dominko T, Simerly C, Schatten G (1999) Ubiquitin tag for sperm mitochondria. Nature 402(6760):371–372
406. Sutovsky P, Moreno RD, Ramalho-Santos J, Dominko T, Simerly C, Schatten G (2000) Ubiquitinated sperm mitochondria, selective proteolysis, and the regulation of mitochondrial inheritance in mammalian embryos. Biol Reprod 63(2):582–590
407. Sutovsky P, Van Leyen K, McCauley T, Day BN, Sutovsky M (2004) Degradation of paternal mitochondria after fertilization: implications for heteroplasmy, assisted reproductive technologies and mtDNA inheritance. Reprod Biomed Online 8(1):24–33
408. Hiendleder S (2007) Mitochondrial DNA inheritance after SCNT. Adv Exp Med Biol 591:103–116
409. St John JC, Lloyd R, El Shourbagy S (2004) The potential risks of abnormal transmission of mtDNA through assisted reproductive technologies. Reprod Biomed Online 8(1):34–44
410. Aitken RJ, De Iuliis GN (2007) Origins and consequences of DNA damage in male germ cells. Reprod Biomed Online 14(6): 727–733
411. Kaneda H, Hayashi J, Takahama S, Taya C, Lindahl KF, Yonekawa H (1995) Elimination of paternal mitochondrial DNA in intraspecific crosses during early mouse embryogenesis. Proc Natl Acad Sci U S A 92(10):4542–4546
412. Shitara H, Hayashi JI, Takahama S, Kaneda H, Yonekawa H (1998) Maternal inheritance of mouse mtDNA in interspecific hybrids: segregation of the leaked paternal mtDNA followed by the prevention of subsequent paternal leakage. Genetics 148(2): 851–857
413. Hayashida K, Omagari K, Masuda J et al (2005) The sperm mitochondria-specific translocator has a key role in maternal mitochondrial inheritance. Cell Biol Int 29(6):472–481
414. Nishimura Y, Yoshinari T, Naruse K et al (2006) Active digestion of sperm mitochondrial DNA in single living sperm revealed by optical tweezers. Proc Natl Acad Sci U S A 103(5):1382–1387
415. Schwartz M, Vissing J (2002) Paternal inheritance of mitochondrial DNA. N Engl J Med 347(8):576–580
416. Marchington DR, Scott Brown MS, Lamb VK et al (2002) No evidence for paternal mtDNA transmission to offspring or extra-embryonic tissues after ICSI. Mol Hum Reprod 8(11):1046–1049
417. Barritt JA, Brenner CA, Malter HE, Cohen J (2001) Rebuttal: interooplasmic transfers in humans. Reprod Biomed Online 3(1):47–48
418. Hiraoka J, Hirao Y (1988) Fate of sperm tail components after incorporation into the hamster egg. Gamete Res 19(4):369–380
419. Simerly CR, Hecht NB, Goldberg E, Schatten G (1993) Tracing the incorporation of the sperm tail in the mouse zygote and early embryo using an anti-testicular alpha-tubulin antibody. Dev Biol 158(2):536–548
420. Sutovsky P, Hewitson L, Simerly CR et al (1996) Intracytoplasmic sperm injection for Rhesus monkey fertilization results in unusual chromatin, cytoskeletal, and membrane events, but eventually leads to pronuclear development and sperm aster assembly. Hum Reprod 11(8):1703–1712
421. Ramalho-Santos J, Sutovsky P, Simerly C et al (2000) ICSI choreography: fate of sperm structures after monospermic rhesus ICSI and first cell cycle implications. Hum Reprod 15(12):2610–2620
422. Ajduk A, Yamauchi Y, Ward MA (2006) Sperm chromatin remodeling after intracytoplasmic sperm injection differs from that of in vitro fertilization. Biol Reprod 75(3):442–451
423. Terada Y, Luetjens CM, Sutovsky P, Schatten G (2000) Atypical decondensation of the sperm nucleus, delayed replication of the male genome, and sex chromosome positioning following intracytoplasmic human sperm injection (ICSI) into golden hamster eggs: does ICSI itself introduce chromosomal anomalies? Fertil Steril 74(3):454–460
424. Battaglia DE, Koehler JK, Klein NA, Tucker MJ (1997) Failure of oocyte activation after intracytoplasmic sperm injection using round-headed sperm. Fertil Steril 68(1):118–122
425. Kim ST, Cha YB, Park JM, Gye MC (2001) Successful pregnancy and delivery from frozen-thawed embryos after intracytoplasmic sperm injection using round-headed spermatozoa and assisted oocyte activation in a globozoospermic patient with mosaic Down syndrome. Fertil Steril 75(2):445–447
426. Rybouchkin AV, Van der Straeten F, Quatacker J, De Sutter P, Dhont M (1997) Fertilization and pregnancy after assisted oocyte activation and intracytoplasmic sperm injection in a case of round-headed sperm associated with deficient oocyte activation capacity. Fertil Steril 68(6):1144–1147
427. Sengoku K, Tamate K, Takaoka Y et al (1999) Requirement of sperm–oocyte plasma membrane fusion for establishment of the plasma membrane block to polyspermy in human pronuclear oocytes. Mol Reprod Dev 52(2):183–188
428. Wortzman-Show GB, Kurokawa M, Fissore RA, Evans JP (2007) Calcium and sperm components in the establishment of the membrane block to polyspermy: studies of ICSI and activation with sperm factor. Mol Hum Reprod 13(8):557–565
429. Morozumi K, Yanagimachi R (2005) Incorporation of the acrosome into the oocyte during intracytoplasmic sperm injection could be potentially hazardous to embryo development. Proc Natl Acad Sci U S A 102(40):14209–14214
430. Morozumi K, Shikano T, Miyazaki S, Yanagimachi R (2006) Simultaneous removal of sperm plasma membrane and acrosome before intracytoplasmic sperm injection improves oocyte activation/embryonic development. Proc Natl Acad Sci U S A 103(47): 17661–17666
431. Katayama M, Sutovsky P, Yang BS et al (2005) Increased disruption of sperm plasma membrane at sperm immobilization promotes dissociation of perinuclear theca from sperm chromatin after intracytoplasmic sperm injection in pigs. Reproduction 130(6):907–916
432. Takeuchi T, Colombero LT, Neri QV, Rosenwaks Z, Palermo GD (2004) Does ICSI require acrosomal disruption? An ultrastructural study. Hum Reprod 19(1):114–117
433. Gomez-Torres MJ, Ten J, Girela JL, Romero J, Bernabeu R, De Juan J (2007) Sperm immobilized before intracytoplasmic

sperm injection undergo ultrastructural damage and acrosomal disruption. Fertil Steril 88(3):702–704
434. Dozortsev D, Rybouchkin A, De Sutter P, Dhont M (1995) Sperm plasma membrane damage prior to intracytoplasmic sperm injection: a necessary condition for sperm nucleus decondensation. Hum Reprod 10(11):2960–2964
435. Pasten C, Morales P, Kong M (2005) Role of the sperm proteasome during fertilization and gamete interaction in the mouse. Mol Reprod Dev 71(2):209–219
436. Wang WH, Day BN, Wu GM (2003) How does polyspermy happen in mammalian oocytes? Microsc Res Tech 61(4): 335–341
437. Sun QY, Fuchimoto D, Nagai T (2004) Regulatory roles of ubiquitin–proteasome pathway in pig oocyte meiotic maturation and fertilization. Theriogenology 62(1–2):245–255
438. Wang H, Song C, Duan C et al (2002) Effects of ubiquitin–proteasome pathway on mouse sperm capacitation, acrosome reaction and in vitro fertilization. Chin Sci Bull 47:127–132

Chapter 26
Advanced Tests of Sperm Function

Joseph P. Alukal and Dolores J. Lamb

Abstract Sperm function tests assess the presence or absence of factors needed for proper fertilization and initiation of embryogenesis; put differently, these tests measure the ability of a sperm to deliver a normal haploid complement of chromosomes to an oocyte. Advanced tests of sperm function have helped us to gain a tremendous understanding of the physiology of sperm capacitation, acrosome reaction, and sperm–ovum interaction. For this reason alone, an understanding of these tests is still vitally important to the practicing andrologist, reproductive endocrinologist, or embryologist. These tests do accurately predict the likelihood of success with IUI (with or without ovarian hyperstimulation) or IVF. Unfortunately, with the increased use of IVF/ICSI, these tests are less widely used by physicians. Despite this, the usage of these tests to properly identify which couples need to proceed to IVF/ICSI (due to a low likelihood of success with IUI or IVF alone) would represent a significant step forward toward a cost-efficient and health-conscious treatment algorithm for couples with infertility.

Keywords Sperm function • Aneuploidy • Capacitation • Acrosome reaction • DNA damage • Sperm penetration assay • Hemizona assay

26.1 Introduction

Despite a growing understanding of the causes of male infertility, as many as 25% of patients never have an underlying etiology for their infertility identified [1]. These patients, whose diagnosis is termed idiopathic male infertility, have an absence of abnormality on standard semen analysis and endocrine evaluation, in addition to a normal physical exam. They represent a complex subset of male infertility, and their evaluation can often be frustrating to even the most experienced practitioners.

The routine semen analysis does not provide a measure of fertility potential. It was theorized that some significant percentage of infertile patients had abnormalities of sperm function that were not readily evident on standard semen analysis. These abnormalities would therefore have to affect such important sperm functions such as cervical mucus penetration, capacitation, sperm–zona pellucida binding, sperm–ova binding, decondensation and fertilization of the oocyte. In order to define these abnormalities, tests assessing these unique functions of spermatozoa were developed. These tests, in addition to their proper utilization and interpretation, are reviewed in this chapter.

Thinking more broadly, sperm function can be considered to be simply summarized as the ability of a single spermatozoon to deliver an appropriate haploid chromosome complement to an ovum. As such, those sperm that have normal motility, cervical mucus penetration, and ova binding, might still be considered functionally deficient if they have an abnormal chromosome complement, or poorly packaged DNA. As such, a brief consideration of both sperm aneuploidy, as assessed by fluorescence in-situ hybridization (sperm FISH), and sperm DNA damage is included in this chapter.

Importantly, the development of intracytoplasmic sperm injection (IVF/ICSI) as an adjunct treatment to in vitro fertilization (IVF) offered patients with abnormal sperm function a renewed hope with regard to having biological children. ICSI enabled otherwise normal spermatozoa to be directly injected into an oocyte, thereby obviating the need for normal sperm function with regard to capacitation and fertilization. As a result of this, the clinical usage of these tests decreased significantly since the onset of ICSI. This is unfortunate as proper evaluation prior to unexpected IVF failure can identify those patients with functional deficiencies and otherwise normal semen parameters who would benefit from the use of ICSI. Thus, the topic of advanced testing of sperm

J.P. Alukal
Scott Department of Urology, Baylor College of Medicine, Houston, TX, USA

D.J. Lamb (✉)
Laboratory for Male Reproductive Research and Testing,
Scott Department of Urology, Baylor College of Medicine,
One Baylor Plaza, N 730/MS 380, Houston, TX 77030, USA
e-mail: dlamb@bcm.edu

D.T. Carrell and C.M. Peterson (eds.), *Reproductive Endocrinology and Infertility: Integrating Modern Clinical and Laboratory Practice*,
DOI 10.1007/978-1-4419-1436-1_26,

function remains vitally important to the understanding of the physiology of fertilization and the many abnormalities that can interfere with this process.

26.1.1 Sperm DNA Damage

A limited consideration of this topic follows here; for a more complete discussion, please see Chap. 30. Taken together, the different tests of sperm DNA damage assess how well the haploid DNA content of each individual sperm is packaged. These tests include acridine orange staining (AO), the sperm chromatin structural assay (SCSA), terminal deoxynucleotidyl transferase-mediated nick end labeling (TUNEL), and the Comet assay (single cell gel electrophoresis – Figs. 26.1 and 26.2). Each test measures sperm DNA integrity in a different fashion; importantly, all of them with the exception of acridine orange staining alone correlate well with each other and with other semen analysis parameters such as density [2]. Moreover, recent work indicates that sperm DNA damage may help predict ART success [3] and predict likelihood of recurrent pregnancy loss [4]. Sperm DNA damage may also serve as a reliable marker of correction of fertility impairing conditions such as varicocele [5]. Clearly, the utility of this test as a measure of sperm function is growing.

26.1.2 Sperm FISH for Chromosomal Aneuploidy

Chromosomal aneuploidy (abnormality in the number of whole chromosomes) results typically from nondisjunction events germ cell meiosis. The result of this is sperm that are either disomic or nullisomic for a particular chromosome. From a reproductive standpoint, this is important in that fertilization with these sperm results in embryos which are either monosomic or trisomic; many of these embryos are spontaneously aborted during pregnancy (resulting in couples presenting with recurrent pregnancy loss) or in offspring which are syndromic (Turner, Down, or Klinefelter Syndromes for example). As such, evaluation of sperm for abnormal numbers of aneuploid cells in couples with normal somatic karyotype presenting with (a) recurrent pregnancy loss (b) prior birth of an infant with a chromosomal disorder of numerical abnormality seems warranted.

To this end, researchers began considering sperm aneuploidy in the 1990s using fluorescent in-situ hybridization in decondensed sperm nuclei [6, 7].

Importantly, normal fertile controls were found to have a relatively standard degree of chromosomal aneuploidy; this included normal values of autosomal disomy of around 0.13% and sex chromosome disomy in 0.37% of sperm [6]. These numbers are in sharp distinction to those observed in infertile men (with normal karyotype). In these men, decrease of aneuploidy increased as standard semen analysis parameters worsened [8].

Other important correlations with sperm aneuploidy have been noted including correlation with higher likelihoods of recurrent pregnancy loss [9]. Work in this laboratory has identified extremely high degrees of sperm aneuploidy in patients with severe oligoasthenoteratozoospermia; these patients also had higher likelihood of failing assisted reproduction. As such, we continue to recommend this test for couples with recurrent pregnancy loss and for couples with history of two or more failed assisted reproductive

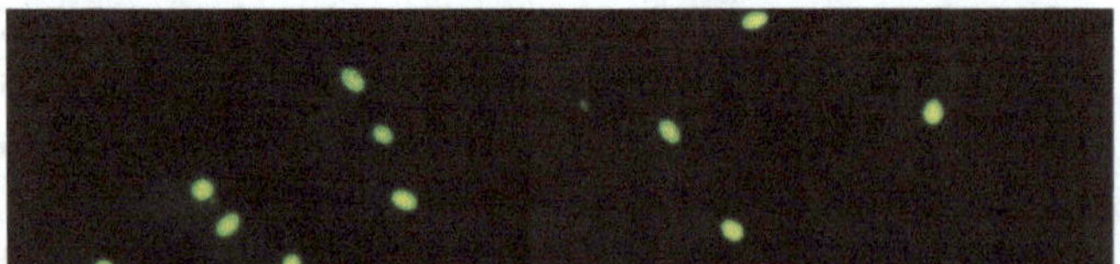

Fig. 26.1 Normal result; sperm DNA damage via modified COMET assay, 40× image

Fig. 26.2 Abnormal result; sperm DNA damage via modified COMET assay, 40× image

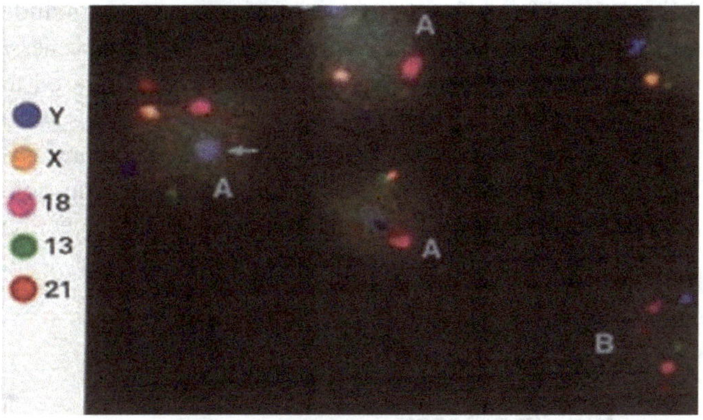

Fig. 26.3 Five color probe fluorescence in-situ hybridization, 100× composite image, Cells marked A have appropriate haploid chromosome complement, Cell marked B is diploid

techniques (ARTs). This is in spite of the labor intensive nature of this test and its relatively high cost.

In our laboratory, multicolor FISH is performed on fixed and decondensed sperm using two sets of probes (tri-color for 18, X, and Y, dual-color for 13 and 21 – Fig. 26.3). Directed probes can be used in cases of known chromosomal abnormality (e.g., abnormal karyotype of fetal remains). FISH results are analyzed by an automated system (Bioview©, Bioview Ltd., Israel) which utilizes computerized cell counting techniques. Results are then confirmed by technicians experienced with manual sperm FISH, and interpreted by qualified personnel. Automation of this process has resulted in an increased efficiency and accuracy in the performance of this difficult and labor intensive test (unpublished data).

26.2 Hypo-osmotic Swelling Test

Possibly the simplest assessment of advanced sperm function is found in the hypo-osmotic swelling test (HOST); this test answers the basic question of whether immotile sperm are alive (with an intact membrane) and are immotile or immotile due to the fact that they are dead. As a test of sperm viability, HOST depends upon the fact that a normal, live spermatozoon can maintain an osmotic gradient when placed in hypo-osmotic conditions. Specifically, when placed in a hypo-osmotic solution (150 mOsm/L or less), living spermatozoon absorb fluid in an effort to maintain an appropriate osmotic condition. The result of this fluid absorption is swelling of the plasma membrane and curling of the tail. Initially described by Jeyendren et al., a normal ejaculated semen sample demonstrates >60% viability when assessed with this test [10].

HOST has a limited list of appropriate uses. It may be helpful in prediction of both IUI and IVF success [11, 12]. Most importantly, the test can be used in the diagnostic evaluation of the infertile male with a question of absent motility due to causes such as immotile cilia syndrome. A normal HOST test in these patients is consistent with viable, but immotile cells, and should prompt genetic testing for causes such as Kartagener's in addition to electron microscopy of sperm tails to identify specific abnormalities in the cytoskeletal architecture of the tail [13, 14]. The other important use of this test is to identify live but immotile sperm obtained at the time of testicular sperm extraction (TESE)-ICSI. Rare sperm found during examination of the testis sample is placed in the hypotonic solution – if swelling occurs, the sperm is immediately placed in injection medium and then used for ICSI. The test has provided a useful adjunct to the TESE-ICSI procedure.

26.3 Cervical Mucus/Sperm Interaction Assay

In much the same way that IVF/ICSI has made many of the tests of sperm–egg interaction less important, intrauterine insemination (IUI), in addition to the ARTs, has minimized the utility of assessments of cervical mucus and sperm. Traditionally assessed using the postcoital test (PCT), assessments of cervical mucus/sperm interaction attempt to quantify the ease with which ejaculated sperm can pass through cervical mucus. Abnormalities of cervical mucus/sperm interaction preventing passage of ejaculated sperm into the uterus from the vagina account for 10% of couples presenting with infertility [15]. As such, even though importance of this test is diminished given modern treatment options in the management of infertile couples, an understanding of the clinical implication of abnormal cervical mucus/sperm interaction is still useful.

Postcoital testing can be performed using numerous protocols; most typically, an aspirate of cervical mucus is taken within one-half hour of intercourse performed at midcycle. The mucus is examined microscopically for such characteristics as ferning, spinnbarkeit and for the number and motility of sperm observed. In a normal test, at least 20 motile sperm are identified per high power field. Causes of abnormal tests can include inappropriately timed coitus, endocrine abnormalities in the female partner, cross-reacting antisperm antibodies, poor semen quality, and coexisting genital tract infection.

Importantly, one of the major limitations of PCT is its inability to distinguish the causes for poor cervical mucus/sperm interaction in the male and female. The TruTrax assay (Humagen) attempted to overcome this limitation by simultaneously assessing sperm interaction with both human and bovine cervical mucus. Studies supported the reliability, reproducibility, and clinical importance of this test [16], however, it is no longer commercially available.

The utilization of PCT has decreased, especially in light of increasing usage of IVF/ICSI. This is despite the data that clearly shows (a) that PCT can predict the likelihood of IUI success [17–20] and (b) that PCT can predict the need for ovarian hyperstimulation in the setting of IUI [21, 22]. Utilization of IVF/ICSI has simply made these questions obsolete.

26.4 Sperm Capacitation Assays and Acrosome Reaction Assays

Capacitation is a series of changes that occurs in the spermatozoon during passage through the female reproductive tract (specifically in fallopian tube) that results in a change in membrane permeability to calcium ions. This in turn results in hypermotility of the spermatozoon in addition to enabling the numerous changes that allow the spermatozoon to proceed through the acrosome reaction and successfully bind the zona pellucida.

While assays to define some aspects of the ability to achieve capacitation have been developed, they are of limited clinical utility. Research in capacitation continues with the goal of interfering with the process for the purposes of contraception [23–25].

If the endpoint of capacitation is the ability of a spermatozoon to undergo the acrosome reaction (AR), it would stand to reason that assessments of the AR are also important. Ejaculated spermatozoa, not having undergone capacitation naturally, do not easily undergo the AR; less than 10% of ejaculated spermatozoa from a normal fertile male can be induced to undergo the AR [26].

In vivo, the AR represents the release of hydrolases that subsequently enable binding and penetration of the zona pellucida by a single spermatozoon. These hydrolases are released from the acrosome itself, which is an organelle unique to spermatozoa. Essentially a modified Golgi apparatus, the acrosome is found in normal spermatozoa between the inner and outer acrosomal membranes, deep to the sperm plasma membrane. Among the many hydrolases found within the acrosome, acrosin is the predominant one. Importantly, the AR occurs specifically when the sperm plasma membrane and the outer acrosomal membrane fuse; again, this process requires capacitation to have occurred.

In vitro assessments of the acrosome reaction included specific stains and antibodies to the acrosomal components [27, 28]; perhaps, the most widely used of these was the triple stain technique [29]. Importantly, in vitro assessments of AR require ejaculated spermatozoa to have undergone ex vivo capacitation [30, 31]. Compounds that induce capacitation ex vivo include progesterone and calcium ionophore A23187 [30, 32, 33]. Again, despite the fact that some studies did correlate abnormal AR assay results with poorer likelihood of successful IVF, the use of the AR assay is increasingly limited. It has fallen out of favor for a number of reasons; these include the development of IVF/ICSI and the labor intensiveness/unreliability of the test at baseline. The test can be used to definitively identify globozoospermia (round headed sperm) with associated total absence of the acrosome; this represents an important genetic defect of spermatogenesis. The gold standard diagnostic test for this condition is also electron microscopy (rarely used in the andrology laboratory).

26.5 Hemizona and Zona-Pellucida Binding Assay

Tests measuring the ability of spermatozoa to bind the zona pellucida with high affinity were first designed by Burkman et al. in 1988 [34]. This built upon the work by Overstreet [35] that considered the nature of sperm–ZP binding in non-viable ova that had been harvested from cancer patients. This, and other, research demonstrated that sperm from IVF-failure couples routinely bound the zona pellucida with less efficacy than sperm taken from fertile controls [36].

Methodologically, the test requires micromanipulation of ovum or ova in question; these ova are bisected, and the two resulting fragments of zona pellucida (hemizona) are removed. These can be stored in preservative without significant rates of loss. Using either fresh or preserved zona, the test is performed using both subject and donor sperm after an isolating wash (either swim-up or Percoll gradient centrifugation). Sperm are incubated with the hemizona for a fixed period of time (41 h) and are then gently washed. Hemizona are then examined using phase-contrast microscopy and the number of sperm bound to each ZP are counted and compared. An index is calculated from this; previous work determined a cutoff of 35% of normal to indicate likelihood of IVF success [37]. The assay requires technical expertise in micromanipulation (cutting the zona pellucida), and it is limited by the fact that it is performed upon ova from failed IVF cycles – ova which may not be normal.

Importantly, modifications to sperm–ZP binding assays have made them more useful. Most specifically, Liu et al. described competitive zona-pellucida binding using fluorescently labeled sperm with different fluors used for the test subject and the donor [36] This simple modification did away with the need to compare hemizona; instead donor and test subject sperm could be incubated with whole ova and allowed to competitively bind. Using standard fluorescence microscopy, an index is again calculated. As a result of this modification, micromanipulation of ova is not necessary to perform the test, which increases the potential of its widespread utilization. In addition, this test allows for the assessment of IVF failed ovum for male versus female factor. When assessing these ova with both control and patient sperm simultaneously, failure to bind the ZP by any sperm implies an egg factor while failure of patient sperm alone to bind implies male factor [36]. This represents a significant step forward in the utility of zona pellucida binding assays.

Interestingly, work from Huszar and colleagues elaborates on this point; these researchers observed that sperm that bound the ZP well also bound hyaluronic acid (HA) beads with an increased affinity [38]. They hypothesized that both ZP and HA binding might be indicative of sperm maturity, and subsequent work confirmed that poor HA binding correlated with poorer strict morphology [39], higher levels of aneuploidy [39], and poorer ICSI outcomes in animal studies [40]. They continue to work along this theory with the hopes of developing a reversible HA binding "trap" that would allow for the selection of mature sperm to be used in IVF/ICSI.

Despite this, usage of ZP binding assays and other related functional tests is still minimal. Increasing usage of IVF/ICSI as a treatment option again plays a significant role; in addition, many labs and clinics did not develop familiarity with the test when it required expertise in micromanipulation (bisection of ova and creation of hemizona), and as such, did not create room for the test in their diagnostic algorithm. In the modern ART lab, this test should be part of a workup of couples that helps direct them to an appropriate reproductive choice. In other words, this test, when properly utilized, can help determine which patients need to proceed to IVF/ICSI, by providing some indication of which patients will fail IVF. If further evolution of this line of testing allows for better selection of mature sperm for ICSI, thereby improving ICSI success rates, this would also represent a significant advance over our current practice.

26.6 Sperm Penetration Assay (or Zona-Free Hamster Oocyte Penetration Assay)

Based upon the observation that human sperm will successfully penetrate zona-free hamster oocytes in vitro, first noted by Yanagamachi et al. in 1976 [41], the sperm penetration assay (SPA), is a test of the ability of spermatozoa to (a) undergo capacitation, (b) fuse with the egg membrane, and (c) disperse sperm DNA content thereby resulting in the formation of the male pronucleus. This complicated test of sperm function was developed in the late 1970s and corresponded with the initial development and utilization of IVF. Practitioners correctly hypothesized that SPA testing might offer useful predictive information regarding IVF success.

Numerous series did correlate normal SPA results with IVF success, with an acceptable number of false-positive results [42, 43]. However, a disproportionate number of false negatives were observed, implying that sperm that failed the SPA were actually able to fertilize oocytes with an acceptable success rate in vitro. Ultimately, this difference was attributed to variability in the rate at which spermatozoa undergo capacitation [44].

With an effort to improving this test, modifications were made to the routine SPA protocol in our laboratory (see Fig. 26.4) [45, 46]. This "optimized SPA" maximized penetration rates through a standardized incubation protocol for spermatozoa (4°C for 42 h in test-yolk buffer followed by a rapid warming protocol); as a result, false negative results were decreased, thereby improving sensitivity. This was

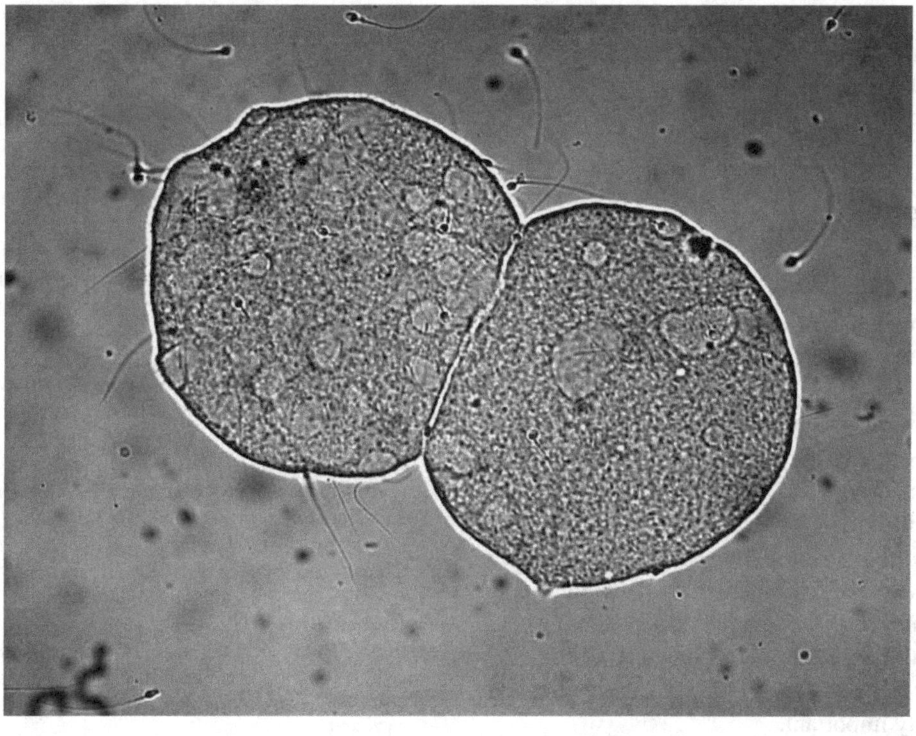

Fig. 26.4 Hamster ovum sperm penetration assay; phase contrast microscopy, 40×. Lighter regions on surface of ovum are decondensed sperm. Some bound sperm that have not yet decondensed are also evident

accomplished while maintaining an appropriate specificity and positive predictive value when used as a predictor of IVF success.

Importantly, the improvement in penetration rates observed as a result of this incubation mandates that sperm penetration is assessed in a different fashion than that which is reported in other descriptions of the test. An average number of penetrations per oocyte is calculated (p/o); this is termed the "sperm capacitation index." Anywhere from 5–50 penetrations per oocyte or more may be observed in a normal result; abnormal results are defined as less than five penetrations per oocyte. Again, these thresholds were successfully validated prospectively using IVF success as the primary outcome [45].

SPA, regardless of the methodology used, is a highly complex bioassay. The important keys to its successful utilization include the stringent use of standards and controls to maintain bioassay control, as well as a laboratory-specific definition of the normal range. The test is highly predictive of a positive outcome in IVF, but cannot predict fertilization failures due to defects in sperm–zona interactions or an egg factor. Its utilization in the evaluation of infertile couples has also decreased significantly since the onset of IVF/ICSI. Again, however, the modern day IVF laboratory should be familiar with this assay, especially as it could be properly used to identify those couples who have a high likelihood for success with IVF alone as opposed to ICSI. Importantly, Gvakharia et al., adapted this test to predict fertilization outcome in IVF–ICSI and successfully predicted those men whose sperm failed to decondense after ICSI [47]. As pressure mounts regarding the safety of IVF/ICSI, proper identification of those patients who truly need ICSI (abnormal SPA assays) remains vitally important.

26.7 Conclusions

The numerous bioassays developed to assess sperm function are complex and somewhat difficult for many practitioners to understand. In this era of increasing utilization of IVF/ICSI, they also seem at first glance to be of limited utility. Instead, these tests offer us vital insight into reproductive and sperm physiology. Moreover, they may again become useful as cost and ethical concerns drive us to reassess the treatment algorithm presented to infertile couples. These tests can identify those men with normal semen parameters (count, motility, morphology), whose sperm are functionally deficient; importantly, this deficiency is NOT evident on standard semen analysis. As practitioners begin to ask themselves the question, "Who should we send for IVF/ICSI?," these tests may again become vitally important.

References

1. Grow DR, Oehninger S, Seltman HJ et al (1994) Sperm morphology as diagnosed by strict criteria: probing the impact of teratozoospermia on fertilization rate and pregnancy outcome in a large in vitro fertilization population. Fertil Steril 62(3):559–567
2. Chohan KR, Griffin JT, Lafromboise M, De Jonge CJ, Carrell DT (2006) Comparison of chromatin assays for DNA fragmentation evaluation in human sperm. J Androl 27(1):53–59
3. Bungum M, Humaidan P, Axmon A et al (2007) Sperm DNA integrity assessment in prediction of assisted reproduction technology outcome. Hum Reprod 22(1):174–179
4. Carrell DT, Liu L, Peterson CM et al (2003) Sperm DNA fragmentation is increased in couples with unexplained recurrent pregnancy loss. Arch Androl 49(1):49–55
5. Zini A, Blumenfeld A, Libman J, Willis J (2005) Beneficial effect of microsurgical varicocelectomy on human sperm DNA integrity. Hum Reprod 20(4):1018–1021
6. Egozcue J, Blanco J, Vidal F (1997) Chromosome studies in human sperm nuclei using fluorescence in-situ hybridization (FISH). Hum Reprod Update 3(5):441–452
7. Downie SE, Flaherty SP, Matthews CD (1997) Detection of chromosomes and estimation of aneuploidy in human spermatozoa using fluorescence in-situ hybridization. Mol Hum Reprod 3(7):585–598
8. Vegetti W, Van Assche E, Frias A et al (2000) Correlation between semen parameters and sperm aneuploidy rates investigated by fluorescence in-situ hybridization in infertile men. Hum Reprod 15(2):351–365
9. Rubio C, Simon C, Blanco J et al (1999) Implications of sperm chromosome abnormalities in recurrent miscarriage. J Assist Reprod Genet 16(5):253–258
10. Jeyendran RS, Van der Ven HH, Perez-Pelaez M, Crabo BG, Zaneveld LJ (1984) Development of an assay to assess the functional integrity of the human sperm membrane and its relationship to other semen characteristics. J Reprod Fertil 70(1):219–228
11. Tartagni M, Schonauer MM, Cicinelli E et al (2002) Usefulness of the hypo-osmotic swelling test in predicting pregnancy rate and outcome in couples undergoing intrauterine insemination. J Androl 23(4):498–502
12. Biljan MM, Buckett WM, Taylor CT et al (1996) Effect of abnormal hypo-osmotic swelling test on fertilization rate and pregnancy outcome in in vitro fertilization cycles. Fertil Steril 66(3): 412–416
13. Jeyendran RS, Van der Ven HH, Zaneveld LJ (1992) The hypoosmotic swelling test: an update. Arch Androl 29(2):105–116
14. Mordel N, Dano I, Epstein-Eldan M, Shemesh A, Schenker JG, Laufer N (1993) Novel parameters of human sperm hypoosmotic swelling test and their correlation to standard spermatogram, total motile sperm fraction, and sperm penetration assay. Fertil Steril 59(6):1276–1279
15. Cohlen BJ, te Velde ER, Habbema JD (1999) Postcoital testing. Postcoital test should be performed as routine infertility test. BMJ 318(7189):1008–1009
16. Niederberger CS, Lamb DJ, Glinz M, Lipshultz LI, Scully NF (1993) Tests of sperm function for evaluation of the male: Penetrak and Tru-Trax. Fertil Steril 60(2):319–323
17. Eggert-Kruse W, Gerhard I, Tilgen W, Runnebaum B (1989) Clinical significance of crossed in vitro sperm-cervical mucus penetration test in infertility investigation. Fertil Steril 52(6): 1032–1040
18. Eggert-Kruse W, Leinhos G, Gerhard I, Tilgen W, Runnebaum B (1989) Prognostic value of in vitro sperm penetration into hormonally standardized human cervical mucus. Fertil Steril 51(2): 317–323

19. Balasch J, Jove I, Ballesca JL et al (1989) Human in vitro fertilization in couples with unexplained infertility and a poor postcoital test. Gynecol Endocrinol 3(4):289–295
20. Hull MG, Joyce DN, McLeod FN, Ray BD, McDermott A (1984) Human in-vitro fertilisation, in-vivo sperm penetration of cervical mucus, and unexplained infertility. Lancet 2(8397):245–246
21. Hull MG (1992) Infertility treatment: relative effectiveness of conventional and assisted conception methods. Hum Reprod 7(6):785–796
22. Forti G, Krausz C (1998) Clinical review 100: evaluation and treatment of the infertile couple. J Clin Endocrinol Metab 83(12): 4177–4188
23. Chiu PC, Chung MK, Tsang HY et al (2005) Glycodelin-S in human seminal plasma reduces cholesterol efflux and inhibits capacitation of spermatozoa. J Biol Chem 280(27):25580–25589
24. Chiu PC, Chung MK, Koistinen R et al (2007) Glycodelin-A interacts with fucosyltransferase on human sperm plasma membrane to inhibit spermatozoa-zona pellucida binding. J Cell Sci 120(Pt 1):33–44
25. Uchida H, Maruyama T, Ohta K et al (2007) Histone deacetylase inhibitor-induced glycodelin enhances the initial step of implantation. Hum Reprod 22(10):2615–2622
26. de Lamirande E, Eiley D, Gagnon C (1993) Inverse relationship between the induction of human sperm capacitation and spontaneous acrosome reaction by various biological fluids and the superoxide scavenging capacity of these fluids. Int J Androl 16(4):258–266
27. Kallajoki M, Virtanen I, Suominen J (1986) The fate of acrosomal staining during the acrosome reaction of human spermatozoa as revealed by a monoclonal antibody and PNA-lectin. Int J Androl 9(3):181–194
28. Sanchez R, Toepfer-Petersen E, Aitken RJ, Schill WB (1991) A new method for evaluation of the acrosome reaction in viable human spermatozoa. Andrologia 23(3):197–203
29. Talbot P, Chacon RS (1981) A triple-stain technique for evaluating normal acrosome reactions of human sperm. J Exp Zool 215(2): 201–208
30. Perry RL, Naeeni M, Barratt CL, Warren MA, Cooke ID (1995) A time course study of capacitation and the acrosome reaction in human spermatozoa using a revised chlortetracycline pattern classification. Fertil Steril 64(1):150–159
31. Lee MA, Trucco GS, Bechtol KB et al (1987) Capacitation and acrosome reactions in human spermatozoa monitored by a chlortetracycline fluorescence assay. Fertil Steril 48(4):649–658
32. Oehninger S, Blackmore P, Morshedi M, Sueldo C, Acosta AA, Alexander NJ (1994) Defective calcium influx and acrosome reaction (spontaneous and progesterone-induced) in spermatozoa of infertile men with severe teratozoospermia. Fertil Steril 61(2):349–354
33. Yovich JM, Edirisinghe WR, Yovich JL (1994) Use of the acrosome reaction to ionophore challenge test in managing patients in an assisted reproduction program: a prospective, double-blind, randomized controlled study. Fertil Steril 61(5):902–910
34. Burkman LJ, Coddington CC, Franken DR, Krugen TF, Rosenwaks Z, Hogen GD (1988) The hemizona assay (HZA): development of a diagnostic test for the binding of human spermatozoa to the human hemizona pellucida to predict fertilization potential. Fertil Steril 49(4):688–697
35. Overstreet JW, Hembree WC (1976) Penetration of the zona pellucida of nonliving human oocytes by human spermatozoa in vitro. Fertil Steril 27(7):815–831
36. Liu DY, Clarke GN, Lopata A, Johnston WI, Baker HW (1989) A sperm-zona pellucida binding test and in vitro fertilization. Fertil Steril 52(2):281–287
37. Oehninger S, Franken D, Alexander N, Hodgen GD (1992) Hemizona assay and its impact on the identification and treatment of human sperm dysfunctions. Andrologia 24(6):307–321
38. Huszar G, Ozenci CC, Cayli S, Zavaczki Z, Hansch E, Vigue L (2003) Hyaluronic acid binding by human sperm indicates cellular maturity, viability, and unreacted acrosomal status. Fertil Steril 79(Suppl 3):1616–1624
39. Huszar G, Ozkavukcu S, Jakab A, Celik-Ozenci C, Sati GL, Cayli S (2006) Hyaluronic acid binding ability of human sperm reflects cellular maturity and fertilizing potential: selection of sperm for intracytoplasmic sperm injection. Curr Opin Obstet Gynecol 18(3):260–267
40. Huszar G, Jakab A, Sakkas D et al (2007) Fertility testing and ICSI sperm selection by hyaluronic acid binding: clinical and genetic aspects. Reprod Biomed Online 14(5):650–663
41. Yanagimachi R, Yanagimachi H, Rogers BJ (1976) The use of zona-free animal ova as a test-system for the assessment of the fertilizing capacity of human spermatozoa. Biol Reprod 15(4): 471–476
42. Aitken RJ, Irvine DS, Wu FC (1991) Prospective analysis of sperm-oocyte fusion and reactive oxygen species generation as criteria for the diagnosis of infertility. Am J Obstet Gynecol 164(2):542–551
43. Margalioth EJ, Feinmesser M, Navot D, Mordel N, Bronson RA (1989) The long-term predictive value of the zona-free hamster ova sperm penetration assay. Fertil Steril 52(3):490–494
44. Perreault SD, Rogers BJ (1982) Capacitation pattern of human spermatozoa. Fertil Steril 38(2):258–260
45. Smith RG, Johnson A, Lamb D, Lipshultz LI (1987) Functional tests of spermatozoa. Sperm penetration assay. Urol Clin North Am 14(3):451–458
46. Johnson A, Bassham B, Lipshultz LI, Lamb DJ (1995) A quality control system for the optimized sperm penetration assay. Fertil Steril 64(4):832–837
47. Gvakharia MO, Lipshultz LI, Lamb DJ (2000) Human sperm microinjection into hamster oocytes: a new tool for training and evaluation of the technical proficiency of intracytoplasmic sperm injection. Fertil Steril 73(2):395–401

Chapter 27
Genetic Testing of Male Infertility

Csilla Krausz

Abstract Patients with severe male factor are more likely to be carriers of chromosomal abnormalities both in their sperm and in their lymphocytes. These abnormalities include numerical alterations, structural alterations, and Y chromosome microdeletions. Gene mutations that cause male infertility and studies identifying polymorphic regions that, in conjunction with environmental factors, may be associated with male infertility have been described. Until further gene mutations are identified, standard genetic testing of infertile men is largely limited to chromosomal karyotyping, Y chromosome analysis, and cystic fibrosis gene mutation analysis.

Keywords Karyotype • Y chromosome microdeletion • Mutation • Polymorphism • CFTR • Gene

27.1 Introduction

27.1.1 Genetic Testing in Male Infertility

Nearly 7% of men are affected by semen anomalies, such as abnormal sperm number, motility, and/or morphology. The etiology of impaired sperm production and function can be related to different factors acting at pretesticular, posttesticular or directly at the testicular level [1]. Genetic factors can be identified in each etiologic category, and some of them can be tested in selected groups of patients (Table 27.1). With the aid of an extensive medical work up (medical history, physical examination, semen analysis, hormone measurement, ultrasound examination of the genital tract, and genetic testing), a diagnosis of the cause of male infertility can be obtained in about 70% of cases, while in the remaining 30%, no clear-cut cause is found, and these cases are referred to as "idiopathic infertility." Currently, unidentified monogenic mutations ("causal factors") or polymorphisms ("genetic risk factors") acting with other undefined cofactors (genetic or environmental) are likely to be involved in the majority of "idiopathic" cases. This chapter deals with routine genetic testing in male infertility (focusing on indications and genetic counseling) and will shortly discuss about new genetic factors with potential clinical interest.

27.1.1.1 When Should We Suspect a Genetic Cause?

Both the medical history and physical examination are of value for orienting doctors toward a genetic cause. Much care should be taken concerning the collection of familial history for infertility, congenital abnormalities, mental retardation, miscarriages, and premature ovarian failure (mother or sisters). Medical history of bronchiectasis, sinusitis, and dextrocardia at the physical examination is typical for the Kartagener syndrome, although situs inversus may be absent in certain cases.

Certain physical features, such as hypoandrogenization and hypospadia, may be due to mutations in the androgen receptor gene. Extremely small firm testes, with typical eunocoid features are indicative of Klinefelter syndrome. On the other hand, an eunocoid habitus with infantile genitalia, sparse or nearly absent body hair, gynecomastia, and low testicular volume is typical of congenital gonadotrophin deficiency, which can be associated with hypo- or anosmia in Kallmann's syndrome.

27.2 Pretesticular (Congenital Endocrine) Forms of Male Infertility Due to Genetic Factors

A fully efficient hypothalamic-pituitary-gonadal axis is requested for both endocrine and reproductive functions of the testis. Genetic factors causing deficit of gonadotrophins (LH, FSH) may act at hypothalamic or pituitary level and are

C. Krausz (✉)
Andrology Unit, Department of Clinical Physiopathology, University of Florence, Viale Pieraccini, 6, Florence 50139, Italy
e-mail: c.krausz@dfc.unifi.it

D.T. Carrell and C.M. Peterson (eds.), *Reproductive Endocrinology and Infertility: Integrating Modern Clinical and Laboratory Practice*, DOI 10.1007/978-1-4419-1436-1_27, © Springer Science+Business Media, LLC 2010

Table 27.1 Diagnostic genetic testing in male infertility. All listed gene and chromosomal anomalies are in direct cause effect relationship with azoo/oligozoospermia, except "gr/gr" deletions and some of the chromosomal anomalies which are considered "risk factors" (i.e., they can be found also in normospermic subjects but at a significantly lower frequency). *CAVD* congenital absence of vas deferens, *AZF* azoospermia factor

Gene or region	Chromosome location	Pattern of inheritance	Indication for testing
Pretesticular			
KAL-1	Xp22.3	X-linked	Kallmann sdr
KAL-2 (FGFR1)	8p12	Autosomal dominant	Kallmann sdr or normosmic IHH
PROK2/PROK2R	3p21.1/20p13	Autosomal recessive	Kallmann sdr or normosmic IHH
FGF8	10q24	Fibroblast growth factor 8 Autosomal dominant	Kallmann sdr
GnRHR	*4q13.2-3*	Autosomal recessive	IHH (normosmic)
KiSS1/GPR54	*1q32/19p13.3*	Autosomal recessive	IHH (normosmic)
FSHB	*11p13*		Isolated FSH deficiency
LHB	*19q13.32*		Isolated LH deficiency
Posttesticular			
CFTR	*7q31.2*	Autosomal recessive	CAVD (bilateral/monolateral) Idiopathic epydidimal obstruction
Testicular			
Chromosomal Anomalies(structural or numerical)*			Oligozoospermia<10 millions spzoa/ml
AZF	*Yq11*	Y-linked	Oligozoospermia<5 millions spzoa/ml
AR	Xq11-12	X-linked	Hypoandrogenized (high ASI) infertile man
*gr/gr**	AZFc	Y-linked	Oligozoospermia

responsible for the congenital forms of hypogonadotropic hypogonadism. Idiopathic hypogonadotropic hypogonadism (IHH) may be an isolated condition or associated with anosmia/hyposmia (Kallmann syndrome). While the list of candidate genes is constantly increasing, the aethiology remains still unidentified in 70–80% of cases [2–5]. The clinical heterogeneity is remarkable in some of these genetic forms of isolated hypogonadotropic hypogonadism, suggesting that environmental factors or epigenetic phenomena and/or modifier genes may influence the phenotype.

27.2.1 Kallmann Syndrome

The Kallmann syndrome is a clinically and genetically heterogeneous disorder, characterized by hypogonadotropic hypogonadism and anosmia or hyposmia. Segregation analysis in familial cases demonstrated diverse inheritance patterns (autosomal dominant, autosomal recessive, X-linked). To date, loss-of-function mutations causing this pathology have been described in two genes: *KAL1,* encoding anosmin-1 [6, 7] and *KAL2* encoding fibroblast growth factor receptor 1 (FGFR1) [8]. Recently, mutations in *PROKR2* encoding G protein-coupled prokineticin receptor-2 and *PROK2* encoding its ligand, prokineticin-2 were also reported [9], and they are two new candidate genes for this disease.

KAL1 is located at Xp22.3, and mutations are responsible for the X-linked form of the disease. Although incomplete penetrance of hypogonadism and/or anosmia within and across families with Kallmann syndrome is frequently described, patients with *KAL1* mutations exhibit an almost uniformly severe and highly penetrant reproductive phenotype. Among nonreproductive and nonolfactory disorders, renal agenesis and bimanual synkinesis show the highest incidence, occurring in approximately 30–40% and 75% of cases, respectively. These mutations have been identified in approximately 8–11% of the sporadic and in 14–50% of the familial cases of X-linked Kallmann syndrome [10, 11]. No correlation has been demonstrated between phenotype and location of the mutations.

The *FGFR1* gene, also called *KAL2*, is located at chromosome 8p12. *FGFR1* abnormalities have been associated with wide variability of sexual maturation from complete absence of puberty to normal reproductive function within families harboring the same mutation [12]. Mutations in the *FGFR1* (*KAL2*) gene occur in approximately 7–10% of patients (male and female) with autosomal dominant IHH, anosmic/hyposmic or normosmic [8, 13, 14]. These patients may also have neurologic abnormalities, midfacial defects, and skeletal anomalies. The similar clinical phenotype shared by *KAL-1* and *FGFR1* mutated patients suggests a putative anosmin-1 and FGFR1 interaction and/or activation of common pathways.

The *PROKR2* gene was mapped to chromosome 20p13, whereas the *PROK2* gene to 3p21.1. There are only few studies about the frequency of PROKR2 and PROK2 mutations. Dode et al. [9] investigated 192 (144 males and 48 females) unrelated individuals affected by Kallmann syndrome and identified 10 different mutations of PROKR2 (one frameshift and nine missense mutations) in 14 patients with variable degrees of olfactory and reproductive dysfunction. The cause–effect relationship between the majority of these mutations and the phenotype is suggested by the site, i.e., in highly conserved amino acids and the lack of these mutations in the control group. However, functional studies are still missing. It is also important to note that some other mutations of the PROK2 and PROKR2 genes were detected in clinically unaffected individuals as well, indicating that additional genetic or nongenetic factors are involved in disease production. At this regard, in a sporadic case of Kallmann syndrome, a heterozygous mutation in both the PROKR2 and the KAL1 gene was detected suggesting digenic inheritance.

27.2.1.1 Idiopathic Hypogonadotropic Hypogonadism

The GnRH-R and GPR54/Kiss1 genes have been implicated in IHH etiology of normosmic patients, and a few mutations of the beta subunits of LH and FSH were described in patients with selective gonadotropin deficiency [2, 3, 5].

The human GnRH receptor gene (*GnRH-R*) has been mapped to chromosome 4q13.2–3, and mutations have been found exclusively in normosmic IHH patients. Approximately, 40% of autosomal recessive and 16% of sporadic IHH cases are due to mutations in this gene [15, 16]. The two most frequent GnRH receptor mutations are Q106R and R262Q, accounting for approximately half of all reported GnRH-R mutations [17]. Both these mutations usually occur in a compound heterozygous state and have been shown to cause partial loss of function in in vitro studies [18]. The phenotypic spectrum of normosmic IHH patients with *GnRH-R* mutations varies from partial to complete hypogonadism. Recently, subtle phenotypes such as apparent constitutional delay of growth and puberty and borderline oligospermia were reported in males with partial loss-of-function mutations of the GnRH receptor [19].

Recently, kisspeptin and its receptor GPR54 have been strongly implicated in the regulation of puberty onset through the regulation of GnRH secretion. The human *GPR54* gene is located at chromosome 19p13.3 while *KiSS1* to 1q32. In 2003, two independent groups described inactivating mutations in the *GPR54* gene in normosmic IHH patients [20, 21]. Since then, only a few loss-of-function mutations have been described in the *GPR54* gene, comprising approximately 5% of all normosmic IHH patients investigated to date. Mutations in *GPR54* cause autosomal recessive IHH in both humans and mice. The phenotype of compound heterozygous patients ranges from partial hypogonadism [20], to a severe phenotype including micropenis, bilateral cryptorchidism and undetectable levels of gonadotropins [22]. Heterozygous carriers of *GPR54* loss-of-function mutations have normal pubertal development. The majority of IHH patients identified with *GPR54* mutations are either familial or sporadic cases with consanguineous parents. Although the *KiSS1* gene is another obvious candidate for genetic screening in cases of IHH, only one homozygous 20 nucleotide insertion in the 3′ terminal end of the coding sequence was described after having tested a relatively large group of patients with sporadic or familial normosmic IHH [23]. The mutation was found in a boy with micropenis and bilateral cryptorchidism diagnosed with IHH at the age of 3 months. However, no functional studies regarding this unique finding have been published so far.

Gonadotrophin deficiency can be also due to mutations of the beta subunits of LH and FSH. To date, only four distinct *FSHB* mutations in five unrelated females and two males with hypogonadism have been described (for review see [24] and references therein). Because of the functional consequences of these mutations, patients were found to have undetectable serum FSH and elevated serum LH levels. Mutations of LHB gene are also very rare and only two have been described so far. In one subject, the homozygous mutation (Q54R missense mutation) leads to delayed puberty, arrested spermatogenesis, low testosterone but elevated serum LH [25]. In the second patient with delayed puberty and infertility due to a homozygous G36D missense mutation serum LH was undetectable [26]. Treatment with hCG in this patient promoted virilization, increased testosterone levels, and enabled normal spermatogenesis [26].

27.2.1.2 Genetic Testing and Counseling

Given that the screening for mutations in all the above described genes provides the identification of mutations only in about 20–30% of IHH cases, additional genetic causes are expected to be discovered in the future. The diagnosis of congenital hypogonadotropic hypogonadism is normally made before adulthood since in the majority of cases it is associated with delayed puberty. However, in some cases, reduced spermatogenesis and mild hypoandrogenism may be the only symptoms, and thus the diagnosis may be delayed till adulthood. From a practical point of view, the selection of genes to be screened in a given individual is on the basis of the presence/absence of hypo/anosmia and the type of inheritance patterns in the family. However, in sporadic cases and in normosmic IHH – because of the lack of a clear cut genotype phenotype correlation – each candidate gene should be tested in a sequential way. Since spermatogenesis can be relatively easily induced by hormonal treatment, genetic screening prior therapy would be strongly suggested. The treatment with gonadotrophins will allow natural conception in the large majority of cases (even with relatively low sperm count), hence the identification of the involved gene (X-linked, autosomal dominant or recessive) can provide a more accurate genetic counseling, i.e., a risk estimation for transmission to the offspring.

For the moment, no relationship between treatment responsiveness and type of genetic defect has been reported. However, it is interesting to note that in some cases of IHH, long term testosterone treatment has lead to spontaneous reversibility of reproductive function [27]. It is therefore plausible that in the future, the identification of mutations will have not only diagnostic but also prognostic value for treatment options and responsiveness.

27.3 Posttesticular Forms of Male Infertility Due to Genetic Factors

The association between *CFTR* (Cystic Fibrosis Transmembrane Conductance Regulator) mutations and congenital agenesia of vas deferens (CAVD), both mono or bilateral, is well established [28, 29]. The CFTR gene [30, 31] is located on cr. 7 (7q31.2) and it is highly mutated with more than 1,500 mutations and variants described in the gene bank (www.genet.sickkids.on.ca/cftr/). A severe reduction in the amount of functional CFTR protein (generally due to the presence of two "severe" mutations) is associated to CF (Cystic Fibrosis) which is the most common fatal autosomal-recessive disorder in the white population (frequency 1:2,500). The combination of less severe mutations, and thus a less severe reduction of functional CFTR protein (below 50% but above 10%) may lead to "mild forms" of cystic fibrosis, including CAVD. The most widely diffused mutation both in CF and CAVD is the delta F508 mutation (about 70% of the total CF mutations in patients). Some mutations are frequently found in CAVD such as G542X, R553X, W1282X (all non sense mutations where X symbolizes a stop codon), N1303K (missense), R117H. The role of intron 8 variants (IVS8-5T, IVS8-7T, IVS8-9T) in the phenotypic expression of mutations is also well established. The three variants includes different numbers of thymidines within the acceptor splice site of intron 8, i.e., 5, 7 and 9, respectively. The length of the T tract affects the spilicing efficiency of exon 9 and thus the percent of normal CFTR mRNA. The 5T tract is the less efficient and allows about 8–10% of CFTR mRNA to be completed with exon 9. The lack of exon 9 leads to a nonfunctional Cl channel, and thus the combination of 5T with other mutations (severe or mild) may cause the development of CF or CAVD. There is a five- to sixfold increase in the frequency of the 5T variant among CAVD chromosomes [29].

The pathophysiological basis of *CFTR* mutation in cystic fibrosis and CAVD is related to the abnormal function of the CFTR-encoded chloride channel that leads to a defective fluid transport [32]. Since azoospermia is due to obstruction, patients with CAVD are assumed to have normal testicular function and spermatozoa can be retrieved for later use in in vitro fertilization cycles. Some studies suggested an association between CFTR mutation and defective testicular function; however, the latest data based on an extensive *CFTR* analysis in infertile individuals versus well selected fertile population definitively excludes the involvement of the *CFTR* gene variants in sperm production [33]. In a mouse model, Xu et al. [34] demonstrated that CFTR protein is involved also in HCO3- membrane transport as well, which is essential for sperm capacitation and thus for sperm fertilizing ability. These data would suggest a possible role for *CFTR* mutations in the aethiology of unexplained couple infertility, but it requires further confirmation.

27.3.1 Genetic Testing and Counseling

Currently the *CFTR* mutation screening should be limited to obstructive defects, which can be correlated to the reduction of functional CFTR protein, i.e., CAVD and idiopathic epydidimal obstruction. Given that the frequency of a particular *CF* mutation is a variable between different geographic areas and shows important ethnic differences, the routine mutation screening is based on a panel of mutations (normally 30), which are the most common for a given population. Since the 5T-tract variant is now considered a mild *CFTR* mutation rather than a polymorphism, it should be analyzed in each CAVD patient. The mutation screening in CAVD patients will lead to the identification of *CFTR* mutations in 80–90% (depending on how extensive is the analysis, i.e., if the entire gene is analyzed), while in patients with idiopathic epydidimal obstruction it will be around 47% of [35]. CAVD with associated renal anomalies is related to another, not yet identified genetic defect, therefore these patients have no additional risk to be *CFTR* mutation carriers in respect to the general population.

Since the carrier frequency of *CFTR* mutations in persons with Northern European descent is high (1:25), the screening for CF gene mutations in the female partners of men with CAVD without congenital kidney anomalies should be performed before assisted reproduction. In most cases, the standard screening panel, containing the 30–50 most common mutations for a given geographic area and ethnic group, may not be sufficient for detecting mutations in both partners. For this reason, a whole gene screening is advised in both, CAVD patient and his partner. If mutations are detected in both partners, the risk of an offspring with CF (or mild forms of CF, depending on the type and combination of mutations) is very high and Preimplantation Genetic Diagnosis (PGD) should be advised to the couple. However, in most cases, it remains difficult to make precise risk estimates due to different degree of penetrance of the same genotype between different individuals [36].

27.4 Testicular Forms Due to Genetic Factors

Although the list of potential genetic factors affecting spermatogenesis directly at the testicular level is progressively expanding, there are only a few diagnostic genetic tests available for clinical purposes (Table 27.1). Given the apparently low prevalence of causative single gene mutations, idiopathic infertility should be regarded as a polygenic disease with complex traits. Data on genetic variants/polymorphisms are promising although highly controversial. Gene sequence variants are likely to be involved in the phenotypic translation of environmental factors, however there are only sporadic studies concerning this specific topic. On the other hand, when more than one study is published on genetic risk factors, data are often contradictory, and in many occasions, the first described positive association is not confirmed in later studies. Discrepancies in the literature are mainly due to biases related to the study design (for example insufficient size of the study population, inadequate selection of controls and patients, lack of matching for ethnic background) or to methodology issues. A comprehensive review about polymorphisms is given in [37, 38].

Genetic anomalies related to primitive testicular failure can be detected in leucocytes or directly in spermatozoa. Among the first, karyotype evaluation and Y chromosome microdeletion screening have become routine genetic tests for men with severe spermatogenic failure. Among the seconds, sperm DNA integrity testing and sperm aneuploidy analysis by FISH should be advised only for distinct pathologies, and they are discussed in the other chapters of this book and in [39, 40].

27.4.1 Chromosomal Abnormalities

Karyotype abnormalities occur in about 0.4% of the general population and can affect the number or the structure of chromosomes. Severely impaired sperm production is associated with a significantly higher frequency of both numerical and structural chromosomopathies [41]. The more severe is the testicular phenotype the higher is the frequency of chromosomal abnormalities. Patients with less than 10 millions spermatozoa/ml show already a ten times higher incidence (4%) of mainly autosomal structural abnormalities in respect to the general population. Among severe oligospermic men (<5 million spermatozoa/ml), the frequency increases to 7–8%, whereas in nonobstructive azoospermic men, the frequency reaches the highest values, 15–16%. Klinefelter syndrome (47, XXY) represents the most common karyotype abnormality in severe male factor infertility, followed by Y chromosome terminal deletions (Yq-) and structural autosomal abnormalities.

27.4.1.1 Klinefelter Syndrome

Klinefelter syndrome is the most common sex chromosome abnormality in humans with an incidence of 1:600 in live births and 1 in 300 in spontaneous abortion [42]. It is also the most frequent chromosomal anomaly in azoospermic men (14%). About 80% of patients bear a 47, XXY karyotype, whereas the other 20% represented either by 47, XXY/46, XY mosaics or higher grade sex chromosomal aneuploidy or structurally abnormal X chromosome [43]. The syndrome is classically characterized by hypergonadotrophic azoospermia, small firm testes and symptoms of androgen deficiency. Patients affected by this syndrome have an average of 30–50% of testicular sperm recovery rate [44–48], however some authors report much higher figures (up to 72%) [49]. Hormone levels (FSH, Inhibin B), testis volume do not seem to predict for the presence or absence of spermatozoa in the testis. Among the predictive factors, younger age is considered a positive predictor since patients at younger age have a higher incidence of testicular sperm recovery. Westlander et al. [46] reported successful sperm recovery in 5/11 patients <34 years, whereas 0/7 patients >34 years old. Rarely, spermatozoa can be found in the ejaculate of mosaic patients or in nonmosaic but young patients [48]. The former indicates the potential importance of an early diagnosis. Although men at their early twenties may not desire immediate conception, a preventive sperm cryopreservation of ejaculated spermatozoa should be a correct way to preserve their fertility. Azoospermic patients affected by Klinefelter syndrome may generate their own genetic children by undergoing to TESE followed by ICSI.

Genetic Counseling

On the basis of sperm FISH studies showing an increased frequency of sex chromosomal abnormalities and increased incidence of autosomal aneuploidies (disomy for chromosomes 13, 18 and 21), concerns have been raised about the chromosomal normality of the embryos generated through ICSI [39]. To date, 49 healthy children have been born using ICSI without PGD and the conception of one 47,XXY fetus has been reported [50, 51]. However, a study based on ICSI combined with PGD on 113 embryos shows that there is a significant fall in the rate of normal embryos for couples with Klinefelter sdr. in respect to controls (54% versus 77.2%). Because of the significant increase of sex chromosomal and autosomal abnormalities in the embryos of Klinefelter patients, PGD should be strongly advised [50].

27.4.1.2 Autosomal Abnormalities

The most frequently found autosomal karyotype abnormalities are Robertsonian translocations, reciprocal translocations, paracentric inversions and marker chromosomes. In 60% of all cases of Robertsonian translocations, a (13;14)-translocation is found. This abnormality is rarely observed in azoospermic men but is often found in oligospermic patients (about nine times higher in infertile men than in newborns). However, since Robertsonian translocations have been found also in normospermic fertile males in the same pedigree [52], the contribution of this chromosomal defect to disturbed spermatogenesis remains to be clarified. Pericentric inversions are 13 times higher in infertile men, and probably interfere with meiosis, leading to a reduced rate of postmeiotic sperm development.

Genetic Counseling

The importance of the detection of these structural chromosomal anomalies is related to the increased risk of aneuploidy or unbalanced chromosomal complements in the fetus. Similarly, for Klinefelter syndrome, sperm FISH analysis and/or PGD should be performed to give a more accurate risk estimation of affected offspring.

27.4.1.3 Other Chromosomal Abnormalities

47,XYY male: The frequency of males with this karyotype is 1:750. Carriers of this abnormality show a great diversity in the degree of spermatogenic impairment, ranging from severe oligozoospermia to apparent normality [53]. Distortion of sex vescicule formation is probably the major cause of disturbed spermatogenesis in these men [54].

XX-male: This is a disorder of sex determination and occurs in about 1:20,000 newborns. In about 80% of cases, XX-maleness can be explained by the translocation of the SRY gene (encoding the testis determining factor, [55]) to the X chromosome. The cause of SRY-negative XX-maleness remains to be elucidated [56, 57]. The phenotypic features of the syndrome are gynecomastia, female hair pattern and small testes with azoospermia. Genital malformations such as hypospadias are rare. In SRY-negative patients, ambiguous genitalia is a frequent finding [58].

Aneuploidies of autosomes: Most numerical aneuploidies of autosomes are lethal. Patients affected by Down's syndrome may be fertile or infertile [59].

27.4.1.4 Y Chromosome Deletions

The first association between azoospermia and microscopically detectable deletions of the long arm of the Y chromosome has been demonstrated by Tiepolo and Zuffardi in 1976 [60]. Since in four patients the deletion was de novo (their fathers were tested and found to carry intact Y chromosome), they proposed the existence of a spermatogenesis factor, the AZoospermia factor (AZF) encoded by a gene on distal Yq. Thanks to the development of molecular genetic tools and large STS based screening in patients affected by azoo/severe oligozoospermia, Vogt et al. [61] were able to define three recurrently deleted nonoverlapping subregions in proximal, middle and distal Yq11, designated AZFa, AZFb and AZFc, respectively. Only several years after the discovery of the three AZF regions, with the precise knowledge of the Y structure in Yq11, it has become evident that the AZFb and AZFc regions are overlapping [62]. New deletion patterns in the AZFb/AZFc regions have been proposed; however, since data in the literature are based on markers, which are unable to distinguish between these subtypes, it is more convenient to refer to the three "classical" deletion intervals (Fig. 27.1). Deletions that are clinically relevant remove partially or in the large majority of cases completely one or more AZF regions, and they represent the most frequent molecular genetic cause of oligo/azoospermia [63]. The complete removal of the AZFa and AZFb regions are associated with severe testicular phenotype, Sertoli Cell Only sdr and spermatogenic arrest, respectively. The complete removal of the AZFc region causes a variable phenotype which may range from azoospermia to oligozoospermia. The above reported genotype/phenotype correlation confers to Y deletion analysis a prognostic value for testicular sperm retrieval [64, 65]. In each region a number of candidate genes have been identified (see Fig. 27.1), however their function in spermatogenesis remains largely unknown [66]. Since deletions occur in block-removing more than one gene- the role of a single AZF gene cannot be extrapolated from the AZF deletion phenotype and thus it is unclear if they are all participating in spermatogenesis. The deletion phenotypes suggest that the AZFa and AZFb regions contain at least one gene with essential spermatogenic function, whereas genes of the AZFc region are more likely to affect the efficiency of spermatogenesis.

To date only three confirmed gene specific deletions have been reported in the literature and were all in the same gene, *USP9Y*, which is located in the AZFa region [67, 68]. Besides *USP9Y*, the AZFa region contains another gene, *DDX3Y* (former *DBY*). The associated oligozoospermia in our two recently reported cases of *USP9Y* deletions [68] indicates that this gene is not essential for the initiation and completion of spermatogenesis, and it probably has a role only in enhancing the quality and efficiency of spermatogenesis. On the other hand, since the removal of both AZFa genes is associated with the complete absence of spermatogenic cells in the testis, a crucial role for DDX3Y gene can be predicted [111].

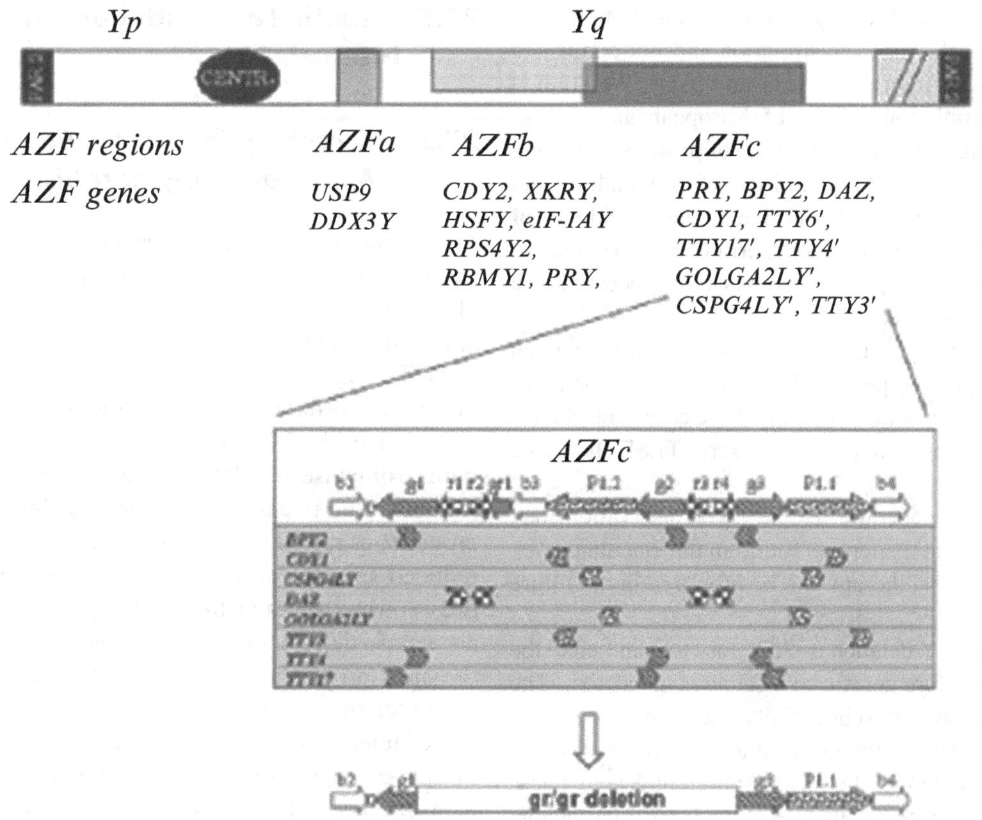

Fig. 27.1 Schematic representation of the Y chromosome with the indication of AZoospermia Factor (AZF) regions and genes located in these regions. The AZFc region is presented in more details: i) the position of multicopy genes inside the AZFc amplicons; ii) the approximate extent of gr/gr deletion are shown
*transcription unit families

The rarity of single AZF gene mutations or deletions is in sharp contrast with the relatively high frequency of AZF deletions. A likely explanation is that the peculiar structure and the sequence organization of the Y chromosome make prone this chromosome to the loss of large regions such as the AZF regions [66].

The clinical significance of Yq deletions have been debated for long time mainly because of the large variability in deletion frequencies reported by different authors and because Yq deletions have also been reported in "fertile" men. The absence of AZF deletions in over 1,000 normospermic men clearly indicate that AZF deletions are specific for spermatogenic disturbances [63, 69]. After more than 10 years of clinical research, it can now be concluded that (1)Y deletions have been found almost exclusively in patients with <1 millions spermatozoa/ml (even in association with other abnormal andrological findings); (2) deletions are extremely rare with a sperm concentration >5 millions of spermatozoa/ml (approximately 0.7%), and in certain cases, deletions removed only single STSs that, without further confirmation by other techniques, such as Southern blotting or breakpoint definition, are of dubious significance; (3) the most frequently deleted region is AZFc (approximately 65–70%), followed by deletions of the AZFb and AZFb+c or AZFa+b+c regions (25–30%), whereas deletions of the AZFa region are extremely rare (5%).

27.4.1.5 Genetic Testing and Counseling

The screening for AZF deletions has a diagnostic, prognostic and preventive value. Thanks to the EAA guidelines [70] and EAA/EMQN external quality control programme (http://www.emqn.org/emqn/) Yq testing has become more homogeneous and reliable in different routine genetic laboratories. Indications for AZF deletions screening are based on sperm count and include azoospermia and severe oligozoospermia (<5 million spermatozoa/ml). The EAA guidelines provide a set of primers (two markers for each region) which is able to detect over 95% of clinically relevant deletions [70]. The initial large variability of deletion frequencies was more likely the consequence of technical problems and the use of unreliable markers rather than an expression of true ethnic differences. Although the composition of the study population is certainly the major factor influencing deletion frequency, the 55% or 37% frequency rate in patients affected by SCOS or severe male factor infertility reported in the late 90th by one Italian group was clearly overestimation and not confirmed by later studies (for review see [71] and [63]). We studied four different populations (three of European and one of non-European origin) with a similar set of primers and using homogeneous criteria for the definition of "idiopathic" and "nonidiopathic" infertility [72–74]. The highest incidence of 15% was found in idiopathic azoospermic men, whereas in the group of severe oligospermic patients, it dropped to 5–7% independently from the ethnic origin [75].

Concerning the prognostic value of this genetic test: given that a genotype phenotype correlation does exist for complete AZFa and AZFb deletions and in these cases, the chance of testicular sperm retrieval is virtually zero, TESE should be avoided [64, 65].

As a preventive procedure, sperm cryoconservation may be advised to patients if sperm is found in the ejaculate [71]. The same "preventive" therapy can be proposed in the future to the son.

After conception, Y deletion is obligatory transmitted to the male offspring therefore genetic counseling is mandatory. The phenotype of son may vary substantially, and the extent of spermatogenic failure (still in the range of azoo/oligozoospermia) cannot be predicted entirely because of different genetic background and the presence or absence of environmental factors with potential toxicity to reproductive function.

We, and others, have reported that a significant proportion of spermatozoa from men with Y microdeletion are nullisomic for sex chromosomes [76, 77]. This result indicates a potential risk for the offspring to develop 45,X0 Turner's syndrome and other phenotypic anomalies associated with sex chromosome mosaicism, including ambiguous genitalia. The screening for Y chromosome microdeletions in patients bearing a mosaic 46XY/45X0 karyotype with sexual ambiguity and/or Turner stigmata has shown a relatively high incidence of AZFc deletions (33%) [78]. Additional data support that Yq microdeletions could be associated with an overall Y chromosomal instability leading to the formation of 45,X0 cell lines [79, 80].

Despite this theoretical risk, the 36 babies (18 male and 18 female) born from fathers affected by Yq microdeletions are phenotypically normal [63]. This could be due to the reduced implantation rate and a likely higher risk of spontaneous abortions of embryos bearing a 45,X0 karyotype. However, only PGD together with the abortion rate would provide a more accurate estimation about the real risks of 46, XY/45,X0 mosaicism and Turner syndrome.

PGD can be offered to the couple both for sex selection and for avoiding the transfer of 45,X0 embryos. The first indication may raise some ethical concerns since infertility may not be considered as a disease, whereas the second remains a theoretical indication in the absence of direct evidences.

27.5 Genetic Tests with Potential Clinical Interest

27.5.1 Screening for Steroid Receptor Mutations/Polymorphisms

The crucial role of androgens and estrogens in the endocrine regulation of spermatogenesis is well known, therefore genes of their receptors are a logical target for mutational analysis in infertile male.

However, in the clinical practice, the situation is rather different. To date, only one patient with an inactivating mutation in the ERα (*ESR1*) gene [81] and four patients with aromatase (CYP19) deficiency have been reported [82–85]. The phenotypes of these patients are rather heterogeneous ranging from normal sperm concentration, but reduced sperm viability in case of the *ESR1* mutation to oligozoospermia and bilateral cryptorchidism in case of aromatase deficiency [83, 85]. Among *ER* polymorphisms, the most promising appear to be the (TA)n repeats in the promoter region of *ESR1* [86], which seems to influence the efficiency of spermatogenesis. However, this polymorphism is not a risk factor for male infertility. Further data are needed on this and other ER polymorphisms, especially in relationship with environmental exposure to xenoestrogens [38, 39].

In contrast to ER, a large number of mutations have been identified in the *AR* gene worldwide and are available at *AR* gene mutation (web: http:/www.mcgill.ca/androgendb) [87]. The androgen receptor (AR) is a ligand activated transcription factor which is encoded by the AR gene located on the long arm of the X chromosome (Xq11-q12). A significant number of the reported mutations have been supported by functional assays to result in lower ligand binding or transactivation potential of the mutant receptor molecule. Mutations in the AR gene results in mild to complete androgen insensitivity [88]. The phenotypic features of complete androgen insensitivity syndrome (CAIS) are female external genitalia and absence of pubic hair (Morris syndrome). In partial androgen insensitivity syndrome (PAIS), several different phenotypes are evident, ranging from predominantly female phenotype (female external genitalia, pubic hair with or without clitoromegaly and partially to completely fused labia) through ambiguous genitalia to predominantly male phenotype with micropenis, perineal hypospadias and cryptorchidism. The later phenotype is also termed as Reifenstein syndrome.

Patients with mild AIS (MAIS) have male infertility as their primary or even sole symptom.

Only a few mutations have been reported in infertile men [87, 89] and most of them resulted in the reduction of transactivation potential of the mutant protein. In a recent screening of 1,517 azoo-oligozoospermic individuals, 26 patients carrying AR mutations (20 different mutations) (1.7%) were found, and none in the control group [89]. There has been no correlation between the type of mutation and the subtype of infertility (azoospermia, oligozoospermia or oligoteratozoospermia) and not all carriers had high Androgen Sensitivity Index (ASI). Apart from the difficulty to preselect patients for the analysis, the need for routine testing in unselected infertile subjects is further questioned by other reports in which none or very few mutations were detected in large series of idiopathic infertile men [90, 91].

The analysis of polymorphic regions in exon 1 of *AR* has been object of a large quantity of publications [92–96]. The polymorphic (CAG)n codes for a polyglutamine, whereas the (GGC)n repeats for a polyglicin stretch. It has been demonstrated for the (CAG)n repeats in in vitro experiments that the length of the polyglutamine tract, while remaining within the polymorphic range, is inversely correlated with the transactivation activity of the receptor [92] Concerning the (GGC) n repeat, a recent report showed that ARs with other GGN repeat length than the most common one of 23 have lower transactivating capacity [97].

Despite promising in vitro data, the initial observations of a significant association between relatively long CAG repeats and impaired sperm production [93] has not been confirmed by subsequent studies ([95], for review see [96] and references therein). Similarly, it is still under question whether (GGC)n repeat has a pathogenic role in abnormal spermatogenesis [38]. Discrepancies in the literature maybe the consequence of: (1) ethnic differences (the association seems to be more consistent in the Asiatic populations); (2) the heterogeneity of the control (unselected men or proven fertile men or normospermic men) and of the infertile (different inclusion criteria) groups; (3) inadequate sample size (especially in the first positive studies).

In conclusion, neither mutation screening of the AR or ER nor analysis of microsatellites (CAG, GGC or TA) in both genes can be proposed as routine diagnostic tests in patients with abnormal spermatogenesis. Mutations of AR are rare in association with idiopathic male infertility and many of the mutations described in infertile men still needs to be characterized for their functional consequences. Consequently, the mutation screening should be limited to infertile patients with altered ASI and/or hypoandrogenization. Concerning the CAG repeat length, this polymorphism is an unlikely risk factor for male infertility if we consider only large studies. However, the role of CAG repeat length in modulating androgen action is more evident in patients affected by hypoandrogenism (for example subjects affected by Klinefelter syndrome) and its analysis could be useful for the definition of thresholds at which testosterone treatment should be initiated, and to personalize the dosage of substitutive testosterone therapy [98]. Similarly, it can be expected that *ESR* polymorphisms are relevant only in association with certain conditions (overweight/obesity for instance) or in case of exposure to environmental endocrine disrupters.

27.5.2 Screening for gr/gr Deletions

Apart from the classical AZF deletions, a new type of Yq deletion has recently attracted the attention of geneticist and andrologist. A partial deletion in the AZFc region, termed "gr/gr," has been described specifically in infertile men with varying degrees of spermatogenic failure [99]. This deletion removes half the AZFc gene content including two copies of the major AZFc candidate gene called DAZ [100]. In the last 3 years an intensive search for "gr/gr" deletions in infertile and control men has started in order to define their frequency and clinical significance (for review see [38] and references therein). It is impossible to perform a reliable meta-analysis because of the extreme heterogeneity of the published data (methodological differences, different inclusion criteria of the controls, lack of ethnic matching of controls and patients). The currently used method for the detection of "gr/gr" deletions is based on STS plus/minus PCR analysis. Importantly, this analysis may also detect false deletions because of rearrangements of the STS containing sequence and is also unable to rule out a duplication of the nondeleted part of the AZFc region. The majority of "gr/gr" studies lack a detailed molecular analysis, i.e., the reduced gene dosage is not confirmed, and the type of deleted gene copies is also unknown. These methodological differences together with the inappropriate control selection (general population or fertile controls with unknown sperm count) may contribute to the contradictory results.

In studies with appropriate control selection and confirmation of deletions, gr/gr deletions are clearly a risk factor for spermatogenic disturbances [99, 101]. Although it is not understood why in certain individuals the deletion does not affect spermatogenesis, it is likely that Y background plays an important modulating role. In fact, certain Y hgrs contains constitutively gr/gr deletions and are diffused in certain populations indicating that other compensatory mechanisms may exist on certain Y backgrounds [102].

27.5.2.1 Genetic Counseling

Given that fathers bearing gr/gr deletion will obligatory transmit this genetic variant (together with their Y background) to the male offspring, it is likely that their sons will have a similar spermatogenic disturbance in the future. gr/gr deletions are more likely to cause oligozoospermia than azoospermia, and in our central Italian population (>1,000 subjects tested), the calculated OR is 7.5 (95% CI: 1.2–32.2). Thus, gr/gr deletion screening should be introduced among genetic diagnostic tests, especially prior assisted reproductive techniques.

27.6 Conclusions

Patients with severe male factor are more likely to be carriers of chromosomal abnormalities both in their sperm and in their lymphocytes. Although, the overall frequency of de novo autosomal karyotype abnormalities does not seem to be increased in ICSI offspring, there is a significant higher incidence of sex chromosome aneuploidies and of minor malformations (mainly urogenital tract) in offspring from fathers affected by severe male factor infertility [103, 104]. The use of male gametes in ICSI or IVF without knowing the genetic basis of testicular failure and of its consequence is an urgent issue to be solved. Although, the estimated number of genes involved in human spermatogenesis ranges between 1,000 and over 4,000, according to different authors [105, 106], the genetic basis of primitive testicular failure remains obscure in the majority of cases [107].

Several strategies can be applied in order to identify new genetic causes of impaired sperm production and/or function. The most commonly used in human genetics is linkage analysis, however, its role in this specific field is limited by the small family sizes in inherited forms of the disease. Another widely successful strategy in complex disorders, such as male infertility, is the candidate gene approach. Candidate genes can be identified: (1) through comparative analysis of genes in several model organisms (cross species approach) which can identify highly conserved genes that share similar spatiotemporal expression profiles and serves analogous roles [108]; (2) gene knock outs in model organisms. Unfortunately, the search for candidate gene mutations in unselected infertile men did not lead to any major advancement. For a higher efficiency, mutation screening in human should be based on a deep knowledge of biological function of candidate genes in order to preselect patients on the basis of the expected phenotype. Since "idiopathic" male infertility is expected to be a genetically heterogeneous disorder, the lack of preselection of patients may be partially responsible for the apparent paucity of monogenic disorders (causative mutations) in male infertility. An alternative option is genome wide association studies using high-throughput genotyping, which should lead to a relatively fast identification of infertility-associated diseases genes in humans. However, this strategy requires large sample's size in order to achieve sufficient statistical power and to

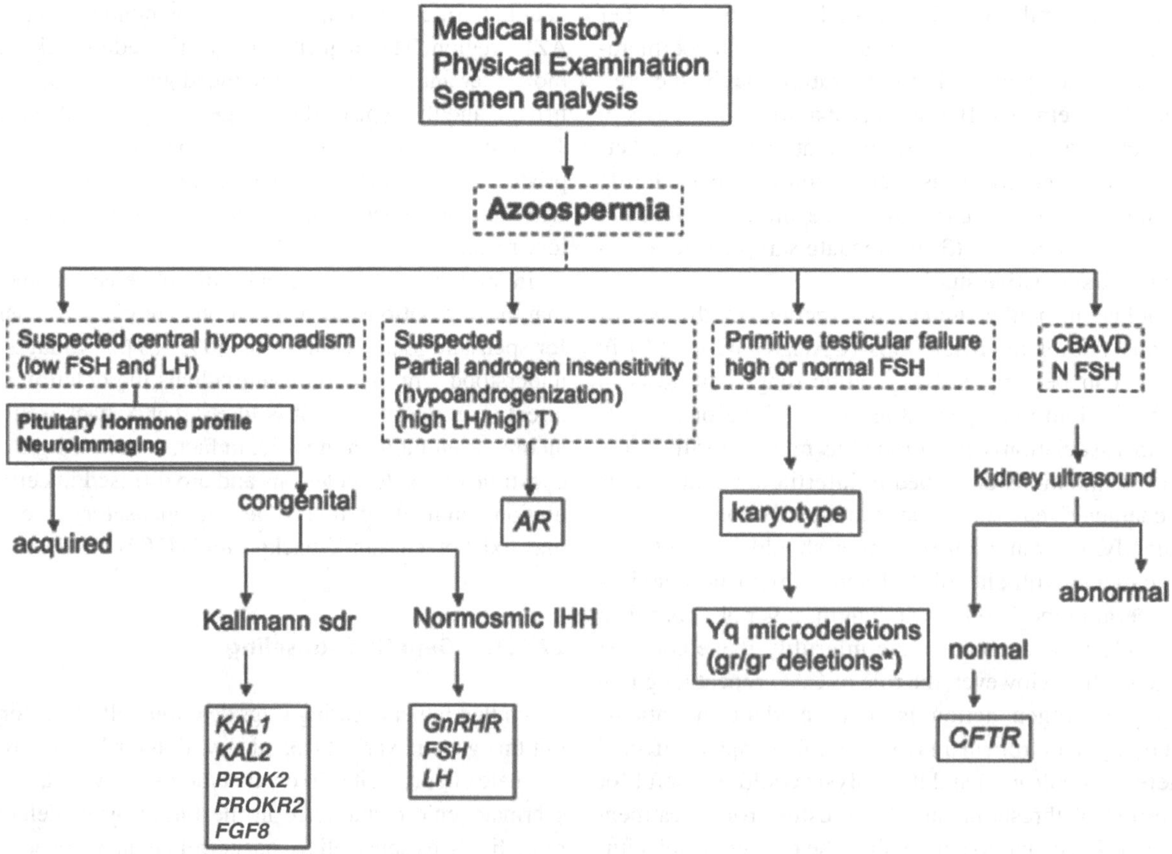

Fig. 27.2 Diagnostic flow chart for the genetic management of azoospermic patients
* the testing for this type of deletion should be restricted to those ethnic groups for which reliable large case-control studies are available with risk estimate

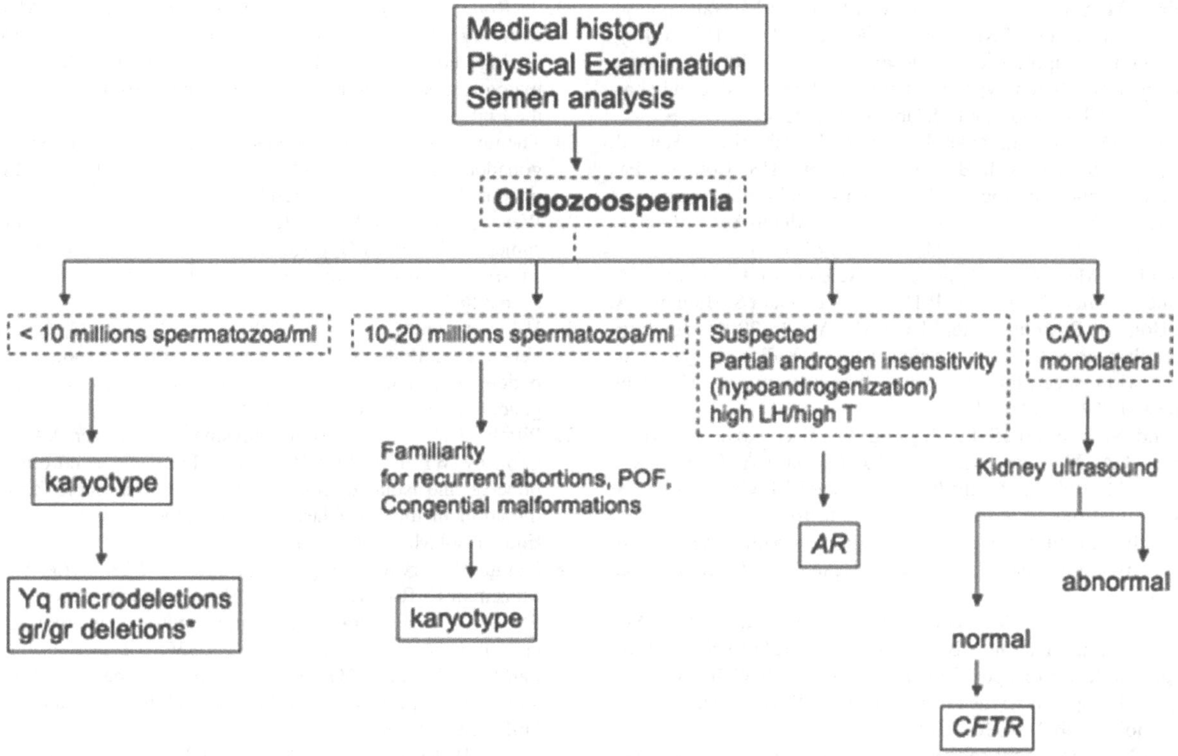

Fig. 27.3 Diagnostic flow chart for the genetic management of oligozoospermic patients
* the testing for this type of deletion should be restricted to those ethnic groups for which reliable large case-control studies are available with risk estimate

avoid population stratification or ethnic admixture in cases and controls. For a substantial advancement in this field, there is an urgent need for large multicenter/multiethnic studies. Finally, postgenomic approaches such as sperm mRNA profiling [109] and proteomics [110] are promising and may potentially lead to a more straight forwarded analysis of selected spermatogenesis genes in groups of patients with similar phenotypes and expression profiles.

In the meantime, until a radical change in the process of identification of new genetic factors is achieved, our clinical practice remains to be based on a few genetic tests such as karyotype analysis, Y chromosome microdeletions (gr/gr deletions), and mutation screening of a few selected genes according to the specific phenotype. Patients should undergo a complete analysis for relevant etiologies, as demonstrated in Figs. 27.2 and 27.3.

References

1. Krausz C, Forti G (2000) Clinical aspects of male infertility. Results Probl Cell Differ 28:1–21
2. Cerrato F, Seminara SB (2007) Human genetics of GPR54. Rev Endocr Metab Disord 8:47–55
3. Huhtaniemi I, Alevizaki M (2007) Mutations along the hypothalamic-pituitary-gonadal axis affecting male reproduction. Reprod Biomed Online 15:622–632
4. Layman LC (2007) Hypogonadotropic hypogonadism. Endocrinol Metab Clin North Am 36:283–296
5. Trarbach EB, Silveira LG, Latronico AC (2007) Genetic insights into human isolated gonadotropin deficiency. Pituitary 10:381–391
6. Franco B, Guioli S, Pragliola A, Incerti B, Bardoni B, Tonlorenzi R, Carrozzo R, Maestrini E, Pieretti M, Taillon-Miller P, Brown CJ, Willard HF, Lawrence C, Persico MG, Camerino G, Ballabio A (1991) A gene deleted in Kallmann's syndrome shares homology with neural cell adhesion and axonal path-finding molecules. Nature 353:529–536
7. Legouis R, Hardelin JP, Levilliers J, Claverie JM, Compain S, Wunderle V, Millasseau P, Le Paslier D, Cohen D, Caterina D et al (1991) The candidate gene for the X-linked Kallmann syndrome encodes a protein related to adhesion molecules. Cell 67:423–435
8. Dodé C, Levilliers J, Dupont JM, De Paepe A, Le Dû N, Soussi-Yanicostas N, Coimbra RS, Delmaghani S, Compain-Nouaille S, Baverel F, Pêcheux C, Le Tessier D, Cruaud C, Delpech M, Speleman F, Vermeulen S, Amalfitano A, Bachelot Y, Bouchard P, Cabrol S, Carel JC, Delemarre-van de Waal H, Goulet-Salmon B, Kottler ML, Richard O, Sanchez-Franco F, Saura R, Young J, Petit C, Hardelin JP (2003) Loss-of-function mutations in FGFR1 cause autosomal dominant Kallmann syndrome. Nat Genet 33(4):463–465
9. Dodé C, Teixeira L, Levilliers J, Fouveaut C, Bouchard P, Kottler ML, Lespinasse J, Lienhardt-Roussie A, Mathieu M, Moerman A, Morgan G, Murat A, Toublanc JE, Wolczynski S, Delpech M, Petit C, Young J, Hardelin JP (2006) Kallmann syndrome: mutations in the genes encoding prokineticin-2 and prokineticin receptor-2. PLoS Genet 2:e175

10. Oliveira LM, Seminara SB, Beranova M, Hayes FJ, Valkenburgh SB, Schipani E, Costa EM, Latronico AC, Crowley WF Jr, Vallejo M (2001) The importance of autosomal genes in Kallmann syndrome: genotype-phenotype correlations and neuroendocrine characteristics. J Clin Endocrinol Metab 86:1532–1538
11. Quinton R, Duke VM, de Zoysa PA, Platts AD, Valentine A, Kendall B, Pickman S, Kirk JM, Besser GM, Jacobs HS, Bouloux PM (1996) The neuroradiology of Kallmann's syndrome: a genotypic and phenotypic analysis. J Clin Endocrinol Metab 81:3010–3017 Erratum in: J Clin Endocrinol Metab. 1996;81:3614
12. Pitteloud N, Meysing A, Quinton R, Acierno JS Jr, Dwyer AA, Plummer L, Fliers E, Boepple P, Hayes F, Seminara S, Hughes VA, Ma J, Bouloux P, Mohammadi M, Crowley WF Jr (2006) Mutations in fibroblast growth factor receptor 1 cause Kallmann syndrome with a wide spectrum of reproductive phenotypes. Mol Cell Endocrinol 254–255:60–69
13. Pitteloud N, Acierno JS Jr, Meysing A, Eliseenkova AV, Ma J, Ibrahimi OA, Metzger DL, Hayes FJ, Dwyer AA, Hughes VA, Yialamas M, Hall JE, Grant E, Mohammadi M, Crowley WF Jr (2006) Mutations in fibroblast growth factor receptor 1 cause both Kallmann syndrome and normosmic idiopathic hypogonadotropic hypogonadism. Proc Natl Acad Sci U S A 103: 6281–6286
14. Trarbach EB, Costa EM, Versiani B, de Castro M, Baptista MT, Garmes HM, de Mendonca BB, Latronico AC (2006) Novel fibroblast growth factor receptor 1 mutations in patients with congenital hypogonadotropic hypogonadism with and without anosmia. J Clin Endocrinol Metab 91:4006–4012
15. de Roux N, Young J, Misrahi M, Genet R, Chanson P, Schaison G, Milgrom E (1997) A family with hypogonadotropic hypogonadism and mutations in the gonadotropin-releasing hormone receptor. N Engl J Med 337(22):1597–1602
16. Beranova M, Oliveira LM, Bédécarrats GY, Schipani E, Vallejo M, Ammini AC, Quintos JB, Hall JE, Martin KA, Hayes FJ, Pitteloud N, Kaiser UB, Crowley WF Jr, Seminara SB (2001) Prevalence, phenotypic spectrum, and modes of inheritance of gonadotropin-releasing hormone receptor mutations in idiopathic hypogonadotropic hypogonadism. J Clin Endocrinol Metab 86:1580–1588
17. Bhagavath B, Podolsky RH, Ozata M, Bolu E, Bick DP, Kulharya A, Sherins RJ, Layman LC (2006) Clinical and molecular characterization of a large sample of patients with hypogonadotropic hypogonadism. Fertil Steril 85:706–713
18. Bedecarrats GY, Linher KD, Kaiser UB (2003) Two common naturally occurring mutations in the human gonadotropin-releasing hormone (GnRH) receptor have differential effects on gonadotropin gene expression and on GnRH-mediated signal transduction. J Clin Endocrinol Metab 88:834–843
19. Lin L, Conway GS, Hill NR, Dattani MT, Hindmarsh PC, Achermann JC (2006) A homozygous R262Q mutation in the gonadotropin-releasing hormone receptor presenting as constitutional delay of growth and puberty with subsequent borderline oligospermia. J Clin Endocrinol Metab 91:5117–5121
20. Seminara SB, Messager S, Chatzidaki EE, Thresher RR, Acierno JS Jr, Shagoury JK, Bo-Abbas Y, Kuohung W, Schwinof KM, Hendrick AG, Zahn D, Dixon J, Kaiser UB, Slaugenhaupt SA, Gusella JF, O'Rahilly S, Carlton MB, Crowley WF Jr, Aparicio SA, Colledge WH (2003) The GPR54 gene as a regulator of puberty. N Engl J Med 349:1614–1627
21. de Roux N, Genin E, Carel J-C, Matsuda F, Chaussain J-L, Milgrom E (2003) Hypogonadotropic hypogonadism due to loss of function of the KiSS1-derived peptide receptor *GPR54*. Proc Natl Acad Sci U S A 100(19):10972–10976
22. Semple RK, Achermann JC, Ellery J, Farooqi IS, Karet FE, Stanhope RG, O'rahilly S, Aparicio SA (2005) Two novel missense mutations in g protein-coupled receptor 54 in a patient with hypogonadotropic hypogonadism. J Clin Endocrinol Metab 3:1849–1855
23. de Roux N, Acierno JS Jr, Houang M, Derbois C, Matsuda M, Meysing AU et al (2004) An unique short 3′ duplication of the coding sequence ligand identified in a large cohort of isolated hypogonadotropic hypogonadism patients. 86th Annual Meeting of the Endocrine Society
24. Themmen AP (2005) An update of the pathophysiology of human gonadotrophin subunit and receptor gene mutations and polymorphisms. Reproduction 130:263–274
25. Weiss J, Axelrod L, Whitcomb RW, Harris PE, Crowley WF, Jameson JL (1992) Hypogonadism caused by a single amino acid substitution in the beta subunit of luteinizing hormone. N Engl J Med 326:179–183
26. Valdes-Socin H, Salvi R, Daly AF, Gaillard RC, Quatresooz P, Tebeu PM, Pralong FP, Beckers A (2004) Hypogonadism in a patient with a mutation in the luteinizing hormone beta-subunit gene. N Engl J Med 351:2619–2625
27. Pitteloud N, Acierno JS Jr, Meysing AU, Dwyer AA, Hayes FJ, Crowley WF Jr (2005) Reversible kallmann syndrome, delayed puberty, and isolated anosmia occurring in a single family with a mutation in the fibroblast growth factor receptor 1 gene. J Clin Endocrinol Metab 90:1317–1322
28. Dumur V, Gervais R, Rigot JM, Lafitte JJ, Manouvrier S, Biserte J, Mazeman E, Roussel P (1990) Abnormal distribution of CF delta F508 allele in azoospermic men with congenital aplasia of epididymis and vas deferens. Lancet 336:512
29. Patrizio P, Leonard DG (2000) Mutations of the cystic fibrosis gene and congenital absence of the vas deferens. Results Probl Cell Differ 28:175–186
30. Kerem B, Rommens JM, Buchanan JA, Markiewicz D, Cox TK, Chakravarti A, Buchwald M, Tsui LC (1989) Identification of the cystic fibrosis gene: genetic analysis. Science 245:1073–1080
31. Riordan JR, Rommens JM, Kerem B, Alon N, Rozmahel R, Grzelczak Z, Zielenski J, Lok S, Plavsic N, Chou JL et al (1989) Identification of the cystic fibrosis gene: cloning and characterization of complementary DNA. Science 245:1066–1073
32. Anderson MP, Gregory RJ, Thompson S, Souza DW, Paul S, Mulligan RC, Smith AE, Welsh MJ (1991) Demonstration that CFTR is a chloride channel by alteration of its anion selectivity. Science 253:202–205
33. Larriba S, Bassas L, Egozcue S, Giménez J, Ramos MD, Briceño O, Estivill X, Casals T (2001) Adenosine triphosphate-binding cassette superfamily transporter gene expression in severe male infertility. Biol Reprod 65:394–400
34. Xu WM, Shi QX, Chen WY, Zhou CX, Ni Y, Rowlands DK, Yi Liu G, Zhu H, Ma ZG, Wang XF, Chen ZH, Zhou SC, Dong HS, Zhang XH, Chung YW, Yuan YY, Yang WX, Chan HC (2007) Cystic fibrosis transmembrane conductance regulator is vital to sperm fertilizing capacity and male fertility. Proc Natl Acad Sci U S A 104:9816–9821
35. Oates RD, Amos JA (1994) The genetic basis of congenital bilateral absence of the vas deferens and cystic fibrosis. J Androl 15:1–8
36. Cuppens H, Cassiman JJ (2004) CFTR mutations and polymorphisms in male infertility. Int J Androl 27:251–256
37. Krausz C (2006) Polymorphisms and male infertility. In: Carrell DT (ed) The genetics of male infertility. Humana Press, Totowa, NJ, pp 275–290
38. Krausz C, Giachini C (2007) Genetic risk factors in male infertility. Arch Androl 53:125–133
39. Martin RH (2006) The clinical relevance of sperm aneuploidy. In: Carrell DT (ed) The genetics of male infertility. Humana Press, Totowa, NJ, pp 129–144
40. Sakkas D, Bizzaro D, Manicardi GC (2006) Chromatin damage and male infertility. In: Carrell DT (ed) The genetics of male infertility. Humana Press, Totowa, NJ, pp 303–316
41. Vincent MC, Daudin M, De MP, Massat G, Mieusset R, Pontonnier F, Calvas P, Bujan L, Bourrouillout G (2002) Cytogenetic investigations

of infertile men with low sperm counts: a 25-year experience. J Androl 23:18–22
42. Nielsen J, Wohlert M (1991) Chromosome abnormalities found among 34, 910 newborn children: results from a 13-year incidence study in Arhus, Denmark. Hum Genet 87:81–83
43. Nieschlag E, Behre HM, Meschede D, Kamischke A (2000) Disorders at the testicular level. In: Nieschlag E, Behre HM (eds) Andrology: male reproductive health and dysfunction, 2nd edn. Springer, Heidelberg, pp 133–159
44. Tournaye H, Staessen C, Liebaers I, Van Assche E, Devroey P, Bonduelle M, Van Steirteghem A (1996) Testicular sperm recovery in nine 47, XXY Klinefelter patients. Hum Reprod 11:1644–1649
45. Okada H, Fujioka H, Tatsumi N, Kanzaki M, Okuda Y, Fujisawa M, Hazama M, Matsumoto O, Gohji K, Arakawa S, Kamidono S (1999) Klinefelter's syndrome in the male infertility clinic. Hum Reprod 14:946–952
46. Westlander G, Ekerhovd E, Granberg S, Hanson L, Hanson C, Bergh C (2001) Testicular ultrasonography and extended chromosome analysis in men with nonmosaic Klinefelter syndrome: a prospective study of possible predictive factors for successful sperm recovery. Fertil Steril 75:1102–1105
47. Westlander G, Ekerhovd E, Bergh C (2003) Low levels of serum inhibin B do not exclude successful sperm recovery in men with nonmosaic Klinefelter syndrome. Fertil Steril 79(Suppl 3): 1680–1682
48. Kamischke A, Baumgardt A, Horst J, Nieschlag E (2003) Clinical and diagnostic features of patients with suspected Klinefelter syndrome. J Androl 24:41–48
49. Rucker GB, Mielnik A, King P, Goldstein M, Schlegel PN (1998) Preoperative screening for genetic abnormalities in men with nonobstructive azoospermia before testicular sperm extraction. J Urol 160:2068–2071
50. Staessen C, Tournaye H, Van Assche E, Michiels A, Van Landuyt L, Devroey P, Liebaers I, Van Steirteghem A (2003) PGD in 47, XXY Klinefelter's syndrome patients. Hum Reprod Update 9:319–330
51. Lanfranco F, Kamischke A, Zitzmann M, Nieschlag E (2004) Klinefelter's syndrome. Lancet 364:273–283
52. Chandley AC, Edmond P, Christie S, Gowans L, Fletcher J, Frackiewicz A, Newton M (1975) Cytogenetics and infertility in man. I. Karyotype and seminal analysis: results of a five-year survey of men attending a subfertility clinic. Ann Hum Genet 39:231–254
53. Skakkebaek NE, Zeuthen E, Nielsen J, Yde H (1973) Abnormal spermatogenesis in XYY Males: a report on 4 cases ascertained through a population study. Fertil Steril 24:390–395
54. Berthelsen JG, Skakkebaek N, Perboll O et al (1981) Electron microscopic demonstration of the extra Y chromosome in spermatocytes from human XYY males. In: Byskov AG, Peters H (eds) Development and function of reproductive organs. Excerpta medica, Amsterdam, pp 328–337
55. Sinclair AH, Berta P, Palmer MS, Hawkins JR, Griffiths BL, Smith MJ, Foster JW, Frischauf AM, Lovell-Badge R, Goodfellow PN (1990) A gene from the human sex-determining region encodes a protein with homology to a conserved DNA-binding motif. Nature 346:240–244
56. MElreaveyMcElreavey K, Barbaux S, Ion A, Fellous M (1995) The genetic basis of murine and human sex determination: a review. Heredity 75:599–611
57. Lalli E, Ohe K, Latorre E, Bianchi ME, Sassone-Corsi P (2003) Sexy splicing: regulatory interplays governing sex determination from Drosophila to mammals. J Cell Sci 116:441–445
58. Abbas NE, Toublanc JE, Boucekkine C, Toublanc M, Affara NA, Job JC, Fellous M (1990) A possible common origin of "Y-negative" human XX males and XX true hermaphrodites. Hum Genet 84:356–360
59. Zühlke C, Thies U, Braulke I, Reis A, Schirren C (1994) Down syndrome and male fertility: PCR-derived fingerprinting, serological and andrological investigations. Clin Genet 46:324–326
60. Tiepolo L, Zuffardi O (1976) Localization of factors controlling spermatogenesis in the nonfluorescent portion of the human Y chromosome long arm. Hum Genet 34:119–124
61. Vogt PH, Edelmann A, Kirsch S, Henegariu O, Hirschmann P, Kiesewetter F, Köhn FM, Schill WB, Farah S, Ramos C, Hartmann M, Hartschuh W, Meschede D, Behre HM, Castel A, Nieschlag E, Weidner W, Gröne HJ, Jung A, Engel W, Haidl G (1996) Human Y chromosome azoospermia factors (AZF) mapped to different subregions in Yq11. Hum Mol Genet 5:933–943
62. Repping S, Skaletsky H, Lange J, Silber S, Van Der Veen F, Oates RD, Page DC, Rozen S (2002) Recombination between palindromes P5 and P1 on the human Y chromosome causes massive deletions and spermatogenic failure. Am J Hum Genet 71:906–922
63. Krausz C, Degl'Innocenti S (2006) Y chromosome and male infertility: update, 2006. Front Biosci 11:3049–3061
64. Brandell RA, Mielnik A, Liotta D, Ye Z, Veeck LL, Palermo GD, Schlegel PN (1998) AZFb deletions predict the absence of spermatozoa with testicular sperm extraction: preliminary report of a prognostic genetic test. Hum Reprod 13:2812–2815
65. Krausz C, Quintana-Murci L, McElreavey K (2000) Prognostic value of Y deletion analysis: what is the clinical prognostic value of Y chromosome microdeletion analysis? Hum Reprod 15:1431–1434
66. Skaletsky H, Kuroda-Kawaguchi T, Minx PJ, Cordum HS, Hillier L, Brown LG, Repping S, Pyntikova T, Ali J, Bieri T, Chinwalla A, Delehaunty A, Delehaunty K, Du H, Fewell G, Fulton L, Fulton R, Graves T, Hou SF, Latrielle P, Leonard S, Mardis E, Maupin R, McPherson J, Miner T, Nash W, Nguyen C, Ozersky P, Pepin K, Rock S, Rohlfing T, Scott K, Schultz B, Strong C, Tin-Wollam A, Yang SP, Waterston RH, Wilson RK, Rozen S, Page DC (2003) The male-specific region of the human Y chromosome is a mosaic of discrete sequence classes. Nature 423:825–837
67. Sun C, Skaletsky H, Birren B, Devon K, Tang Z, Silber S, Oates R, Page DC (1999) An azoospermic man with a de novo point mutation in the Y-chromosomal gene USP9Y. Nat Genet 23:429–432
68. Krausz C, Degl'Innocenti S, Nuti F, Morelli A, Felici F, Sansone M, Varriale G, Forti G (2006) Natural transmission of USP9Y gene mutations: a new perspective on the role of AZFa genes in male fertility. Hum Mol Genet 15:2673–2681
69. Krausz C, McElreavey K (2001) Y chromosome microdeletions in 'fertile' males. Hum Reprod 16:1306–1307
70. Simoni M, Bakker E, Krausz C (2004) EAA/EMQN best practice guidelines for molecular diagnosis of y-chromosomal microdeletions. State of the art. Int J Androl 27:240–249
71. Krausz C, McElreavey K (1999) Y chromosome and male infertility. Front Biosci 15:1–8
72. Krausz C, Bussani-Mastellone C, Granchi S, McElreavey K, Scarselli G, Forti G (1999) Screening for microdeletions of Y chromosome genes in patients undergoing ICSI procedure. Hum Reprod 14:1717–1721
73. Krausz C, Rajpert-De Meyts E, Frydelund-Larsen L, Quintana-Murci L, McElreavey K, Skakkebaek NE (2001) Double-blind Y chromosome microdeletion analysis in men with known sperm parameters and reproductive hormone profiles: microdeletions are specific for spermatogenic failure. J Clin Endocrinol Metab 86:2638–2642
74. Krausz C, Quintana-Murci L, Barbaux S, Siffroi JP, Rouba H, Delafontaine D, Souleyreau-Therville N, Arvis G, Antoine JM, Erdei E, Taar JP, Tar A, Jeandidier E, Plessis G, Bourgeron T, Dadoune JP, Fellous M, McElreavey K (1999) A high frequency of Y chromosome deletions in males with nonidiopathic infertility. J Clin Endocrinol Metab 84:3606–3612
75. Krausz C, Forti G, McElreavey K (2003) The Y chromosome and male fertility and infertility. Int J Androl 26:70–75
76. Siffroi JP, Le Bourhis C, Krausz C, Barbaux S, Quintana-Murci L, Kanafani S, Rouba H, Bujan L, Bourrouillou G, Seifer I, Boucher D, Fellous M, McElreavey K, Dadoune JP (2000) Sex chromosome

mosaicism in males carrying Y chromosome long arm deletions. Hum Reprod 15:2559–2562
77. Jaruzelska J, Korcz A, Wojda A, Jedrzejczak P, Bierla J, Surmacz T, Pawelczyk L, Page DC, Kotecki M (2001) Mosaicism for 45, X cell line may accentuate the severity of spermatogenic defects in men with AZFc deletion. J Med Genet 38:798–802
78. Patsalis PC, Sismani C, Quintana-Murci L, Taleb-Bekkouche F, Krausz C, McElreavey K (2002) Effects of transmission of Y chromosome AZFc deletions. Lancet 360:1222–1224
79. Patsalis PC, Skordis N, Sismani C, Kousoulidou L, Koumbaris G, Eftychi C, Stavrides G, Ioulianos A, Kitsiou-Tzeli S, Galla-Voumvouraki A, Kosmaidou Z, Hadjiathanasiou CG, McElreavey K (2005) Identification of high frequency of Y chromosome deletions in patients with sex chromosome mosaicism and correlation with the clinical phenotype and Y-chromosome instability. Am J Med Genet 135:145–149
80. Le Bourhis C, Siffroi JP, McElreavey K, Dadoune JP (2000) Y chromosome microdeletions and germinal mosaicism in infertile males. Mol Hum Reprod 6:688–693
81. Smith EP, Boyd J, Frank GR, Takahashi H, Cohen RM, Specker B, Williams TC, Lubahn DB, Korach KS (1994) Estrogen resistance caused by a mutation in the estrogen-receptor gene in a man. N Engl J Med 331:1056–1061
82. Morishima A, Grumbach MM, Simpson ER, Fisher C, Qin K (1995) Aromatase deficiency in male and female siblings caused by a novel mutation and the physiological role of estrogens. J Clin Endocrinol Metab 80:3689–3698
83. Carani C, Qin K, Simoni M, Faustini-Fustini M, Serpente S, Boyd J, Korach KS, Simpson ER (1997) Effect of testosterone and estradiol in a man with aromatase deficiency. N Engl J Med 337:91–95
84. Deladoey J, Fluck C, Bex M, Yoshimura N, Harada N, Mullis PE (1999) Aromatase deficiency caused by a novel P450arom gene mutation: impact of absent estrogen production on serum gonadotropin concentration in a boy. J Clin Endocrinol Metab 84:4050–4054
85. Maffei L, Murata Y, Rochira V, Tubert G, Aranda C, Vazquez M, Clyne CD, Davis S, Simpson ER, Carani C (2004) Dysmetabolic syndrome in a man with a novel mutation of the aromatase gene: effects of testosterone, alendronate, and estradiol treatment. J Clin Endocrinol Metab 89:61–70
86. Guarducci E, Nuti F, Becherini L, Rotondi M, Balercia G, Forti G, Krausz C (2006) Estrogen receptor alpha promoter polymorphism: stronger estrogen action is coupled with lower sperm count. Hum Reprod 21:994–1001
87. Gottlieb B, Beitel LK, Wu JH, Trifiro M (2004) The androgen receptor gene mutations database (ARDB). Hum Mutat 23:527–533
88. Quigley CA, De Bellis A, Marschke KB, el-Awady MK, Wilson EM, French FS (1995) Androgen receptor defects: historical, clinical, and molecular perspectives. Endocr Rev 16:271–321
89. Ferlin A, Vinanzi C, Garolla A, Selice R, Zuccarello D, Cazzadore C, Foresta C (2006) Male infertility and androgen receptor gene mutations: clinical features and identification of seven novel mutations. Clin Endocrinol 65:106–160
90. Singh R, Deepa SR, Madhavi S, Gupta NJ, Chakravarty B, Singh L, Thangaraj K (2006) Male infertility: no evidence of involvement of androgen receptor gene among Indian men. J Androl 27:102–105
91. Rajender S, Singh L, Thangaraj K (2007) Phenotypic heterogeneity of mutations in androgen receptor gene. Asian J Androl 9:147–179
92. Tut TG, Ghadessy FJ, Trifiro MA, Pinsky L, Yong EL (1997) Long polyglutamine tracts in the androgen receptor are associated with reduced trans-activation, impaired sperm production, and male infertility. J Clin Endocrinol Metab 82:3777–3782
93. Dowsing AT, Yong EL, Clark M, McLachlan RI, de Kretser DM, Trounson AO (1999) Linkage between male infertility and trinucleotide repeat expansion in the androgen-receptor gene. Lancet 354:640–643
94. von Eckardstein S, Syska A, Gromoll J, Kamischke A, Simoni M, Nieschlag E (2001) Inverse correlation between sperm concentration and number of androgen receptor CAG repeats in normal men. J Clin Endocrinol Metab 86:2585–2590
95. Rajpert-De Meyts E, Leffers H, Petersen JH, Andersen AG, Carlsen E, Jorgensen N, Skakkebaek NE (2002) CAG repeat length in androgen-receptor gene and reproductive variables in fertile and infertile men. Lancet 359:44–46
96. Asatiani K, von Eckardstein S, Simoni M, Gromoll J, Nieschlag E (2003) CAG repeat length in the androgen receptor gene affects the risk of male infertility. Int J Androl 26:255–261
97. Lundin KB, Giwercman A, Dizeyi N, Giwercman YL (2007) Functional in vitro characterisation of the androgen receptor GGN polymorphism. Mol Cell Endocrinol 264:184–187
98. Zitzmann M, Depenbusch M, Gromoll J, Nieschlag E (2004) X-chromosome inactivation patterns and androgen receptor functionality influence phenotype and social characteristics as well as pharmacogenetics of testosterone therapy in Klinefelter patients. J Clin Endocrinol Metab 89:6208–6217
99. Repping S, Skaletsky H, Brown L, van Daalen SK, Korver CM, Pyntikova T, Kuroda-Kawaguchi T, de Vries JW, Oates RD, Silber S, van der Veen F, Page DC, Rozen S (2003) Polymorphism for a 1.6-Mb deletion of the human Y chromosome persists through balance between recurrent mutation and haploid selection. Nat Genet 35:247–251
100. Reijo R, Lee TY, Salo P, Alagappan R, Brown LG, Rosenberg M, Rozen S, Jaffe T, Straus D, Hovatta O et al (1995) Diverse spermatogenic defects in humans caused by Y chromosome deletions encompassing a novel RNA-binding protein gene. Nat Genet 10:383–393
101. Giachini C, Laface I, Guarducci E, Balercia G, Forti G, Krausz C (2008) Partial AZFc deletions and duplications: clinical correlates in the Italian population. Hum Genet 124:399–410.
102. Repping S, van Daalen SK, Brown LG, Korver CM, Lange J, Marszalek JD, Pyntikova T, van der Veen F, Skaletsky H, Page DC, Rozen S (2006) High mutation rates have driven extensive structural polymorphism among human Y chromosomes. Nat Genet 38:463–467
103. Sutcliffe AG, Taylor B, Saunders K, Thornton S, Lieberman BA, Grudzinskas JG (2001) Outcome in the second year of life after in-vitro fertilisation by intracytoplasmic sperm injection: a UK case-control study. Lancet 357:2080–2084
104. Foresta C, Ferlin A (2001) Offspring conceived by intracytoplasmic sperm injection. Lancet 358:1270
105. Venables JP, Cooke HJ (2000) Lessons from knockout and transgenic mice for infertility in men. J Endocrinol Invest 23:584–591
106. Hochstenbach R, Hackstein JH (2000) The comparative genetics of human spermatogenesis: clues from flies and other model organisms. Results Probl Cell Differ 28:271–298
107. Nuti F, Krausz C (2008) Gene polymorphisms/mutations relevant to abnormal spermatogenesis. Reprod Biomed Online 16:504–513
108. Roy A, Lin Y-N, Matzuk MM (2006) Genetics of idiopathic male infertility. In: Carrell DT (ed) The genetics of male infertility. Humana Press, Totowa, NJ, pp 99–114
109. Ostermeier GC, Goodrich RJ, Diamond MP, Dix DJ, Krawetz SA (2005) Toward using stable spermatozoal RNAs for prognostic assessment of male factor fertility. Fertil Steril 83: 1687–1694
110. de Mateo S, Martínez-Heredia J, Estanyol JM, Domíguez-Fandos D, Vidal-Taboada JM, Ballescà JL, Oliva R (2007) Marked correlations in protein expression identified by proteomic analysis of human spermatozoa. Proteomics 7:4264–4277
111. Tyler-Smith C, Krausz C (2009) The will-o'-the-wisp of genetics--hunting for the azoospermia factor gene. N Engl J Med 360:925–927

Chapter 28
Varicocele and Male Infertility

Cigdem Tanrikut and Peter N. Schlegel

Abstract Varicocele is the most common treatable issue in male factor infertility. Although varicocele is also detected in the general population, it is more prevalent in the infertile male, and treatment may be of benefit for some infertile couples. Corrective techniques that optimize testicular function and minimize potential morbidities are important. Future research endeavors should focus on elucidating the mechanism of varicocele effects on spermatogenesis to better identify men who will benefit from treatment and to refine treatment approaches.

Keywords Varicocele • Varicocelectomy • Infertility • Hypogonadism • Male

28.1 Introduction

28.1.1 Historical Perspective

Varicocele is an abnormal dilatation of the veins that comprise the pampiniform plexus. The first narrative of varicocele, and its oft-noted ipsilateral testicular atrophy, dates back to the second century AD, as described by the Roman writer Celsus: "the veins are swollen and twisted over the testicle, which becomes smaller than its fellow…." Despite this accurate physical description many centuries ago, the association between varicocele and male factor infertility went unmentioned until the turn of the nineteenth century, at which time Bennet demonstrated improvement in semen quality after correcting bilateral varicoceles in a patient [1]. Similarly, three decades later, Macomber and Sanders described an infertile patient with oligospermia who became normospermic and fertile after undergoing varicocele repair [2]. Since that time, multiple studies of series of patients have documented an improvement in semen parameters and fertility status after varicocele repair [3–7].

28.1.2 Incidence

Varicoceles are found in up to 15% of the general population [8–10], in approximately one-third of men who present with primary infertility [4, 5], and in as many as 80% of those patients with secondary infertility [11, 12]. Although varicoceles may be unilateral or bilateral, the vast majority are left-sided. Isolated right varicoceles are rather uncommon and, if encountered, warrant further evaluation to eliminate the possibility of a causative retroperitoneal pathology.

28.2 Pathophysiology

Deficient or absent valves within the internal spermatic vein are likely an underlying issue contributing to the development of varicocele. Valvular anomalies, together with the anatomy of the spermatic vein system, may explain the preponderance of left-sided varicoceles. As compared with the right internal spermatic vein, the left internal spermatic vein has a longer course and higher insertion. In addition, it empties into the left renal vein at an acute angle in contrast to the right side's oblique insertion into the inferior vena cava.

A venographic study, published in 1994, of more than 650 patients under evaluation for left varicocele demonstrated that 73% did not have internal spermatic vein valves [13]. This finding corroborates previous results of an autopsy series performed by Ahlberg et al., in which cadavers with varicoceles did not have valves within the left internal spermatic vein, whereas cadavers without varicoceles were noted to have multiple valves within the internal spermatic vein [14]. Deficient or absent valves coupled with a single long

C. Tanrikut (✉)
Department of Urology, Massachusetts General Hospital, MGH Fertility Center, 55 Fruit Street, YAW 10A, Boston, MA 02114, USA
e-mail: ctanrikut@partners.org

P.N. Schlegel
Departments of Urology and Reproductive Medicine, Weill Medical College of Cornell University, New York, NY

D.T. Carrell and C.M. Peterson (eds.), *Reproductive Endocrinology and Infertility: Integrating Modern Clinical and Laboratory Practice*,
DOI 10.1007/978-1-4419-1436-1_28,

vein would result in increased hydrostatic pressure transmitted along the spermatic vein to the pampiniform plexus of the testis, leading to venous dilatation and thus varicocele formation. This hypothesis is supported by evidence indicating that men with varicocele have higher mean internal spermatic venous pressures when upright and during Valsalva maneuver than the same measures in a control group without varicocele [15].

28.2.1 Hypothesized Mechanisms of Varicocele-Induced Dysfunction

Several hypotheses have been proposed to explain the impact of varicocele on testicular function. The most widely propagated of these relates to an alteration of the thermal environment within the testis. Optimal sperm production occurs at temperatures cooler than core body temperature and, under normal conditions, a countercurrent heat exchange mechanism between the pampiniform plexus and testicular inflow supports this ideal environment [16]. Several studies indicate that this cooling mechanism is disturbed in patients with varicocele, leading to elevated scrotal and testicular temperatures [17, 18]. Additional studies reflect a reduction in testicular temperature after varicocele repair [16, 19].

A second hypothesis is based on the idea that venous stasis within the varicocele might create a relatively hypoxic milieu within the testis and/or dilution of intratesticular testosterone. However, via testicular venous blood sampling, neither the presence of testicular hypoxia nor lower internal spermatic vein testosterone concentrations has been demonstrated in men with varicocele or in rodent models [20, 21].

Another theory suggests that renal and/or adrenal metabolites may reflux into the spermatic vein and these may, in turn, detrimentally affect spermatogenesis either by direct or indirect effects. Catecholamines and cortisol produced by the adrenal gland had been identified as potential deleterious substances [22]. This concept was not confirmed through further investigation, though; levels of catecholamines and cortisol obtained from the internal spermatic veins of patients with varicoceles and those without were not significantly different [23].

28.2.1.1 Clinical and Histologic Effects

Varicoceles are associated with lower sperm concentration, reduced motility, and/or abnormal morphology on semen analysis [1, 24–26] although not all patients with varicocele will exhibit changes in semen parameters. Larger varicoceles cause more severe impairment of testis function [27]. In addition, varicocele may induce a progressive, duration-dependent deleterious effect on spermatogenesis as demonstrated by the increased incidence of varicocele in men with secondary infertility [28, 29].

Recent prospective controlled studies point to greater levels of sperm DNA damage as determined by higher DNA fragmentation indices in infertile men with varicocele. Elevated levels of oxidative stress were also evident in these patients [30, 31].

Many infertile patients with varicocele also display some degree of ipsilateral testicular atrophy on physical examination [32, 33]. Histologic changes noted in testis biopsy samples of subfertile patients with varicocele reveal a range of abnormalities: tubular thickening, interstitial fibrosis, decreased spermatogenesis, or maturation arrest [33–35].

28.3 Diagnosis

Clinically relevant varicocele should typically be detectable on physical examination. A thorough physical examination should be carried out in a warm room or with the aid of a heating pad in order to relax the scrotum; this allows for careful palpation of the spermatic cord and accurate identification of varicocele. Scrotal examination is performed with the patient both standing and supine in order to fully assess varicocele size. Varicocele is most readily apparent when the patient stands and performs a Valsalva maneuver. If readily visible on initial inspection, the varicocele is considered a grade 3 (large) varicocele (Fig. 28.1) according to the original classification system established by Dubin and Amelar [36]. If the so-called "Bags of worms" is palpable without Valsalva maneuver, the varicocele is classified as grade 2 (moderate). Grade 1 (small) varicoceles are perceptible only

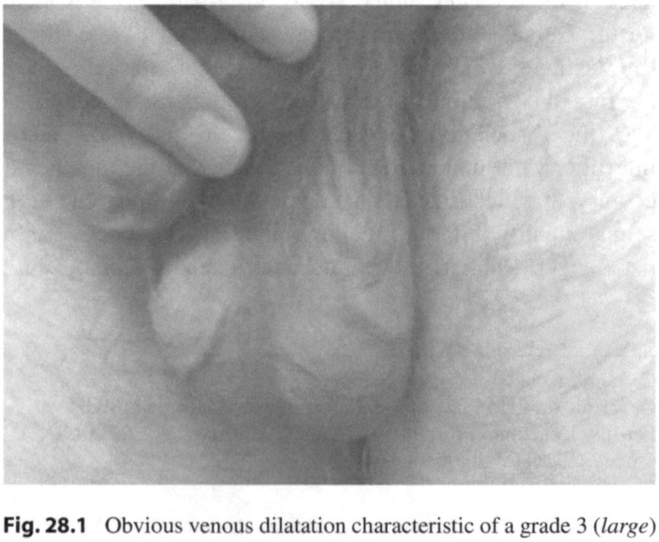

Fig. 28.1 Obvious venous dilatation characteristic of a grade 3 (*large*) varicocele

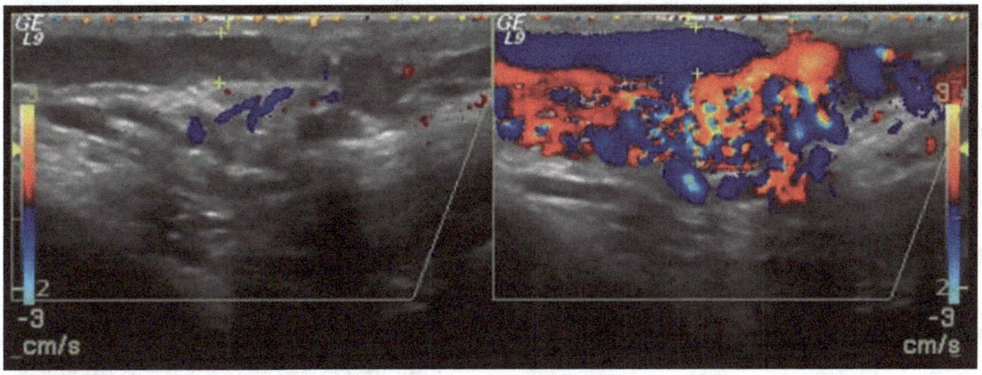

Fig. 28.2 Sonographic representation of dilated pampiniform plexus during Valsalva maneuver

with Valsalva maneuver. Upon reclining to the supine position, a varicocele should decrease in size. If spermatic cord fullness persists in this position, the spermatic cord thickening is more likely due to cord lipoma or inguinal hernia. Measurement of testicular volume may be obtained via orchidometer or calipers in order to determine if atrophy is present.

Scrotal sonogram with Doppler flow (Fig. 28.2) may provide a useful adjunct to varicocele identification if physical examination is indeterminate or difficult due to a “tight” scrotum or the patient’s body habitus. Ultrasonographic detection of veins greater than 2.7–3 mm in diameter suggests the presence of a clinically relevant varicocele. Ultrasound evaluation also helps identify presence of a subclinical, or nonpalpable, varicocele on the contralateral side to a clinical varicocele [37].

Venography provides detailed information regarding spermatic venous anatomy, but is not indicated for routine diagnosis of varicocele given its invasive nature. It may be used as a therapeutic modality as discussed below.

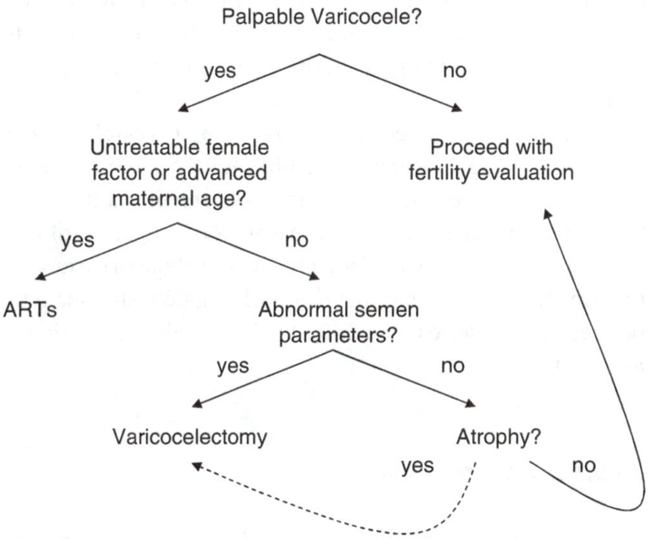

Fig. 28.3 Treatment algorithm for varicocele repair

28.4 Indications for Treatment

As previously stated, not all men with varicocele have clinical problems, so the determination of appropriate candidates for varicocele repair in the fertility setting is warranted (Fig. 28.3). Patients with palpable varicocele and abnormal semen parameters should be considered for repair, provided the female partner does not have mitigating factors that would require assisted reproductive techniques regardless of the male partner’s semen parameters. In addition, the presence of a clinically detectable varicocele with concomitant mild testis atrophy may be considered for repair, even with normal semen parameters, in an effort to preserve testicular function. Although most varicoceles do not cause pain, the presence of pain alone may be an indication for varicocele repair. Other causes of testicular pain should be carefully considered before surgical treatment of scrotal pain.

Varicocele size is a key variable associated with extent of improvement in semen parameters after repair [27, 28]. However, there is controversy regarding the clinical utility of correcting nonpalpable, ultrasound-detected varicoceles [38]. Recent research efforts have aimed to define criteria by which one may determine whether to repair subclinical varicocele. Consideration of varicocele repair for subclinical varicocele greater than 2.7–3 mm with reversal of flow on color Doppler ultrasound is reasonable [38, 39].

28.5 Modalities of Treatment

A number of different techniques exist to correct varicocele, each with the goal of preventing reflux of blood into the aberrant dilated veins of the pampiniform plexus.

With any approach, one should make an effort to spare the artery in order to optimally preserve testicular function [40]. No identifiable differences in fertility outcomes have yet been identified with any of the various approaches [41, 42].

28.5.1 Surgery

28.5.1.1 Retroperitoneal

Palomo first described retroperitoneal ligation of the internal spermatic vein in 1949 [43]. A transverse incision is made medial to the anterior superior iliac spine over the level of the internal inguinal ring. The underlying fascia and muscle fibers are split, and the peritoneum is bluntly retracted medially to expose the internal spermatic vein that is ligated and divided.

At this level, the vein is usually a single vessel and can readily be ligated to prevent reflux into the aberrant veins, contributing to varicocele [6]. However, repair via this technique does not lend itself to assessment and ligation of cremasteric veins, which may potentially contribute to varicocele recurrence [44] and may inadvertently ligate testicular lymphatics and arteries (leading to hydrocele or testicular atrophy).

28.5.1.2 Laparoscopic

Laparoscopic varicocelectomy is achieved via transperitoneal access to the internal inguinal ring. Similar to the retroperitoneal approach, the spermatic vein is ligated high, superior to the internal inguinal ring. Postoperative hydrocele development may be as high as 30% [45] with this type of repair. In addition, laparoscopic repair carries with it the potential for serious morbidity because of its transperitoneal approach.

28.5.1.3 Inguinal

An inguinal approach to varicocele repair was first described by Ivanissevich in 1960 [46]. An incision is made overlying the inguinal canal. The external oblique aponeurosis is incised to expose the spermatic cord, taking care to preserve the ilioinguinal nerve. Spermatic veins within the cord are ligated and divided.

Modifications to the original procedure may provide assistance: (1) Doppler ultrasound can be used to help identify the testicular artery and (2) Optical loupe magnification or an operating microscope can be used. This procedure not only allows for spermatic vein ligation close to the internal inguinal ring where fewer branches are likely, but also provides access to cremasteric vessels that may contribute to varicocele.

28.5.1.4 Microsurgical Approach

The modified inguinal technique may be further enhanced with use of an operating microscope. The added benefit of 8–15 times magnification [47, 48] allows for easier identification and preservation of the testicular arteries, sparing of lymphatic drainage of the scrotum, and recognition and ligation of all internal and external spermatic veins in order to achieve a complete repair with minimal morbidity [49].

The subinguinal approach is similar to the inguinal technique; however, after making a small incision overlying the external inguinal ring, the spermatic cord is mobilized without opening the external oblique aponeurosis. Due to the small incision and lack of muscle-splitting, the subinguinal technique may be less morbid and better-tolerated by patients [50].

28.5.2 Percutaneous Embolization

The only nonsurgical option for varicocele repair is a percutaneous transvenous approach with real-time fluoroscopy [51]. Access to the internal spermatic vein is achieved by a catheter placed in the right femoral vein via the standard Seldinger technique. Under fluoroscopic guidance, the catheter is manipulated into the internal spermatic vein associated with the varicocele. Occlusion of the aberrant veins may be accomplished with coils, fibrin glue, deployable balloons [52], or sclerosing agents [53]. Adequate venous occlusion is confirmed via repeat venography. In patients with anomalous venous anatomy, transvenous access may be complicated or impossible such that failure to correct varicocele at the time of procedure is approximately 27% [54]. In those who achieve correction at the time of procedure recurrence rates range from 11 to 16% [55, 56]. For these reasons, percutaneous embolization is often used as a second-line intervention for those patients who recur after surgical repair or have had extensive prior inguinal surgery.

28.5.3 Complications

Known risks of varicocele repair include hydrocele formation, recurrence of varicocele, and testicular atrophy. Postoperative hydrocele development secondary to ligation of scrotal lymphatic drainage may occur after any of the surgical interventions. Hydrocele almost never occurs after percutaneous embolization as the lymphatic vessels are unaffected in this transvenous approach.

Varicocele may recur if adequate ligation or occlusion of spermatic veins has not been accomplished. The microsurgical approach has by far the lowest recurrence rate (<1%) credited to the advantage magnification affords [47, 49]. As long as the testicular artery and vasal venous outflow are preserved, testicular atrophy should not occur.

28.6 Outcomes of Varicocele Repair

From a fertility perspective, the goal of repair should be to improve semen parameters and pregnancy rates in couples with male-factor infertility associated with varicocele. A significant improvement of semen parameters is seen after varicocele repair in most men [57, 58]. When a small varicocele is found in conjunction with a larger contralateral varicocele, bilateral repair results in greater improvement of semen parameters as compared with unilateral repair of the larger varicocele alone [59, 60].

Pregnancy outcomes are a bit more difficult to assess due to small studies, lack of a control arm in most studies, and mixed cohorts of male partners with palpable or nonpalpable varicoceles. These confounding factors make it difficult to compose a definitive statement with respect to fertility as an outcome measure; reported pregnancy rates after varicocele repair range from 20 to 69%. A recent meta-analysis, including studies of men with palpable varicoceles and abnormal semen parameters who underwent surgical repair, reported on rates of "natural" pregnancy [7]. The results indicate that spontaneous pregnancy rates after varicocelectomy are significantly better than for men who were managed conservatively, with an odds ratio of 2.63 (95% confidence interval 1.60–4.33, fixed effects model).

In azoospermic or severely oligospermic men with palpable varicocele, varicocelectomy has been performed in an effort to improve semen quality. In those men with nonobstructive azoospermia and varicocele, 22–58% had sperm reported on postvaricocelectomy semen analysis [61–64]. It is not clear if histologic diagnosis of testis biopsy samples at the time of varicocelectomy predicts return of sperm to the ejaculate [62, 64]. Although spontaneous pregnancies have been reported in previously oligospermic patients [61, 63], men with nonobstructive azoospermia only occasionally have adequate sperm in the ejaculate after varicocele repair to avoid testicular sperm extraction. In addition, previous varicocelectomy does not appear to enhance sperm retrieval rates at the time of testicular sperm extraction [63, 65]. Although varicocele repair in the man with nonobstructive azoospermia may optimize testicular function, it is relatively unlikely to avoid the need for testicular sperm extraction.

As noted before, varicocele may be associated with abnormal DNA integrity. Preliminary data suggest the potential of varicocelectomy to improve DNA integrity [65, 66]. Given the measurable effect of DNA fragmentation (abnormal DNA integrity) on fertility outcomes – including IVF and ICSI results – varicocele repair may be considered even for couples who undergo IVF-ICSI. Undoubtedly, additional larger-scale studies are indicated to further clarify this aspect of varicocele research.

28.7 Conclusions

Varicocele is a significant correctable condition for many infertile couples who have male factor infertility. A thorough examination to adequately assess for varicocele and meticulous surgical technique for correction of varicocele lead to improved semen parameters and fertility outcomes in comparison with nonoperative management. Additional studies are needed to further evaluate the mechanism(s) by which a varicocele adversely affects fertility.

In summary, a varicocele is a risk factor for impaired spermatogenesis and male-factor infertility. Larger (palpable) varicoceles are more likely to be clinically significant, and abnormal semen parameters with a palpable varicocele is an indication for varicocele repair. Microsurgical varicocelectomy has the least morbidity and lowest recurrence rate of any of the repair options. Varicocele repair has been shown to effect an improvement in semen parameters, pregnancy outcomes, and possibly DNA integrity.

28.8 Summary: Evidence-Based Guidelines

- Varicocele is a risk factor for impaired spermatogenesis and male-factor infertility
- Larger (palpable) varicoceles are more likely to be clinically significant
- Abnormal semen parameters in the setting of palpable varicocele is an indication for varicocele repair
- Microsurgical varicocelectomy has the least morbidity and lowest recurrence rate of any of the repair options
- Varicocele repair has been shown to effect an improvement in semen parameters, pregnancy outcomes, and possibly DNA integrity

References

1. Bennet W (1889) Varicocele, particularly with reference to its radical cure. Lancet 1:261–262
2. Macomber D, Sanders M (1929) The spermatozoa count: its value in the diagnosis, prognosis and treatment of sterility. N Engl J Med 200:981

3. Russell JK (1954) Varicocele in groups of fertile and subfertile males. Br Med J 1(4873):1231–1233
4. Dubin L, Amelar RD (1977) Varicocelectomy: 986 cases in a twelve-year study. Urology 10(5):446–449
5. Greenberg SH, Lipshultz LI, Wein AJ (1978) Experience with 425 subfertile male patients. J Urol 119(4):507–510
6. Madgar I, Weissenberg R, Lunenfeld B, Karasik A, Goldwasser B (1995) Controlled trial of high spermatic vein ligation for varicocele in infertile men. Fertil Steril 63(1):120–124
7. Marmar JL, Agarwal A, Prabakaran S et al (2007) Reassessing the value of varicocelectomy as a treatment for male subfertility with a new meta-analysis. Fertil Steril 88(3):639–648
8. Mecham R, Twonsend R, Rademacher D, Drose J (1994) The incidence of varicoceles in the general population when ealuated by physical examination, gray scale sonography and color Doppler sonography. J Urol 151:1535–1538
9. Handelsman DJ, Conway AJ, Boylan LM, Turtle JR (1984) Testicular function in potential sperm donors: normal ranges and the effects of smoking and varicocele. Int J Androl 7(5):369–382
10. Johnson DE, Pohl DR, Rivera-Correa H (1970) Varicocele: an innocuous condition? South Med J 63(1):34–36
11. Jarow JP, Coburn M, Sigman M (1996) Incidence of varicoceles in men with primary and secondary infertility. Urology 47(1):73–76
12. Gorelick JI, Goldstein M (1993) Loss of fertility in men with varicocele. Fertil Steril 59(3):613–616
13. Braedel HU, Steffens J, Ziegler M, Polsky MS, Platt ML (1994) A possible ontogenic etiology for idiopathic left varicocele. J Urol 151(1):62–66
14. Ahlberg NE, Bartley O, Chidekel N (1966) Right and left gonadal veins. An anatomical and statistical study. Acta Radiol Diagn 4(6):593–601
15. Shafik A, Bedeir GA (1980) Venous tension patterns in cord veins. I. In normal and varicocele individuals. J Urol 123(3):383–385
16. Zorgniotti AW, Macleod J (1973) Studies in temperature, human semen quality, and varicocele. Fertil Steril 24(11):854–863
17. Tessler AN, Krahn HP (1966) Varicocele and testicular temperature. Fertil Steril 17(2):201–203
18. Lewis RW, Harrison RM (1979) Contact scrotal thermography: application to problems of infertility. J Urol 122(1):40–42
19. Wright EJ, Young GP, Goldstein M (1997) Reduction in testicular temperature after varicocelectomy in infertile men. Urology 50(2):257–259
20. Donohue RE, Brown JS (1969) Blood gases and pH determinations in the internal spermatic veins of subfertile men with varicocele. Fertil Steril 20(2):365–369
21. Turner TT, Jones CE, Roddy MS (1987) Experimental varicocele does not affect the blood-testis barrier, epididymal electrolyte concentrations, or testicular blood gas concentrations. Biol Reprod 36(4):926–932
22. Comhaire F, Vermeulen A (1974) Varicoceles: cortisol and catecholamines. Fertil Steril 25:88–95
23. Steeno O, Koumans J, De Moor P (1976) Adrenal cortical hormones in the spermatic vein of 95 patients with left varicocele. Andrologia 8(2):101–104
24. World Health Organization (1992) The influence of varicocele on parameters of fertility in a large group of men presenting in infertility clinics. Fertil Steril 57:1289–1293
25. Nagao R, Playmate S, Berger R, Perin E, Paulsen C (1986) Comparison of gonadal function between fertile and infertile men with varicoceles. Fertil Steril 46:930–933
26. Macleod J (1965) Seminal cytology in the presence of varicocele. Fertil Steril 16:735–757
27. Steckel J, Dicker AP, Goldstein M (1993) Relationship between varicocele size and response to varicocelectomy. J Urol 149(4):769–771
28. Chehval MJ, Purcell MH (1992) Deterioration of semen parameters over time in men with untreated varicocele: evidence of progressive testicular damage. Fertil Steril 57(1):174–177
29. Witt MA, Lipshultz LI (1993) Varicocele: a progressive or static lesion? Urology 42(5):541–543
30. Saleh RA, Agarwal A, Sharma RK, Said TM, Sikka SC, Thomas AJ Jr (2003) Evaluation of nuclear DNA damage in spermatozoa from infertile men with varicocele. Fertil Steril 80(6):1431–1436
31. Smith R, Kaune H, Parodi D et al (2006) Increased sperm DNA damage in patients with varicocele: relationship with seminal oxidative stress. Hum Reprod 21(4):986–993 (Oxford, England)
32. Sigman M, Jarow JP (1997) Ipsilateral testicular hypotrophy is associated with decreased sperm counts in infertile men with varicoceles. J Urol 158(2):605–607
33. Agger P, Johnsen SG (1978) Quantitative evaluation of testicular biopsies in varicocele. Fertil Steril 29(1):52–57
34. Kass EJ, Chandra RS, Belman AB (1987) Testicular histology in the adolescent with a varicocele. Pediatrics 79(6):996–998
35. Hadziselimovic F, Herzog B, Liebundgut B, Jenny P, Buser M (1989) Testicular and vascular changes in children and adults with varicocele. J Urol 142(2 Pt 2):583–585 discussion 603–605
36. Dubin L, Amelar RD (1970) Varicocele size and results of varicocelectomy in selected subfertile men with varicocele. Fertil Steril 21(8):606–609
37. Kondoh N, Meguro N, Matsumiya K, Namiki M, Kiyohara H, Okuyama A (1993) Significance of subclinical varicocele detected by scrotal sonography in male infertility: a preliminary report. J Urol 150(4):1158–1160
38. Jarow JP, Ogle SR, Eskew LA (1996) Seminal improvement following repair of ultrasound detected subclinical varicoceles. J Urol 155(4):1287–1290
39. Schiff JD, Li PS, Goldstein M (2006) Correlation of ultrasound-measured venous size and reversal of flow with Valsalva with improvement in semen-analysis parameters after varicocelectomy. Fertil Steril 86(1):250–252
40. Chan PT, Wright EJ, Goldstein M (2005) Incidence and postoperative outcomes of accidental ligation of the testicular artery during microsurgical varicocelectomy. J Urol 173(2):482–484
41. Shlansky-Goldberg RD, VanArsdalen KN, Rutter CM et al (1997) Percutaneous varicocele embolization versus surgical ligation for the treatment of infertility: changes in seminal parameters and pregnancy outcomes. J Vasc Interv Radiol 8(5):759–767
42. Nieschlag E, Behre HM, Schlingheider A, Nashan D, Pohl J, Fischedick AR (1993) Surgical ligation vs. angiographic embolization of the vena spermatica: a prospective randomized study for the treatment of varicocele-related infertility. Andrologia 25(5): 233–237
43. Palomo A (1949) Radical cure of varicocele by a new technique; preliminary report. J Urol 61(3):604–607
44. Murray RR Jr, Mitchell SE, Kadir S et al (1986) Comparison of recurrent varicocele anatomy following surgery and percutaneous balloon occlusion. J Urol 135(2):286–289
45. Hassan JM, Adams MC, Pope JC, Demarco RT, Brock JW 3rd (2006) Hydrocele formation following laparoscopic varicocelectomy. J Urol 175(3 Pt 1):1076–1079
46. Ivanissevich O (1960) Left varicocele due to reflux; experience with 4,470 operative cases in forty-two years. J Int Coll Surg 34:742–755
47. Silber SJ (1979) Microsurgical aspects of varicocele. Fertil Steril 31(2):230–232
48. Wosnitzer M, Roth JA (1983) Optical magnification and Doppler ultrasound probe for varicocelectomy. Urology 22(1):24–26
49. Goldstein M, Gilbert BR, Dicker AP, Dwosh J, Gnecco C (1992) Microsurgical inguinal varicocelectomy with delivery of the testis: an artery and lymphatic sparing technique. J Urol 148(6): 1808–1811
50. Marmar JL, Kim Y (1994) Subinguinal microsurgical varicocelectomy: a technical critique and statistical analysis of semen and pregnancy data. J Urol 152(4):1127–1132

51. Gazzera C, Rampado O, Savio L, Di Bisceglie C, Manieri C, Gandini G (2006) Radiological treatment of male varicocele: technical, clinical, seminal and dosimetric aspects. Radiol Med 111(3):449–458
52. Walsh PC, White RI Jr (1981) Balloon occlusion of the internal spermatic vein for the treatment of varicoceles. JAMA 246(15):1701–1702
53. Gat Y, Bachar GN, Zukerman Z, Belenky A, Gornish M (2004) Varicocele: a bilateral disease. Fertil Steril 81(2):424–429
54. Pryor JL, Howards SS (1987) Varicocele. Urol Clin North Am 14(3):499–513
55. Halden W, White RI Jr (1987) Outpatient embolotherapy of varicocele. Urol Clin North Am 14(1):137–144
56. Keoghane SR, Jones L, Wright MP, Kabala J (2001) Percutaneous retrograde varicocele embolisation using tungsten embolisation coils: a five year audit. Int Urol Nephrol 33(3):517–520
57. Schlesinger MH, Wilets IF, Nagler HM (1994) Treatment outcome after varicocelectomy. A critical analysis. Urol Clin North Am 21(3):517–529
58. Agarwal A, Deepinder F, Cocuzza M et al (2007) Efficacy of varicocelectomy in improving semen parameters: new meta-analytical approach. Urology 70(3):532–538
59. Scherr D, Goldstein M (1999) Comparison of bilateral versus unilateral varicocelectomy in men with palpable bilateral varicoceles. J Urol 162(1):85–88
60. Libman J, Jarvi K, Lo K, Zini A (2006) Beneficial effect of microsurgical varicocelectomy is superior for men with bilateral versus unilateral repair. J Urol 176(6 Pt 1):2602–2605 discussion 5
61. Matthews GJ, Matthews ED, Goldstein M (1998) Induction of spermatogenesis and achievement of pregnancy after microsurgical varicocelectomy in men with azoospermia and severe oligoasthenospermia. Fertil Steril 70(1):71–75
62. Kim ED, Leibman BB, Grinblat DM, Lipshultz LI (1999) Varicocele repair improves semen parameters in azoospermic men with spermatogenic failure. J Urol 162(3 Pt 1):737–740
63. Schlegel PN, Kaufmann J (2004) Role of varicocelectomy in men with nonobstructive azoospermia. Fertil Steril 81(6): 1585–1588
64. Pasqualotto F, Sobreiro B, Hallak J, Pasqualotto E, Lucon A (2006) Induction of spermatogenesis in azoospermic men after varicocele repair: an update. Fertil Steril 85:635–639
65. Zini A, Blumenfeld A, Libman J, Willis J (2005) Beneficial effect of microsurgical varicocelectomy on human sperm DNA integrity. Hum Reprod 20(4):1018–1021 (Oxford, England)
66. Werthman P, Wixon R, Kasperson K, Evenson DP (2008) Significant decrease in sperm deoxyribonucleic acid fragmentation after varicocelectomy. Fertil Steril 90:1800–1804

Chapter 29
Sperm Retrieval Techniques

Paul J. Turek

Abstract Sperm retrieval procedures are integral to the care of men with obstructive and nonobstructive azoospermia. In men with obstruction, depending on the condition, sperm may be retrieved from the vas deferens, epididymis, or testis. In men with nonobstructive azoospermia, the testis is the only reliable source of sperm for ICSI. The various sperm retrieval techniques and reported success rates are reviewed in this chapter. In addition, an evidence-based review of the differences in ICSI outcomes among the different sperm sources is presented. Finally, important details regarding the timing of sperm and oocyte retrieval, sperm cryopreservation, and the efficient use of laboratory staff effort are discussed.

Keywords Azoospermia • ICSI • Testis • Epididymis • Vas deferens • Sperm • Vasectomy • Obstruction • Sperm aspiration • Microsurgery • Mapping

29.1 Introduction

Sperm retrieval techniques are procedures designed to collect sperm from organs within the male genital tract. First developed in 1985 [1], 10 years before the description of intracytoplasmic sperm injection (ICSI), sperm retrieval combined with in vitro fertilization (IVF) and ICSI have become invaluable techniques to allow infertile men without ejaculated sperm the opportunity for biological fatherhood. These procedures are largely performed in anejaculatory or azoospermic men who are either unable to produce an ejaculate or produce an ejaculate without sperm, respectively. Sperm retrieval techniques are based on acquiring sperm from the reproductive tract, including the vas deferens, epididymis, and testicle (Fig. 29.1). They are indicated for men in whom the transport of sperm is not possible because the ductal system that normally carries sperm to the ejaculate is either absent or unreconstructable, or if sperm production is low, as in nonobstructive azoospermia. An evidence-based discussion of these techniques is presented in this chapter.

Several evidence-based principles can be used to guide clinical care in sperm retrieval cases:

1. A recent Cochrane meta-analysis has determined that there is insufficient data from randomized trials to recommend any particular surgical sperm retrieval technique for either obstructive or nonobstructive azoospermia [2]. Indeed, many different approaches are taken for sperm retrieval.
2. Although it is not difficult to retrieve sperm from azoospermic men with obstruction, it can be very difficult to find sperm in men with testicular failure and nonobstructive azoospermia.
3. Since assisted reproduction (IVF-ICSI) does not have a 100% success rate, it behooves reproductive urologists to develop and use sperm retrieval techniques that are not only reliable and of low morbidity, but that also have the potential to harvest sufficient sperm to enable multiple IVF-ICSI attempts without repeat surgery [3].

It is also important to realize that sperm retrieved from the male reproductive tract requires assisted reproductive technologies for success. Indeed, sperm retrieval is intimately tied to the complementary procedures on the female partner that are listed in Table 29.1.

29.1.1 Vasal Sperm Aspiration

Patients with congenital or acquired obstruction of the excurrent ductal system at the level of the prostate, or abdominal or pelvic portions of the vas deferens are candidates for this technique. Men with ejaculatory failure due to diabetes or spinal cord injury are also candidates for this approach to sperm retrieval. Obstruction can result from abdominal or pelvic trauma, surgery such as a vasectomy or, occasionally, severe infections that obliterate the vas deferens lumen.

P.J. Turek (✉)
Director, The Turek Clinic,
San Francisco, CA, USA
e-mail: PaulTurek@gmail.com

D.T. Carrell and C.M. Peterson (eds.), *Reproductive Endocrinology and Infertility: Integrating Modern Clinical and Laboratory Practice*,
DOI 10.1007/978-1-4419-1436-1_29,

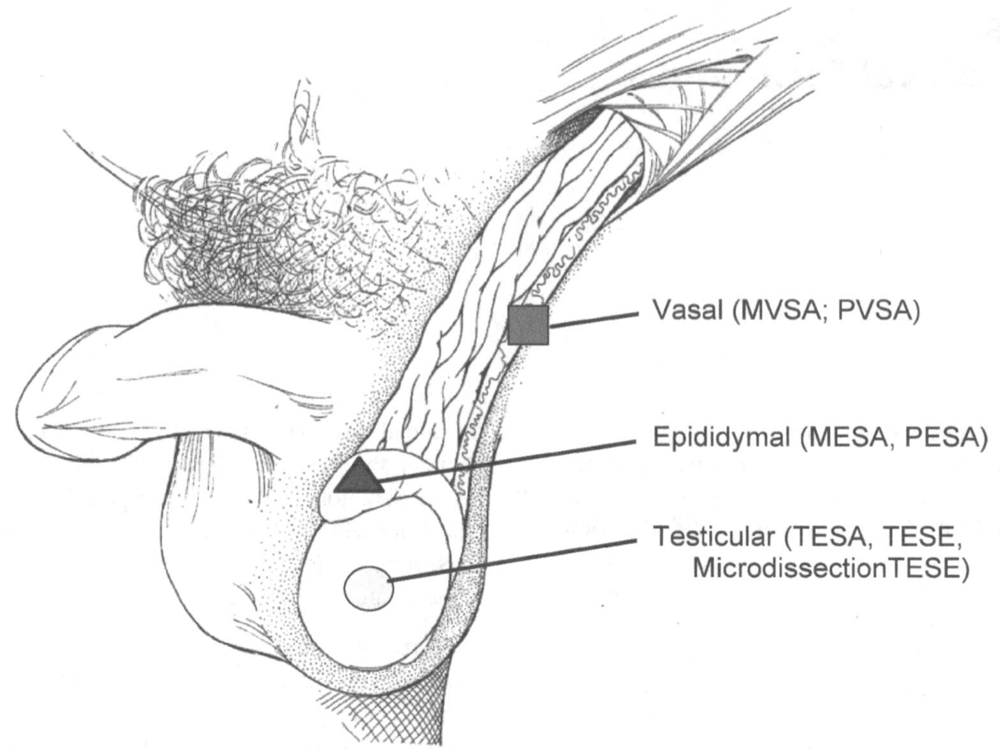

Fig. 29.1 Sperm retrieval techniques involve finding sperm in three reproductive tract organs: the vas deferens, epididymis, and testicle. Seminal vesicle sperm aspiration is also possible but not widely used. *MVSA* microscopic vasal sperm aspiration, *PVSA* percutaneous vasal sperm aspiration, *MESA* microscopic epididymal sperm aspiration, *PESA* percutaneous epididymal sperm aspiration, *TESA* testicular sperm aspiration, *TESE* testis sperm extraction by biopsy, *Microdissection TESE* microscopic testis sperm extraction by biopsy

Table 29.1 Levels of assisted reproduction required for sperm retrieval

Procedure	Source organ	IUI	IVF	ICSI
Vasal aspiration (MVSA, PVSA)	Vas deferens	Yes	Yes	Maybe
Epididymal aspiration (MESA, PESA)	Epididymis	Maybe	Yes	Yes
Testis (TESA, TESE, MicroTESE)	Testicle	No	Yes	Yes

A prerequisite for successful vasal sperm aspiration is the presence of normal sperm production. This is evaluated indirectly with the findings of (a) normal testis volume and (b) normal serum follicle-stimulating hormone (FSH) and testosterone levels. The most direct way to verify normal sperm production is with a diagnostic testis biopsy.

Vasal aspiration is performed either coincident with the day of the wife's ovulation or in advance of ovulation and frozen and thawed for use. It involves a brief, same-day procedure under local anesthesia, often accompanied by intravenous sedation, and performed in the manner of a no-scalpel vasectomy. Through a scrotal puncture the vas deferens is identified. Using either a microscope in the operating room or loupe magnification, a small incision or a puncture is made in the delicate muscular wall of the vas deferens until the lumen is entered (Fig. 29.2). Fine-tipped (24 gauge) 1 mL syringes charged with 0.1 mL of Earles (or other) culture medium are used to aspirate the clear fluid leaking from the vas. More fluid can be expressed from the vas deferens with gentle massaging of the testis vas deferens. After sufficient sperm are obtained (>10–20 million), the wall of the vas deferens is closed with microscopic sutures if a hemivasotomy is performed (Fig. 29.3). No closure is needed for a puncture vasotomy. The recovery period is about 24 h. Complications of the procedure include low risks of bleeding (1%) and infection (1%) that accompany scrotal surgery in general, and the potential that a scar will form in the lumen vas deferens and occlude it (5%).

Among the three sources of retrieved sperm, vasal sperm is the most "mature" or fertilizable sperm, as this sperm has already passed through the epididymis, where sperm maturation occurs. Although most commonly used in conjunction with IVF-ICSI, the maturity of this sperm is reflected by the fact that pregnancies have been achieved with vasal sperm

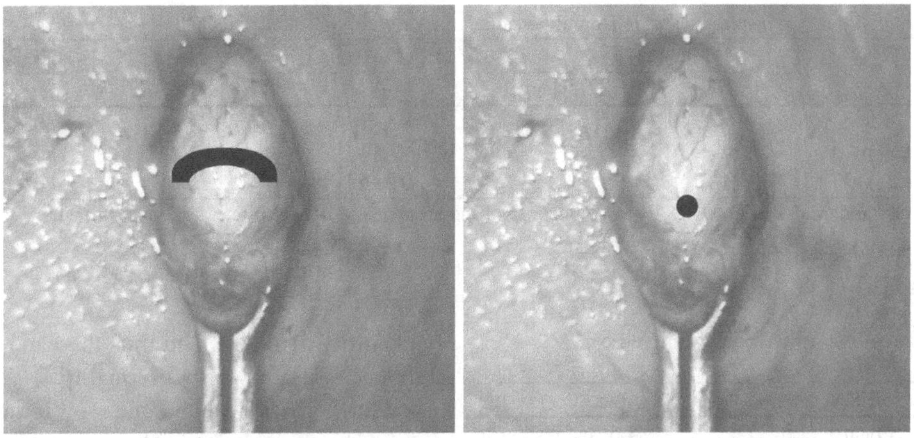

Fig. 29.2 Two approaches to vasal sperm aspiration. The vas deferens is delivered with a no-scalpel approach. Vasal sperm is aspirated by either a small incision in the vas deferens wall that is closed microscopically (hemivasotomy, left panel) or through a small puncture (27–30 gauge) into the lumen (puncture vasotomy, right panel)

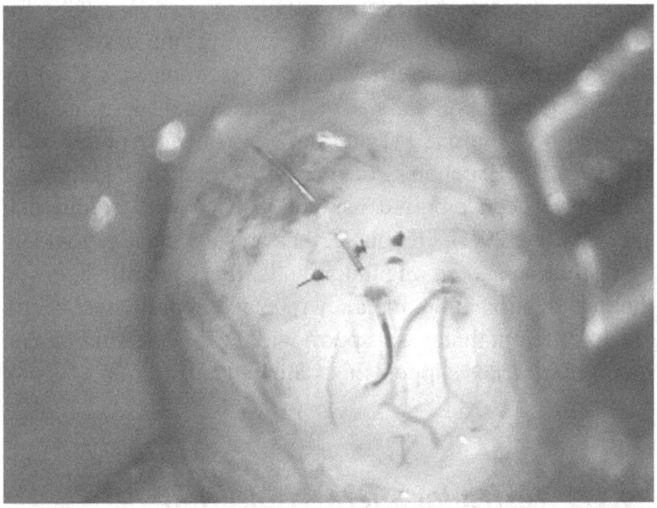

Fig. 29.3 Closure of formal hemivasotomy. The incision in the vas deferens lumen is closed microsurgically in two layers. The inner layer is complete with three suture knots visible and the outer layer has been started with the needle perforating the serosal layer of the vas on each side of the incision

and intrauterine insemination (IUI) [4, 5] and IVF [6] as well. Excellent sperm motility can be expected, depending on the condition for which vasal aspiration is performed. In our study of vasal aspiration in fertile men undergoing vasectomy, a mean sperm motility of 71% was observed (Table 29.2) [7]. Two pronuclear fertilization rates equivalent to that obtained with ejaculated sperm can be expected with aspirated vasal sperm.

29.1.2 Epididymal Sperm Aspiration

Epididymal sperm aspiration is performed when the vas is either absent such as with congenital absence of the vas deferens (CAVD) or is scarred from prior surgery, trauma, or infection. It is also performed in cases of anejaculation due to diabetes or spinal cord injury. Epididymal sperm aspiration is performed in a manner similar to vasal sperm aspiration and can also be undertaken either coincident with the wife's ovulation for IVF or in advance of IVF and frozen and thawed for use. These techniques are also useful for intraoperative sperm retrieval during microsurgical reconstructive procedures such as epididymovasostomy after vasectomy. Similar to vasal sperm aspiration, epididymal sperm retrieval is most successful when sperm production in the testis is normal. Although originally described as a procedure done under general anesthesia, it is now most commonly performed under local anesthesia with or without intravenous sedation [8]. The recovery period after this same day procedure is also about 24 h.

Two different approaches to epididymal sperm aspiration are commonly taken: microscopic epididymal sperm aspiration (MESA) in which the epididymis is explored microsurgically and sperm aspirated from individual epididymal tubules, or percutaneous epididymal sperm aspiration (PESA) in which sperm are aspirated blindly from the epididymis without an incision. The differences between the two techniques are outlined in Table 29.3. The most important difference between these techniques is that individual epididymal tubules are sampled for sperm with MESA, but multiple

Table 29.2 Motility and viability of aspirated sperm from the vas deferens, epididymis and testis [7]

	Motility (%)		Vital stain (% viable)		HOS (% viable)	
Aspirated sperm	Fresh	Thawed	Fresh	Thawed	Fresh	Thawed
Testis ($n=5$, NOA)	5±3.6	0.2±1	86±5	46±12	60±12	31±6
Epididymis ($n=8$, obstructive)	22±18	7±0.7	57±20	24±13	40±14	17±10
Vas deferens ($n=5$, fertile)	71±16	38±13	91±6	51±11	80±11	39±15

Note: Values are mean±standard deviation; *HOS* hypo-osmotic swelling assay, *NOA* nonobstructive azoospermia

Table 29.3 Comparison of two epididymal sperm retrieval techniques [3]

Parameter	MESA	PESA
Anesthesia	Local anesthesia±sedation	Local anesthesia
Operating microscope	Needed	Not needed
Successful retrieval	90–95%	67–90%
Sperm banked	Excellent	Good
Days to work	2	1–2
Patient satisfaction	High	High
Complications	<1%	<1%
Need to repeat for more sperm	Low	Moderate
Cost	More	Less

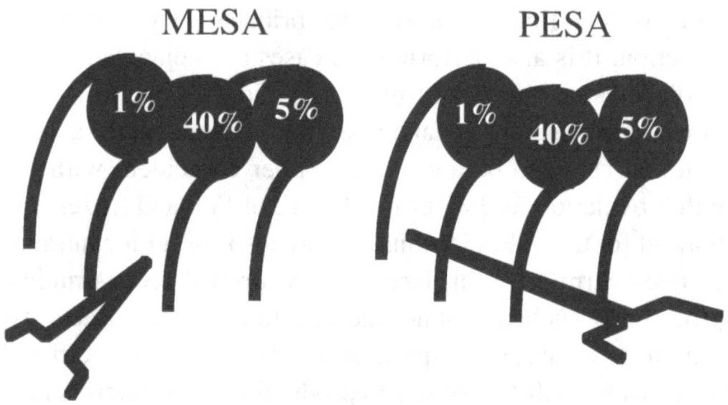

Fig. 29.4 Essential difference between MESA and PESA techniques. Physiologically, not all epididymal tubules will contain sperm with similar motility. Values represent the percent sperm motility within an individual epididymal tubule. With MESA, individual epididymal tubules are sampled, which allows for the capture of sperm with maximum motility for use or thaw. With PESA, multiple epididymal tubules are sampled simultaneously which results in an aspirated sperm specimen with an average motility that is generally lower than with MESA, as the sampling is blind and less selective. This difference can translate into lower quality sperm for banking and increase the need for repeat surgical procedures

epididymal tubules are sampled blindly with PESA (Fig. 29.4). This fact underlies important differences in epididymal sperm quality that can affect the overall yield and bankability of sperm, and thus the need to repeat the procedure because of poor sperm quality.

With the MESA technique, sperm are directly collected from a single, isolated epididymal tubule in much the same manner as the vasal procedure (Fig. 29.5). Depending on the length of the epididymis available for aspiration, multiple, separate aspiration sites can be made progressing from the corpus to the cauda epididymis to find sperm with motility. When 10–20 million sperm are obtained, the epididymal tubule is closed with microscopic suture, and the sperm are processed for assisted reproduction.

Epididymal sperm are not as "mature" as vasal sperm that have traversed the entire length of the epididymis. As a consequence, epididymal sperm usually require IVF-ICSI for pregnancy success (Table 29.1). However, the development of epididymal sperm retrieval techniques preceded ICSI by 10 years [1] and pregnancies with epididymal sperm are possible with IVF alone [1] and have also been reported with IUI [9, 10]. Excellent oocyte fertilization and pregnancy rates have been reported using IVF-ICSI with epididymal sperm (Table 29.4). Of course, these results may vary widely by institution and among individuals. It is generally believed that fertilization and pregnancy rates with epididymal sperm are no different than vasal sperm with IVF-ICSI, although no randomized trials support this statement.

29.1.3 Testicular Sperm Aspiration and Extraction

The newest of the three sperm aspiration techniques, testicular sperm retrieval, was first reported in 1993, 1 year after ICSI [11]. It is a breakthrough in the sense that it demonstrates that sperm do not have to "mature" and pass through the epididymis to be able to fertilize an egg. Because of their immaturity, however, testicular sperm require IVF-ICSI for success (Table 29.1).

Testicular sperm extraction is indicated for "obstructed" patients in whom sperm production is normal and there is a blockage in the epididymis (either from prior surgery, infection or due to congenital absence), or a blockage within the ducts that conduct sperm out of the testicle (efferent ductules).

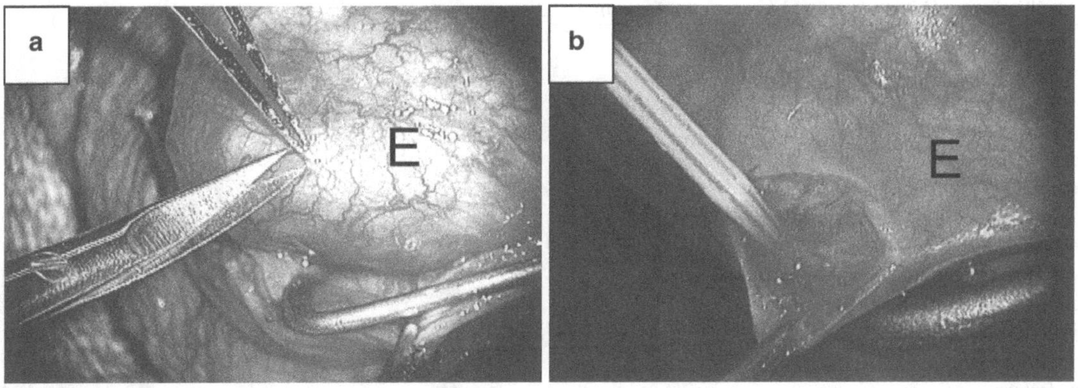

Fig. 29.5 MESA Technique. (**a**) The epididymis (E) is exposed through a 1 cm incision and explored under low power microscopy. The epididymal tunic or covering is then incised overlying a dilated epididymal tubule, as shown here. (**b**) After opening the isolated epididymal tubule under high power magnification, epididymal fluid and sperm are aspirated into syringes or microneedles

Table 29.4 Published ICSI outcomes with fresh and frozen-thawed epididymal sperm

	Fertilization rate (%)		Pregnancy rate (%)	
Unpaired controls	Fresh	Frozen-thawed	Fresh	Frozen-thawed
Nagy et al. (1995)	56	56	30	33
Oates et al. (1996)	20	37	0	29
Cha et al. (1997)	68.4	72.4	44.4	63.6
Holden et al. (1997)	73[a]	47	27[a]	18.4
Van Steirteghem et al. (1998)	64.8	54.7	44.3	33.8
Shibahara et al. (1999)	68.6	45.3	60	23.1
Paired controls				
Friedler et al. (1998)	56	53	32	37
Hutchon et al. (1998)	64	66	34.5[a]	26.7
Tournaye et al. (1999)	60.1	53	32.1	35.2
Cayan et al. (2001)	58.4	62	31.6	36.8

[a]Fresh ejaculated sperm was compared with frozen-thawed epididymal sperm

It is also useful for men in whom sperm production is severely compromised within the testis, such that so few sperm are produced that they cannot reach the ejaculate through the excurrent ducts ("nonobstructive azoospermia"). Men with nonobstructive azoospermia generally have testis atrophy, an elevated FSH and no sperm on centrifuged pellet analysis of the ejaculate. The definitive diagnosis of nonobstructive azoospermia requires that the testis biopsy show abnormal or absent spermatogenesis. The etiology of this condition varies widely and it occurs in about 1–5% of all infertile men. Conditions that can result in nonobstructive azoospermia are listed in Table 29.5.

29.1.3.1 Testis Sperm Retrieval with Obstructive Azoospermia

Patients with congenital or acquired obstruction of the excurrent ductal system at the level of the epididymis or vas deferens are candidates for this technique. Men with ejaculatory failure due to diabetes, spinal cord injury, other neurologic diseases, or performance anxiety are also candidates for this approach to sperm retrieval. By definition, obstructive azoospermia implies normal sperm production, as suggested by hormonal or testis biopsy findings. In men with obstruction, sperm from the testis can be retrieved by needle aspiration (TESA) or percutaneous or open surgical biopsy (TESE).

Testis sperm aspiration is performed either coincident with the day of the wife's ovulation or in advance of ovulation and frozen and thawed for use. Similar to other sperm retrieval techniques, it is a same-day procedure under local anesthesia, with or without intravenous sedation. TESA involves stabilization of the testis in the surgeon's hand with the epididymis held posteriorly followed by insertion of a hollow needle (16–23 gauge) into the testis through the stretched skin of the scrotum [12]. Research has shown that sperm in obstructed testes will be found throughout the

Table 29.5 Conditions associated with nonobstructive azoospermia

Congenital or genetic
Karyotype abnormality (e.g. Klinefelter syndrome)
Y chromosome microdeletion
Germ cell late maturation arrest
Cryptorchidism
Congenital anorchia
Hypothalamic-pituitary-gonadal dysfunction (e.g. Kallmann syndrome)
Androgen excess (e.g. congenital adrenal hyperplasia)
Androgen receptor abnormalities
Estrogen or prolactin excess
Thyroid abnormalities
Idiopathic testis failure
Acquired
Torsion
Epididymoorchitis
Ischemic atrophy (e.g. after hernia repair)
Ionizing radiation (e.g. cancer radiotherapy)
Chemotherapy (e.g. cyclophosphamide)
Heat or thermal exposure
Hypothalamic or pituitary tumor (e.g. hyperprolactinemia)
Drug induced (e.g. anabolic steroids, alcohol, glucocorticoids)
Severe systemic illness (e.g. cancer, diabetes, renal failure)
Pesticide or toxin exposure
Sperm autoimmunity
Varicocele

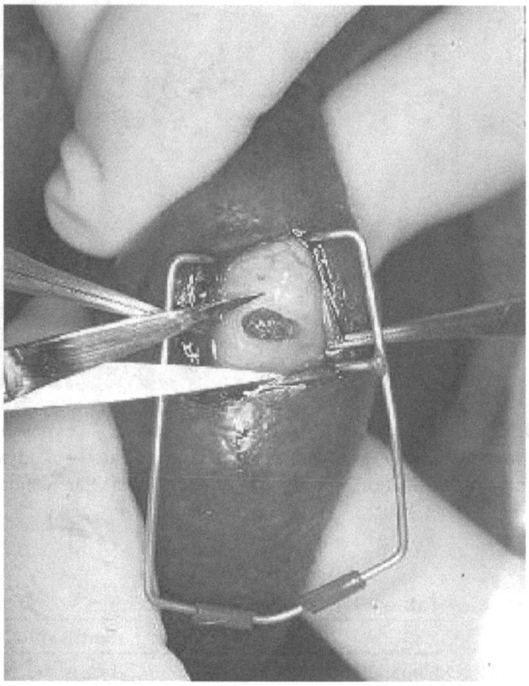

Fig. 29.6 "Window" technique for open testis biopsy for sperm retrieval. After the scrotal incision is made and the tunical vaginalis space entered, a self-retaining eyelid retractor is used to create a "window" into the space. The testis is incised and tissue transected. Multiple different incisions are possible with this approach, but the blood supply to the testis can be compromised by using multiple incisions

testicular parenchyma and therefore the location of sperm aspiration matters little [13]. Once within the testis, negative pressure is applied to the needle through its connection with plastic intravenous tubing and a 20 mL syringe with the plunger fully pulled back. The negative pressure is maintained by clamping the tubing near its attachment to the syringe. Several excursions of the needle (butterfly or angiocath) are then made within the substance of the testis until testis tissue is observed within the intravenous tubing attached to the needle. After sampling is complete, the suction is removed from the system and the tissue within the needle and tubing expelled with positive pressure into one inch Petri dishes or test tubes containing sperm wash medium for processing by the andrology laboratory. Manual pressure is applied to the aspiration site for two minutes for hemostasis. This procedure can be repeated on the same or opposite side until sufficient sperm are obtained for IVF-ICSI. The recovery period is also about 24 h. Complications of the procedure include low risks of bleeding (1%) and infection (1%).

Alternatively, percutaneous or open surgical biopsies (TESE) can be performed to obtain testis sperm in obstructive azoospermia [14, 15]. Percutaneous core biopsies are obtained in a manner similar to the aspiration procedure described earlier, except that a Biopty gun (Monopty no.14; Bard Inc, Covington, USA) with a 14-gauge needle is used. The needle is placed into the testis at the lower pole directed to the upper pole and the gun is fired, producing a tissue core that is then placed in sperm wash medium for processing. There is a 1–5% chance of intratesticular hematoma when percutaneously biopsied testes are examined with ultrasound after the procedure. Open surgical biopsies are performed according to the "window technique" illustrated in Fig. 29.6 and described by Coburn and Lipshultz [15]. A small incision is made in the scrotal skin and the tunica vaginalis space entered sharply. A second incision is made in the tunica albuginea of the testis, parallel to the small, visible vessels on the tunic surface, and testis tissue extruded through the incision, sharply transected and placed in sperm wash medium for processing. Both incisions are closed with absorbable suture. With this approach, recovery takes 24–48 h, substantial amounts of tissue can be biopsied and bleeding and hematoma minimized because it can be visibly controlled during the procedure.

Among the three sources of retrieved sperm, testicular sperm is the least "mature" or fertilizable sperm. For this reason, IVF-ICSI is used with testicular sperm in both obstructive and nonobstructive conditions (Table 29.1). Fresh testis sperm has a mean motility of 5% (Table 29.2), which is generally satisfactory for ICSI [7]. Normal oocyte fertilization

Table 29.6 Comparison of ICSI oocyte fertilization rates among sperm from different sources at a single IVF center

Descriptor	Normal ejaculate (≥20 × 10⁶/ml)	Severe oligospermia (≤1 × 10⁶/ml)	Epididymal sperm	Obstructed testis sperm	Nonobstructive testis sperm
# Cycles	185	60	35	12	22
# Patients	144	57	34	10	19
Egg age (yrs)	*36.1 ± 3.8	35.5 ± 4.9	**33.3 ± 4.8	33.9 ± 4.0	**32.7 ± 3.9
Day 3 FSH	8.1 ± 6.3	7.3 ± 2.7	6.6 ± 2.0	10.0 ± 3.7	6.6 ± 1.8
# Eggs	*12.9 ± 8.4	16.0 ± 8.0	**20.2 ± 9.3	13.4 ± 7.3	**20.5 ± 10.5
# Eggs injected	1801	760	593	129	358
2PN	+75.7%	++70.5%	74.5%	76.7%	+++70.4%
1PN	*2.4%	*1.3%	**5.9%	4.7%	3.9%

Note: * and ** significantly different by one way Anova ($P < 0.001$)
+ and ++ significantly different by one way Anova ($P = 0.007$)
+ and +++significantly different by one way Anova ($P = 0.039$)

rates with ICSI using testis sperm are generally thought to be 5–10% lower than with epididymal or vasal sperm, but this has not been our experience at UCSF where ICSI fertilization rates of 70–75% are typically observed with sperm from all sources (Table 29.6) [16]. A recent meta-analysis concluded that there is no evidence to suggest that any IVF-ICSI outcome, including pregnancy rate, differs between testis and epididymal sperm in cases of obstruction [17].

29.1.3.2 Testis Sperm Retrieval with Nonobstructive Azoospermia

Although testis sperm retrieval in obstructed men with normal sperm production is not difficult, there is a failure to obtain sperm for ICSI in 25–50% of men with nonobstructive azoospermia [18, 19]. In addition, clinical features, including testicular size, history of ejaculated sperm, serum FSH or inhibin levels, or biopsy histology, do not accurately predict whether or not sperm will be recovered during testicular exploration [19]. Because of this, several strategies have been developed to more accurately determine which men with nonobstructive azoospermia are candidates for ICSI and surgical techniques refined to minimize trauma to the testis during sperm harvest procedures. Several evidence-based points should precede a discussion of the various sperm retrieval strategies used for nonobstructive azoospermia:

1. Although TESA is generally sufficient for sperm retrieval from obstructed men, it is much less reliable in cases of nonobstructive azoospermia. As such, TESE is the preferred method for harvesting sperm in this condition.
2. Sperm production in cases of nonobstructive azoospermia can be "patchy" or "focal" in nature [13], and it is precisely this problem that makes reliable sperm retrieval difficult in these patients. It appears that as the sample size increases, the chance of finding sperm also increases (Fig. 29.7) [20–22]. However, the optimal number of samples for sperm detection in nonobstructive azoospermia has not been determined.
3. To date, no randomized controlled trial has compared the efficiency of all strategies for sperm retrieval for nonobstructive azoospermia. A recent systematic review analyzed 24 descriptive studies reporting results of sperm retrieval for nonobstructive azoospermia and concluded that there may be advantages to certain strategies in terms of sperm retrieval success, but there is no relationship between the technique used to find sperm and clinical pregnancy or live birth rates obtained with testis sperm [23].

To minimize procedures and maximize the likelihood of finding sperm in nonobstructive azoospermia, several approaches have been taken for sperm harvesting which are reviewed here.

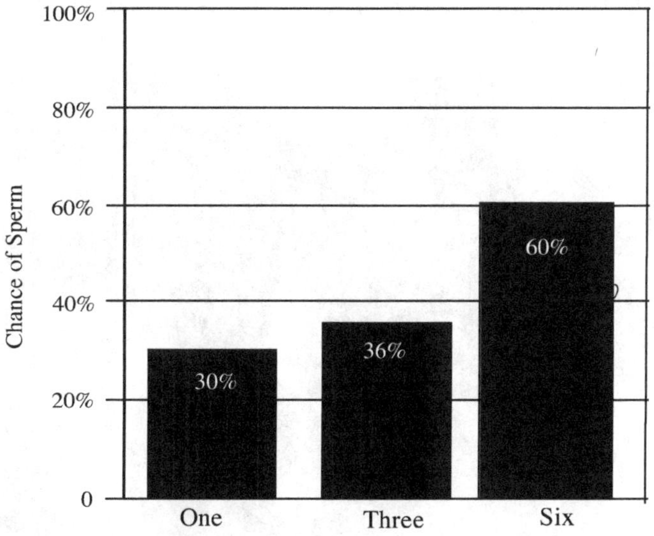

Fig. 29.7 Chances of finding sperm in nonobstructive azoospermia increase with sample size. Here, reported sperm retrieval rates are compared when one, three, and six biopsies are made in series' of individual testes. It is likely that a point exists in which further sampling does not appreciably improve sperm retrieval rates, although this sample size is unknown. Data from references [20–22]

Multibiopsy TESE

One of the first strategies reported [19], this approach involves straightforward TESE as described earlier for obstructive azoospermia and is performed at the time of oocyte retrieval. Unlike the approach for obstruction however, more biopsies are taken until enough sperm are obtained for ICSI, as sperm may not be present on all biopsies. This approach will produce sufficient sperm in 49.5% (95% CI 49.0–49.9) as assessed by systematic review, and may require 15 biopsies or more from a testis to find sperm [19, 23]. It is generally performed after a prior diagnostic biopsy has shown nonobstructive azoospermia, and is considered the most invasive strategy with the highest risk of permanent injury to the testis because of its random nature and the need for multiple incisions in the testis.

Simultaneous Diagnostic Biopsy and Multibiopsy TESE with Cryopreservation

Advocated by Mulhall et al. in Boston [24], this approach involves taking testis tissue by biopsy for both diagnostic assessment and sperm retrieval at the same time. This approach eliminates the need for a separate diagnostic procedure before the TESE. In general, this procedure is performed *in advance* of ICSI to avoid potential cancellation of IVF-ICSI cycles if sperm harvest fails. Similar to the multibiopsy method, multiple biopsies are taken from the testis and the procedure terminated when satisfactory numbers of sperm are obtained for ICSI. All sperm are cryopreserved and then thawed for a future IVF cycle. The issues that surround the use of frozen-thawed testis sperm will be discussed separately below. The surgical risks of this approach are similar to the multibiopsy method.

Microdissection TESE

First reported by Schlegel in 1999 [25], this technique is conceptually similar to the multibiopsy TESE but has important differences, including the use of an operating room microscope. This technique is based on the concept that seminiferous tubules that contain sperm are larger in diameter and more opaque or whiter, than tubules without active spermatogenesis because of the larger number of intratubular germ cells in these tubules. This difference can be detected with optical magnification of 20–25× that is possible with an operating room microscope. For this approach, a single large incision is made in the testis and the organ is "clam shelled" open (Fig. 29.8a). Under microscopy, selected enlarged tubules are biopsied, thus reducing the volume of tissue excised (Fig. 29.8b). With operative microscopy, the arterial anatomy within the testis is better identified, theoretically reducing the risk of serious testis injury. Schlegel and others have shown that less tissue is excised with this method and that better sperm retrieval rates (43–63% of cases) are obtained with this method compared to the multibiopsy method (17–45% of cases) [25–30]. However, on systematic review of seven published series using microdissection, it was concluded that this technique performs better than conventional TESE only in histologic cases of Sertoli cell-only, where tubules containing active foci of spermatogenesis can be identified [23].

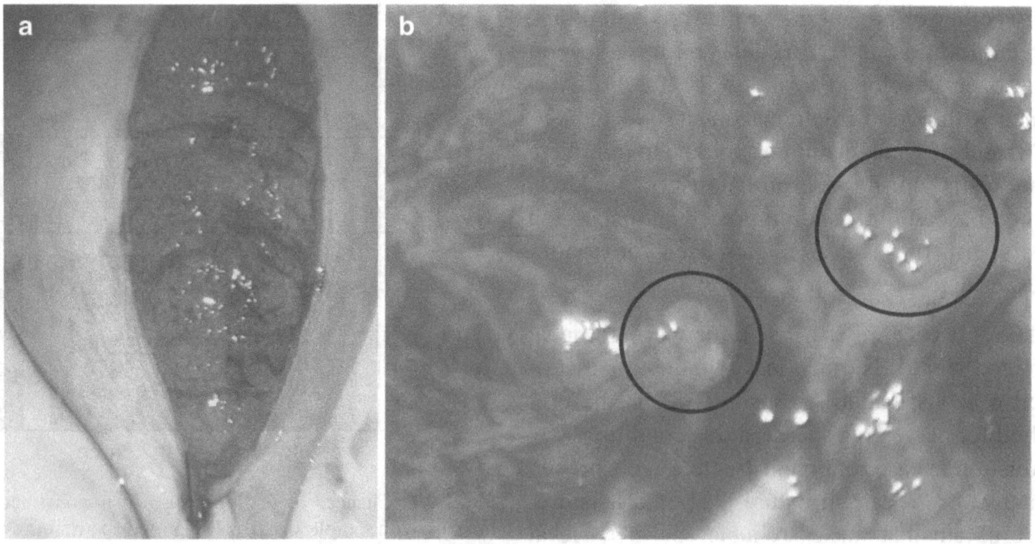

Fig. 29.8 Microdissection TESE. (**a**) A large, full-length incision is made in the testis (either vertical or longitudinal) under low power (6–8×) microscopy; (**b**) The seminiferous tubules are easily identified under high power microscopy (20–25×) and the larger, white, more opaque tubules (*circled in black*) are selectively biopsied for TESE. Photo courtesy of C. Niederberger

Given the level of surgical invasiveness with microdissection, the issue of testis injury has been a concern with TESE procedures. Studies have addressed changes in testosterone production or structural changes to the testis after TESE and microdissection TESE. In a study by Ramasamy et al., testosterone levels had dropped by 20% of pre-microdissection levels 3–6 months after sperm retrieval surgery, achieving 85% of baseline levels at 12 months and 95% at 18 months [30]. A histological study of the testis following TESE procedures revealed a 7% decrease in seminiferous tubule volume and a 5% decrease in germ cell density within tubules, suggesting that sperm retrieval procedures may have lasting effects on testis function [31]. Schlegel and Su found that 82% of men had abnormal ultrasonographic findings 3 months after TESE procedures, which resolved by 6 months [32], suggesting that 6 months is needed for the testis to fully recover after sperm retrieval procedures. Finally, a systemic review of the complications of sperm retrieval noted that microdissection TESE appears to be at least as safe as any other sperm retrieval procedure [23].

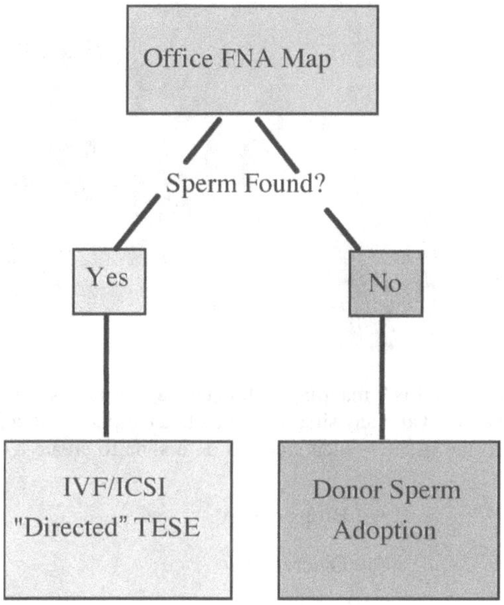

Fig. 29.9 Schematic clinical pathway for nonobstructive azoospermic patients who undergo testis FNA mapping

Fine Needle Aspiration Mapping and Map-Directed TESE

This is our current approach to nonobstructive azoospermia [33]. It involves performing a small non-surgical procedure termed fine needle aspiration (FNA) "mapping" in the office before IVF-ICSI to determine patient candidacy for successful future sperm retrieval. Information obtained from the map, including if, where, and how much sperm is present in the testis, is then used to "direct" TESE at the time of egg retrieval. By having a "map" ahead of time, fewer and smaller biopsies are required to harvest sufficient sperm for ICSI [33] (Fig. 29.9) and the variable of whether or not sperm will be found in nonobstructive azoospermic men is well defined in advance of IVF-ICSI.

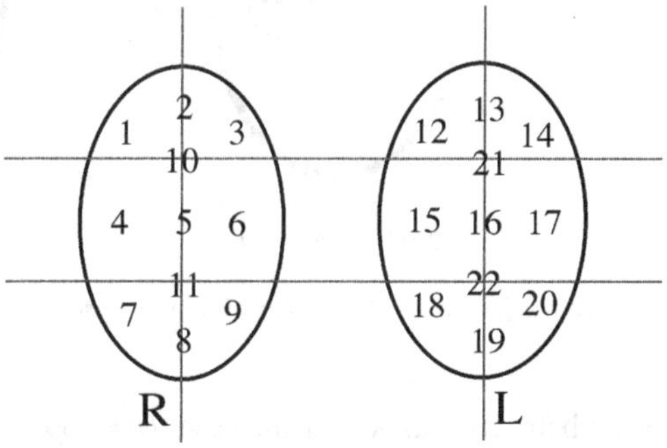

Fig. 29.10 Systematic template of fine needle aspiration (FNA) sites used to detect sperm in men with nonobstructive azoospermia

Applying FNA to the testis is not a new idea, having been performed since the early 1900s as a diagnostic alternative to open testis biopsy [34]. What's new is the concept of "mapping" testes to specifically locate sperm for IVF-ICSI. FNA mapping involves a systematic, templated, non-surgical approach to define the focality of sperm production within nonobstructive azoospermic testes. An example of an FNA map template typically used for nonobstructive azoospermia is illustrated in Fig. 29.10. Systematic FNA is an outpatient procedure performed under local anesthesia. The scrotal skin is stretched taut over the testis and wrapped with sponge. The "wrap" serves as a convenient handle to manipulate the testis and also fixes the scrotal skin over the testis, as shown in Fig. 29.11a. Using a marking pen, the planned sites of aspiration are marked on the scrotal skin overlying the testis. FNA is performed with a 23 gauge fine needle attached to a 10 mL syringe and held with a Cameco syringe holder. The needle is placed into the testis at a marked site and moved in-and-out. After the needle is withdrawn from the testis, the aspirated seminiferous tubules (1–5 mg) are gently smeared on the slide and immediately immersed into 95% ethyl alcohol fixative (Fig. 29.11b). The procedure is well-tolerated by patients with no reported complications (yet), with a mean of two pain pills taken and a recovery time of <24 h. After Papaniculaou staining, the cytology slides are reviewed by an experienced cytologist who can identify the presence or absence of sperm or other germ cells at each site. If sperm are found on the map, patients are advised to proceed with IVF-ICSI at which time fresh testis sperm retrieval is performed.

Based on sperm quantity and distribution in the testes as assessed by the map, sperm are retrieved by TESA, TESE or microdissection, proceeding in this sequence from the least to most invasive procedure. From a review of 3 years of

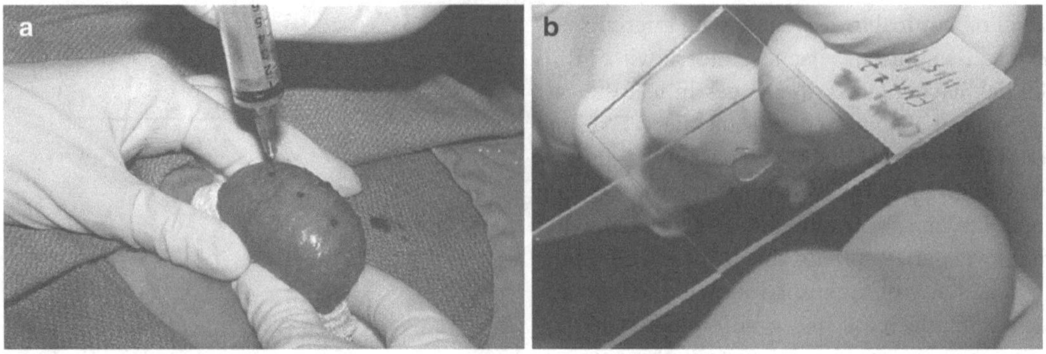

Fig. 29.11 The FNA mapping technique. (**a**) Testis tissue is percutaneously aspirated at many sites according to a template with a 23 gauge needle; (**b**) the tissue is then smeared on a slide to create a cytologic specimen before fixing in alcohol and undergoing a routine Papanicolaou (PAP) stain to identify sperm

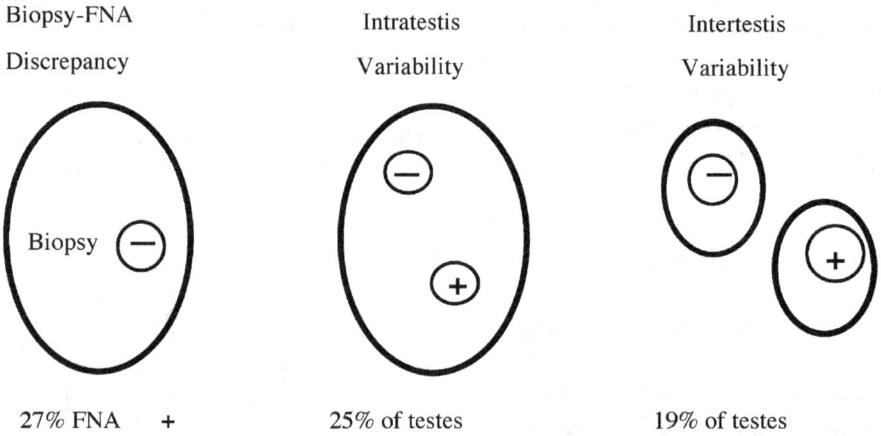

Fig. 29.12 Geographic variation in sperm findings based on FNA maps in 96 men with nonobstructive azoospermia (from reference [13])

mapped nonobstructive azoospermia cases ($n = 159$) at UCSF, 44% required only TESA, 33% required TESE, and only 23% needed microdissection–TESE for sperm retrieval. In addition, the majority (78%) of these sperm retrieval cases were performed unilaterally [35]. Overall, sufficient sperm for all oocytes retrieved was possible in 95% of cases, with 100% of TESA/TESE cases and 80% of microdissection cases. In addition, among men who underwent a second sperm retrieval procedure, sperm was retrieved in 91% of attempts, and in all patients who had a third sperm retrieval ($n = 6$). This suggests that knowledge of sperm location with FNA mapping can simply and streamline sperm retrieval procedures in difficult cases of nonobstructive azoospermia.

Also interesting is the information garnered from FNA mapping about the biology and geography of sperm production in nonobstructive azoospermia [13]. As shown in Fig. 29.12, there is a significant likelihood that FNA map will show sperm despite a biopsy negative for sperm, and there are also reasonable likelihoods (19–25%) of intratesticular and intertesticular variability in sperm production. This type of information can be useful to guide clinicians through the care of patients with this challenging clinical condition.

Outcomes From Testis Sperm Retrieval in Obstructive vs. Nonobstructive Azoospermia

A recent systemic meta-analysis of 1103 ICSI cycles and 998 embryo transfers from published non-randomized studies compared the outcomes of sperm retrieval in obstructive and nonobstructive azoospermic cases [17]. In a fixed model analysis, there was a significantly higher normal fertilization rate (RR 1.18; CI 1.13–1.23) and clinical pregnancy rate (RR 1.36; CI 1.1–1.69) in obstructive vs. nonobstructive cases. A nonsignificant increase in ongoing pregnancy rate was also detected (RR 1.19; CI 0.87–1.61). Importantly, there was no difference in implantation rates (1.01; 0.87–1.61) or miscarriage rates (RR 0.84; CI 0.48–1.48) between these two male factor groups.

29.1.4 Laboratory Effort and Timing of Sperm Retrieval

To achieve excellent outcomes in sperm retrieval cases, clinical care must be carefully timed and orchestrated between procedures on both partners. Several issues should be mentioned regarding the andrology laboratory effort needed to obtain sperm and the timing of sperm and oocyte retrieval, especially in cases of nonobstructive azoospermia. Regarding the technical effort needed to find surgically retrieved sperm, at UCSF, we use a sliding scale for the andrology laboratory: one to two man- hours of processing time needed for TESA procedures, 2–4 h for TESE procedures and 4–6 h for microdissection procedures. In this way, the andrology laboratory staff can gauge the level of difficulty of the sperm retrieval procedure and be prepared in advance for the task based simply on proposed procedure. In addition, since it is clear that testis sperm motility will remain stable or increase with incubation in vitro for 24–48 h after sperm retrieval, the delayed use of fresh testis sperm retrieved in advance of IVF-ICSI is now commonly undertaken to simplify the timing of the procedures on both infertile partners [36].

29.1.5 Sperm Cryopreservation

The ability to freeze and thaw surgically retrieved sperm is a significant advance in the care of men with azoospermia. It has simplified the timing and orchestration of fertility procedures performed on both infertile partners, added convenience to the schedules of reproductive urologists who perform surgical sperm retrieval procedures, and allowed couples who require IVF-ICSI to have multiple opportunities to conceive without repeating surgical sperm retrieval. The literature supports the idea that motile, frozen-thawed epididymal sperm is associated with ICSI outcomes equal to fresh epididymal sperm (Table 29.4) [17], and thus epididymal sperm retrieval procedures are commonly performed in advance of IVF-ICSI cycles and frozen and thawed for later use. One caveat that we have found using this sperm concerns epididymal sperm retrieved from the high caput or efferent ductule region [37]. Although fresh efferent duct sperm has excellent motility (35%), it exhibits the cryobiological behavior more reflective of testicular sperm than epididymal sperm and thaws with very low motility (1.5%). ICSI fertilization rates, however, do not differ between these two kinds of epididymal sperm (66% efferent duct; 71% other epididymal sperm). In summary, sperm cryopreservation has become an invaluable addition to the care of men with epididymal sperm.

Cryopreservation of testicular sperm presents a slightly more complicated scenario. In most centers, fresh testis sperm is preferred to frozen-thawed testis sperm. This preference is largely driven by the large decrease in motility observed after testis sperm is thawed (see Table 29.2), but it is also driven by the generally low or the occasional complete lack of motility observed in fresh testis sperm, depending on the case. Our experience has been to use motile testis sperm whenever possible, which often requires that it be retrieved fresh. However, given that fresh testis sperm has viability rates that approach 90% (Table 29.2), we do not require that fresh testis sperm be motile for ICSI. As Table 29.2 suggests, however, when nonmotile, frozen-thawed testis sperm is used for ICSI, a lower fertilization rate should be expected, as only 50% of sperm are viable [7]. Regardless, a meta-analysis of the literature on the outcomes of fresh and frozen-thawed testis sperm suggests that fertilization rates, clinical pregnancy rates, and ongoing clinical pregnancy rates do not differ between these groups [17]. However, a significant decrease in implantation rates (RR 1.75; CI 1.1–2.80) was observed with frozen thawed compared to fresh testis sperm, possibility reflecting differences in sperm viability between these two groups. Thus, each center should develop its own algorithm regarding the handling of fresh or frozen-thawed testis sperm.

29.2 Conclusions

1. A meta-analysis has determined that there is insufficient data from randomized trials to recommend any particular surgical sperm retrieval technique for either obstructive or nonobstructive azoospermia. A variety of procedures exist for sperm retrieval in these conditions.
2. Although it is not difficult to retrieve sperm from azoospermic men with obstruction, it can be very difficult to find sperm in men with testicular failure and nonobstructive azoospermia. Sperm production in cases of nonobstructive azoospermia can be "patchy" or "focal" in nature, and this problem makes reliable sperm retrieval difficult with this condition. As such, TESA is generally sufficient for sperm retrieval from obstructed men, but TESE is the preferred method for harvesting sperm in nonobstructive azoospermia.
3. To date, no randomized controlled trial has compared the efficiency of all strategies for sperm retrieval for nonobstructive azoospermia. A systematic review concluded that there may be advantages to certain strategies in terms of sperm retrieval success, but there is no relationship between the retrieval technique and clinical outcomes with testis sperm.
4. Since IVF-ICSI does not have a 100% success rate, it behooves reproductive urologists to develop and use sperm retrieval techniques that are not only reliable and of low morbidity, but that also have the potential to harvest sufficient sperm to enable multiple IVF-ICSI attempts without repeat surgery.
5. Sperm cryopreservation is an invaluable addition for epididymal sperm retrieval. The literature suggests that motile, frozen-thawed epididymal sperm has ICSI outcomes

equal to fresh epididymal sperm, and thus these procedures are commonly performed in advance of IVF-ICSI cycles and frozen and thawed for later use.

6. A meta-analysis reviewing outcomes of fresh and frozen-thawed testis sperm suggests that fertilization rates, clinical pregnancy rates, and ongoing clinical pregnancy rates do not differ between these groups. However, a significant decrease in implantation rates was observed with frozen thawed compared to fresh testis sperm, possibility reflecting differences in sperm viability between these groups.

References

1. Temple-Smith PD, Southwick GJ, Yates CA et al (1985) Human pregnancy by IVF using sperm aspirated from the epididymis. J In Vitro Fert Embryo Transf 2:119–122
2. Van Peperstraten A, Proctor ML, Johnson NP, Philipson G (2006) Techniques for surgical retrieval of sperm prior to ICSI for azoospermia review. Cochrane Database Syst Rev 3:CD002807
3. Turek PJ, Conaghan J, Nudell DM (1999) Methods of epididymal sperm retrieval: a urologic perspective. Assist Reprod Rev 9:60–64
4. Qiu Y, Wang SM, Yang DT, Wang LG (2003) Percutaneous vasal sperm aspiration and intrauterine insemination for infertile males with anejaculation. Fertil Steril 79:618–620
5. Saito K, Kinoshita Y, Suzuki K, Kawakami Y, Sato D, Matsuura K (2002) Successful pregnancy with intrauterine insemination using vasal sperm retrieved by electric stimulation. Fertil Steril 77: 621–623
6. Chiang H, Liu C, Tzeng C, Wei H (2000) No-scalpel vasal sperm aspiration and in vitro fertilization for the treatment of anejaculation. Urology 55:918–921
7. Bachtell N, Conaghan J, Turek PJ (1999) The relative viability of human spermatozoa from the testis, epididymis and vas deferens before and after cryopreservation. Hum Reprod 14:101–104
8. Nudell DM, Conaghan J, Pedersen RA, Givens CR, Schriock ED, Turek PJ (1998) The mini-MESA for sperm retrieval: a study of urological outcomes. Hum Reprod 13:1260–1265
9. Qiu Y, Yang DT, Wang SM, Sun HQ, Jia YF (2003) Successful pregnancy and birth after intrauterine insemination using caput epididymal sperm by percutaneous aspiration. Asian J Androl 5:73–75
10. Qiu Y, Yang DT, Wang SM (2004) Restoration of fertility in vasectomized men using percutaneous vasal or epididymal sperm aspiration. Contracept 69:497–500
11. Schoysman R, Segal L, Van der Zwalmen P, Nijs M, Bertin G, Cittadini E, Cimino C, Ruvolo G, Cefalù E, Palermo R (1993) Fertilization of oocytes by testicular spermatozoa and pregnancy in the human. Acta Eur Fertil 24:103–105
12. Gorgy A, Podsiadly BT, Bates S, Craft IL (1998) Testicular sperm aspiration (TESA): the appropriate technique. Hum Reprod 13: 1111–1114
13. Turek PJ, Cha I, Ljung B-M, Conaghan J (2000) Diagnostic findings from testis fine needle aspiration mapping in obstructed and non-obstructed azoospermic men. J Urol 163:1709–1716
14. Tuuri T, Moilanen J, Kaukoranta S, Makinen S, Kotola S, Hovatta O (1999) Testicular biopty gun needle biopsy in collecting spermatozoa for intracytoplasmic injection, cryopreservation and histology. Hum Reprod 14:1274–1278
15. Coburn M, Wheeler TM (1991) Testicular biopsy in male infertility evaluation. In: Lipshultz LI, Howards SS (eds) Infertility in the male, 2nd edn. Mosby Year Book, Philadelphia, pp 223–253
16. Shen S, Wong C, Fujimoto VY, Cedars MI, Turek PJ (2003) Do different sperm types influence Intracytoplasmic Sperm Injection (ICSI) fertilization rates? Fertil Steril 80:211
17. Nicopoullos JDM, Gilling-Smith C, Almeida PA, Norman-Taylor J, Grace I, Ramsay JWA (2004) Use of surgical sperm retrieval in azoospermic men: a meta-analysis. Fertil Steril 82:691–701
18. Kahraman S, Ozgur S, Alatas C, Aksoy S, Taşdemir M, Nuhoğlu A, Taşdemir I, Balaban B, Biberoğlu K, Schoysman R, Nijs M, Vanderzwalmen P (1996) Fertility with testicular sperm extraction and intracytoplasmic sperm injection in non-obstructive azoospermic men. Hum Reprod 11:756–760
19. Tournaye H, Verheyen G, Nagy P, Ubaldi F, Goossens A, Silber S, Van Steirteghem AC, Devroey P (1997) Are there predictive factors for successful testicular sperm recovery in azoospermic patients? Hum Reprod 12:80–86
20. Kim E, Gilbaugh J, Patel VR, Turek PJ, Lipshultz LI (1997) Testis biopsies frequently demonstrate sperm in men with azoospermia and significantly elevated follicle-stimulating hormone levels. J Urol 157:144–146
21. Weiss DB, Gottschalk-Sabag S, Bar-On E (1997) Seminiferous tubule cytological pattern in infertile, azoospermic men in diagnosis and therapy. Harefuah 132:614–618
22. Altay B, Hekimgil M, Cikili N, Turna B, Soydan S (2001) Histopathological mapping of open testicular biopsies in patients with unobstructive azoospermia. BJU Int 87:834–837
23. Donoso P, Tournaye H, Devroey P (2007) Which is the best sperm retrieval technique for non-obstructive azoospermia? A systematic review. Hum Reprod Update 13:539–549
24. Mulhall JP, Burgess CM, Cunningham D, Carson R, Harris D, Oates RD (1997) Presence of mature sperm in testicular parenchyma of men with nonobstructive azoospermia: prevelance and predictive factors. Urology 49:91–96
25. Schlegel PN (1999) Testicular sperm extraction: microdissection improves sperm yield with minimal tissue excision. Hum Reprod 14:131–135
26. Amer M, Ateyah A, Hany R, Zohdy W (2000) Prospective comparative study between microsurgical and conventional testicular sperm extraction in non-obstructive azoospermia: follow-up by serial ultrasound examinations. Hum Reprod 15:653–656
27. Okada H, Dobashi M, Yamazaki T, Hara I, Fujisawa M, Arakawa S, Kamidono S (2002) Conventional versus microdissection testicular sperm extraction for nonobstructive azoospermia. J Urol 168: 1063–1067
28. Okubo K, Ogura K, Ichioka K, Terada N, Matsuta Y, Yoshimura K, Arai Y, Honda T, Umeoka K, Nakahori T, Takahashi A, Umaoka Y (2002) Testicular sperm extraction for non-obstructive azoospermia: results with conventional and microsurgical techniques. Hinyokika Kiyo 48:275–280
29. Tsujimura A, Matsumiya K, Miyagawa Y, Tohda A, Miura H, Nishimura K, Koga M, Takeyama M, Fujioka H, Okuyama A (2002) Conventional multiple or microdissection testicular sperm extraction: a comparative study. Hum Reprod 17:2924–2929
30. Ramasamy R, Yagan N, Schlegel PN (2005) Structural and functional changes to the testis after conventional versus microdissection testicular sperm extraction. Urology 65:1190–1194
31. Tash JA, Schlegel PN (2001) Histologic effects of testicular sperm extraction on the testicle in men with nonobstructive azoospermia. Urology 57:334–337

32. Schlegel PN, Su LM (1998) Physiological consequences of testicular sperm extraction. Hum Reprod 13:505–506
33. Turek PJ, Givens C, Schriock ED, Meng M, Pederson RA, Conaghan J (1999) Testis sperm extraction and intracytoplasmic sperm injection guided by prior fine needle aspiration mapping in nonobstructive azoospermia. Fertil Steril 71:552–558
34. Ljung B-M (12) Techniques of aspiration and smear preparation. In: Koss LG, Woyke S, Olszewski W (eds) Aspiration biopsy: cytologic interpretation and histologic bases, 2nd edn. Igaku-Shoin, New York, pp 34–1992
35. Jad AM, Turek PJ (2002) Experience with testis FNA mapping and microdissection (M & M) in difficult nonobstructive azoospermia cases. Fertil Steril 78:S71
36. Morris DS, Dunn RL, Schuster TG, Ohl DA, Smith GD (2007) Ideal culture time for improvement in sperm motility from testicular sperm aspirates of men with azoospermia. J Urol 178:2087–91 Discussion 2091
37. Zenke U, Jalalian L, Suthar A, Turek PJ (2004) The difficult MESA: findings from tubuli recti sperm aspiration. J Assist Reprod Genet 21:31–35

Chapter 30
The Clinical Utility of the Evaluation of Sperm Chromatin

Sergey I. Moskovtsev and Brendan M. Mullen

Abstract Interest in the use of sperm DNA integrity as a predictor of fertility potential is on the rise. Clear differences in the levels of sperm DNA damage have been observed between fertile and infertile men. Sperm DNA damage has been found to be adversely affected by age. Men with a high percentage of DNA fragmentation have very low potential for in vitro and in vivo fertility. Moreover, DNA fragmentation is linked to effects on embryonic development, implantation and risk of recurrent miscarriages, and the health of offspring. The potential causes of sperm DNA damage are complex with multiple factors acting at both the intratesticular and post-testicular levels. Oxidative stress, defective sperm chromatin packaging, and disordered abortive apoptosis, are the three putative mechanisms most commonly associated with DNA damage. Sperm DNA damage can occur and can be assessed at different levels in the reproductive tract. Several methods have been developed to evaluate sperm DNA damage as well as assess DNA maturity, quality of packaging, and protamination of the chromatin. The challenge in the management of patients with elevated DNA damage increases proportionately with the rise of such damage. Positive effect of oral antioxidants has been reported. Several methods designed to separate superior spermatozoa from normal DNA have shown promising results, but await further evaluation and confirmation.

Keywords Sperm chromatin • Male infertility • Sperm DNA damage • Sperm DNA integrity

30.1 Introduction

Approximately 15% of couples attempting to have children are unable to conceive within 1 year [1]. Significant male factor alone accounts for 20% of these cases with a further 30–40% due to a combination of both male and female factors. In nearly one third of male factor infertility, the cause remains unexplained and is considered idiopathic [2]. The semen values needed for successful conception are much lower than the values for normality of a fertile population. The most recent World Health Organization (WHO) manual for semen evaluation has recognized these limitations and changed "normal" to reference values [3]. These semen parameter guidelines, such as concentration, motility and morphology, are somewhat artificial due to a significant overlap between the parameters of infertile and fertile men [4, 5]. In fact, for a sperm to fertilize an oocyte in vivo, it must be capable of successfully completing a sequence of events: from normal spermatogenesis and maturation to embryo development. If any one of the steps is defective, the sperm will not fertilize, and if most of the sperm are defective, fertilization may not occur [6].

The laboratory investigation of male infertility includes semen analysis, tests of sperm function, and DNA integrity assessment [7, 8]. Many studies have attempted to predict the utility of selected semen parameters and tests of sperm function, but it is not clear which tests have the most prognostic or diagnostic value, and there is no single laboratory test that can assess the total fertility potential of spermatozoa [7, 9].

Since the introduction of intracytoplasmic sperm injection (ICSI), many traditional diagnostic algorithms have been underutilized because of their apparent poor prognostic value in predicting fertilization [10]. However, there has been renewed interest in the use of tests beyond semen analysis due, in part, to the increase in the number of studies, indicating an elevated risk of anomalies in children born after ICSI [11–15]. This could be explained, in part, by the lack of spermatozoa selection, procedure related hazards, and genetic and epigenetic alterations [11, 12].

There is increasing interest in the use of DNA integrity as a predictor of fertility potential [16, 17]. Clear differences in the levels of sperm DNA damage have been observed between fertile and infertile men [18, 19]. Men with a high percentage of DNA fragmentation have very low potential for in vitro [20] and in vivo fertility [17, 21–23]. Moreover, DNA fragmentation has been linked to defective embryonic development [24, 25]; implantation failure and risk of recurrent miscarriages [26].

S.I. Moskovtsev (✉) and B.M. Mullen
Andrology Laboratory, Department of Pathology and Laboratory Medicine, Mount Sinai Hospital, Toronto, Ontario, Canada
e-mail: smoskovtsev@mtsinai.on.ca

D.T. Carrell and C.M. Peterson (eds.), *Reproductive Endocrinology and Infertility: Integrating Modern Clinical and Laboratory Practice*,
DOI 10.1007/978-1-4419-1436-1_30,

30.2 Sperm DNA Structure

The structure of sperm chromatin is very complex with some organizational features unique to germ cells. While sperm chromatin organization remains a subject of extensive research, evidence from several laboratories suggests that sperm DNA is folded into loop domains in specific sequences [27, 28]. During normal spermatogenesis, endogenous nicks develop, which if not repaired, result in decreased fertility potential [29]. The spermatozoa-specific organization of DNA loop domains is very different from somatic cell DNA looping and is not associated with chromosome function or DNA replication as it would be in somatic cells, since mature spermatozoa are genetically inactive [30]. It has been suggested that loop-domain organization contributes to the function of the paternal genome [31, 32].

Several levels of complex DNA organization, each with specific characteristics, have been proposed. The primary level of the chromatin organization, often referred to as chromosomal anchoring by the nuclear annulus; two strands of histone-free nucleic acids attach to a bent-shaped ring about 2 μm in length, called the "nuclear annulus" [33]. This annulus is specific to spermatozoa; the point of its formation during spermatogenesis is unknown. The nuclear annulus has nonrandom DNA sequences, which initiate aggregation at specific sites of each chromosome to chromatin condensation, play a role in packaging of chromosomes, and determine the shape of the sperm nucleus [34].

At the next level of sperm DNA organization, anchored chromosomes are arranged into DNA loop domains of ~30–50 kb connected at their bases to the sperm nuclear matrix attachment regions [28]. Spermatozoa are highly differentiated cells that result from a multistep process of spermatogenesis. After meiosis, histones are gradually removed from the chromosomes and replaced by highly basic transitional proteins, and then by protamines [35]. Protamines play an essential role in the normal sperm chromatin packaging [36]. In the "donut-loop model" proposed by Ward, [37] each loop domain is folded into one protamine toroid connected by a DNAase sensitive region. It has been suggested that DNA present in toroid-linker regions is organized differently than the rest of the sperm DNA, and may remain organized into nucleosomes by residual histones [28]. Almost 10% of the DNA in human spermatozoa is bound to residual histones, the majority of which are sperm-specific variants of H2B localized in the near telomere or telomere regions with smaller amounts of histone H4 distributed throughout the sperm nucleus [38, 39]. The function of these histones in human sperm remains unknown. The retained histones may mark genes for early embryo gene expression [40] and bind the chromosomal domains required for the initial stages of male pronucleus formation [41]. Sperm containing different quantities of H2B may have different patterns of chromosomal packaging, which would impact fertilization and early embryo development [42].

Recent studies have demonstrated nonrandom positioning and arrangement of chromosomes in the sperm nucleus. In the interphase nucleus, the chromosomes occupy specific nonoverlapping territories according to their mass and gene density [43]. The chromosomes fold into hairpin-like structures with the centromeres located in the centre of the nucleus, where centromeres of nonhomologous chromosomes form chromocenters [29, 34]. In spermatozoa, telomeres localize in the nuclear periphery where they interact with each other by forming dimers and tetramers [44]. In human spermatozoa, p- and q-subtelomeres belonging to one chromosome are notably closer than subtelomeres from different chromosomes [45]. Chromosome looping could be the result of specific associations between terminal chromatin structures of chromosome arms and dependent on chromosome arm-specific subtelomeric sequences with the involvement of some protein complexes, such as sperm telomere binding protein [44]. During fertilization, the sperm chromosomes are withdrawn from the nucleus and remodeled. If the topology of the chromosomes is altered, it would lead to a shift in the ordered chromosome removal, disruption of the sequence of events involved in fertilization and early embryo development [41].

30.3 Mechanisms of Sperm DNA Damage

The pathophysiology of DNA damage may be due to a number of factors acting at the testicular and posttesticular levels [46]. The etiology of this process is still the subject of extensive research and debate. It is unknown whether a single factor or multiple factors acting in concert are responsible for the DNA damage. Sperm DNA damage has been found to be increased in individuals with a history of smoking and drug use, exposure to environmental and occupational toxins as well as in patients with varicoceles, history of testicular trauma or cancer [47–49]. The rapidly dividing germinal epithelium of the seminiferous tubules is a target for drugs and irradiation, both of which are associated with DNA damage influenced by the duration and the dose of the exposure [50]. Although spermatogenesis may recover months to years after cessation of therapy, evidence of sperm DNA damage may persist.

Several theories have been proposed to explain sperm DNA fragmentation including, disordered apoptosis, oxidative stress, and defective sperm chromatin packaging.

30.3.1 Apoptosis

Testicular germ cell apoptosis occurs normally and continuously throughout life. It is the end result of various pathological conditions leading to deregulation of the spermatogenesis control system, and may be triggered by an internal clock or by extra-cellular mediators, such as cytokines, hormones, viruses, chemicals or physical factors [48, 51]. Both apoptosis and necrosis has been reported in ejaculated human spermatozoa [52, 53]. However, it is unsettled whether ejaculated spermatozoa retain the ability to activate the apoptotic signaling cascade, or whether the detected apoptotic markers merely reflect an apoptotic process that started before ejaculation [54]. In the absence of an apoptotic pathway, necrosis has been cited as the main source of elimination of spermatozoa in normozoospermic samples [55]. However, Blanc-Layrac and associates reported both necrosis and apoptosis in ejaculated samples obtained from 30 normozoospermic patients presenting for infertility evaluation [56]. Apoptosis during spermatogenesis is responsible for the removal of up to 75% of potential spermatozoa and may be responsible for the selective depletion of DNA damaged germ cells [57, 58]. This serves to maintain a Sertoli cell to germ cell ratio adequate to support normal spermatogenesis. It has been proposed that some of the spermatozoa with DNA damage that have initiated apoptosis subsequently escape apoptosis (abortive apoptosis) [58]. The cell-surface protein Fas may mediate apoptosis in sperm [59]. The percentage of Fas-positive spermatozoa is small in men with normal semen parameters, while it may reach 50% in men with abnormal semen parameters. The combination of DNA damage and spermatozoa with apoptotic markers may indicate the presence of abortive apoptosis [54]. In contrast, some reported no correlation between apoptotic markers and sperm DNA damage [60].

30.3.2 Oxidative Stress

Human spermatozoa are susceptible to oxidative stress because of a high content of polyunsaturated fatty acids in their plasma membranes [61]. Although reactive oxygen species (ROS) at low concentrations have an important physiological effect on hyperactivation, capacitation, and acrosome reaction of spermatozoa, in high concentration, they have a pathological effect [62]. High levels of ROS can adversely affect sperm DNA integrity as well as other sperm functions [63]. Kodama and coworkers found a 1.5-fold increase in the level of oxidated DNA derivatives in infertile men compared with fertile men [17]. It has been reported that approximately 25–40% of infertile men have high levels of ROS detectable in their semen [64]. Leukocytes derived ROS generation may be responsible for the DNA damage in patients with genital tract infection or idiopathic genital tract inflammation [65]. However, other sources of ROS or other factors not related to ROS may be responsible for the DNA damage [66].

Antioxidants present in seminal plasma may control ROS generation to some degree, but the production of excessive amounts of ROS may overcome the antioxidant protective activities of seminal plasma leading to oxidative stress [67, 68].

30.3.3 Defective Sperm Chromatin Packaging

Normal chromatin packaging is essential for proper DNA organization; as histones are replaced by transitional proteins and then by protamines, DNA becomes more condensed and genetically inactive [35]. It has been postulated that the endogenous nicks that develop during normal spermatogenesis relieve torsional stress and aid chromatin rearrangement during the replacement of the histones by protamines. Chromatin remodeling steps during spermatozoal maturation have been associated with spontaneous transient DNA double strand breaks [69]. Moreover, the presence of endogenous nicks in spermatozoa may indicate the presence of disorders during spermatogenesis and an incomplete maturation. A transient increase in the nuclear histone to protamine ratio has been reported following febrile illness [70]. Protamine deficiency, either relative or complete, is a relatively frequent sperm chromatin abnormality. Approximately, 5–15% of infertile men demonstrate a complete protamine deficiency [71]. An endogenous nuclease (topoisomerase II) is required to create and ligate nicks that facilitate protamination during spermiogenesis [72]. Topoisomerase II appears to be the only enzyme responsible for the transient DNA double-strand break repair during the spermatid stage of spermatogenesis [73]. Altered topoisomerase II activity during spermatogenesis maybe responsible for persistent endogenous nicks and residual breaks in the DNA of ejaculated spermatozoa, and point to incomplete maturation of germ cells [74]. Bannister and Schimenti have proposed a defective checkpoint in the meiotic prophase as the cause of sperm DNA fragmentation in ejaculated spermatozoa, as the recombination checkpoint does not allow meiotic division I to proceed until the DNA is fully repaired or the defective spermatocytes removed [75]. Sperm protamine deficiency has been implicated in male infertility, in particular, aberrant P1/P2 ratios significantly correlate with fertility status [71]. Abnormal ratios of P1/P2 in ejaculated spermatozoa have been reported to inversely correlate with DNA fragmentation, suggesting a protective role of the protamines in sperm DNA damage [76].

30.4 Methods of Sperm DNA Evaluation

Sperm DNA damage can occur and can be assessed at different stages of development. Several methods have been developed to evaluate sperm DNA damage (Table 30.1).

30.4.1 Assessment of Sperm DNA Damage or Fragmentation

The direct evaluation of DNA damage or fragmentation in the form of single- or double-strand DNA breaks can be evaluated by Sperm Chromatin Structure Assay (SCSA®)/DNA Integrity Assay, Acridine Orange Test (AOT), Terminal Deoxynucleotidyl Transferase-mediated Deoxyuridine Triphosphate Nick End Labeling (TUNEL) assay, In Situ Nick Translation (ISNT) assay, or measured and quantified by Comet assay. Base modification can be assessed by the measurement of oxidative DNA damage biomarkers, such as 8-hydroxydeoxyguanosine (8-OHdG).

30.4.1.1 Sperm Chromatin Structure Assay/DNA Integrity Assay

The SCSA/DNA Integrity Assay is the most widely used method of direct sperm DNA assessment and is currently the only DNA integrity test with statistically sound normative values [77]. This assay measures the susceptibility of sperm DNA to acid induced partial DNA denaturation in situ [78]. The extent of denaturation is determined by a metachromatic

Table 30.1 Methods of sperm DNA evaluation

Test	Principle	Detection method	Advantage	Disadvantage
Assessment of DNA damage or fragmentation				
Sperm Chromatin Structure Assay® (SCSA) or DNA Integrity Assay	Susceptibility to DNA denaturation	Flow cytometry	Correlation to other tests Standardized High sensitivity Clinically significant Large number of cells analyzed	Special equipment
Acridine Orange Test (AOT)	Susceptibility to DNA denaturation	Fluorescent microscopy	Simple Inexpensive	Indistinct colors Poor correlation with other test Interlaboratory variations
Terminal Deoxynucleotidyl Transferase-mediated Deoxyuridine Triphosphate Nick End Labeling (TUNEL)	Single- and double-strand breaks	Fluorescent microscopy-Bright field microscopy Flow cytometry	Correlation to other tests High sensitivity Clinically significant	Special equipment Interlaboratory variations
In Situ Nick Translation (ISNT)	Single-strand breaks		Specific to endogenous breaks	Clinically not proven
Comet assay (neutral and alkaline)	Single- and double-strand breaks (double-strand breaks for neutral)	Single-cell gel electrophoresis Fluorescent microscopy	High specificity Quantification of DNA damage in individual cell	Interlaboratory variations Time consuming Not standardized
8-Hydroxy-deoxyguanosine (8-OHdG) Assay	Measurement of DNA oxidation Detecting 8-OHdG	High performance liquid chromatography Flow cytometry	Quantitative High specificity	Special equipment Artifactual oxidation
Assessment of DNA packaging or condensation				
Aniline Blue stain	Staining lysine residues of remaining histones	Bright field microscopy	Simple Inexpensive	Interlaboratory variations Heterogeneous slide staining
Toluidine blue stain	Staining phosphate residues of chromatin	Bright field microscopy	Simple Inexpensive Correlation to other tests	Interlaboratory variations Heterogeneous slide staining
Chromomycin A_3 stain (CMA_3)	Protamination of mature sperm	Fluorescent microscopy	Simple High sensitivity	Interlaboratory variations

shift of acridine orange (AO); under acid conditions, AO intercalated with double-stranded DNA emits green fluorescence and AO associated with single-stranded DNA emits red fluorescence [79]. The assay measures several parameters, including the DNA fragmentation index (DFI), which assesses sperm with single-strand DNA breaks. DFI is calculated as the ratio of red fluorescing sperm to the total amount of red plus green fluorescing sperm in an individual sperm sample. Three levels of DNA fragmentation have been reported to be associated with excellent (low DFI ≤ 15%), good (moderate DFI >15 to <30%) and fair to poor (high DFI ≥ 30%) fertility potential respectively [79]. Another parameter calculated by this assay is the high DNA stainable cells (HDS) representing the percentage of immature spermatozoa with incomplete chromatin condensation. The clinical significance of HDS has not been established [23].

Spermatozoa from infertile patients exhibit higher DNA damage compared to a fertile population [80]. Strong correlation between DFI results and semen parameters have been reported by some [8, 19, 81], while others have observed only weak or no correlation [20, 82]. High DNA damage showed a strong correlation to intrauterine insemination (IUI) pregnancy rates and to independently predict IUI failure [23, 80]. For conventional In vitro fertilization (IVF) outcome, some studies have reported no pregnancies if the DFI is above the 27% threshold [77]. It is presumed that DFI does not affect fertilization rates, as paternal effects on the embryo have not been observed till the second cleavage division or day three of embryo development [8]. The relationship between embryo quality and development is not established, as some have observed an inverse correlation between DFI and embryo quality [83], while others were unable to demonstrate this relationship [20].

Since ICSI bypasses all means of natural selection of sperm by an egg, it is interesting that some have observed a significant positive predictive value of SCSA for fertilization by ICSI [20], an observation not confirmed by others [80]. DFI has also been shown to correlate to disordered implantation and may indicate involvement of a damaged paternal genome [20]. It has been suggested that couples with unexplained infertility and patients treated with assisted reproductive techniques (ART) would be the groups of patients most likely to benefit from assessment of sperm DNA integrity [23, 84].

30.4.1.2 Acridine Orange Test

The acridine orange test is a slide-based version of SCSA that measures the susceptibility of sperm DNA to acid induced denaturation by means of the metachromatic property of acridine orange. The dye intercalated into native double-stranded DNA fluoresces green and fluoresces orange–red when associated with single-stranded DNA or RNA, when exposed to blue light [85]. Correlation of AOT to standard semen parameters as well as IVF and ICSI outcomes have been reported [86, 87]. Others have reported that the test is insufficiently reliable for clinical use, because of the poor condition for the metachromatic shift of AO from green to orange-red, leading to indistinct color and difficulties in discriminating between normal and damaged cells [80]. Moreover, rapidly fading fluorescence and heterogeneous slide staining exacerbate the problems with interpreting the AOT results [88].

30.4.1.3 Terminal Deoxynucleotidyl Transferase-Mediated Deoxyuridine Triphosphate Nick End Labeling Assay

TUNEL is another assay for the direct assessment of sperm DNA fragmentation. The test is based on the detection of DNA precursor deoxyuridine triphosphate (dUTP) at both single- and double- stranded DNA breaks by enzymatic reaction. The number of incorporated dUTP at the 3′-OH ends of DNA increases with the number of strand breaks [52]. The incorporated labeled nucleotides can be detected in spermatozoa by fluorescence or light microscopy as well as by flow cytometry, making it possible to evaluate a large number of spermatozoa [89]. The TUNEL is widely used as low intra and interobserver variability for this assay, and good correlation to SCSA has been reported [60, 80]. Several studies have shown that abnormal TUNEL results correlate to abnormal standard semen parameters and predict the outcomes of IVF and ICSI [54, 90]. Reference values vary between different research groups: a threshold of 12% TUNEL-positive spermatozoa was suggested to have a predictive value for IUI [21] and 20% for ICSI [90]. However, Henkel and colleague reported numbers much higher, 36.5% for IVF and 24.3% ICSI [91]. The rate of subsequent spontaneous abortion was also linked to increased DNA damage as assessed by TUNEL [26].

30.4.1.4 In Situ Nick Translation Assay

The ISNT assay is a modified TUNEL assay that is only able to detect single-stranded DNA breaks. The test utilizes incorporation of labeled dUTP in a reaction catalyzed by the template dependent enzyme DNA polymerase I. The assay identifies spermatozoa with variable levels of endogenous DNA damage [92]. Unfortunately, this technique has been shown to be less sensitive in comparison to other assays [18, 63].

30.4.1.5 Comet Assay

The Comet assay uses single-cell gel electrophoresis to evaluate single- and double- stranded breaks. The test is performed by in situ lysis of sperm membranes and DNA denaturation within an agarose gel [93]. The assay is based on the principle of a faster rate of migration of smaller fragmented DNA towards an anode in an electrophoretic field as compared to larger nonfragmented DNA. Damaged DNA is visualized by DNA-specific fluorescent dye and gives the appearance of a comet, with double-stranded, undamaged DNA remaining in the comet head. Comet parameters, such as fluorescence intensity, comet tail length, and comet moment, are analyzed by an imaging software [94]. The intensity of staining of the tail is compared to the comet head intensity and expressed as a percentage of damaged DNA within the total DNA of the spermatozoon. The Comet assay can be performed in neutral or alkaline ($pH > 13$) conditions. Under neutral conditions, only double-stranded breaks are identified [54], however, in an alkaline environment, single- and double- strand breaks, and alkali-labile sites, are detectable [95]. The Comet assay is considered the most sensitive technique available to measure the magnitude of DNA damage in an individual cell. However, overestimation of DNA breaks in spermatozoa has been linked to induced DNA damage and alkali-labile sites [95]. High interlaboratory variation of Comet assay results has also been cited as a disadvantage of this technique [96]. Good correlation to TUNEL assay results [97], standard semen parameters, and embryo development and pregnancy rates in IVF and ICSI programs, have been reported [24, 98].

30.4.1.6 8-Hydroxydeoxyguanosine Assay

The 8-OHdG assay uses one of the biomarkers of oxidative injury that occur with oxidative base modification of DNA [99]. DNA damage is mediated via free radicals formed by some environmental toxins, radiation, xenobiotics or even as a part of physiological metabolism [100]. The mutagenic quality of 8-OHdG has been reported to be a possible cause of malformations, genetic diseases, and cancer [101]. High performance liquid chromatography, following electrochemical or gas chromatography detection, is used to identify this biomarker. This method requires extraction and enzymatic digestion of sperm DNA followed by extraction of 8-OHdG. The assay requires special equipment and a large number of spermatozoa [102]. More recently, direct detection of 8-oxoguanine using flow cytometry has been employed [103]. High levels of 8-OHdG have been shown to correlate with sperm motility and function as well as with male infertility [16, 104]. A positive correlation has been found between sperm DNA damage assessed but SCSA and DNA oxidation measured by 8-OHdG [105].

30.4.2 Assessment of Sperm DNA Packaging or Condensation

During spermatogenesis, histones are replaced by protamines, resulting in a highly condensed sperm chromatin occupying over 90% of the spermatozoa's nuclear volume. If the chromatin package is disturbed, DNA decondensation can occur due to persistence of histones or an abnormal ratio of protamines [33]. Several tests have been developed to directly assess DNA maturity, quality of packaging and protamination of the chromatin.

30.4.2.1 Aniline Blue Stain

Aniline blue is an acidic dye binding to chromatin proteins in spermatozoa with abnormally loosely packaged DNA. This test is based on the presence of lysine-rich histones in spermatozoa with impaired chromatin packaging or immature forms, in comparison to arginine–cysteine rich protamines of spermatozoa with intact DNA. In an acid based reaction, aniline blue binds to the basic lysine residues causing blue staining [106]. This test has been correlated to semen parameters [107] and outcome of IVF [108]; however, the relationship to ICSI outcome is contradictory [109, 110].

30.4.2.2 Toluidine Blue Stain

Toluidine blue is a basic thiazine nuclear stain incorporated into loosely packed or damaged chromatin where it binds to the phosphate residues of DNA showing a deep violet color [111]. The test has been shown to correlate to standard semen parameters [112]. Results are calculated as a percentage of stained spermatozoa and expressed as abnormal DNA Index, with 35% recommended as an infertility threshold. Significant correlation between this test and TUNEL results has been reported [113].

30.4.2.3 Chromomycin A_3 Stain

Chromomycin A_3 is a guanine–cytosine fluorochrome directly competing with protamines for association with DNA. The staining relates to the degree of protamination of mature spermatozoa [74]. It has been correlated with semen analysis results [114] with good predictive value for the outcomes of IVF and ICSI [109, 115].

30.5 The Clinical Utility of Sperm DNA Assessment

30.5.1 Age and DNA Integrity

The basis of the relationship between age and male fertility involves several potential factors including decline in sex hormone production, accessory gland function, testicular function, semen quality, sperm DNA integrity, and genetic alterations.

The effect of age on male fertility and specifically on DNA integrity is of particular interest because of the growth in the number of men choosing to father children at older ages. For example, in the United States, the birthrate for fathers older than 35 years increased up to 40% from 1980 [116]. A Canadian study confirmed this observation, as men older than 40 years of age constituted almost 25% of the patient population presenting for fertility evaluation [81]. The increase in average parental age at the time of attempted first pregnancy is attributed to socioeconomic factors in modern society, changes in reproductive behavior, prolonged life expectancy, and improvement in assisted reproductive techniques.

In the largest study to date of the effect of age on sperm DNA damage, 1,125 men presenting for fertility evaluation underwent assessment of DNA damage as measured by the DFI [81]. Sperm DNA damage was significantly increased in men older than 45 years compared to all other age groups. DFI was high, corresponding to fair to poor fertility potential, in the oldest age group, and moderate, corresponding to good fertility potential, in the younger age groups. Our current observations have confirmed these data; to date in our laboratory, 4,655 patients have undergone sperm DNA damage assessment (Table 30.2).

These data support the observation of Spano and colleagues, that DNA damage almost doubled from about age 25 years to age 55 years (10.0% and 18.0% respectively) [117]. Of interest, DFI values in our study [81] were 50% higher at both time points, as our data included results from patients presenting for fertility investigation in comparison to Spano's study, which selected subjects from an occupational hazard study with no known history of infertility. Similar results were observed in a study of 97 healthy men [118].

Other investigators, employing different assays to evaluate sperm chromatin or DNA fragmentation, have reported a similar negative effect of age on sperm DNA quality. DNA fragmentation, as measured by TUNEL assay, was inversely related to male age in gonadotrophin-stimulated IUI cycles [21] as well as in 508 men of unselected couples attending a clinic for infertility investigation [119]. DNA damage assessed by the Comet assay increased with age, in a study of unselected men undergoing IVF treatment [24], this observation was confirmed in subsequent studies [120, 121]. Schmid and coworkers [122] using the Comet assay in 80 nonsmokers with no known fertility problems found a significant correlation between male age and sperm single-stranded DNA breaks under alkaline conditions, but not under neutral conditions.

In addition to the postulated mechanisms of DNA damage (disordered apoptosis, oxidative stress, and defective sperm chromatin packaging) discussed earlier, other mechanisms may be operative in older men. One possibility is age-dependent accumulation of DNA damage coupled with a less efficient apoptotic cell selection system [120]. Alternatively, the DNA damage may be attributable to age-related damage to the genes involved in the apoptotic pathway [123]. An age-related, cumulative birth cohort effect resulting from changing pre or perinatal exposures with altered testicular development may also be operative [124]. Likewise, chromosomal breaks and point mutations in germ cells are also known to increase with male age [125], which may reflect a decrease in the overall efficiency of DNA repair with age. Alternatively, DNA integrity of ejaculated spermatozoa may be more stable in younger, fertile sperm donors than in older patients with reduced semen quality [55]. It has been reported that prolonged incubation of density gradient selected sperm adversely affects sperm survival in older patients and patients with extensive sperm DNA damage [126].

30.5.2 Semen Analysis and Sperm DNA Damage

Many studies using different methods of sperm DNA assessment in different patient populations have produced a variety of results. Although some studies have reported either only a weak or no correlation between the conventional semen parameters and sperm DNA damage, most indicate that spermatozoa from patients with abnormal sperm count, morphology, and motility have increased levels of DNA damage. It is clear that semen analysis and DNA evaluation measure different aspects of the spermatozoa's fertilizing capacity [18].

Table 30.2 Relationship of DNA fragmentation to age

Age	Group I≤30 (*n*=322)	Group II. >30 to ≤35 (*n*=1456)	Group III >35 to ≤40 (*n*=1635)	Group IV >40 to ≤45 (*n*=844)	Group V >45 to ≤50 (*n*=269)	Group VI >50 (*n*=129)
DFI	15.2±10*	17.1±10.6*	18.7±12.2*	22.2±13.7*	26.1±16.1*	33.9±18.2

Note: *$P<0.05$

Table 30.3 Relationship of DNA fragmentation to semen parameter

Parameter	Means ± SD (n=2,451)	R value	P value
Volume (mL)	2.9±1.5	0.003	NS
Concentration (sperm[a]/mL)	63.7±58.9	−0.220	<0.01
Motile Concentration (sperm[a]/mL)	24.5±30.17	−0.414	<0.01
Motility (%)	31.9±16.6	−0.627	<0.01
Linearity[b]	60.1±12.4	−0.154	<0.01
VSL (μm/s)[b]	45.1±12.2	−0.392	<0.01
VCL (μm/s)[b]	75.3±22.6	−0.379	<0.01
ALH (μm)[b]	3.0±0.9	−0.167	<0.01
Normal Morphology (%)[c]	22.1±12.0	−0.450	<0.01
Vitality (%)[d]	70.8±13.1	−0.695	<0.01

NS not significant, *VSL* Curvilinear velocity, *VCL* Straight-line velocity, *ALH* Amplitude of lateral head displacement
[a] Number of sperm × 10^6
[b] Number of subjects: 2,414
[c] Number of subjects: 2,379
[d] Number of subjects: 1,942

Significant correlation to sperm motility only was reported in the studies of sperm donor [127] and infertility patients [83] when SCSA was employed. Similar results involving comparable DNA damage assessment (DFI) were reported by others, with significant correlations observed between DFI and motility and normal morphology [128]; as well as concentration, motility and normal morphology [129–131]. However, others have reported no relationship between DNA damage assessed by SCSA and semen parameters [20, 79].

In a study of 1,230 unselected nonazoospermic patients presenting to our laboratory for infertility evaluation and DNA integrity assessment, DFI was significantly correlated to sperm concentration, motility, normal morphology and vitality [66]. By now, we have doubled the number of analyzed subjects and can confirm our privies report (Table 30.3).

TUNEL assay was also reported to correlate to semen parameters. Sperm DNA fragmentation rates assessed by TUNEL assay were significantly higher in patients with abnormal sperm parameters than in those with normal parameters [132]. In another study, increased DNA fragmentation was associated with a decrease in sperm concentration and motility [48]. Other TUNEL studies reported significant correlations to concentration only [18]; morphology only [26], motility and morphology [63, 133]; concentration, motility and normal morphology [90, 134]. However, others have reported no correlation between TUNEL assessments and standard semen parameters [135].

Taking into account that DNA damage may occur at either the testicular or post-testicular level, it is understandable that studies using different methods of DNA assessment would have found various correlation levels with the standard semen parameters [46]. The differences could also be explained by the origin of the DNA damage: in patients with failure to repair DNA breaks during spermatogenesis, changes would likely be related to abnormal spermatogenesis and present as oligozoospermia or teratozoospermia. However, if the sperm DNA damage was mostly due to oxidative damage, the changes would most likely present in the form of asthenozoospermia. Abnormal spermatogenesis would lead to the presence in the ejaculate of spermatozoa with altered maturation, defective chromatin packaging and condensation, which would be more susceptible to ROS induced damage [136].

30.5.3 Natural Conception and Sperm DNA Damage

Several studies, using a variety of detection techniques, have shown significant differences in sperm DNA damage levels between fertile and infertile men [18, 19, 48]. In a study involving patients attempting natural conception, the probability of fertilization was close to zero in patients with DFI>30% [137]. This was confirmed by a later study, as patients with DFI lower than 40% had a ten times better chance of achieving pregnancy than subjects with higher levels of DNA damage [17].

30.5.4 ART and Sperm DNA Damage

While demand for ART treatment, which includes both in vitro (IUI) and in vivo (IVF, ICSI) procedures, is increasing every year, the overall live birth rates following this type of treatment remains below 30% [137]. Many studies have attempted to predict the utility of selected semen parameters and tests of sperm function, but it is not clear which tests have the most prognostic or diagnostic value for ART procedures [7, 9]. Several studies have suggested that the standard semen parameters have low prognostic value in predicting ART outcomes [4, 5]. Maternal age, related to oocyte quality, is the only established prognostic factor for ART outcome [138].

Interest in the use of DNA integrity as a predictor of fertility potential is increasing [16, 17], as clear differences in the levels of sperm DNA damage have been observed between fertile and infertile men [18, 19, 48, 139]. Normal sperm DNA structure is essential for correct transmission of the paternal genome. It has been reported that one third of patient seeking ART have high rates of DNA damage [83]. In laboratory, we have evaluated 4,655 patients presenting for fertility investigation, which included both fertile and infertile subjects; DFI ranged from 2.2 to 97.8% (19.4% ± 12.8), in 720 patients (15%) DFI was above 30%.

30.5.4.1 IUI and Sperm DNA Damage

The results of several IUI studies have shown similarities to the studies of natural conception and the effect of DNA damage. The chance of fertilization by IUI is very low if DFI reaches 30% [131]. Bungum and coworkers found that in couples undergoing IUI, the chance of live birth was 8.7 times more likely if the male partner had a DFI ≤ 27% [83]. The significant correlation between DFI and IUI was confirmed by the same group in a larger study of 387 IUI cycles [23]. A meta-analysis of four studies indicated that patients were 7.1 times more likely to achieve a pregnancy or delivery in vivo after IUI procedures with DFI < 30% [80].

Good correlation between TUNEL assay and IUI was also reported, when semen samples containing 12% sperm with fragmented DNA were used for insemination; no pregnancies were achieved [21].

30.5.4.2 IVF/ICSI and Sperm DNA Damage

Fertilization and Embryo Development

While high sperm DNA damage for patients with natural conception or IUI is clearly related to pregnancy odds, the results of ART involving in vitro fertilization techniques, such as IVF and ICSI, are controversial. While a few studies have identified a good correlation between fertilization rates and DNA damage [53, 131], a majority of them have reported no clear correlation between sperm DNA damage and fertilization rates using a variety of assessment techniques such as SCSA [140, 141]; TUNEL assay [90, 91], and Comet assay [24, 98]. The lack of correlation between fertilization rates and DNA damage is not surprising since maternal regulation is responsible for early embryo cleavage with the paternal effect starting after the second cleavage division [8]. In a study by Tesarik and coworkers [25], high DNA damage was associated with repeated ART treatment failures even when normal early embryo morphology was present. These results were similar to other studies; sperm DNA damage was negatively correlated to embryo quality in IVF only [142], and IVF and ICSI cycles [131]. Significant correlation between sperm DNA damage and blastocyst development has been reported [143]. Virro et al. showed that men with DFI > 30% were at risk of low blastocyst formation rates when IVF or ICSI were performed [141].

Pregnancies

Several studies employing SCSA have reported a strong correlation of high DFI and IVF treatment outcome, with no pregnancies achieved when DFI reaches 27–30% [77, 79]. A recent meta-analysis of six studies using IVF or ICSI procedures confirmed this report; patients were 1.8 times more likely to achieve a pregnancy or delivery if the DFI was <30% [80]. Virro et al. using the same DNA damage assessment showed that men with DFI > 30% had no ongoing pregnancies following IVF or ICSI [141]. In contrast, others have reported no differences in SCSA parameters between patients with or without pregnancies in IVF and ICSI cycles [140]. Successful pregnancies in IVF/ICSI cycles can even be obtained using semen samples with a high proportion of DNA damage [23, 144, 145].

Other studies using different methods to assess DNA fragmentation have examined the relationship of DNA status and pregnancies following both IVF and ICSI. Some studies have shown that abnormal TUNEL results predict the outcome of IVF and ICSI [54, 90]. No pregnancies were achieved when DNA damage was more than 20% for ICSI cycles [90]. Henkel and colleague, using TUNEL, reported a higher threshold for DNA damage with 36.5% for IVF and 24.3% for ICSI [91]. Lewis et al. also reported a close relationship between DNA damage assessed by the Comet assay and pregnancies in ICSI cycles [98].

The value of sperm DNA fragmentation tests in predicting pregnancy rates may be different in IVF and ICSI treatments. It appears that the predictive value of DNA assessment is decreased in ICSI compared to IVF [23, 83, 144]. This may be partially explained by the etiology of the infertility as it has been shown that the highest level of DNA damage is usually found in patients with severe semen abnormalities, for whom, ICSI treatment would be the treatment of choice [18, 24, 90]. Patients referred for ICSI would mostly represent the male infertility group, whereas in an IVF group, female factor might predominate. It has also been suggested that the effect of DNA damage may be related to the ability of the oocyte to repair such damage and to the extent of the damage in a particular spermatozoon [140]. The difference in predictive value in IVF and ICSI treatment may also relate to the type of assay being used as well as the nature of DNA damage. For TUNEL and Comet assays, the predictive value appears to be stronger in ICSI patients compared with IVF [24, 90]. This is not true for SCSA as this assay identifies susceptibility to acid-induced DNA denaturation of spermatozoa [146].

Since ICSI bypasses all means of natural selection of sperm by the oocyte, it is interesting that some observed better results with ICSI than IVF in patients with high DFI [20, 144]. Bungum et al. found significantly better results with ICSI than with routine IVF in patients with DFI>27%. In a study including 223 IVF and 388 ICSI cycles, the same group found better pregnancy results for ICSI treatment than for IVF when DFI was >30% [23]. The results may be explained, in part, by technical differences between the two procedures as well as by different culture conditions, as spermatozoa injected into oocytes usually has a shorter incubation time during which it may be exposed to ROS [144].

Host and colleagues suggested that technical differences in ICSI may influence the relationship to DNA integrity as attempts are usually made to choose spermatozoa with normal morphology. This might be one of the reasons for the reduced predictive value of SCSA in ICSI [147].

Miscarriage and Spontaneous Abortion

The low correlation between sperm DNA damage and fertilization rates indicates that genetically damaged spermatozoa may be able to fertilize an oocyte and lead to adverse effects on the health of the embryo and fetus [23, 26, 137, 140, 141, 148]. Several studies have examined the relationship between sperm DNA damage and rates of spontaneous abortion. In a study by Gandini and associates, sperm DNA damage >30% assessed by SCSA was associated with increased miscarriage rates [140]. In another study, almost 40% of miscarriages were related to a DFI>30% [137]. Others have reported a higher rate of spontaneous abortions at 12 weeks of gestation in those with DFI>30% [141]. In contrast, Bungum and coworkers showed no statistically significant association between high DFI and early pregnancy loss when DFI was >30%, however, they could not exclude the fact that DFI levels >60% were associated with a higher risk of early pregnancy loss [23].

Using TUNEL assay, repeat pregnancy loss patients had higher DNA damage in comparison to the general population (22% vs.11%) [26]. The close link between sperm DNA fragmentation assessed by TUNEL and pregnancy loss was also observed with ICSI treatment; 62.5% of miscarriages were reported in the group with high DNA damage compared to no miscarriages in the group with low DNA damage. However, this correlation was not confirmed in IVF cycles in the same study [148].

The oocyte has the capacity to repair DNA damage to some extent; however, this process could be incomplete or unsuitable due to oocyte's defective repair mechanisms, and also due to advanced maternal age [8, 138]. The correlation between sperm DNA damage and pregnancy loss also related to paternal genome anomalies blocking the correct embryo development [148]. It was also suggested that, since the IGF2 gene present in human spermatozoa is involved in the formation of the placenta, impairment of this gene by DNA damage would increase the risk of early pregnancy loss [149].

30.5.5 Effect of DNA Quality on Offspring

A major area of concern is the effect of sperm DNA damage on the fetus and offspring [11, 12]. With the increasing use of ICSI, which bypasses normal egg–sperm interactions and allows even very low quality sperm to initiate a successful pregnancy, the negative effect of the DNA damage may present more frequently and more severely [10–15]. In these situations, the extent of DNA damage with its promutagenic effect may overpower the oocyte's capacity to repair the DNA damage. This will increase the risk of mutations after fertilization, as the oocyte attempts to repair the DNA damage and escalate the chance of imprinting disorders [150]. Two thirds of the of 25 studies included in a recent meta-analysis revealed a 25% or greater increase in risk of birth defects in infants conceived through IVF and/or ICSI compared with naturally conceived children [151]. The link between ART and the birth of children exhibiting diseases may be due to defects in the pattern of DNA methylation leading to imprinting disorders and some epigenetic errors [152].

There is a four to five time increased risk of childhood cancer in the offspring of men with a high proportion of sperm DNA fragmentation caused by extensive smoking [153]. Another possible consequence of sperm DNA damage is infertility in the form of Y chromosome microdeletions. These deletions arise de novo in the germ line of the infertile male's father and likely due to the fact that the Y chromosome contains a high number of repetitive DNA sequences that are targets for homologous intrachromosomal recombination [150].

30.6 Reduction of Sperm DNA Damage

In the light of findings regarding the impact of sperm DNA fragmentation on embryonic development, implantation and risk of recurrent miscarriages, as well as the health of offspring, several strategies have been recommended to reduce damage. Recently, some positive progress has been made in the management of patients with high sperm DNA damage.

30.6.1 Oral Antioxidants

Antioxidants present in seminal plasma may control ROS generation to some degree, but the production of excessive amounts of ROS may overcome the antioxidant protective activities of seminal plasma leading to oxidative stress [67, 68]. Many antioxidants play an important role in various biological processes: enzyme production, DNA synthesis, testicular development and sperm maturation are microelement and vitamin dependent [154]. The protective effect of several antioxidants on sperm DNA integrity has been reported both in in vitro studies and in patients with moderately elevated DNA damage [155–157]. Greco and colleagues reported a decrease in DNA damage in 76% of patients with moderately increased DNA fragmentation (≥15%) after oral treatment with vitamins C and E [156]. Siver and associates were unable to demonstrate a beneficial effect of high antioxidant intake (vitamins C, E, beta-carotene) on sperm chromatin integrity in men with infertility [158]. The same group, however, reported a beneficial effect of higher antioxidant consumption on sperm concentration and motility in the same patient population [159]. The differences in the effects of antioxidant treatment among studies are likely related to the type, dosage and duration of the treatment as well as to differences in patient populations and different nature of DNA damage [155]. Antioxidant therapy would only be of benefit to patients whose DNA damage is due, primarily, to oxidative stress [160]. The variation in response may also be related to individual differences in nutrient absorption and metabolism of the antioxidants [158], as well as to failure of the antioxidant system or enzyme production in some patients [161]. Multiple antioxidants acting through different mechanisms on diverse free radicals have been suggested as a therapeutic approach in the treatment of male infertility [155].

30.6.2 Sperm Separation

A single ejaculate is heterogeneous in terms of semen and DNA quality. Several methods designed to separate superior spermatozoa have been recommended. Some of these methods are used routinely in the preparation of ejaculate prior to ART treatment; both swim-up and density gradient centrifugation methods were evaluated for DNA damage. The swim-up procedure was shown to better eliminate defective spermatozoa. DFI dropped from 12 to 5.5% after swim-up [140], however, in a different study, gradient density preparation also showed a decrease in DFI from 28 to 24% after treatment [142]. It has been suggested that the elevated SCSA values in neat spermatozoa reflect chromatin abnormalities within the entire sperm population that may not be eliminated by sperm preparation techniques [137].

Several novel techniques to separate "best" spermatozoa have been introduced. One of these is the separation of spermatozoa by magnetic-activated cell sorting (MACS). The technique is based on the spermatozoa's ability to express the apoptotic marker of phosphatidylserine, which would bind to Annexin-V-conjugated micro-beads and separated by a magnetic field into Annexin-V positive and negative fractions [162]. While the nonapoptotic sperm fraction contains morphologically normal spermatozoa, no assessment of it DNA content has been yet reported [163].

Another new method is the electrophoretic separation of sperm. The method is based on the observation that mature spermatozoa are more electronegative due to negatively charged glycocalyx rich in sialic acid residues. Sperm are separated by traveling toward the positively charged cathode and away from the negatively charged anode [164]. It has been shown that electrophoretically isolated spermatozoa have low DNA damage revealed by TUNEL assay. The first pregnancy and normal birth after ICSI using electrophoretically isolated spermatozoa has been reported [165].

30.6.3 High-Magnification ICSI

ICSI with spermatozoa selected through the use of a high-magnification digitally enhanced optical system allowing ×6,600 magnification been reported [164]. This magnification reveals intranuclear vacuoles possibly associated with alterations in chromatin packaging [166]. ICSI performed by this system has been shown to significantly increase pregnancy rates compared with conventional ICSI in patients with both high and low sperm DNA fragmentation [167].

30.6.4 ICSI with Testicular Spermatozoa

It has been suggested that some sperm DNA damage may occur in the epididymis where exposure of the sperm to ROS is longer in duration [91]. Retrieval of testicular spermatozoa, which generally has lower levels of DNA damage, has been suggested for patients with markedly increased DNA damage [168]. The reproductive outcome of ICSI using ejaculated and testicular spermatozoa in 18 patients was compared. The pregnancy rate using testicular spermatozoa was 44% vs. 6% using ejaculated spermatozoa and the implantation rate was 22% vs. 2% or one pregnancy, which spontaneously aborted. In contrast, a meta-analysis of several studies could not find any differences in the outcomes of ICSI when epididymal, testicular and neat spermatozoa were compared [169].

30.7 Conclusions

While data regarding sperm DNA damage is somewhat conflicting, some clinical results have been confirmed by several research groups and should be considered in the management of infertility patients. An evaluation/treatment algorithm, for the use of sperm chromatin assessment in male infertility, is presented in Fig. 30.1.

The recommendations must be assessed in the context of the couple's fertility history and other clinical parameters as sperm DNA damage has only a relative and not absolute clinical value.

1. Reliable, robust, clinically proven assays have to be employed in the evaluation of sperm DNA damage. SCSA or DNA Integrity Assay are good examples of such assays with accumulated clinical data supported by clinical cut-off levels.
2. Sperm DNA damage is relatively common in infertile males, especially in men with disordered spermatogenesis characterized by severely abnormal semen parameters. However, since the relationship between standard semen parameters and DNA damage is not strong, sperm DNA

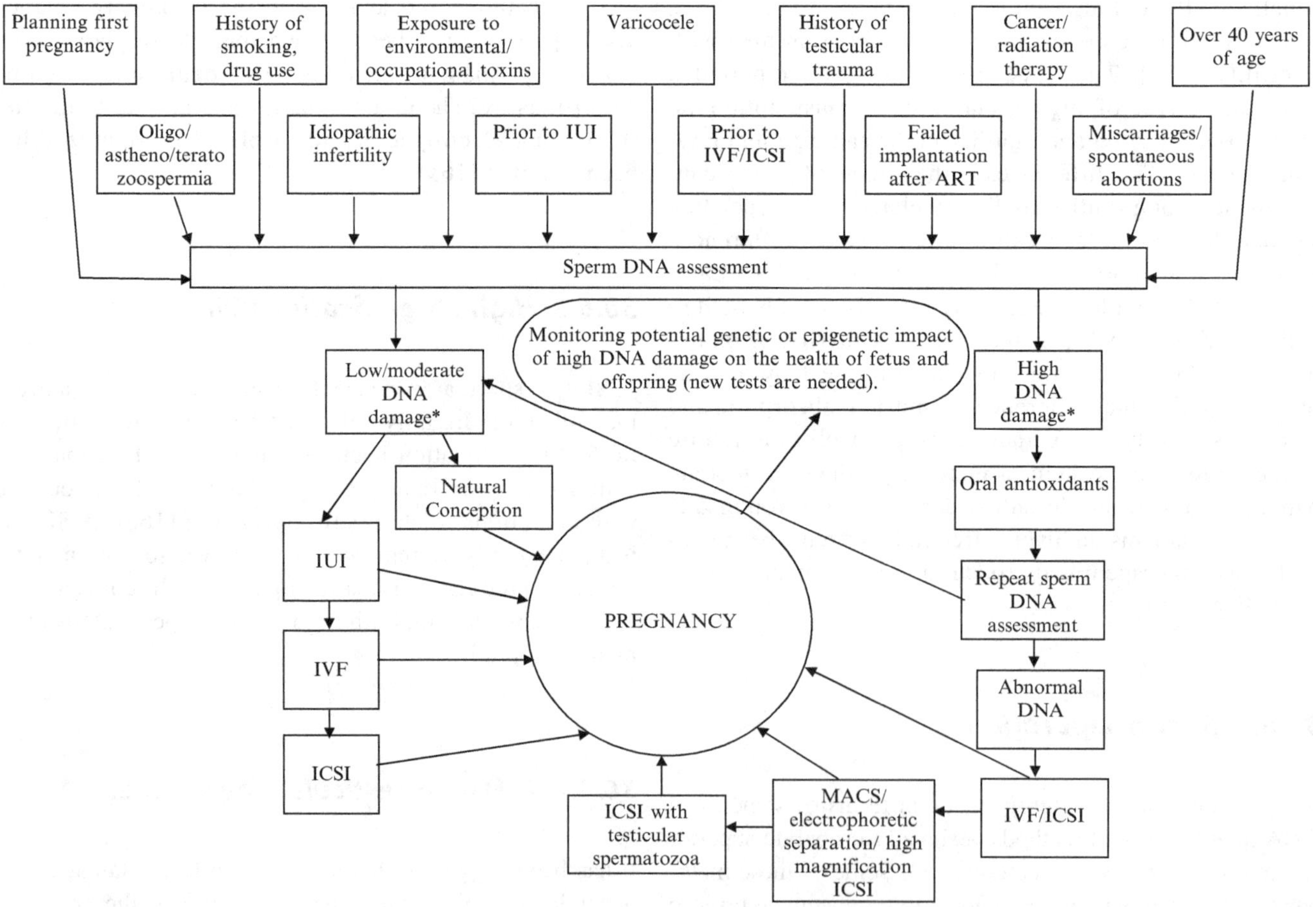

Fig. 30.1 Evaluation/treatment algorithm for the use of sperm chromatin assessment in male infertility Note: * Based on value of clinical cut-off levels for DFI

assessment should be recommended for patients with abnormal semen parameters as well as for normozoospermic patients as part of the investigation of male infertility.

3. Assessment of sperm DNA damage in patients with idiopathic infertility may clarify the cause of infertility.
4. Sperm DNA assessment should be offered to patients undergoing infertility evaluation or treatment with a history of smoking and drug use, exposure to environmental and occupational toxins, as well as in patients with varicoceles, history of testicular trauma and cancer patients, as all will have a negative effect on sperm DNA damage.
5. There is a strong correlation between male age and sperm DNA damage. This is of particular concern as older men tend to reproduce with older women. Age related diminished capacity of the oocyte to repair DNA damage must also be considered. DNA assessment should be included in the fertility evaluation of men over 40 years of age.
6. Sperm DNA damage has been established as a good predictor of negative pregnancy outcomes in patients with natural conception. DNA assessment should be offered to patients planning a first pregnancy.
7. Sperm DNA damage has been established as a good predictor of negative pregnancy outcomes in patients undergoing IUI treatment. Normally, several IUI cycles would be offered to the couple; however, if high sperm DNA damage is present, IVF or ICSI treatment should be recommended.
8. DNA assessment should be offered to couples undergoing IVF or ICSI even though it offers only a moderate prediction of pregnancy outcome. Several reports indicate that ICSI would be preferable to IVF as better pregnancy results were achieved in patients with high DNA damage with ICSI.
9. Although the impact of DNA damage on fertilization is probably small, the negative effect on embryo development and the fetus could be severe. Patients with a history of failed implantation after ART, miscarriages and spontaneous abortions should be evaluated to exclude a contribution of the paternal genome.
10. In patients with known elevated DNA damage, oral antioxidant therapy could be offered for 2–3 months prior to the ART treatment, as a beneficial effect of oral antioxidants has been shown on sperm DNA damage and ART outcomes.
11. Several novel methods designed to isolate spermatozoa with normal DNA have been recommended including MACS, electrophoretic spermatozoa separation, and high-magnification ICSI. However, further evaluation and confirmation is necessary before these are introduced into general practice.
12. In cases where all efforts to reduce sperm DNA damage have failed, ICSI with testicular spermatozoa should be considered.
13. ART treatment in general and ICSI in particular bypasses the natural selection of spermatozoa and increases the chance of introducing unbalanced or damaged DNA into the oocyte. Because the treatment might influence the health of the fetus and offspring, monitoring of the risk of using potentially damaged spermatozoa is necessary and development of specific screening tests is essential.
14. Properly designed research studies and specifically randomized controlled trials are necessary to obtained deeper clinical evidence and to satisfy demanding interest for evidence-based guidelines of the management of patient with elevated DNA damage.

References

1. Greenhall E, Vessey M (1990) The prevalence of subfertility: a review of the current confusion and a report of two new studies. Fertil Steril 54:978–983
2. Mosher WD, Pratt WF (1991) Fecundity and infertility in the United States: incidence and trends. Fertil Steril 56:192–193
3. World Health Organization (1999) WHO laboratory manual for the examination of human semen and sperm-cervical mucus interaction, 4th edn. Cambridge University Press, Cambridge, UK
4. Tomlinson MJ, Kessopoulou E, Barratt CLR (1999) The diagnostic and prognostic value of traditional semen parameters. J Androl 20:588–593
5. Guzick DS, Overstreet JW, Factor-Litvak P et al (2001) Sperm morphology, motility, and concentration in infertile and fertile men. N Engl J Med 345:1388–1393
6. Liu DY, Baker HW (2002) Evaluation and assessment of semen for IVF/ICSI. Asian J Androl 4:281–285
7. Carrell DT (2000) Semen analysis at the turn of the century: an evaluation of potential uses of new sperm function assays. Arch Androl 44:65–75
8. Lewis SEM, Aitken RJ (2005) DNA damage to spermatozoa has impacts on fertilization and pregnancy. Cell Tissue Res 322:33–41
9. Sherins RJ (1995) Are semen quality and male fertility changing? N Engl J Med 332:327–328
10. Nagy ZP, Verheyen G, Tournaye H, Van Steirteghem AC (1998) Special applications of intracytoplasmic sperm injection: the influence of sperm count, motility, morphology, source and sperm antibody on the outcome of ICSI. Hum Reprod 13:143–154
11. Bonduelle M, Aytoz A, Van Assche E, Devroey P, Liebaers I, Van Steirteghem A (1998) Incidence of chromosomal aberrations in children born after assisted reproduction through intracytoplasmic sperm injection. Hum Reprod 13:781–782
12. In't Veld P, Brandenburg H, Verhoeff A, Dhont M, Los F (1995) Sex chromosomal abnormalities and intracytoplasmic sperm injection. Lancet 346:773
13. Bonduelle M, Van Assche E, Joris H, Keymolen K, Devroey P, Van Steirteghem A, Liebaers I (2002) Prenatal testing in ICSI pregnancies: incidence of chromosomal anomalies in 1586 karyotypes and relation to sperm parameters. Hum Reprod 17:2600–2614

14. Verpoest W, Tournaye H (2006) ICSI: hype or hazard? Hum Fertil 9:81–92
15. The ESHRE Capri Workshop Group (2007) Intracytoplasmic sperm injection (ICSI) in 2006: Evidence and Evolution. Hum Reprod Update 13:515–526
16. Kodama H, Yamaguchi R, Fukuda J, Kasai H, Tanaka T (1997) Increased oxidative deoxyribonucleic acid damage in the spermatozoa of infertile male patients. Fertil Steril 68:519–524
17. Spano M, Bonde JP, Hjollund HI, Kolstad HA, Cordelli E, Leter G (2000) Sperm chromatin damage impairs human fertility. The Danish First Pregnancy Planner Study Team. Fertil Steril 73:43–50
18. Irvine DS, Twigg JP, Gordon EL, Fulton N, Milne PA, Aitken RJ (2000) DNA integrity in human spermatozoa: relationships with semen quality. J Androl 21:33–44
19. Zini A, Bielecki R, Phang D, Zenzes MT (2001) Correlations between two markers of sperm DNA integrity, DNA denaturation and DNA fragmentation, in fertile and infertile men. Fertil Steril 75:674–677
20. Larson-Cook KL, Brannian JD, Hansen KA, Kasperson KM, Aamold ET, Evenson DP (2003) Relationship between the outcomes of assisted reproductive techniques and sperm DNA fragmentation as measured by the sperm chromatin structure assay. Fertil Steril 80:895–902
21. Duran EH, Morshedi M, Taylor S, Oehninger S (2002) Sperm DNA quality predicts intrauterine insemination outcome – a prospective cohort study. Hum Reprod 17:3122–3128
22. Benchaib M, Lornage J, Mazoyer C, Lejeune H, Salle B, Francois Guerin J (2007) Sperm deoxyribonucleic acid fragmentation as a prognostic indicator of assisted reproductive technology outcome. Fertil Steril 87:93–100
23. Bungum M, Humaidan P, Axmon A, Spano M, Bungum L, Erenpreiss J, Giwercman A (2007) Sperm DNA integrity assessment in prediction of assisted reproduction technology outcome. Hum Reprod 22:174–179
24. Morris ID, Ilott S, Dixon L, Brison DR (2002) The spectrum of DNA damage in human sperm assessed by single cell electrophoresis (COMET assay) and its relationship to fertilization and embryo development. Hum Reprod 17:990–998
25. Tesarik J, Greco E, Mendoza C (2004) Late, but not early, paternal effect on human embryo development is related to sperm DNA fragmentation. Hum Reprod 19:611–615
26. Carrell DT, Liu L, Peterson CM et al (2003) Sperm DNA fragmentation is increased in couples with unexplained recurrent pregnancy loss. Arch Androl 49:49–55
27. Ward WS, Partin AW, Coffey DS (1989) DNA loop domains in mammalian spermatozoa. Chromosoma 98:153–159
28. Ward MA, Ward WS (2004) A model for the function of sperm DNA degradation. Reprod Fertil Dev 16:547–554
29. Hoyer-Fender S, Singh PB, Motzkus D (2000) The murine heterochromatin protein M31 is associated with the chromocenter in round spermatids and Is a component of mature spermatozoa. Exp Cell Res 254:72–79
30. Ward WS, Zalensky AO (1996) The unique, complex organization of the transcriptionally silent sperm chromatin. Crit Rev Eukaryot Gene Expr 6:139–147
31. Sotolongo B, Ward WS (2001) DNA loop domain organization: the three dimensional genomic code. J Cell Biochem Suppl 35:23–26
32. Barone JG, De Lara J, Cummings KB, Ward WS (1994) DNA organization in human spermatozoa. J Androl 15:139–144
33. Ward WS, Coffey DS (1989) Identification of a sperm nuclear annulus: a sperm DNA anchor. Biol Reprod 41:361–370
34. Zalensky AO, Allen MJ, Kobayashi A, Zalenskaya IA, Balhorn R, Bradbury EM (1995) Well-defined genome architecture in the human sperm nucleus. Chromosoma 103:577–590
35. Wouters-Tyrou D, Martinage A, Chevaillier P, Sautiere P (1998) Nuclear basic proteins in spermiogenesis. Biochimie 80:117–128
36. Balhorn R (1982) A model for the structure of chromatin in mammalian sperm. J Cell Biol 93:298–305
37. Ward WS (1993) Deoxyribonucleic acid loop domain tertiary structure in mammalian spermatozoa. Biol Reprod 48:1193–1201
38. Gineitis AA, Zalenskaya IA, Yau PM, Bradbury EM, Zalensky AO (2000) Human sperm telomere-binding complex involves histone H2B and secures telomere membrane attachment. J Cell Biol 151:1591–1598
39. Zalensky AO, Siino JS, Gineitis AA et al (2002) Human testis/sperm-specific histone H2B (hTSH2B). Molecular cloning and characterization. J Biol Chem 277:43474–43480
40. Gardiner-Garden M, Ballesteros M, Gordon M, Tam PP (1998) Histone- and protamine-DNA association: conservation of different patterns within the beta-globin domain in human sperm. Mol Cell Biol 18:3350–3356
41. Zalenskaya IA, Bradbury EM, Zalensky AO (2000) Chromatin structure of telomere domain in human sperm. Biochem Biophys Res Commun 279:213–218
42. Singleton S, Zalensky A, Doncel GF, Morshedi M, Zalenskaya IA (2007) Testis/sperm-specific histone 2B in the sperm of donors and subfertile patients: variability and relation to chromatin packaging. Hum Reprod 22:743–750
43. Zalenskaya IA, Zalensky AO (2004) Non-random positioning of chromosomes in human sperm nuclei. Chromosome Res 12:163–173
44. Solov'eva L, Svetlova M, Bodinski D, Zalensky AO (2004) Nature of telomere dimers and chromosome looping in human spermatozoa. Chromosome Res 12:817–823
45. Zalensky AO, Tomilin NV, Zalenskaya IA, Teplitz R, Bradbury EM (1997) Telomere-telomere interactions and telomere binding proteins in mammalian sperm. Exp Cell Res 232:29–41
46. Fischer MA, Willis J, Zini A (2003) Human sperm DNA integrity: correlation with sperm cytoplasmic droplets. Urology 61:207–211
47. Agarwal A, Said TM (2003) Role of sperm chromatin abnormalities and DNA damage in male infertility. Hum Reprod Update 9:331–345
48. Gandini L, Lombardo F, Paoli D et al (2000) Study of apoptotic DNA fragmentation in human spermatozoa. Hum Reprod 15:830–839
49. Stahl O, Eberhard J, Jepson K et al (2006) Sperm DNA integrity in testicular cancer patients. Hum Reprod 21:3199–3205
50. Morris ID (2002) Sperm DNA damage and cancer treatment. Int J Androl 25:255–261
51. Wyllie AH, Kerr JFR, Currie AR (1980) Cell death: the significance of apoptosis. Int Rev Cytol 68:251–306
52. Gorczyca W, Traganos F, Jesionowska H, Darzynkiewicz Z (1993) Presence of DNA strand breaks and increased sensitivity of DNA in situ to denaturation in abnormal human sperm cells: analogy to apoptosis of somatic cells. Exp Cell Res 207:202–205
53. Lopes S, Sun JG, Jurisicova A, Meriano J, Casper RF (1998) Sperm deoxyribonucleic acid fragmentation is increased in poor-quality semen samples and correlates with failed fertilization in intracytoplasmic sperm injection. Fertil Steril 69:528–532
54. Sakkas D, Moffatt O, Manicardi GC, Mariethoz E, Tarozzi N, Bizzaro D (2002) Nature of DNA damage in ejaculated human spermatozoa and the possible involvement of apoptosis. Biol Reprod 66:1061–1067
55. Lachaud C, Tesarik J, Canadas ML, Mendoza C (2004) Apoptosis and necrosis in human ejaculated spermatozoa. Hum Reprod 19:607–610
56. Blanc-Layrac G, Bringuier AF, Guillot R, Feldmann G (2000) Morphological and biochemical analysis of cell death in human ejaculated spermatozoa. Cell Mol Biol (Noisy-le-grand) 46:187–197

57. Sinha Hikim AP, Swerdloff RS (1999) Hormonal and genetic control of germ cell apoptosis in the testis. Rev Reprod 4:38–47
58. Sakkas D, Seli E, Bizzaro D, Tarozzi N, Manicardi GC (2003) Abnormal spermatozoa in the ejaculate: abortive apoptosis and faulty nuclear remodelling during spermatogenesis. Reprod Biomed Online 7:428–432
59. Lee J, Richburg JH, Younkin SC, Boekelheide K (1997) The Fas system is a key regulator of germ cell apoptosis in the testis. Endocrinology 138:2081–2088
60. Barroso G, Morshedi M, Oehninger S (2000) Analysis of DNA fragmentation, plasma membrane translocation of phosphatidylserine and oxidative stress in human spermatozoa. Hum Reprod 15:1338–1344
61. Aitken RJ, Clarkson JS, Fishel S (1989) Generation of reactive oxygen species, lipid peroxidation, and human sperm function. Biol Reprod 41:183–197
62. Beckman KB, Ames BN (1997) Oxidative decay of DNA. J Biol Chem 272:19633–19636
63. Twigg J, Fulton N, Gomez E, Irvine DS, Aitken RJ (1998) Analysis of the impact of intracellular reactive oxygen species generation on the structural and functional integrity of human spermatozoa: lipid peroxidation, DNA fragmentation and effectiveness of antioxidants. Hum Reprod 13:1429–1436
64. Zini A, de Lamirande E, Gagnon C (1993) Reactive oxygen species in semen of infertile patients: levels of superoxide dismutase- and catalase-like activities in seminal plasma and spermatozoa. Int J Androl 16:183–188
65. Alvarez JG, Sharma RK, Ollero M et al (2002) Increased DNA damage in sperm from leukocytospermic semen samples as determined by the sperm chromatin structure assay. Fertil Steril 78:319–329
66. Moskovtsev SI, Willis J, White J, Mullen JB (2007) Leukocytospermia: relationship to sperm deoxyribonucleic acid integrity in patients evaluated for male factor infertility. Fertil Steril 88:737–740
67. Griveau JF, Le Lannou D (1997) Reactive oxygen species and human spermatozoa: physiology and pathology. Int J Androl 20:61–69
68. Sikka SC (2004) Role of oxidative stress and antioxidants in andrology and assisted reproductive technology. J Androl 25:5–18
69. Marcon L, Boissonneault G (2004) Transient DNA strand breaks during mouse and human spermiogenesis new insights in stage specificity and link to chromatin remodeling. Biol Reprod 70:910–918
70. Evenson DP, Jost LK, Corzett M, Balhorn R (2000) Characteristics of human sperm chromatin structure following an episode of influenza and high fever: a case study. J Androl 21:739–746
71. Carrell DT, Liu L (2001) Altered protamine 2 expression is uncommon in donors of known fertility, but common among men with poor fertilizing capacity, and may reflect other abnormalities of spermiogenesis. J Androl 22:604–610
72. Laberge RM, Boissonneault G (2005) On the nature and origin of DNA strand breaks in elongating spermatids. Biol Reprod 73:289–296
73. McPherson SM, Longo FJ (1992) Localization of DNase I-hypersensitive regions during rat spermatogenesis: stage-dependent patterns and unique sensitivity of elongating spermatids. Mol Reprod Dev 31:268–279
74. Bianchi PG, Manicardi GC, Bizzaro D, Bianchi U, Sakkas D (1993) Effect of deoxyribonucleic acid protamination on fluorochrome staining and in situ nick-translation of murine and human mature spermatozoa. Biol Reprod 49:1083–1088
75. Bannister LA, Schimenti JC (2004) Homologous recombinational repair proteins in mouse meiosis. Cytogenet Genome Res 107:191–200
76. Aoki VW, Moskovtsev SI, Willis J, Liu L, Mullen JB, Carrell DT (2005) DNA integrity is compromised in protamine-deficient human sperm. J Androl 26:741–748
77. Spano M, Seli E, Bizzaro D, Manicardi GC, Sakkas D (2005) The significance of sperm nuclear DNA strand breaks on reproductive outcome. Curr Opin Obstet Gynecol 17:255–260
78. Evenson DP, Darzynkiewicz Z, Melamed MR (1980) Relation of mammalian sperm chromatin heterogeneity to fertility. Science 210:1131–1133
79. Evenson DP, Larson KL, Jost LK (2002) Sperm chromatin structure assay: its clinical use for detecting sperm DNA fragmentation in male infertility and comparisons with other techniques. J Androl 23:25–43
80. Evenson D, Wixon R (2006) Meta-analysis of sperm DNA fragmentation using the sperm chromatin structure assay. Reprod Biomed Online 12:466–472
81. Moskovtsev SI, Willis J, Mullen JB (2006) Age-related decline in sperm deoxyribonucleic acid integrity in patients evaluated for male infertility. Fertil Steril 85:496–499
82. Saleh RA, Agarwal A, Nelson DR et al (2002) Increased sperm nuclear DNA damage in normozoospernic infertile men: a prospective study. Fertil Steril 78:313–318
83. Bungum M, Humaidan P, Spano M, Jepson K, Bungum L, Giwercman A (2004) The predictive value of sperm chromatin structure assay (SCSA) parameters and the outcome of intrauterine insemination, IVF and ICSI. Hum Reprod 19:1401–1408
84. Zini A, Libman J (2006) Sperm DNA damage: Clinical significance in the era of assisted reproduction. CMAJ 175:495–500
85. Tejada RI, Mitchell JC, Norman A, Marik JJ, Friedman S (1984) A test for the practical evaluation of male fertility by acridine orange (AO) fluorescence. Fertil Steril 42:87–91
86. Ibrahim ME, Pedersen H (1988) Acridine orange fluorescence as male fertility test. Arch Androl 20:125–129
87. Virant-Klun I, Tomazevic T, Meden-Vrtovec H (2002) Sperm single-stranded DNA, detected by acridine orange staining, reduces fertilization and quality of ICSI-derived embryos. J Assist Reprod Genet 19:319–328
88. Katayose H, Yanagida K, Hashimoto S, Yamada H, Sato A (2003) Use of diamide–acridine orange fluorescence staining to detect aberrant protamination of human-ejaculated sperm nuclei. Fertil Steril 79:670–676
89. Sergerie M, Laforest G, Boulanger K, Bissonnette F, Bleau G (2005) Longitudinal study of sperm DNA fragmentation as measured by terminal uridine nick end-labelling assay. Hum Reprod 20:1921–1927
90. Benchaib M, Braun V, Lornage J et al (2003) Sperm DNA fragmentation decreases the pregnancy rate in an assisted reproductive technique. Hum Reprod 18:1023–1028
91. Henkel R, Kierspel E, Hajimohammad M et al (2003) DNA fragmentation of spermatozoa and assisted reproduction technology. Reprod Biomed Online 7:477–484
92. Manicardi GC, Tombacco A, Bizzaro D, Bianchi U, Bianchi PG, Sakkas D (1998) DNA strand breaks in ejaculated human spermatozoa: comparison of susceptibility to the nick translation and terminal transferase assays. Histochem J 30:33–39
93. Steele EK, McClure N, Maxwell RJ, Lewis SE (1999) A comparison of DNA damage in testicular and proximal epididymal spermatozoa in obstructive azoospermia. Mol Hum Reprod 5:831–835
94. Collins AR, Dobson VL, Dusinska M, Kennedy G, Stetina R (1997) The comet assay: what can it really tell us? Mutat Res 375:183–193
95. Singh NP, Danner DB, Tice RR, McCoy MT, Collins GD, Schneider EL (1989) Abundant alkali-sensitive sites in DNA of human and mouse sperm. Exp Cell Res 184:461–470
96. Olive PL, Durand RE, Banath JP, Johnston PJ (2001) Analysis of DNA damage in individual cells. Methods Cell Biol 64:235–249

97. Aravindan GR, Bjordahl J, Jost LK, Evenson DP (1997) Susceptibility of human sperm to in situ DNA denaturation is strongly correlated with DNA strand breaks identified by single-cell electrophoresis. Exp Cell Res 236:231–237
98. Lewis SE, O'Connell M, Stevenson M, Thompson-Cree L, McClure N (2004) An algorithm to predict pregnancy in assisted reproduction. Hum Reprod 19:1385–1394
99. Wiseman H, Halliwell B (1996) Damage to DNA by reactive oxygen and nitrogen species: role in inflammatory disease and progression to cancer. Biochem J 313:17–29
100. Halliwell B (1998) Can oxidative DNA damage be used as a biomarker of cancer risk in humans? Problems, resolutions and preliminary results from nutritional supplementation studies. Free Radic Res 29:469–486
101. Fraga CG, Motchnik PA, Shigenaga MK, Helbock HJ, Jacob RA, Ames BN (1991) Ascorbic acid protects against endogenous oxidative DNA damage in human sperm. Proc Natl Acad Sci USA 88:11003–11006
102. Shen HM, Chia SE, Ong CN (1999) Evaluation of oxidative DNA damage in human sperm and its association with male infertility. J Androl 20:718–723
103. Schaaf GJ, Nijmeijer SM, Maas RF, Roestenberg P, de Groene EM, Fink-Gremmels J (2002) The role of oxidative stress in the ochratoxin A-mediated toxicity in proximal tubular cells. Biochim Biophys Acta 1588:149–158
104. Chen CS, Chao HT, Pan RL, Wei YH (1997) Hydroxyl radical-induced decline in motility and increase in lipid peroxidation and DNA modification in human sperm. Biochem Mol Biol Int 43:291–303
105. Oger I, Da Cruz C, Panteix G, Menezo Y (2003) Evaluating human sperm DNA integrity: relationship between 8-hydroxydeoxyguanosine quantification and the sperm chromatin structure assay. Zygote 11:367–371
106. Chevaillier P, Mauro N, Feneux D, Jouannet P, David G (1987) Anomalous protein complement of sperm nuclei in some infertile men. Lancet 2:806–807
107. Colleu D, Lescoat D, Boujard D, Le Lannou D (1988) Human spermatozoal nuclear maturity in normozoospermia and asthenozoospermia. Arch Androl 21:155–162
108. Haidl G, Schill WB (1994) Assessment of sperm chromatin condensation: an important test for prediction of IVF outcome. Arch Androl 32:263–266
109. Razavi S, Nasr-Esfahani MH, Mardani M, Mafi A, Moghdam A (2003) Effect of human sperm chromatin anomalies on fertilization outcome post-ICSI. Andrologia 35:238–243
110. Hammadeh ME, Strehler E, Zeginiadou T, Rosenbaum P, Schmidt W (2001) Chromatin decondensation of human sperm in vitro and its relation to fertilization rate after ICSI. Arch Androl 47:83–87
111. Krzanowska H (1982) Toluidine blue staining reveals changes in chromatin stabilization of mouse spermatozoa during epididymal maturation and penetration of ova. J Reprod Fertil 64:97–101
112. Andreetta AM, Stockert JC, Barrera C (1995) A simple method to detect sperm chromatin abnormalities: cytochemical mechanism and possible value in predicting semen quality in assisted reproductive procedures. Int J Androl 18:23–28
113. Erenpreiss J, Jepson K, Giwercman A, Tsarev I, Erenpreisa J, Spano M (2004) Toluidine blue cytometry test for sperm DNA conformation: comparison with the flow cytometric sperm chromatin structure and TUNEL assays. Hum Reprod 19:2277–2282
114. Franken DR, Franken CJ, de la Guerre H, de Villiers A (1999) Normal sperm morphology and chromatin packaging: comparison between aniline blue and chromomycin A3 staining. Andrologia 31:361–366
115. Esterhuizen AD, Franken DR, Lourens JG, Prinsloo E, van Rooyen LH (2000) Sperm chromatin packaging as an indicator of in-vitro fertilization rates. Hum Reprod 15:657–661
116. Martin JA, Hamilton BE, Sutton PD, Ventura SJ, Menacker F, Munson ML (2005) Births: final data for 2003. Natl Vital Stat Rep 54:1–116
117. Spano M, Kolstad AH, Larsen SB et al (1998) The applicability of the flow cytometric sperm chromatin structure assay in epidemiological studies. Asclepios. Hum Reprod 13:2495–2505
118. Wyrobek AJ, Eskenazi B, Young S et al (2006) Advancing age has differential effects on DNA damage, chromatin integrity, gene mutations, and aneuploidies in sperm. Proc Natl Acad Sci USA 103:9601–9606
119. Vagnini L, Baruffi RL, Mauri AL et al (2007) The effects of male age on sperm DNA damage in an infertile population. Reprod Biomed Online 15:514–519
120. Singh NP, Muller CH, Berger RE (2003) Effects of age on DNA double-strand breaks and apoptosis in human sperm. Fertil Steril 80:1420–1430
121. Trisini AT, Singh NP, Duty SM, Hauser R (2004) Relationship between human semen parameters and deoxyribonucleic acid damage assessed by the neutral comet assay. Fertil Steril 82:1623–1632
122. Schmid TE, Eskenazi B, Baumgartner A et al (2007) The effects of male age on sperm DNA damage in healthy non-smokers. Hum Reprod 22:180–187
123. Martin RH, Rademaker AW (1987) The effect of age on the frequency of sperm chromosomal abnormalities in normal men. Am J Hum Genet 41:484–492
124. Sharpe RM, Skakkebaek NE (1993) Are oestrogens involved in falling sperm counts and disorders of the male reproductive tract? Lancet 341:1392–1395
125. Crow JF (1997) The high spontaneous mutation rate: is it a health risk? Proc Natl Acad Sci USA 94:8380–8386
126. Moskovtsev SI, Willis J, White J, Mullen JB (2007) Sperm survival: relationship to age-related sperm DNA integrity in infertile men. Arch Androl 53:29–32
127. Giwercman A, Richthoff J, Hjollund H et al (2003) Correlation between sperm motility and sperm chromatin structure assay parameters. Fertil Steril 80:1404–1412
128. Apedaile AE, Garrett C, Liu DY, Clarke GN, Johnston SA, Baker HW (2004) Flow cytometry and microscopic acridine orange test: relationship with standard semen analysis. Reprod Biomed Online 8:398–407
129. Moskovtsev SI, Willis J, Azad A, Mullen JB (2005) Sperm DNA integrity: correlation with sperm plasma membrane integrity in semen evaluated for male infertility. Arch Androl 51:33–40
130. Erenpreiss J, Bars J, Lipatnikova V, Erenpreisa J, Zalkalns J (2001) Comparative study of cytochemical tests for sperm chromatin integrity. J Androl 22:45–53
131. Saleh RA, Agarwal A, Nada EA et al (2003) Negative effects of increased sperm DNA damage in relation to seminal oxidative stress in men with idiopathic and male factor infertility. Fertil Steril 79:1597–1605
132. Huang CC, Lin DP, Tsao HM, Cheng TC, Liu CH, Lee MS (2005) Sperm DNA fragmentation negatively correlates with velocity and fertilization rates but might not affect pregnancy rates. Fertil Steril 84:130–140
133. Muratori M, Piomboni P, Baldi E et al (2000) Functional and ultrastructural features of DNA-fragmented human sperm. J Androl 21:903–912
134. Erenpreisa J, Erenpreiss J, Freivalds T et al (2003) Toluidine blue test for sperm DNA integrity and elaboration of image cytometry algorithm. Cytometry A 52:19–27

135. Host E, Lindenberg S, Kahn JA, Christensen F (1999) DNA strand breaks in human sperm cells: a comparison between men with normal and oligozoospermic sperm samples. Acta Obstet Gynecol Scand 78:336–339
136. Erenpreiss J, Spano M, Erenpreisa J, Bungum M, Giwercman A (2006) Sperm chromatin structure and male fertility: biological and clinical aspects. Asian J Androl 8:11–29
137. Evenson DP, Jost LK, Marshall D et al (1999) Utility of the sperm chromatin structure assay as a diagnostic and prognostic tool in the human fertility clinic. Hum Reprod 14:1039–1049
138. Andersen AN, Gianaroli L, Felberbaum R et al (2005) Assisted reproductive technology in Europe, 2001. Hum Reprod 20: 1158–1176
139. Hull MG, Fleming CF, Hughes AO, McDermott A (1996) The age-related decline in female fecundity: a quantitative controlled study of implanting capacity and survival of individual embryos after in vitro fertilization. Fertil Steril 65:783–790
140. Gandini L, Lombardo F, Paoli D et al (2004) Full-term pregnancies achieved with ICSI despite high levels of sperm chromatin damage. Hum Reprod 19:1409–1417
141. Virro MR, Larson-Cook KL, Evenson DP (2004) Sperm chromatin structure assay (SCSA) related to blastocyst rate, pregnancy rate and spontaneous abortion in IVF and ICSI cycles. Fertil Steril 81:1289–1295
142. Tomlinson MJ, Moffatt O, Manicardi GC, Bizzaro D, Afnan M, Sakkas D (2001) Interrelationships between seminal parameters and sperm nuclear DNA damage before and after density gradient centrifugation: implications for assisted conception. Hum Reprod 16:2160–2165
143. Seli E, Gardner DK, Schoolcraft WB, Moffatt O, Sakkas D (2004) Extent of nuclear DNA damage in ejaculated spermatozoa impacts on blastocyst development after in vitro fertilization. Fertil Steril 82:378–383
144. Boe-Hansen GB, Fedder J, Ersboll AK, Christensen P (2006) The sperm chromatin structure assay as a diagnostic tool in the human fertility clinic. Hum Reprod 21:1576–1582
145. Payne JF, Raburn DJ, Couchman GM, Price TM, Jamison MG, Walmer DK (2005) Redefining the relationship between sperm deoxyribonucleic acid fragmentation as measured by the sperm chromatin structure assay and outcomes of assisted reproductive techniques. Fertil Steril 84:356–364
146. Tarozzi N, Bizzaro D, Flamigni C, Borini A (2007) Clinical relevance of sperm DNA damage in assisted reproduction. Reprod Biomed Online 14:746–757
147. Host E, Lindenberg S, Smidt-Jensen S (2000) The role of DNA strand breaks in human spermatozoa used for IVF and ICSI. Acta Obstet Gynecol Scand 79:559–563
148. Borini A, Tarozzi N, Bizzaro D et al (2006) Sperm DNA fragmentation: paternal effect on early post-implantation embryo development in ART. Hum Reprod 21:2876–2881
149. Fowden AL, Sibley C, Reik W, Constancia M (2006) Imprinted genes, placental development and fetal growth. Horm Res 65:50–58
150. Aitken RJ, Krausz C (2001) Oxidative stress, DNA damage and the Y chromosome. Reproduction 122:497–506
151. Hansen M, Bower C, Milne E, de Klerk N, Kurinczuk JJ (2005) Assisted reproductive technologies and the risk of birth defects-a systematic review. Hum Reprod 20:328–338
152. DeBaun MR, Niemitz EL, Feinberg AP (2003) Association of in vitro fertilization with Beckwith-Wiedemann syndrome and epigenetic alterations of LIT1 and H19. Am J Hum Genet 72:156–160
153. Ji BT, Shu XO, Linet MS et al (1997) Paternal cigarette smoking and the risk of childhood cancer among offspring of nonsmoking mothers. J Natl Cancer Inst 89:238–244
154. Ebisch IM, Thomas CM, Peters WH, Braat DD, Steegers-Theunissen RP (2007) The importance of folate, zinc and antioxidants in the pathogenesis and prevention of subfertility. Hum Reprod Update 13:163–174
155. Agarwal A, Nallella KP, Allamaneni SS, Said TM (2004) Role of antioxidants in treatment of male infertility: an overview of the literature. Reprod Biomed Online 8:616–627
156. Greco E, Iacobelli M, Rienzi L, Ubaldi F, Ferrero S, Tesarik J (2005) Reduction of the incidence of sperm DNA fragmentation by oral antioxidant treatment. J Androl 26:349–353
157. Menezo YJ, Hazout A, Panteix G et al (2007) Antioxidants to reduce sperm DNA fragmentation: an unexpected adverse effect. Reprod Biomed Online 14:418–421
158. Silver EW, Eskenazi B, Evenson DP, Block G, Young S, Wyrobek AJ (2005) Effect of antioxidant intake on sperm chromatin stability in healthy non-smoking men. J Androl 26:550–556
159. Eskenazi B, Kidd SA, Marks AR, Sloter E, Block G, Wyrobek AJ (2005) Antioxidant intake is associated with semen quality in healthy men. Hum Reprod 20:1006–1012
160. Tesarik J, Ubaldi F, Rienzi L et al (2004) Caspase-dependent and -independent DNA fragmentation in Sertoli and germ cells from men with primary testicular failure: relationship with histological diagnosis. Hum Reprod 19:254–261
161. Aitken RJ, Gordon E, Harkiss D et al (1998) Relative impact of oxidative stress on the functional competence and genomic integrity of human spermatozoa. Biol Reprod 59:1037–46
162. Said TM, Grunewald S, Paasch U et al (2005) Advantage of combining magnetic cell separation with sperm preparation techniques. Reprod Biomed Online 10:740–746
163. Aziz N, Said T, Paasch U, Agarwal A (2007) The relationship between human sperm apoptosis, morphology and the sperm deformity index. Hum Reprod 22:1413–1419
164. Ainsworth C, Nixon B, Aitken RJ (2005) Development of a novel electrophoretic system for the isolation of human spermatozoa. Hum Reprod 20:2261–2270
165. Ainsworth C, Nixon B, Jansen RP, Aitken RJ (2007) First recorded pregnancy and normal birth after ICSI using electrophoretically isolated spermatozoa. Hum Reprod 22:197–200
166. Bartoov B, Berkovitz A, Eltes F et al (2003) Pregnancy rates are higher with intracytoplasmic morphologically selected sperm injection than with conventional intracytoplasmic injection. Fertil Steril 80:1413–1419
167. Hazout A, Dumont-Hassan M, Junca AM, Cohen Bacrie P, Tesarik J (2006) High-magnification ICSI overcomes paternal effect resistant to conventional ICSI. Reprod Biomed Online 12:19–25
168. Greco E, Scarselli F, Iacobelli M et al (2005) Efficient treatment of infertility due to sperm DNA damage by ICSI with testicular spermatozoa. Hum Reprod 20:226–230
169. Nicopoullos JD, Ramsay JW, Almeida PA, Gilling-Smith C (2004) Assisted reproduction in the azoospermic couple. BJOG 111:1190–1203

Part IV
Assisted Reproductive Therapies: Artificial Insemination

Chapter 31
Artificial Insemination: Intrauterine Insemination

Pieternel Steures, Ben W.J. Mol, and Fulco van der Veen

Abstract Artificial insemination has been used to treat infertility since the eighteenth century, and continues to be commonly performed. This chapter explores the medical indications for use of artificial insemination and provides evidence-based recommendations for therapeutic use.

Keywords Artificial insemination • Controlled ovarian hyperstimulation • Gonadotropins • Intrauterine insemination • Clomiphene citrate

31.1 Introduction

In couples with unexplained subfertility, cervical factor subfertility and male subfertility intrauterine insemination (IUI) is often the first step in the treatment cascade. IUI is easy to perform, inexpensive, and a minor burden to the couples. For these reasons, it is probably the most frequently performed treatment in daily fertility practice. In an IUI cycle, semen is processed in the laboratory and the motile spermatozoa are concentrated in a small volume. This is inseminated directly into the uterine cavity. Thus, the quintessence of IUI is based on three steps. Firstly, semen processing based on the theory that by this process the number of motile sperms is increased at the site of fertilization. Secondly, bypassing the possibly "hostile" cervical mucus and bringing the semen in closer proximity of the oocyte. Thirdly, optimizing the timing by monitoring or inducing ovulation. All these steps should theoretically increase the probability of conception, especially in the case of compromised semen parameters.

Intrauterine insemination can be performed with or without controlled ovarian hyperstimulation. The aim of controlled ovarian hyperstimulation is to correct subtle cycle disorders, to increase the number of available oocytes for fertilization and to improve the timing of insemination.

P. Steures (✉), B.W.J. Mol, and F. van der Veen
Centre for Reproductive Medicine, Academic Medical Centre, Amsterdam, The Netherlands
e-mail: pn.steures@amc.uva.nl

In this chapter, we will give an overview of the history of IUI, various treatment modalities, and the effectiveness of IUI. We will also discuss the occurrence of multiple pregnancy after IUI, patients' preferences, and we will make a plea for the use of prognostic models.

31.2 History

Insemination with semen of the partner developed from vaginal insemination via intracervical insemination to intrauterine insemination. The first homologous insemination was described in the mid fifteenth century by the French doctor de Villeneuve. His patient was the second wife of King Henry IV of Castile. King Henry had divorced his first wife on the grounds that their marriage had never been consummated. With his second wife, he continued his desperate efforts and even tried insemination [1, 2]. A German physician, Hieronymus Munzer, who examined the king, later wrote that he could not have an erection [3]. Retrospective analysis from chronicles and manuscripts seem to show that King Henry was suffering from hypogonadism or a pituitary tumor and was probably sterile [4]. Around 1550, Bartholomeus Eustachius advised a woman to bring the semen up with her finger after intercourse [2].

The first scientifically described homologous insemination was performed in London by the Scottish physiologist and surgeon, John Hunter in 1790 [5]. He advised a man with severe perineal hypospadias to collect his semen directly after coitus in a syringe and to introduce it into the vagina of his wife, while the female organs were still under the influence of the coitus, and in the proper state for accepting the semen. The woman conceived after this procedure. Numerous scientific reports have since then been published disclosing that between 1850 and 1900 artificial insemination was practised by medical experts in France, England, Germany and the United States [2]. Initially, insemination techniques were rather curious, and the success rates of the treatment were amazingly high. Homologous insemination was practised in France by Girault as early as 1838, and appeared to be

D.T. Carrell and C.M. Peterson (eds.), *Reproductive Endocrinology and Infertility: Integrating Modern Clinical and Laboratory Practice*,
DOI 10.1007/978-1-4419-1436-1_31,

successful in eight out of ten cases [2]. The technique described the manual introduction of a probe filled with husband's semen through the cervical canal and emptying it by blowing. Gigon, a surgeon in Paris in 1848, guided a rubber tube into the cervical canal and let the husband empty a semen filled glass syringe through it. At this time, there was no knowledge about the need of an ovum for fertilization, the existence of an ovulation, or about the time of ovulation. The time chosen for this procedure by both French authors was shortly after the end of the menstrual period, probably in the mid follicular phase which would be too early for ovulation, but Gigon repeated the insemination 5 days later.

Intrauterine insemination was generally favored over vaginal insemination as it was considered to be more efficacious [6]. Between 1900 and World War II a small number of scientific reports were published about homologous inseminations. In that period, scientific interest shifted to artificial insemination with donor semen. Methods of freezing and thawing sperm were developed. In World War II, homologous semen was also frozen to inseminate spouses at home; the so called "distance indication" [5]. After World War II most studies dealt with fine tuning of the technical aspects of IUI. For instance, it had been observed that spermatozoa in the first part of the ejaculate were more vigorous and moved in a more progressive manner than those in the second part. To assess the results of insemination of partitioned ejaculates, a study was performed which concluded that separation of the ejaculate into two portions and introduction of the best portion appeared to be useful in IUI [7]. A second study assessed the results after the insemination of isolated motile sperm into the uterine cavity [8].

The first publication of a randomized clinical trial of intrauterine insemination was in 1984, and it dealt with men with poor semen quality [9]. Since then, many randomized clinical trials that addressed the effectiveness of IUI were performed. From 1996 onwards, guidelines on IUI were developed. In these clinical guidelines, IUI with or without controlled ovarian hyperstimulation (COH) was recommended as treatment of first choice for couples with unexplained subfertility, cervical factor and male subfertility [10–13].

31.3 Techniques of Intrauterine Insemination

There is a wide variation in the practice of performing IUI. This variation is due to the fact that an IUI cycle is a cascade of interventions with several modifications of manipulating the normal menstrual cycle, i.e., ovarian hyperstimulation, use of GnRH analogs, monitoring of the follicular growth, and timing and/or induction of the ovulation. These interventions in the follicular phase are then followed by techniques in the second phase of the IUI cycle, i.e., semen preparation, timing of insemination, number of inseminations per cycle and bed rest or not after insemination, which may also vary considerably from center to center. We will discuss these treatment modalities in the following paragraphs.

31.3.1 Controlled Ovarian Hyperstimulation

Intrauterine insemination can be performed in a natural cycle or can be combined with controlled ovarian hyperstimulation. The two most frequently used drugs are clomiphene citrate and gonadotropins.

31.3.1.1 Clomiphene Citrate

Clomiphene citrate (Clomid, Serophene) is used extensively. It is cheap (€ 0.46 per tablet, 50 mg), easy to use and effective. Clomiphene citrate blocks the estrogen receptors of the hypothalamus. This altered feedback information causes the hypothalamus to make and release more gonadotropin releasing hormone (GnRH), which in turn causes the pituitary to make and release more FSH and LH. Clomiphene citrate is taken orally for approximately 5 days early in the menstrual cycle. Protocols include early start from cycle day 3 or as late as from cycle day 5. For IUI, mostly two tablets (100 mg) are given per day.

Clomiphene citrate is generally very well tolerated. Some side effects are relatively common, i.e., vasomotor flushes, mood swings, and nausea, but they are rarely persistent or severe enough to threaten the completion of the 5-day course or next cycle of treatment [14]. Limited endometrial proliferation has been observed in some women treated with clomiphene citrate [15], but the effect is minor or not at all evident in the large majority of women [16–18]. Although some studies have suggested that fecundity may relate to endometrial thickness, others have failed to demonstrate any significant correlation [14]. Two epidemiological studies published in the last decade suggested that the risk of ovarian cancer might be significantly increased in women exposed to clomiphene citrate [19, 20], but subsequent studies have failed to corroborate those findings [21–24]. The authors of a recent pooled analysis of eight case-control studies concluded that neither fertility drug use (odds ratio (OR): 1.60, 95% CI 0.90–2.87) nor use for more than 12 months was associated with ovarian cancer (OR: 1.54, 95% CI 0.45–5.27) [25]. Although the confidence intervals are not significant, these point estimates should in our view not be taken too lightly and more studies, preferably large cohort studies, are needed. In any case, prolonged treatment with clomiphene citrate is generally futile and should therefore be avoided.

31.3.1.2 Gonadotropins

The gonadotropins Follicle Stimulating Hormone (FSH) and Luteinizing Hormone (LH) are released under the control of gonadotropin-releasing hormone (GnRH) produced in the hypothalamus. FSH directly affects the production and maturation of follicles by stimulating the granulosa cells of ovarian follicles. LH stimulates the thecal cells to produce testosterone (and indirectly estradiol), and an LH surge is obligatory for the rupture of the dominant follicle. The first FSH preparation used in fertility practice was extracted from postmenopausal urine (human menopausal gonadotropin, hMG). Although the extraction and purification of hMG had been developed in Italy in the late 1940s, clinical interest in gonadotropins did not grow until 1960, when the first hMG-assisted human birth was reported [26]. Improvements in purification techniques led to increasing relative amounts of the active ingredients and the first urine-derived preparation containing only urinary FSH (uFSH) became available in 1983 [27]. The large quantities of urine required and the massive increase in worldwide demand for FSH for fertility treatment put pressure on production and availability. In the 1990s, recombinant DNA technology led to the development and clinical introduction of human recombinant FSH (rFSH).

Meta-analysis of data from three studies in a total of 132 couples showed a non significant difference in favour of hMG above FSH on the effectiveness of IUI (OR 2.2, 95% CI 0.91–5.1). This benefit of hMG compared to rFSH has also been seen in a meta-analysis of seven randomized trials, consisting of a total of 2159 women in IVF. [28]. This review showed a significant increase in live birth rate for hMG (relative risk, RR = 1.2, 95% CI 1.0–1.4). The reason that the data in IUI do not reach significance that might be due to the scarcity of data on this comparison in IUI and the lower pregnancy chances after IUI, which makes the number needed to find a difference between these stimulation protocols even larger [29].

FSH is taken by subcutaneous injections daily, usually by the woman herself. Because of the individual variety of the follicular response, it is prudent to begin with a low starting dose like 50–75 IE per day. If this dosage does not lead to multifollicular growth, the dose can be increased in the next cycle. FSH injections are started on cycle day 3, 4 or 5 and continued until a dominant follicle of at least 18 mm in diameter has developed.

Different dosage regimens for gonadotropins have been described, ranging from 75 IE to 150 IE daily or alternating schemes, but data on effectiveness are limited. A meta-analysis of these dosage regimens was based on small numbers of patients in only two studies and showed that doubling the daily dose of gonadotropins per day from 75 IU to 150 IU did not improve pregnancy rates (OR 1.2, 95% CI 0.69–1.9), but tended to increase the risk of achieving a multiple pregnancy (OR 3.4, 95% CI 0.46–25) [29].

No side-effects are known other than irritation at the side of injection [30]. The theoretical longterm risk of transmission of prion proteins from urine in hMG is still a debate. Although infections by urine prions has never been identified in its 40 years of use, some advise against the use of hMG [31], whereas others consider the risk to be minimal and no reason to prescribe recombinant preparations over urinary ones [32].

Two randomized studies showed that in couples with unexplained subfertility or male subfertility there is no difference in the effectiveness of IUI after ovarian hyperstimulation with clomiphene citrate compared to the use of follicle stimulating hormone (Relative risk of 1.1, confidence interval 0.51 to 2.3) [33].

31.3.2 Analogs

Gonadotropin-Releasing Hormone (Gn-RH) stimulates the pituitary gland, thereby causing secretion of FSH and LH. After the discovery of the amino acid sequence of GnRH in 1967, several synthetic gonadotropin releasing agonists and antagonists were developed to control pituitary FSH and LH secretion. The GnRH agonists induce FSH and LH release after binding, but under continuous administration they induce pituitary desensitization by a mechanism still far from understood, leading to strong suppression of LH and to a lesser extent of FSH. In the 1980s, the first reports were published using GnRH agonists in IVF to suppress FSH and LH and to prevent premature LH surges [34]. It took nearly 10 more years to develop GnRH antagonists, agents which are able to suppress gonadotropin release directly by competitive receptor binding [35]. The effectiveness of these agonists or antagonists in preventing a premature LH surge and thereby increasing pregnancy rates has been proven in in vitro fertilization [35, 36]. The interest for the use of GnRH-agonists or -antagonists in IUI cycles with ovarian hyperstimulation was kindled after the finding of premature LH surges, which were thought to interfere with adequate timing of IUI [37]. However, meta-analysis of four studies with in a total of 391 couples showed no benefit of the addition of agonists compared to gonadotropins alone (OR 0.98, 95% CI 0.60–1.6) [29]. Three studies compared the addition of an antagonist to gonadotropins alone and also did not find a significant beneficial effect (OR 1.5, 95% CI 0.83–2.8).

31.3.3 Monitoring, Timing, and/or Induction of Ovulation

In IUI cycles without ovarian hyperstimulation, monitoring of the follicle growth by sonography is usually considered a matter of taste. In IUI cycles with ovarian hyperstimulation, the follicular growth is always monitored by sonography, since uncontrolled multifollicular growth may lead to (high order) multiple pregnancies.

For the detection of ovulation, either LH-surge tests can be used or ovulation can be induced by human chorionic gonadotropin (hCG). A meta-analysis of three trials that compared hCG administration with LH monitoring in couples undergoing IUI for male subfertility showed clinical pregnancy rates of 10% vs. 12% per couple (OR 0.77, 95% CI 0.40–1.5). In couples undergoing IUI for unexplained subfertility the clinical pregnancy rates were 7 and 8%, respectively (OR 0.84, 95% CI 0.39–1.8) [38].

31.3.4 Modalities of Insemination

Various preparation processes for semen have been described (see Chap. 24). A wide range in the timing of the insemination is described in literature. IUI is commonly performed between 36 and 42 h after a positive LH surge test, but evidence on the effectiveness of timing is scarce. IUI 33 or 39 h after the administration of hCG resulted in the same pregnancy results, and therefore the timing of the insemination may depend on local convenience of the hospital [39].

Insemination has to be performed only once per cycle, since a systematic review showed no difference in the effect between one insemination compared to two inseminations [40].

A 10-min interval of bed rest after IUI has a positive effect on the pregnancy rate. In a randomized trial, which compared immediate mobilization to supine position for 10 min after insemination in 95 couples, 16 couples out of 55 (29%) who had bed rest and four couples out of 40 (10%) couples who mobilized immediately became pregnant (RR:1.2, 95% CI 1.1–2.1) [41]. This important aspect of IUI has only been investigated in one trial with less than 100 patients and deserves more attention.

31.4 Effectiveness of Intrauterine Insemination

Intrauterine insemination is the treatment of first choice in unexplained subfertility, cervical factor subfertility and male subfertility [10–13]. However, the question whether this choice is based on valid and precise effect estimates of IUI relative to expectant management and to other treatment modalities like IVF, is often overlooked. To provide evidence on this issue, the next paragraphs show meta-analyses after a systematic review of the available literature for each indication. The trials that were included in these meta-analyses adhered to present quality standards for design, conduct and report. For each indication, IUI was compared with intercourse (expectant management) or IVF. The comparison IUI without controlled ovarian hyperstimulation versus IUI with controlled ovarian hyperstimulation was also made for the indications unexplained subfertility, cervical factor subfertility, and male subfertility.

31.4.1 Intrauterine Insemination in Unexplained Subfertility

Unexplained subfertility is defined as subfertility without any demonstrable cause after the basic fertility work-up.

Fourteen randomized clinical trials have reported on the effectiveness of IUI in couples with unexplained subfertility that adhered to today's quality standards [42–55].

Twelve studies were included in a Cochrane review and two additional studies were published since the publication of this Cochrane review [45, 55, 56].

The outcomes of the meta-analysis for the various comparisons are summarized in Fig. 31.1.

IUI without COH was associated with higher ongoing pregnancy rates than expectant management and timed intercourse with COH, but these effects were not statistically significant with relative risks (RR) of 1.3 (95% CI 0.84–1.9) and 1.5 (95% CI 0.95–2.3), respectively.

IUI with COH offered no benefit over expectant management (RR 1.0, 95% CI 0.67–1.5). In line with the comparison IUI with COH versus expectant management, IUI with COH had also no beneficial effect over timed intercourse with COH (RR for clinical pregnancies: 1.1 (95% CI 0.90–1.5)).

One study compared IUI versus IVF. This study did not show a significant beneficial effect (RR for IUI without COH compared to IVF: 0.60 (95% CI 0.35–1.1) and RR for IUI with COH compared to IVF: 0.92 (95% CI 0.58–1.5)).

The comparison IUI with COH vs. IUI without COH was made in four studies and showed that IUI with COH was significantly more effective than IUI without COH for live birth rates (RR 1.8, 95% CI 1.2–2.7).

31.4.2 Intrauterine Insemination in Cervical Factor Subfertility

Cervical factor subfertility is defined as the absence of progressive motile spermatozoa in cervical mucus of good quality and normal semen parameters. The rationale of intrauterine insemination in couples with a cervical factor subfertility is to bypass the "hostile" cervical mucus.

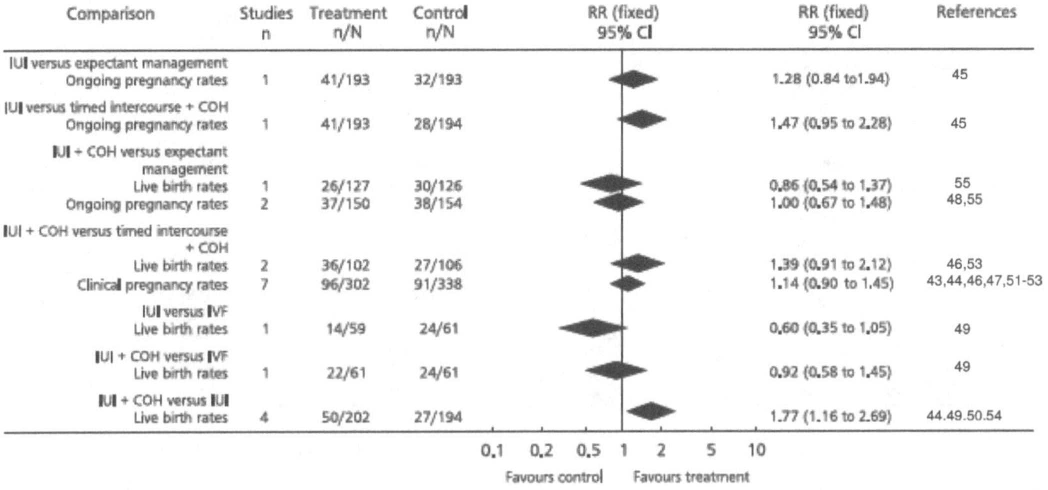

Fig. 31.1 Summary of pregrancy resuts per couple for unexplained subfertility

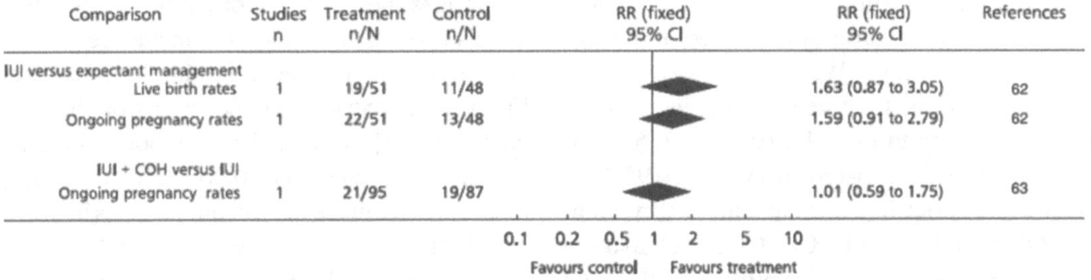

Fig. 31.2 Summary of pregnancy results per couple for cervical factor subfertility

Although it seems logical to perform IUI in these cases, evidence is scarce. In a Cochrane review, five randomized clinical trials were reported [57–61]. These studies all compared IUI without COH with timed intercourse. The quality of these five trials was poor, and therefore we do not include these studies in the meta-analyses described in these paragraphs. Since the publication of the Cochane review, two new studies have been published [62, 63]. Only a trend towards any effectiveness of IUI in these couples is seen. Addition of COH did not further improve the pregnancy rates (Fig. 31.2). Data of IUI in comparison with IVF are not available. More randomized studies are needed before definite conclusions can be drawn.

31.4.3 Intrauterine Insemination in Male Subfertility

Over time, different definitions of male subfertility have been used with different cut-off values for sperm parameters. The definition for male subfertility defined by the World Health Organization (WHO) is semen quality below the normal standards, i.e., sperm concentration $<20\times10^6$ per ml, and/or total motility <50% and/or normal morphology <15% and/or >50% anti-sperm antibodies [64]. Nine randomized clinical trials that adhered to today's quality standards reported on the effectiveness of IUI in couples with male subfertility [44, 49, 50, 53, 63, 65–68]. Eight studies were included in a Cochrane review and one additional study was published since the publication of this Cochrane review [63, 69]. The outcomes of the meta-analysis of the various comparisons are summarized in Fig. 31.3.

The effectiveness of IUI without COH was only investigated in one study in which IUI without COH was almost five times more effective than timed intercourse. However, due to the small numbers the confidence interval is very wide (RR 4.5, 95% CI 0.52–39).

One study found IUI with COH equally effective as timed intercourse with COH in terms of live birth (RR 0.91, 95% CI 0.39–2.1). For the outcome clinical pregnancies, two more studies could be included. The summary estimate indicated a beneficial effect of IUI with COH, but this was not statistically significant (RR 1.4, 95% CI 0.79–2.4).

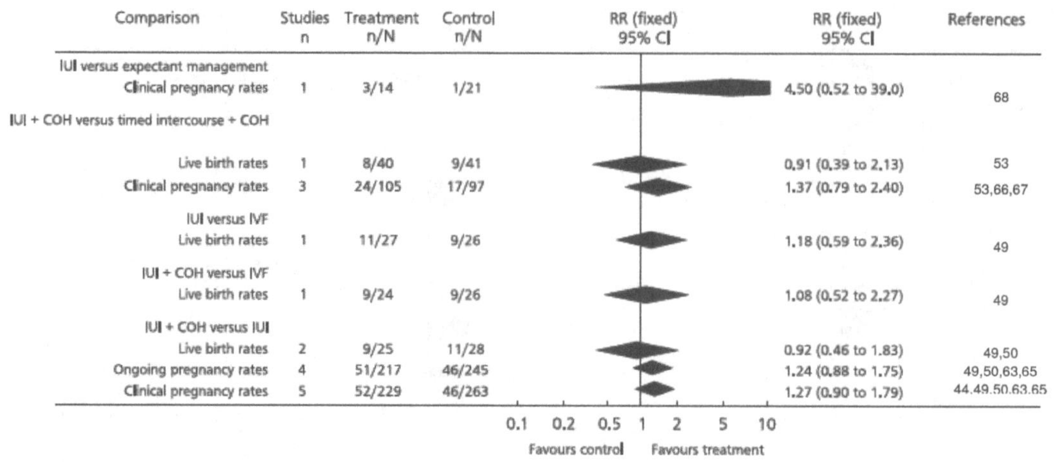

Fig. 31.3 Summary of pregnancy results per couple for male subfertility

Only one randomized trial compared IUI with or without COH with IVF. This study was already discussed in the section on unexplained subfertility. We found no significant beneficial effect of any of the treatment modalities (RR for IUI without COH compared to IVF: 1.2 (95% CI 0.59–2.4) and RR for IUI with COH compared to IVF: 1.1 (95% CI 0.52–2.3)). Most trials about IUI in male subfertility compared IUI with COH to IUI without COH. COH had no additional effect in these couples (RR for live birth: 0.92 (95% CI 0.46–1.8), RR ongoing pregnancies 1.2 (95% CI 0.88–1.8)).

In conclusion, the number of randomized trials assessing the effectiveness of IUI is limited and that most of these studies have small sample sizes. Overall, this results in imprecise effect estimates, as demonstrated by relatively large confidence intervals. Only one comparison was significant in this meta-analysis: IUI with COH improved pregnancy rates compared to IUI without COH in unexplained subfertility. However, this data is of limited clinical value as we do not know whether IUI without COH is of any benefit compared to expectant management.

31.5 Risks of Intrauterine Insemination

Although IUI is a simple concept, the addition of COH carries the risk of multiple pregnancies. Eight of the above described randomized trials on the effectiveness of IUI compared IUI with COH to treatment without COH, be it as expectant management or as IUI without COH, and reported on multiple pregnancy rates. The multiple pregnancy rates after IUI with COH varied in these studies from two out of 37 ongoing pregnancies (5.4%) [48, 55] to 10 out of 66 clinical pregnancies (15%) [43, 46, 52, 53].

Besides the limited information provide by the trials, there are also data available on the incidence of multiple pregnancies after IUI collected in the National Registries of 15 European countries and one survey on the IUI results in The Netherlands [70, 71]. These reports present data on over 50,000 IUI cycles and 20,000 IUI cycles, respectively. The reported percentage of twin pregnancies in the European report and the Dutch report were 9.9 and 9.0% per (ongoing) pregnancy, respectively. Even though these registrations do not provide a complete overview of the IUI results in Europe, this percentage of multiple pregnancies probably mimics reality.

It seems reasonable to assume that the probability of achieving a multiple pregnancy is correlated with the aggressiveness of the ovarian hyperstimulation and the applied cancelation criteria (see ovarian hyperstimulation) [72]. In a Cochrane review on different dosage regimens, two trials were included [40]. In the high dosage group (gonadotrophins >75 IU per day) 4 multiple pregnancies out of 46 pregnancies (9%) were found and in the low dosage group (gonadotropins 75 IU or less) 1 multiple pregnancy out of 42 pregnancies (2%) (OR 3.35, 95% CI 0.46–24.58).

Although most individual studies describe their cancel criteria, there are no studies on the relation of these criteria and multiple pregnancy rates. At the moment, it is therefore not possible to provide evidencebased cancel criteria in the prevention of multiple pregnancy.

31.6 Patients' Preferences for Intrauterine Insemination

Nowadays patients' preferences are incorporated into medical decision making. The preferences of couples suffering from subfertility for IUI compared to expectant management and to IVF have been investigated in interviews [73, 74]. In the interviews that compared IUI to expectant management, couples were offered scenarios in which the chance on a spontaneous pregnancy was varied against a fixed pregnancy chance after IUI with or without controlled ovarian hyperstimulation. The results showed that even when the spontaneous pregnancy chances are still reasonable, couples prefer IUI with or without controlled ovarian hyperstimulation over expectant management (probability of a spontaneous pregnancy 41 and 51% or lower, respectively). The risk of a multiple pregnancy did not affect patients' preferences. Instead, 77% of the couples continued IUI with controlled ovarian hyperstimulation even at a 100% certainty of having a multiple pregnancy.

For the preferences of IUI compared to IVF, the majority of couples prefer continuation of IUI over IVF before they start IUI and after three cycles of IUI. After six cycles the preferences shift towards IVF.

31.7 Intrauterine Insemination or Expectant Management

Until recently, the main emphasis in reproductive medicine has been on finding causal diagnoses for the couples' subfertility and to treat accordingly. In couples classified with unexplained subfertility, mild male subfertility, cervical factor subfertility, mild endometriosis, or one-sided tubal pathology such a strict causal diagnosis has not been found and in these couples IUI can be considered.

As IUI is a burden to couples, generates costs and bears the risk of multiple pregnancy, it should only be offered to a couple if the success rate after treatment clearly exceeds the probability of a spontaneous pregnancy in that couple [75, 76]. This implicates that the fertility work-up also has to include a prognostic dimension [77]. To be able to make adequate and reliable predictions in clinical practice, formal prediction models, in which the contribution of each factor is quantified, were developed in the recent past.

At the moment, there are nine prediction models for spontaneous pregnancy, but only one model has been validated in an external population. This is an extremely important issue, because most prediction models tend to be overoptimistic when applied to other populations than the one in which they were developed [78]. This validated prediction model predicts accurately the chances of a spontaneous pregnancy among subfertile ovulatory couples [79, 80].

This model can be used by computer with the following URL: http://www.amc.nl/index.cfm?sid = 1602.

If the model predicts a low spontaneous pregnancy chance, IUI can be considered, but first the chance of an ongoing pregnancy after IUI should be calculated to determine whether benefit may be expected from IUI. At the moment, there is one IUI prediction model that has been externally validated and has shown to be accurate [81, 82].

By using these models and comparing the prognoses generated by the models for the couple, they can be counseled on an individual base. Such an approach can prevent overtreatment, decreases the misuse of facilities and other resources and minimizes the risk of multiple pregnancy, which can be avoided by an expectant management [55].

31.8 Conclusion

Intrauterine insemination has a long history and is probably worldwide the most performed treatment in subfertility. There are various modalities in the performance of IUI as well as various strategies for the stimulation of the ovaries. However, the evidence on the effectiveness of intrauterine insemination is still surprisingly scarce and does not allow us to provide firm recommendations. Only two conclusions can be drawn on the effectiveness of IUI; IUI with COH improves pregnancy rates over IUI without COH in couples with unexplained subfertility and IUI with COH has not been shown to be effective in couples with unexplained subfertility and a good prognosis. Therefore, the prognosis of the couples should be taken into account in clinical decision making. This enables us to distinguish those couples who may benefit from treatment from those who are unlikely too. Couples with an intermediate to good prognosis of a treatment independent pregnancy may be encouraged for expectant management and to postpone IUI for a while.

31.9 Cases

31.9.1 Case 1

A couple who have a wish for a second child for 3 years. The woman is 29 years old. After the basic fertility work-up no cause for their subfertility has been found.

What do you do?

Expectant management or IUI?

Based on prognostic models their spontaneous pregnancy chance, resulting in a live-born child, in the next 12 months is 52%, whereas their chance of an ongoing pregnancy after 6 cycles of IUI with FSH is 40%.

Recommendation: Expectant management.

31.9.2 Case 2

A couple who have a wish for a child for 3 years. They have not been pregnant before. The woman is 36 years old. After the basic fertility work-up no cause for their subfertility has been found.

What do you do?

Expectant management or IUI?

Based on prognostic models their spontaneous pregnancy chance, resulting in a live born child, in the next 12 months is 24%, whereas their chance of an ongoing pregnancy after 6 cycles of IUI with FSH is 34%.

Recommendation: IUI with FSH.

References

1. Maganto PE (2003) [Henry IV of Castilla (1454–1474). An exceptional urologic patient. An endocrinopathy causing the uro-andrological problems of the Monarch. Artificial insemination attempts (IV)]. Arch Esp Urol 56(3):245–254
2. Schellen AMCM (1957) Artificial insemination in the Human. Elsevier, Amsterdam
3. Maganto PE (2003) [Henry IV of Castilla (1454-1474). An exceptional urologic patient. An endocrinopathy causing the uro-andrological problems of the monarch. Impotence and penile malformation (III)]. Arch Esp Urol 56(3):233–241
4. Maganto PE (2003) [Henry IV de Castilla (1454–1474). An exceptional urologic patient. Morphological and personality portrait of Henry IV "The impotent" in contemporary chronicles and manuscripts (I)]. Arch Esp Urol 56(3):211–220
5. Schellen AMCM (1960) Artificial Insemination in the Human, The social aspects of society. Utrecht, Antwerpen, Het Spectrum. Ref Type: Serial (Book, Monograph)
6. Gérard J (1888) Nouvelles Causes de Stérilité. Paris, Marpon & Flammarion. Ref Type: Serial (Book, Monograph)
7. Farris EJ, Murphy DP (1960) The characteristics of the two parts of the partitioned ejaculate and the advantages of its use for intrauterine insemination. A study of 100 ejaculates. Fertil Steril 11:465–469
8. Glass RH, Ericsson RJ (1978) Intrauterine insemination of isolated motile sperm. Fertil Steril 29(5):535–538
9. Kerin JF, Kirby C, Peek J, Jeffrey R, Warnes GM, Matthews CD et al (1984) Improved conception rate after intrauterine insemination of washed spermatozoa from men with poor quality semen. Lancet 1(8376):533–535
10. Danish Society of Obstetrics and Gynaecology (DSOG) and Danish Fertility Society (DFS) (1997) Guideline-Homologous intrauterine insemination. Danish Guideline
11. Dutch Society of Obstetrics and Gynaecology (2000) Guideline – Intra-uterine insemination (IUI). NVOG-richtlijn nr 29:29
12. National Agency for Accreditation and Evaluation in Healthcare (ANAES) (1996) Guideline-Infertility of a couple. French Guideline
13. National Collaborating Centre for Women's and Children's Health cbN (2004) Fertility guideline: assessment and treatment for people with fertility problems. http://www nice org uk/pdf/ CG011fullguideline pdf
14. The Practice Committee of the American Society for Reproductive Medicine (2006) Use of clomiphene citrate in women. Fertil Steril 86:S187–S193
15. Greenblatt RB (1961) Chemical induction of ovulation. Fertil Steril 12:402–404
16. Dickey RP, Olar TT, Taylor SN, Curole DN, Matulich EM (1993) Relationship of endometrial thickness and pattern of fecundity in ovulation cycles: effect of clomiphene citrate alone and with human menopausal gonadotropin. Fertil Steril 59:756–760
17. Eden JA, Place J, Carter GD, Jones J, Alaghband-Zadeh J, Pawson ME (1989) The effect of clomiphene citrate on follicular phase increase in endometrial thickness and uterine volume. Obstet Gynecol 73:187–190
18. Randall JM, Templeton A (1991) Transvaginal sonographic assessment of follicular and endometrial growth in spontaneous and clomiphene citrate cycles. Fertil Steril 56:208–212
19. Whittemore AS, Harris R, Itnyre J (1992) Collaborative Ovarian Cancer Group. Characteristics relating to ovarian cancer risk: collaborative analysis of 12 US case-control studies II. Invasive epithelial ovarian cancers in white women. Am J Epidemiol 136:1184–1203
20. Rossing MA, Daling JR, Weiss NS, Moore DE, Self SG (1994) Ovarian tumors in a cohort of infertile women. N Engl J Med 331:771–776
21. Venn A, Watson L, Lumley J, Giles G, King C, Healy D (1995) Breast and ovarian cancer incidence after infertility and in vitro fertilisation. Lancet 346:995–1000
22. Modan B, Ron E, Lerner-Geva L, Blumstein T, Menczer J, Rabinovici J et al (1998) Cancer incidence in a cohort of infertile women. Am J Epidemiol 147:1038–1042
23. Mosgaard BJ, Lidegaard O, Kjaer SK, Schou G, Andersen AN (1997) Infertility, fertility drugs, and invasive ovarian cancer: a case-control study. Fertil Steril 67:1005–1012
24. Potashnik G, Lerner-Geva L, Genkin L, Chetrit A, Lunenfeld E, Porath A (1999) Fertility drugs and the risk of breast and ovarian cancers: results of a long-term follow-up study. Fertil Steril 71:853–859
25. Ness RB, Cramer DW, Goodman MT, Kjaer SK, Mallin K, Mosgaard BJ (2002) Infertility, fertility drugs, and ovarian cancer: a pooled analysis of case-control studies. Am J Epidemiol 155:217–224
26. Lunenfeld B, Sulmovici S, Rabau E et al (1962) L'induction de l'ovulation dans les amenorrhees hypophysaires pas an traitment combine de gonadotrophines urinaires menopausiques et de gonadotropines chorioniques. R Soc Franc Gynecol 32:346–351
27. Huirne JAF, Lambalk CB, van Loenen ACD, Schats R, Hompes PGA, Fauser BCJM, Macklon NS (2004) Contemporary pharmacological manipulation in assisted reproduction. Drugs 64:297–322
28. Coomarasamy A, Afnan M, Cheema D, van der Veen F, Bossuyt PM, van Wely M (2008) Urinary hMG versus recombinant FSH for controlled ovarian hyperstimulation following an agonist long down-regulation protocol in IVF or ICSI treatment: a systematic review and meta-analysis. Hum Reprod 23(2):310–315
29. Cantineau AEP, Cohlen BJ, Heineman MJ (2007) Ovarian stimulation protocols (anti-oestrogens, gonadotropins with and without GnRH agonist/antagonist) for intrauterine insemination (IUI) in women with subfertility (Review). Cochrane Database Syst Rev CD005356
30. Albano C, Smitz J, Camus M et al (1996) Pregnancy and birth in an in-vitro fertilization cycle after controlled ovarian hyperstimulation in a woman with a history of allergic reaction to human menopausal gonadotropin. Hum Reprod 11:1632–1634
31. Matorras R, Rodriquez-Escudero FJ (2002) Bye-bye urinary gonadotrophins? the use of urinary gonadotrophins should be discouraged. Hum Reprod 17:1675
32. Balen A (2002) Bye-bye urinary gonadotrophins? is there a risk of prion disease after the administration of urinary-derived gonadotrophins? Hum Reprod 17:1676–1680
33. Dankert T, Kremer JAM, Cohlen BJ, Hamilton CJCM, Pasker-de Jong PCM, Straatman H et al (2007) A randomized clinical trial of

clomiphene citrate versus low dose recombinant FSH for ovarian hyperstimulation in intrauterine insemination cycles for unexplained and male subfertlity. Hum Reprod 22:792–797
34. Hughes EG, Fedorkow DM, Daya S, Sagle MA, van de Koppel P, Collins JA (1992) The routine use of gonadotropin-releasing hormone agonists prior to in vitro fertilization and gamete intrafallopian transfer: a meta-analysis of randomized controlled trials. Fertil Steril 58:888–896
35. Shapiro DB, Mitchell-Leef D (2003) GnRH antagonist in in vitro fertilization: where we are now. Minerva Ginecol 55:373–388
36. Barlow DH (1998) GnRH agonists and in vitro fertilization. J Reprod Med 43:245–251
37. Loumaye E (1990) The control of endogenous secretion of LH by gonadotrophinreleasing hormone agonists during ovarian hyperstimulation for in-vitro fertilization and embryo transfer. Hum Reprod 5:357–376
38. Kosmas IP, Tatsioni A, Musavi Fatemi H, Kolibianakis EM, Tournaye H, Devroey P (2006) Human chorionic gonadotropin administration vs. luteinizing monitoring for intrauterine insemination timing, after administration of clomiphene citrate: a meta-analysis. Fertil Steril 87:607–612
39. Claman P, Wilkie V, Collins D (2004) Timing intrauterine insemination either 33 or 39 hours after administration of human chorionic gonadotropin yields the same pregnancy rates as after superovulation therapy. Fertil Steril 82:13–16
40. Cantineau AE, Heineman MJ, Cohlen BJ (2003) Single versus double intrauterine insemination in stimulated cycles for subfertile couples: a systematic review based on a Cochrane review. Hum Reprod 18:941–946
41. Saleh A, Lin Tan S, Biljan MM, Tulandi T (2000) A randomized study of the effect of 10 min of bed rest after intrauterine insemination. Fertil Steril 74:509–511
42. Agarwal S, Mittal S (2004) A randomised prospective trial of intrauterine insemination versus timed intercourse in superovulated cycles with clomiphene. Indian J Med Res 20(6):519–522
43. Arcaini L, Bianchi S, Baglioni A, Marchini M, Tozzi L, Fedele L (1996) Superovulation and intrauterine insemination vs superovulation alone in the treatment of unexplained infertility – A randomized study. J Reprod Med 41(8):614–618
44. Arici A, Byrd W, Bradshaw K, Kutteh WH, Marshburn P, Carr BR (1994) Evaluation of clomiphene citrate and human chorionic-gonadotropin treatment – a prospective, randomized, crossover study during intrauterine insemination cycles. Fertil Steril 61(2):314–318
45. Bhattacharya S, Harrild A, Harrold H, Lyall D, McQueen C, Tay C (2006) A randomised trial of expectant management, clomifene and intrauterine insemination (IUI) in the treatment of infertility. Fertil Steril 86(Suppl 2):S43–S44. Ref Type: Abstract
46. Chung CC, Fleming R, Jamieson ME, Yates RWS, Coutts JRT (1995) Randomized comparison of ovulation induction with and without intrauterine insemination in the treatment of unexplained infertility. Hum Reprod 10(12):3139–3141
47. Crosignani PG, Walters DE, Soliani A (1991) The ESHRE multicentre trial on the treatment of unexplained infertility: a preliminary report. European Society of Human Reproduction and Embryology. Hum Reprod 6(7):953–958
48. Deaton JL, Gibson M, Blackmer KM, Nakajima ST, Badger GJ, Brumsted JR (1990) A randomized, controlled trial of clomiphene citrate and intrauterine insemination in couples with unexplained infertility or surgically corrected endometriosis. Fertil Steril 54(6):1083–1088
49. Goverde AJ, McDonnell J, Vermeiden JP, Schats R, Rutten FF, Schoemaker J (2000) Intrauterine insemination or in-vitro fertilisation in idiopathic subfertility and male subfertility: a randomised trial and cost-effectiveness analysis. Lancet 355(9197):13–18
50. Guzick DS, Carson SA, Coutifaris C, Overstreet JW, Factor-Litvak P, Steinkampf MP et al (1999) Efficacy of superovulation and intrauterine insemination in the treatment of infertility. National Cooperative Reproductive Medicine Network. N Engl J Med 340(3):177–183
51. Janko P, Hruzik P, Saliba H, Zidzik J (1998) Induction of ovulation with or without intrauterine insemination in cases of unexplained sterility. Fertil.Steril 70(3):S442
52. Karlstrom PO, Bergh T, Lundkvist O (1993) A prospective randomized trial of artificial insemination versus intercourse in cycles stimulated with human menopausal gonadotropin or clomiphene citrate. Fertil Steril 59:554–559
53. Melis GB, Paoletti AM, Ajossa S, Guerriero S, Depau GF, Mais V (1995) Ovulation induction with gonadotropins as sole treatment in infertile couples with open tubes – a randomized prospective comparison between intrauterine insemination and timed vaginal intercourse. Fertil Steril 64(6):1088–1093
54. Murdoch AP, Harris M, Mahroo M, Williams M, Dunlop W (1991) Gamete intrafallopian transfer (gift) compared with intrauterine insemination in the treatment of unexplained infertility. Br J Obstet Gynaecol 98(11):1107–1111
55. Steures P, van der Steeg JW, Hompes PG, Habbema JD, Eijkemans MJ, Broekmans FJ et al (2006) Intrauterine insemination with controlled ovarian hyperstimulation versus expectant management for couples with unexplained subfertility and an intermediate prognosis: a randomised clinical trial. Lancet 368(9531):216–221
56. Verhulst SM, Cohlen BJ, Hughes E, te Velde E, Heineman MJ (2006) Intra-uterine insemination for unexplained subfertility (review). Cochrane Database Syst Rev 4:CD001838
57. Check JH, Bollendorf A, Zaccardo M, Lurie D, Vetter B (1995) Intrauterine insemination for cervical and male factor without superovulation. Arch Androl 35(2):135–141
58. Glazener CM, Coulson C, Lambert PA, Watt EM, Hinton RA, Kelly NJ et al (1987) The value of artificial insemination with husband's semen in infertility due to failure of postcoital sperm-mucus penetration – controlled trial of treatment. Br J Obstet Gynaecol 94(8):774–778
59. Kirby CA, Flaherty SP, Godfrey BM, Warnes GM, Matthews CD (1991) A prospective trial of intrauterine insemination of motile spermatozoa versus timed intercourse. Fertil Steril 56(1):102–107
60. Martinez AR, Bernardus RE, Voorhorst FJ, Vermeiden JPW, Schoemaker J (1990) Intrauterine insemination does and clomiphene citrate does not improve fecundity in couples with infertility due to male or idiopathic factors – a prospective, randomized, controlled-study. Fertil Steril 53(5):847–853
61. te Velde ER, van Kooy RJ, Waterreus JJ (1989) Intrauterine insemination of washed husband's spermatozoa: a controlled study. Fertil Steril 51(1):182–185
62. Steures P, van der Steeg JW, Hompes PG, Bossuyt PM, Habbema JD, Eijkemans MJ et al (2007) Effectiveness of intrauterine insemination in subfertile couples with an isolated cervical factor: a randomized clinical trial. Fertil Steril 88:1692–1696
63. Steures P, van der Steeg JW, Hompes PG, Bossuyt PM, Habbema JD, Eijkemans MJ et al (2007) The additional value of ovarian hyperstimulation in intrauterine insemination for couples with an abnormal postcoital test and a poor prognosis: a randomized clinical trial. Fertil Steril 88:1618–1624
64. World Health Organization (1999) WHO laboratory manual for the examination of human semen and semen-cervical mucus interaction, 4th edn. Cambridge University Press, Cambridge, England
65. Cohlen BJ, te Velde ER, van Kooij RJ, Looman CW, Habbema JD (1998) Controlled ovarian hyperstimulation and intrauterine insemination for treating male subfertility: a controlled study. Hum Reprod 13:1553–1558
66. Gregoriou O, Vitoratos N, Papadias C, Konidaris S, Gargaropoulos A, Rizos D (1996) Pregnancy rates in gonadotrophin stimulated cycles with timed intercourse or intrauterine insemination for the treatment of male subfertility. Eur J Obstet Gynecol Reprod Biol 64:213–216

67. Nan PM, Cohlen BJ, te Velde ER, van Kooij RJ, Eimers JM, van Zonneveld P et al (1994) Intra-uterine insemination or timed intercourse after ovarian stimulation for male subfertility? A controlled study. Hum Reprod 9:2022–2026
68. Kerin J, Quinn P (1987) Washed intrauterine insemination in the treatment of oligospermic infertility. Semin Reprod Endocrinol 5:23–33
69. Bensdorp AJ, Cohlen BJ, Heineman MJ, Vandekerckhove P (2007) Intra-uterine insemination for male subfertility. Cochrane Database Syst Rev 4:CD000360
70. Andersen AN, Gianaroli L, Felberbaum R, de Mouzon J, Nygren KG (2005) Assisted reproductive technology in Europe, 2001. Results generated from European registers by ESHRE. Hum Reprod 20:1158–1176
71. Steures P, van der Steeg JW, Hompes PG, van der Veen F, Mol BW (2007) Intrauterine insemination in The Netherlands. Reprod Biomed Online 14:110–116
72. Cohlen BJ (2005) Should we continue performing intrauterine inseminations in the year 2004? Gynecol Obstet Invest 59:3–13
73. Steures P, Berkhout JC, Hompes PGA, van der Steeg JW, Bossuyt PMM, van der Veen F, Habbema JDF, Eijkemans MJC, Mol BWJ (2005) Patients' preferences in deciding between intrauterine insemination and expectant management. Hum Reprod 20: 752–755
74. van Weert JM, van den Broek J, van der Steeg JW, van der Veen F, Flierman PA, Mol BWJ, Steures P (2007) Patients' preferences for intrauterine insemination or in-vitro fertilization. Reprod Biomed Online 15:422–427
75. Wasson JH, Sox HC, Neff RK, Goldman L (1985) Clinical prediction rules. Applications and methodological standards. N Engl J Med 313(13):793–799
76. te Velde ER, Cohlen BJ (1999) The management of infertility. N Engl J Med 340(3):224–226
77. Habbema JDF, Collins J, Leridon H, Evers JLH, Lunenfeld B, Velde ERT (2004) Towards less confusing terminology in reproductive medicine: a proposal. Fertil Steril 82(1):36–40
78. Stolwijk AM, Zielhuis GA, Hamilton CJ, Straatman H, Hollanders JM, Goverde HJ et al (1996) Prognostic models for the probability of achieving an ongoing pregnancy after in-vitro fertilization and the importance of testing their predictive value. Hum Reprod 11(10):2298–2303
79. Hunault CC, Habbema JD, Eijkemans MJ, Collins JA, Evers JL, te Velde ER (2004) Two new prediction rules for spontaneous pregnancy leading to live birth among subfertile couples, based on the synthesis of three previous models. Hum Reprod 19:2019–2026
80. van der Steeg JW, Steures P, Eijkemans MJC, Habbema JDF, Hompes PGA, Broekmans FJ, van Dessel HJHM, Bossuyt PMM, van der Veen F, Mol BWJ (2007) Pregnancy is predictable a large-scale prospective external validation of the prediction of spontaneous pregnancy in subfertile couples. Hum Reprod 22:536–542
81. Steures P, van der Steeg JW for CECERM, Mol BWJ, Eijkemans MJC, van der Veen F, Habbema JDF, Hompes PGA, Bossuyt PMM, Verhoeve HR, van Kasteren YM, van Dop PA (2004) Prediction of an ongoing pregnancy after intrauterine insemination. Fertil Steril 82:45–51
82. Custers IM, Steures P, van der Steeg JW, van Dessel HJHM, Bernardus RE, Bourdrez P, Koks CA, Riedijk WJ, Burggraaff JM, van der Veen F, Mol BWJ (2007) External validation of a prediction model for an ongoing pregnancy after intrauterine insemination. Fertil Steril 88:425–431

Chapter 32
Sperm Preparation for Artificial Insemination

Greg L. Christensen

Abstract Intrauterine insemination (IUI) is a common treatment for couples with infertility issues. In order to operate a good IUI program, several elements are necessary. This chapter attempts to provide a comprehensive description of these elements including: aspects of patient education, communication between the laboratory and the referring physician, employee training, safety, sample identification, and documentation procedures. It also describes supplies and reagents needed for IUI, multiple techniques for the preparation of sperm, and advantages of the different preparations. A discussion of special considerations such as the use of positive samples for infectious disease, use of sex-selected sperm, and chemical motility enhancement is included.

Keywords Artificial insemination • Intrauterine insemination • IUI • Density gradient • Swim-up • Sperm wash • Sperm quality

32.1 Introduction

Due to increased social acceptance and the successful range of infertility therapies now available, more people than ever are seeking treatment for infertility. A broad range of conditions, affecting both the male and female, contribute to infertility. Many circumstances, such as severe oligozoospermia or blocked fallopian tubes, are immediate indications that more aggressive therapies, such as in vitro fertilization (IVF), are needed to be pursued for a reasonable chance of success. However, the majority of patients with less severe or unexplained forms of infertility have a reasonable chance of success with less invasive intrauterine insemination (IUI). While the decision of which infertility therapy to pursue depends on a number of factors including infertile pathologies, age, and finances, for many couples IUI will be the first and only therapy needed.

Several factors can contribute to the success rates of IUI, including sperm quality, insemination timing and number of inseminations, age, and the use of ovarian stimulation [1–3]. One of the major male factors influencing the rates is the concentration of motile sperm in the prepared sample used for insemination, with pregnancy rates falling off quickly when less than 5 million motile sperm are inseminated [4, 5]. Normal sperm morphology has also been evaluated, though the correlation with pregnancy rates is less clear. On average, the pregnancy rate per IUI cycle is about 10–15% when motile sperm are available, though higher rates have been reported, especially when combined with the use of gonadotropins [6].

Under normal circumstances, sperm must pass through the cervical mucus to reach the uterus, a process that limits uterine entrance to only the healthiest sperm and prevents dead sperm, debris, and seminal fluid from getting in. Due to the presence of prostaglandins and microbes in the seminal fluid, semen cannot be placed directly into the uterus without the potential of inducing painful cramping and infection. With the advent of sperm preparation techniques to remove seminal fluids, nonmotile cells, and debris, sperm can be placed directly into the uterus with minimal risk. In instances where sperm quality is less than optimal or adverse mucus or cervical conditions exist, IUI can be highly advantageous in achieving pregnancy.

Besides removing prostaglandins, processing semen samples prior to IUI has other advantages. Sperm from semen samples can be concentrated and reduced to a volume that is consistent with what the uterine cavity can hold. Decapacitation factors present in the semen are removed, increasing the sperm's fertilization ability. Processing semen samples can also select for fractions of sperm with the best motility and improve overall motility. Finally, the prepared sample of sperm can be placed in preparation media known to support sperm capacitation and survival.

The purpose of this chapter is to relay practical information concerning the preparation of sperm for IUI. Besides protocols for sperm preparation, information will be given on laboratory communication, training, safety, equipment, records, and other topics relevant to sperm preparation.

G.L. Christensen (✉)
The Fertility Center at University Women's Healthcare,
University of Louisville, Louisville, KY, USA
e-mail: Gregchristensen.phd@gmail.com

D.T. Carrell and C.M. Peterson (eds.), *Reproductive Endocrinology and Infertility: Integrating Modern Clinical and Laboratory Practice*,
DOI 10.1007/978-1-4419-1436-1_32,

32.2 Patient Education

Prior to visiting the laboratory for sperm preparation, it is important that a couple be educated on the insemination process. Educating the patients on the correct timing and protocol for scheduling sperm preparations, semen collection, and the specific requirements of the laboratory preparing the sample will reduce the patients' stress. In addition to resulting in a more positive experience for the patients, it will also allow the staff to work more efficiently.

Many patients undergoing insemination have questions concerning the interpretation of home ovulation test kits and when to schedule their insemination. The laboratory and office staff responsible for scheduling inseminations should be trained and knowledgeable on assisting patients in this regard. In some instances, sperm preparations require the collection of more than one sample, and the patient's chart should always be consulted when advising the patient on insemination timing. The staff should also be aware of the requirement for a physician's order on the type of sperm preparation wanted, and in the event the patient has a responsibility to provide the order prior to the procedure, that information should be communicated to him. Depending on the ordering physician and source of sperm to be used, there may also be requirements for STD testing on the part of the male and/or female partner. It is important that staff be trained and able to communicate these requirements to current or potential patients.

Patients should also be instructed on several points concerning sample collection. Male partners are often uncomfortable with the collection process and they should be informed on whether home collection is allowed and what to expect of the collection facilities if they collect the semen sample onsite. In the event the patient is going to bring the sample in, they should be told what type of container to use, how the sample should be collected and labeled, how to transport the sample to the clinic, and who is allowed to drop off the sample. For onsite collection, it is important to review the collection and sample identification process with the patient and have a clear system to document that the instruction has been given.

32.3 Laboratory and Physician Communication

Prior to processing a semen sample for insemination, the laboratory needs to receive an order from the patient's physician authorizing the laboratory to prepare the sample and specifying the type of sperm preparation requested. In the event that several attempts at conception will be made using IUI, a standing order can be provided by the physician. In some cases, the physician may want recommendations for how to prepare the sample, based on a semen analysis or sperm function test data. Documentation should be available, and the staff educated on who is authorized to give this information. Staff should also be educated on who is authorized and how to discuss the results of a sperm preparation with a physician. Protocols should also be in place on how to communicate adverse findings, such as high numbers of white blood cells in the final sample or very low motile sperm counts, to the physician in a timely fashion.

32.4 Employee Training

Before a technician is allowed to independently prepare a sample, they should be trained and demonstrate proficiency with each of the different types of sperm preparations used by the laboratory (see Chap. 5 by Keel and Schalue). Documentation of this training should be kept in the employee's file as well as documentation that they have reviewed the written sperm preparation protocols at least yearly and have maintained their proficiency.

Another important aspect of educating staff is making sure that each technician is following the written protocol. This ensures that insemination samples are treated the same, regardless of the technician, and helps reduce variability between technicians. Participation in a quality control program to verify that laboratory employees can obtain comparable results for motilities and counts is also important for identifying training needs and providing reliable results. Technicians should also be trained to note any unusual observations about an insemination sample and call it to the attention of the supervisor.

32.5 Sample Handling and Safety

The laboratory needs to have written protocols in place that provide for a safe working environment and protect the lab staff from potential exposure risks. In addition to protocols detailing how samples are to be handled, the protocols should also address the bigger picture of the working environment and a laboratory technician's ability to process a sample safely on a given day.

Regardless of the donor or origin, all semen samples must be treated as a source of transmissible disease and handled with care. Because of this risk, one of the most important aspects of handling and processing semen safely is the use of appropriate personal protective equipment. Lab staff should have access to gloves, scrubs or lab coats, and gear to protect the face while working on samples. Gloves should be changed regularly and hands washed frequently. Any contaminated waste needs to be disposed of properly in a biohazardous waste container. Only closed-toe shoes should be worn in the lab and hairstyles and jewelry should be modified if they present a hazard to safety.

With regards to the lab environment, trash cans, chairs, or other items should be placed so that they are out of the way when samples are being processed. Clutter on work surfaces should be eliminated to prevent spills or accidents. The use of syringes with sharp needles should be avoided, blunt needles or pipettes are a much safer alternative. The standard practice of not eating, drinking, or applying cosmetics in the lab also needs to be observed.

As a final note, it is important that the technician be capable of safely handling the sample. Only technicians who have been trained on safety procedures and passed off by a supervisor should prepare samples for IUI. It is also important that on any given day, a technician should not be impaired due to lack of sleep, medication, sickness or otherwise, that they cannot safely work in the lab setting.

32.6 Sample Identification and Documentation

The correct identification of a sperm sample, from initial receipt until the actual insemination takes place, is absolutely critical. The consequences of misidentifying a sample can result in significant psychological and monetary expenses for all parties involved. For this reason, undertaking a careful, systematic approach to sample identification is crucial.

Regardless of whether a sample is collected at home or onsite, a system should be in place to positively identify a patient and make sure an accurate label, confirmed by the patient, is placed on the sample container in their presence, with a minimum of two unique identifiers. Once accepted by the lab, the sperm sample and materials used to process the sample should be kept completely separate from those used for other samples. Some strategies that have been used include labeling and/or color-coding all materials used for a sample and physically separating the materials used into a separate workstation. Before releasing the sample to the patient for the insemination, all materials should be reviewed and documentation made to confirm the correct materials were used. The final sample released to the patient should be clearly labeled with the patient's name and identifiers, and the patient should be requested to confirm the information is accurate. Prior to insemination, the care provider performing the procedure should also confirm the information on the sample with the patient.

32.7 Equipment and Reagents

The following table lists the general supplies needed to prepare sperm for IUI.

Equipment for sperm preparation	
Nondisposable	Disposable
Microscope	Specimen containers
Centrifuge	15 mL Centrifuge tubes
Incubator	Culture tubes
Refrigerator	Sterile plastic pipettes
Dry heating blocks	Sterile 3 mL syringes
Sperm counting chambers	Blunt 18 GA needles
Test tube racks	Personal protective equipment
	Biohazardous waste containers
	Sperm preparation media
	Packaging materials

A good microscope and centrifuge are the core elements of preparing sperm for IUI, and care should be taken to select good equipment. Centrifuges can have either a fixed or swinging rotor, though swinging rotors are more effective at pelleting the sperm sample in the bottom of the tube. They should be capable of spinning the sample at 300 × g; however, higher speeds may be necessary for some applications related to semen analysis. As a quality control measure, the centrifuge should be calibrated at least every 6 months. A compound microscope with phase contrast and 20×, 40×, and 100× objectives is ideal. In general, only the 20× and 40× objectives will be used for preparing the sample, but the 100× is useful for evaluating for contaminating cells or looking at fixed slides generated from the sperm preparation.

Temperature control is an important aspect of sperm preparation. A refrigerator is necessary to store media, and a dry incubator set at 37°C to maintain semen samples, the media needed each day, and sperm counting chambers at the correct temperature. As a complement to the incubator, heating blocks containing metal tube blocks can be placed at each workstation, to keep the specimen, media and counting chambers for an individual separate from other samples being processed. As a part of daily QC, the temperatures of the equipment used should be recorded daily, and adjustments made as necessary.

A number of disposable items are required, and it should be emphasized that all materials coming in contact with the sample be sterile. Several suppliers provide sterile specimen containers, and patients should be discouraged from trying to use a container they "sterilized" at home in the dishwasher. For aspirating and moving the sample between containers, either sterile pipettes or a sterile syringe and blunt needle can be used. To save on the cost of centrifuge tubes and decrease the potential for contamination, media needed for the day can be aliquoted into culture tubes and kept in the incubator or heating block until needed.

There are now several good, commercially available medias for sperm washing. The majority of these media is buffered with HEPES ((N-(2-hydroxyethyl) piperazine-N′-(2-ethanesulfonic acid);(N-(2-hydroxyethyl)piperazine-1-ethanesulfonic acid)), which allows them to maintain a pH of 7.3–7.5 without the need for a CO_2-controlled environment. In addition to sperm wash media, refrigeration media and density gradient medias are also readily available from different suppliers of ART products.

Regardless of which medias are used, good quality control dictates that the new lots of media and any other disposables that will contact the semen or sperm sample be tested for sperm toxicity. The simplest way to do this is to wash a good quality donor semen sample and evaluate the motility of the sample over the course of several hours during exposure to the material or media being tested. As a control, a previously tested media of known quality can be used for comparison.

32.8 Sperm Preparation Worksheets and Records

An important component of sperm preparation for IUI is having a well-designed sperm preparation worksheet to record the details of a sperm preparation. A universal worksheet can be created that works well for all different types of preparation. There are several necessary aspects to the worksheet, the first being information about the patient and the visit. This should include the patient's name and partner's name, unique identifiers, the date, the referring physician, and type of preparation being performed. General information concerning the semen sample should include the source (husband, donor), days of abstinence, collection site, and type of collection container used. The results section should document the semen sample's initial characteristics: volume, motility, concentration if desired, viscosity, and agglutination. There should also be space to record the sample's final volume and characteristics. Worksheets should document when preparations were started and finished, which staff received, prepared, and released the sample, and any unusual observations about the sample or preparation. In addition to the patient's worksheet, a log ought to be maintained of reagents and lot numbers used to prepare samples. Another log should be maintained of the daily patient visits and sperm preparations.

32.9 Overview of Sperm Preparations

Over the years, several different techniques for sperm preparation have been developed and tested for efficacy. Many of the techniques are no longer in use or used in only a few laboratories. The preparation techniques presented in this chapter represent those that have proven effective, simple to perform, or useful for special circumstances.

32.9.1 Basic Wash Preparation

32.9.1.1 Overview

The basic wash is the simplest and least expensive sperm preparation to perform. It is able to concentrate the sperm into a workable volume for insemination, removing the seminal fluid with its associated decapacitation factors and prostaglandins. Besides its simplicity, the advantage of a basic wash is that essentially all of the sperm in the ejaculate will be recovered. This is especially useful for samples with a low concentration of motile sperm. It is also beneficial for cryopreserved samples, or other fragile samples that would benefit from reduced processing and increased recovery. The disadvantage of a basic wash is that it concentrates all of the live sperm, dead sperm, white blood cells, red blood cells, and seminal debris together. As a result, the healthy sperm are exposed to higher levels of reactive oxygen species (ROS), which can decrease sperm function and negatively affect fertilization [7, 8]. Therefore, the basic wash is not recommended for regular samples when there are a lot of cellular contaminants or dead cells present.

32.9.1.2 Protocol

1. Label all materials used in the processing of the sperm sample, including paperwork and specimen container, with the patient's name and additional unique identifiers.
2. Once the sample has liquefied, gently swirl the container several times to mix the sample and perform a motility assessment and concentration estimate. Record the results on the patient's worksheet. Record any unusual observations regarding the sample.
3. Aspirate the sample, record the volume, and place it in a labeled, sterile centrifuge tube.
4. Dilute the semen sample with sperm wash media, using at least two parts wash media to one part semen. Mix the semen and wash media by gently inverting the tube several times. Use additional centrifuge tubes if necessary.
5. Centrifuge the sample for 10 min at 300 × g.
6. Gently decant the supernatant into an approved waste container as soon as the sample has finished spinning.
7. Resuspend the sperm pellet with 0.5–0.7 mL of fresh media until the sample appears homogenous.
8. Load 0.6–0.8 mL of the sample into the syringe that will be used for the insemination and maintain the sample at 37°C until time for the insemination.

9. Use the remainder of the sample to evaluate the final motility, concentration, and morphology, according to lab protocol. Record the results on the patient's worksheet.
10. Release the sample to the patient or care provider performing the insemination, according to lab protocol.

Note: For cryopreserved samples, decrease the centrifuge time to 7–8 min. For samples with a known high titer of anti-sperm antibodies, the sample can be collected into a container with 10 mL of sperm wash media and immediately processed to help improve motility in the final sample.

32.9.2 Density Gradient Preparation

32.9.2.1 Overview

The density gradient preparation consists of filtering sperm by centrifugal force through either one or multiple layers of increasingly concentrated silane-coated silica particles. Typically, semen is placed directly on top of the density gradient layers, and during centrifugation, the most motile sperm pass through the different layers, making a soft pellet at the bottom. The seminal fluids, dead or nonmotile sperm, and cellular debris are held up at the interfaces between the layers. The sperm that have successfully pelleted at the bottom can then be recovered, washed to remove the density gradient media, and used for IUI.

For samples with a high concentration of motile sperm, good results can be obtained by using a single layer of 90% gradient media. However, by using an additional layer on top of the 90% layer, the seminal debris can be distanced from the final pellet, more sperm can enter the first layer and by passing through two interfaces the final sample may contain a higher percentage of clean, motile sperm. The ability to select for a population of clean, motile sperm makes it very useful for samples with a lot of dead sperm, round cells, or debris. Unless it is necessary to remove WBCs, it is not advisable to use density gradient preparations for samples with low concentrations of progressively motile sperm, as recovery may be limited.

32.9.2.2 Protocol

1. Prepare a density gradient column by placing 1.5 mL of 90% sperm gradient media in the bottom of a sterile centrifuge tube. Gently layer an additional 1.5 mL of 35% sperm gradient media on top of the 90% layer. Maintain the column at 37°C until ready for use.
2. Label all materials used in the processing of the sperm sample, including paperwork and specimen container, with the patient's name and additional unique identifiers.
3. Once the sample has liquefied, gently swirl the container several times to mix the sample and perform a motility assessment and concentration estimate. Record the results on the patient's worksheet. Record any unusual observations regarding the sample.
4. Aspirate the sample, record the volume, and gently layer it on top of the prepared gradient column. If the semen volume is greater than 4 mL, the sample can be divided and layered on separate gradient columns.
5. Centrifuge the sample at 300 × g for 15 min.
6. Gently aspirate the supernatant, 35% layer, and upper surface of the 90% layer and discard. Combine 90% layers if more than one gradient column was used.
7. Dilute the 90% layers with sperm wash media, using at least two parts wash media to one part sperm gradient media. Gently invert the centrifuge tube to mix the sample.
8. Centrifuge the sample for 10 min at 300 × g.
9. Gently decant the supernatant into an approved waste container as soon as the sample has finished spinning.
10. Resuspend the sperm pellet with 0.5–0.7 mL of fresh media until the sample appears homogenous.
11. Load 0.6–0.8 mL of the sample into the syringe that will be used for the insemination and maintain the sample at 37°C until time for the insemination.
12. Use the remainder of the sample to evaluate the final motility, concentration, and morphology, according to lab protocol. Record the results on the patient's worksheet.
13. Release the sample to the patient or care provider performing the insemination, according to lab protocol.

Note: To avoid contaminating the final sample with cells or debris present in the semen or upper layers of the gradient, it is advisable to use a new syringe to resuspend the final sample with fresh media and load for insemination.

32.9.3 Swim-Up Preparation

32.9.3.1 Overview

First described in 1984 [9], the swim-up preparation is a cost-effective way to separate a clean fraction of sperm with good motility. A major disadvantage is that sperm yields tend to be low, especially if the initial sample has a low concentration or decreased progressive motility. Therefore, when being used for IUI, only samples with a high initial concentration and good progressive motility should be prepared with this technique.

The swim-up preparation relies on the ability of sperm with good motility to migrate into a clean layer of media. Several variations on the swim-up exist. Fresh media can be layered directly on top of the semen, over the top of a washed pellet, or over the top of a resuspended pellet. In the event there is a large volume of semen, the first variation may require several centrifuge tubes to obtain adequate surface area between the semen and media. The media layers would then need to be combined and centrifuged to concentrate the collected sperm. Layering fresh media over a sperm pellet has the double disadvantage of reducing the surface area between the sperm and clean media and concentrating the healthy sperm with the dead cells and contaminating cells, greatly increasing the potential for ROS damage. For these reasons, a protocol using the third technique is described, which limits the need for extra supplies, reduces the potential for ROS damage, and to a certain degree increases the surface area between the washed sperm and the clean media into which they are migrating.

32.9.3.2 Protocol

1. Label all materials used in the processing of the sperm sample, including paperwork and specimen container, with the patient's name and additional unique identifiers.
2. Once the sample has liquefied, gently swirl the container several times to mix the sample and perform a motility assessment and concentration estimate. Record the results on the patient's worksheet. Record any unusual observations regarding the sample.
3. Aspirate the sample, record the volume, and place it in a labeled, sterile centrifuge tube.
4. Dilute the semen sample with sperm wash media, using at least two parts wash media to one part semen. Mix the semen and wash media by gently inverting the tube several times. Use additional centrifuge tubes if necessary.
5. Centrifuge the sample for 10 min at 300 × g.
6. Gently decant the supernatant into an approved waste container as soon as the sample has finished spinning.
7. Resuspend the sperm pellet with 0.6–0.7 mL of fresh media until the sample appears homogenous.
8. Using a clean pipette, gently layer 1.0 mL of fresh sperm wash media on top of the resuspended pellet.
9. Without disturbing the layers, incubate the sample at 37°C for 60 min.
10. After the incubation period and without disturbing the bottom layer, load 0.6–0.8 mL of the upper layer into the syringe that will be used for the insemination and maintain the sample at 37°C until time for the insemination.
11. Use the remainder of the sample to evaluate the final motility, concentration, and morphology, according to lab protocol. Record the results on the patient's worksheet.
12. Release the sample to the patient or care provider performing the insemination, according to lab protocol.

Note: During the incubation step, the surface area between the layers can be increased, therefore increasing the sperm yield, if the tube can be safely placed in the incubator at an angle, rather than vertical. A glass beaker or Styrofoam rack, for instance, might be used for this purpose.

32.9.4 Refrigeration Incubation Preparation

32.9.4.1 Overview

While not a standard preparation, in certain circumstances the refrigeration incubation can be very useful. By mixing semen with refrigeration media, similar to the media used for sperm cryopreservation, the sperm can be stored for up to 48 h. This is useful when the male cannot be available on the day of insemination or for storing a sample for a short term to be combined with a fresh sample collected on the day of insemination. The refrigeration process also promotes sperm capacitation and increases fertilization as measured by the sperm penetration assay (SPA) in patients with poor initial SPA scores [10].

32.9.4.2 Protocol

1. Label all materials used in the processing of the sperm sample, including paperwork and specimen container, with the patient's name and additional unique identifiers.
2. Once the sample has liquefied, gently swirl the container several times to mix the sample and perform a motility assessment and concentration estimate. Record the results on the patient's worksheet. Record any unusual observations regarding the sample.
3. Aspirate the sample, record the volume, and place it in a labeled, sterile centrifuge tube.
4. Add a commercial refrigeration media, warmed to room temperature, in a one-to-one ratio to the semen. Use additional tubes if necessary.
5. Place the tube(s) containing the mixture into a beaker filled with enough ambient temperature water to be just above the level of the semen – refrigeration media mixture in the tubes.
6. Place the beaker with the sample in a refrigerator (2–6°C) and allow the samples to incubate up to 48 h. At very minimum, the samples should incubate long enough to reach the temperature of the refrigerator.
7. Remove the sample from the refrigerator and the beaker of water and allow it to sit at room temperature for 10 min.
8. Dilute the semen – refrigeration media mixture with sperm wash media, using at least two parts wash media

to one part semen. Mix gently by inverting the tube several times. Use additional centrifuge tubes if necessary.
9. Centrifuge the sample for 10 min at 300 × g.
10. Gently decant the supernatant into an approved waste container as soon as the sample has finished spinning.
11. Resuspend the sperm pellet with 0.5–0.7 mL of fresh media until the sample appears homogenous.
12. Load 0.6–0.8 mL of the sample into the syringe that will be used for the insemination and maintain the sample at 37°C until time for the insemination.
13. Use the remainder of the sample to evaluate the final motility, concentration, and morphology, according to lab protocol. Record the results on the patient's worksheet.
14. Release the sample to the patient or care provider performing the insemination, according to lab protocol.

Note: If a refrigerated sample is going to be combined with a fresh sample, it can be washed and combined with the fresh sample after each sample has been washed once. The combined samples can then be washed together with fresh media to concentrate the sperm together. If desired, the refrigerated sample can also be washed and placed on a density gradient column and then combined with a fresh sample that has also gone through a gradient column, prior to the final wash.

32.9.5 Heparin Incubation Preparation

32.9.5.1 Overview

In vitro, heparin stimulates the movement of calcium across the sperm cell membrane, which promotes capacitation of the sperm and can increase motility. Low doses of heparin can also improve the SPA results of patients who have a poor SPA result without heparin [10]. Patients with decreased motility or concentration may benefit from the use of heparin during sperm preparation. However, it is advisable to base the use of heparin on an SPA, rather than on semen analysis data alone.

32.9.5.2 Protocol

1. Label all materials used in the processing of the sperm sample, including paperwork and specimen container, with the patient's name and additional unique identifiers.
2. Prepare the heparin-sperm wash media by adding 1% clinical grade heparin, by volume, to the warmed sperm wash media.
3. Once the sample has liquefied, gently swirl the container several times to mix the sample and perform a motility assessment and concentration estimate. Record the results on the patient's worksheet. Record any unusual observations regarding the sample.
4. Aspirate the sample, record the volume, and place it in a labeled, sterile centrifuge tube.
5. Dilute the semen sample with the heparin-sperm wash media, using at least two parts wash media to one part semen. Mix the semen and wash media by gently inverting the tube several times. Use additional centrifuge tubes if necessary.
6. Centrifuge the sample for 10 min at 300 × g.
7. Gently decant the supernatant into an approved waste container as soon as the sample has finished spinning.
8. Resuspend the sperm pellet with 1.0 mL of fresh heparin-sperm wash media until the sample appears homogenous.
9. Place the sample in a 37°C block or incubator for 1 h and incubate for 60 min.
10. Add 5–7 mLs of fresh sperm wash media, without heparin, to the incubated sperm sample.
11. Centrifuge the sample for 10 min at 300 × g.
12. Gently decant the supernatant into an approved waste container as soon as the sample has finished spinning.
13. Resuspend the sperm pellet with 0.5–0.7 mL of fresh sperm wash media until the sample appears homogenous.
14. Load 0.6–0.8 mL of the sample into the syringe that will be used for the insemination and maintain the sample at 37°C until time for the insemination.
15. Use the remainder of the sample to evaluate the final motility, concentration, and morphology, according to lab protocol. Record the results on the patient's worksheet.
16. Release the sample to the patient or care provider performing the insemination, according to lab protocol.

32.9.6 Retrograde Wash Preparation

32.9.6.1 Overview

Retrograde ejaculation occurs when semen moves into the bladder rather than passing out through the urethra. Retrograde ejaculation can result from a variety of conditions such as diabetes, surgery, medication, spinal cord injury, or congenital malformations. The condition is encountered frequently in the Andrology setting, and laboratories preparing sperm should be prepared to work with retrograde samples.

32.9.6.2 Patient Preparation and Semen Collection

When a patient calls to set up an appointment for a retrograde sperm wash, they should be instructed on additional collection procedures unique to retrograde sperm preparation. Because sperm do not survive well in urine, collection should only be considered at the facility preparing the sample. Under the direction of his care provider, the patient may also be instructed to take sodium bicarbonate orally, prior to collection, to regulate the pH of the urine [11]. The patient should come to the appointment well hydrated. Immediately prior to having the patient attempt collecting a semen sample and subsequent urine sample, have them void their bladder. The patient should be given two containers, one for attempting to collect an antegrade semen sample and a second to collect the retrograde urine sample.

32.9.6.3 Antegrade Sample Processing

Dependent upon the pathology, a patient with retrograde ejaculation may, on occasion, produce an antegrade semen sample. In the event this happens, the sample should be processed using a standard wash or density gradient protocol, depending on the sample quality. If a good quality antegrade sample is produced, the lab may choose to forgo preparing the retrograde sample. If a poor antegrade sample is produced, it can be prepared and combined with the retrograde sample.

32.9.6.4 Retrograde Wash Protocol

1. Label all materials used in the processing of the sperm sample, including paperwork and specimen container, with the patient's name and additional unique identifiers.
2. Immediately upon receipt of the collected sample, note the volume and divide the urine into several labeled centrifuge tubes.
3. Centrifuge the sample for 8 min at 300 × g.
4. Gently decant the supernatant from each tube into an approved waste container as soon as the sample has finished spinning.
5. Add 0.5 mL of sperm wash media to each pellet, resuspend, and combine the pellets into a single tube.
6. Dilute the recombined pellets with 5–7 mLs of sperm wash media. Mix by gently inverting the tube several times.
7. Centrifuge the sample for 10 min at 300 × g.
8. Gently decant the supernatant into an approved waste container as soon as the sample has finished spinning.
9. Resuspend the sperm pellet with 0.5–0.7 mL of fresh media until the sample appears homogenous.
10. Load 0.6–0.8 mL of the sample into the syringe that will be used for the insemination and maintain the sample at 37°C until time for the insemination.
11. Use the remainder of the sample to evaluate the final motility, concentration, and morphology, according to lab protocol. Record the results on the patient's worksheet.
12. Release the sample to the patient or care provider performing the insemination, according to lab protocol.

Notes: When aliquoting the original retrograde sample into different centrifuge tubes, it may be immediately apparent that a few tubes contain the majority of the coagulated semen sample. For best results, these tubes should be further diluted with sperm wash media before the initial wash.

32.9.7 Preparation of Cryopreserved Sperm

32.9.7.1 Patient Samples

In many instances, patients choose to use cryopreserved sperm that was stored prior to chemotherapy or military duty, or for other personal reasons. As cryopreserved sperm are less robust than those in fresh samples, extra precaution should be taken when they are prepared. Generally, cryopreserved samples should not be subjected to more than a single wash in sperm wash media. The centrifugation time should also be reduced to 6–8 min. Patients should be educated that cryopreserved samples will have reduced sperm motility compared to the fresh state of the sample before freezing. Depending on the circumstances and the number of frozen vials a patient has stored, a plan should be made to thaw a sufficient number of vials to give the patients a reasonable chance of achieving pregnancy.

32.9.7.2 Donor Samples

Many patients now choose to take advantage of the easy access to sperm donor profiles provided by the Internet and order donor sperm from sperm banks across the country. The sperm samples are typically shipped just prior to their anticipated use and stored in the shipping dewar until needed. Whenever a donor sample arrives, it is important to confirm it has arrived in good condition, and is the correct sample. If the sample is not going to be used right away, measures should be taken to place it in a more permanent storage container. Most sperm banks are now providing donor samples that are prewashed. Under these circumstances, all that is necessary is to thaw the vial, check a drop of the warmed sample to confirm if it meets the sperm bank's standards, and load it into the insemination syringe. If the sample was not washed prior to freezing, it will be necessary to wash the sample using the simple wash procedure, shortened to 6–8 min of centrifugation, prior to intrauterine insemination.

32.9.8 *Sample Handling After Preparation*

Once a final sample has been prepared, care should be taken to protect the sample from extreme shifts in temperature. If the insemination is to take place at the same facility at which the sperm was prepared, an arrangement could be made to keep the sample in the laboratory incubator until it is time for the procedure. If the insemination will take place at a location away from the preparation facility, the sperm sample should be packaged in an insulated container for transport. It is also important that the insemination time be scheduled to coincide with the completion of the sperm preparation to avoid any untimely delays that could compromise the sample.

32.10 Special Considerations

32.10.1 *Preparation of Sperm for IUI Collected by PVS or EEJ*

In the United States alone, there are 11,000 new spinal cord injuries (SCIs) every year. The majority of these injuries occur in men between the ages of 16 and 30 for whom reproductive health is still an important issue [12]. Only a small percentage of these men will be able to conceive without the help of assisted reproductive therapies. While some centers choose to collect sperm from anejaculatory SCI patients only through surgical methods to be used with ICSI, IUI is still a valid and less obtrusive method for many.

According to a recent study, semen can be successfully collected 95% of the time by penile vibratory stimulation (PVS) or electroejaculation (EEJ). In 70% of the collections, the total motile sperm count is high enough to proceed with intrauterine insemination, according to the standards of 94% of the survey respondents [13]. In many instances, PVS can be performed at home, making it even more attractive to SCI patients.

Due at least in part to the relatively low frequency of ejaculations in SCI patients, sperm motility is often reduced. In many instances, the samples can also contain large amounts of red blood cells, white blood cells, and debris. Another issue that can make the preparation of SCI samples more challenging is the increased occurrence of retrograde ejaculation. Because of these special circumstances, technicians preparing semen samples collected by PVS or EEJ should be prepared for the different possibilities.

If a normal appearing antegrade sample is collected, the choice of preparations can be based on the sperm parameters. If the sample contains excessive debris, round cells, or dead sperm, a density gradient preparation may be necessary to "clean it up." If the sample is retrograde, then steps should be taken accordingly to quickly remove the sperm from any urine present. If the sample is to be collected by a physician in a clinical setting, the physician may wish to flush the bladder with sperm wash media, which could produce different samples to analyze, depending on the presence of an antegrade sample and the number of flushes. In this event, a clear method of labeling each container should be established between the physician and the laboratory, so the content of each container is clear.

32.10.2 *Infectious Disease Processing*

Preparation of sperm for IUI in HIV-1 serodiscordant couples remains highly controversial, despite the accumulated evidence of more than 3,000 cycles, resulting in more than 360 births with no reported cases of seroconversion [14]. Laboratories that prepare sperm for IUI from HIV positive or hepatitis C positive men typically subject the sample to density gradient centrifugation followed by swim-up migration [14] to remove the nonmotile CD4 macrophages and lymphocytes that harbor the bulk of the viral load [15, 16]. It is also typical for HIV positive men in a serodiscordant relationship seeking to conceive through IUI to be under the care of an infectious disease specialist to monitor the patient's viral load and treat it accordingly. Developments in highly sensitive polymerase chain reaction techniques have recently demonstrated that low viral loads of HIV-1 can still be present in samples processed through gradient columns where all nonmotile cells have been removed [17]. For this reason, it is important to continue developing techniques to validate the absence of HIV and other transmissible viruses in semen samples processed for IUI [18].

32.10.3 *Posthumous Collected Sperm*

A few reports have now documented pregnancies and live births using sperm retrieved posthumously [19, 20]. However, in all cases, the pregnancies were achieved through ICSI. Due to the poor quality and quantity of posthumous collected sperm, it is unrealistic to use these samples for IUI.

32.10.4 *Sperm Preparation for Sex Selection*

During the preceding decades, different strategies to sort sperm based on the content of an X or Y sperm have been implemented. Ericcson first described the use of human serum albumin columns to produce a sample with an increased proportion of Y-bearing sperm [21]. The use of Sephadex columns to increase the concentration of X-bearing sperm has also been described [22]. While the initial findings of these and subsequent studies were very promising, the results have become controversial [23, 24], and if the samples do produce a higher number of male or female offspring, the result is not due to an increase of X- or Y-bearing sperm in the sample [25]. Currently, flow cytometry based methods are being offered commercially to separate sperm for sex selection in humans and a broad range of domestic species [26, 27]. Fluorescent in-situ hybridization confirms that following separation, sperm fractions can be enriched to 90 and 75% for the X and Y chromosome, respectively [26, 28], for human sperm. When the initial sample concentration is sufficiently high, the sorted samples are adequately concentrated for IUI.

32.10.5 Chemical Motility Enhancement

The most commonly used agent for sperm motility enhancement is pentoxifylline, a methylxanthine derivative that inhibits phosphodiesterase and increases cellular levels of cAMP. Several reports have been published documenting improved motility parameters in both fresh and frozen sperm samples when exposed to pentoxifylline [29–31]. However, the improvements appear limited to those individuals who have poor initial motility, and it should be used with discrimination [32]. The use of pentoxifylline to improve recovery of motile sperm for ICSI is an accepted practice, but the use of pentoxifylline in connection with human IUI is less common, and the benefits unclear [33]. Until further data are available, the use of pentoxifylline for preparing sperm for IUI should be approached cautiously.

Another methylxanthine phosphodiesterase inhibitor that has been evaluated for its benefits in improving sperm motility parameters is caffeine [34, 35]. However, a recent review on the topic indicates that caffeine has negative effects on the sperm plasma membrane and fertilization [36]. There is also no current data on the use of caffeine in connection with IUI.

32.11 Conclusions

Intrauterine insemination will continue to be used widely for treatment of infertility. In order to provide the highest level of care, a successful IUI program should take many factors into consideration. Besides having good sperm preparation protocols, it is necessary to educate and prepare patients, train staff on safety, documentation, and sample management, and be aware of the special considerations associated with IUI.

References

1. Agarwal SK, Buyalos RP (1996) Clomiphene citrate with intrauterine insemination: is it effective therapy in women above the age of 35 years? Fertil Steril 65(4):759–763
2. Osuna C, Matorras R, Pijoan JI, Rodriguez-Escudero FJ (2004) One versus two inseminations per cycle in intrauterine insemination with sperm from patients' husbands: a systematic review of the literature. Fertil Steril 82(1):17–24
3. Guzick DS, Sullivan MW, Adamson GD et al (1998) Efficacy of treatment for unexplained infertility. Fertil Steril 70(2):207–213
4. Ombelet W, Deblaere K, Bosmans E et al (2003) Semen quality and intrauterine insemination. Reprod Biomed Online 7(4):485–492
5. Wainer R, Albert M, Dorion A et al (2004) Influence of the number of motile spermatozoa inseminated and of their morphology on the success of intrauterine insemination. Hum Reprod 19(9): 2060–2065
6. Guzick DS, Carson SA, Coutifaris C et al (1999) Efficacy of superovulation and intrauterine insemination in the treatment of infertility. National Cooperative Reproductive Medicine Network. N Engl J Med 340(3):177–183
7. Aitken RJ, Clarkson JS (1987) Cellular basis of defective sperm function and its association with the genesis of reactive oxygen species by human spermatozoa. J Reprod Fertil 81(2):459–469
8. Mortimer D (1991) Sperm preparation techniques and iatrogenic failures of in-vitro fertilization. Hum Reprod 6(2):173–176
9. Mahadevan M, Baker GH (1984) Assesment and preparation of semen for in vitro fertilization. Springer-Verlag, Berlin
10. Carrell DT, Bradshaw WS, Jones KP, Middleton RG, Peterson CM, Urry RL (1992) An evaluation of various treatments to increase sperm penetration capacity for potential use in an in vitro fertilization program. Fertil Steril 57(1):134–138
11. Aust TR, Brookes S, Troup SA, Fraser WD, Lewis-Jones DI (2008) Development and in vitro testing of a new method of urine preparation for retrograde ejaculation; the Liverpool solution. Fertil Steril 89(4):885–891
12. National Spinal Cord Injury Statistical Center (2006) University of Alabama at Birmingham, Annual Statistical Report, June 2006
13. Kafetsoulis A, Brackett NL, Ibrahim E, Attia GR, Lynne CM (2006) Current trends in the treatment of infertility in men with spinal cord injury. Fertil Steril 86(4):781–789
14. Sauer MV (2005) Sperm washing techniques address the fertility needs of HIV-seropositive men: a clinical review. Reprod Biomed Online 10(1):135–140
15. Quayle AJ, Xu C, Mayer KH, Anderson DJ (1997) T lymphocytes and macrophages, but not motile spermatozoa, are a significant source of human immunodeficiency virus in semen. J Infect Dis 176(4):960–968
16. Van Voorhis BJ, Martinez A, Mayer K, Anderson DJ (1991) Detection of human immunodeficiency virus type 1 in semen from seropositive men using culture and polymerase chain reaction deoxyribonucleic acid amplification techniques. Fertil Steril 55(3):588–594
17. Muciaccia B, Corallini S, Vicini E et al (2007) HIV-1 viral DNA is present in ejaculated abnormal spermatozoa of seropositive subjects. Hum Reprod 22(11):2868–2878
18. Lesage B, Vannin AS, Emiliani S, Debaisieux L, Englert Y, Liesnard C (2006) Development and evaluation of a qualitative reverse-transcriptase nested polymerase chain reaction protocol for same-day viral validation of human immunodeficiency virus type 1 ribonucleic acid in processed semen. Fertil Steril 86(1):121–128
19. Shefi S, Raviv G, Eisenberg ML et al (2006) Posthumous sperm retrieval: analysis of time interval to harvest sperm. Hum Reprod 21(11):2890–2893

20. Land S, Ross LS (2002) Posthumous reproduction: current and future status. Urol Clin North Am 29(4):863–871
21. Ericsson RJ, Langevin CN, Nishino M (1973) Isolation of fractions rich in human Y sperm. Nature 246(5433):421–424
22. Steeno O, Adimoelja A, Steeno J (1975) Separation of X- and Y-bearing human spermatozoa with the sephadex gel-filtration method. Andrologia 7(2):95–97
23. Martin RH (1994) Human sex pre-selection by sperm manipulation. Hum Reprod 9(10):1790–1791
24. Sills ES, Kirman I, Thatcher SS 3rd, Palermo GD (1998) Sex-selection of human spermatozoa: evolution of current techniques and applications. Arch Gynecol Obstet 261(3):109–115
25. Vidal F, Moragas M, Catala V et al (1993) Sephadex filtration and human serum albumin gradients do not select spermatozoa by sex chromosome: a fluorescent in-situ hybridization study. Hum Reprod 8(10):1740–1743
26. Schulman JD, Karabinus DS (2005) Scientific aspects of preconception gender selection. Reprod Biomed Online 10(Suppl 1): 111–115
27. Maxwell WM, Evans G, Hollinshead FK et al (2004) Integration of sperm sexing technology into the ART toolbox. Anim Reprod Sci 82–83:79–95
28. Vidal F, Fugger EF, Blanco J et al (1998) Efficiency of MicroSort flow cytometry for producing sperm populations enriched in X- or Y-chromosome haplotypes: a blind trial assessed by double and triple colour fluorescent in-situ hybridization. Hum Reprod 13(2):308–312
29. Yovich JM, Edirisinghe WR, Cummins JM, Yovich JL (1990) Influence of pentoxifylline in severe male factor infertility. Fertil Steril 53(4):715–722
30. Sharma RK, Agarwal A (1997) Influence of artificial stimulation on unprocessed and Percoll-washed cryopreserved sperm. Arch Androl 38(3):173–179
31. Paul M, Sumpter JP, Lindsay KS (1995) Action of pentoxifylline directly on semen. Hum Reprod 10(2):354–359
32. Tesarik J, Thebault A, Testart J (1992) Effect of pentoxifylline on sperm movement characteristics in normozoospermic and asthenozoospermic specimens. Hum Reprod 7(9):1257–1263
33. Negri P, Grechi E, Tomasi A, Fabbri E, Capuzzo A (1996) Effectiveness of pentoxifylline in semen preparation for intrauterine insemination. Hum Reprod 11(6):1236–1239
34. Mbizvo MT, Johnston RC, Baker GH (1993) The effect of the motility stimulants, caffeine, pentoxifylline, and 2-deoxyadenosine on hyperactivation of cryopreserved human sperm. Fertil Steril 59(5):1112–1117
35. Rees JM, Ford WC, Hull MG (1990) Effect of caffeine and of pentoxifylline on the motility and metabolism of human spermatozoa. J Reprod Fertil 90(1):147–156
36. Henkel RR, Schill WB (2003) Sperm preparation for ART. Reprod Biol Endocrinol 1:108

Chapter 33
Sperm Banking, Donation, and Transport in the Age of Assisted Reproduction: Federal and State Regulation

Grace M. Centola

Abstract Cryopreservation of semen is a common procedure, both for autologous sperm banking and for donor sperm insemination. Additionally, new techniques employing semen banking are now common, including the use of epididymal aspirates and testicular biopsy specimens used for assisted reproductive therapies (ART). This chapter explores the regulatory, scientific, and practical aspects of sperm cryopreservation and banking.

Keywords Sperm banking • Sperm donation • Artificial insemination • Donor sperm • Sperm cryopreservation • Regulation of reproductive tissue banking

33.1 Introduction

Cryopreservation of semen is a routine procedure for preserving male gametes for subsequent use in artificial insemination or assisted reproduction (ART). Semen cryopreservation is also mandated for anonymous donor sperm, which must be frozen and quarantined for a minimum of 6 months with initial and pre-release testing prior to use [1–3].

Semen cryopreservation is not a new procedure, with the earliest reports of sperm freezing from the eighteenth century by Spallanzani and Mantegazza in 1866 [4]. The first report of the survival of human sperm after cooling to −269°C and storage at −79°C occurred in 1938, and in 1949 the use of glycerol as a cryoprotectant, making possible large-scale freezing and banking of mammalian sperm was reported [4]. The landmark reports of human semen cryobanking and subsequent successful insemination were published in the 1950s [6]. The use of nitrogen vapor for freezing and storage of sperm was described in 1962 by Sherman, with normal offspring resulting in 1972 following 10 years storage of cryopreserved sperm [4]. At present, normal offspring have been known to result from the use of human semen cryopreserved for more than 28 years [7].

33.2 Sperm Banking

Semen is cryopreserved for autologous use as well as for use in therapeutic donor insemination. Autologous semen cryopreservation is indicated prior to surgical sterilization or vasectomy, prior to treatment for malignant and nonmalignant diseases, as well as intraoperative freezing during exploratory testicular biopsy for infertility in cases of obstructive or nonobstructive azospermia. Although more uncommon, premortem and postmortem cryopreservation of semen, testicular tissue, and/or epididymal or seminal vesicle aspirates are also indications for preservation of the male gametes. With the advent of assisted reproduction, particularly intracytoplasmic sperm injection (ICSI), which requires only one spermatozoon for fertilization of the oocyte, sperm banking is worthwhile even if only one ejaculate can be cryopreserved prior to initiation of cancer treatment [8]. More commonly, ART programs will store a male partner's semen in the event that sperm are not available on the day of oocyte retrieval for use in oocyte insemination or ICSI. ART fertilization and pregnancy rates in men with less than 10^3 spermatozoa per ml were similar if fresh or frozen sperm were used although results for fresh sperm were lower than controls while men demonstrating 10^3–10^5 spermatozoa/ml demonstrated rates similar to controls [8]. This data confirms the utility of banking sperm even in the severely oligozoospermic male.

Intraoperative cryopreservation of microsurgically retrieved epididymal sperm and testicular sperm in men with obstructive azospermia yields pregnancy rates comparable to those using fresh sperm [9, 10]. Intraoperative cryopreservation is also useful in cases of reconstructive surgery such as vasovasostomy or epididymovasostomy. However, sperm retrieval and cryopreservation at the time of vasectomy reversal may not be a cost-effective treatment strategy as compared to

G.M. Centola (✉)
Cryobank compliance Services, 5125 Delfa Lane, Macedon, NY, USA
e-mail: centolag@yahoo.com

D.T. Carrell and C.M. Peterson (eds.), *Reproductive Endocrinology and Infertility: Integrating Modern Clinical and Laboratory Practice*,
DOI 10.1007/978-1-4419-1436-1_33,

fresh harvest of sperm at the time of ART in the persistent azoospermic patient [11].

Sperm banking is strongly recommended for men as well as postpubertal teens with malignant disease who may someday desire biological children, even though a small but significant percentage of these men later use the stored semen [9, 12]. The cumulative percentage of use of banked sperm was shown to be above 10% in a 15 year cryopreservation study [13]. A diagnosis of testicular cancer was associated with a lower use of the banked sperm as compared to men with other cancers [13]. Sperm banks are increasingly used for fertility preservation in the event of disease or surgical treatment, especially for men with Hodgkin's disease or testicular cancer [14–17]. Walchaerts and colleague [17] also demonstrated an average annual increase of 7.5% in the number of men using sperm banking for testicular cancer during the period 1990–2004 in the 22 French CECOS centers. For Hodgkin's disease, the increase was also observed, but not as striking as for testicular cancer. Oncologists are advised to strongly urge their patients to preserve sperm prior to cancer treatment to safeguard future fertility [8, 17].

There is concern about transfer of genetically damaged sperm after cryopreservation; however, there has been no proven increase in genetic or phenotypic abnormalities in offspring conceived using banked sperm from men treated for malignant or nonmalignant diseases [9]. In fact, studies have shown that the DNA from prepared spermatozoa from fertile men was unaffected by cryopreservation, whereas spermatozoa from infertile men were significantly damaged by cryopreservation and thawing [18]. Other reports have demonstrated no excessive fetal losses in over 11,000 pregnancies conceived by insemination with donor sperm [19], as well as normal offspring from use of frozen testicular spermatozoa [20], and frozen epididymal sperm [21] in assisted reproduction. In a review of two prospective and large population-based studies, one in France and one in Australia, the general characteristics of children born after ART with frozen spermatozoa were not different from the general population in regards to weight, prematurity, stillbirths, sex ratio, overall health, and psychosocial development [22]. However, more recently, cryopreservation was shown to decrease overall sperm quality as assessed by the sperm chromatin structure assay (SCSA), with subsequent improvement in nuclear maturity after swim-up of the thawed semen [23].

33.3 Donor Sperm

It has been over 20 years since there was a shift to use of frozen and quarantined donor sperm for artificial insemination. With the advent of increased concerns regarding the transmission of sexually transmissible diseases (STDs), particularly acquired immune deficiency syndrome (AIDS), the practice of artificial insemination with donated semen shifted in the late 1980s to the exclusive use of cryopreserved donor semen [1]. In 1989, the French Federation CECOS sperm banks reported that since 1973, approximately 17,000 pregnancies resulted from the use of frozen donor sperm in artificial insemination or for in vitro fertilization [24]. In a survey conducted by the United States Congress Office of Technology Assessment in1988, [25], 30,000 births annually occurred as a result of artificial insemination with donor sperm. By 1988, only cryopreserved semen was recommended for donor insemination, although clearly not all physicians adopted these recommendations [4]. Similarly, in the late 1980s, the American Association of Tissue Banks published standards and the American Fertility Society (now American Society for Reproductive Medicine) published practice recommendations for the sole use of frozen, quarantined donor semen. Similarly, the advent of HIV and serious sequelae of HIV infection has resulted in reassessment of artificial insemination practice in the United Kingdom [26].

State regulations, and now federal regulations, have mandated the sole use of cryopreserved donor semen that has been quarantined for a minimum of 6 months with rigorous initial and prerelease testing after the quarantine. The Food and Drug Administration (FDA) published specific regulations requiring testing, cryopreservation, and quarantine of anonymous donor semen (FDA 21 CFR 1271) collected after May 2005. The FDA regulations do not require testing and quarantine of semen from sexually intimate partners, and allow the use of directed or known semen donor specimens as long as the donor has been tested within 7 days of the donations. For known sperm donors, the semen does not have to be quarantined for 6 months. On the other hand, for anonymous donors, the semen must be quarantined for 6 months followed by retesting prior to release for insemination.

New York State has specific regulations for donors of reproductive tissue (NYS Part 52-8). Similarly, California has detailed regulations for reproductive tissue donors, while Maryland, Florida, and Georgia statutes refer to the FDA regulations. The general recommendation is to follow the more strict regulations, which may be the FDA or specific state regulations for use of donated semen. At a minimum, the FDA regulations for testing of reproductive tissue donors must be followed by all tissue banks and ART programs in the US, or for any facility shipping specimens into the US. The FDA regulations must also be followed for any tissue originating in the US and being shipped to a foreign country.

It is interesting to note that a recent publication recommended that guidelines be changed to allow the use of fresh sperm for insemination [27]. In this study, a computer model of 80,000 women undergoing artificial insemination with donor sperm showed that if all women chose to use fresh sperm from donors that were tested but where sperm was not frozen and quarantined, there would be over 8,000 more births per year with a mean cost of $15,501 less than with use of banked donor sperm. Furthermore, the model suggests that one recipient would become infected with HIV every 5.1 years, during which time 180,000 noninfected children would be borne [27].

33.4 Sperm Donor Testing

Both federal and state regulations require testing for HIV 1 and 2, HTLVI/II, Hepatitis B and C, and other sexually transmitted infections (i.e., syphilis, N. gonorrhea, and Chlamydia trachomatis). Nucleic acid tests (NAT) must be used if FDA-approved tests are available for a particular analyte. Currently, NAT testing is available for HIV-1, Hepatitis C and most recently, N. gonorrhea. Donors must also undergo rigorous review of medical, family, and social histories, and have a physical examination focusing on the urogenital system. Sperm must then be frozen and quarantined for 6 months, followed by retesting prior to release for artificial insemination. Statutes also regulate who can be a sperm donor, that is, sperm donors must be at low risk for STDs, particularly HIV and hepatitis.

The FDA requires all facilities that process, store, and distribute donor sperm, oocytes, or embryos to be registered with the Center for Biologics (CBER) of the FDA. New York State requires that all facilities processing, storing, and distributing donor sperm be licensed by the state as a tissue bank. Furthermore, NYS requires that any NYS physician or ART program utilizing donor sperm for artificial insemination acquire the donor sperm from an NYS licensed sperm bank. This insures that the donors would be screened and sperm quarantined according to the NYS regulations. Although the state and federal regulations may appear cumbersome and often confusing, the regulations are aimed at protecting the public health and minimizing the risk of communicable disease transmission.

The FDA regulations (21CFR 1271) address only communicable disease testing, and does not refer to any additional testing such as genetic testing or general health testing of the donors or recipients. On the other hand, NYS for example does require testing for certain nontrivial genetic malformations for which genetic tests are available such as cystic fibrosis deletion testing, Tay Sach's disease, sickle cell anemia, thalassemia, and hemoglobinopathies. Karyotyping is not required by any regulations, and has not been recommended [28].

Both federal and state regulations define anonymous and directed sperm donors. Commercially available donor sperm is acquired from donors who wish to remain anonymous to the recipients as well as to the child. Many sperm banks offer identity release programs where the donor can agree to have their identity released, once the offspring has reached the age of maturity (i.e., 18 years of age). Only the offspring can request the donor identity from the participating sperm bank where the donor has agreed to identity release. Not all sperm donors agree to identity release, and regulations do not require identity release. In fact, current NYS regulations require that the sperm donors remain anonymous. Recently, a review of US donor insemination programs demonstrated that an increasing number of programs are offering open-identity donors, particularly with oocyte donation [29]. In Canada, studies have shown that sperm donors who are more likely to be identified to the offspring are more likely to donate sperm altruistically [30]. The Canadian Assisted Human Reproduction Act of 2004 prohibited the payment of donors of sperm or oocytes for their donation. In the UK, sperm donors must agree to identity release, with their identity being on a national registry [31]. The Human Fertilization and Embryology Act of 1990 established a registry of children born from donor insemination, mandated donor identity release, set standards for semen storage, as well as standards for donor selection and screening, consent, counseling, and legal issues [31]. Any US sperm bank transporting donor sperm into the UK must accompany the shipment with a donor identity release authorization.

Donor insemination has been used in greater numbers to provide for biological children to single women, as well as women in same-sex committed relationships. Reports of single women who choose to become mothers using a sperm donor are scarce [32]. One report demonstrated that in 62 families headed by a single woman, the socio-economic development of the children seems to be within the normal range, while about one-fifth of the women gave birth to twins, the health conditions of the mothers and children and difficulties encountered by the mothers raised some concerns [32]. The incidence of birth defects and health problems in the offspring conceived with frozen sperm has been shown to be similar to that in the general population [22]. The psychosocial development of these children, however, is not as well reported due to the confidentiality concerning sperm donation, and the desire of these parents not to tell anyone about the circumstances of their children's conception [22].

33.5 Laboratory Procedures for Sperm Cryopreservation

Cryopreservation is cell-specific, is dependent upon the cells' water permeability and the amount of intracellular water, as well as the type of cryopreservative medium used in the process. Spermatozoa are ideal cells to cryopreserve since they have a relatively small volume, a large surface area, and very little cytoplasm (hence very little intracellular water) than many other cells. Human semen has been successfully cryopreserved since 1953, with glycerol as the most widely used cryoprotectant [5].

Following cryopreservation, there is a significant decrease in sperm motility, velocity, and viability upon thaw [33], with a TEST-yolk buffered medium with 10% glycerol faring better than straight glycerol as the cryoprotectant. There is a significant variability between samples in sperm motility, motion characteristics, and survival rate compared to variability in prefreeze sperm parameters [34]. However, Agarwal et al. [14] have shown that the effect of cryopreservation on sperm quality was identical to its effect on sperm from normal fertile men, and this and other reports demonstrated that normal fertile sperm survived significantly better than semen specimens from infertile men or the poorer quality semen specimens from cancer patients [35]. Regardless of the methodology used for sperm cryopreservation, a 40–60% decrease in sperm motility and viability is expected, although certain methods, cryopreservatives, packaging, freeze rate, storage, and thawing technique will affect that survival. Cryopreservation of sperm is much easier, and more successful than embryo or oocyte cryopreservation, and it is probably due to the differences in the sperm cell anatomy, and the fact that the concentration of sperm allows loss of cells with a relatively low decrease in fertility as compared to the similar effects on oocytes or embryos.

Glycerol is the cryoprotectant of choice for human spermatozoa, and is used at a concentration of 5–10%. Cryosurvival rates improve with the addition of glycerol to more complex buffering systems [36]. An early study compared the effects of eight different media on postthaw sperm motility [37]. Two extenders combining zwitterions, TES and TRIS with sodium citrate and egg yolk, were superior to others and were considered to be the optimal extenders for maintaining sperm viability after thawing. Hallak and coworkers [12] compared sperm motility, morphology, and membrane integrity in sperm frozen with TEST-yolk-glycerol and glycerol alone media and showed that TEST-yolk-glycerol resulted in significantly better motility, morphology, and sperm membrane integrity. An egg yolk-based freezing medium has been commercialized, and has been the cryoprotectant of choice for freezing of human sperm [38]. Another medium developed by Mahadevan and Trounson known as Human Sperm Preservation Medium (HSPM) containing Tyrode's buffer and glycerol but no egg yolk showed a higher yield of motile sperm than an egg yolk containing medium [39]. However, in other studies, TEST-yolk medium showed a significantly higher recovery of motile sperm as compared to HSPM, particularly when slow freezing was done as compared to rapid vapor freezing [40]. Although morphology was the same using all methods, these authors concluded that TEST-yolk buffer was the superior cryopreservative. Furthermore, in specimens where more than 50% of sperm were normal morphologically, the best postthaw recovery of motile sperm was achieved. Chromatin packaging and morphology, as well as membrane integrity and viability of human sperm decrease significantly after freezing and thawing [23], whether slow programmable freezing is used or rapid vapor freezing, although those with a normal morphology prior to freezing seem to withstand the freeze-thaw procedure better than low-quality specimens [41]. The egg yolk-based "TEST-yolk" buffer freezing medium is routinely used for preparation of ICI ready sperm.

Recently, Hossain and Osuamkpe [38] demonstrated that a 100 mM concentration of sucrose with rapid freezing showed a satisfactory postthaw motility and viability as compared with higher concentrations of sucrose. Many cryopreservatives have been evaluated for effects on sperm survivability, including dimethlysufoxide (DMSO), which was proven to be superior to propanediol and glycerol for maintenance of structure and function of frozen testicular tissue [42, 43]. Similarly, ethylene glycol was shown to be better than glycerol or DMSO for acrosome preservation of human spermatozoa [44]. Since both egg yolk and serum albumin are of animal origin and thus risk human exposure to animal viruses, others have utilized lecithin along with DMSO and glycerol with promising results (Reed, M.; Jeyendran, RS. personal communication). A novel intrauterine insemination (IUI)-ready cryoprotectant has been developed using HEPES-buffered human tubal fluid, with 1% human serum albumin, 4% sucrose, and 6% glycerol for semen samples prefreeze processed by gradient separation [45, 46]. Similar buffering systems have been commercialized to prepare washed sperm for cryopreservation.

33.6 Laboratory Techniques for Sperm Cryopreservation

The simplest method for freezing spermatozoa involves addition of glycerol to a final concentration of 7.5–8.0%. However, glycerol alone has been replaced by more sophisticated cryopreservatives that result in better sperm survival after freezing and thaw. TEST-yolk buffer medium contains a 15% concentration of glycerol and is added at a ratio of 1:1 semen to yolk buffer. Any cryopreservative is added in a very slow, dropwise fashion so as to minimize osmotic shock to the spermatozoa. Following thorough mixing, the semen-cryopreservative mixture can be aliquoted into cryovials or straws, usually at a volume of 0.5 ml per vessel.

Semen can also be processed by either gradient centrifugation or centrifugation wash procedure prior to cryopreservation to prepare an IUI-ready specimen. In these instances, the sperm can be processed or washed using the laboratory's standard protocol using media, such as an HEPES-buffered human tubal fluid or Ham's F-10 medium, all commercially available. The resulting sperm pellet would then be resuspended in nutrient medium, and the appropriate cryopreservative added to a final concentration of 7.5–8.0% glycerol.

Vials or straws of semen can either be frozen using a controlled rate freezer, which slowly reduces the temperature of the specimen, or a manual method. Once again, regardless of the technique utilized, sperm appear to be hearty enough with adequate survival after freezing and thawing, to suggest the use of the simplest and most cost effective method for cryopreservation. In the age of assisted reproduction using ICSI, even the lowest sperm counts, and testicular tissue or epididymal aspirates can be successfully frozen, thawed, and utilized to achieve fertilization and pregnancy.

Once the vials or straws are filled, if a programmable freezer is to be used, the specimens are placed into the freezer and the preprogrammed freezing cycle is initiated. A common freezing program begins with the specimen at room temperature, followed by cooling at a rate of −50°C per minute to 4°C, then at a rate of −10°C per minute to −80°C. The specimens are held at −80°C for 10 min, and then plunged into liquid nitrogen (LN). Other programs have also been successful for freezing sperm, and each should be validated for any individual laboratory.

For manual freezing, a test tube of the semen can be placed first into a beaker of room temperature water, which is then held in a refrigerator for 30–45 min. This allows slow cooling of the sperm. The semen is then aliquoted into cooled vials or straws, loaded onto a cryo cane, then suspended for 10 min approximately 1 in. above the LN level in a tank (approximately −75°C). The cane is then plunged into the LN for storage. A second manual method involves placing the vials onto a metal cane at room temperature, followed by placing the cane directly into an LN-charged dry shipper for 30 min. This dry shipper is presumably at LN temperature. The cane on which the vials are suspended can then be plunged directly into the liquid phase of an LN storage tank.

It is important that a test vial of semen be thawed approximately 24–48 h after initial freezing to determine the rate of sperm survival. This is a routine procedure with fertile donor sperm. However, with client sperm prior to disease treatment, a test vial may not be possible since the sperm parameters are initially poor, and it is necessary to freeze as much of the sperm as possible.

33.7 Storage of Cryopreserved Semen

The storage container, either vial or straw, should be able to be withstand the temperatures of freezing, storage, and thawing without loss of integrity. It should also be sealed after packaging to remain impervious to microbial particles during the entire cryopreservation and thawing process.

Specimens are generally stored directly in liquid nitrogen in special dewars. It is important that cells are stored at less than −135°C, because it is at this temperature that all molecular activity ceases. At higher temperatures, water may re-crystallize, inducing cellular injury. In the past, mechanical freezers were available that presumably maintained the specimens at less than this temperature. However, these methods for semen storage did not gain favor, and thus, LN storage tanks have continued to be the accepted method for semen storage.

33.8 Cross Contamination

Donors of semen for artificial insemination are chosen from the low risk population and are rigorously tested for sexually transmitted diseases, thus posing a relatively low risk of transmission between vials in a cryo storage tank. Sperm bankers or client depositors, from the general population, are not screened for sexually transmitted infections, and thus there may be more of a risk that vials from such men might carry disease. For the risk, however, to become an effective danger, the microorganisms in semen must be capable of transmitting disease, and most importantly, must survive the freezing and thawing procedure [47]. N. gonorrhea has been known to survive storage in LN for 18 months [48], and the addition of antibiotics do not appear to eliminate the risk of transmission [47, 49]. In addition, both mycoplasma hominis and ureaplasma urealyticum have survived freezing and thawing [50], as did Chlamydia [51], herpes simplex virus-2 [52], cytomegalovirus [53], and hepatitis C [54, 55]. On the other hand, yeasts and Trichomonas vaginalis [50] did not survive cryopreservation. In one notable study, Matz et al. [56] reported an HIV-1 infection after insemination with fresh semen. However, those women who received frozen semen from the same donor did not show any signs of HIV infection, presumably because cryopreservation led to a decline in viral titer [47, 56]. Mazzilli et al. [47] recommend the use of quarantine tanks to store specimens for 6 months before placing specimens in a main storage system, once retesting results are negative for STDs. They suggest, correctly however, that because of the long incubation periods for viruses, such as HIV and hepatitis and the impossibility of covering all pathogens, that use of quarantine holding tanks is not realistic.

The actual risk of transmission of pathogens in an LN tank, therefore, is not known and can only be theoretically assumed. Several cases of hepatitis B transmission have been reported following leakage of blood bags in a storage tank [57]. Several organisms have been identified in semen and embryos stored for 6–35 years, although none were pathogenic to humans [47, 58]. Some of the organisms were found in the samples, others in the liquid nitrogen, none were cross contaminated. Although there have been no reported cases of cross contamination in tanks of reproductive tissue, there is a theoretical risk. For reasons such as this, many regulatory bodies mandate separate storage of donor semen (from tested donors) and client semen (nontested patients).

There are several ways to minimize the risk of cross contamination within an LN storage dewar. Straws and vials must be sealed properly. Vials must have intact "O" rings, and caps must be secure. Labs should utilize vials or straws guaranteed to withstand LN temperatures. Ionomeric resin straws currently available commercially appear to be one of the most secure types of containers [59].

There has been controversy over storage of reproductive tissue either in the liquid phase or vapor phase of LN not only to maintain cell viability, but also most importantly to reduce or eliminate the possibility of microbial cross contamination between vials or straws in the liquid phase of LN [60]. There are protocols for storage in LN vapor as opposed to the liquid phase. These involve setting the level of liquid such that the specimen level is located where the stored specimens would be maintained at LN temperature or at least lower than −135°C. Special thermometers or thermocouples inserted into an LN tank can be employed to record the temperature at the specimen level in the tank, and set off alarms in the event that the temperature rises above a set level.

The manufacturer's recommendations for the care of the LN tanks should be followed carefully. For liquid storage, LN levels should be closely monitored to make sure they continually cover stored specimens. Tanks should be examined regularly for the presence of frost or defects on the exterior. An increase in the filling frequency or exterior frost build up could indicate that a dewar may be in the process of failing. Replacement or repair is warranted. At a minimum, however, specimens should be removed to a different tank to prevent loss of specimens. The laboratory's quality control program should include recording the liquid nitrogen levels and filling activities of each liquid nitrogen refrigerator. NYS regulations require tank LN levels to be measured at least twice in a 7-day period of time. Many facilities employ monitored alarms for automatic tank filling and to detect low liquid levels or out of range vapor temperatures for additional measure of safety for specimen storage.

33.9 Transport of Cryopreserved Semen

Transportation of cryopreserved sperm must be at LN temperature to maintain the specimens in the frozen state. Shifts in temperature above the threshold of −135°C can be detrimental to cell survival. TEST-yolk buffer was able to maintain postthaw sperm motility during shipping and handling better than glycerol alone as the cryopreservative [61]. Furthermore, motility was significantly compromised in specimens stored more than 2 days in an LN shipping dewar if frozen in glycerol vs. yolk buffer [61]. Thus, it is imperative that specimens be handled and transported using very careful and validated methods.

Specimens should be shipped or transported using "dry shippers". These are dewars, which have an inner core that absorbs the LN, maintaining the chamber at LN temperature. All of the LN is absorbed into the tank lining, and thus liquid is not present in the central chamber. The liquid phase of LN is considered a hazardous substance and as such is not allowed to be transported by airplane. However, dry shippers do not contain liquid nitrogen, and thus are able to be shipped by major carriers.

Dry shippers can maintain LN temperature for several days. It is imperative that tanks containing frozen semen or embryos be shipped by priority overnight shipping. Shippers used for transport must be appropriately validated to insure that they are functioning properly and will hold temperature for the stated interval of days. Tanks should be handled according to the manufacturer's requirements to insure that the tanks maintain temperature, do not leak, and maintain the specimens in a frozen state. Use of a reputable facility for storage and transport of reproductive specimens, many of which are irreplaceable, is strongly recommended.

33.10 Clinical Aspects of use of Frozen Semen in Artificial Insemination and Art

Use of frozen-thawed semen is now a routine procedure in clinical ART. The question arises, however, which type of artificial insemination – intrauterine insemination (IUI) or intracervical insemination (ICI) is most efficacious. Most if not all commercial sperm banks provide semen specimens, which are "ICI" (intracervical) or "IUI" (intrauterine) ready.

The choice of whether to perform an ICI or IUI with thawed semen is left to the reproductive endocrinologist. For cervical insemination, results have shown that insemination should be performed two consecutive days based on ovulation timing [62]. Many studies, however, have demonstrated that IUI is superior to ICI, and most physicians will perform an IUI for two consecutive days as well. The monthly fecundity rate for IUI has been shown to be significantly higher as compared to ICI [63–65]. These results were confirmed by subsequent meta-analysis [66]. The results were similar in a study of ICI vs. IUI in single women with no known fertility problems [67].

Recently, Wolf et al. [46] demonstrated similar IUI fecundity rates using IUI-ready donor sperm as compared to conventional cryopreserved sperm based on both prospective and retrospective assessments. Since ICI specimens are frozen as whole semen plus cryopreservative, this specimen must be processed to remove the seminal contaminants and cryopreservative prior to an intrauterine insemination. Generally, thawed ICI vials should be minimally manipulated to reduce spermatozoa loss due to the shock of processing. Thawed semen can be diluted slowly with nutrient medium, preferably HEPES-buffered human tubal medium (HTF) [68], centrifuged at 280–300×g for 10 min, and the sperm pellet resuspended in HTF for the insemination. The only concern is that centrifugation of the whole thawed semen concentrates in the pellet both motile and nonmotile sperm, cells, and debris for placement into the uterus. Gradient centrifugation of thawed semen results in a significant loss of sperm numbers, but a clean specimen relatively devoid of dead cells and debris. A low concentration of motile sperm can be used for IVF/ICSI, so this is not of concern, but a low recovery of motile sperm is not favorable for standard insemination. It appears that gradient preparation prior to cryopreservation might be superior to washing after thawing for the IUI, particularly for high-quality donor sperm specimens. Low sperm count specimens, such as from client depositors, would still be frozen as raw semen with TEST-yolk buffer.

References

1. Centers for Disease Control (1988) Semen Banking, organ and tissue transplantation and HIV antibody testing. In: Morbidity and Mortality Weekly Report 37:58–59
2. Meirow D, Schenker JG (1993) Sperm donation – should the use of frozen-thawed semen alter treatment modalities? Int J Fertil 38:325–331
3. Merino G, Murrieta S, Rodriguez L, Sandoval C (1994) Semen cryopreservation/artificial insemination. Mol Androl 6:170–175
4. Ginsburg KA, Montgomery-Rice V (1996) Therapeutic donor insemination: screening, indications and technique. In: Centola GM, Ginsburg KA (eds) Evaluation and treatment of the infertile male. Cambridge University Press, Cambridge, pp 171–193
5. Bunge RG, Sherman JK (1953) Fertilizing capacity of frozen human spermatozoa. Nature 172:767
6. Sherman JK (1973) Synopsis fo the use of frozen semen since 1964: State of the art of human semen banking. Fertil Steril 24:397–412
7. Clarke GN, Liu deY, Baker HW (2006) Recovery of human sperm motility and ability to interact with the human zona pellucida after more than 28 years of storage in liquid nitrogen. Fertil Steril 86:721–722
8. Schover LR, Brey K, Lichtin A, Lipshultz LI, Jeha S (2002) Oncologists' attitudes and practices regarding banking sperm before cancer treatment. J Clin Oncol 20:1890–1897
9. Anger JT, Gilbert BR, Goldstein M (2003) Cryopresrvation of sperm: indications, methods and results. J Urol 170:1079–1084
10. Ben Rhouma K, Marrakchi H, Khouja H, Attalah K, Ben Miled E, Sakly M (2003) Outcome of intracytoplasmic injection of fresh and frozen-thawed testicular spermatozoa. A comparative study. J Reprod Med 48:349–354
11. Boyle KE, Thomas AJ, Marmar JL, Hirschberg S, Belker AM, Jarow JP (2006) Sperm harvesting and cryopreservation during vasectomy reversal is not cost effective. Fertil Steril 85:961–964
12. Hallak J, Sharma RK, Wellstead C, Agarwal A (2000) Cryopreservation of human spermatozoa: comparison of TEST-yolk buffer and glycerol. Int J Fertil Women's Med 45:38–42
13. Ragni G, Somigliana E, Restelli L, Salvi R, Arnoldi M, Paffoni A (2003) Sperm banking and rate of assisted reproduction treatment: insights from a 15-year cryopreservation program for male cancer patients. Cancer 97:1624–1629
14. Agarwal A, Tolentino MV Jr, Sidhu RS, Avzman I, Lee JC, Thomas AJ Jr, Shekarriz M (1995) Effect of cryopreservation on semen quality in patients with testicular cancer. Urology 46:382–389
15. Agarwal A (2000) Semen banking in patients with cancer: 20 year experience. Int J Androl 23:16–19
16. Chung K, Irani J, Knee G, Efymow B, Blasco L, Patrizio P (2004) Sperm cryopreservation for male patients with cancer: an epidemiological analysis at the University of Pennsylvania. Eur J Obstet Gynecol Reprod Biol 113:S7–S11
17. Walschaerts M, Muller A, Daudin M, Hennebicq S, Eric H, Thonneau P (2007) Sperm cryopreservation: Recent and marked increase in use for testicular cancer compared with hodgkin disease. J Androl 28:801–803
18. Donnelly ET, Steele EK, McClure N, Lewis SEM (2001) Assessment of DNA integrity and morphology of ejaculated sperm from fertile and infertile men before and after cryopreservation. Hum Reprod 16:1191–1199
19. Thepot F, Mayaux MJ, Czyglick F, Wack T, Selva J, Jalbert P (1996) Incidence of birth defects after artificial insemination with frozen donor spermatozoa: a collaborative study of the French CECOS federation on 11535 pregnancies. Hum Reprod 11:2319–2323
20. Rives N, Sibert L, Clavier B, Delabroye V, Marpeau L, Mace B (1998) Full-term delivery following intracytoplasmic sperm injection with frozen-thawed immotile testicular spermatozoa. Hum Reprod 13:3399–3401
21. Patrizio P, Ord T, Balmaceda JP, Asch R (1995) Successful fertilization, pregnancy and birth using epididymal sperm frozen 24 hours after conventional oocyte insemination. Fertil Steril 64:863–865
22. Lansac J, Royere D (2001) Follow-up studies of children born after frozen sperm donation. Hum Reprod 7:33–37
23. Gandini L, Lombardo F, Lenzi A, Spano M, Dondero F (2006) Cryopreservaiton and sperm DNA integrity. Cell Tiss Bank 7:91–98
24. David G, Czyglick F, DaLage C, Alnot MO, Dadoune JP, Auger J, Thepot F, Boulanger JC, Bugnon C, Clavequin MC, Meunier J, Berjeon J, Izard J, Sauvalle A, Boucher D, Janny J, Jalbert P, Servoz-Gavin M, Delecour M (1989) Artificial procreation with frozen donor semen: Experience of the French Federation CECOS. Hum Reprod 4:757–761
25. U.S. Congress OTA (1988) Artificial insemination practice in the United States: Summary of a 1987 survey: background paper. OTA-BP-BA-48. Washington, DC. U.S. Government Printing Office
26. McLaughlin EA (2002) Cryopreservation, screening and storage of sperm the challenges for the twenty-first century. Hum Fertil 5:S61–S65
27. Payne MA, Lamb EJ (2004) Use of frozen semen to avoid human immunodeficiency virus type 1 transmission by donor insemination: A cost effective analysis. Fertil Steril 81:80–92
28. del Mar Perez M, Marina S, Egozcue J (1990) Karyotype screening of potential sperm donors for artificial insemination. Hum Reprod 5:282–285
29. Scheib JE, Cushing RA (2007) Open-identity donor insemination in the United States. Is it on the rise? Fertil Steril 88:231–232
30. Daniels K, Feyles V, Nisker J, perez-v-Perez M, Newton C, Parker JA, Tekpetev F, Haase J (2006) Sperm donation: implications of Canada's assisted human reproduction act 2004 for recipients,

donors, health professionals and institutions. J Obstet Gynaecol Can 28:608–615
31. HFEA (1997) Sixth Annual Report, Human fertilisation and embryology Authority, London
32. Weissenberg R, Landau R, Madgar I (2007) Older single mothers assisted by sperm donation and their children. Hum Reprod 22:2784–2791
33. Keel BA, Webster BW (1989) Semen analysis data from fresh and cryopreserved donor ejaculated: Comparison of cryoprotectants and pregnancy rates. Fertil Steril 52:100–105
34. Nallella KP, Sharma RK, Said TM, Agarwal A (2004) Inter-sample variability in post-thaw human spermatozoa. Cryobiology 49:195–199
35. Centola GM, Raubertas RF, Mattox JH (1992) Cryopreservation of human semen: Comparison of cryopreservatives, sources of variability and prediction of post-thaw survival. J Androl 13:283–288
36. Mazur P (1993) Fundamental cryobiology. In: 1993 Regional Postgraduate Course. Cryopreservation of spermatozoa and embryos. The American Fertility Society, Birmingham, AL, pp 1–32
37. Prins GS, Weidel L (1986) A comparative study of buffer systems as cryoprotectants for human spermatozoa. Fertil Steril 46:147
38. Hossain AM, Osuamkpe CO (2007) Sole use of sucrose in human sperm cryopreservation. Arch Androl 53:99–103
39. Mahadevan M, Trouson AO (1983) Effect of cryopreservative media and dilution methods on the preservation of human spermatozoa. Andrologia 15:355–366
40. Stanic P, Tandara M, Sonicki Z, Simunic V, Radakovic B, Suchanek E (2000) Comparison of protective media and freezing techniques for cryopreservation of human semen. Eur J Obstet Gynecol Reprod Biol 91:65–70
41. Hammadeh ME, Dehn C, Hippach M, Zeginiadou T, Steiber M, Georg T, Rosenbaum P, Schmidt W (2001) Comparison between computerized slow-stage and static liquid nitrogen vapour freezing methods with respect to the deleterious effect on chromatin and morphology of spermatozoa from fertile and subfertile men. Int J Androl 24:66–72
42. Keros V, Rosenlund B, Hultenby K, Aghajanova L, Levkov L, Hovatta O (2005) Optimizing cryopreservation of human testicular tissue: Comparison of protocols with glycerol, propanediol and dimethylsulphoxide as cryoprotectants. Hum reprod 20:1676–1687
43. Keros V, Hultenby K, Borgstron B, Fridstrom M, Jahnukainen K, Hovatto O (2007) Methods of cryopreservation of testicular tissue with viable spermatogonia in pre-pubertal boys undergoing gonadotoxic cancer treatment. Hum Reprod 22:1384–1395
44. Ortloff C, Deppe M, Schill WB, Sanchez R (2006) A new technique to evaluate the ability of cryoprotectors to prevent premature acrosome reaction in human spermatozoa. Andrologia 38:230–232
45. Larson JM, McKinney KA, Mixon BA, Burry KA, Wolf DP (1997) An intrauterine insemination-ready cryopreservation method compared with sperm recovery after conventional freezing and post-thaw processing. Fertil Steril 68:143–148
46. Wolf DP, Patton PE, Burry KA, Kaplan PF (2001) Intrauterine insemination-ready versus conventional semen cryopreservation for donor insemination: a comparison of retrospective results and a prospective, randomized trial. Fertil Steril 76:181–185
47. Mazzilli F, Delfino M, Imbrogno N, Elia J, Dondero F (2006) Survival of micro-organisms in cryostorage of human sperm. Cell Tissue Banking 7:75–79
48. Sherman JK, Rosenfeld J (1975) Importance of frozen-stored human semen in the spread of gonorrhea. Fertil Steril 26:1043–1047
49. Glander HJ, Schonborn C, Rytter M (1983) Microbiolocial investigations on cryopreserved human semen. Int J Androl 6:358–366
50. Glander HJ, Schonborn C, Rytter M (1983) Microbioligcal investigations on cryopreserved human semen. Int J Androl 6:358–366
51. Thorsen P, Moller BR, Halkier-Sorensen L, From E, Nielson NC (1991) Survival of Chlamydia in human semen prepared for artificial insemination by donor. Acta Obstet Gynecol Scand 70:133–135
52. Sherman JK, Menna JH (1986) Cryosurvival of herpes simplex virus-2 during cryopreservation of human spermatozoa. Cryobiology 23:383–385
53. Mansat A, Mengelle C, Chalet M, Boumzebra A, Mieusset R, Puel J, Prouheze C, Segondy M (1997) Cytomegalovirus detection in cryopreserved semen samples collected for therapeutic donor insemination. Hum Reprod 12:1663–1666
54. McKee TA, Avery S, Majid A, Brindsen PR (1996) Risks for transmission of hepatitis C virus during artificial insemination. Fertil Steril 66:161–163
55. Massey EJ, Dasani H, Jones P, Saleem AK (1996) Storage of sperm and embryos. Storage facility exists for sperm from patients positive for antibody to hepatitis C virus. BMJ 313:1078
56. Matz B, Kupfer B, Ko Y, Walger P, Vetter H, Eberle J, Gurtler L (1998) HIV-1 infection by artificial insemination. Lancet 351:728
57. Tedder RS, Gilson RJ, Briggs M, Loveday C, Cameron CH, Garson JA, Kelly GE, Weller IV (1991) Hepatitis C virus: evidence for secual transmission. BMJ 302:1299–1302
58. Bielanski A, Bergeron H, Lau PC, Devenish J (2003) Microbial contamination of embryos and semen during long term banking in liquid nitrogen. Cryobiology 46:146–152
59. Lwtur-Konirsch H, Collin G, Sifer C, Devaux A, Kurttenn F, Madelanat P, Brun-Vezinet F, Feldmann F, Benifla JL (2003) Safety of cryopreservation straws for human gametes or embryos: a study with human immunodeficiency virus-1 under cryopreservation conditions. Hum Reprod 18:140–144
60. Tomlinson M, Sakkas D (2000) Is a review of standard procedures for cryopreservation needed? Safe and effective cryopreservation-should sperm banks and fertility centers move toward storage in liquid nitrogen vapour? Hum Reprod 12:2460–2463
61. Carrell DT, Wilcox AL, Urry RL (1996) Effect of fluctuations in temperature encountered during handling and shipment of human cryopreserved semen. Andrologia 28:315–319
62. Centola GM, Mattox J, Raubertas R (1990) Pregnancy rates after double versus single insemination with frozen semen. Fertil Steril 54:1089–1092
63. Patton PE, Burry KA, Thurmond A, Novy MJ, Wolf DP (1992) Intrauterine insemination outperforms intracervical insemination in a randomized, controlled study with frozen, donor semen. Fertil Steril 57:559–564
64. Matorras R, Pijoan JI, Gorostiaga A, Ramon O, Diez J, Rodriguez-Escudero FJ, Corcostegui B (1996) Intrauterine insemination with frozen sperm increases pregnancy rates in donor insemination cycles under gonadotropin stimulation. Fertil Steril 65:620–625
65. Patton PE (2005) Optimizing success in a donor insemination program. In: Patton PE, Battaglia DE (eds) Office andrology, Humana Press, Totowa, NJ, pp 91–108
66. Goldberg JM, Mascha E, Falcone T, Attaran M (1999) Comparision of intrauterine and intracervical insemination with frozen donor sperm: A meta-analysis. Fertil Steril 72:792–795
67. Carroll N, Palmer JR (2001) A comparison of intrauterine versus intracervical insemination in fertile single women. Fertil Steril 75:656–660
68. Byrd W, Ackerman GE, Bradshaw KD, Maddox MA, Svendsen BA, Carr BR (1991) Comparison of bicarbonate and HEPES-buffered media on pregnancy rates after intrauterine insemination with cryopreserved donor sperm. Fertil Steril 56:540–546

Chapter 34
Reproductive Treatment of HIV-1 Discordant Couples

Valeria Savasi and Enrico Ferrazzi

Abstract The total number of people living with HIV had reached 39.5 million. In developed countries, the major risk for HIV transmission is by heterosexual intercourse. The general conditions and life expectancy of many patients with HIV infection are very good, and three-quarters of these individuals are in their reproductive years. For these reasons, a significant percentage of young couples with HIV in one partner can be expected to make plans for the future and to desire children. Clinicians practicing assisted reproduction should become familiar with guidelines for care in HIV-1 discordant couples in order to prevent HIV-1 transmission.

Recent findings: The main themes covered by this chapter include: epidemiology of HIV-1 in the world; biology of the virus and its presence in the various parts of the sperm; recently published guidelines from the American Society for Reproductive Medicine; ethics and recommendations concerning assisted reproduction in people infected by virus; and clinical practices and evidence-based guidelines that allow assisted reproduction in HIV-serodiscordant couples.

Summary: This chapter will review the safety, counselling points, and outcomes of HIV-1 serodiscordant couples undergoing assisted reproduction with sperm washing and other advanced reproductive technologies used to prevent HIV transmission in our center.

Keywords Assisted reproductive technique • HIV • Sperm washing • Serodiscordant couple

34.1 Introduction

According to the latest UNAIDS/World Health Organization (WHO) [1] update (December 2006), the total number of people living with HIV-1 infection had reached 39.5 million. We know that early diagnosis of HIV-1 infection [2] and timely access to medical care can improve treatment outcomes and potentially decrease the risk of transmission [3]. In developed countries, the major risk for HIV-1 transmission is by heterosexual intercourse, and the number of contaminations is increasing [4]. In the past, the drug users were the biggest reserve of the virus, and the majority of the subjects addicted to drugs were men. For these reasons, women today are at risk to be infected by heterosexual intercourse. Male-to-female transmission of HIV-1 is now estimated to be 1 per 1,000 acts of unprotected intercourses [5–9], and it depends on many factors, such as viremia, virospermia, $CD4^+$ count, and genital infections, etc. Major advances in pharmaceutical research have greatly improved the prognosis of patients with HIV-1 infection. Correct clinical and therapeutic management of these patients enables the disease to be maintained in a chronic state, and, in most cases, avoid fatal progression. The general conditions and life expectancy of many patients with HIV infection are very good, and three-quarters of these individuals are in their reproductive years. For these reasons, a significant percentage of young couples with HIV in one partner can be expected to make plans for the future and to desire children [10]. This desire for children in serodiscordant couples is at variance with recommendations that encourage the condom use in vaginal and anal contacts. Many of them now express the desire for parenthood as a fundamental part of healthy family life and a return to normalcy. Guidelines from the American Society for Reproductive Medicine (ASRM) and ethical recommendations concerning assisted reproduction in people infected by HIV have recently been modified to allow assisted reproduction in HIV-serodiscordant couples.

34.2 HIV in Semen

Araneta et al. [11] and Matz et al. [12] reported that semen used for donor artificial inseminations can transmit HIV-1 infection. However, studies on the presence of HIV in sperm have yielded contradictory results. Using different approaches, Baccetti et al. [13] detected HIV-1 particles and HIV-1 DNA in ejaculated sperm of HIV-seropositive patients. The same group identified a specific HIV receptor,

V. Savasi (✉) and E. Ferrazzi
Department of Obstetrics and Gynaecology, Sacco Clinical Sciences Institute, University of Milan Medical School, Milan, 74 20157, Italy
e-mail: valeria.savasi@unimi.it

DOI 10.1007/978-1-4419-1436-1_34,

alternative to CD4+, on the sperm membrane. This HIV receptor molecule is a galactosyl-alkyl-acylglycerol (GalAAG), a glycolipid structurally related to galactosylceramide and consistent with the receptor for HIV identified in CD4+ cells [13, 14]. At the same time, other authors report the total absence of HIV particles and nucleic acids in sperm [15–17], demonstrating that separation of seminal fluid and cellular elements from sperm by washing techniques, reduces the viral load of semen detected by PCR and RT-PCR. Semprini et al. [18] were the first to use washed sperm of HIV-1-infected men for intrauterine inseminations (IUI). There are several reports indicating that HIV-1 DNA cannot be found in washed spermatozoa separated from associated non-spermatozoa seminal cells and seminal plasma [16, 19, 20]. In contrast to these reassuring epidemiological and laboratory findings, there are reports indicating the possibility that HIV-1 virions are found attached to the sperm cells surface and even within its cytoplasm, by transmission electronic microscopy. Other papers report that proviral HIV-1 DNA can be detected in spermatozoa of men with acquired immune deficiency syndrome (AIDS), by extraction PCR, or found in spermatozoa of men infected with HIV-1, by in situ PCR (IS-PCR) [13, 21–36]. To investigate these contradictory findings and to assess the role of sperm-washing technique in eliminating both HIV-1 RNA and HIV-1 DNA from semen infected with HIV-1, we tested the ejaculates of men infected with HIV-1 before and after processing semen into the three main seminal fractions – nonspermatozoa cells, cell-free seminal plasma, and spermatozoa – by highly sensitive extractive nested PCR, and by IS-PCR. All samples of spermatozoa recovered after separation by gradient centrifugation and swim-up (sperm washing) were free of HIV-1 RNA (above our threshold of 50 copies/ml) and of proviral DNA (Table 34.1). This confirms findings of previous reports in which nested PCR [20, 37, 38] was used to assess the efficacy of sperm washing in HIV-infected semen. Although other more recent methodologies of sperm washing [39] confirm the validity of the general principle of removing the cellular component of semen, contradictory reports could be due to: the inaccuracy of PCR techniques in older studies [40]; a minimum threshold (one viral copy) of the PCR assay used to detect viral copies, which is set too low [38, 41, 42]; or, an improper use of the definition of sperm washing [43], without the final swim-up of spermatozoa. Of the seven seminal plasma samples that tested positive for HIV-1 RNA, six were from patients on HAART. Four men had elevated blood viral load and three had an undetectable viremia. These findings confirm previous findings reporting discrepancies between hematologic and seminal HIV-1 concentrations [20, 44], either due to subtherapeutic concentrations of antiretroviral drugs in the male seminal tract or due to local production of HIV-1 RNA from localized cells, which poorly respond to antiretroviral treatment. The false-positive detection of HIV-1 DNA by IS-PCR in semen of HIV-1-noninfected men confirm that this technique is not adequate for studying the presence of provirus in semen fractions. The presence of the virus in spermatozoa pellet samples could be due to the presence of nonspecific contaminants not completely eliminated during semen separation by discontinuous gradient centrifugation before swim-up. Alternatively, these could be real false-positive results due to nonspecific hybridization of IS-PCR. Bagasra et al. [23], Nuovo et al. [34] and Muciaccia et al. [35] showed the presence of provirus, through IS-PCR, in spermatozoa and germ cells at all stages of differentiation, from spermatogonium to round spermatids. However, in none of these studies were proper standards for IS-PCR specificity assessed in noninfected males. These methodological limitations of IS-PCR probably explain why in recent studies this technique has been abandoned. Fiore et al evaluated the relationship between the seminal HIV-1 viral load and the efficiency of a standardized sperm-washing procedure in removing HIV-1 RNA from semen samples. The results of his paper indicate that the amount of virus present in the original sample affects the efficiency of the procedure and that previous studies on sperm washing were performed on semen samples containing limited amounts of virus (generally less than 5×10^4 copies/mL). The bias of his study was that he used eight semen samples from eight healthy HIV-1 seronegative men and he tested semen for HIV-1 RNA after adding a different dilution of the virus. He hypothesized that the genital tract represents a distinct compartment compared with the blood and that viral loads in semen are variable irrespective

Table 34.1 Detection of HIV-1 RNA and HIV-1 DNA in semen compartments and in blood

	Whole semen	Seminal plasma	Non sperm cells	Washed-separated spermatozoa before swim-up	Washed-separated spermatozoa after swim-up	Peripheral blood
Number of sample	48	53	38	46	46	55
HIV-1 RNA positive tests N° (%)	2 (4%)	7 (13%)	1 (3%)	1 (2%)	0 (0%)	42 (76%)
Number of samples	54	–	52	46	46	55
HIV-1 DNA positive tests N° (%)	0 (0%)	–	8 (15%)	0 (0%)	0 (0%)	55 (100%)

of plasma loads and/or antiretroviral treatment. On the contrary, Vernazza holds that the risk of HIV-1 virus transmission depends exclusively on the viral load of the HIV-infected partner and proposes "an HIV-infected person on anti-retroviral therapy with completely suppressed viremia cannot propagate HIV through sexual contact."

34.2.1 Algorithm for Semen Processing and Sperm Washing with Swim Up

34.3 Semen Processing and Sperm Washing with Swim-Up

The following section describes the semen processing technique used in our work. (Algorithm for semen processing and sperm washing with swim-up) Semen analyses were performed and samples were processed using a 40–80% density gradient (Pureception Kit, Sage) to separate motile spermatozoa from nonsperm cells, immotile spermatozoa, and seminal plasma. The ejaculate was layered over the gradient and centrifuged at 400 g for 30 min. After centrifugation, the supernatant was removed and the sperm pellet recovered and resuspended in 3 ml of fresh medium (Sperm washing medium, Sage). A washing at 400 g for 10 min was performed and the supernatant was discarded. (Algorithm for sperm washing with swim-up) One ml of medium was subsequently gently layered on the pellet and the tube was incubated at 37° for 1 h. After swim-up, a supernatant volume of about 500 µl was recovered and an aliquot of this volume (100 µl) was tested for detectable HIV-1 RNA using a Real time PCR assay (Biomerieux), according to the manufacturer's instructions. The remaining washed sperm (400 µl) was stored at 4°for about 22 h and used for IUI, or IVF, IVF-ICSI (FIVET/ICSI) procedures, if the PCR test for HIV-1 was negative Fig. 34.1.

34.3.1 Algorithm for Sperm Washing with Swim-Up

ICSI/FIVET refers to FIVET with microdropelet insemination or ICSI using fresh or frozen spermatoza.

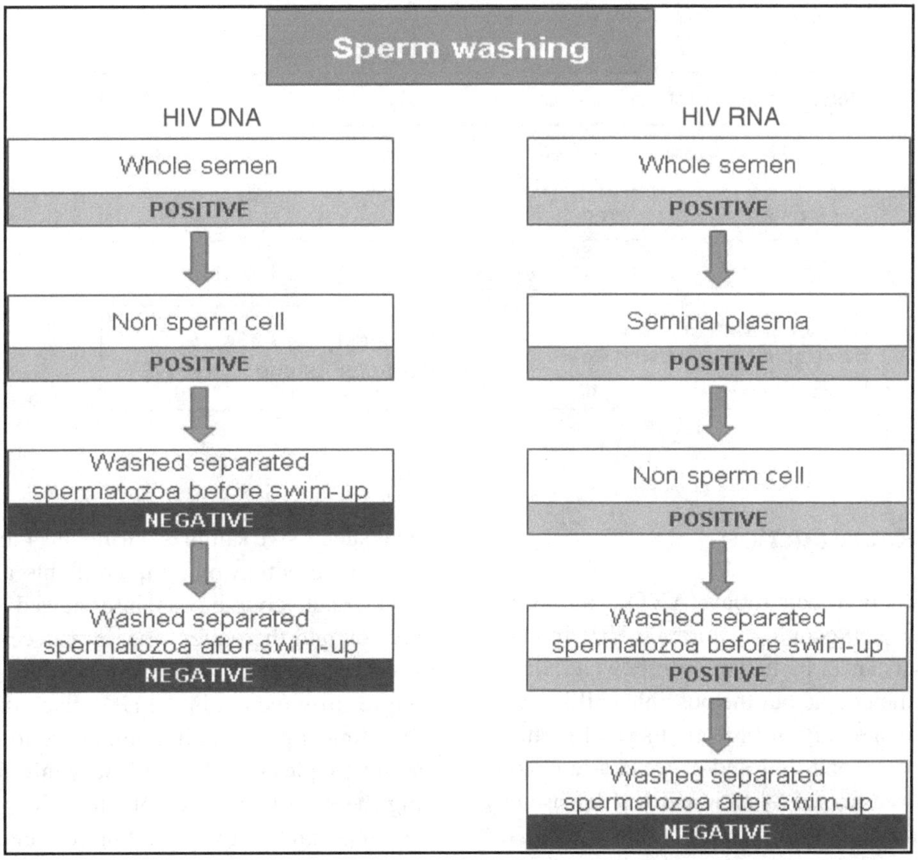

Fig. 34.1 Semen processing

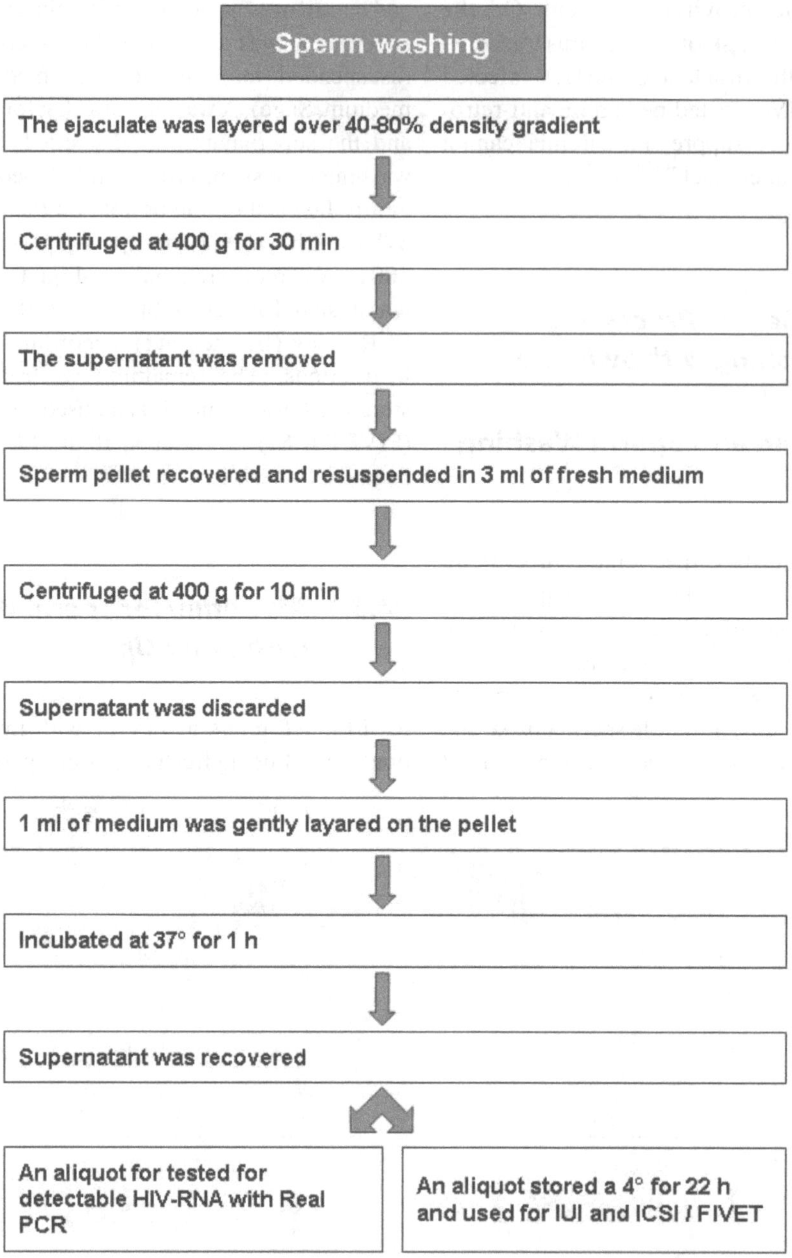

34.4 Assisted Reproduction

The assisted reproduction technology (ART) program was offered to serodiscordant couples with male HIV infection seeking medical assistance. Inclusion criteria were adopted to protect not only the couple but the possible child as well. Partners were to engage only in protected sexual relations. HIV status had to be monitored and/or treated, and long-term compliance was assessed by an infectious disease physician. Standard laboratory criteria were adopted: (1) CD4$^+$ lymphocytes >200/mm^3 at least twice in the 4 months prior to treatment; (2) stable viral load, with no increase >0.5 log in two successive samples during the 4 months prior to treatment; (3) infection by an quantifiable amplifiable strain of HIV-1. Each couple was interviewed by psychologist at inclusion and thereafter whenever necessary. Female fertility was assessed by standard procedures. Table 34.2 shows the infertility factors in the HIV discordant couples.

In clinical practice, it is important to screen the HIV discordant couples in order to identify infertility factors, considering the high prevalence of subfertility factors. One of the most important factors is testing for genital tract infection in both males and females. The exact mechanisms involved in male-to-female transmission of HIV-1 are as yet undefined,

Table 34.2 Infertility factors in HIV-1 discordant couples

Infertility factors	(%)
<1.5 m/ml motile spermatozoa after processing	16.5
Male genital tract infections	47
Female genital tract infections	29
Monolateral or bilateral tubal damage	12
Abnormalities of the uterine cavity	7
Endometriosis	1.5
Hyperprolactinaemia	14
Anovulatory cycles	0

Table 34.3 Microorganism isolated from urethra in HIV-1 positive men and their control HIV-1 negative men

Microorganism isolated from the urethra	HIV-positive subjects n 236 (%)	HIV-negative subjects n 202 (%)
Enterobacteriacee	10 (4.2)	23 (11.3)
Streptococci	13 (5.5)	38 (18.8)
Staphilococci	6 (2.5)	1 (0.5)
Enterobacter + Streptococci	–	5 (2.5)
Haemophilus	2 (0.8)	0
Corynebacterium	1 (0.4)	0
Chlamydia	10 (4.2)	0
Mycoplasma	45 (19)	2 (1)
Gardnerella	1 (0.4)	0
Trichomonas	1(0.4)	0
Candida Albicans	2 (0.8)	0
None	169 (71)	133 (66)

but circumstantial evidence indicates that genital tract infections may act as facilitating factors. In sub-Saharan and Latino American countries, where heterosexual transfer of the virus is the leading cause of infection, there is a high prevalence of carriers of genital infections. The presence of a sexually transmitted pathogen recruits inflammatory cells in both the male and female genital tract. This may increase the number of HIV-1 infected cells in the semen or vaginal fluid of the seropositive subject, leading to a higher risk of infection for the seronegative partner. Conversely, when the infection is present in the seronegative partner, the uninfected inflammatory cells may become a specific target for the virus. For all these reasons, we studied the prevalence of genital tract infections in a large cohort of heterosexual HIV-positive males who acquired the infection through drug addiction. To understand whether genital tract infections in these subjects were a consequence of their seropositivity and immunodeficiency or originated from their previous life style, we similarly tested for genital tract infections in a cohort of previously drug-addicted males who did not acquire HIV. The results are reported in Table 34.3. The data we report indicate that HIV-positive subjects who acquired HIV through drug-addiction have a high prevalence of genital tract infections. In the urethral samples of seropositive males, Mycoplasma hominis was isolated in 19% of cases and in only 1% of the seronegative subjects ($p<0.001$). As genital tract infections may facilitate male-to-female transmission of HIV, and HIV-infected subjects often ignore the recommendation for condom-protected intercourse, their detection and eradication may have an impact on the reduction of male-to-female sexual transfer of the virus.

The assisted reproductive technology laboratory used for the procedure was considered a "viral risk" area, and was separated from laboratory facilities used for couples negative for HIV, HBV and HCV. The ART laboratory complied with standard recommended safety precautions [1]. Specific precautions were implemented against the risk of HIV, HCV and HBV contamination as recommended by the French decree of May 10, 2001 [45], and the potentially infected gametes and embryos were handled separately. A special biosafety cabinet workstation was used for all tasks that involved handling sperm, oocytes, and embryos.

The reproductive technique of choice in serodiscordant couples for HIV-positive male partner, with no other infertility problem, is AIH after sperm washing. It is efficient, safe, and relatively low cost. The efficiency of the sperm-washing technique [62] was proven by a large number of AIH ($n=3{,}000$) performed with safe pregnancies published in 2007. A previous review [46] reported 3,221 cycles worldwide, most of them in Europe. In the September 2007 issue of AIDS [61], a paper was presented where eight European centres offering assisted reproduction with sperm washing to HIV-1 serodiscordant couples combined their results. A total of 1,036 couples underwent 3,390 assisted reproduction cycles resulting in 580 pregnancies. No transmission of HIV to the female partner was observed after 3,272 cycles with complete follow-up information. The upper level of the 95% CI of the transmission risk was thus 0.09%. This multicentric, retrospective study, included centres with different clinical approaches beginning as early as 1992 resulting in possible bias.

Some Reproductive Centres for HIV-1 discordant couple used frozen semen [37] for IUI, resulting in a negative impact on the number of available motile sperm after freezing [43] and the pregnancy rate per IUI. In agreement with Nicopoullos et al. [48] we found a positive trend also between IUI outcome and total motile cells inseminated, and for these reasons, it would be better use fresh semen after Real PCR.

This number of successful pregnancies after sperm washing now adds up to more than 3,000 reported cases attesting to the safety and efficacy of sperm washing [46]. The experience of our laboratory recommends that IUI should be performed only when the semen processing includes sperm washing with a swim-up phase for sperm cell selection [49, 50]. In socioeconomic areas, where HIV infection does no longer represent a terminal illness [10], the desire for fathering a child has become a legitimate, ethical, and medical issue [46, 51, 52]. Counselling to have unprotected intercourse on the day of ovulation reduces the risk of horizonatal transmission of HIV, but would condemn about 5% of women to be infected by their partners according to Mandelbrot et al. [53]. This is an unacceptable option when considered epidemiologically scale and not as a single medical practice risk-perception. Adoption and heterologous insemination are alternatives [20].

The efficiency of IUI, with its safe outcome after semen separation, sperm washing, including swim-up, and its relatively low cost make this the technique of choice in serodiscordant couples for an HIV positive male partner, when no other infertility problems are involved. When the female partner is suffering from infertility factors, or the male partner had less than 1×10^6 total motile cells in the final fraction after sperm washing, or both partners have a combination of subfertility conditions, we performed IVF/IVF-ICSI. The pregnancy rate per embryo transfer during IVF/IVF-ICSI was in agreement with similar small HIV series [37] and larger non-HIV series [54]. Savasi [62] recently reported their experience on a large group of patients (500 fresh IVF/IVF-ICSI cycles) without HIV-1 transmission to the female partners with an adequate follow-up. Other markers of outcome were as good in these couples treated after sperm washing as in other infertility series of comparable age. The fertilization rate was 65% by IVF and 88% by ICSI [38]. The major problem with IVF/IVF-ICSI in all serodiscordant couples is the high multiple pregnancy rate and the associated obstetrical and neonatal complications associated with these high risk pregnancies (14% for Garrido et al. (38), and 57.1% for Pena et al. [55]. The additional costs of prenatal and neonatal care in multiple pregnancies must also be considered [56, 57]. In our personal experience, the multiple pregnancy rate by IVF/ICSI was only ten percent reflecting our caution in ovulation induction and embryo transfer. It is prudent to extend testing for HIV-1 by PCR after semen processing and sperm washing with swim-up not only for IUI but IVF and IVF-ICSI until a final biological marker is provided. So far, we agree with Garrido et al. [58] and Gilling-Smith [47] that, in order to protect patient from technical errors during semen washing, viral detection sampling prior to any assisted reproduction technique is the method of choice [59, 60]. (Algorithm for HIV discordant couple (Male infected)).

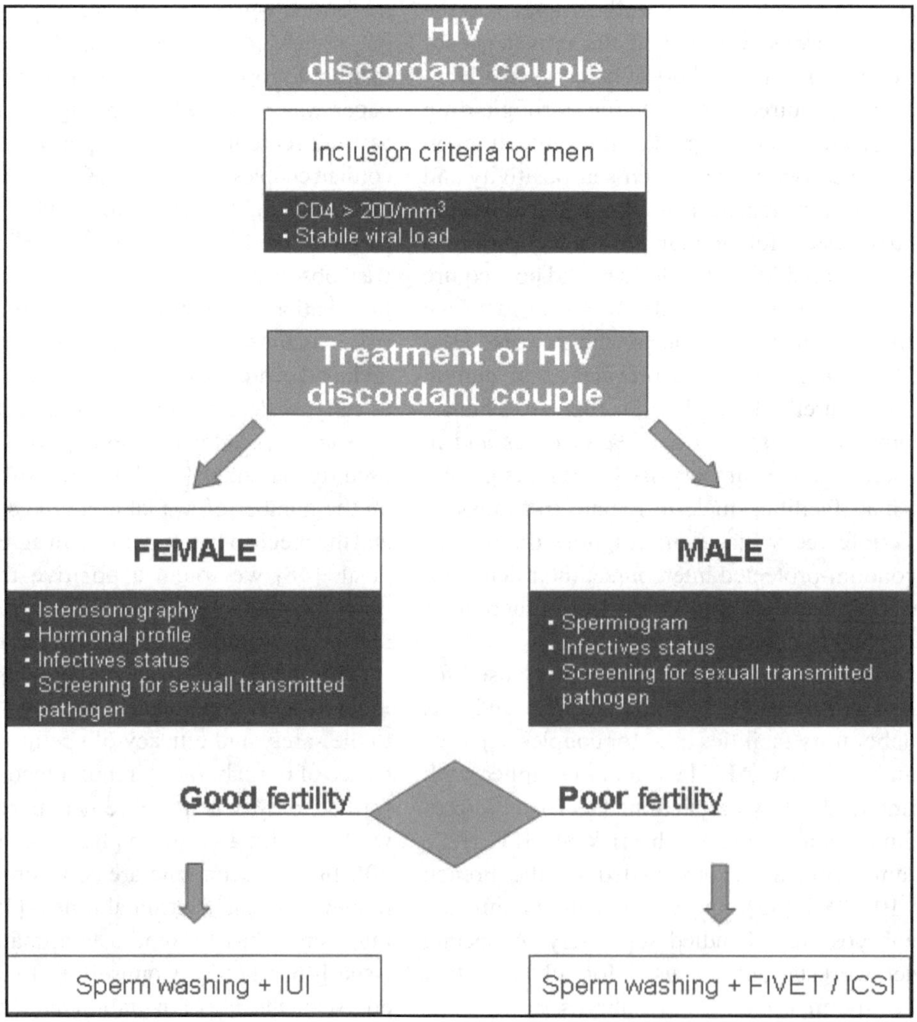

34.4.1 Algorithm for HIV Discordant Couple (Male Infected)

*FIVET/ICSI refers to fresh IVF (microdroplet insemination) or IVF-ICSI with embryo transfer.

34.5 Conclusion

Healthcare policymakers should be made aware of the changing pattern of HIV infected patients in western countries in order to allocate resources that will prevent HIV transmission within serodiscordant couples who desire to participate in a significant part of human life: childbearing. In western countries, we recommend that assisted reproductive programmes, using techniques such as IUI with semen processing with sperm washing and swim-up, should be integrated into the global public health initiative against HIV.

References

1. World Health Organization (1999) WHO Laboratory Manual for the Examination of Human Semen and Semen ± Cervical Mucus Interaction, 4th edn. Cambridge University Press, Cambridge
2. May M, Sterne JA, Sabin C et al (2007) Prognosis of HIV-1-infected patients up to 5 years after initiation of HAART: collaborative analysis of prospective studies. AIDS 21:1185–1197
3. Barroso PF, Schechter M, Gupta P et al (2000) Effect of antiretroviral therapy on HIV shedding in semen. Ann Intern Med 15:280–284
4. Ethics Committee of the American Society for Reproductive Medicine (2002) Human immunodeficiency virus and infertility treatment. Fertil Steril 77:218–222
5. De Vincenzi I (1994) A longitudinal study of immunodeficiency virus transmission by heterosexual partners. European Study Group on Heterosexual Transmission of HIV. New Engl J Med 33:341–346
6. Downs AM, De Vincenzi I (1996) Probability of heterosexual transmission of HIV: relationship to the number of unprotected sexual contacts European Study Group in Heterosexual Transmission of HIV. J Acquir Immune Defic Syndr Hum Retrovirol 11:388–395
7. Mandelbrot L, Heard I, Henrion-Geant E et al (1997) R Natural conception in HIV-negative women with HIV-infected partners. Lancet 349:850–851
8. Padian NS, Shiboski SC, Glass SO et al (1997) Heterosexual transmission of human immunodeficiency virus (HIV) in northern California: results from a ten-year study. Am J Epidemiol 146:350–357
9. Pena JE, Thornton MH II, Sauer MV (2003) Assessing the clinical utility of in vitro fertilization with intracytoplasmic sperm injection in human immunodeficiency virus type 1 serodiscordant couples: report of 113 consecutive cycles. Fertil Steril 80:356–362
10. Englert Y, Van Vooren JP, Place I et al (2001) ART in HIV-infected couples. Hum Reprod 16:1309–1315
11. Araneta MR, Mascola L, Eller A et al (1995) HIV transmission through donor artificial insemination. J Am Med Assoc 273:854–858
12. Matz B, Kupfer B, Ko Y et al (1998) HIV-1 infection by artificial insemination. Lancet 351:728
13. Baccetti B, Benedetto A, Burrini AG et al (1994) HIV-particles in spermatozoa of patients with AIDS and their transfer into the oocyte. J Cell Biol 127:903–914
14. Brogi A, Presentini R, Moretti E et al (1998) New insights into the interaction between the gp120 and the HIV receptor in human sperm. J Reprod Immunol 41:213–231
15. Lasheeb AS, King J, Ball JK et al (1997) Semen characteristics in HIV-1 positive men and the effect of semen washing. Genitourin Med 73:303–305
16. Quayle AJ, Xu C, Mayer KH et al (1997) T lymphocytes and macrophages, but not motile spermatozoa are a significant source of human immunodeficiency virus in semen. J Infect Dis 176:960–968
17. Pudney J, Nguyen H, Xu C et al (1998) Microscopic evidence against HIV-1 infection of germ cells or attachment to sperm. J Reprod Immunol 4:105–125
18. Semprini AE, Levi-Setti P, Bozzo M et al (1992) Insemination of HIV-negative women with processed semen of HIV-positive partners. Lancet 28:1317–1319
19. Borzy MS, Connell RS, Kiessling AA (1988) Detection of human immunodeficiency virus in cell-free seminal fluid. J Acquir Immune Defic Syndr 1:419–424
20. Bujan L, Pasquier C, Labeyrie E et al (2004) Insemination with isolated and virologically tested spermatozoa is a safe way for human immunodeficiency type 1 virus-serodiscordant couples with an infected male partner to have a child. Fertil Steril 82:857–862
21. Bagasra O, Freund M, Weidmann J et al (1988) Interaction of human immunodeficiency virus with human sperm in vitro. J Acquir Immune Defic Syndr 1:431–435
22. Bagasra O et al (1990) Presence of HIV-1 in sperm of patients with HIV-1/AIDS. Mol Androl 2:109–125
23. Bagasra O, Farzadegan H, Seshamma T et al (1994) Detection of HIV-1 proviral DNA in sperm from HIV-1 infected men. AIDS 8:1669–1674
24. Anderson DJ et al (1990) Presence of HIV-1 in semen. In: Alexander NJ, Gabelnick HL, Spieler JM (eds) Heterosexual transmission of AIDS. Proceedings of the second contraceptive research and development (CONRAD) program international workshop, Held in Norfolk, Virginia, February 1–3, 1989. Wiley-Liss, New York, pp 167–180
25. Baccetti B, Benedetto A, Burrini AG et al (1991) HIV particles detected in spermatozoa of patients with AIDS. J Submicrosc Cytol Pathol 23:339–345
26. Baccetti B, Benedetto A, Collodel G et al (1998) The debate on the presence of HIV-1 in human gametes. J Reprod Immunol 41:41–67
27. Gobert B, Amiel C, Tang JQ et al (1990) CD4-like molecules in human sperm. FEBS Lett 261:339–342
28. Miller VE, Scofield VL (1990) Transfer of HIV-1 by semen: role of sperm. In: Alexander NJ, Gabelnick HL, Spieler JM (eds) Heterosexual transmission of AIDS. Proceedings of the second contraceptive research and development (CONRAD) program international workshop, Held in Norfolk, Virginia, February 1–3, 1989. Wiley-Liss, New York, pp 147–154
29. Pudney J (1990) Caveats associated with identifying HIV-1 using transmission electron microscopy. In: Alexander NJ, Gabelnick HL, Spieler JM (eds) Heterosexual transmission of AIDS. Proceedings of the second contraceptive research and development (CONRAD) program international workshop, Held in Norfolk, Virginia, February 1–3, 1989. Wiley-Liss, New York, pp 197–204
30. Mermin JH, Holodniy M, Katzenstein DA et al (1991) Detection of human immunodeficiency virus DNA and RNA in semen by the polymerase chain reaction. J Infect Dis 164:769–772
31. Van Voorhis BJ, Martinez A, Mayer K et al (1991) Detection of HIV-1 in semen from seropositive men using culture and polymerase chain detection deoxyribonucleic acid amplification techniques. Fertil Steril 55:588–594

32. Scofield VL, Rao B, Broder S et al (1994) HIV interaction with sperm. AIDS 8:1733–1736
33. Dussaix E, Guetard D, Dauget C et al (1993) Spermatozoa as potential carriers of HIV-1. Res Virol 144:487–495
34. Nuovo GJ, Becker J, Simsir A et al (1994) HIV-1 nucleic acids localize to the spermatogonia and their progeny. A study by polymerase chain reaction in situ hybridization. Am J Pathol 144:1142–1148
35. Muciaccia B, Uccini S, Filippini A et al (1998) Presence and cellular distribution of HIV-1 in the testes of seropositive subjects: an evaluation by in situ PCR hybridization. FASEB J 12:151–163
36. Shevchuk MM, Nuovo GJ, Khalife G (1998) HIV-1 in testis: quantitative histology and HIV-1 localization in germ cells. J Reprod Immunol 41:69–79
37. Ohl J, Partisani M, Wittemer C et al (2003) Assisted reproduction techniques for HIV serodiscordant couples: 18 months of experience. Hum Reprod 18:1244–1249
38. Garrido N, Meseguer M, Bellver J et al (2004) A Report of the results of a 2 year programme of sperm wash and ICSI treatment human immunodeficiency virus and hepatitis C virus serodiscordant couples. Hum Reprod 19:2581–2586
39. Politch JA, Xu C, Tucker L, Anderson DJ (2004) Separation of human immunodeficiency virus type 1 from motile sperm by the double tube gradient method versus other methods. Fertil Steril 81:440–447
40. Marina S, Marina F, Alcolea R et al (1998) Human immunodeficiency virus type 1-serodiscordant couples can bear healthy children after undergoing intrauterine insemination. Fertil Steril 70:35–39
41. Garrido N, Meseguer M, Bellver J (2002) In vitro fertilization with intracytoplasmic sperm injection for human immunodeficiency virus-1 serodiscordant couples. Am J Obstet Gynecol 187:1121
42. Meseguer M, Garrido N, Gimeno C et al (2002) Comparison of polymerase chain reaction-dependent methods for determining the presence of human immunodeficiency virus and hepatitis C virus in washed sperm. Fertil Steril 78:1199–1202
43. Leruez-Ville M, de Almeida M, Tachet A et al (2002) Assisted reproduction in HIV-1-serodifferent couples: the need for viral validation of processed semen. AIDS 16:2267–2273
44. Xu C, Politch JA, Mayer KH, Anderson DJ (2005) Human immunodeficiency virus type-1 episomal cDNA in semen. AIDS Res Ther 2:9
45. Decree of May 10 (2001). Prise en charge en assistance médicale à la procréation des patients à risque viral. Page 7735. Arrêté du 10 mai 2001. Journal Officiel de la République Française, 15 mai 2001
46. Sauer MV (2005) Sperm washing techniques address the fertility needs of HIV-seropositive men: a clinical review. Reprod Biomed Online 1:135–140
47. Gilling-Smith C (2000) Assisted reproduction in HIV-discordant couples. AIDS Read 10:581–587
48. Nicopoullos JD, Almeida PA, Ramsay JWA, Gilling-Smith C (2004) The effect human immunodeficiency virus on sperm parameters and the outcome of intrauterine insemination following sperm washing. Hum Reprod 19:2289–2297
49. Hanabusa H, Kuji N, Kato S et al (2000) An evaluation of semen processing methods for eliminating HIV-1. AIDS 14:1611–1616
50. Persico T, Savasi V, Ferrazzi E et al (2006) Detection of human immunodeficiency virus-1 RNA and DNA by extractive and in situ PCR in unprocessed semen and seminal fractions isolated by semen-washing procedure. Hum Reprod 21:1525–1530
51. Barreiro P (2004) Benefit of antiretroviral therapy for serodiscordant couples willing to be parents. Late breakers Seventh International Congress on Drug Therapy in HIV Infection, 14–18 November, Abstract number *PL*13.3, Glasgow, Scotland
52. Klein J, Pena JE, Thornton MH, Sauer MV (2003) Understanding the motivations, concerns, and desires of human immunodeficiency virus 1-serodiscordant couples wishing to have children through assisted reproduction. Obstet Gynecol 101:987–994
53. Mandelbrot L, Heard I, Henrion-Geant E, Henrion R (1997) Natural conception in HIV-negative women with HIV-infected partners. Lancet 349:850–851
54. ESHRE (2006) Assisted reproductive technology in Europe, 2002. Results generated from European registers by ESHRE. Hum Reprod 21:1680–1697
55. Pena JE, Thornton MH, Sauer MV (2003) Assessing the clinical utility of in vitro fertilization with intracytoplasmic sperm injection in human immunodeficiency virus type 1 serodiscordant couples: report of 113 consecutive cycles. Fertil Steril 80:356–362
56. Nakhuda GS, Sauer MV (2005) Addressing the growing problem of multiple gestations created by assisted reproductive therapies. Semin Perinatol 29:355–362
57. Oliviennes F (2000) Double trouble: yes a twin pregnancy is an adverse outcome. Hum Reprod 15:1663–1665
58. Garrido N, Remohí J, Pellicer A, Meseguer M (2006) The effectiveness of modified sperm washes in severely oligoasthenozoospermic men infected with human immunodeficiency and hepatitis C viruses. Fertil Steril 86:1544–1546
59. Garrido N, Meseguer M (2006) Use of washed sperm for assisted reproduction in HIV-positive males without checking viral absence. A risky business? Hum Reprod 21:567–568 (Letter)
60. Piomboni P, Mencaglia L, De Leo V (2006) Reply to: Use of washed sperm for assisted reproduction in HIV-positive males without checking viral absence. A risky business? Hum Reprod 21:568 (Letter)
61. Bujan L, Hollander L, Coudert M, Gilling-Smith C, Vucetich A, Guibert J, Vernazza P, Ohl J, Weigel M, Englert Y, Semprini AE (2007) CREAThE network. Safety and efficacy of sperm washing in HIV-1-serodiscordant couples where the male is infected: results from the European CREAThE network. AIDS 12: 1909–1914
62. Savasi V, Ferrazzi E, Lanzani C, Oneta M, Parrilla B, Persico T (2007) Safety of sperm washing and ART outcome in 741 HIV-1-serodiscordant couples. Hum Reprod 22:772–777

Chapter 35
Ovulation Induction

Mark Gibson

Abstract Induction of ovulation is primarily used for treatment of infertility in anovulatory women. Long-term management of anovulatory states may result in incidental or intended establishment of regular ovulation when fertility is not a goal, for example, when insulin-enhancing agents or dopamine agonists are administered to women with polycystic ovary syndrome (PCOS) or hyperprolactinemia, respectively. This chapter will focus specifically on induction of ovulation for women who desire restoration of ovulation for the purpose of becoming pregnant.

Induction of ovulation for fertility treatment should be undertaken with awareness of other potential fertility factors affecting the likelihood of conception. Most important among these are tubal patency and semen quality, and ideally these should be evaluated prior to therapy. This is certainly true in the case of treatments entailing substantial cost and disruption for the patient such as administration of gonadotropins. In practice, when the history is convincing that the male and tubal factors are very likely normal, and treatment is of lesser intensity and cost, evaluation of male and tubal factors may be delayed until after a few cycles of successful ovulation have occurred without conception.

Keywords Ovulation induction • Anovulation • Gonadotropin • Clomiphene citrate • Luteinizing hormone • Obesity • PCOS • Cancer

M. Gibson (✉)
Utah Center for Reproductive Medicine, Department of Obstetrics and Gynecology, University of Utah School of Medicine, Salt Lake City, UT, USA
e-mail: mark.gibson@hsc.utah.edu

35.1 Induction of Ovulation for Specific Disorders

35.1.1 *Women with Normal Gonadotropin and Prolactin Levels*

This category generally corresponds to WHO group II ovulatory disorders and includes women designated as having polycystic ovary syndrome. It also includes women with absent or infrequent ovulation not reaching criteria for PCOS because of lack of clinical or biochemical evidence for increased androgen production and normal ovarian imaging. Subsets of women in this diagnostic group can be defined in terms of a number of criteria (hirsutism, insulin resistance, ovarian morphology, steroid and gonadotropin levels), but there is little evidence that these characteristics, or combinations of them, usefully predict response to different treatments. The exception to this statement is obesity, as several studies have suggested that elevated BMI is a risk factor for decreased response to oral ovulation induction medications, insulin-enhancing agents, and gonadotropins [1–4].

35.1.1.1 Weight Loss

Because it is often effective as a primary therapy, and facilitates medical therapy if required, and because of risks of obesity to health in pregnancy and in general, it could be argued that efforts to achieve weight loss should precede medical induction of ovulation when obesity accompanies anovulation [5–7]. Although obesity alone is not a cause of anovulation or PCOS among most women, and although PCOS may exist in the absence of elevated body mass index, the resumption of normal cycles among obese anovulatory women who lose weight through lifestyle measures or bariatric surgery is striking. Weight loss achieved through alteration of lifestyle may restore ovulation and regular cycles among a large proportion of overweight or obese women with PCOS and enhance response to medical therapies in

D.T. Carrell and C.M. Peterson (eds.), *Reproductive Endocrinology and Infertility: Integrating Modern Clinical and Laboratory Practice*, DOI 10.1007/978-1-4419-1436-1_35, © Springer Science+Business Media, LLC 2010

those remaining anovulatory [5, 8, 9]. Bariatric surgery has been shown to be highly effective in ameliorating metabolic and endocrine features of PCOS and restoring ovulation in morbidly obese anovulatory women [10]. Together these observations show that expression of features comprising PCOS appears conditional to elevation of BMI in some women. In addition to a requirement of higher dosing of ovulation-inducing drugs, obesity has been associated with higher rates of early pregnancy loss in general and among women with PCOS treated with ovulation induction [11–13]. Additionally, because elevated BMI is a risk factor for gestational diabetes and cesarean section, and has long-term adverse consequences to general health, a program of weight loss is a highly appropriate and often effective approach not only to restoration of ovulation, but improvement in pregnancy outcomes among obese, anovulatory women desiring pregnancy [5].

35.1.1.2 Triphenylethylene Derivatives: Clomiphene and Tamoxifen

Clomiphene citrate has been used for over 40 years to induce ovulation in normogonadotropic anovulatory women and remains the first line drug of choice [14]. Overall success rates for establishment of ovulation in unselected series are typically in the vicinity of three quarters of patients or more, pregnancy rates per ovulation may be lower than in normal spontaneously ovulatory women, and likelihood of pregnancy in treatment series is a function of number of cycles studied, patient age, and other fertility factors [15]. Obesity may predict a lower likelihood of response to clomiphene, or need for higher dosing, but other clinically useful prognostic factors have not been identified [1, 3]. Clomiphene's companion triphenylethylene derivative, Tamoxifen, is used similarly to Clomiphene in European practice at slightly lower dosing and achieves comparable results [16, 17].

Pharmacology

Clomiphene citrate is marketed as a racemic mixture of two steroisomers, with different activities and rates of clearance. The *cis* isomer, enclomiphene, is the most antiestrogenic, and the shortest lived in the circulation, while much less activity is attributed to the *trans* isomer, zuclomiphene, which has a half-life sufficiently long that it may accumulate in the circulation over successive cycles of use [18–20]. No pharmacologically important or teratogenic influence has been attributed to the persistence of zuclomiphene in the circulation, and physiologic and endocrine responses to clomiphene are similar across successive cycles of administration [21]. Both isomers can be considered selective estrogen receptor modulators, exerting weak estrogen agonist effects, which are dominated by antagonistic effects against a background of normal circulating estrogen levels in the reproductive-aged woman [22]. Following association of clomiphene with estrogen receptor, its dissociation is delayed, reducing estrogen receptor levels available for estrogen action within the cell. Its primary mechanism of action is central, at the hypothalamus, where loss of estrogen feedback results in increased GnRH pulse frequency and amplitude, although other sites of action may contribute to its ovulation restoring effect [23–26]. In anovulatory women with a competent hypothalamic pituitary unit the resultant increase in gonadotropin levels is often sufficient to initiate folliculogenesis for one or more susceptible ovarian follicles. Folliculogenesis in clomiphene-induced ovulation is characterized by slightly greater follicle size at the time of the LH surge than in spontaneous cycles among normal women [27–29]. Multiple follicular development is common, and dose requirements for acceptable numbers of mature follicles are difficult to predict. Doses as low as 25 mg daily for achievement of numerically safe folliculogenesis may be necessary in some women using clomiphene either for ovulation induction or superovulation.

Dosing and Administration

Clomiphene is usually given daily doses over 5 days beginning shortly after the onset of ovulatory menses or progestin-induced withdrawal bleeding. No significant differences in ovulation and pregnancy rates are associated with drug initiation on the second through fifth days from onset of menses, though earlier start days may improve pregnancy rates when clomiphene is used for superovulation therapy [30, 31]. Therapy is commonly initiated at 50 mg/day for 5 days and titrated upward in 50 mg/day increments until an ovulatory response is achieved. Response to clomiphene remains consistent over sequential cycles of therapy [21]. The maximal approved dosage is 150 mg/day, and failure to respond at this dose commonly defines "clomiphene failure," though a few patients unresponsive to this dose will respond to doses as high as 250 mg/day in some reported clinical series [1, 15]. Lengthening the period of clomiphene administration has been reported to elicit an ovulatory response among some patients failing at the standard doses and durations of therapy [32, 33]. Adjunctive medications, including insulin-enhancing agents and glucocorticoids, and pretreatment with oral contraceptives may result in ovulation among patients failing with standard clomiphene regimens and are discussed further below.

An endogenous LH-surge occurs highly reliably if adequate folliculogenesis occurs. In settings where insemination is part of the treatment, administration of hCG, based on ultrasound measurements of follicular diameters is often given in order to time insemination [34]. Ovulation occurs on an average of 38 h after hCG administration but with a range of intervals of over 12 h [35, 36].

Monitoring

Response to clomiphene can be documented inexpensively and conveniently by one or combinations of the following: detection of an LH surge using commercially available kits, basal temperature records, progesterone determinations timed to the anticipated midluteal phase, and the subsequent occurrence of timely, normal menses. Addition of midcycle ultrasound monitoring of numbers of follicles of mature size to assure adequate but not excessive response may add safety and shorten the time to achievement of an appropriate dose. In cycles without follicular response, upward dose adjustment that follows a short course of progestin can be planned at the time of ultrasound. In the event that excessive numbers of responsive follicles are found, interruption of the cycle and prevention of pregnancy with high-dose progestins can be instituted. If ultrasound is used, ultrasound monitoring in subsequent cycles is likely unnecessary in future cycles once a clomiphene dose providing an effective, yet safe response is seen.

Adverse Effects

Clomiphene's antiestrogenic effects are considered an explanation for poor estrogenization and reduced endometrial growth during the follicular phase of the cycle; most observers have found increased rates of attenuated preovulatory changes in cervical mucus and reduced thickness of proliferative phase endometrium when clomiphene is used for superovulation or ovulation induction [15, 28, 37–39]. Some of these effects may be attributable to the elevation of preovulatory progesterone levels seen in clomiphene cycles [40]. These effects are variable, with little evidence for a dose–response relationship, and for cervical mucus, are difficult to quantify reliably [41]. They do not appear to worsen over successive cycles of therapy, and studies have not confirmed an adverse effect of these changes on likelihood of pregnancy in clomiphene-treated cycles [21, 42, 43]. On the other hand, it has been shown that estrogen supplementation may increase endometrial thickness in clomiphene cycles, and that this effect is associated with improved probabilities of pregnancy [44, 45]. This observation is difficult to reconcile with the observation that estrogen levels are appropriately elevated in the preovulatory period (often greatly so and in proportion to the number of follicles matured) in women with poor cervical mucus quality or endometrial development. The alterations in cervical mucus and endometrial development have been proposed to account for the "discrepancy" between ovulation rates and pregnancy rates among clomiphene-treated women. However, when expressed as events per ovulatory cycle, pregnancy rates among anovulatory women treated with clomiphene are not greatly discrepant with rates for fertile populations and do not take into account other factors that may affect fecundity in infertile couples for whom clomiphene is prescribed.

Residual ovarian cysts are seen after cycles of ovulation induction, though it is not clear that the likelihood of residual structures is greater for clomiphene-stimulated than spontaneously ovulatory follicles [46]. Resolution of these occurs similarly with expectant management or use of hormonal suppression [47, 48]. Conduct of induction of ovulation with clomiphene despite persistent cyst may result in slightly lower rates of ovulation, though a difference in rates of conception has not been shown [49].

Side Effects

Principal side effects for patients using clomiphene are vasomotor symptoms and mood changes, usually limited to the time around administration of the medication. Both are variable in intensity, and common, but careful studies of their prevalence, severity, and impact of quality of life for infertile patients are needed [50, 51]. Less commonly patients may experience visual symptoms. Because there are rare reports of long-term persistence of visual symptoms or optic neuropathy, clomiphene should be discontinued when visual complaints are prominent or persistent [52, 53].

Pregnancy Outcomes

Although some reports have suggested an increase in the rate of spontaneous abortion among pregnancies resulting from clomiphene induction of ovulation, most case series and clinical trials do not find evidence for such an effect [54–56]. Numerous series [57–59] show little evidence for a teratogenic influence of the drug [59–61]. Small increases in risks for specific birth defects (neural tube defect and hypospadius) have been reported in some series, but these are inconsistently reported, and the subfertile state itself appears to confer such risks independent of treatment [57–59, 62, 63]. Several pregnancy complications are reported to be increased among women with PCOS who have undergone induction of ovulation, findings that are may be attributable to the comorbidities of PCOS, including increased BMI and insulin resistance or other unknown factors associated with infertility [64, 65].

The most important risk associated with the use of medical agents for induction of ovulation and superovulation is multiple pregnancy and particularly high-order multiple pregnancy.

The contribution to the burden of multiple pregnancy in the USA is roughly equivalent for ovulation induction treatments and ART [66]. Risk of multiple pregnancy is related to age and to the number of follicles achieved. Judicious dosing, use of ultrasound monitoring, and willingness to interrupt cycles at risk are mainstays in reducing risk of multiple pregnancy. High-order multiple pregnancy is related not only to follicles at diameters commonly thought to indicate maturity, but to numbers of intermediate (12 mm or more) sized follicles [67, 68]. Measurements of serum estradiol levels are complementary to ultrasound for indicating follicular maturity and risks for multiple gestation and OHSS [69].

Adjunctive Measures

Because treatment of patients failing to respond to clomiphene has until recently presented only the choice between surgical management (laparoscopic ovarian ablative therapies) or the complex and expensive administration of gonadotropins, a variety of adjunctive medical regimens to increase ovulation rates associated with clomiphene therapy have been evaluated [17]. Clomiphene resistance is not clearly defined in the literature, but most studies of alternative methods for ovulation induction define clomiphene resistance among their subjects as failure to ovulate at a clomiphene dose of 150 mg given for 5 days. The advent of aromatase inhibitors for ovulation induction can be added to the alternatives to progression to surgical or gonadotropin therapy, and these are discussed separately later following discussion of adjunctive measures.

Clomiphene with Dexamethasone

Dexamethasone administration augments responsiveness to clomiphene and is an effective adjunct when clomiphene alone does not achieve ovulation [17]. Initial observations suggested that the benefit from dexamethasone related to the presence of increased levels of circulating DHEAS [70–73]. Other series and recent randomized clinical trials show a benefit of dexamethasone without respect to DHEAS levels [74–76]. The mechanism for the observed benefit of glucocorticoids is obscure, particularly in view of their effectiveness without regard to levels of circulating androgens. They increase insulin resistance and must act quite differently than insulin-enhancing agents. Two studies have shown that approximately half of patients failing to ovulate at clomiphene doses of 150 mg for 5 days will ovulate if dexamethasone at a dose of 1-mg BID is initiated with clomiphene and continued for 10 days [75, 76].

Insulin-Enhancing Agents

Insulin-enhancing agents alone result in restoration of ovulation for women with WHO group II anovulation and have been shown to enhance responsiveness to clomiphene [77–83]. Response to metformin has not been consistently correlated with obesity or measures of insulin resistance, suggesting mechanisms of action other than correction of hyperinsulinemia [84, 85]. Several studies have shown ovulation rates greater than 50% among women with PCOS using metformin in doses of 1,500 mg/day as a primary therapy [77, 82, 86, 87]. Other insulin-enhancing agents have shown similar activity, but the majority of studies concern metformin [88–90]. The likelihood of establishing regular ovulation with these agents increases over a period of several months of drug administration [82]. Some studies have supported primary or adjunctive use of metformin with clomiphene as a first line therapy for PCOS [77, 82]. More recent evidence from multicenter clinical trials does not support use of metformin as a first line agent either alone, or with clomiphene for induction of ovulation in PCOS patients. Metformin alone or in combination with clomiphene does not increase rates of ovulation, conceptions per ovulation, or rates of ongoing pregnancy among subjects that conceived [7, 55, 56, 82, 91]. Metformin does not reduce the threshold dose for Clomid effectiveness when used as a first line therapy [56, 92]. Metformin does represent an alternative to clomiphene for those intolerant of it, or as an adjunctive measure when clomiphene alone does not induce ovulation [81, 93–95]. Its effectiveness appears greater when its use is accompanied by loss of weight [9]. The effect of differing durations of metformin therapy prior to clomiphene administration remains uncertain and dose–response characteristics are not well elucidated [96]. Metformin has been held to reduce the risk of spontaneous abortion among women with PCOS [82, 97]. Where shown effective in this respect, spontaneous abortion rates in control groups not receiving metformin were exceptionally high, and an abortion-sparing effect of metformin is not confirmed in large, multicenter, randomized trials [55, 56].

Suppression of Ovarian Function as a Pretreatment

Treatment with long-acting GnRH agonists or with oral contraceptives may result in subsequent resumption of regular ovulation, at least for a time, for some women with chronic anovulation. In line with this effect, it has been shown as well that likelihood of ovulation among clomiphene-resistant women is increased from 8 to 71% by pretreatment with 6–7 weeks of continuously administered combined oral contraceptives. Subsequent treatment cycles are more often ovulatory, and pregnancy rates substantially increased as a result of pretreatment with hormonal contraceptives [98, 99].

Other Adjunctive Agents

Bromocriptine has been employed with limited success as an adjunct to clomiphene, and there is insufficient evidence to support its use [17]. Pulsatile gonadotropin releasing hormone administration may be effective, but clinical evidence is insufficient to support its use in clinical practice [100, 101].

35.1.1.3 Aromatase Inhibitors: Letrozole and Anastrozole

Transient inhibition of estrogen production with aromatase inhibitors (AIs) appears to act similarly to the transient estrogen receptor modulation effected by clomiphene and tamoxifen in causing a rise in levels of FSH and initiation of folliculogenesis. Both agents have shorter half-lives than clomiphene (approximately 2 days, and 3 days for Anastrozole and Letrozole, respectively) [102]. Use of AIs for ovulation induction has a much briefer history than use of clomiphene, but there is substantial evidence for efficacy.

Letrozole has been studied at doses of 2.5–7.5 mg per day, and Anastrozole at doses of 1 mg, both given for 5 days early in the cycle, and both have been used to induce ovulation in normogonadotropic, normoprolactinemic anovulation, with no evidence in a difference in effectiveness [17, 103, 104]. For induction of ovulation, rates of ovulation and conception compare favorably with outcomes seen with clomiphene [105–110], and outcomes when either clomiphene or Letrozole are used in protocols for superovulation and insemination are similar as well [111, 112]. The two agents appear equivalently effective in inducing ovulation in more than half of women with PCOS deemed clomiphene resistant [13, 104, 113]. These agents differ from clomiphene in their effects in several respects, however. Successful ovulation induction with aromatase inhibitors rarely results in more than two preovulatory follicles, reducing the concern for high-order multiple pregnancies as seen with clomiphene [105, 109, 114]. Because of this, there appears to be less need to avert multiple gestation with ultrasound monitoring. There is evidence in some studies for a less frequent problem with the reduced endometrial proliferation seen with clomiphene when aromatase inhibitors are used [105]. These differences may owe to the shorter half-life of aromatase inhibitors or more fundamental aspects of their mechanism of action.

Aromatase inhibition during pregnancy may be teratogenic. A single unpublished report has linked induction of ovulation with aromatase inhibitor to birth defects among resulting offspring. This concern is mitigated by a large cohort study in which the frequency and types birth defects after aromatase inhibitor induction of ovulation were found equivalent to those after induction of ovulation with clomiphene, and within expectations for the birth population at large [61]. Moreover, such teratogenesis lacks biologic plausibility owing to the brief half-lives of these agents, since exposures of any type that occur prior to ovulation have not been shown teratogenic. Because of concerns for teratogenesis, and despite this reassurance, Letrozole (as Femara) is labeled with a black box warning regarding use in women anticipating pregnancy. Clinicians who do use aromatase inhibitors are impelled nevertheless to make patients aware of these concerns and to assure that they understand them. Informed consent is commonly advised. Most importantly, use of aromatase inhibitors should be accompanied by precautions to administration to patients who are unknowingly pregnant.

Aromatase inhibitors may offer advantages over clomiphene in efficacy for both ovulation and achievement of pregnancy, but this inference is not supported by substantive head-to-clinical trials. Moreover, the cloud of imputed teratogenesis will linger and be difficult to dispel with finality. Hence, aromatase inhibitors at present, in most practices, remain second-line agents, to be used for clomiphene-resistant women or women intolerant of clomiphene [14].

Surgical Methods

Surgical reduction of ovarian volume is an alternative to gonadotropin administration if antiestrogens, aromatase inhibitors, adjunctive dexamethasone, and insulin-enhancing agents have failed. Following on the original observations of Stein and Leventhal, numerous contemporary studies have shown that various measures for reduction of ovarian volume restore ovulation. Various new methods for ovarian volume reduction result in rates of ovulation and pregnancy comparable to those achieved for PCOS patients with gonadotropins, and some of these indicate a favorable comparison with respect to cost of treatment [17, 115–122]. Even though oocyte retrieval during ART may confer this effect and increase the likelihood of subsequent resumption of ovulation in women with PCOS [99], one trial has found that metformin is as effective as ovarian diathermy in restoring ovulation in clomiphene-resistant women, suggesting that this should be tried before resorting to surgery. Those not ovulating after ovarian volume-reducing procedures may nevertheless become more responsive to medical measures for ovulation induction [119]. Newly reported success using ultrasound-guided methods offers lower cost and less invasiveness [121]. Despite conclusions in some quarters that use of surgical methods should precede resorting to gonadotropins, most centers in the USA favor the latter for clomiphene-resistant patients [123]. It is likely that widespread use of ovarian volume-reducing interventions has not occurred because of surgical risks related to procedures, the poorly characterized risk of significant adnexal adhesions, and unknown long-term effects on ovarian reserve [124]. Many clinicians never or rarely use surgical approaches for ovulation induction in PCOS patients, while others appear to use this approach liberally and in preference over use of gonadotropins.

Gonadotropins

Gonadotropin administration is the medical therapy of last resort for normogonadotropic, normoprolactinemic anovulation because of cost, intensiveness of monitoring, and attendant risks. Moreover, these patients present unique difficulties in the achievement of ovulation that is both safe and effective. Management of these patients with gonadotropins is discussed as a separate topic in the section on use of gonadotropins for ovulation induction in hypogonadotropic hypogonadism.

35.1.2 Hyperprolactinemia

Evaluation and treatment of disorders of prolactin excess is the subject of a separate chapter in this volume. When prolactin elevation is not due to medications or hypothyroidism, dopamine agonists are the primary and specific therapy for restoration of ovulation. Agents currently in use include bromocriptine, use of which is supported by 30 years of experience, and cabergoline, which offers less-frequent administration, often greater tolerability, and possibly a greater likelihood of effecting long-term resolution of hyperprolactinemic disorders after a course of therapy.

Characterization of hyperprolactinemic disorders awaited the development of sensitive and specific radioimmunoassays for human prolactin and advances in imaging the pituitary and its vicinity [125–129]. Although spontaneous or clomiphene-induced ovulation and conception can occur when prolactin levels are substantially less than 100 ng/ml, most patients were found to require specific treatment to normalize prolactin levels [130–133]. Dopaminergic therapy with bromocriptine initially competed with transphenoidal surgery as a primary therapy [134, 135]. Three principal lines of evidence led to the contemporary treatment paradigm that recognizes medical therapy as the primary management tool for restoration of ovulation for hyperprolactinemic states. First, idiopathic and microadenoma-related hyperprolactinemic exhibits a generally benign natural history, and spontaneous regression is not uncommon with or without intercedent pregnancy [100, 136–141]. Second, although adenomas may enlarge during pregnancy, clinically important progression is uncommon and can more often than not be managed medically [142–146]. Finally, surgical therapy, in addition to costs and risks is often followed by frank tumoral or biochemical recurrence of hyperprolactinemia [147]. Symptomatic enlargement may occur in as many as one sixth to one fourth of pregnancies complicated by macroprolactinomas, and prepregnancy debulking decreases this risk substantially, such that surgery continues to have a place for management of large prolactin-secreting tumors [146, 148].

Bromocriptine remains the agent of choice for restoration of ovulation for fertility in hyperprolactinemic states [149–151]. Bromocriptine administration is given daily and is often effective at very low doses (e.g., 1.25 mg). Bromocriptine use is frequently accompanied by gastrointestinal side effects, headache, and orthostatic hypotension. Slow progression of dosing to levels required to restore ovulation reduces prevalence and severity of side effects, as does vaginal administration [152–157]. Vaginal admininstration is associated with enhanced pharmacokinetics, and dose requirements should be correspondingly lower [158]. Monitoring is usually based on establishment of menses and clinical measures of ovulatory response. Prolactin levels can guide therapy, but it is notable that regular ovulation may occur when prolactin levels are suppressed, but remain above the normal range. Monitoring adenomas with imaging during therapy to restore ovulation is only of utility when the status of large lesions is a concern. No teratogenic effect of bromocriptine has been demonstrated, and its use in pregnancy is widely held safe, but it is usually discontinued once pregnancy is recognized [138, 159]. Because of much greater and longer experience with its use in pregnancy, bromocriptine is the drug of choice for symptomatic enlargement of prolactinomas during pregnancy; this is rare and occurs almost exclusively when macroprolactinomas are present at the outset of treatment [148, 150, 160, 161]. Bromocriptine is preferred over cabergoline for management of symptomatic adenoma progression in pregnancy. Continuation of bromocriptine during pregnancy when macroadenoma is present as a preventive for symptomatic enlargement has been reported, but evidence does not support this approach in favor of observation with reservation of use of medication if enlargement occurs [148, 162].

Cabergoline shows greater efficacy and tolerability than bromocriptine and is often effective for patients not responding to bromocriptine [150, 151]. Use and monitoring are similar to bromocriptine, but dosing is lower and less frequent; therapy is initiated at 0.5 mg twice weekly. Cabergoline appears more likely than bromocriptine to cause induction of long-term remission of prolactinomas and hyperprolactinemia [163–166]. It is generally now regarded as the first line medical agent for treatment of hyperprolactinemia when pregnancy is not desired. There is no evidence of teratogenicity for cabergoline, but its long half-life and limited data regarding safety in pregnancy lead most authors to recommend bromocriptine as a first line agent when fertility is sought, or advise suspension of cabergoline in the cycle prior to conception [151, 167, 168].

Clomiphene may be effective in some patients with modest elevations of prolactin who are intolerant of dopaminergic medications or when dopaminergic therapy results in incomplete normalization of prolactin levels [130, 149, 169]. The addition of hCG administration once follicle development occurs may be helpful in assuring ovulation when clomiphene is used in these circumstances, as estrogen-mediated positive feedback on LH secretion is blunted in the presence of elevations in prolactin levels [170].

35.1.3 Hypogonadotropic Hypogonadism

Induction of ovulation for women with hypogonadotropic hypogonadism ordinarily requires administration of gonadotropins. A trial of antiestrogen or aromatase inhibitor therapy may occasionally be successful for patients with functional hypothalamic amenorrhea, but most women in this diagnostic category have insufficient hypothalamic and or pituitary competence to respond to these agents [171]. Direct stimulation of folliculogenesis with gonadotropins bypasses the need for hypothalamic–pituitary competence and is also effective in patients with PCOS who are unresponsive to antiestrogens, aromatase inhibitors, and insulin-enhancing agents. Administration of gonadotropins is not a first line therapy for anovulation, except in situations where inadequacy of endogenous gonadotropin secretion is known to exist, because use of gonadotropins is expensive and entails greater risks. Costs attendant to gonadotropin therapy include the high costs of the agents themselves and the need for frequent ultrasound and or laboratory assessment of response. Complications associated with gonadotropin use include ovarian hyperstimulation syndrome (OHSS) and multiple pregnancy.

Gonadotropins were first used prior to the availability of ultrasound or rapid assays for determination of serum or urinary estrogens. Response was monitored by cervical mucus changes (reflecting estrogen production), and later with the addition of assays of 24-h urinary estrogens. The advent of RIA technology for assay for serum estradiol and ultrasound imaging have improved the precision of monitoring patients during therapy and have added increased ability to avoid OHSS and high-order multiple pregnancy.

Gonadotropin preparations have undergone considerable evolution since the use of initial products prepared from the urine of postmenopausal women. Newer gonadotropin products of (human) biologic origin benefit from improved purification as well as selective purification methods for FSH. Subsequent advances have led to development of recombinant methodologies for synthesis of both FSH and LH, though only the former is in current clinical use.

FSH and LH both have important roles in natural folliculogenesis, but in patients with even nominal background LH secretion, FSH is sufficient for induction of functional preovulatory follicles. In patients with profoundly suppressed or absent gonadotropins, folliculogenesis may occur without sufficient accompanying estrogen synthesis, and in these patients use of LH, even in low amounts, corrects this abnormality and presumably improves the chance of pregnancy. LH activity alone can drive folliculogenesis in follicles of intermediate size and greater, and LH (or hCG) can be substituted for FSH without consequence to ongoing follicular maturation once mid-sized follicles are achieved [172]. There is good evidence that inclusion of LH activity in the gonadotropin preparation used results in selective stimulation of lead follicles, with reduction in the number of intermediate sized follicles present in the course of ovulation induction or superovulation [173–176]. Inclusion of low-dose hCG in protocols using FSH preparations has been shown to create this outcome as well. Use of preparations including LH, or low-dose hCG provides equivalent effectiveness in achieving pregnancy, but the predicted concomitant reduction in the risk of multiple pregnancy and OHSS has not been shown in clinical trials.

35.1.3.1 Pharmacology of Gonadotropin Preparations

Gonadotropins are secreted and circulated as populations of glycoprotein hormones that are heterogeneous in pharmacokinetics and bioactivity by virtue of variation in degrees and nature of glycosylation and sulfonation [177]. Circulating isoforms are separable by isoelectric focusing, have differing pharmacokinetics and biologic activities, and are present in different proportions in different commercial preparations [178–181]. Preparations derived from purification of urine contain inactive and unrelated proteins [182].

Preparations containing both FSH and LH are prepared so that the two gonadotropins have equal numbers of international units activity per unit volume. Because human menopausal urinary FSH bioactivity exceeds FSH activity in purified preparations, hCG is added to achieve the desired unit equivalency of FSH and LH activity. hCG may account for most of the LH activity in such preparations [182, 183]. Owing to the long half-life of hCG, preparations including hCG to confer LH activity will confer an increase in LH activity over successive days [184]. Since LH activity can contribute to follicular growth in intermediate and larger follicles, this characteristic likely has pharmacodynamic implications when comparing FSH only to FSH/LH preparations [172, 174].

FSH, by virtue of greater glycosylation, persists longer in the circulation than LH, and with a terminal half-life of approximately one and one-half days can accumulate during a course of therapy whereas this is less so for LH [185–188]. Preparations of FSH that utilize modifications of the FSH molecule that confer a substantially longer half-life and require less-frequent dosing have been studied, but are not in current production for use [184, 189].

FSH and LH in clinically used products are standardized against recognized reference preparations using in vivo bioassay, and because of molecular heterogeneity that differs according to the method of preparation or synthesis these show differences in bio- and immmunoreactivity according to the method of measurement [190–192]. Despite differences in FSH pharmacokinetics and measures of bio- vs. immunoreactivity between traditional, highly purified urinary preparations and recombinant products, clear evidence for practical clinical significance for these differences is limited [193–198]. Some trials and metanalyses of trials do show small differences in clinical outcomes according to the gonadotropin preparation used [176, 199–202]. Whether or not advances in production of gonadotropins have led to improvements in clinical outcomes, newer more purified products allow for subcutaneous, rather than intramuscular administration [203], and recombinant techniques allow for easier control of purity and consistency of preparations. In practice, cost, access, and route of administration required are often factors in choice of product.

Daily dosing, which is usual practice, results in patterns of gonadotropin levels markedly dissimilar from those seen in the course of normal ovulatory physiology (lack of pulsatility, achievement of single maximum over 24 h approximately 12 h after injection, and gradual accumulation of levels over the days of follicle recruitment). Despite this, daily injection has not been shown inferior to or been replaced by regimens using more frequent or pulsatile administration [204–206]. Pharmacokinetics after intramuscular or subcutaneous administration of recombinant preparations are similar, even in obese women [203]. Obesity is associated with an increase in dose requirements in WHO type II patients that is not related to differences in pharmacokinetics [2, 203, 207].

35.1.3.2 Administration

Typical regimens for gonadotropin administration initiate gonadotropins after withdrawal bleeding (postovulatory or progestin-induced) of the endometrium, and superovulation regimens typically commence on day 3 of menses. Dosing in each cycle seeks to achieve a response providing a desirable number of mature oocytes without incurring the risk of multiple gestation or OHSS. Patients vary considerably with respect to the effective threshold dose for initiation and maintenance of follicular maturation, and this dose is generally inversely related to ovarian reserve and hence age. FSH receptor polymorphisms and as-yet-undetermined factors contribute to interindividual responsiveness to gonadotropin preparations, such that dosing is empiric and individualized based on response [208].

Monitoring for a follicular response predicting fertile ovulation, but not excessive response is essential. Achievement of ovulation is not the principal challenge with induction of ovulation using gonadotropins; rather, it is the achievement of a response that is safe with regard to the risks of multiple gestation and OHSS. Monitoring to prevent OHSS and multiple gestation relies on an integration of biophysical and hormonal data. Typical monitoring, therefore, utilizes ultrasound after 5 days of daily administration at the initially selected dose, with subsequent dosing and intervals for repeat assessments based on ultrasound findings and estradiol levels.

Ultrasound monitoring is used for measurement of endometrial thickness, and determination of numbers and size of ovarian follicles, and ovarian volume. Because follicle maturity and competence for ovulation may occur over a wide range of diameters, serum levels of estradiol provide complementary data that aid importantly in assessment of functional maturity of follicles on the one hand and of the risks of multiple gestation and OHSS on the other [209, 210]. Circulating estradiol levels peak approximately half day after the preceding dose of gonadotropins, and standardization of times for drug administration and serum draw for determination of estradiol response (usually evening and morning, respectively) is a common practice for this reason [211]. Current practice views the complementary use of utlrasound and estrogen measurement essential for effectiveness and safety of therapy [34, 69, 212–215]. It is important to note that numbers of intermediate (9–15 mm) as well as mature follicles contribute to the prediction of OHSS and multiple gestation [67, 68, 216–219]. Interpretation of estradiol levels assumes that competent mature follicle accounts for 200–400 pg/ml of circulating estradiol and that risks for OHSS and multiple gestation increase as levels approach 1,000 pg/ml [209, 216, 219]. Reliance on estradiol levels alone can be misleading, however, and numbers of dominant as well as intermediate-sized follicles are more predictive of multiple gestation than estradiol levels [218, 220–222]. Younger age increases risks for OHSS and multiple gestation and should be factored into assessment of risk as predicted by ultrasound and estradiol levels [216, 221].

Serum anti-Mullerian hormone level at baseline has been shown to be a predictor of OHSS among women undergoing controlled ovarian stimulation for ART, as has free serum vascular endothelial growth factor concentration on the day of hCG administration [223, 224]. These may achieve usefulness in selection of type and dose of gonadotropin agents and monitoring procedures to prevent OHSS in women undergoing ovulation induction with gonadotropins.

Follicles with diameters of 16 mm are viewed as capable of release of a mature oocyte, though smaller follicles do contribute to the risk of multiple gestation. When lead follicles reach a mean diameter of 18 mm, and if measures of risk for multiple gestation and OHSS are permissive, ovulation is triggered with administration of 10,000 international units of hCG subcutaneously or intramuscularly [225]. Reducing risk for development of OHSS by using lower (5,000 IU) doses of hCG, or by using recombinant LH, with its much shorter half-life has been proposed. Such approaches lack validation with significant numbers of subjects, and a commercially available preparation of recombinant LH is not currently available [194, 226].

Luteal function may be truncated in patients without sufficient endogenous LH, and this is typically corrected either with supplemental progesterone or a booster injection of hCG several days after the ovulatory dose of hCG is given. Extending luteal function with additional hCG can increase the risk of OHSS.

35.1.3.3 Use of Gonadotropins for WHO Group II Anovulation

The therapeutic window for gonadotropin dosing for patients with WHO group II anovulation is notoriously narrow. Increased follicular responsiveness in these patients is attributable to the size of the cohort of responsive follicles, not to a difference in sensitivity to gonadotropins at the level of the follicle [227]. Dose increases that are too frequent or too great in magnitude can lead to sudden generalized folliculogenesis that threatens the development of OHSS and high-order multiple pregnancy that necessitate cycle cancellation. Baseline ovarian volume in these patients is a predictor for difficulty in achieving safe follicular development for both ovulation and conception, and increased body weight predicts higher dose requirements [2, 228]. Formulas for prediction of a safe and effective initial dose of gonadotropin have been attempted, but management in most centers is empiric and based on observation for response as dose is increased [229]. Low initial dosing followed by gradual dose increases as dictated by response has been repeatedly affirmed as a superior strategy for eliciting safe ovulatory responses for these patients [160, 203, 207, 230–240]. Decreased frequency of dosing is another version of this approach and has shown promise [241]. A 3-day initiation at high doses of FSH followed by chronic low-dose strategies may offer advantages over conventional chronic low-dose protocols [242]. The chronic low-dose regimen appears safer and is more likely to result in pregnancy than a clomiphene–menotropin sequential regimen [243]. Chronic low-dosing protocols vary somewhat, but typically initiate therapy at 75 IU or less and space dosing increments of 37.5 IU, if required, initially by 7–14 days and thereafter by 7 days [244]. Use of preparations with LH activity may aid in achieving focused rather than generalized follicular development, and regimens converting from FSH to LH activity alone (as low-dose hCG) may enhance this desired effect further [174, 245–247]. There is evidence that the adjunctive use metformin reduces the risk for excessive follicular recruitment by FSH [248, 249].

Numerous studies have shown that the total dose of gonadotropins required for ovulation induction in clomiphene-resistant patients can be reduced by following administration of clomiphene with gonadotropins [250–252]. A similar benefit has shown that Letrozole is used at the initiation of cycles of gonadotropin therapy [253]. Pulsatile subcutaneous administration of FSH has been used for induction of ovulation with success, but offers no advantage over daily administration [205]. Addition of GnRHa suppression to pulsatile administration regimens is clinically effective, but it has not been shown to be superior [254].

35.1.4 Hypergonadotropic Hypogonadism

Premature ovarian failure is a heterogeneous entity, and it is frequently difficult to assign an etiologic diagnosis for women with these disorders. Efforts to afford ovulation and fertility have very low success rates, and these are hampered by poor understanding of how to characterize subgroups of these patients with respect to response to treatment. Karyotype abnormalities and premutations for fragile X syndrome in *FMR-1* gene are frequently associated with premature ovarian failure and have reproductive implications for women with these disorders. Evaluation of women with premature ovarian failure should also include assessment for evidence of polyglandular autoimmunity prior to any efforts to restore ovulation.

Case reports of successful therapy have in common the strategy of suppressing gonadotropin secretion with pharmacologic doses of estrogen or suppression of gonadotropins with long-acting agonists, or antagonists of GnRH, with or without subsequent administration of gonadotropins [42, 255, 256]. Evaluation of isolated case reports must be tempered by appreciation of the fact that many women with this diagnosis exhibit occasional and unpredictable spontaneous ovulation. Ovulation-restoring strategies designed to capitalize on ultrasound evidence of such episodes have not yet been shown effective [257].

Systematic evaluation of treatment to restore ovulation in premature ovarian failure has centered on strategies that administer gonadotropins, with or without prior suppression of endogenous hypergonadotropism. Results of most trials have shown very low response rates [258]. One randomized trial, in which the overall response rate was 10%, did not find that prior suppression of gonadotropins increased the likelihood of an ovulatory response to gonadotropin administration [258]. More recent trials suggest that gonadotropin stimulation following suppression of endogenous gonadotropins may be helpful. Long-acting GnRH agonist pretreatment has been shown in one study to achieve modest success rates (10–20%), which may be more effective if gonadotropin administration is accompanied by glucocorticoid therapy [259]. Use of high-dose estrogen for suppression of endogenous gonadotropins prior to gonadotropin administration has shown promising results as well [260].

Notwithstanding encouraging results in recent trials, it is important to recognize that restoration of ovulation is doubtful for the patient with hypergonadotropic hypogonadism with any known treatment strategy, and that pregnancies are even more unlikely. Moreover, the profile of pregnancy outcomes for women treated with these new protocols is unknown. Therefore, it is preferable, when possible, that ovulation induction for women with these disorders be conducted in the setting of formal clinical investigation.

35.1.5 Cancer and Ovulation Induction Treatments

Initial investigations linked use of ovulation induction agents with development of ovarian malignancies; early investigations found such an effect, specifically with long-term use of clomiphene [261, 262]. Several subsequent studies have not confirmed an association with ovulation induction although several studies identify infertility, the altered anthropometrics and endocrinology of anovulation, and reduced parity in particular to be potential confounding risks factors for gynecologic malignancies [263–267]. Biases (ascertainment, recall) and associations of ovulation induction underlying conditions favoring ovarian malignancy cloud this issue considerably. Recent analyses of data available from the several case control studies to date suggest that there may be a small increase in the relative risk of ovarian tumors of low malignant potential related to ovulation treatments, but not invasive epithelial ovarian cancers or other cancers of the reproductive system [268–272]. Although the current synthesis of available data is reassuring, it would discourage casual or protracted use of clomiphene and other modalities for ovulation induction or superovulation. In addition, patients should be made aware of concerns regarding ovulation induction agents and malignancy as a routine part of education about therapeutic alternatives.

35.1.6 Summary

35.1.6.1 Women with Normal Gonadotropin and Prolactin Levels

Weight loss achieved through alteration of lifestyle may restore ovulation and regular cycles among a large proportion of overweight or obese women with PCOS and enhance response to medical therapies in those remaining anovulatory [5,8,9]. Bariatric surgery has been shown to be highly effective in ameliorating metabolic and endocrine features of PCOS and restoring ovulation in morbidly obese anovulatory women [10]. Obesity has been associated with higher rates of early pregnancy loss in general and among women with PCOS treated with ovulation induction [11–13]. Additionally, because elevated BMI is a risk factor for gestational diabetes and cesarean section and has long-term adverse consequences to general health, a program of weight loss is a highly appropriate and often effective approach not only to restoration of ovulation, but improvement in pregnancy outcomes among obese, anovulatory women desiring pregnancy [5].

Clomiphene Citrate

Clomiphene citrate is marketed as a racemic mixture of two steroisomers, with different activities and rates of clearance. The *cis* isomer, enclomiphene, is the most antiestrogenic, and the shortest lived in the circulation, while much less activity is attributed to the *trans* isomer, zuclomiphene, which has a half-life sufficiently long that it may accumulate in the circulation over successive cycles of use [18–20]. No pharmacologically important or teratogenic influence has been attributed to the persistence of zuclomiphene in the circulation, and physiologic and endocrine responses to clomiphene are similar across successive cycles of administration [21]. Following association of clomiphene with estrogen receptor, its dissociation is delayed, reducing estrogen receptor levels available for estrogen action within the cell. Clomiphene's primary mechanism of action is central, at the hypothalamus, where loss of estrogen feedback results in increased GnRH pulse frequency and amplitude, although other sites of action may contribute to its ovulation-restoring effect [23–26]. In anovulatory women with a competent hypothalamic pituitary unit the resultant increase in gonadotropin levels is often sufficient to initiate folliculogenesis for one or more susceptible ovarian follicles. Folliculogenesis in clomiphene-induced ovulation is characterized by slightly greater follicle size at the time of the LH surge than in spontaneous cycles among normal women [27–29]. Multiple follicular development is common, and dose requirements for acceptable numbers of mature follicles are difficult to predict. Doses as low as 25 mg daily for achievement of numerically safe folliculogenesis may be necessary in some women using clomiphene either for ovulation induction or superovulation. The maximal approved dosage is 150 mg/day, and failure to respond at this dose commonly defines "clomiphene failure," though a few patients unresponsive to this dose will respond to doses as high as 250 mg/day in some reported clinical series [1, 15]. Response to clomiphene can be documented inexpensively and conveniently by one or combinations of the following: detection of an LH surge using commercially available kits, basal temperature records, progesterone determinations timed to the anticipated midluteal phase, and the subsequent occurrence of timely, normal menses. Addition of midcycle ultrasound monitoring of numbers of follicles of mature size to assure adequate but not excessive response may add safety and shorten the time to achievement of an appropriate dose. In cycles without follicular response, upward dose adjustment that follows a short course of progestin can be planned at the time of ultrasound. In the event excessive numbers of responsive follicles are found, interruption of the cycle and prevention of pregnancy with high-dose progestins can be instituted. If ultrasound is used, ultrasound monitoring in subsequent cycles is likely unnecessary in future cycles once a clomiphene dose providing an effective, yet safe response is seen.

Clomiphene's antiestrogenic effects are considered an explanation for poor estrogenization and reduced endometrial growth during the follicular phase of the cycle; most observers have found increased rates of attenuated preovulatory changes in cervical mucus and reduced thickness of proliferative phase endometrium when clomiphene is used for superovulation or ovulation induction [15, 28, 37–39]. Clomiphene should be discontinued when visual complaints are prominent or persistent [52, 53]. Although some reports have suggested an increase in the rate of spontaneous abortion among pregnancies resulting from clomiphene induction of ovulation, most case series and clinical trials do not find evidence for such an effect [54–56]. Numerous series [57–59] show little evidence for a teratogenic influence of the drug [59–61]. The most important risk associated with the use of medical agents for induction of ovulation and superovulation is multiple pregnancy, particularly high-order multiple pregnancy. The contribution to the burden of multiple pregnancy in the USA is roughly equivalent for ovulation induction treatments and ART [66].

Clomiphene Resistance

Two studies have shown that approximately half of patients failing to ovulate at clomiphene doses of 150 mg for 5 days will ovulate if dexamethasone at a dose of 1 mg BID is initiated with clomiphene and continued for 10 days [72]. Several studies have shown ovulation rates greater than 50% among women with PCOS that take metformin in doses of 1,500 mg/day as a primary therapy [77, 86, 87].

It has been shown that likelihood of ovulation among clomiphene-resistant women is increased from 8 to 71% by pretreatment with 6–7 weeks of continuously administered combined oral contraceptives. Subsequent treatment cycles are more often ovulatory, and pregnancy rates substantially increased as a result of pretreatment with hormonal contraceptives [98, 99].

Letrozole has been studied in doses of 2.5–7.5 mg per day and Anastrozole at doses of 1 mg, both given for 5 days early in the cycle, and both have been used to induce ovulation in normogonadotropic, normoprolactinemic anovulation, with no evidence in a difference in effectiveness [17, 103]. Concerns over teratogenesis are mitigated by a large cohort study [61]. However, because of concerns for teratogenesis, Letrozole (as Femara) is labeled with a black box warning regarding its use in women anticipating pregnancy. Clinicians who do use aromatase inhibitors are impelled to make patients aware of these concerns. Informed consent is commonly advised. Most importantly, use of aromatase inhibitors should be accompanied by clear precautions to avoid use in patients who are unknowingly pregnant.

Widespread use of ovarian volume-reducing interventions has not occurred because of surgical risks related to procedures, the poorly characterized risk of significant adnexal adhesions, and unknown long-term effects on ovarian reserve [124].

35.1.6.2 Hyperprolactinemia

Bromocriptine remains the agent of choice for restoration of ovulation for fertility in hyperprolactinemic states [149–151]. Bromocriptine administration is daily and is often effective at very low doses (e.g., 1.25 mg). Slow progression of dosing to levels required to restore ovulation reduces prevalence and severity of side effects, as does vaginal administration [152–157]. No teratogenic effect of bromocriptine has been demonstrated, and its use in pregnancy is widely held safe, but it is usually discontinued once pregnancy is recognized [159, 138]. Cabergoline shows greater efficacy and tolerability than bromocriptine and is often effective in patients not responding to bromocriptine [150, 151]. There is no evidence of teratogenicity for cabergoline, but its long half-life and limited data regarding safety in pregnancy lead most authors to recommend bromocriptine as a first line agent when fertility is sought or advise suspension of cabergoline in the cycle prior to conception [151, 157, 168].

35.1.6.3 Hypogonadotropic Hypogonadism

FSH and LH both have important roles in natural folliculogenesis, but in patients with even nominal background LH secretion, FSH is sufficient for induction of functional preovulatory follicles. In patients with profoundly suppressed or absent gonadotropins, folliculogenesis may occur without sufficient accompanying estrogen synthesis, and in these patients use of LH, even in low amounts, corrects this abnormality and presumably improves the chance of pregnancy. LH activity alone can drive folliculogenesis in follicles of intermediate size and greater, and LH (or hCG) can be substituted for FSH without consequence to ongoing follicular maturation once mid-sized follicles are achieved [172].

Whether or not advances in production of gonadotropins have led to improvements in clinical outcomes, newer more purified products allow for subcutaneous, rather than intramuscular administration [203], and recombinant techniques allow for easier control of purity and consistency of preparations. In practice, cost, access, and route of administration required are often factors in choice of product. Typical monitoring utilizes ultrasound after 5 days of daily administration at the initially selected dose, with subsequent dosing and intervals for repeat assessments based on ultrasound findings and estradiol levels. Typical monitoring, therefore, utilizes ultrasound after 5 days of daily administration at the initially selected dose, with subsequent dosing and intervals for repeat assessments based on ultrasound findings and estradiol levels. Follicles with diameters of 16 mm are viewed as capable of release of a mature oocyte, though smaller follicles do contribute to the risk of multiple gestation. The therapeutic window for gonadotropin dosing for patients with WHO group II anovulation is notoriously narrow. The chronic low-dose regimen appears safer and more likely to result in pregnancy than a clomiphene–menotropin sequential regimen [243]. Chronic low-dosing protocols vary somewhat, but typically initiate therapy at 75 IU or less and space dosing increments of 37.5 IU, if required, initially by 7–14 days and thereafter by 7 days [244].

35.1.6.4 Hypergonadotropic Hypogonadism

Karyotype abnormalities and premutations for fragile X syndrome in *FMR-1* gene are frequently associated with premature ovarian failure and have reproductive implications for women with these disorders. Evaluation of women with premature ovarian failure should also include assessment for evidence of polyglandular autoimmunity prior to any efforts to restore ovulation. Long-acting GnRH agonist pretreatment has been shown in one study to achieve modest success rates (10–20%), which may be more effective if gonadotropin administration accompanied by glucocorticoid therapy. Pretreatment with 0.05-mg ethinyl estradiol prior to gonadotropin administration resulted in ovulation for one-third of subjects administered with high-dose gonadotropins, while no subjects given gonadotropins without estrogen pretreatment ovulated. Response to gonadotropins was predicted by the degree of FSH suppression attained with estrogen administration [260].

35.1.6.5 Cancer and Ovulation Induction Treatments

Recent analyses of data available from the several case control studies to date suggest that there may be a small increase in the relative risk of ovarian tumors of low malignant potential related to ovulation treatments, but not invasive epithelial ovarian cancers or other cancers of the reproductive system [268–272].

References

1. Shepard MK, Balmaceda JP, Leija CG (1979) Relationship of weight to successful induction of ovulation with clomiphene citrate. Fertil Steril 32(6):641–645
2. Balen AH, Platteau P, Andersen AN et al (2006) The influence of body weight on response to ovulation induction with gonadotrophins in 335 women with World Health Organization group II anovulatory infertility. BJOG 113(10):1195–1202
3. Galtier-Dereure F, Pujol P, Dewailly D, Bringer J (1997) Choice of stimulation in polycystic ovarian syndrome: the influence of obesity. Hum Reprod 12 Suppl 1:88–96
4. Palomba S, Falbo A, Orio F Jr, Tolino A, Zullo F (2009) Efficacy predictors for metformin and clomiphene citrate treatment in anovulatory infertile patients with polycystic ovary syndrome. Fertil Steril 91(6):2557–2567
5. Clark AM, Thornley B, Tomlinson L, Galletley C, Norman RJ (1998) Weight loss in obese infertile women results in improvement in reproductive outcome for all forms of fertility treatment. Hum Reprod 13(6):1502–1505
6. Guzick DS (2004) Polycystic ovary syndrome. Obstet Gynecol 103(1):181–193
7. Guzick DS (2007) Ovulation induction management of PCOS. Clin Obstet Gynecol 50(1):255–267
8. Clark AM, Ledger W, Galletly C et al (1995) Weight loss results in significant improvement in pregnancy and ovulation rates in anovulatory obese women. Hum Reprod 10(10):2705–2712
9. Hoeger KM, Kochman L, Wixom N, Craig K, Miller RK, Guzick DS (2004) A randomized, 48-week, placebo-controlled trial of intensive lifestyle modification and/or metformin therapy in overweight women with polycystic ovary syndrome: a pilot study. Fertil Steril 82(2):421–429
10. Escobar-Morreale HF, Botella-Carretero JI, Alvarez-Blasco F, Sancho J, San Millan JL (2005) The polycystic ovary syndrome associated with morbid obesity may resolve after weight loss induced by bariatric surgery. J Clin Endocrinol Metab 90(12):6364–6369

11. Hamilton-Fairley D, Kiddy D, Watson H, Paterson C, Franks S (1992) Association of moderate obesity with a poor pregnancy outcome in women with polycystic ovary syndrome treated with low dose gonadotrophin. Br J Obstet Gynaecol 99(2):128–131
12. Lashen H, Fear K, Sturdee DW (2004) Obesity is associated with increased risk of first trimester and recurrent miscarriage: matched case-control study. Hum Reprod 19(7):1644–1646
13. Metwally M, Ledger WL, Li TC (2008) Reproductive endocrinology and clinical aspects of obesity in women. Ann N Y Acad Sci 1127:140–146
14. Thessaloniki ESHRE/ASRM-Sponsored PCOS Consensus Workshop Group (2008) Consensus on infertility treatment related to polycystic ovary syndrome. Fertil Steril 89(3):505–522
15. Gysler M, March CM, Mishell DR Jr, Bailey EJ (1982) A decade's experience with an individualized clomiphene treatment regimen including its effect on the postcoital test. Fertil Steril 37(2):161–167
16. Gerhard I, Runnebaum B (1979) Comparison between tamoxifen and clomiphene therapy in women with anovulation. Arch Gynecol 227(4):279–288
17. Beck JI, Boothroyd C, Proctor M, Farquhar C, Hughes E (2005) Oral anti-oestrogens and medical adjuncts for subfertility associated with anovulation. Cochrane Database Syst Rev 1:CD002249
18. Glasier AF, Irvine DS, Wickings EJ, Hillier SG, Baird DT (1989) A comparison of the effects on follicular development between clomiphene citrate, its two separate isomers and spontaneous cycles. Hum Reprod 4(3):252–256
19. Mikkelson TJ, Kroboth PD, Cameron WJ, Dittert LW, Chungi V, Manberg PJ (1986) Single-dose pharmacokinetics of clomiphene citrate in normal volunteers. Fertil Steril 46(3):392–396
20. Turner RT, Evans GL, Sluka JP et al (1998) Differential responses of estrogen target tissues in rats including bone to clomiphene, enclomiphene, and zuclomiphene. Endocrinology 139(9):3712–3720
21. Opsahl MS, Robins ED, O'Connor DM, Scott RT, Fritz MA (1996) Characteristics of gonadotropin response, follicular development, and endometrial growth and maturation across consecutive cycles of clomiphene citrate treatment. Fertil Steril 66(4):533–539
22. Clark JH, Guthrie SC (1981) Agonistic and antagonistic effects of clomiphene citrate and its isomers. Biol Reprod 25(3):667–672
23. Adashi EY (1984) Clomiphene citrate: mechanism(s) and site(s) of action – a hypothesis revisited. Fertil Steril 42(3):331–344
24. Olsson JH, Granberg S (1990) Effect of clomiphene isomers on oestradiol synthesis in cultured human granulosa cells. Hum Reprod 5(8):928–932
25. Zhuang LZ, Adashi EY, Hsuch AJ (1982) Direct enhancement of gonadotropin-stimulated ovarian estrogen biosynthesis by estrogen and clomiphene citrate. Endocrinology 110(6):2219–2221
26. Schwartz LB, Brezinski A, Laufer N (1993) The effect of clomiphene citrate isomers on human granulosa-lutein cells in culture. Gynecol Endocrinol 7(4):229–233
27. Hata T, Yoshino K, Nagahara Y, Matsunaga I, Kitao M (1983) Precise day of ovulation determined by real-time ultrasound evidence of graafian follicular development. Int J Gynaecol Obstet 21(6):435–438
28. Haritha S, Rajagopalan G (2003) Follicular growth, endometrial thickness, and serum estradiol levels in spontaneous and clomiphene citrate-induced cycles. Int J Gynaecol Obstet 81(3): 287–292
29. Fossum GT, Vermesh M, Kletzky OA (1990) Biochemical and biophysical indices of follicular development in spontaneous and stimulated ovulatory cycles. Obstet Gynecol 75(3 Part 1):407–411
30. Wu CH, Winkel CA (1989) The effect of therapy initiation day on clomiphene citrate therapy. Fertil Steril 52(4):564–568
31. Dehbashi S, Vafaei H, Parsanezhad MD, Alborzi S (2006) Time of initiation of clomiphene citrate and pregnancy rate in polycystic ovarian syndrome. Int J Gynaecol Obstet 93(1):44–48
32. Adams R, Mishell DR Jr, Israel R (1972) Treatment of refractory anovulation with increased dosage and prolonged duration of cyclic clomiphene citrate. Obstet Gynecol 39(4):562–566
33. Fluker MR, Wang IY, Rowe TC (1996) An extended 10-day course of clomiphene citrate (CC) in women with CC-resistant ovulatory disorders. Fertil Steril 66(5):761–764
34. O'Herlihy C, Evans JH, Brown JB, de Crespigny LJ, Robinson HP (1982) Use of ultrasound in monitoring ovulation induction with human pituitary gonadotropins. Obstet Gynecol 60(5):577–582
35. Andersen AG, Als-Nielsen B, Hornnes PJ, Franch Andersen L (1995) Time interval from human chorionic gonadotrophin (HCG) injection to follicular rupture. Hum Reprod 1995;10(12): 3202–3205
36. Fischer RA, Nakajima ST, Gibson M, Brumsted JR (1993) Ovulation after intravenous and intramuscular human chorionic gonadotropin. Fertil Steril 60(3):418–422
37. Eden JA, Place J, Carter GD, Jones J, Alaghband-Zadeh J, Pawson ME (1989) The effect of clomiphene citrate on follicular phase increase in endometrial thickness and uterine volume. Obstet Gynecol 73(2):187–190
38. Dehbashi S, Parsanezhad ME, Alborzi S, Zarei A (2003) Effect of clomiphene citrate on endometrium thickness and echogenic patterns. Int J Gynaecol Obstet 80(1):49–53
39. Palomba S, Russo T, Orio F Jr et al (2006) Uterine effects of clomiphene citrate in women with polycystic ovary syndrome: a prospective controlled study. Hum Reprod 21(11):2823–2829
40. Fedele L, Brioschi D, Marchini M, Dorta M, Parazzini F (1989) Enhanced preovulatory progesterone levels in clomiphene citrate-induced cycles. J Clin Endocrinol Metab 69(3):681–683
41. Dickey RP, Taylor SN, Curole DN, Rye PH, Lu PY, Pyrzak R (1997) Relationship of clomiphene dose and patient weight to successful treatment. Hum Reprod 12(3):449–453
42. Check JH, Dietterich C, Lurie D (1995) The effect of consecutive cycles of clomiphene citrate therapy on endometrial thickness and echo pattern. Obstet Gynecol 86(3):341–345
43. Kolibianakis EM, Zikopoulos KA, Fatemi HM et al (2004) Endometrial thickness cannot predict ongoing pregnancy achievement in cycles stimulated with clomiphene citrate for intrauterine insemination. Reprod Biomed Online 8(1):115–118
44. Unfer V, Costabile L, Gerli S, Papaleo E, Marelli G, Di Renzo GC (2001) Low dose of ethinyl estradiol can reverse the antiestrogenic effects of clomiphene citrate on endometrium. Gynecol Obstet Invest 51(2):120–123
45. Gerli S, Gholami H, Manna C, Di Frega AS, Vitiello C, Unfer V (2000) Use of ethinyl estradiol to reverse the antiestrogenic effects of clomiphene citrate in patients undergoing intrauterine insemination: a comparative, randomized study. Fertil Steril 73(1): 85–89
46. Frattarelli JL, Dempsey MS (2004) Characteristics of baseline ovarian cysts in clomiphene citrate ovulation cycles. Fertil Steril 82(4):979–981
47. Ben-Ami M, Geslevich Y, Battino S, Matilsky M, Shalev E (1993) Management of functional ovarian cysts after induction of ovulation. A randomized prospective study. Acta Obstet Gynecol Scand 72(5):396–397
48. MacKenna A, Fabres C, Alam V, Morales V (2000) Clinical management of functional ovarian cysts: a prospective and randomized study. Hum Reprod 15(12):2567–2569
49. Csokmay JM, Frattarelli JL (2006) Basal ovarian cysts and clomiphene citrate ovulation induction cycles. Obstet Gynecol 107(6):1292–1296
50. Blenner JL (1991) Clomiphene-induced mood swings. J Obstet Gynecol Neonatal Nurs 20(4):321–327
51. Choi SH, Shapiro H, Robinson GE et al (2005) Psychological side-effects of clomiphene citrate and human menopausal gonadotrophin. J Psychosom Obstet Gynaecol 26(2):93–100

52. Purvin VA (1995) Visual disturbance secondary to clomiphene citrate. Arch Ophthalmol 113(4):482–484
53. Lawton AW (1994) Optic neuropathy associated with clomiphene citrate therapy. Fertil Steril 61(2):390–391
54. Dickey RP, Taylor SN, Curole DN, Rye PH, Pyrzak R (1996) Incidence of spontaneous abortion in clomiphene pregnancies. Hum Reprod 11(12):2623–2628
55. Legro RS, Barnhart HX, Schlaff WD et al (2007) Clomiphene, metformin, or both for infertility in the polycystic ovary syndrome. N Engl J Med 356(6):551–566
56. Moll E, Bossuyt PM, Korevaar JC, Lambalk CB, van der Veen F (2006) Effect of clomifene citrate plus metformin and clomifene citrate plus placebo on induction of ovulation in women with newly diagnosed polycystic ovary syndrome: randomised double blind clinical trial. BMJ 332(7556):1485
57. Whiteman D, Murphy M, Hey K, O'Donnell M, Goldacre M (2000) Reproductive factors, subfertility, and risk of neural tube defects: a case-control study based on the Oxford Record Linkage Study Register. Am J Epidemiol 152(9):823–828
58. Zhu JL, Basso O, Obel C, Bille C, Olsen J (2006) Infertility, infertility treatment, and congenital malformations: Danish national birth cohort. BMJ 333(7570):679
59. Ahlgren M, Kallen B, Rannevik G (1976) Outcome of pregnancy after clomiphene therapy. Acta Obstet Gynecol Scand 55(4):371–375
60. Correy JF, Marsden DE, Schokman FC (1982) The outcome of pregnancy resulting from clomiphene-induced ovulation. Aust N Z J Obstet Gynaecol 22(1):18–21
61. Tulandi T, Martin J, Al-Fadhli R et al (2006) Congenital malformations among 911 newborns conceived after infertility treatment with letrozole or clomiphene citrate. Fertil Steril 85(6):1761–1765
62. Elizur SE, Tulandi T (2008) Drugs in infertility and fetal safety. Fertil Steril 89(6):1595–1602
63. Wu YW, Croen LA, Henning L, Najjar DV, Schembri M, Croughan MS (2006) Potential association between infertility and spinal neural tube defects in offspring. Birth Defects Res A Clin Mol Teratol 76(10):718–722
64. Thatcher SS, Jackson EM (2006) Pregnancy outcome in infertile patients with polycystic ovary syndrome who were treated with metformin. Fertil Steril 85(4):1002–1009
65. Basso O, Baird DD (2003) Infertility and preterm delivery, birthweight, and Caesarean section: a study within the Danish National Birth Cohort. Hum Reprod 18(11):2478–2484
66. Dickey RP (2007) The relative contribution of assisted reproductive technologies and ovulation induction to multiple births in the United States 5 years after the Society for Assisted Reproductive Technology/American Society for Reproductive Medicine recommendation to limit the number of embryos transferred. Fertil Steril 88(6):1554–1561
67. Dickey RP, Taylor SN, Lu PY, Sartor BM, Rye PH, Pyrzak R (2005) Risk factors for high-order multiple pregnancy and multiple birth after controlled ovarian hyperstimulation: results of 4, 062 intrauterine insemination cycles. Fertil Steril 83(3):671–683
68. Dickey RP, Taylor SN, Lu PY, Sartor BM, Rye PH, Pyrzak R (2001) Relationship of follicle numbers and estradiol levels to multiple implantation in 3, 608 intrauterine insemination cycles. Fertil Steril 75(1):69–78
69. Hull ME, Moghissi KS, Magyar DM, Hayes MF, Zador I, Olson JM (1986) Correlation of serum estradiol levels and ultrasound monitoring to assess follicular maturation. Fertil Steril 46(1):42–45
70. Lobo RA, Paul W, March CM, Granger L, Kletzky OA (1982) Clomiphene and dexamethasone in women unresponsive to clomiphene alone. Obstet Gynecol 60(4):497–501
71. Daly DC, Walters CA, Soto-Albors CE, Tohan N, Riddick DH (1984) A randomized study of dexamethasone in ovulation induction with clomiphene citrate. Fertil Steril 41(6):844–848
72. Singh KB, Dunnihoo DR, Mahajan DK, Bairnsfather LE (1992) Clomiphene-dexamethasone treatment of clomiphene-resistant women with and without the polycystic ovary syndrome. J Reprod Med 37(3):215–218
73. Diamant YZ, Evron S (1981) Induction of ovulation by combined clomiphene citrate and dexamethasone treatment in clomiphene citrate nonresponders. Eur J Obstet Gynecol Reprod Biol 11(5):335–340
74. Trott EA, Plouffe L Jr, Hansen K, Hines R, Brann DW, Mahesh VB (1996) Ovulation induction in clomiphene-resistant anovulatory women with normal dehydroepiandrosterone sulfate levels: beneficial effects of the addition of dexamethasone during the follicular phase. Fertil Steril 66(3):484–486
75. Parsanezhad ME, Alborzi S, Motazedian S, Omrani G (2002) Use of dexamethasone and clomiphene citrate in the treatment of clomiphene citrate-resistant patients with polycystic ovary syndrome and normal dehydroepiandrosterone sulfate levels: a prospective, double-blind, placebo-controlled trial. Fertil Steril 78(5):1001–1004
76. Elnashar A, Abdelmageed E, Fayed M, Sharaf M (2006) Clomiphene citrate and dexamethazone in treatment of clomiphene citrate-resistant polycystic ovary syndrome: a prospective placebo-controlled study. Hum Reprod 21(7):1805–1808
77. Neveu N, Granger L, St-Michel P, Lavoie HB (2007) Comparison of clomiphene citrate, metformin, or the combination of both for first-line ovulation induction and achievement of pregnancy in 154 women with polycystic ovary syndrome. Fertil Steril 87(1):113–120
78. Khorram O, Helliwell JP, Katz S, Bonpane CM, Jaramillo L (2006) Two weeks of metformin improves clomiphene citrate-induced ovulation and metabolic profiles in women with polycystic ovary syndrome. Fertil Steril 85(5):1448–1451
79. Kocak M, Caliskan E, Simsir C, Haberal A (2002) Metformin therapy improves ovulatory rates, cervical scores, and pregnancy rates in clomiphene citrate-resistant women with polycystic ovary syndrome. Fertil Steril 77(1):101–106
80. Lord JM, Flight IH, Norman RJ (2003) Insulin-sensitising drugs (metformin, troglitazone, rosiglitazone, pioglitazone, D-chiro-inositol) for polycystic ovary syndrome. Cochrane Database Syst Rev 3:CD003053
81. Nestler JE, Jakubowicz DJ, Evans WS, Pasquali R (1998) Effects of metformin on spontaneous and clomiphene-induced ovulation in the polycystic ovary syndrome. N Engl J Med 338(26): 1876–1880
82. Palomba S, Orio F Jr, Falbo A et al (2005) Prospective parallel randomized, double-blind, double-dummy controlled clinical trial comparing clomiphene citrate and metformin as the first-line treatment for ovulation induction in nonobese anovulatory women with polycystic ovary syndrome. J Clin Endocrinol Metab 90(7): 4068–4074
83. Palomba S, Orio F Jr, Nardo LG et al (2004) Metformin administration versus laparoscopic ovarian diathermy in clomiphene citrate-resistant women with polycystic ovary syndrome: a prospective parallel randomized double-blind placebo-controlled trial. J Clin Endocrinol Metab 89(10):4801–4809
84. Kumari AS, Haq A, Jayasundaram R, Abdel-Wareth LO, Al Haija SA, Alvares M (2005) Metformin monotherapy in lean women with polycystic ovary syndrome. Reprod Biomed Online 10(1):100–104
85. Liu KE, Tataryn IV, Sagle M (2006) Use of metformin for ovulation induction in women who have polycystic ovary syndrome with or without evidence of insulin resistance. J Obstet Gynaecol Can 28(7):595–599
86. De Leo V, la Marca A, Petraglia F (2003) Insulin-lowering agents in the management of polycystic ovary syndrome. Endocr Rev 24(5):633–667

87. Heard MJ, Pierce A, Carson SA, Buster JE (2002) Pregnancies following use of metformin for ovulation induction in patients with polycystic ovary syndrome. Fertil Steril 77(4):669–673
88. Azziz R, Ehrmann D, Legro RS et al (2001) Troglitazone improves ovulation and hirsutism in the polycystic ovary syndrome: a multicenter, double blind, placebo-controlled trial. J Clin Endocrinol Metab 86(4):1626–1632
89. Rouzi AA, Ardawi MS (2006) A randomized controlled trial of the efficacy of rosiglitazone and clomiphene citrate versus metformin and clomiphene citrate in women with clomiphene citrate-resistant polycystic ovary syndrome. Fertil Steril 85(2):428–435
90. Ghazeeri G, Kutteh WH, Bryer-Ash M, Haas D, Ke RW (2003) Effect of rosiglitazone on spontaneous and clomiphene citrate-induced ovulation in women with polycystic ovary syndrome. Fertil Steril 79(3):562–566
91. Barbieri RL (2003) Metformin for the treatment of polycystic ovary syndrome. Obstet Gynecol 101(4):785–793
92. Cataldo NA, Barnhart HX, Legro RS et al (2008) Extended-release metformin does not reduce the clomiphene citrate dose required to induce ovulation in polycystic ovary syndrome. J Clin Endocrinol Metab 93(8):3124–3127
93. Vandermolen DT, Ratts VS, Evans WS, Stovall DW, Kauma SW, Nestler JE (2001) Metformin increases the ovulatory rate and pregnancy rate from clomiphene citrate in patients with polycystic ovary syndrome who are resistant to clomiphene citrate alone. Fertil Steril 75(2):310–315
94. Siebert TI, Kruger TF, Steyn DW, Nosarka S (2006) Is the addition of metformin efficacious in the treatment of clomiphene citrate-resistant patients with polycystic ovary syndrome? A structured literature review. Fertil Steril 86(5):1432–1437
95. Creanga AA, Bradley HM, McCormick C, Witkop CT (2008) Use of metformin in polycystic ovary syndrome: a meta-analysis. Obstet Gynecol 111(4):959–968
96. Sinawat S, Buppasiri P, Lumbiganon P, Pattanittum P (2008) Long versus short course treatment with metformin and clomiphene citrate for ovulation induction in women with PCOS. Cochrane Database Syst Rev 1:CD006226
97. Jakubowicz DJ, Iuorno MJ, Jakubowicz S, Roberts KA, Nestler JE (2002) Effects of metformin on early pregnancy loss in the polycystic ovary syndrome. J Clin Endocrinol Metab 87(2):524–529
98. Branigan EF, Estes MA (1999) Treatment of chronic anovulation resistant to clomiphene citrate (CC) by using oral contraceptive ovarian suppression followed by repeat CC treatment. Fertil Steril 71(3):544–546
99. Branigan EF, Estes MA (2003) A randomized clinical trial of treatment of clomiphene citrate-resistant anovulation with the use of oral contraceptive pill suppression and repeat clomiphene citrate treatment. Am J Obstet Gynecol 188(6):1424–1428; discussion 9–30
100. Martin TL, Kim M, Malarkey WB (1985) The natural history of idiopathic hyperprolactinemia. J Clin Endocrinol Metab 60(5):855–858
101. Bayram N, van Wely M, van der Veen F (2006) Pulsatile gonadotrophin releasing hormone for ovulation induction in subfertility associated with polycystic ovary syndrome (review). Cochrane Collab 4:1–18
102. Buzdar AU (2003) Pharmacology and pharmacokinetics of the newer generation aromatase inhibitors. Clin Cancer Res 9(1 Part 2):468S–472S
103. Mitwally MF, Biljan MM, Casper RF (2005) Pregnancy outcome after the use of an aromatase inhibitor for ovarian stimulation. Am J Obstet Gynecol 192(2):381–386
104. Badawy A, Mosbah A, Shady M (2008) Anastrozole or letrozole for ovulation induction in clomiphene-resistant women with polycystic ovarian syndrome: a prospective randomized trial. Fertil Steril 89(5):1209–1212
105. Atay V, Cam C, Muhcu M, Cam M, Karateke A (2006) Comparison of letrozole and clomiphene citrate in women with polycystic ovaries undergoing ovarian stimulation. J Int Med Res 34(1):73–76
106. Begum MR, Ferdous J, Begum A, Quadir E (2009) Comparison of efficacy of aromatase inhibitor and clomiphene citrate in induction of ovulation in polycystic ovarian syndrome. Fertil Steril 92(3):853–857
107. Casper RF (2009) Letrozole versus clomiphene citrate: which is better for ovulation induction? Fertil Steril 92(3):858–859
108. Bayar U, Basaran M, Kiran S, Coskun A, Gezer S (2006) Use of an aromatase inhibitor in patients with polycystic ovary syndrome: a prospective randomized trial. Fertil Steril 86(5):1447–1451
109. Badawy A, Aal IA, Abulatta M (2009) Clomiphene citrate or anastrozole for ovulation induction in women with polycystic ovary syndrome? A prospective controlled trial. Fertil Steril 92(3): 860–863
110. Badawy A, Metwally M, Fawzy M (2007) Randomized controlled trial of three doses of letrozole for ovulation induction in patients with unexplained infertility. Reprod Biomed Online 14(5):559–562
111. Fisher SA, Reid RL, Van Vugt DA, Casper RF (2002) A randomized double-blind comparison of the effects of clomiphene citrate and the aromatase inhibitor letrozole on ovulatory function in normal women. Fertil Steril 78(2):280–285
112. Bayar U, Tanriverdi HA, Barut A, Ayoglu F, Ozcan O, Kaya E (2006) Letrozole vs. clomiphene citrate in patients with ovulatory infertility. Fertil Steril 85(4):1045–1048
113. Elnashar A, Fouad H, Eldosoky M, Saeid N (2006) Letrozole induction of ovulation in women with clomiphene citrate-resistant polycystic ovary syndrome may not depend on the period of infertility, the body mass index, or the luteinizing hormone/follicle-stimulating hormone ratio. Fertil Steril 85(2):511–513
114. Wu HH, Wang NM, Cheng ML, Hsieh JN (2007) A randomized comparison of ovulation induction and hormone profile between the aromatase inhibitor anastrozole and clomiphene citrate in women with infertility. Gynecol Endocrinol 23(2):76–81
115. Farquhar CM, Williamson K, Brown PM, Garland J (2004) An economic evaluation of laparoscopic ovarian diathermy versus gonadotrophin therapy for women with clomiphene citrate resistant polycystic ovary syndrome. Hum Reprod 19(5):1110–1115
116. Farquhar CM, Williamson K, Gudex G, Johnson NP, Garland J, Sadler L (2002) A randomized controlled trial of laparoscopic ovarian diathermy versus gonadotropin therapy for women with clomiphene citrate-resistant polycystic ovary syndrome. Fertil Steril 78(2):404–411
117. Kaya H, Sezik M, Ozkaya O (2005) Evaluation of a new surgical approach for the treatment of clomiphene citrate-resistant infertility in polycystic ovary syndrome: laparoscopic ovarian multi-needle intervention. J Minim Invasive Gynecol 12(4):355–358
118. Armar NA, Lachelin GC (1993) Laparoscopic ovarian diathermy: an effective treatment for anti-oestrogen resistant anovulatory infertility in women with the polycystic ovary syndrome. Br J Obstet Gynaecol 100(2):161–164
119. Farhi J, Soule S, Jacobs HS (1995) Effect of laparoscopic ovarian electrocautery on ovarian response and outcome of treatment with gonadotropins in clomiphene citrate-resistant patients with polycystic ovary syndrome. Fertil Steril 64(5):930–935
120. Api M, Gorgen H, Cetin A (2005) Laparoscopic ovarian drilling in polycystic ovary syndrome. Eur J Obstet Gynecol Reprod Biol 119(1):76–81
121. Badawy A, Khiary M, Ragab A, Hassan M, Sherief L (2009) Ultrasound-guided transvaginal ovarian needle drilling (UTND) for treatment of polycystic ovary syndrome: a randomized controlled trial. Fertil Steril 91(4):1164–1167
122. Malkawi HY, Qublan HS, Hamaideh AH (2003) Medical vs. surgical treatment for clomiphene citrate-resistant women with polycystic ovary syndrome. J Obstet Gynaecol 23(3):289–293

123. Saleh AM, Khalil HS (2004) Review of nonsurgical and surgical treatment and the role of insulin-sensitizing agents in the management of infertile women with polycystic ovary syndrome. Acta Obstet Gynecol Scand 83(7):614–621
124. Kandil M, Selim M (2005) Hormonal and sonographic assessment of ovarian reserve before and after laparoscopic ovarian drilling in polycystic ovary syndrome. BJOG 112(10):1427–1430
125. Seppala M, Hibroven E, Ranta T, Virkkunen P, Leppaluoto J (1975) Raised serum prolactin levels in amenorrhoea. Br Med J 2(5966):305–306
126. L'Hermite M, Hotton F, Kleiner S, Caufriez A, Robyn C (1977) Amenorrhoea, sterility and hyperprolactinaemia. Importance of complex movement tomographic x-ray study and follow-up of the sella turcica. Ann Endocrinol 38(4):327–332
127. Davajan V, Kletzky O, March CM, Roy S, Mishell DR Jr (1978) The significance of galactorrhea in patients with normal menses, oligomenorrhea, and secondary amenorrhea. Am J Obstet Gynecol 130(8):894–904
128. Marrs RP, Kletzky OA, Teal J, Davajan V, March C, Mishell DR Jr (1979) Comparison of serum prolactin, plain radiography, and hypocycloidal tomography of the sella turcica in patients with galactorrhea. Am J Obstet Gynecol 135(4):467–469
129. Keye WR, Jr., Chang RJ, Wilson CB, Jaffe RB (1980) Prolactin-secreting pituitary adenomas. III. Frequency and diagnosis in amenorrhea-galactorrhea. JAMA 244(12):1329–1332
130. Crosignani PG, Ferrari C, Scarduelli C, Picciotti MC, Caldara R, Malinverni A (1981) Spontaneous and induced pregnancies in hyperprolactinemic women. Obstet Gynecol 58(6):708–713
131. Bergh T, Nillius SJ, Wide L (1978) Bromocriptine treatment of 42 hyperprolactinaemic women with secondary amenorrhoea. Acta Endocrinol 88(3):435–451
132. Franks S, Murray MA, Jequier AM, Steele SJ, Nabarro JD, Jacobs HS (1975) Incidence and significance of hyperprolactinaemia in women with amenorrhea. Clin Endocrinol 4(6):597–607
133. Mroueh AM, Siler-Khodr TM (1977) Bromocryptine therapy in cases of amenorrhea-galactorrhea. Am J Obstet Gynecol 127(3):291–298
134. Hardy J (1979) The transsphenoidal surgical approach to the pituitary. Hosp Pract 14(6):81–89
135. Franks S (1979) Use of bromocriptine in hyperprolactinaemic anovulation and related disorders. Drugs 17(5):337–348
136. Ampudia X, Puig-Domingo M, Schwarzstein D et al (1992) Outcome and long-term effects of pregnancy in women with hyperprolactinaemia. Eur J Obstet Gynecol Reprod Biol 46(2–3):101–107
137. Schlechte J, Dolan K, Sherman B, Chapler F, Luciano A (1989) The natural history of untreated hyperprolactinemia: a prospective analysis. J Clin Endocrinol Metab 68(2):412–418
138. Weil C (1986) The safety of bromocriptine in hyperprolactinaemic female infertility: a literature review. Curr Med Res Opin 10(3):172–195
139. Pepperell RJ, Martinez C, Dickinson A (1983) Natural history of patients with hyperprolactinaemia. Clin Reprod Fertil 2(4): 237–247
140. Bergh T, Nillius SJ, Larsson SG, Wide L (1981) Effects of bromocriptine-induced pregnancy on prolactin-secreting pituitary tumours. Acta Endocrinol 98(3):333–338
141. Isaacs AJ (1979) Resolution of hyperprolactinaemia after bromocriptine-induced pregnancy. Lancet 1(8119):784–785
142. Zarate A, Canales ES, Alger M, Forsbach G (1979) The effect of pregnancy and lactation on pituitary prolactin-secreting tumours. Acta Endocrinol 92(3):407–412
143. Jewelewicz R, Vande Wiele RL (1980) Clinical course and outcome of pregnancy in twenty-five patients with pituitary microadenomas. Am J Obstet Gynecol 136(3):339–343
144. Weinstein D, Yarkoni S, Schenker JG et al (1981) Conservative management of suspected prolactin secreting pituitary adenoma during pregnancy. Eur J Obstet Gynecol Reprod Biol 11(5):305–312
145. Maeda T, Ushiroyama T, Okuda K, Fujimoto A, Ueki M, Sugimoto O (1983) Effective bromocriptine treatment of a pituitary macroadenoma during pregnancy. Obstet Gynecol 61(1):117–121
146. Molitch ME (1996) Evaluation and management of pituitary tumors during pregnancy. Endocr Pract 2(4):287–295
147. Serri O, Rasio E, Beauregard H, Hardy J, Somma M (1983) Recurrence of hyperprolactinemia after selective transsphenoidal adenomectomy in women with prolactinoma. N Engl J Med 309(5):280–283
148. Molitch ME (1999) Management of prolactinomas during pregnancy. J Reprod Med 44(12 Suppl):1121–1126
149. al-Suleiman SA, Najashi S, Rahman J, Rahman MS (1989) Outcome of treatment with bromocriptine in patients with hyperprolactinaemia. Aust N Z J Obstet Gynaecol 29(2):176–179
150. Verhelst J, Abs R (2003) Hyperprolactinemia: pathophysiology and management. Treat Endocrinol 2(1):23–32
151. Molitch ME (2002) Medical management of prolactin-secreting pituitary adenomas. Pituitary 5(2):55–65
152. Acarturk F, Altug N (2001) In-vitro and in-vivo evaluation of a matrix-controlled bromocriptine mesilate-releasing vaginal ring. J Pharm Pharmacol 53(12):1721–1726
153. Darwish AM, Farah E, Gadallah WA, Mohammad II (2007) Superiority of newly developed vaginal suppositories over vaginal use of commercial bromocriptine tablets: a randomized controlled clinical trial. Reprod Sci 14(3):280–285
154. Ricci G, Giolo E, Nucera G, Pozzobon C, De Seta F, Guaschino S (2001) Pregnancy in hyperprolactinemic infertile women treated with vaginal bromocriptine: report of two cases and review of the literature. Gynecol Obstet Invest 51(4):266–270
155. Darwish AM, Hafez E, El-Gebali I, Hassan SB (2005) Evaluation of a novel vaginal bromocriptine mesylate formulation: a pilot study. Fertil Steril 83(4):1053–1055
156. Ginsburg J, Hardiman P, Thomas M (1992) Vaginal bromocriptine – clinical and biochemical effects. Gynecol Endocrinol 6(2):119–126
157. Vermesh M, Fossum GT, Kletzky OA (1988) Vaginal bromocriptine: pharmacology and effect on serum prolactin in normal women. Obstet Gynecol 72(5):693–698
158. Katz E, Weiss BE, Hassell A, Schran HF, Adashi EY (1991) Increased circulating levels of bromocriptine after vaginal compared with oral administration. Fertil Steril 55(5):882–884
159. Krupp P, Monka C (1987) Bromocriptine in pregnancy: safety aspects. Klin Wochenschr 65(17):823–827
160. Calaf Alsina J, Ruiz Balda JA, Romeu Sarrio A et al (2003) Ovulation induction with a starting dose of 50 IU of recombinant follicle stimulating hormone in WHO group II anovulatory women: the IO-50 study, a prospective, observational, multicentre, open trial. BJOG 110(12):1072–1077
161. Chiodini I, Liuzzi A (2003) PRL-secreting pituitary adenomas in pregnancy. J Endocrinol Invest 26(1):96–99
162. de Wit W, Coelingh Bennink HJ, Gerards LJ (1984) Prophylactic bromocriptine treatment during pregnancy in women with macroprolactinomas: report of 13 pregnancies. Br J Obstet Gynaecol 91(11):1059–1069
163. Mattei AM, Ferrari C, Ragni G et al (1984) Serum prolactin and ovarian function after discontinuation of drug treatment for hyperprolactinaemia: a study with bromocriptine and metergoline. Br J Obstet Gynaecol 91(3):244–250
164. Ferrari C, Mattei A, Melis GB et al (1989) Cabergoline: long-acting oral treatment of hyperprolactinemic disorders. J Clin Endocrinol Metab 68(6):1201–1206
165. Ferrari C, Paracchi A, Mattei AM, de Vincentiis S, D'Alberton A, Crosignani P (1992) Cabergoline in the long-term therapy of hyperprolactinemic disorders. Acta Endocrinol 126(6):489–494
166. Ferrari C, Piscitelli G, Crosignani PG (1995) Cabergoline: a new drug for the treatment of hyperprolactinaemia. Hum Reprod 10(7):1647–1652

167. Rains CP, Bryson HM, Fitton A (1995) Cabergoline. A review of its pharmacological properties and therapeutic potential in the treatment of hyperprolactinaemia and inhibition of lactation. Drugs 49(2):255–279
168. Colao A, Lombardi G, Annunziato L (2000) Cabergoline. Expert Opin Pharmacother 1(3):555–574
169. Radwanska E, McGarrigle HH, Little V, Lawrence D, Sarris S, Swyer GI (1979) Induction of ovulation in women with hyperprolactinemic amenorrhea using clomiphene and human chorionic gonadotropin of bromocriptine. Fertil Steril 32(2):187–192
170. Aono T, Miyake A, Yasuda TS, Koike K, Kurachi K (1979) Restoration of oestrogen positive feedback effect on LH release by bromocriptine in hyperprolactinaemic patients with galactorrhoea-amenorrhoea. Acta Endocrinol 91(4):591–600
171. Borges LE, Morgante G, Musacchio MC, Petraglia F, De Leo V (2007) New protocol of clomiphene citrate treatment in women with hypothalamic amenorrhea. Gynecol Endocrinol 23(6): 343–346
172. Sullivan MW, Stewart-Akers A, Krasnow JS, Berga SL, Zeleznik AJ (1999) Ovarian responses in women to recombinant follicle-stimulating hormone and luteinizing hormone (LH): a role for LH in the final stages of follicular maturation. J Clin Endocrinol Metab 84(1):228–232
173. Platteau P, Andersen AN, Balen A et al (2006) Similar ovulation rates, but different follicular development with highly purified menotrophin compared with recombinant FSH in WHO Group II anovulatory infertility: a randomized controlled study. Hum Reprod 21(7):1798–1804
174. Filicori M, Cognigni GE, Pocognoli P et al (2003) Comparison of controlled ovarian stimulation with human menopausal gonadotropin or recombinant follicle-stimulating hormone. Fertil Steril 80(2):390–397
175. Filicori M, Cognigni GE, Gamberini E, Parmegiani L, Troilo E, Roset B (2005) Efficacy of low-dose human chorionic gonadotropin alone to complete controlled ovarian stimulation. Fertil Steril 84(2):394–401
176. Kilani Z, Dakkak A, Ghunaim S et al (2003) A prospective, randomized, controlled trial comparing highly purified hMG with recombinant FSH in women undergoing ICSI: ovarian response and clinical outcomes. Hum Reprod 18(6):1194–1199
177. Wide L, Naessen T, Sundstrom-Poromaa I, Eriksson K (2007) Sulfonation and sialylation of gonadotropins in women during the menstrual cycle, after menopause, and with polycystic ovarian syndrome and in men. J Clin Endocrinol Metab 92(11):4410–4417
178. Barrios-De-Tomasi J, Timossi C, Merchant H et al (2002) Assessment of the in vitro and in vivo biological activities of the human follicle-stimulating isohormones. Mol Cell Endocrinol 186(2):189–198
179. Andersen CY, Leonardsen L, Ulloa-Aguirre A, Barrios-De-Tomasi J, Kristensen KS, Byskov AG (2001) Effect of different FSH isoforms on cyclic-AMP production by mouse cumulus-oocyte-complexes: a time course study. Mol Hum Reprod 7(2):129–135
180. Matikainen T, De Leeuw R, Mannaerts B, Huhtaniemi I (1994) Circulating bioactive and immunoreactive recombinant human follicle stimulating hormone (Org 32489) after administration to gonadotropin-deficient subjects. Fertil Steril 61(1):62–69
181. D'Antonio M, Borrelli F, Datola A et al (1999) Biological characterization of recombinant human follicle stimulating hormone isoforms. Hum Reprod 14(5):1160–1167
182. van de Weijer BH, Mulders JW, Bos ES, Verhaert PD, van den Hooven HW (2003) Compositional analyses of a human menopausal gonadotrophin preparation extracted from urine (menotropin). Identification of some of its major impurities. Reprod Biomed Online 7(5):547–557
183. Stokman PG, de Leeuw R, van den Wijngaard HA, Kloosterboer HJ, Vemer HM, Sanders AL (1993) Human chorionic gonadotropin in commercial human menopausal gonadotropin preparations. Fertil Steril 60(1):175–178
184. Klein J, Lobel L, Pollak S et al (2003) Development and characterization of a long-acting recombinant hFSH agonist. Hum Reprod 18(1):50–56
185. Balasch J, Fabregues F, Casamitjana R, Penarrubia J, Vanrell JA (2003) A pharmacokinetic and endocrine comparison of recombinant follicle-stimulating hormone and human menopausal gonadotrophin in polycystic ovary syndrome. Reprod Biomed Online 6(3):296–301
186. Duijkers IJ, Klipping C, Mulders TM, Out HJ, Coelingh Bennink HJ, Vemer HM (1997) Pharmacodynamics and pharmacokinetics after repeated subcutaneous administration of three gonadotrophin preparations. Hum Reprod 12(11):2379–2384
187. Voortman G, van de Post J, Schoemaker RC, van Gerven JM (1999) Bioequivalence of subcutaneous injections of recombinant human follicle stimulating hormone (Puregon(R)) by Pen-injector and syringe. Hum Reprod 14(7):1698–1702
188. Duijkers IJ, Beerens MC, Coelingh Bennink HJ, Huisman JA, Rombout F, Vemer HM (1995) Pharmacokinetics of two human menopausal gonadotrophin preparations after single intravenous administration during pituitary suppression. Hum Reprod 10(6):1367–1372
189. Duijkers IJ, Klipping C, Boerrigter PJ, Machielsen CS, De Bie JJ, Voortman G (2002) Single dose pharmacokinetics and effects on follicular growth and serum hormones of a long-acting recombinant FSH preparation (FSH-CTP) in healthy pituitary-suppressed females. Hum Reprod 17(8):1987–1993
190. Olivares A, Cardenas M, Timossi C, Zarinan T, Diaz-Sanchez V, Ulloa-Aguirre A (2000) Reactivity of different LH and FSH standards and preparations in the world health organization matched reagents for enzyme-linked immunoassays of gonadotrophins. Hum Reprod 15(11):2285–2291
191. Fauser BC (1998) Developments in human recombinant follicle stimulating hormone technology: are we going in the right direction? Hum Reprod 13 Suppl 3:36–46; discussion 7–51
192. Rose MP, Gaines-Das RE (1998) Characterisation, calibration and comparison by international collaborative study of international standards for the calibration of therapeutic preparations of FSH. J Endocrinol 158(1):97–114
193. Mannaerts BM, Rombout F, Out HJ, Coelingh Bennink H (1996) Clinical profiling of recombinant follicle stimulating hormone (rFSH; Puregon): relationship between serum FSH and efficacy. Hum Reprod Update 2(2):153–161
194. le Cotonnec JY, Loumaye E, Porchet HC, Beltrami V, Munafo A (1998) Pharmacokinetic and pharmacodynamic interactions between recombinant human luteinizing hormone and recombinant human follicle-stimulating hormone. Fertil Steril 69(2):201–209
195. le Cotonnec JY, Porchet HC, Beltrami V, Khan A, Toon S, Rowland M (1994) Clinical pharmacology of recombinant human follicle-stimulating hormone (FSH). I. Comparative pharmacokinetics with urinary human FSH. Fertil Steril 61(4):669–678
196. van Wely M, Bayram N, van der Veen F (2003) Recombinant FSH in alternative doses or versus urinary gonadotrophins for ovulation induction in subfertility associated with polycystic ovary syndrome: a systematic review based on a Cochrane review. Hum Reprod 18(6):1143–1149
197. Balen A, Platteau P, Andersen AN, Devroey P, Helmgaard L, Arce JC (2007) Highly purified FSH is as efficacious as recombinant FSH for ovulation induction in women with WHO Group II anovulatory infertility: a randomized controlled non-inferiority trial. Hum Reprod 22(7):1816–1823
198. van Wely M, Bayram N, van der Veen F, Bossuyt PM (2005) Predicting ongoing pregnancy following ovulation induction with recombinant FSH in women with polycystic ovary syndrome. Hum Reprod 20(7):1827–1832

199. Daya S, Gunby J (2000) Recombinant versus urinary follicle stimulating hormone for ovarian stimulation in assisted reproduction cycles. Cochrane Database Syst Rev 4:CD002810
200. Strowitzki T, Seehaus D, Korell M, Hepp H (1998) Low-dose FSH stimulation in polycystic ovary syndrome: comparison of 3 FSH-preparations. Exp Clin Endocrinol Diab 106(5):435–439
201. Szilagyi A, Bartfai G, Manfai A, Koloszar S, Pal A, Szabo I (2004) Low-dose ovulation induction with urinary gonadotropins or recombinant follicle stimulating hormone in patients with polycystic ovary syndrome. Gynecol Endocrinol 18(1):17–22
202. Daya S (2002) Updated meta-analysis of recombinant follicle-stimulating hormone (FSH) versus urinary FSH for ovarian stimulation in assisted reproduction. Fertil Steril 77(4):711–714
203. Steinkampf MP, Hammond KR, Nichols JE, Slayden SH (2003) Effect of obesity on recombinant follicle-stimulating hormone absorption: subcutaneous versus intramuscular administration. Fertil Steril 80(1):99–102
204. Rossmanith WG, Sterzik K, Wolf AS (1987) Initial experiences with subcutaneous pulsatile human menopausal gonadotropin administration: successful induction of ovulation in patients with polycystic ovarian disease. Int J Fertil 32(6):460–466
205. Quartero HW, Dixon JE, Westwood O, Hicks B, Chapman MG (1989) Ovulation induction in polycystic ovarian disease by pure FSH (Metrodin). A comparison between chronic low-dose pulsatile administration and i.m. injections. Hum Reprod 4(3):247–249
206. Yuen BH, Pride SM, Callegari PB, Leroux AM, Moon YS (1989) Clinical and endocrine response to pulsatile intravenous gonadotropins in refractory anovulation. Obstet Gynecol 74(5):763–768
207. Dale O, Tanbo T, Lunde O, Abyholm T (1993) Ovulation induction with low-dose follicle-stimulating hormone in women with the polycystic ovary syndrome. Acta Obstet Gynecol Scand 72(1):43–46
208. Achrekar SK, Modi DN, Desai SK, Mangoli VS, Mangoli RV, Mahale SD (2009) Follicle-stimulating hormone receptor polymorphism (Thr(307)Ala) is associated with variable ovarian response and ovarian hyperstimulation syndrome in Indian women. Fertil Steril 91(2):432–439
209. Navot D, Margalioth EJ, Laufer N, Brzezinski A, Birkenfeld A, Schenker JG (1987) Periovulatory 17 beta-estradiol pattern in conceptional and nonconceptional cycles during menotropin treatment of anovulatory infertility. Fertil Steril 47(2):234–237
210. Muechler EK, Kohler D, Huang KE (1981) Monitoring of ovulation induction with HMG-HCG therapy by plasma estrogen and progesterone. Int J Fertil 26(4):273–278
211. Haning RV Jr, Levin RM, Behrman HR, Kase NG, Speroff L (1979) Plasma estradiol window and urinary estriol glucuronide determinations for monitoring menotropin induction of ovulation. Obstet Gynecol 54(4):442–447
212. Diamond MP, Wentz AC (1986) Ovulation induction with human menopausal gonadotropins. Obstet Gynecol Surv 41(8):480–490
213. Smith DH, Picker RH, Sinosich M, Saunders DM (1980) Assessment of ovulation by ultrasound and estradiol levels during spontaneous and induced cycles. Fertil Steril 33(4):387–390
214. Aboulghar M (2003) Prediction of ovarian hyperstimulation syndrome (OHSS). Estradiol level has an important role in the prediction of OHSS. Hum Reprod 18(6):1140–1141
215. D'Angelo A, Davies R, Salah E, Nix BA, Amso NN (2004) Value of the serum estradiol level for preventing ovarian hyperstimulation syndrome: a retrospective case control study. Fertil Steril 81(2):332–336
216. Tur R, Barri PN, Coroleu B, Buxaderas R, Martinez F, Balasch J (2001) Risk factors for high-order multiple implantation after ovarian stimulation with gonadotrophins: evidence from a large series of 1878 consecutive pregnancies in a single centre. Hum Reprod 16(10):2124–2129
217. Blankstein J, Shalev J, Saadon T et al (1987) Ovarian hyperstimulation syndrome: prediction by number and size of preovulatory ovarian follicles. Fertil Steril 47(4):597–602
218. Navot D, Goldstein N, Mor-Josef S, Simon A, Relou A, Birkenfeld A (1991) Multiple pregnancies: risk factors and prognostic variables during induction of ovulation with human menopausal gonadotrophins. Hum Reprod 6(8):1152–1155
219. Reuter KL, Cohen S, Furey L, Baker S (1996) Sonographic appearance of the endometrium and ovaries during cycles stimulated with human menopausal gonadotropin. J Reprod Med 41(7):509–514
220. Levy T, Orvieto R, Homburg R, Peleg D, Dekel A, Ben-Rafael Z (1996) Severe ovarian hyperstimulation syndrome despite low plasma oestrogen concentrations in a hypogonadotrophic, hypogonadal patient. Hum Reprod 11(6):1177–1179
221. Navot D, Relou A, Birkenfeld A, Rabinowitz R, Brzezinski A, Margalioth EJ (1988) Risk factors and prognostic variables in the ovarian hyperstimulation syndrome. Am J Obstet Gynecol 159(1):210–215
222. Orvieto R (2003) Prediction of ovarian hyperstimulation syndrome. Challenging the estradiol mythos. Hum Reprod 18(4):665–667
223. Lee TH, Liu CH, Huang CC et al (2008) Serum anti-Mullerian hormone and estradiol levels as predictors of ovarian hyperstimulation syndrome in assisted reproduction technology cycles. Hum Reprod 23(1):160–167
224. Ludwig M, Jelkmann W, Bauer O, Diedrich K (1994) Prediction of severe ovarian hyperstimulation syndrome by free serum vascular endothelial growth factor concentration on the day of human chorionic gonadotrophin administration. Hum Reprod 14(10):2437–2441
225. O'Herlihy C, Pepperell RJ, Robinson HP (1982) Ultrasound timing of human chorionic gonadotropin administration in clomiphene-stimulated cycle. Obstet Gynecol 59(1):40–45
226. Emperaire JC, Edwards RG (2004) Time to revolutionize the triggering of ovulation. Reprod Biomed Online 9(5):480–483
227. Van Der Meer M, Hompes PG, De Boer JA, Schats R, Schoemaker J (1998) Cohort size rather than follicle-stimulating hormone threshold level determines ovarian sensitivity in polycystic ovary syndrome. J Clin Endocrinol Metab 83(2):423–426
228. Lass A, Vassiliev A, Decosterd G, Warne D, Loumaye E (2002) Relationship of baseline ovarian volume to ovarian response in World Health Organization II anovulatory patients who underwent ovulation induction with gonadotropins. Fertil Steril 78(2):265–269
229. Imani B, Eijkemans MJ, Faessen GH, Bouchard P, Giudice LC, Fauser BC (2002) Prediction of the individual follicle-stimulating hormone threshold for gonadotropin induction of ovulation in normogonadotropic anovulatory infertility: an approach to increase safety and efficiency. Fertil Steril 77(1):83–90
230. Shoham Z, Patel A, Jacobs HS (1991) Polycystic ovarian syndrome: safety and effectiveness of stepwise and low-dose administration of purified follicle-stimulating hormone. Fertil Steril 55(6):1051–1056
231. Hamilton-Fairley D, Kiddy D, Watson H, Sagle M, Franks S (1991) Low-dose gonadotrophin therapy for induction of ovulation in 100 women with polycystic ovary syndrome. Hum Reprod 6(8):1095–1099
232. Grigoriou O, Antoniou G, Antonaki V, Patsouras C, Zioris C, Karakitsos P (1996) Low-dose follicle-stimulating hormone treatment for polycystic ovarian disease. Int J Gynaecol Obstet 52(1):55–59
233. Ergur AR, Yergok YZ, Ertekin A, Kucuk T, Mungen E, Tutuncu L (1998) Clomiphene citrate-resistant polycystic ovary syndrome. Preventing multifollicular development. J Reprod Med 43(3):185–190
234. Homburg R, Levy T, Ben-Rafael Z (1995) A comparative prospective study of conventional regimen with chronic low-dose administration of follicle-stimulating hormone for anovulation associated with polycystic ovary syndrome. Fertil Steril 63(4):729–733
235. Hedon B, Hugues JN, Emperaire JC et al (1998) A comparative prospective study of a chronic low dose versus a conventional ovulation stimulation regimen using recombinant human follicle stimulating hormone in anovulatory infertile women. Hum Reprod 13(1O):2688–2692

236. Strowitzki T, Seehaus D, Korell M, Hepp H (1994) Low-dose follicle stimulating hormone for ovulation induction in polycystic ovary syndrome. J Reprod Med 39(7):499–503
237. Andoh K, Mizunuma H, Liu X, Kamijo T, Yamada K, Ibuki Y (1998) A comparative study of fixed-dose, step-down, and low-dose step-up regimens of human menopausal gonadotropin for patients with polycystic ovary syndrome. Fertil Steril 70(5):840–846
238. Balasch J, Fabregues F, Creus M, Casamitjana R, Puerto B, Vanrell JA (2000) Recombinant human follicle-stimulating hormone for ovulation induction in polycystic ovary syndrome: a prospective, randomized trial of two starting doses in a chronic low-dose step-up protocol. J Assist Reprod Genet 17(10):561–565
239. Gorry A, White DM, Franks S (2006) Infertility in polycystic ovary syndrome: focus on low-dose gonadotropin treatment. Endocrine 30(1):27–33
240. Christin-Maitre S, Hugues JN (2003) A comparative randomized multicentric study comparing the step-up versus step-down protocol in polycystic ovary syndrome. Hum Reprod 18(8):1626–1631
241. Buckler HM, Robertson WR, Anderson A, Vickers M, Lambert A (1999) Ovulation induction with low dose alternate day recombinant follicle stimulating hormone (Puregon). Hum Reprod 14(12):2969–2973
242. Balasch J, Fabregues F, Creus M, Puerto B, Penarrubia J, Vanrell JA (2001) Follicular development and hormone concentrations following recombinant FSH administration for anovulation associated with polycystic ovarian syndrome: prospective, randomized comparison between low-dose step-up and modified step-down regimens. Hum Reprod 16(4):652–656
243. Yong EL, Ng SC, Chan CL, Kumar J, Teo LS, Ratnam SS (1997) Chronic low-dose follicle-stimulating hormone compared with clomiphene/human menopausal gonadotropin for induction of ovulation. Gynecol Endocrinol 11(1):35–42
244. Hugues JN, Cedrin-Durnerin I, Howles CM et al (2006) The use of a decremental dose regimen in patients treated with a chronic low-dose step-up protocol for WHO Group II anovulation: a prospective randomized multicentre study. Hum Reprod 21(11):2817–2822
245. Filicori M, Cognigni GE, Pocognoli P et al (2002) Modulation of folliculogenesis and steroidogenesis in women by graded menotrophin administration. Hum Reprod 17(8):2009–2015
246. Filicori M, Cognigni GE, Samara A et al (2002) The use of LH activity to drive folliculogenesis: exploring uncharted territories in ovulation induction. Hum Reprod Update 8(6):543–557
247. Lee KL, Couchman GM, Walmer DK (2005) Successful pregnancies in patients with estrogenic anovulation after low-dose human chorionic gonadotropin therapy alone following hMG for controlled ovarian hyperstimulation. J Assist Reprod Genet 22(1):37–40
248. De Leo V, la Marca A, Ditto A, Morgante G, Cianci A (1999) Effects of metformin on gonadotropin-induced ovulation in women with polycystic ovary syndrome. Fertil Steril 72(2):282–285
249. Palomba S, Falbo A, Orio F Jr et al (2005) A randomized controlled trial evaluating metformin pre-treatment and co-administration in non-obese insulin-resistant women with polycystic ovary syndrome treated with controlled ovarian stimulation plus timed intercourse or intrauterine insemination. Hum Reprod 20(10):2879–2886
250. Kistner RW (1976) Sequential use of clomiphene citrate and human menopausal gonadotropin in ovulation induction. Fertil Steril 27(1):72–82
251. March CM, Tredway DR, Mishell DR Jr (1976) Effect of clomiphene citrate upon amount and duration of human menopausal gonadotropin therapy. Am J Obstet Gynecol 125(5):699–704
252. Kemmann E, Jones JR (1983) Sequential clomiphene citrate-menotropin therapy for induction or enhancement of ovulation. Fertil Steril 39(6):772–779
253. Mitwally MF, Casper RF (2004) Aromatase inhibition reduces the dose of gonadotropin required for controlled ovarian hyperstimulation. J Soc Gynecol Investig 11(6):406–415
254. Nakamura Y, Yamada H, Yoshida K et al (1990) Induction of ovulation with pulsatile subcutaneous administration of human menopausal gonadotropin in patients with polycystic ovary syndrome. Horm Res 33(Suppl 2):43–48
255. Check JH, Katsoff B (2008) Ovulation induction and pregnancy in a woman with premature menopause following gonadotropin suppression with the gonadotropin releasing hormone antagonist, cetrorelix – a case report. Clin Exp Obstet Gynecol 35(1):10–12
256. Check ML, Check JH, Kaplan H (2004) Pregnancy despite imminent ovarian failure and extremely high endogenous gonadotropins and therapeutic strategies: case report and review. Clin Exp Obstet Gynecol 31(4):299–301
257. Bidet M, Bachelot A, Touraine P (2008) Premature ovarian failure: predictability of intermittent ovarian function and response to ovulation induction agents. Curr Opin Obstet Gynecol 20(4):416–420
258. van Kasteren YM, Hoek A, Schoemaker J (1995) Ovulation induction in premature ovarian failure: a placebo-controlled randomized trial combining pituitary suppression with gonadotropin stimulation. Fertil Steril 64(2):273–278
259. Badawy A, Goda H, Ragab A (2007) Induction of ovulation in idiopathic premature ovarian failure: a randomized double-blind trial. Reprod Biomed Online 15(2):215–219
260. Tartagni M, Cicinelli E, De Pergola G, De Salvia MA, Lavopa C, Loverro G (2007) Effects of pretreatment with estrogens on ovarian stimulation with gonadotropins in women with premature ovarian failure: a randomized, placebo-controlled trial. Fertil Steril 87(4):858–861
261. Rossing MA, Daling JR, Weiss NS, Moore DE, Self SG (1994) Ovarian tumors in a cohort of infertile women. N Engl J Med 331(12):771–776
262. Whittemore AS (1994) The risk of ovarian cancer after treatment for infertility. N Engl J Med 331(12):805–806
263. Whittemore AS, Harris R, Itnyre J (1992) Characteristics relating to ovarian cancer risk: collaborative analysis of 12 US case-control studies. II. Invasive epithelial ovarian cancers in white women. Collaborative Ovarian Cancer Group. Am J Epidemiol 136(10):1184–1203
264. Dor J, Lerner-Geva L, Rabinovici J et al (2002) Cancer incidence in a cohort of infertile women who underwent in vitro fertilization. Fertil Steril 77(2):324–327
265. Klip H, Burger CW, Kenemans P, van Leeuwen FE (2000) Cancer risk associated with subfertility and ovulation induction: a review. Cancer Causes Control 11(4):319–344
266. Rossing MA, Tang MT, Flagg EW, Weiss LK, Wicklund KG (2004) A case-control study of ovarian cancer in relation to infertility and the use of ovulation-inducing drugs. Am J Epidemiol 160(11):1070–1078
267. Meirow D, Schenker JG (1996) The link between female infertility and cancer: epidemiology and possible aetiologies. Hum Reprod Update 2(1):63–75
268. Kashyap S, Moher D, Fung MF, Rosenwaks Z (2004) Assisted reproductive technology and the incidence of ovarian cancer: a meta-analysis. Obstet Gynecol 103(4):785–794
269. Ayhan A, Salman MC, Celik H, Dursun P, Ozyuncu O, Gultekin M (2004) Association between fertility drugs and gynecologic cancers, breast cancer, and childhood cancers. Acta Obstet Gynecol Scand 83(12):1104–1111
270. Brinton L (2007) Long-term effects of ovulation-stimulating drugs on cancer risk. Reprod Biomed Online 15(1):38–44
271. Brinton LA, Lamb EJ, Moghissi KS et al (2004) Ovarian cancer risk after the use of ovulation-stimulating drugs. Obstet Gynecol 103(6):1194–1203
272. Brinton LA, Moghissi KS, Scoccia B, Westhoff CL, Lamb EJ (2005) Ovulation induction and cancer risk. Fertil Steril 83(2):261–274; quiz 525–526

Chapter 36
Transvaginal Sonography in Reproductive Endocrinology and Infertility

Anne Kennedy and C. Matthew Peterson

Abstract Transvaginal sonogram (TVS) is now the gold standard for the evaluation of infertility and assisted reproduction, early pregnancy, ectopic pregnancy, and first trimester pregnancy-related abnormalities. Additionally, identification of fetal abnormalities is also performed via TVS. The primary advantage of TVS over transabdominal sonography lies in its ability to place a high-frequency transducer next to the regions of interest. This chapter reviews the methodology and applications of transvaginal ultrasound usage in the practice of reproductive medicine, including its use in conjunction with in vitro fertilization. Specific guidelines are presented for optimal use of transvaginal ultrasound.

Keywords Transvaginal sonography • TVS • Doppler effect • 3D ultrasound • 4D ultrasound • Transducers • Bioeffects • Uterus • Congenital uterine anomalies • Leiomyoma • Endometrium • Pregnancy • Gestational age assessment • Multifetal pregnancies • Adenexae • Stroma • Functional ovarian cysts • Paraovarian/paratubal cysts • Epithelial ovarian tumor • Endometrioma • Pelvic inflammatory disease • Tubal ovarian abscess • Dermoid • Malignant neoplasms • Embryo transfer

36.1 History of Transvaginal Sonography

The first transvaginal sonogram (TVS) reported was attributed to Kratochwil in 1969 [1]. In the mid-1980s, transvaginal sonography was initially utilized to evaluate infertility problems in Japan as well as the United States [2–5]. Subsequently, applications for TVS have rapidly expanded [6–9].

TVS is now the gold standard for the evaluation of infertility and assisted reproduction [10, 11], early pregnancy [12–19], ectopic pregnancy, and first trimester pregnancy-related abnormalities [20–30]. Additionally, identification of fetal abnormalities is also performed via TVS [31–33].

The primary advantage of TVS over transabdominal sonography lies in its ability to place a high-frequency transducer next to the regions of interest. This allows optimal visualization of the uterus, cervix, ovaries, adnexal regions, and cul-de-sac, as well as the urinary bladder and bowel. It is particularly useful in the evaluation of an obese patient [34, 35], and in the evaluation of the retroverted or retroflexed uterus.

36.2 Limitations of TVS

While TVS is considered the gold standard in assisted reproduction, it must be remembered that transabdominal scans provide a global overview of pelvic anatomy. Lesions outside the relatively short range of the intravaginal probe could be missed when transabdominal scanning is omitted. Because of the high frequency of the transducer, resolution is optimal, but the field of view is small, and tissue penetration is limited [6, 22, 36]. Additionally, it must be remembered that transvaginal access limits maneuverability. In rare circumstances, TVS may be contraindicated. In prepubertal and virginal patients, translabial scanning may provide additional information. This technique can also be utilized in postmenopausal patients and patients in whom acute pelvic pain precludes the use of TVS. There are also other patients, who refuse transvaginal examination because of psychological or personal reasons.

36.3 Practical Physics

36.3.1 Ultrasound

Sound is a waveform of energy. Ultrasound utilizes high-frequency sound waves (2–10 MHz) to create a visual image [37]. The transvaginal ultrasound probe both generates

A. Kennedy
Department of Radiology, University of Utah, Health Sciences Center, Salt Lake City, UT, USA

C.M. Peterson (✉)
Utah Center for Reproductive Medicine, Department of Obstetrics and Gynecology, University of Utah School of Medicine, 30 N. Medical Drive, 2B200, Salt Lake City, UT, USA
e-mail: c.matthew.peterson@hsc.utah.edu

D.T. Carrell and C.M. Peterson (eds.), *Reproductive Endocrinology and Infertility: Integrating Modern Clinical and Laboratory Practice*,
DOI 10.1007/978-1-4419-1436-1_36,

sound waves capable of penetrating organic tissue and receives the reflected sound wave energy. Received waves are converted into an electrical signal. These signals are then used to generate a 3D image on an oscilloscope (the ultrasound monitor).

36.3.2 Doppler Effect

When a source generating sound waves moves relative to the observer, or when an observer moves relative to a source, there is a shift in frequency of the reflected waves. If the distance between the observer and the source is increasing, the frequency decreases, whereas the frequency increases if the distance between the observer and the source is decreasing. This phenomenon is called the Doppler Effect (or Doppler Shift) named after Austrian Physicist Christian Johann Doppler (1803–1853). The formula describing the Doppler Shift for a moving source is given by:

$$f_2 = f_1 v/(v \pm v_s)$$

Where, f_2 is the apparent frequency, f_1 is the actual frequency emitted by the source, v is the speed of sound in the medium, and v_s is the speed of the source through the medium (a negative sign is used if the source is moving toward the observer). The formula that describes Doppler Shift for a moving observer is:

$$f_o = f_s(v \pm v_o)/v$$

Where, f_o is the observed frequency, f_s is the source frequency, v is the speed of sound, and v_o is the speed of the observer (negative if the observer is receding from the source).

Examples of the Doppler effect include the change in pitch of a passing automobile, and the red shift of a star moving from the earth (a change in light's wavelength not sound wavelength). Applications include short range radar devices, which capture a change in frequency between the emitted and returning pulses showing the relative speed of an object.

Modern transvaginal systems now include color flow imaging and duplex Doppler technology, as well as 3D and 4D imaging. Color flow imaging identifies the potential areas of vascularity, while duplex Doppler is used to characterize the waveform pattern and resistivity [38–40]. It should be remembered that vascular conditions with slow flow may not be detected with color flow Doppler. One of the utilities of color flow Doppler or duplex Doppler techniques is in identifying vascular structures and distinguishing them from nonvascular entities, such as dilated fallopian tubes or fluid-filled bowel loops. This can be particularly helpful prior to transvaginal oocyte retrieval in order to identify vascular structures which should be avoided and in evaluating dilated tubes and complex ovarian masses. The utility of color flow imaging and Doppler technology is being advanced with regards to adnexal and uterine masses [41–43] and in the evaluation of infertility, early pregnancy and its complications.

The practical application and nuances of Doppler ultrasound application in gynecology are beyond the scope of this chapter and are best covered in texts dedicated to the subject: Kurjak A, Fleischer AC (Editors). Doppler Ultrasound in Gynecology, Parthenon Pub Group, London UK 1997, ISBN: 1850706239 and Kurak A (Editor) An Atlas of Transvaginal Color Doppler (Second Edition), Taylor and Francis, London UK, 2000, ISBN: 1850700931.

36.3.3 3D Ultrasound

Three-dimensional US images can be obtained by two methods: freehand or automated. The freehand method requires operator movement of the transducer through the region of interest. The main drawback of freehand systems is that that of the image quality proves to be worse than the automated 3D ultrasound. All sonographers perform this freehand activity in their minds as they scan. Automated acquisition uses a dedicated 3D transducer that sweeps through the region of interest selected by the operator (the "volume box") as the probe is held in a stationary position. The operator selects a constant speed of sweep with lower speeds providing a higher resolution and higher speeds the converse. A large "volume box" leads to longer acquisition time. The digitally stored 3D data can be manipulated and differentially displayed: multiplanar display, niche mode or surface rendering mode. For gynecologic applications, many prefer the multiplanar display, which shows three perpendicular planes (axial, sagittal and coronal) and allows navigation through these three planes. Three-dimensional US volume calculation using the Virtual Organ Computer-aided Analysis (VOCAL) is more accurate than 2D volume calculations [44]. Vascularization of tissues within the region of interest can also be assessed using 3D Power-Doppler ultrasound (3D PD) and the VOCAL program [45]. Three vascular indexes can be calculated. The Vascularization Index (VI) expressed as a percentage, measures the number of color voxels in the studied volume, and represents the number of blood vessels within the tissue. The Flow Index (FI) is the average color value of all color voxels, representing the average color intensity. The Vascular–Flow Index (VFI) is the average color value of all gray and color voxels and represents both blood flow and vascularization, and is a surrogate for "perfusion." An excellent review of the utility

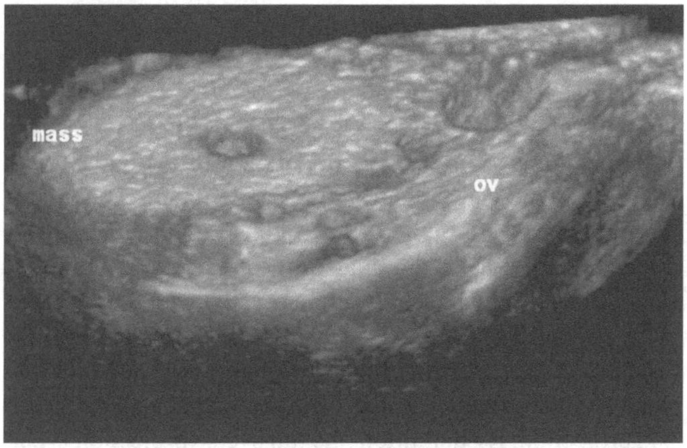

Fig. 36.1 Three-dimensional image of ovary with a mass (dermoid)

of 3D ultrasound is found in the review by Alcazar [46]. 4D or dynamic 3D scanners are now available and allow not only a depiction of volume but movement as well. Experts feel that 3D and 4D ultrasound are not essential, but represent an additional tool allowing multiplanar demonstration of anatomy e.g. demonstration of the fundal contour in cases of müllerian duct anomalies thus allowing a more specific diagnosis than is possible on 2D alone (Fig. 36.1).

36.4 Ultrasound Equipment

36.4.1 Transducers

Transvaginal transducers are either mechanical or electronically focused sector probes [47, 48]. The mechanical sector probe consists of one or more crystals that rotate or oscillate in an oil medium. Electronic transvaginal transducers have an array of crystals, which are sequentially triggered to produce an ultrasound beam (phased array), or utilize a set of crystals shaped to produce the sector image (curvilinear). Multiple variations of these basic configurations are available in the marketplace.

Mechanical transducers are less expensive, and can provide a wide field of view. However, the near-field resolution of mechanical transducers is less than that of the electronically focused transducers. Mechanical probes usually have fixed focal zones. The electronically focused probes are more expensive and have either fixed or multiple focal zones. Transducers vary in shape, size, frequency, and sector angles used [39, 40, 49, 50].

The transducer can be either rounded or rectangular in shape, and ranges from 1.5 to 3 cm in their longest dimensions. The tips are either straight or angulated in relationship to the shaft of the probe. The ability to insert the probe is affected by contour and configuration of the tip. Large rectangular tips may be somewhat difficult to introduce in some women and the application should be considered before purchase. Transvaginal probes are end firing with the beam projected symmetrically from the center of the face of the transducer in a straight probe, or angulated with the beam projected asymmetrically in an angulated probe. Both designs have advantages and disadvantages to be considered. Angulated probes can image structures that might otherwise be difficult to reach without patient discomfort. However, the angulated tip sometimes requires reversing the transducer 180° and inverting the image on the screen. Scan angles, depending on the manufacturer, vary from 90 to 115°. Scanning angles as wide as 240° may be obtained.

Transvaginal transducers are available in frequencies of 5, 6.5, 7, 7.5 and 8 MHz. The transducers may be of a single frequency, but dual-frequency and multiple-frequency probes are available. The probe with the highest frequency transducer that allows adequate tissue penetration provides the best resolution. The 5 MHz transducer provides appropriate images in most clinical situations. However, careful scanning of the endometrium may require a 7.5 MHz transducer. The physics of ultrasound is such that the higher the frequency, the better the resolution, but increased resolution is obtained at the cost of decreased tissue penetration. The selection of the transducer frequency balances these two competing properties [49].

36.5 The Examination

36.5.1 Patient Preparation

TVS for follicular monitoring and anatomy scan can usually be completed within 10 min. All patients should be advised of the reason for this technique and its utility [51]. The majority of women accept transvaginal scanning and prefer it over the uncomfortable, full-bladder, transabdominal approach. Written informed consent is rarely required; however, under unusual circumstances, it may be advisable. The pediatric virginal patient or patients with psychological or social issues may be best managed with informed consent documentation. A chaperone is always advisable and has proven crucial in numerous circumstances. This individual can also be helped with the recording of information or pointing out findings during the study. The majority of women who will undergo TVS are familiar with pelvic exams and are able to correlate the insertion of the transvaginal probe with that of the placement of a speculum. Patient advocacy suggests that the patient should be offered the opportunity to insert the probe herself should she so desire.

The patient is asked to empty her bladder immediately before the examination and she is placed in the supine position with thighs maximally abducted and knees flexed. Occasionally, elevation of the buttocks by a pillow or a wedge may be required. Visualization of lateral structures requires the patient to completely abduct her thighs. When visualization is difficult, it is imperative to remind the patient to let her knees fall out to the side in a near frog leg-lithotomy position (Fig. 36.2).

The TV probe should be covered with a condom containing a small amount of gel to insure good sound conduction between the transducer face and the overlying condom. Absence of the gel is a common cause of inadequate visualization. Once the transducer has been covered, additional gel should be placed on the outside of the sheath tip. Sterile gel is used in most facilities; however, any uncontaminated coupling gel agent is acceptable. In patients where probe insertion is difficult, assistance can be provided by placing a gloved finger with gel on it at the introitus and pushing inferiorly against the pubococcygeus muscle. The patient is then advised to bear down which will relax the pubococcygeus muscle for easy insertion of a finger or the transvaginal probe. Once the patient understands this process of bearing down to relax the pubococcygeus muscle and open the vagina, insertion of the transvaginal probe is greatly facilitated. It is important for novice sonographers to remember the posterior angulation of the vagina with the perineum.

Papilloma virus can remain infectious for 48 h outside the body; therefore, a condom and gloves should be utilized and disinfection of the probe should occur after each use. Manufacturers provide individual instructions for appropriate decontamination.

36.5.2 Image Planes

Standard anatomic planes are termed sagittal, transverse, and coronal. Ultrasound projections have been defined by the path of the entering beam and the orientation of the patient with reference to the viewer. During transabdominal scanning, the common planes are sagittal (longitudinal) and transverse. By convention in transabdominal ultrasound, the longitudinal view places the transducer beam in parallel with the long axis of the patient. The long-axis view of a structure represents the structure displayed in its longest dimension. The short-axis plane section is defined as the view perpendicular to the long-axis projection. By definition, the transverse projection is perpendicular to the longitudinal view in the axial plane.

The display of TVS images is not standard worldwide. There are four ways to display TV images: The apex of the ultrasound beam oriented up, down, to the right, or to the left. U.S. sonographers display the apex of the sector wedge at the top of the screen while, in contrast, European sonographers prefer to display the image with the apex of the beam at the bottom. Both of these are in contrast to the convention for abdominal sonography. In abdominal sonography, anatomic convention places the head at the left of the image, the anterior aspect of the patient at the top of the image, the posterior aspect at the bottom of the image, and the patient's feet are at the right of the image. If TV ultrasound images were displayed using the same convention as abdominal scans, the apex of the sector wedge would be placed at the right of the screen, requiring a shift from the top of the screen to 90° to the right. An awareness of the arbitrary differences between European and U.S. imaging will help to avoid confusion. Because of the difference, however, labeling is required, particularly for publication.

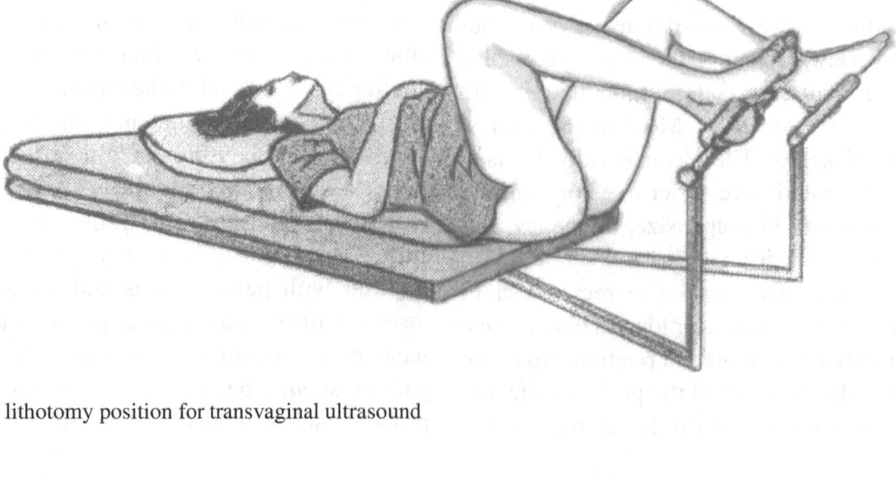

Fig. 36.2 Frog legged lithotomy position for transvaginal ultrasound

36.5.3 Basic Maneuvers

Basic maneuvers with transvaginal scanning include advancing or withdrawing the transducer along the axis of the vagina to provide a clear view of the uterus, angling the transducer by pointing the tip from side to side or anterior to posterior in order to evaluate adnexal structures, or to view the cul-de-sac. When introducing the transducer, the cervix and lower uterine segment of the uterus are usually visualized initially and then the uterine fundus becomes apparent. The transducer should be oriented to obtain a long-axis view of the uterus including the endometrium. Thereafter, the endometrial thickness is measured and the myometrium and endometrium are scanned anterior-to-posterior and side-to-side to look for any abnormalities (fibroids, polyps, etc.). The probe is then angulated laterally to examine the ovaries and adnexae in both a long-axis and short-axis view. The long-axis view of the ovary represents the structure displayed in its longest dimension. The short-axis plane section is defined as the view perpendicular to the long-axis projection. While looking for the ovaries, it is common to visualize the internal iliac vessels immediately posterior to the ovary. It is important not to confuse pelvic veins for ovarian follicles in various images of the ovaries. This is particularly important during transvaginal oocyte retrieval. Color flow Doppler is helpful in avoiding these errors in interpretation. Thereafter, follicles are measured. After completing ovarian measurements and follicle count and dimension(s) on the basis of clinic preferences, attention is placed on the cul-de-sac to assess the presence of simple or echogenic fluid [52]. Echogenic fluid usually correlates with hemorrhage (e.g. from a ruptured ectopic pregnancy), pus from an inflammatory process, or proteinaceous fluid.

36.5.4 Examination Bioeffects

The low acoustic energy required in diagnostic ultrasound has never been proven to cause an adverse fetal outcome [53]. The potential adverse effects of ultrasound are based only on extrapolation from experimental data. Growth retardation has been shown in the fetal mouse [54]. Intensities 100–1000 times used for diagnostic ultrasound can cause cavitational damage [53, 55, 56]. Conceivably, the death of an organism might result from such very high intensity levels [57]. Dose effects could be calculated from known output levels and exposure time, but because of the variability and exposure time, it is difficult to perform studies with adequate statistical power. Color flow imaging has lower power output than Doppler interrogation and this should be considered when flow evaluation is utilized during early pregnancy. Despite its apparent safety and widespread use, sonographers should be aware that higher-frequency transducers, highly selected focal zones, and continuous observation all increase the local deposition of energy. A guiding principal for all sonographers is to reduce the power output "as low as reasonably achievable" (ALARA) [58].

36.5.5 Pelvic Structures

36.5.5.1 Uterus

Using TVS, the uterus is evaluated in three scanning planes: long axis, semiaxial (oblique semicoronal), and short axis. The long axis image is obtained when the transducer is introduced into the vagina (Fig. 36.3). For anteflexed uteri, the probe handle is held inferiorly with a beam directed anteriorly. The opposite position is utilized for the retroflexed uterus. The semiaxial view is obtained by rotating the transducer 90° to the long axis, with the uterus imaged in its width (Fig. 36.4). The short axis view is obtained by retracting the transducer into the mid-vagina and directing it anteriorly through the fornix. Variations of uterine position include an anteflexed uterus, a retroverted uterus, and a retroflexed uterus. A retroverted uterus is defined as a posterior angulation of the uterus and cervix relative to the vagina. The retroflexed uterus is defined as a posterior angulation of the uterine body relative to the cervix.

Normal uterine size is based on the patient's parity and menopausal status [44, 45, 59]. Nulliparous, postpubertal women have uterine sizes measuring approximately 6 cm in length and 3–4 cm in the AP and transverse dimensions. A parous patient has a uterine long axis measuring

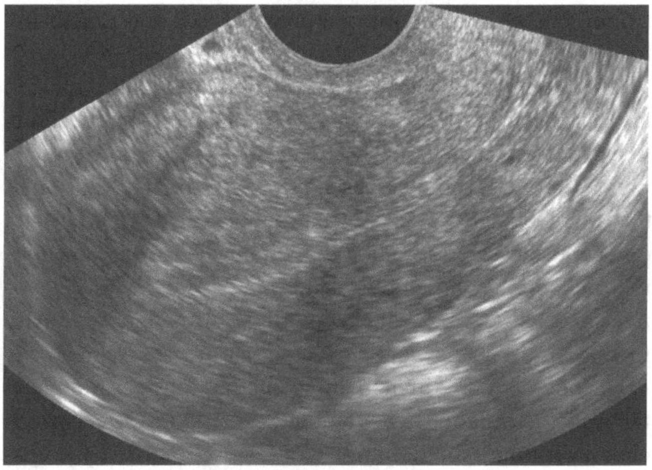

Fig. 36.3 Long axis view of uterus

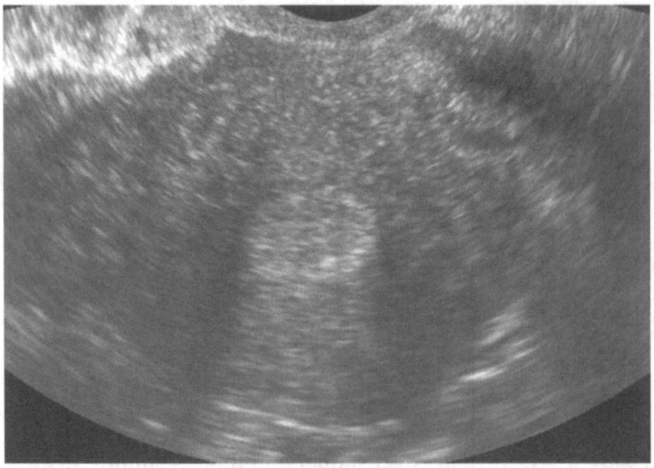

Fig. 36.4 Transverse or semiaxial view of a normal uterus

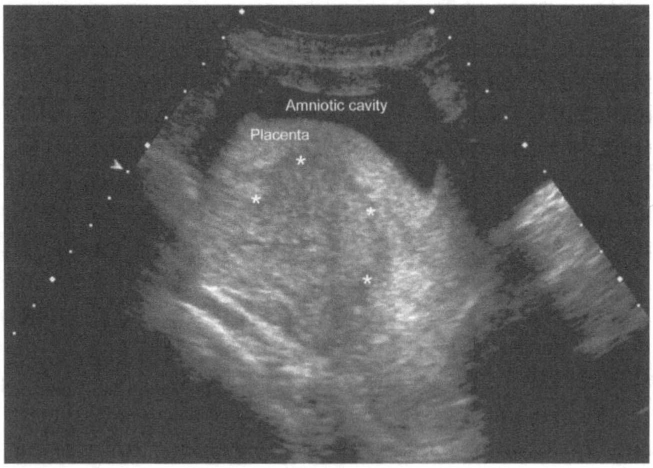

Fig. 36.5 Focal myometrial contraction in pregnant uterus

approximately 8 cm with 4 cm in AP dimension and 5 cm in transverse dimension. In the postmenopausal population the uterus is smaller, approximately 4–6 cm in the longitudinal axis.

Uterine contractions in the medial and outer muscle layers are often observed and typically appear as hypoechoic, thickened myometrium. They occasionally can be confused with a fibroid. Continued observation will show resolution of this thickening (Fig. 36.5). Contractions of the medial and outer muscle layers should be distinguished from subendometrial uterine contractions, which arise from the inner myometrial layer [60–62]. Subendometrial contractions gradually increase in frequency and intensity after menses, with a peak frequency of approximately three contractions per minute at the time of ovulation. The frequency of contractions is associated with the estradiol level. Contractions normally propagate toward the fundus at the time of ovulation and have been hypothesized to participate in sperm transport. Contractions propagate in the opposite direction toward the cervix during menses. The vasculature of the pelvis is demonstrated in Figs. 36.6 and 36.7. Doppler velocities of uterine arteries vary according to the stage of the menstrual cycle [63].

Congenital Uterine Anomalies

Congenital uterine anomalies may be subcategorized into seven major groups:

1. Hypoplasia/agenesis.
2. Unicornuate uteri.
3. Uterine didelphys.
4. Bicornuate uterus.
5. Septate uterus.
6. Arcuate Uterus
7. Anomalies related to DES exposure.

Imperforate hymen or vaginal atresia may cause hematometrocolpos at puberty [64]. Sonographically, hematometrocolpos appears as a distended uterus and vagina filled with fluid. Echogenic clotted blood will appear in dependent portions of the vagina and uterus (Fig. 36.8).

Uterine failed formation/canalization/fusion/resorption abnormalities are best evaluated during the secretory phase of the menstrual cycle because of the prominence of the endometrial lining at this time [65, 66]. Sonohysterography or 3D ultrasound are often extremely helpful in determining unicornuate with a nonfunctional or absent contralateral uterine horn, uterine didelphys, bicornuate uteri, or septate uteri [65, 66]. MRI remains the gold standard for the determination of the fundal configuration, when there is a question between unicornuate, didelphys, bicornuate, or septate uteri (Figs. 36.9–36.14). DES-exposed T-shaped uteri are smaller and lack a characteristic bulbous expansion of the fundus (Fig. 36.15).

Leiomyomas

Leiomyomas represent the most common tumor in the female pelvis, occurring in over 25% of women over age 35 [67]. Leiomyomas are most commonly found in the myometrium, and rarely in cervical tissue. Leiomyomas are described as subserosal, intramural, or submucosal in location. Leiomyomas may cause menorrhagia, dysmenorrhea, or irregular uterine bleeding, and may be associated with infertility. However, many of them are asymptomatic. Leiomyomas are the most common cause of uterine enlargement. The location of the myoma should be documented, and whether it appears to deform, distort or displace the endometrial cavity should be determined. Saline-infusion sonohysterography

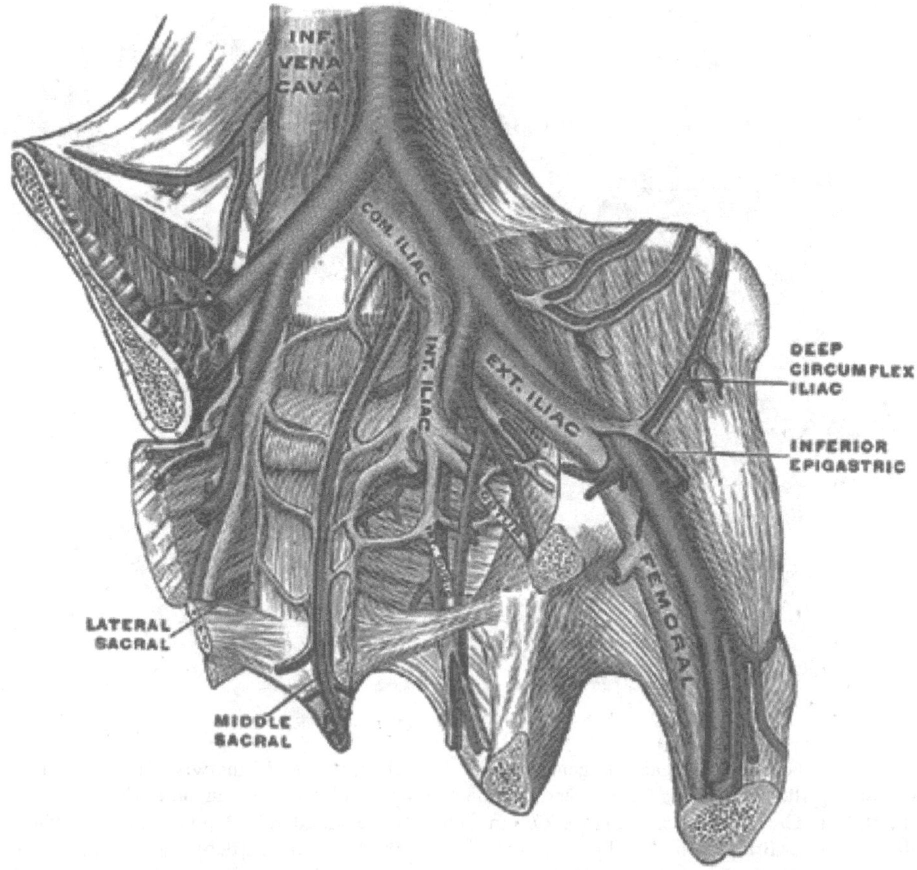

Fig. 36.6 The iliac veins. (Poirier and Charpy) This faithful reproduction of a lithograph plate (586) from Gray's Anatomy, a 2D work of art, is not copyrightable in the U.S. as per Bridgeman Art Library v. Corel Corp.; the same is also true in many other countries, including Germany. Unless stated otherwise, it is from the 20th U.S. edition of Gray's Anatomy of the Human Body, originally published in 1918 and therefore lapsed into the public domain. Other copies of Gray's Anatomy can be found on Bartleby and also on Yahoo! This image is in the public domain because its copyright has expired. This applies worldwide

(SIS) is best suited to determine any abnormalities of the endometrial cavity caused by a leiomyoma. Leiomyomas may be hypoechoic, echoic, or isoechoic, depending on the composition of smooth muscle, calcifications, and connective tissue (Figs. 36.16–36.19).

The differential diagnosis when evaluating a submucosal myoma includes blood, mucus, or endometrial polyps. When multiple leiomyomas are detected, transabdominal ultrasound should be included in the evaluation to better describe the size and extent of these myomas. Endometrial polyps may be difficult to distinguish from small submucosal myomas [68]. Vascular leiomyomas can be identified with color flow Doppler. A diffusely enlarged uterus without clearly definable fibroids and a normal endometrium is suggestive of adenomyosis [69]. In some severe cases, there is a disordered echogenicity of the middle layer of the myometrium. MRI is more accurate than sonography in distinguishing adenomyosis from diffuse leiomyoma [70].

Pelvic varicosities and arteriovenous malformations may be detected by pelvic sonography [38, 71]. Color flow imaging and/or duplex Doppler are helpful in confirming the vascular nature of these abnormalities.

Uterine Vascular Status

The uterine artery pulsatility index (measured from the flow velocity waveforms as the systolic peak velocity minus end-diastolic velocity divided by the mean) has been suggested as a prognostic factor for uterine receptivity and pregnancy from IVF. The impedance blood flow through the uterine artery is classified as low, medium, or high and based on numerical values of 0–1.99, 2–2.99, and greater than or equal to 3, respectively. Increased uterine impedance of blood flow has been associated with lower pregnancy rates in IVF cycles [72]. In these studies, a pulsatility index cutoff value between 2.5 and 3.3 predicts poor endometrial receptivity. Power Doppler to measure blood flow in the uterine arteries and spiral arteries has not demonstrated the ability to predict implantation [73].

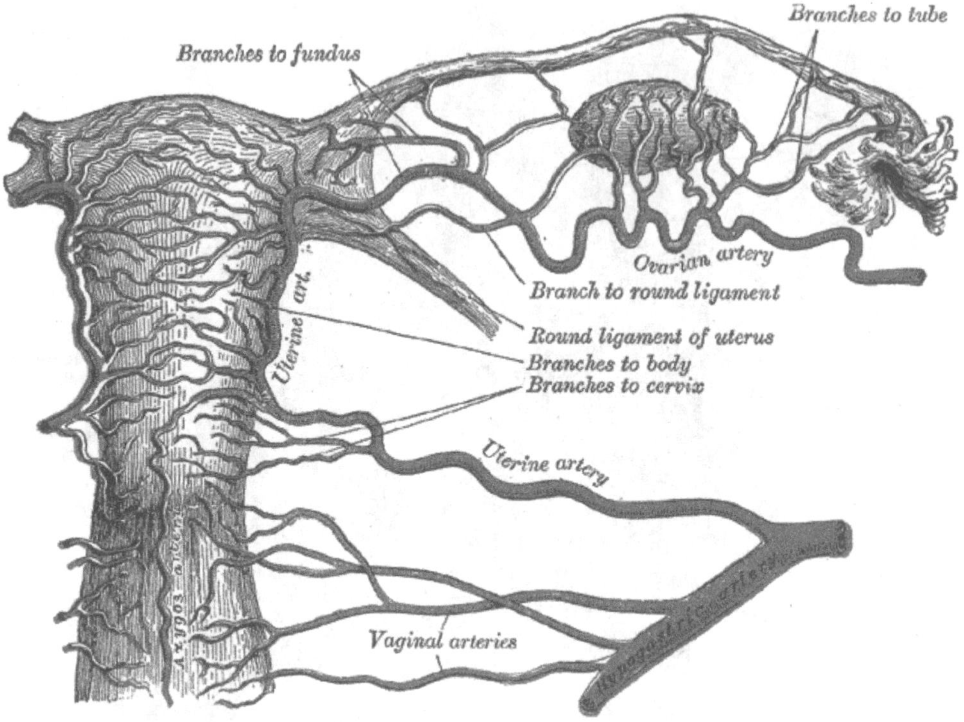

Fig. 36.7 The arteries of the internal organs of generation of the female, seen from behind. (After Hyrtl) This faithful reproduction of a lithograph plate (1170) from Gray's Anatomy, a 2D work of art, is not copyrightable in the U.S. as per Bridgeman Art Library v. Corel Corp.; the same is also true in many other countries, including Germany. Unless stated otherwise, it is from the 20th U.S. edition of Gray's Anatomy of the Human Body, originally published in 1918 and therefore lapsed into the public domain. Other copies of Gray's Anatomy can be found on Bartleby and also on Yahoo! This image is in the public domain because its copyright has expired. This applies worldwide

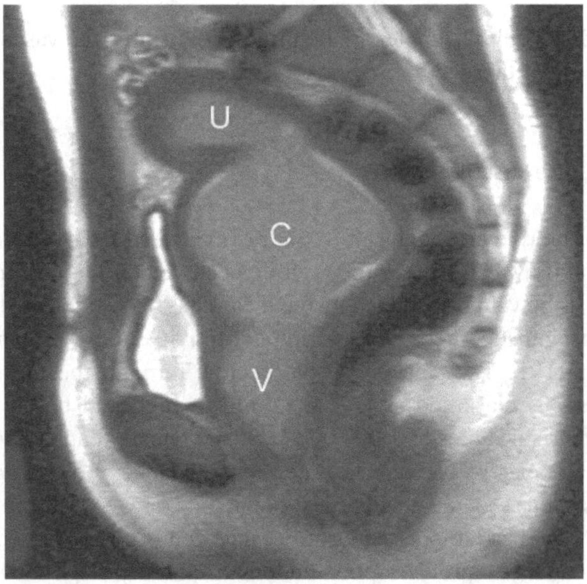

Fig. 36.8 Hematometrocolpos by MR. Both MR and ultrasound reveal distended distal vagina (V) inferior to the bladder (*white*), upper vagina and cervix distended with blood (C), and distended uterus (U)

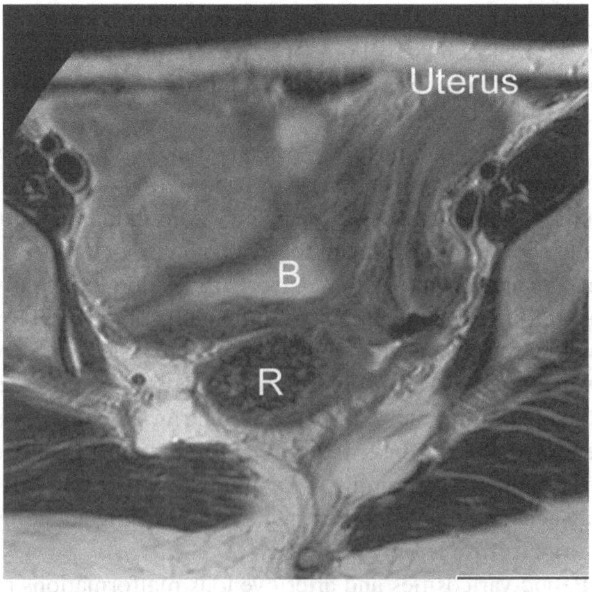

Fig. 36.9 Unicornuate uterus on right by MR (*B* bladder, *R* rectum)

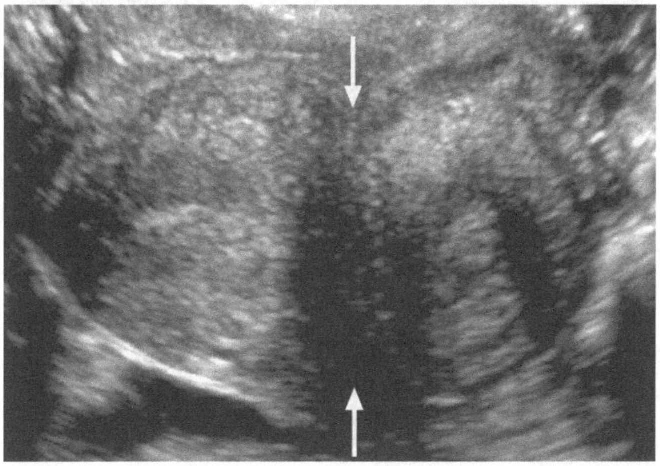

Fig. 36.10 Uterine didelphys by 2D ultrasound showing midline echolucency indicating failed fusion of the uterine horns

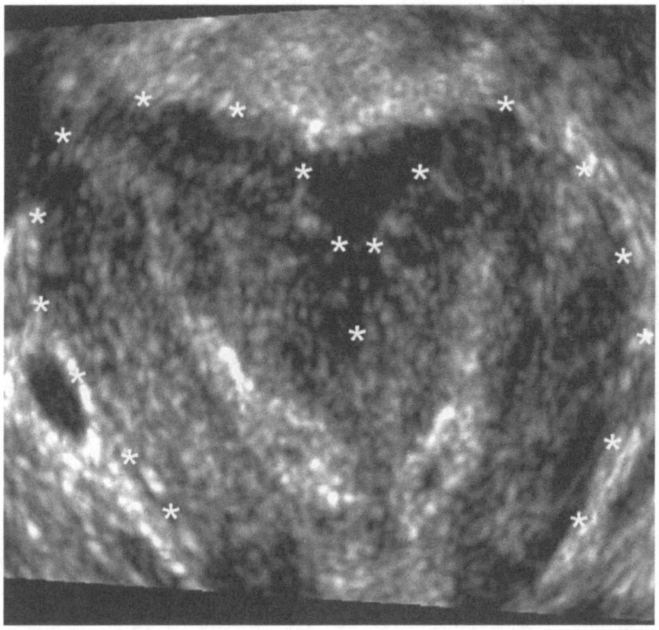

Fig. 36.11 Uterine didelphys by 3D ultrasound showing outline of didelphys uterus (*) and bright endometrial stripes

36.5.5.2 Endometrium

The endometrium is an echogenic interface in the central uterus [74, 75]. Sonographic measurements of endometrial thickness correlates well with actual anatomic endometrial thickness [76, 77] (Fig. 36.20). Proliferative phase endometrium ranges from 3 to 8 mm with secretory phase endometrium measuring 7–14 mm. Postmenopausal endometrial thickness averages 4–8 mm, while postmenopausal endometrium on hormonal replacement therapy ranges from 6 to 10 mm in thickness. The measurement should include both opposing layers of the endometrium, but should not include the hypoechoic halo seen surrounding the more echogenic endometrium [78]. Endometrial fluid, if present, should be excluded from the endometrial measurement, thus a separate measurement of the intrauterine fluid dimension should be obtained. The endometrial thickness and texture are influenced by circulating estrogen and progesterone [79, 80]. During menses, the endometrium appears as a thin echogenic layer. During the early proliferative phase, it thickens and becomes isoechoic, measuring 3–8 mm in AP width. The organization of the glandular elements within the endometrium is related to the hypoechogenicity seen. When ovulation approaches, the endometrium becomes more echogenic secondary to the development of secretions in the endometrial glands, and the various interfaces that develop from distended and tortuous glands [81]. A hypoechoic halo arising from the inner layer of the myometrium surrounds the endometrium. During the periovulatory

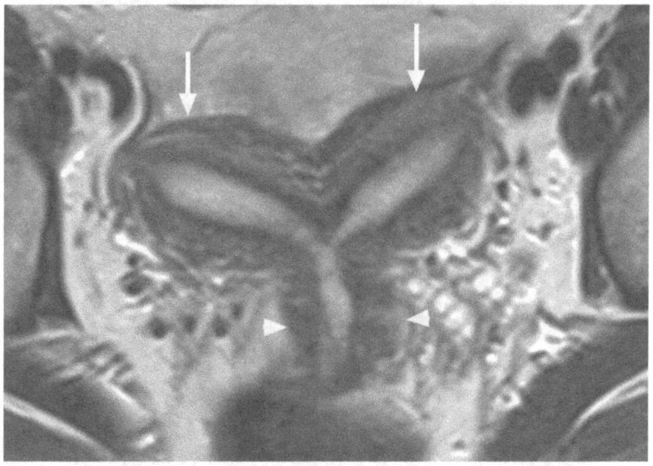

Fig. 36.12 Bicornuate uterus by MR demonstrating wide separation of uterine horns

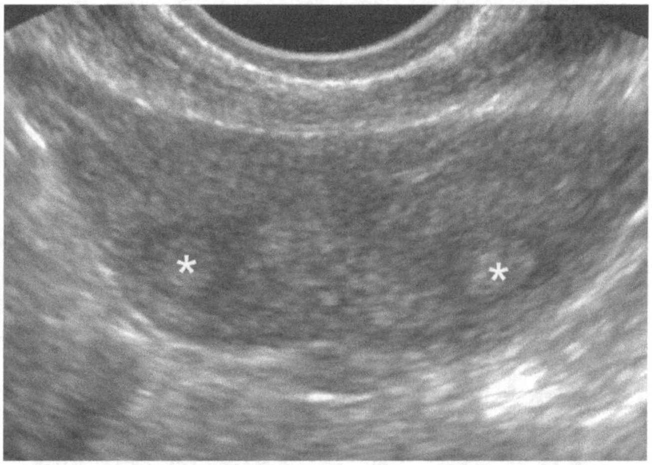

Fig. 36.13 Septate uterus by 2D ultrasound (transverse view)

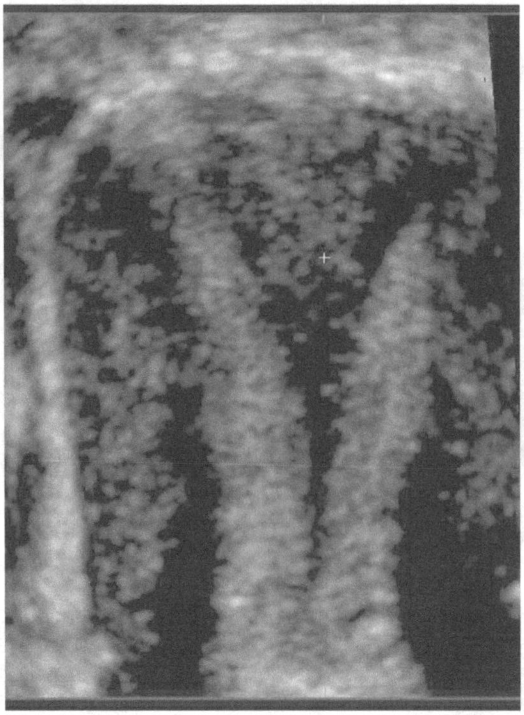

Fig. 36.14 Septate uterus by 3D ultrasound

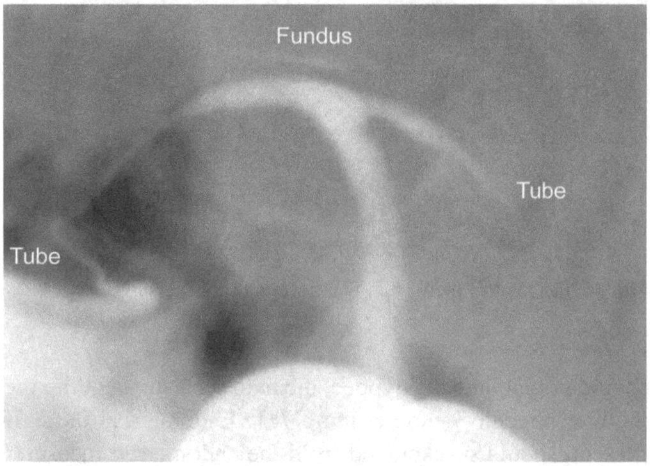

Fig. 36.15 T-shaped uterus by hysterosalpingogram

period, a hypoechoic area develops within the inner endometrium. This is thought to be a representation of edema of the compactum layer. A multilayer appearance of the endometrium (inner hypoechoic layer with outer echogenic layers-trilaminar appearance) has been associated with a higher pregnancy rate in ovulation induction regimens [47, 82]. During the secretory phase, the endometrium achieves its greatest thickness and echogenicity (6–14 mm). When comparing a gonadotropin cycle to a natural cycle, the endometrial lining is slightly thicker in the gonadotropin cycle [83]. Endometrial thickness and echogenicity are negatively

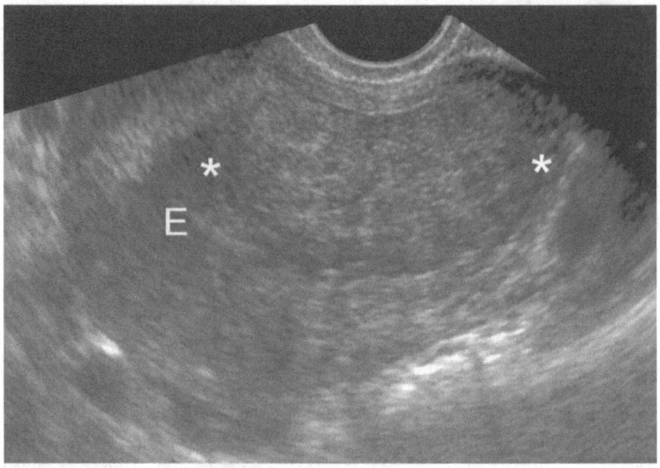

Fig. 36.16 Uterine fibroid – intramural (*) anterior to endometrium (E)

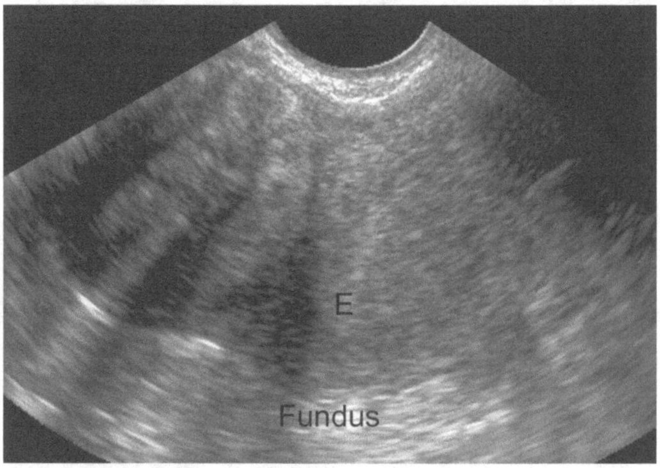

Fig. 36.17 Uterine fibroid – subserosal anterior to endometrium (E) and seen best via abdominal scan

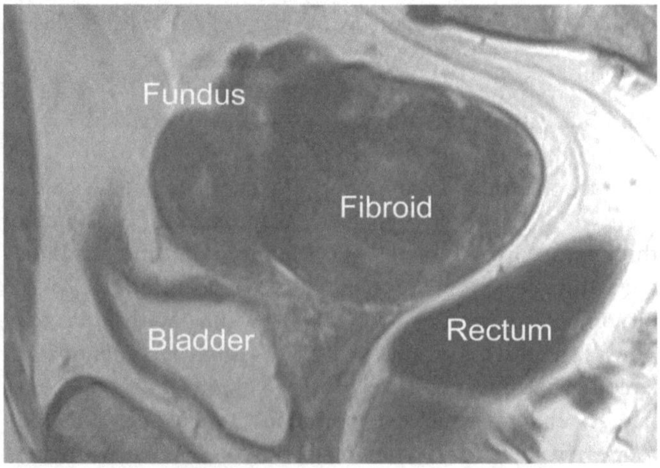

Fig. 36.18 Uterine fibroid – subserosal via MR

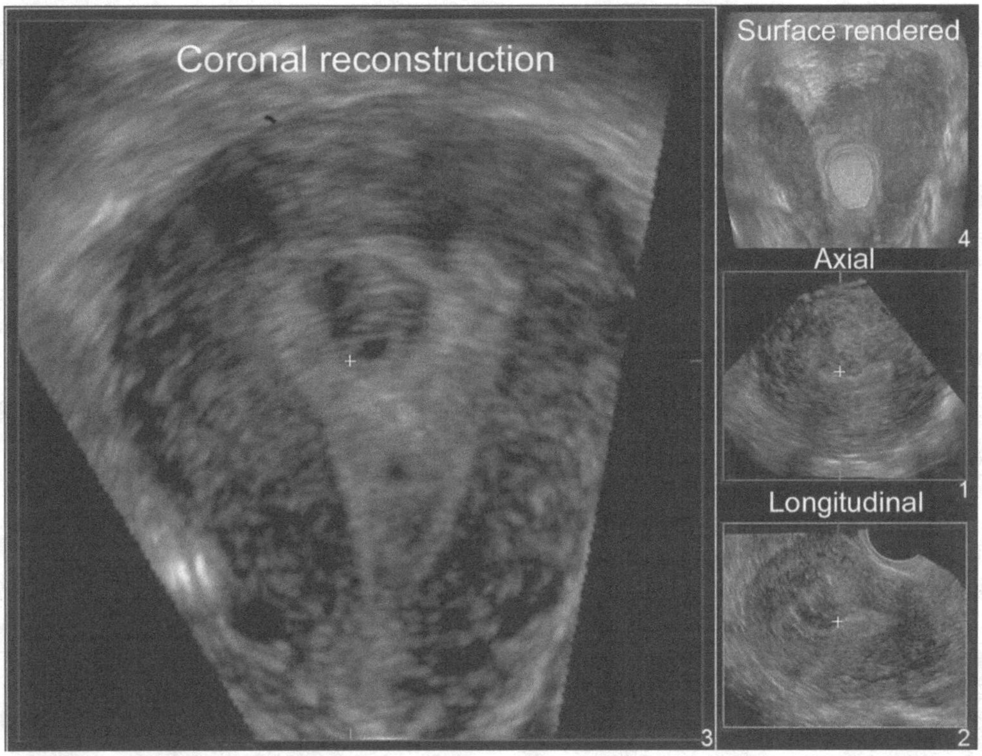

Fig. 36.19 Uterine fibroid – submucosal via 3D ultrasound

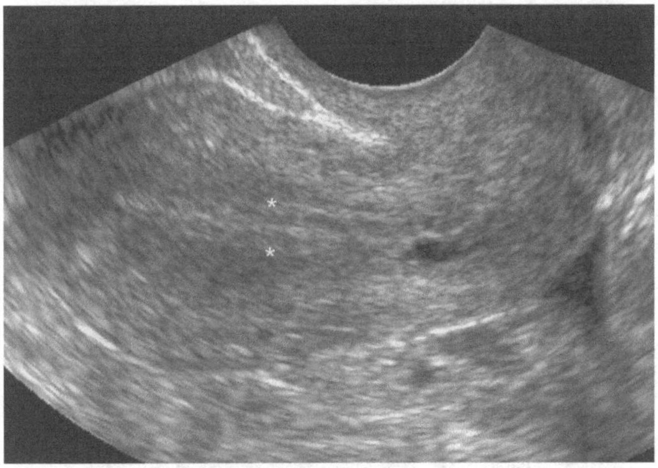

Fig. 36.20 Endometrial thickness measurement

affected by increasing age [84, 85]. Endometrial thickness >14 mm has not been found to consistently affect pregnancy rates. In a large study of women with endometrial thicknesses greater than 14 mm, there was no difference in implantation pregnancy or miscarriage rates when compared with women who had endometrial thicknesses <14 mm [86]. Presently, the pattern and thickness of the endometrial measurement is only marginally predictive of implantation during IVF [87–89]. Endometrial thickness measurement and pregnancy rates from IVF do not show a consistent correlation [83, 85, 90]. While most prefer an endometrial thickness greater than 6 mm, pregnancies have occurred with endometrial thicknesses measured at 4 mm [90–94]. Some investigators have proposed that endometrial echogenicity is a more reliable predictor of pregnancy after IVF [84]. An optimal echogenicity pattern is characterized by a multilayered hypoechoic triple line pattern that has also been referred to as a "ring." However, no consensus as to the predictive nature of an echogenicity pattern and pregnancy with IVF has been established to date [90, 95].

Endometrial Abnormalities

Endometrial thickening may be associated with endometrial hyperplasia, polyps or endometrial carcinoma. In a series of patients with endometrial carcinoma detected by sonography, the average thickness was 17.7 ± 5.8 mm [96]. Endometrial biopsy is required in those patients who are suspected of endometrial hyperplasia or carcinoma. Patients utilizing OCPs routinely show a single hyperechoic line representing the endometrial cavity. A very thin endometrium may indicate the need for additional estrogen in the regimen in women with dysfunctional uterine bleeding.

Endometrial polyps may range in size from microscopic to as large as several centimeters. They typically appear as a diffuse or focal thickening of the endometrium greater than that expected for a woman of comparable age. Polyps are best characterized by sonohysterography (Fig. 36.21).

Endometrial adhesions are best diagnosed by sonohysterography or hysteroscopy. They may be seen during menstruation, where intracavitary fluid outlines the abnormality, or following distention of the uterine cavity with fluid [67] (Fig. 36.22).

Fluid is occasionally seen in the endometrial cavity. It can be associated with pyometra due to pelvic inflammatory disease, normal secretions, congenital vaginal or cervical atresia, cervical strictures or fibrosis, uterine synechiae, or endometrial or cervical carcinoma [97–101] (Fig. 36.23).

Intrauterine conceptive devices are highly echogenic and reflective within the endometrial interface. Metallic and nonmetallic IUDs are best visualized via TVS. TVS has been used to diagnose perforation, malposition, and incomplete removal of the IUD. Myometrial implantation should be suspected when a portion of the IUD extends from the endometrial surface into the surrounding myometrium. Ultrasound can be used to remove the IUD when a coexisting pregnancy is located (Fig. 36.24).

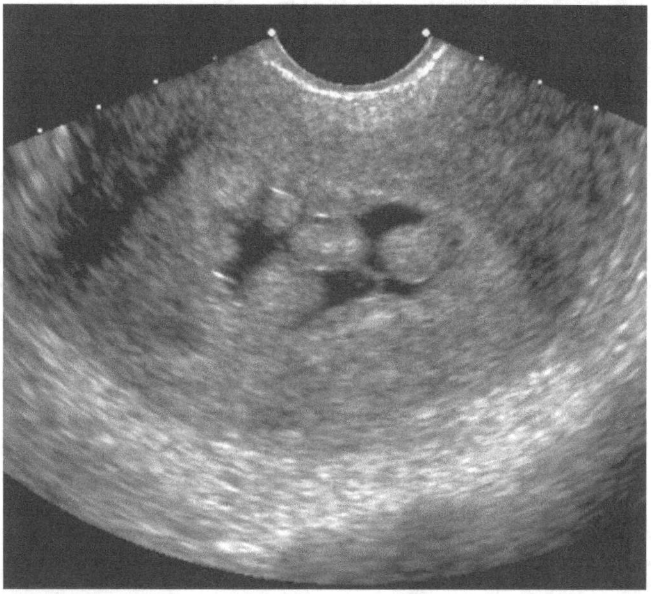

Fig. 36.21 Sonohysterography of polyp

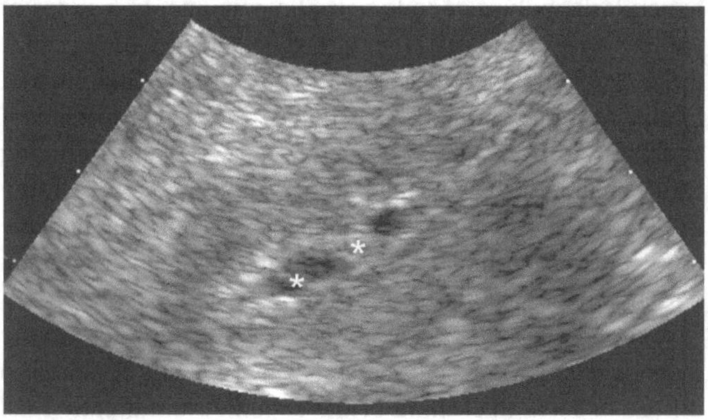

Fig. 36.22 Sonohysterography of adhesions

36.5.5.3 Early Pregnancy

In the context of assisted reproductive technologies, transvaginal ultrasound of an early pregnancy may be problematic. The discriminatory level of human chorionic

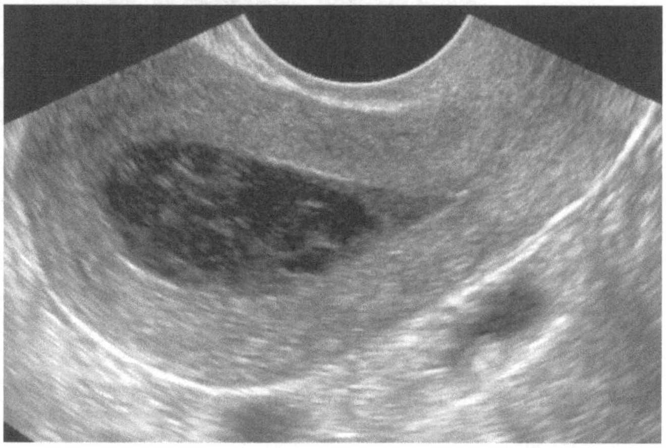

Fig. 36.23 Endometrial fluid pocket

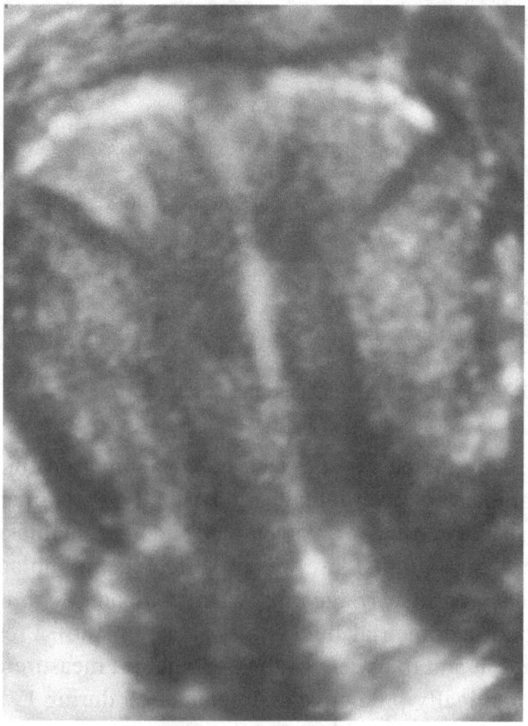

Fig. 36.24 IUD by 3D ultrasound. Three-dimensional reformatted image shows the IUD centrally located within the endometrial cavity. The sidearms are open, directed toward the cornua

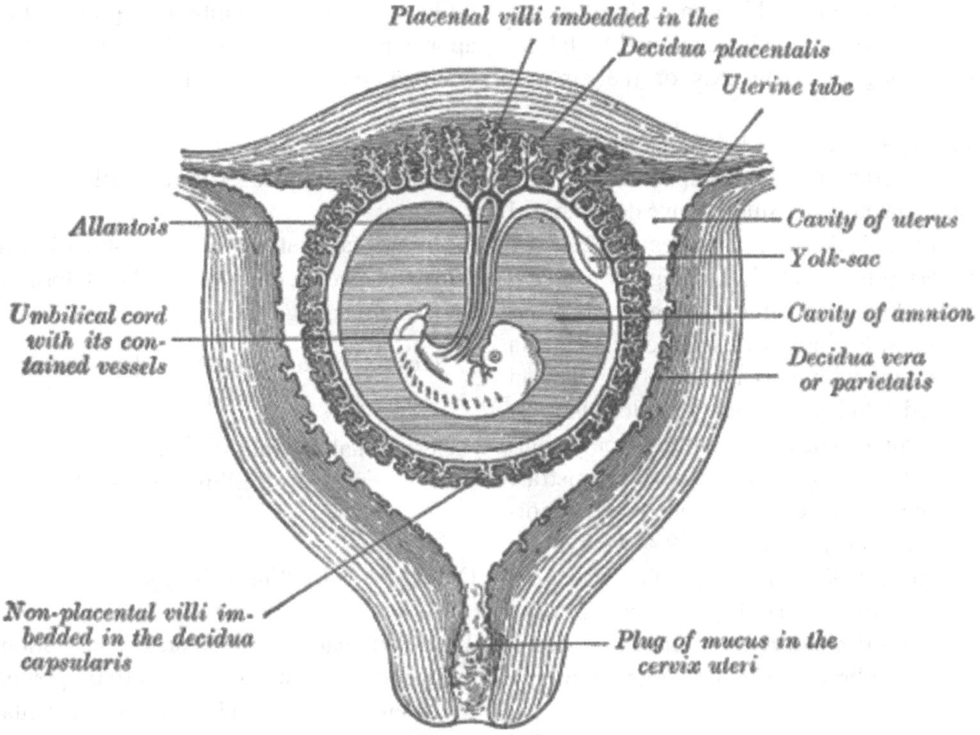

Fig. 36.25 Sectional view of the gravid uterus showing deciduas capsularis, deciduas vera or deciduas parietalis and decidua placentalis. Additionally, the location of the yolk sac and embryo are depicted. This faithful reproduction of a lithograph plate from Gray's Anatomy, a 2D work of art, is not copyrightable in the U.S. as per Bridgeman Art Library v. Corel Corp.; the same is also true in many other countries, including Germany. Unless stated otherwise, it is from the 20th U.S. edition of Gray's Anatomy of the Human Body, originally published in 1918 and therefore lapsed into the public domain. Other copies of Gray's Anatomy can be found on Bartleby and also on Yahoo! This image is in the public domain because its copyright has expired. This applies worldwide

gonadotropin (hCG) for documenting a normal intrauterine gestation is approximately 4,000 mU/mL via the transabdominal approach, and 2,000 mU/mL transvaginally. (Third International Reference Preparation) [12, 15].

In ART patients, multiple gestations may cause the hCG to be above the discriminatory zone before they can be seen. Concurrent problems such as fibroids, obesity, or previous uterine surgery may also affect the ability to image an early intrauterine pregnancy. In the absence of situations described earlier, ultrasound during early pregnancy demonstrates a gestational sac that appears as a thick echogenic rind surrounding a sonolucent center. The gestational sac when it first becomes apparent is surrounded by a thickened decidua. This perimeter then becomes a distinct "double ring" (also known as the "double decidual sac sign"). The inner ring corresponds to the decidua capsularis and the chorion laeve, and the outer ring corresponds to the decidua vera or deciduas parietalis [102] (Figs. 36.25and 36.26).

The gestational sac grows at approximately 1 mm per day in mean diameter during early pregnancy [103]. The yolk sac within the gestational sac has a bright echogenic rim and echolucent center. Published discriminatory levels for the presence of a yolk sac is between 5 and 13 mm in mean gestational sac diameter [104]. The embryo is first recognized as a thickening along the edge of the yolk sac.

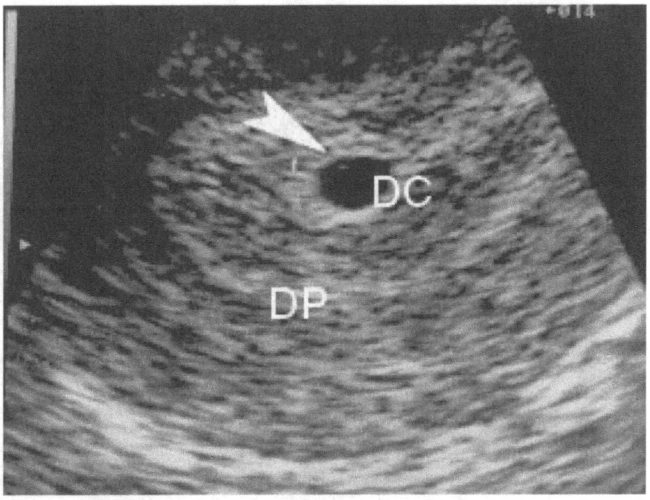

Fig. 36.26 The double decidual sac sign refers to the gestational sac when it first becomes apparent and is surrounded by a thickened decidua. This perimeter then becomes a distinct "double ring" (also known as the "double sac sign"). The inner ring corresponds to the decidua capsularis (DC) and the chorion laeve, and the outer ring corresponds to the decidua vera or decidual parietalis (DP)

The embryo is initially a linear structure of 2–3 mm in length. As it grows, it develops a C-shaped tadpole-like configuration. There is a recognizable crown rump length when the embryo measures between 17 and 22 mm. Before 17 mm, the measurement of embryonic size is performed by taking the greatest length along the long axis of the embryo (Fig. 36.27).

A chemical pregnancy is defined as a pregnancy detected by the measurement of serum hCG, but not proceeding on to clinical recognition of an embryo. Studies have documented that, in one population, 22% of pregnancies detected by hCG assays were lost prior to clinical recognition [105]. Despite this high rate of loss, a chemical pregnancy is prognostic for future success. Patients with such losses have an 83% chance of conception within six cycles [105]. Once an embryo is documented (clinical pregnancy), a loss is most commonly due to a chromosome abnormality. Some studies have documented that 70% of early losses demonstrate abnormal chromosomes [106]. Of the chromosome abnormalities, 64% were autosomal trisomies, 9% were polyploid, 7% were monosomy X, and 6% revealed structural rearrangements. The embryonic heart begins to beat 21 days after conception. The discriminatory level for cardiac activity appears to be at an embryonic size of 5 mm or greater [16, 107].

Great caution should be used when diagnosing a failed pregnancy and serial examinations are often required and prudent. The definition of a failed pregnancy includes: (1) Failure to image a yolk sac within the gestational sac by the time the gestational sac has reached a mean sac diameter of 10 mm; (2) Failure to image an embryo within the gestational sac by the time the mean sac diameter reaches 18 mm; (3) Failure of the sac or embryo to grow at the expected rate – approximately 1 mm per day; or, (4) Loss of previously documented cardiac activity.

Gestational Age Assessment (Table 36.1)

Accurate calculations using on-board software should be utilized; however, quick rule of thumb formulae for calculating the gestational age are:

Gestational age (days) ± 3 days = (mean sac diameter [millimeters] + 30) [108]

Gestational age (days) ± 3 days = (embryo size diameter [millimeters] + 42) [109]

Detection of Multifetal Pregnancies

The determination of amnionicity and chorionicity of multifetal pregnancies is critical. All multifetal pregnancies are at risk for preterm labor and delivery, placental abnormalities, intrauterine growth restriction, and malformations. Monochorionic twins/higher order multiples are at risk for twin-to-twin transfusion syndrome and twin reversed arterial perfusion sequence. Monoamniotic pregnancies carry the additional risks of cord entanglement, and conjoined twinning. The number of gestational sacs can be accurately determined by 5 weeks gestation. The chorionic sac count

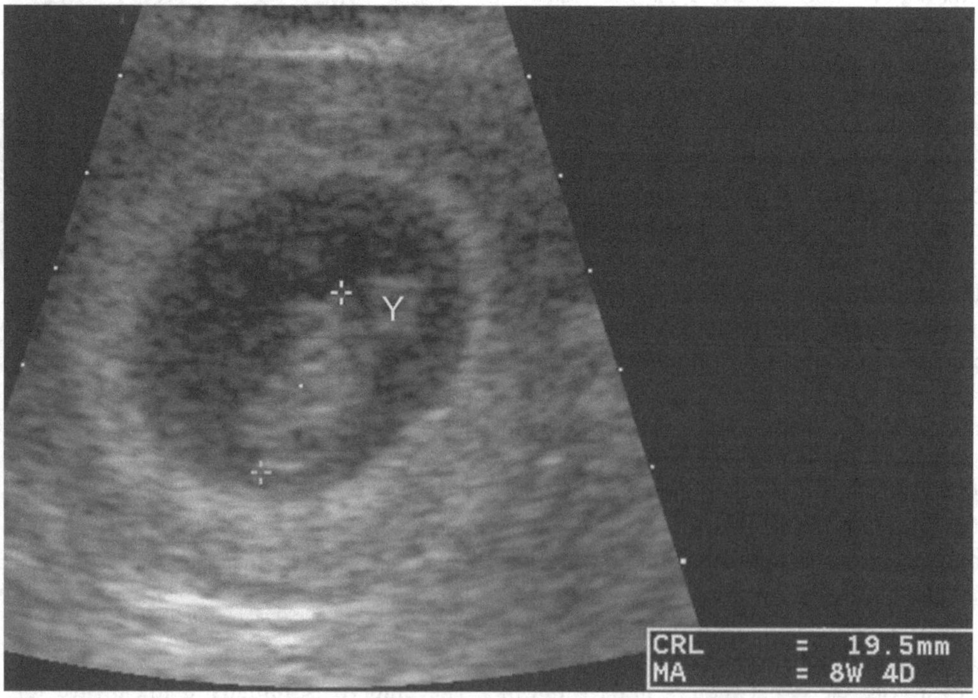

Fig. 36.27 Measuring CRL of early embryo

Table 36.1 Menstrual age, gestational age, crown-rump length, and human chorionic gonadotropin levels (hCG) in early gestation. (hCG values are based on the Third International Reference Preparation)

Menstrual age		Gestational sac size (mm)	Crown-rump length (cm)	hCG Level (first IRP), mean IU/U
Days	Weeks	–	–	–
30	4.3	–	–	–
31	4.4	–	–	–
32	4.6	3	–	1,710
33	4.7	4	–	2,320
34	4.9	5	–	3,100
35	5	5.5	–	4,090
36	5.1	6	–	5,340
37	5.3	7	–	6,880
38	5.4	8	–	8,770
39	5.6	9	–	11,040
40	5.7	10	0.2	13,730
41	5.9	11	0.3	15,300
42	6	12	0.35	16,870
43	6.1	13	0.4	20,480
44	6.3	14	0.5	24,560
45	6.4	15	0.6	29,110
46	6.6	16	0.7	34,100
47	6.7	17	0.8	39,460
48	6.9	18	0.9	45,120
49	7	19	0.95	50,970
50	7.1	20	1	56,900
51	7.3	21	1.1	62,760
52	7.4	22	1.2	68,390
53	7.6	23	1.3	73,640
54	7.7	24	1.4	78,350
55	7.9	25	1.5	82,370
56	8	26	1.6	85,560
57	8.1	26.5	1.7	–
58	8.3	27	1.8	–
59	8.4	28	1.9	–
60	8.6	29	2	–
61	8.7	30	2.1	–
62	8.9	31	2.2	–
63	9	32	2.3	–
64	9.1	33	2.4	–
65	9.3	34	2.5	–
66	9.4	35	2.6	–
67	9.6	36	2.8	–
68	9.7	37	2.9	–
69	9.9	38	3	–
70	10	39	3.1	–
71	10.1	40	3.2	–
72	10.3	41	3.4	–
73	10.4	42	3.5	–
74	10.6	43	3.7	–
75	10.7	44	3.8	–
76	10.9	45	4	–
77	11	46	4.1	–
78	11.1	47	4.2	–
79	11.3	48	4.4	–
80	11.4	49	4.6	–
81	11.6	50	4.8	–
82	11.7	51	5	–
83	11.9	52	5.2	–
84	12	53	5.4	–

is best assessed when embryos can be seen. The number of embryos is determined by the number of embryonic heartbeats. From 8 weeks on, the amnion within the chorionic cavity should be visualized.

36.5.5.4 Adnexae

Ovaries and adnexae are evaluated in both a long-axis and short-axis view. The long-axis view displays the longest dimension. The short-axis plane section is the view perpendicular to the long-axis. The ovarian volume in cubic centimeters is calculated using the following formula: D1 × D2 (in the long axis) × D3 (in the short or perpendicular axis) × 0.52. The ovary is easily recognized by its characteristic oval shape and peripherally placed follicles. It is routine to visualize the internal iliac vessels immediately posterior to the ovary. Follicles are measured according to the convention of each clinic (longest dimension or two dimensions in one plane). After completing ovarian measurements and the follicle count and follicular dimension(s), the cul-de-sac is inspected. Echogenic fluid usually correlates with hemorrhage e.g. in ectopic pregnancy, pus from an inflammatory process, or proteinaceous fluid.

Stromal to Ovarian Area Measurements

A recent study compared ovarian morphologic findings (stroma to ovarian ratio) with serum androgen levels [110]. The ovarian area was calculated by outlining with an ultrasound caliper the external limits of the ovary in the maximal longitudinal axis. The stromal area was determined by outlining with the caliper the outer peripheral profile of the stroma, identified as a hyperechoic area devoid of follicles. The stroma to ovarian area ratio was determined. The mean ovarian area, stromal area, and stroma to ovarian area ratio for each patient was determined by adding the sizes of each ovary and then dividing by 2. Patients with polycystic ovary syndrome showed a significantly higher ovarian volume, ovarian area, and stromal area when compared with control and patients with multifollicular ovaries. Additionally, the PCOS group had higher androstenedione, testosterone, 17-alpha hydroxyprogesterone, and free androgen index when compared with the other groups. A cutoff for the stroma to ovarian area ratio of 0.34 showed a sensitivity of 100% and a specificity of 100% for the PCOS diagnosis. Subsequent studies show reproducibility and defined a cutoff of 0.32. Three-dimensional ultrasound may provide a tool which will further refine stroma to ovarian measurements through the use of computer programs (VOCAL) which allow better quantification of ovarian compartmental volumes (Figs. 36.28 and 36.29).

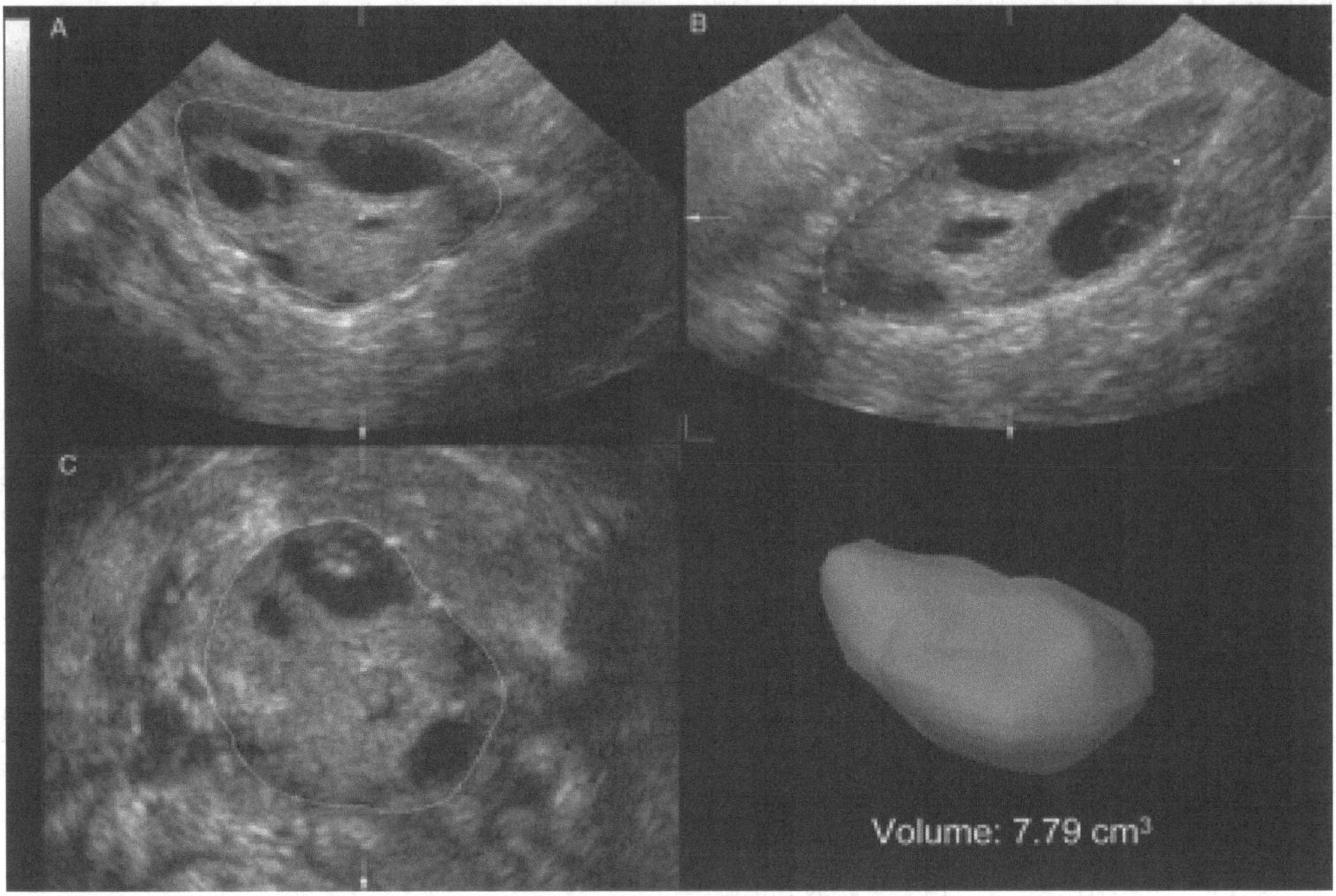

Fig. 36.28 VOCAL technique to display 3D model of ovary (lower right) before the application of "inversion mode" to demonstrate the antral follicles within the ovary. Reprinted with permission from K. Jayaprakasan, et al. Does 3D ultrasound offer any advantage in the pretreatment assessment of ovarian reserve and prediction of outcome after assisted reproduction treatment? Reprinted with permission from Human Reproduction 2007 22(7):1932–1941; doi:10.1093/humrep/dem104

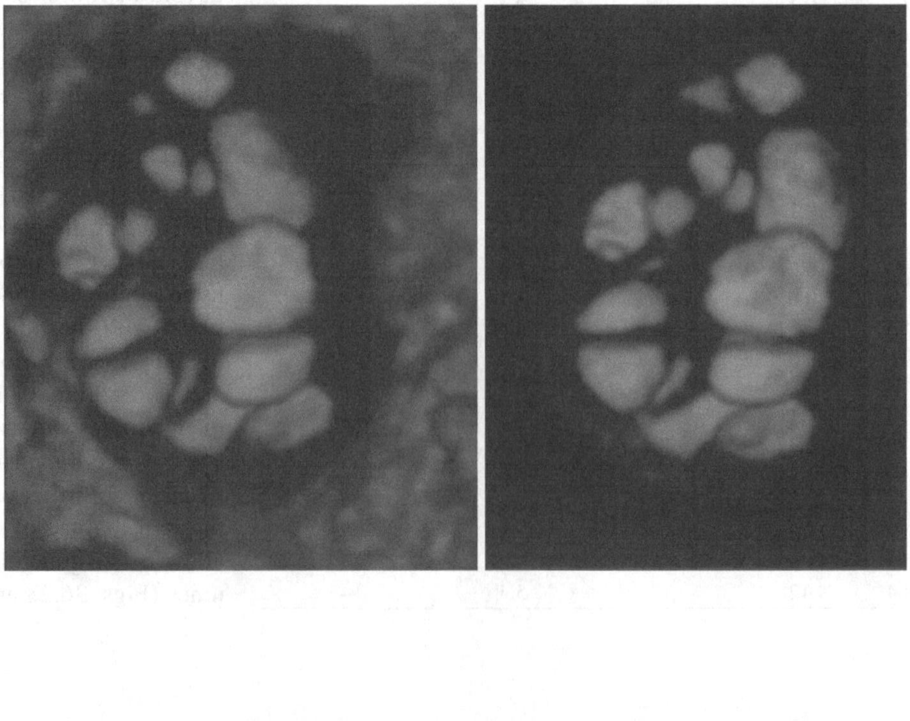

Fig. 36.29 Application of "inversion mode" to a 3D ultrasonographic data set allows immediate demonstration of antral follicles with in an ovary and its surrounding tissue (*left*). Use of VOCAL helps to remove the extra ovarian tissue and to display only the antral follicles (*right*). Reprinted with permission from K. Jayaprakasan, et al. Does 3D ultrasound offer any advantage in the pretreatment assessment of ovarian reserve and prediction of outcome after assisted reproduction treatment? Reprinted with permission from Human Reproduction 2007 22(7):1932–1941; doi:10.1093/humrep/dem104

Common Adnexal Findings

Adnexal Masses

A morphologic scoring system has been defined for the evaluation of adnexal masses [111]. A morphologic score >9 was more likely associated with malignant adnexal masses. These morphologic criteria provide a foundation for the ultrasound assessment of adnexal masses.

Functional Ovarian Cysts

Normal follicles measure between 5 and 24 mm depending on the phase of the cycle. If ovulation does not occur, a persistent follicular cyst may develop. This thin-walled, anechoic, unilocular cyst can be anywhere from 3 to 8 cm in size. They routinely resolve over a period of months.

Paraovarian/Paratubal Cysts

These cysts are usually an incidental finding, but occasionally they may cause symptoms if they grow significantly or undergo torsion. They are usually unilocular, anechoic, thin-walled cysts. They can be discriminated from the ovary by gently advancing the vaginal probe and demonstrating a separation of the cyst from its neighboring ovary. Three-dimensional ultrasound is particularly useful in demonstrating separate structures (Fig. 36.30).

Benign Epithelial Ovarian Tumors

Serous cyst adenomas are routinely unilocular, anechoic cysts, which persists over many months. They are bilateral in 20% of patients. They can be discovered in all age groups. Unilocular anechoic cysts can be monitored over a longer period of time, as nearly 70% of such cysts, even up to 10 cm in size, will resolve with observation [112]. The risk of malignancy in such cysts is estimated at 0.9%. Mucinous cyst adenomas are usually larger than serous cyst adenomas and occasionally can be as large as 30 cm. They routinely contain internal, low-level echoes due to mucin. They often have septations, which can be thick and somewhat bizarre.

Endometrioma

Power Doppler studies show no vascular supply to the central region of the cystic mass, with vessels confined to the periphery of the mass. Endometriomas typically contain low level internal echoes from blood products and show enhanced through transmission of sound. They often have bright punctate echoes within the wall (Fig. 36.31).

Pelvic Inflammatory Disease/Tubal Ovarian Abscess

Patients with pelvic inflammatory disease routinely present with symptoms of pelvic pain, purulent vaginal discharge, and pelvic tenderness. Ultrasound may reveal a dilated tube, which can be better imaged if there is purulent cul-de-sac fluid present. Motion of the transvaginal probe produces exquisite tenderness (Fig. 36.32).

Dermoids

Mature cystic teratomas, or dermoids, are the most common ovarian neoplasm in the reproductive age range. They account for 40–50% of benign ovarian neoplasms and are bilateral in 10–15% of the cases [113]. They are often detected incidentally (Fig. 36.33).

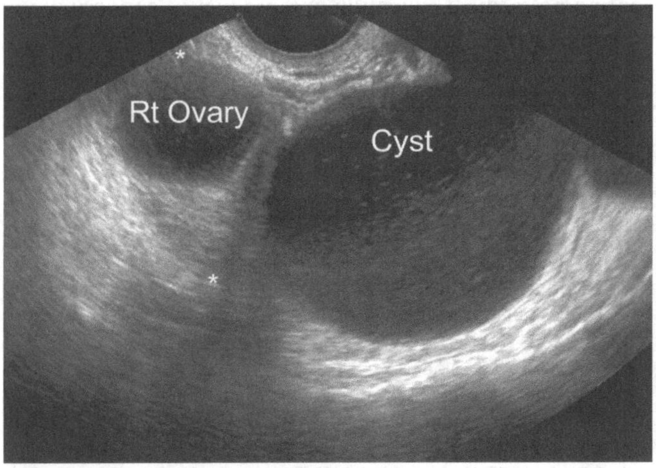

Fig. 36.30 Paratubal-paraovarian cyst

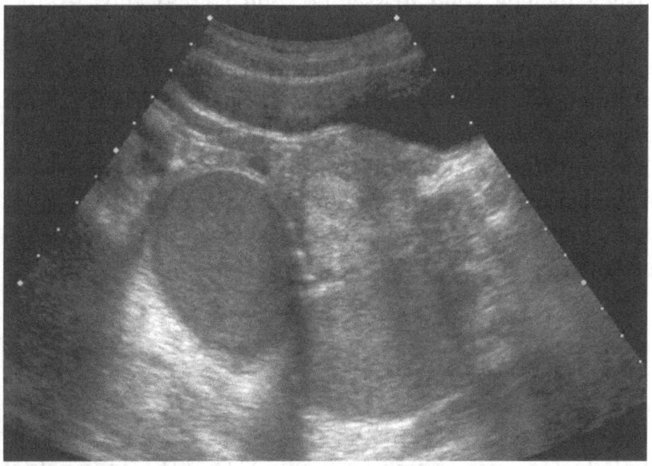

Fig. 36.31 Endometrioma

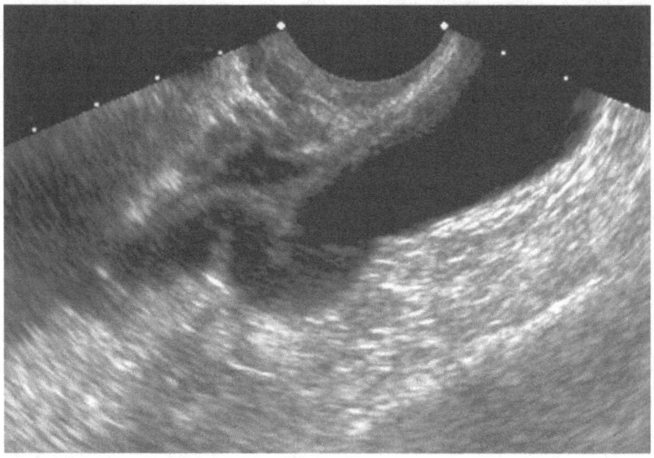

Fig. 36.32 Dilated fallopian tube

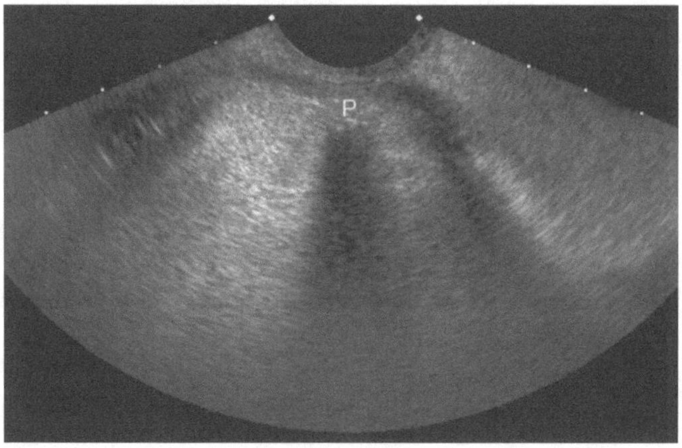

Fig. 36.33 TVS shows highly echogenic fatty content with extensive distal acoustic shadowing. This is known as the "tip of the iceberg" sign in that it is hard to tell how large the lesion may be. The densely shadowing dermoid plug (P) is a characteristic feature of a dermoid

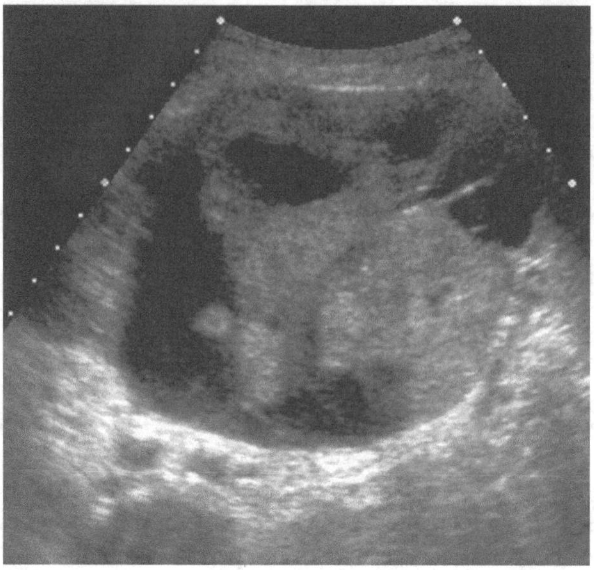

Fig. 36.34 Malignant ovarian cyst with solid components

Malignant Neoplasms

Transvaginal ultrasonographic features suggestive of malignancy include solid masses or solid components, excrescences and papillary projections arising from a cyst wall [114]. Doppler studies have been advocated for discriminating malignant from benign masses, with malignancies showing a resistance index less than 0.4. It should be remembered, however, that many early stage ovarian carcinomas have Doppler indices above the threshold for presumed malignancy and Doppler studies cannot confirm or refute malignancy (Fig. 36.34).

36.5.5.5 Embryo Transfer

Pregnancy rates after embryo transfer are dependent on multiple factors such as embryo quality [115, 116], endometrial receptivity [117], and the transfer technique. It has been documented that an experienced operator utilizing the clinical touch method of embryo transfer affords excellent pregnancy rates. Meta-analyses also suggest the benefits of using 2D transabdominal ultrasound in guiding catheter placement. Theories to explain this possible increase in desired pregnancy outcomes may be increasing the ease of embryo transfer by documenting the uterocervical angle [118], positioning the tip within the miduterine cavity, avoiding the fundus [119], and decreasing the need for instrumentation [120]. A recent meta-analysis found a significantly increased chance of clinical pregnancy (odds ratio 1.5; 95% confidence interval, 1.34–1.68), live birth rate (odds ratio 1.78; 95% CI, 1.19–2.67), and ongoing pregnancy rates (odds ratio 1.51; 95% CI, 1.31–1.74) using transabdominal ultrasound guidance when compared with the standard clinical touch method. Certainly, training in TVS will remain an important aspect of continuing medical education in reproductive endocrinology as well as gynecology.

References

1. Kratochwil A (1969) A new vaginal method of ultrasonotomography. Geburtshilfe Frauenheilkd 29(4):379–385
2. Meldrum DR, Chetkowski RJ, Steingold KA, Randle D (1984) Transvaginal ultrasound scanning of ovarian follicles. Fertil Steril 42(5):803–805
3. Morimoto N, Noda Y, Takai I, Yamada I, Tojo S (1983) Ultrasonographic observation of ovarian follicular development via vaginal route. Nippon Sanka Fujinka Gakkai zasshi 35(2):151–158
4. Schwimer SR, Lebovic J (1984) Transvaginal pelvic ultrasonography. J Ultrasound Med 3(8):381–383

5. Schwimer SR, Lebovic J (1985) Transvaginal pelvic ultrasonography: accuracy in follicle and cyst size determination. J Ultrasound Med 4(2):61–63
6. Lande IM, Hill MC, Cosco FE, Kator NN (1988) Adnexal and cul-de-sac abnormalities: transvaginal sonography. Radiology 166(2):325–332
7. Leibman AJ, Kruse B, McSweeney MB (1988) Transvaginal sonography: comparison with transabdominal sonography in the diagnosis of pelvic masses. AJR Am J Roentgenol 151(1):89–92
8. Mendelson EB, Bohm-Velez M, Joseph N, Neiman HL (1988) Gynecologic imaging: comparison of transabdominal and transvaginal sonography. Radiology 166(2):321–324
9. Nyberg DA, Mack LA, Jeffrey RB Jr, Laing FC (1987) Endovaginal sonographic evaluation of ectopic pregnancy: a prospective study. AJR Am J Roentgenol 149(6):1181–1186
10. Fleischer AC, Herbert CM 3rd, Hill GA, Kepple DM (1990) Transvaginal sonography: applications in infertility. Semin Ultrasound CT MR 11(1):71–81
11. Schulman JD, Dorfmann AD, Jones SL, Pitt CC, Joyce B, Patton LA (1987) Outpatient in vitro fertilization using transvaginal ultrasound-guided oocyte retrieval. Obstet Gynecol 69(4):665–668
12. Bree RL, Edwards M, Bohm-Velez M, Beyler S, Roberts J, Mendelson EB (1989) Transvaginal sonography in the evaluation of normal early pregnancy: correlation with HCG level. AJR Am J Roentgenol 153(1):75–79
13. Cullen MT, Green JJ, Reece EA, Hobbins JC (1989) A comparison of transvaginal and abdominal ultrasound in visualizing the first trimester conceptus. J Ultrasound Med 8(10):565–569
14. Fossum GT, Davajan V, Kletzky OA (1988) Early detection of pregnancy with transvaginal ultrasound. Fertil Steril 49(5):788–791
15. Goldstein SR, Snyder JR, Watson C, Danon M (1988) Very early pregnancy detection with endovaginal ultrasound. Obstet Gynecol 72(2):200–204
16. Levi CS, Lyons EA, Zheng XH, Lindsay DJ, Holt SC (1990) Endovaginal US: demonstration of cardiac activity in embryos of less than 5.0 mm in crown-rump length. Radiology 176(1):71–74
17. Neiman HL (1990) Transvaginal ultrasound embryography. Semin Ultrasound CT MR 11(1):22–33
18. Rempen A (1990) Diagnosis of viability in early pregnancy with vaginal sonography. J Ultrasound Med 9(12):711–716
19. Timor-Tritsch IE, Farine D, Rosen MG (1988) A close look at early embryonic development with the high-frequency transvaginal transducer. Am J Obstet Gynecol 159(3):676–681
20. Bohm-Velez M, Mendelson EB, Freimanis MG (1990) Transvaginal sonography in evaluating ectopic pregnancy. Semin Ultrasound CT MR 11(1):44–58
21. Cacciatore B, Stenman UH, Ylostalo P (1989) Comparison of abdominal and vaginal sonography in suspected ectopic pregnancy. Obstet Gynecol 73(5 Pt 1):770–774
22. Dashefsky SM, Lyons EA, Levi CS, Lindsay DJ (1988) Suspected ectopic pregnancy: endovaginal and transvesical US. Radiology 169(1):181–184
23. Jain KA, Hamper UM, Sanders RC (1988) Comparison of transvaginal and transabdominal sonography in the detection of early pregnancy and its complications. AJR Am J Roentgenol 151(6):1139–1143
24. Mendelson EB, Bohm-Velez M, Saker M (1990) Transvaginal sonography in the abnormal first trimester. Semin Ultrasound CT MR 11(1):34–43
25. Nyberg DA, Mack LA, Laing FC, Jeffrey RB (1988) Early pregnancy complications: endovaginal sonographic findings correlated with human chorionic gonadotropin levels. Radiology 167(3):619–622
26. Pennell RG, Baltarowich OH, Kurtz AB et al (1987) Complicated first-trimester pregnancies: evaluation with endovaginal US versus transabdominal technique. Radiology 165(1):79–83
27. Rempen A (1988) Vaginal sonography in ectopic pregnancy. A prospective evaluation. J Ultrasound Med 7(7):381–387
28. Shapiro BS, Cullen M, Taylor KJ, DeCherney AH (1988) Transvaginal ultrasonography for the diagnosis of ectopic pregnancy. Fertil Steril 50(3):425–429
29. Thorsen MK, Lawson TL, Aiman EJ et al (1990) Diagnosis of ectopic pregnancy: endovaginal vs. transabdominal sonography. AJR Am J Roentgenol 155(2):307–310
30. Timor-Tritsch IE, Yeh MN, Peisner DB, Lesser KB, Slavik TA (1989) The use of transvaginal ultrasonography in the diagnosis of ectopic pregnancy. Am J Obstet Gynecol 161(1):157–161
31. Benacerraf BR (1990) Examination of the second-trimester fetus with severe oligohydramnios using transvaginal scanning. Obstet Gynecol 75(3 Pt 2):491–493
32. Benacerraf BR, Estroff JA (1989) Transvaginal sonographic imaging of the low fetal head in the second trimester. J Ultrasound Med 8(6):325–328
33. Weber TM, Hertzberg BS, Bowie JD (1990) Use of endo-vaginal ultrasound to optimize visualization of the distal fetal spine in breech presentations. J Ultrasound Med 9(9):519–524
34. Timor-Tritsch IE, Bar-Yam Y, Elgali S, Rottem S (1988) The technique of transvaginal sonography with the use of a 6.5 MHz probe. Am J Obstet Gynecol 158(5):1019–1024
35. Timor-Tritsch IE, Rottem S, Thaler I (1988) Review of tansvaginal ultrasonography: a description with clinical application. Ultrasound Q 6:1–34
36. Vilaro MM, Rifkin MD, Pennell RG, et al (1987) Endovaginal ultrasound. A technique for evaluation of nonfollicular pelvic masses. J Ultrasound Med 6(12):697–701
37. Chervenak FA, Gabbe SG (1991) Obstretic ultrasound: assessment of fetal growth and anatomy. In: Gabbe SG, Niebyl JR, Simpson JL (eds) Obstretics, normal and problem pregnancies, 2nd edn. Churchill Livingstone, New York, pp 329–376
38. Jain KA, Jeffrey RB Jr, Sommer FG (1991) Gynecologic vascular abnormalities: diagnosis with Doppler US. Radiology 178(2):549–551
39. Taylor KJ, Burns PN, Wells PN, Conway DI, Hull MG (1985) Ultrasound Doppler flow studies of the ovarian and uterine arteries. Br J Obstet Gynaecol 92(3):240–246
40. Taylor KJ, Ramos IM, Feyock AL et al (1989) Ectopic pregnancy: duplex Doppler evaluation. Radiology 173(1):93–97
41. Baber RJ, McSweeney MB, Gill RW et al (1988) Transvaginal pulsed Doppler ultrasound assessment of blood flow to the corpus luteum in IVF patients following embryo transfer. Br J Obstet Gynaecol 95(12):1226–1230
42. Kurjak A, Zalud I, Jurkovic D, Alfirevic Z, Miljan M (1989) Transvaginal color Doppler for the assessment of pelvic circulation. Acta Obstet Gynecol Scand 68(2):131–135
43. Schaaps JP, Soyeur D (1989) Pulsed Doppler on a vaginal probe. Necessity, convenience, or luxury? J Ultrasound Med 8(6):315–320
44. Goldstein SR, Horii SC, Snyder JR, Raghavendra BN, Subramanyam B (1988) Estimation of nongravid uterine volume based on a nomogram of gravid uterine volume: its value in gynecologic uterine abnormalities. Obstet Gynecol 72(1):86–90
45. Platt JF, Bree RL, Davidson D (1990) Ultrasound of the normal nongravid uterus: correlation with gross and histopathology. J Clin Ultrasound 18(1):15–19
46. Alcazar J (2005) Three dimensional ultrasound in gynecology: current status and future perspectives. Curr Women's Health Rev 1:1–14
47. Fleischer AC, Herbert CM, Hill GA, Kepple DM, Worrell JA (1991) Transvaginal sonography of the endometrium during induced cycles. J Ultrasound Med 10(2):93–95
48. Price R, Fleischer A (eds) (1991) Sonographic instrumentation. Appleton & Lange, Norwalk, CT
49. Kremkau F (1989) Tranducers. In: Diagnostic ultrasound principles: instruments and exercise. 3rd edn. WB Saundres, Philadelphia, pp 65–94
50. Platt LD (1987) New look in ultrasound: the vaginal probe. Contemp Obstet Gynecol 30:99–105

51. Laing FC (1990) Technical aspects of vaginal ultrasound. Semin Ultrasound CT MR 11(1):4–11
52. Nyberg DA, Hughes MP, Mack LA, Wang KY (1991) Extrauterine findings of ectopic pregnancy of transvaginal US: importance of echogenic fluid. Radiology 178(3):823–826
53. Lele PP (1979) Safety and potential hazards in the current applications of ultrasound in obstetrics and gynecology. Ultrasound Med Biol 5(4):307–320
54. O'Brien WD Jr (1983) Dose-dependent effect of ultrasound on fetal weight in mice. J Ultrasound Med 2(1):1–8
55. Lizzi F (1988) Thermal mechanism: American Institute of Ultrasound in Medicine Bioeffects Reprot. J Ultrasound Med 7(suppliment):S8–S17
56. Carstensen EL, Gates AH (1984) The effects of pulsed ultrasound on the fetus. J Ultrasound Med 3(4):145–147
57. Clarke PR, Hill CR (1970) Physical and chemical aspects of ultrasonic disruption of cells. J Acoust Soc Am 47(2):649–653
58. Merritt CR (1989) Ultrasound safety: what are the issues? Radiology 173(2):304–306
59. Warwick W (1973) Gray's anatomy. WB Saunders, Philadelphia
60. Lyons EA, Taylor PJ, Zheng XH, Ballard G, Levi CS, Kredentser JV (1991) Characterization of subendometrial myometrial contractions throughout the menstrual cycle in normal fertile women. Fertil Steril 55(4):771–774
61. de Vries K, Lyons EA, Ballard G, Levi CS, Lindsay DJ (1990) Contractions of the inner third of the myometrium. Am J Obstet Gynecol 162(3):679–682
62. Abramowicz JS, Archer DF (1990) Uterine endometrial peristalsis – a transvaginal ultrasound study. Fertil Steril 54(3):451–454
63. Scholtes MC, Wladimiroff JW, van Rijen HJ, Hop WC (1989) Uterine and ovarian flow velocity waveforms in the normal menstrual cycle: a transvaginal Doppler study. Fertil Steril 52(6):981–985
64. Radman HM, Askin JA, Kolodner LJ (1966) Hydrometrocolpos and hematometrocolpos. Obstet Gynecol 27(1):2–6
65. Nicolini U, Bellotti M, Bonazzi B, Zamberletti D, Candiani GB (1987) Can ultrasound be used to screen uterine malformations? Fertil Steril 47(1):89–93
66. Funk A, Fendel H (1988) Ultrasonic diagnosis of congenital uterine abnormalities. Z Geburtshilfe Perinatol 192(2):77–82
67. Robbins SL (1974) Pathologic basis of disease. WB Saunders, Philadelphia
68. Fedele L, Bianchi S, Dorta M, Brioschi D, Zanotti F, Vercellini P (1991) Transvaginal ultrasonography versus hysteroscopy in the diagnosis of uterine submucous myomas. Obstet Gynecol 77(5):745–748
69. Siedler D, Laing FC, Jeffrey RB, Jr, Wing VW (1987) Uterine adenomyosis. A difficult sonographic diagnosis. J Ultrasound Med 6(7):345–349
70. Togashi K, Ozasa H, Konishi I et al (1989) Enlarged uterus: differentiation between adenomyosis and leiomyoma with MR imaging. Radiology 171(2):531–534
71. Eberhardt H, Cyr DR, Easterling TR, Nyberg DA, Mack LA (1988) Diagnosis of a uterine arteriovenous malformation by duplex sonography. J Diagn Med Sonogr 4:130–132
72. Tur-Kaspa I, Gal M, Hartman M, Hartman J, Hartman A (2006) A prospective evaluation of uterine abnormalities by saline infusion sonohysterography in 1,009 women with infertility or abnormal uterine bleeding. Fertil Steril 86(6):1731–1735
73. Schild RL, Knobloch C, Dorn C, Fimmers R, van der Ven H, Hansmann M (2001) Endometrial receptivity in an in vitro fertilization program as assessed by spiral artery blood flow, endometrial thickness, endometrial volume, and uterine artery blood flow. Fertil Steril 75(2):361–366
74. Callen PW, DeMartini WJ, Filly RA (1979) The central uterine cavity echo: a useful anatomic sign in the ultrasonographic evaluation of the female pelvis. Radiology 131(1):187–190
75. Mendelson EB, Bohm-Velez M, Joseph N, Neiman HL (1988) Endometrial abnormalities: evaluation with transvaginal sonography. AJR Am J Roentgenol 150(1):139–142
76. Fleischer AC, Kalemeris GC, Entman SS (1986) Sonographic depiction of the endometrium during normal cycles. Ultrasound Med Biol 12(4):271–277
77. Fleischer AC, Kalemeris GC, Machin JE, Entman SS, James AE Jr (1986) Sonographic depiction of normal and abnormal endometrium with histopathologic correlation. J Ultrasound Med 5(8):445–452
78. Deichert U, Hackeloer BJ, Daume E (1986) The sonographic and endocrinologic evaluation of the endometrium in the luteal phase. Hum Reprod 1(4):219–222
79. Demas BE, Hricak H, Jaffe RB (1986) Uterine MR imaging: effects of hormonal stimulation. Radiology 159(1):123–126
80. Giorlandino C, Gleicher N, Nanni C, Vizzone A, Gentili P, Taramanni C (1987) The sonographic picture of endometrium in spontaneous and induced cycles. Fertil Steril 47(3):508–511
81. Salm R (1962) Mucin production of normal and abnormal endometrium. Arch Pathol 73:30–39
82. Welker BG, Gembruch U, Diedrich K, al-Hasani S, Krebs D (1989) Transvaginal sonography of the endometrium during ovum pickup in stimulated cycles for in vitro fertilization. J Ultrasound Med 8(10):549–553
83. De Geyter C, Schmitter M, De Geyter M, Nieschlag E, Holzgreve W, Schneider HP (2000) Prospective evaluation of the ultrasound appearance of the endometrium in a cohort of 1,186 infertile women. Fertil Steril 73(1):106–113
84. Sher G, Herbert C, Maassarani G, Jacobs MH (1991) Assessment of the late proliferative phase endometrium by ultrasonography in patients undergoing in-vitro fertilization and embryo transfer (IVF/ET). Hum Reprod 6(2):232–237
85. Noyes N, Liu HC, Sultan K, Schattman G, Rosenwaks Z (1995) Endometrial thickness appears to be a significant factor in embryo implantation in in-vitro fertilization. Hum Reprod 10(4):919–922
86. Dietterich C, Check JH, Choe JK, Nazari A, Lurie D (2002) Increased endometrial thickness on the day of human chorionic gonadotropin injection does not adversely affect pregnancy or implantation rates following in vitro fertilization-embryo transfer. Fertil Steril 77(4):781–786
87. Kupesic S, Bekavac I, Bjelos D, Kurjak A (2001) Assessment of endometrial receptivity by transvaginal color Doppler and three-dimensional power Doppler ultrasonography in patients undergoing in vitro fertilization procedures. J Ultrasound Med 20(2):125–134
88. Noyes N, Hampton BS, Berkeley A, Licciardi F, Grifo J, Krey L (2001) Factors useful in predicting the success of oocyte donation: a 3-year retrospective analysis. Fertil Steril 76(1):92–97
89. Remohi J, Ardiles G, Garcia-Velasco JA, Gaitan P, Simon C, Pellicer A (1997) Endometrial thickness and serum oestradiol concentrations as predictors of outcome in oocyte donation. Hum Reprod 12(10):2271–2276
90. Friedler S, Schenker JG, Herman A, Lewin A (1996) The role of ultrasonography in the evaluation of endometrial receptivity following assisted reproductive treatments: a critical review. Hum reprod update 2(4):323–335
91. Coulam CB, Bustillo M, Soenksen DM, Britten S (1994) Ultrasonographic predictors of implantation after assisted reproduction. Fertil Steril 62(5):1004–1010
92. Gonen Y, Casper RF (1990) Prediction of implantation by the sonographic appearance of the endometrium during controlled ovarian stimulation for in vitro fertilization (IVF). J In Vitro Fert Embryo Transf 7(3):146–152
93. Gonen Y, Casper RF, Jacobson W, Blankier J (1989) Endometrial thickness and growth during ovarian stimulation: a possible predictor of implantation in in vitro fertilization. Fertil Steril 52(3):446–450

94. Sundstrom P (1998) Establishment of a successful pregnancy following in-vitro fertilization with an endometrial thickness of no more than 4 mm. Hum Reprod 13(6):1550–1552
95. Sharara FI, Lim J, McClamrock HD (1999) Endometrial pattern on the day of oocyte retrieval is more predictive of implantation success than the pattern or thickness on the day of hCG administration. J Assist Reprod Genet 16(10):523–528
96. Granberg S, Wikland M, Karlsson B, Norstrom A, Friberg LG (1991) Endometrial thickness as measured by endovaginal ultrasonography for identifying endometrial abnormality. Am J Obstet Gynecol 164(1 Pt 1):47–52
97. Breckenridge JW, Kurtz AB, Ritchie WG, Macht EL Jr (1982) Postmenopausal uterine fluid collection: indicator of carcinoma. AJR Am J Roentgenol 139(3):529–534
98. Chambers CB, Unis JS (1986) Ultrasonographic evidence of uterine malignancy in the postmenopausal uterus. Am J Obstet Gynecol 154(6):1194–1199
99. Laing FC, Filly RA, Marks WM, Brown TW (1980) Ultrasonic demonstration of endometrial fluid collections unassociated with pregnancy. Radiology 137(2):471–474
100. McCarthy KA, Hall DA, Kopans DB, Swann CA (1986) Postmenopausal endometrial fluid collections: always an indicator of malignancy? J Ultrasound Med 5(11):647–649
101. Scott WW Jr, Rosenshein NB, Siegelman SS, Sanders RC (1981) The obstructed uterus. Radiology 141(3):767–770
102. Nyberg DA, Laing FC, Filly RA, Uri-Simmons M, Jeffrey RB Jr (1983) Ultrasonographic differentiation of the gestational sac of early intrauterine pregnancy from the pseudogestational sac of ectopic pregnancy. Radiology 146(3):755–759
103. Daya S, Woods S, Ward S, Lappalainen R, Caco C (1991) Early pregnancy assessment with transvaginal ultrasound scanning. CMAJ 144(4):441–446
104. Rowling SE, Langer JE, Coleman BG, Nisenbaum HL, Horii SC, Arger PH (1999) Sonography during early pregnancy: dependence of threshold and discriminatory values on transvaginal transducer frequency. AJR Am J Roentgenol 172(4):983–988
105. Wilcox AJ, Weinberg CR, O'Connor JF et al (1988) Incidence of early loss of pregnancy. N Engl J Med 319(4):189–194
106. Ohno M, Maeda T, Matsunobu A (1991) A cytogenetic study of spontaneous abortions with direct analysis of chorionic villi. Obstet Gynecol 77(3):394–398
107. Goldstein SR (1992) Significance of cardiac activity on endovaginal ultrasound in very early embryos. Obstet Gynecol 80(4): 670–672
108. Rossavik IK, Torjusen GO, Gibbons WE (1988) Conceptual age and ultrasound measurements of gestational sac and crown-rump length in in vitro fertilization pregnancies. Fertil Steril 49(6):1012–1017
109. Goldstein SR, Wolfson R (1994) Endovaginal ultrasonographic measurement of early embryonic size as a means of assessing gestational age. J Ultrasound Med 13(1):27–31
110. Fulghesu AM, Ciampelli M, Belosi C, Apa R, Pavone V, Lanzone A (2001) A new ultrasound criterion for the diagnosis of polycystic ovary syndrome: the ovarian stroma/total area ratio. Fertil Steril 76(2):326–331
111. Sassone AM, Timor-Tritsch IE, Artner A, Westhoff C, Warren WB (1991) Transvaginal sonographic characterization of ovarian disease: evaluation of a new scoring system to predict ovarian malignancy. Obstet Gynecol 78(1):70–76
112. Modesitt SC, Pavlik EJ, Ueland FR, DePriest PD, Kryscio RJ, van Nagell JR, Jr (2003) Risk of malignancy in unilocular ovarian cystic tumors less than 10 centimeters in diameter. Obstet Gynecol 102(3):594–599
113. Comerci JT Jr, Licciardi F, Bergh PA, Gregori C, Breen JL (1994) Mature cystic teratoma: a clinicopathologic evaluation of 517 cases and review of the literature. Obstet Gynecol 84(1):22–28
114. Valentin L, Hagen B, Tingulstad S, Eik-Nes S (2001) Comparison of "pattern recognition" and logistic regression models for discrimination between benign and malignant pelvic masses: a prospective cross validation. Ultrasound Obstet Gynecol 18:357–365
115. De Neubourg D, Gerris J, Mangelschots K, Van Royen E, Vercruyssen M, Elseviers M (2004) Single top quality embryo transfer as a model for prediction of early pregnancy outcome. Hum Reprod 19(6):1476–1479
116. Roseboom TJ, Vermeiden JP, Schoute E, Lens JW, Schats R (1995) The probability of pregnancy after embryo transfer is affected by the age of the patient, cause of infertility, number of embryos transferred and the average morphology score, as revealed by multiple logistic regression analysis. Hum Reprod 10(11):3035–3041
117. Hoozemans DA, Schats R, Lambalk CB, Homburg R, Hompes PG (2004) Human embryo implantation: current knowledge and clinical implications in assisted reproductive technology. Reprod Biomed Online 9(6):692–715
118. Sallam HN, Agameya AF, Rahman AF, Ezzeldin F, Sallam AN (2002) Ultrasound measurement of the uterocervical angle before embryo transfer: a prospective controlled study. Hum Reprod 17(7):1767–1772
119. Schoolcraft WB, Surrey ES, Gardner DK (2001) Embryo transfer: techniques and variables affecting success. Fertil Steril 76(5):863–870
120. Abou-Setta AM, Mansour RT, Al-Inany HG, Aboulghar MM, Aboulghar MA, Serour GI (2007) Among women undergoing embryo transfer, is the probability of pregnancy and live birth improved with ultrasound guidance over clinical touch alone? A systemic review and meta-analysis of prospective randomized trials. Fertil Steril 88(2):333–341

Part V
Assisted Reproductive Therapy: In Vitro Fertilization

Chapter 37
Establishing the IVF Laboratory: A Systems View

Antonia V. Gilligan

Abstract The modern IVF laboratory is an integral part of the system used to support human embryo growth. The laboratory must be designed to provide the essential maternal supports for fertilization and development to the blastocyst stage. The laboratory must provide a physical barrier to microbial contamination and chemical degradation. This is done by using a high level of pressurization and isolation. Air supplied to the IVF laboratory is both filtered for particulates and chemical contaminates. Selecting "clean" materials for construction complements our efforts to remove embryotoxic materials from the IVF laboratory. If successfully done, the isolation, pressurization, plus particulate and chemical filtration will result in higher pregnancy and implantation rates.

Keywords Laboratory construction • Air quality • Construction materials • Volatile organic compounds • Laboratory equipment

37.1 Introduction

Since 1978, because of the pioneering work of Drs. Edwards and Steptoe, human embryo development has occurred in laboratories. The miracle is that human embryos and gametes can be made to function *outside* the body. The early laboratories were poorly designed largely because we knew very little about this new, complex technology. Often the location of these laboratories was determined by the space available. These laboratories were constructed using the methods employed for constructing similar research laboratories or common operating rooms. If it was a "closet" located next to a pathology laboratory, it would be made to function. The historical view was that the laboratory used to manipulate gametes and culture embryos was a passive partner in the process. Only recently has the laboratory been seen as more than the locus of Assisted Reproductive Technologies (ART) procedures. Historically, the laboratory was not an integral factor in the success of ART procedures.

The evolution of the modern ART laboratory can be compared to the changes that have taken place in the production of integrated circuit products by the microprocessor industry. These wonders of electrical engineering are based upon the use of photolithography. To get a high density of components, particulates must be removed from the air as they interfere with the ability to photographically print the integrated circuits. An industrial product with clearly defined requirements for cleanliness should not be done in a nineti-eth century mill. The same is true of twenty-first century ART facilities. The embryo culture laboratory is a key ingredient in the systems we design to replace the maternal systems for the first 3–5 days of the prospective child's life.

37.2 Key Parameters of Maternal Systems

Most practitioners are in awe of the complexity and refinement of the maternal systems mammals use to nurture their offspring. However, they fail to fully comprehend the need to design corresponding systems into their laboratories. These systems must compensate for the artificial environment we use for embryo culture. Therefore, it is informative to consider the differences and the way we can design systems to compensate for our laboratories. These comments are aimed at the embryo laboratory and not the Andrology laboratories used to analyze and process semen for diagnosis or reproduction.

37.2.1 Temperature

Maternal systems define normal as 98.6°F. The mother surrounds the gametes and embryo with a large mass of tissue actively respiring, insuring a constant temperature. This is done regardless of the temperatures experienced by the mother. In the IVF laboratory, we rely primarily on the incubator as

A.V. Gilligan (✉)
Alpha Environmental, Inc, 11 Ackerman Avenue, Emerson, NJ, 07630, USA

D.T. Carrell and C.M. Peterson (eds.), *Reproductive Endocrinology and Infertility: Integrating Modern Clinical and Laboratory Practice*,
DOI 10.1007/978-1-4419-1436-1_37,

the regulator of temperature. Yet, we must examine the embryos under a number of circumstances. The temperatures experienced by the embryo will range from typical room temperatures to the heat of a microscope illuminator. The laboratory design must comprehend the variations and the manner in which they can be managed. Undue cooling of eggs has been implicated in damage to the miotic spindle.

The modern IVF laboratory is designed to maintain an ambient temperature comfortable for the laboratory staff and also for the embryo. Therefore, careful attention to incubator temperatures are a given, but often times this attention is absent for the auxiliary systems used to maintain temperatures for the cultures when they are outside the incubator.

Routinely, we used heated stages on our microscopes, in our isolates and laminar flow hoods. The heated stage on our microscopes is often set at 98°F, but rarely has the laboratory staff understood that 98.6° at the top of the heated stage will result in a temperature of less than 98°F. This is because of poor heat transference through a plastic dish and mineral oil. To maintain the correct temperature, the stages need to be set based upon an actual measurement of the temperature inside the culture dish.

The next common reason for the degradation of temperature is the issue of incubator location and air supply. Incubators below air supply diffusers will be cooled. Each opening causes the cultures at the top and front of the incubator to be cooled every time. Ideally, the laboratories' design should have the diffusers remote from the incubators. This can be done by using directional diffusers so that incoming air is directed away from the incubators.

The blocks used to heat tubes during retrieval cause a similar issue. They are commonly in the procedure room or just inside the ART laboratory. They should not be chilled by poor placement. Frequent temperature checks and calibration are required.

37.2.2 pH Control

The control of pH is crucial if we are to maximize the productivity of our facilities. Maternal systems use a similar carbonate and bicarbonate as we do in the IVF laboratory but the environment of the fallopian tubes also has a number of secondary systems that can modulate pH. The fluid has a wide assortment of amino acids and proteins that can also adsorb or release hydrogen ions bolstering the simple carbonate bicarbonate buffer.

Our culture system of laboratory incubator and media attempt to reach this level of control. Measuring and controlling this system is usually based upon a Fyrite determination of carbon dioxide concentration that is accurate to ±0.5%. Even there, we are monitoring the pH in the media and not the more critical pH internal to the cells of the embryo.

37.2.3 Waste Products

The topic of nutrimental supports is far too complex to summarize here, but we do know that our procedures to manage the embryo's environment are at best a working compromise. Our methods fail to comprehend the depth of the maternal systems. The abiotic and biological breakdown on amino acids to produce the ammonium ion is well known. However, we do not have a satisfactory solution to remove this metabolic waste. We just periodically decant the old media and replace it with new media, thereby eliminating any growth factor the embryos make.

37.2.4 Detoxification Mechanism

In vivo development is done in an environment which is complemented by a wide variety of detoxification mechanisms, as well as excretory routes. It is this deficiency that is poorly controlled in most IVF facilities. Maternal systems include a fully functional liver, whose biochemical sophistication is backed by millions of years of evolution. The Fallopian tube environment is supported by a chemical plant of exquisite sophistication, the liver. The kidney effectively removes nitrogen wastes selectively. The lungs provide not only oxygen and carbon dioxide but also act as an excretory mechanism for gases and volatile organics. The IVF laboratory using micro drop culture relies not only on the mineral oil overlay to buffer changes in media osmality but also to sequester exogenous pollutants. It is this deficiency that has become our unwitting collaborator in embryo culture. The traditional IVF lab ignores the role of the uncontrolled environment. In this regard, each traditional IVF lab is an uncontrolled experiment in embryo toxicology. These exposures occur at the same time the embryo is initiating development, differentiation through gene activation and transcription.

37.2.5 Sterilizing and Fixing Agents

Aseptic technique cleaning, sterilizing and in some cases, fixing of specimens, can challenge the embryos in ART facilities. Glutaraldehyde, *ortho*-pathaldehyde, ethylene oxide, peroxyacetic acid and formaldehyde all have the potential to be used in or around the IVF laboratories. To avoid these agents disrupting the process of embryo development, they must be used outside the lab. Ethylene oxide [1, 2] has been reported to be a residue on culture dishes and cryogenic supplies which can adversely affect embryos if the plasticware is not fully aired-out prior to use. The dirty utility area should never be included inside the IVF laboratory envelope.

37.2.6 Pollutants as Possible Biological Signals

Nitric oxide (NO) is a common air pollutant. It is also a short lived messenger molecule related to apoptosis in embryo development.

At this time, we have no analogy to the systems used by the maternal embryo system to compensate for this exposure. Therefore, the designer of the IVF laboratory for clinical applications must devise methods to inhibit or remove these potentially offending substances. The balance of this article will be directed to outlining methods to do this.

37.2.7 Mineral Oil and Embryo Culture System

The manipulation of gametes and fertilization in water-based media without a mineral oil overlay should be considered to be substandard. The mineral oil overlay prevents the micro drops used in culture from evaporating, causing an increase in the osmality of the media resulting in the migration of water from the embryonic cells into the media. This is well established, but the mineral oil overlay also acts as a sink for a number of toxic materials. Just as PCB's are sequestered in the fatty tissues of the body, similarly the mineral oil overlay will remove toxic materials from the culture.

Styrene is the raw monomer used in the plastic dishes and flasks used for culture. Styrene is highly reactive. It is sold with a stabilizer to prevent its spontaneous polymerization into polystyrene. From chamber studies, we know that highly reactive material is released from new plasticware. The following experiment underscores how useful mineral oil is in controlling chemical exposure. Mouse embryos were grown in culture with KSOM media. Half of the embryos were exposed to KSOM equilibrated with styrene and grown in organ well dishes. The other half were grown in the same media with a mineral oil overlay. The concentration of styrene was approximately 300 ppm. This is an extremely high level of such a reactive substance. None of the mouse embryos in open culture survived past the two cell stage. Those grown in styrene saturated KSOM with the mineral oil overlay did develop with over 90%+ achieving blastocyst stage. The explanation is fairly simple. The mineral oil has a 1,000 times higher solubility for system when compared with the aqueous media. The result is that 999 of very styrene molecule was hidden in the mineral oil.

Similarly, mineral oil was shown to be protective in an AAAB proficiency test in differentiating between a good media and a bad media [3]. The toxicant added was formaldehyde, a known human carcinogen and very reactive chemically. The vast majority of labs doing the tests using mineral oil microdrop culture correctly identified the good media and the failed media. However, as reported by Miller et al. those doing their culture in open organ well dishes had *both* media failing. The reason is simple and goes to formaldehydes' high volatile nature and high level of reactivity. The concentration of formaldehyde in the bad media slowly fell as it sat in open culture at 98.6° in the incubator. Then, this allowed it to partition to the other "compartments" of the incubator, such as the water pan and the other good cultures. Formaldehyde is highly water soluble. It was then adsorbed by the aqueous media allowing the mouse embryos to be exposed to it.

Mineral oil's ability to sequester oil soluble components is not an absolute barrier [4]. Remember that the mineral oil media air interface has series of equilibriums between each phase as a material.

Having set the stage for understanding some of the challenges facing a laboratory designer, let us now expand the key functions the laboratory must do if exogenous toxic materials are to be removed from our ART facilities. This is done by erecting solid barriers, pressurizing the space and using chemical and particulate filtration.

37.3 Key Characteristics of Modern IVF Facilities

The modern ART laboratory provides a physical barrier to exterior pollutants. Since we are incapable of detoxifying small molecules reliably without degrading the embryos, the only alternative is to develop a set of redundant barriers to the physical transport of the potentially toxic materials.

The modern ART or IVF laboratory's construction is based upon multiple barriers to provide a durable barrier as the facility is used for a 10–15 year working life.

1. The facility has a significant level of positive pressurization and this is used as a supplement to the physical barriers.
2. The air supply is drawn from the cleanest environment possible.
3. The air supply changes rapidly, continually flushing clean air into the lab and displacing the "old" air that may have been contaminated by activities performed in and around the laboratory.
4. Use of chemical filtration to remove airborne pollutants before they enter the ART laboratory.
5. Use of inert building materials and construction techniques to select materials with a zero or low probability of releasing potentially toxic materials.

While many organizations have some of these factors in their design, they are often incomplete or compromised by poor execution.

There are no standards for IVF construction nor are there even generally recognized guidelines. The default standards are based upon the ART facility being an operating or procedure room. The closest engineering standards for these laboratories can be found in the joint publications of the American Institute of Architects and the United States government's Department of Health and Human Services in their guidelines for Health Care Facilities. Tables 2.1 and 2.2 of the 2006 Guidelines [5] is summarized below Table 37.1.

The problems with this *lassie faire* approach are legion. Let us examine the reasons in detail. Pressurization is the differential pressure between two rooms or compartments. Pressurization is *not* an absolute barrier. It means that the average force of the air molecules on one side of a barrier is higher than the other side. It says nothing as to the velocity and direction of any particular molecule. The resistance to infiltration is a complex relationship of temperature and pressure and the number of penetrations. All other factors being equal, the higher the difference between the labs internal air pressure and the external air pressure, the lower the potential that a toxic material can enter the laboratory.

The extensive use of exhaust air or return air ensures a high level of volatile organics in hospital settings. Commonly, people think the air outside is dirtier than the inside air. The reverse is true [6–8]. Indoor air is dirtier than outside except when unusual exterior circumstances are operating. Such disturbances include air pollution alerts accompanied with temperature inversions which trap pollutants close to ground level. High ozone levels combining with high levels of Poly Aromatic Hydrocarbons (PAH) can cause a similar decline in outdoor air quality. Fires, or road paving operations should also be added to this listing.

The traditional laboratory with typical medical construction erects walls and ceilings with numerous large penetrations. The historic method of pressurization is supplying an excess of air into the room when compared to what is exhausted. The problem is that most IVF labs have rooms with so many holes that the level of pressurization is at 0.01 in. of water (2.5 Pa). This is not an effective barrier. The poor design is rendered worse by the typical access to the lab through one door. Open the door and the pressure differential disappears instantaneously. To be effective at a reasonable cost, the room must be sealed. Access should be provided by the use of a double door vestibule arrangement or, for passage of cathers and tubes, double doors pass through used integrated circuit fabrication. A realistic level of pressurization is at least 0.1 in. (25 Pa) of water. This can be easily met by building walls where all penetrations are sealed with gaskets and silicone caulking. Ceiling lighting can be suspended from the ceiling. The most common types of lighting mounted in the ceiling have numerous holes from running wires but also from cooling the lamps. Use of these fixtures will degrade the level of pressurization very quickly.

In evaluating the quality of construction, it is instructive to know that leakage from a vessel is proportional to the square of the radius of the sum of the penetrations. So, if poor building techniques are used, the sum of all the voids in penetrations will be several square feet. In a modern ART facility, all outlets are gasketed and the medical gas outlets are gasketed or sealed. The video lines and data links are sealed. All lighting is sealed or suspended from the ceiling in a way where all penetrations are closed. The sole leaks are at the doorway. These are reduced by the use of elastomeres seals, which are compressed when the door is closed. The leakage is controlled when the doors are opened by the use of redundant doors. Modern ART facilities have open penetrations on the order of square inches.

37.3.1 HEPE Filtration

The use of High Efficiency Particle Elimination (HEPE) filtration is a common feature of most ART laboratories. In many cases, the users of these filters are under a profound misunderstanding of their function. The typical HEPE filter is rated as being 99.97% effective in the removal of particles that are >0.3 μ. The filter is made by compressing a meshwork of fiberglass with binders and then is sealed into a pleated arrangement with a metal frame. The diagram below is a typical illustration.

The filter is not an effective barrier to embryo toxic materials that could enter the laboratory. An SEM view of

Table 37.1 Guidelines for Healthcare Facility

	Specified range	Comments
Temperature	68–73°F (20–23°C)	No requirements for stability
Relative humidity	30–60%	
Pressurization	Air movement is out	Generally this level is positive and is routinely called out as 0.01 in. of water (2.5 Pa)
Minimum air changes of outdoor air/hour	3	Since most facilities have a total of 15 total air changes this means that 12 air changes per hour are just re-air-conditioned without any VOC removal since chemical filters are not required. In practice, to control airborne transmission of infectious agents, High Efficiency Particle elimination (HEPE) is used
Filtration	HEPE	Stops molds, bacteria and some large viruses plus large >0.3 μ particulates

the filter clearly illustrates the reason. The holes inside the filter are 0.3 μ or 30,000 nm in size. The typical volatile organic is on the order of 1–10 nm in size. The target molecular population is in orders of magnitude smaller than the holes in the HEPE filter.

37.3.2 Material Selection for Construction

The materials used in building the laboratory have a significant and long term potential to degrade the environment. Many common building materials and practices are contraindicated for ART facilities.

37.3.2.1 Oil Based Paints

These materials use mineral oil, linseed oil and turpentine to act as carriers for pigments. They work very well and in professional painters hands, can produce wonderful and durable finishes. However, they do not dry by the mere evaporation of the solvents. Rather, by a slow oxidation of the oils to bind the pigments. This drying process takes months to be fully cured. In the meantime, the paint is off-gassing oxidation products of the oils which are toxic.

37.3.2.2 Linoleum

This traditional product is often marketed as being "Green" in the sense that this common flooring product is made from renewable materials grown on farms. Linseed produces linseed oil and the Jute provides the fiber backing. In some products, natural or recycled rubber is added to the linseed oil jute overlay. All of these materials are problematic in that, in a manner similar to oil based paints, they will release a bewildering array of organics.

37.3.2.3 Particleboard

This is a common byproduct of lumber production where wood chips and sawdust are bound together with adhesives and pressure. The problem is that the materials will off-gas a human carcinogen and mutagen formaldehyde. The literature is replete with references for this source of the most commonly found embryotoxic material [9].

37.3.2.4 Urethane Foam Insulation

This is a two-part mixture that is sprayed into walls and voids to seal and insulate but even low VOC formulations outgas a wide variety of aldehydes, most commonly including formaldehyde and acetaldehyde. Its use has declined because of these difficulties, but structures still exist with this material in place.

37.3.2.5 Urea Formaldehyde Resins

These are plastic resins that found their way into plastic laminates for particleboard or for our plastic applications. Often, their use isn't obvious unless the architect and laboratory operator fully examine every technical sheet or Material Safety Data Sheet (MSDS) to ascertain if they are constituents of a particular product.

37.4 Performance of Traditional IVF Laboratory Architecture

With the above as preface, let us examine how these laboratories function at the level of chemical exposure to the embryos. Cohen et al. [10–12]. These papers detail the various sources of volatile organic compounds and some of their sources and impacts. The table below shows the level of VOC's from seven traditional IVF facilities Table 37.2.

The table shows the sum of the VOC found in seven traditional IVF laboratories as determined by an established gas chromatography/mass spectroscopy (GC/MS) known as Toxic Organics-15 (TO-15) as listed in the US EPA methods of environmental analysis [13].

The situation was clarified by one laboratory built in the manner described below which suddenly experiences a reduction of 1/3 in their productivity as measured by their ongoing pregnancy rate. Before the incident, their ongoing pregnancy rate was 35% and fell to 23%. The analysis of the air from this facility compared to other facilities is shown below Table 37.3:

Laboratory # 7 is the case in point. To remove the aldehydes that were produced by a paving of the parking lot during the summertime, a chemical filter using activated carbon and potassium permanganate was installed in the Heating Ventilation and Air Conditioning (HVAC) serving the laboratory. The chemical filter materials would adsorb some

Table 37.2 Volatile organic compound (VOC) levels from a survey of seven laboratories

Location	Range of VOC's μg/m^3	Mean VOC levels μg/m^3	Standard deviation
Outside air	128–1,830	533	705
Air supply	303–2,797	1,152	1,110
IVF lab	310–4,404	2,862	1,818
Incubator	717–9,485	2,769	3,054
Adjacent to the IVF lab	473–7,141	4,372	2,419

Table 37.3 Aldehydes in several traditional IVF laboratories

The total below are the sum of the following species
Acrolien, acetaldehyde, butanal, pentanal, hexanal, heptanal, octanal, nonanal

Laboratory	Outside air $\Sigma\ \mu g/m^3$	Incubator air $\Sigma\ \mu g/m^3$
1	0	0
2	1.6	N/A
3	0	17.1
4	0	0
5	35	3.5
7	57.6	75.7

of the higher molecular weight aldehydes such as Heptanal, Hexanal, etc. The potassium permanganate media is an oxidizer and reacts with the smaller aldehydes such as formaldehyde and acetaldehyde by breaking them down to carbon dioxide and water. With the installation of the equipment, the pregnancy rate rebounded to its previous level of productivity. The diagram above illustrates schematically the type of labs described earlier.

37.5 Modern IVF Facilities

IVF laboratories are now being built worldwide with the following general specifications Table 37.4:

The above specifications are offered as guidelines and should be evaluated upon the potential size of the facility, the budget available and the expected future size of the facility. Some of the design features have trade-offs.

37.5.1 100% Outside Air vs. 50% Outside Air

Modern IVF laboratories can be considered to be a biological clean room with microbial control and a particular emphasis on the control of volatile organic compounds and a particularly toxic subset of VOC's, namely aldehydes.

As stated earlier, the outside air is cleaner than air drawn from the interior of the building. Therefore, using outside air provides the cleanest air and allows the chemical filters to last longer since they are removing a low concentration of pollutants. Having a large amount of fresh air coming into the laboratory causes a flushing action to quickly remove any pollutant or toxicant, which is generated inside the IVF laboratory.

The use of outside air is also favored by a design philosophy. If the chemical filters aren't properly maintained and eventually exhausted, a 100% outside air system will perform better than one with a 50% return air provision.

Table 37.4 Guidelines for IVF laboratories

Parameter	Minimal requirements measured by	Preferred requirements measured by
Ventilation rate	7.5 fresh air changes per hour are a minimal standard-tracer gas exchange	15–25 fresh air changes per hour are the higher standard-tracer gas exchange
Relative humidity	30–60%	30–55%
Pressurization	0.200 "of water from the IVF lab to outside-micromanometer accurate to 0.001" of water	0.250 "of water from the IVF lab to outside-micromanometer accurate to 0.001" of water
VOC	Supplied air <500 $\mu g/m^3$ US EPA TO-14/TO-15	<80% with MW > 100 amu of the outside air supplied air <350 $\mu g/m^3$ US EPA TO-14/15
Aldehyde	Supplied air <3.0 $\mu g/m^3$ US EPA T0-11	<outside air <2.0 $\mu g/m^3$ US EPA TO-11
Particle counts	<100, 000 Cu Ft 0.5–10 μ Fed Spec 209 E	<10,000 Cu Ft 0.5–10 μ Fed Spec 209 E

IVF laboratories using 50% outside air and 50% return air are very workable. They tend to have a shorter filter life. They have reduced the cost of operations because of a lower energy use. While both systems are energy hogs when compared with traditional IVF labs, a 50:50 system is cheaper to run. It is also the preferred option for laboratories where summer temperatures are above 90+°F (32+°C) combined with very high levels of relative humidity of 90%+.

Humidity control in the IVF laboratory is essential to inhibit mold growth. Mold is a common contaminant in IVF labs and is often carried in by the laboratory staff because of poor scrub control, such as when the scrubs are routinely worn outside the lab. For 100% outside air systems, the ideal HVAC system will use deep cooling coils to aid in fully cooling the air in an effort to wring out the humidity. The ability to cool the air is dependent on the length of time the air is in contact with the coil but also how cold the cooling coils are. One hundred percent of laboratories in hot, very humid climates call for the use of a mechanical chiller or large scale coolant loop with a cooling tower.

37.5.2 Chemical Filtration

We have already mentioned the use of activated carbon as a media to remove a variety of organic compounds. Activated carbon works best on large organics that have numerous conjugate double bonds. The carbon provides a surface with a cloud of free electrons which interact with the VOC and hold them by van der Walls forces. Its hold is tenuous for smaller molecules, but becomes very large and significant as the organic molecule's molecular weight increases.

The materials that are not absorbed well by activated carbon are usually small, water soluble molecules. These are oxidized by exposing them to potassium permanganate on an alumina or zeolites matrix. The material is oxidized to carbon dioxide and water with the permanganate reduced to manganese dioxide.

In designing the chemical filter, the time the air spends in intimate contact with the media is crucial. A minimum residence time of 0.2 s is acceptable. A typical "z" type tray filter is shown.

Longer residence times are better, but economics eventually forces a compromise. The chemical filter should be located immediately in front of the HEPE filter. Keeping the chemical filter in a cool air stream promotes its removal efficiency. High summertime temperatures will reduce the carbons ability to hold a VOC contaminant.

37.5.3 Laboratory Layout

Each IVF laboratory design has elements that require compromises, but the following arrangements have been shown to be highly desirable. The access to the IVF laboratory and rooms inside it should be through air-locks or vestibules which maintain a constant level of pressurization in the lab. The area in the lab doing gamete manipulation and embryo examination and culture should have the highest level of pressurization with the level dropping to zero as you go through the IVF lab micromanipulation and incubators to the vestibule.

The gas supply room should be adjoining the IVF laboratory, but should be on a different ventilation system and should be at least 0.2 in. of water (5 Pa) lower in pressure than the IVF laboratory.

Liquid nitrogen supplies should be placed as close as possible to the lab without being in the lab. A set of dedicated gas and liquid nitrogen should be provided. Long pipe runs of vacuum insulate nitrogen lines will be expensive and will cause a high percentage of the liquid nitrogen to evaporate before it is used. Gas lines for incubator and laminar flow hoods should be run via the above ceiling space or walls.

37.5.4 Casework for IVF Laboratories

As detailed earlier, particleboard is not an option because of its off-gassing potential. While many labs have particle board casework or Formica, it is no guarantee that new laboratories will get a lot of particleboard with a low aldehyde release potential. Metal casework, either stainless steel or powder coated steel, is recommended. In this product, a polymer coat is applied to the metal while it is charged and then baked at elevated temperatures. The result is casework that is largely inert. Countertops can be either the common epoxy top, Corian, a synthetic marble composite or metal.

37.5.5 Flooring

Carpet, linoleum and tiles are not acceptable. Sheet vinyl works very well. It should be glued to the floor with sections heat-welded together, eliminating cracks where dirt or microbial material can accumulate.

37.5.6 Paint

Low VOC formulations of water based alkyd paint are acceptable. Epoxy paints can be used if they are applied in the manner ordained by the manufacturer.

37.5.7 Lighting

The laboratory should be equipped with two types of lighting. Typically, fluorescent lighting is provided, so full illumination is available for routine operations such as cleaning and equipment maintenance when the embryos are inside the incubators. Fluorescent lighting when embryos are out in the open is contraindicated. Hirao et al. was the first to show that light with a wavelength of <480 nm could damage hamster oocytes [14]. For those times when the embryos are outside the incubator, low level lighting from incandescent, halogen or LEDs should be considered. The reason is that these forms of illumination have a lower potential to generate potentially damaging ultraviolet light which could degrade the embryos.

37.6 The Modern IVF Laboratory

The schematic below illustrates the concepts described subsequently:

The schematic above illustrates a 100% outside air system. It has been applied to a number of IVF practices and found to provide a stable environment resulting in increased productivity. As mentioned earlier, there are alternative arrangements. Some laboratories have added a duct which can carry the exhausted air back to the air handler so that if an environmental emergency occurs outside, the air inside the IVF laboratory can be recycled.

The illustration shows a solid ceiling of sheet rock. Some laboratories have substituted a suspended tile ceiling. The suspended tile ceiling, if used, must be carefully selected. If suspended tiles are used, they must be of the type used in clean rooms and not the typical medical suspended ceilings. Cleanroom ceilings use suspended panels that have robust frames using aluminum extrusions. The frames are bolted together and have a closed cell gasket usually made of a silicone rubber, which is sealed by pushing the rigid honeycombed panels onto the frames which have a knife-type edge into the silicone rubber gasket. The panel is then locked into place with a mechanical clamp. These ceilings are more expensive than a solid gypsum ceiling.

Some firms make a "cleanroom type ceiling" with the same frames used in commercial spaces with an open cell urethane foam gasket. The panels are gypsum board with a vinyl covering. These ceilings, even when properly installed, still leak significantly and will degrade the efforts to pressurize the IVF laboratory.

37.6.1 Supplementary Air Cleaning Utilities

The types of laboratories described above will eliminate many of the sources of embryotoxic materials but not all of them because they have several ways of entering the laboratory. We have already described the use of carbon dioxide to control pH in embryo cultures. The carbon dioxide used is generally USP grade. As the cylinder is used, it gradually changes from liquid carbon dioxide to compressed carbon dioxide gas. At this point, any impurity in the carbon dioxide will be released to the incubator. A carbon filter is used to absorb this slug of pollutants.

Small portable air cleaners are often used inside the incubator itself to remove impurities that can be released by the plasticware used in the incubator plus fugitive emissions from the incubator, particularly from new equipment. Mayer et al. [15] has reported their beneficial affects.

Larger room air cleaners are often placed at the entrance of the facility in a way to reduce the level of VOC's at the entry point.

37.7 The Reality of Building an IVF Laboratory

To this point, we have been dealing with the laboratory's design as an exercise in science and engineering. However, while these principals are clearly important, there are procedural and business issues that need to be raised. The process of design and construction should be explained.

1. The practice must peer into the future and consider the growth potential and the way the laboratory should be arranged. Build too large a laboratory and you will waste costly resources. Build it too small and you will regret the project in 5 years as the area served by your practice hopefully widens.
2. Involve the staff of the laboratory in its design and lay it out before you enter into the design process.
3. Will a full operating room be desired? Does the practice want to perform other surgical procedures besides the typical retrieval and embryo transfer?
4. What local or state codes are you dealing with and how will it affect your operating room or procedure room?
5. Will general gas anesthesia be used as an option or will the practice only use intravenous sedation?
6. How will retrievals be done? Some practices use isolets with a separate carbon dioxide supply and stereo microscope to collect ovum. Other practices use laminar flow hoods with a blood gas supply and water heated table held at 98.6°F. Both methods work well.
7. Incubator atmospheres must be provided which brings the questions of normal levels of oxygen or reduced oxygen. The modern trend is to use a reduced oxygen atmosphere. The fallopian tube has a lower level of oxygen (a nominal 18% vs. a reduced 6%). If a reduced oxygen atmosphere is to be used, then more nitrogen will be required. It can be supplied by compressed gases or from liquid nitrogen. In this arrangement, a large tank of liquid nitrogen is used to supply both the liquid nitrogen from cryogenic gamete and embryo storage. The liquid nitrogen is heated when needed to generate a sufficient volume of gaseous nitrogen to the incubators.
8. Alternative gas supply arrangements can also be considered. For very large practices with ample space, it may be wise to use gas storage tanks outside the building. These centralized tank systems allow bulk deliveries by truck, freeing the embryology staff from the job of changing tanks and shuffling large liquid nitrogen tanks. This is an option for large practices and should be evaluated based upon the labor savings and lower cost of bulk gas delivery.
9. Avoid design changes as they will delay the project and increase the cost of the project. When negotiating a project with a contractor, he should be aware that he will be forced to provide a "competitive bid" for his services when the project first starts up. However, once selected, he will consider any changes as an opportunity to reconfigure his costs. Change notices, the document that covers the changes, will not be based upon a competitive cost since you are

not likely to dismiss him and start with a new contractor. This is why it is so important that your design be resolved in detail before you start building. Involve the entire team that will use the facility. Ideally, walk through each procedure and figure out the equipment needed and where it will be located.

10. Test the final product and verify that the laboratory meets the design specifications. A complex construction project such as an IVF lab rarely is completed without some defect. It may be as simple as door seals that result in allowed level of pressurization or a high level of resistance in the ductwork because of a poor layout of the supply ducts with more turns than originally planned. The laboratories performance should be tested and the tests should include VOC sampling to check the performance of the chemical filter. The ventilation rates must be verified independently from the contractors testing. Particle counts are also advisable.
11. Final payments for the construction *must* be based upon satisfactory completion of the IVF laboratory testing verifying that the practice has received what was designed and paid for. Failure to make the final 10–20% payment contingent on passing the final test will leave the practice with a motivator for repairs in the highly likely event the new facility has a defect.

37.7.1 Design Flexibility and Options

The designs discussed here should be considered as part of a spectrum of options. Alternatives are available which have a slightly different arrangement of components. They still have the same basic elements. The work of Boone [16] and Worilow [17, 18] have reported their level of success with this approach. They both report independently an increase in productivity and implantation rates.

37.8 Performance of Modern IVF Laboratories

The table below summarizes the chemical testing results of 11 facilities built according to the general guidelines discussed earlier. Not every lab has every feature, but they all adhere to the general intent of having robust chemical and particulate filtration, a real level of effective pressurization and correct material selection Table 37.5.

37.8.1 IVF Productivity and Modem Laboratories

A reasonable person will ask "so with all this effort, what is the payoff?" Modern IVF laboratories will have variations in productivity, but these fluctuations should be driven by variations in patient factors and treatment decisions and not the intrusion of embryo toxic materials entering the laboratory. With three facilities, a limited retrospective study was done. The practices agreed not to change their embryo culture system and to use the same procedures for a year(s) after the new laboratory was brought on stream. The results were statistically significant increases in pregnancy rates in two practices. Three practices reported a statistically significant increase in implantation rate. The results of the study are below.

The practice of Dr. James Goldfarb, Medical Director, and Dr. Nina Desai, Laboratory Director of the Cleveland Clinic Foundation in Beachwood, Ohio has gone from an

Table 37.5 Chemical testing results of 11 laboratories built using modern guidelines

Lab #	Outside or pre-filter VOC μg/m³	Post-filter or IVF lab VOC μg/m³	Outside or pre-filter aldehyde μg/m³	IVF lab aldehyde μg/m³	Ventilation rate (fresh air changes/h)
1	12,014	227	17.2	0.0	5.0
2	286	141	12.2	2.2	12.6
3	447	402	3.4	2.2	11.4
4	597	387	17.3	8.4	9.1
5	10,711	701	11.8	0.0	14.8
6	4,199	614	6.3	0.0	7.2
7	57,670	606	6.1	1.8	14.4
8	647	298	17.1	1.9	5.1
9	113	126	4.3	0.0	15.2
10	2,462	369	9.1	3.8	7.3
11	134.8	101.4	5.0	1.3	Undetermined
Mean of all modern IVF labs	8,116	361	10	2	10

Table 37.6 Comparison of IVF data before and after laboratory remodel at the Cleveland Clinic

Year	Retrievals	Pregnancy	(%)	ET	Implant IR	(%)
1997–1998 traditional IVF lab	445	159	35.7	1,567	243	15.5
1999–2002 modern IVF lab	1,194	593	49.6	3,448	907	32.6

Table 37.7 Comparison of IVF data before and after laboratory remodel at Reproductive Medicine and Fertility Associates

Year	Retrievals	Pregnancy	(%)	ET	Implant IR	(%)
2000–2001 traditional IVF lab	346	159	45.95	952	240	25.2
2001–2002 modern IVF lab	329	166	50.5	1,119	357	31.9

Table 37.8 Comparison of IVF data before and after laboratory remodel at The Institute for Reproductive Medicine and Health

Year	Retrievals	Pregnancy	(%)	ET	Implant IR	(%)
2002 traditional IVF lab	200	66	33.0	616	94	15.2
2003 modern IVF lab	185	83	44.9	531	110	20.9

uncontrolled IVF laboratory in a busy surgical suite, to an isolated, modern IVF laboratory. The results showed a statistically significant increase in their pregnancy rates and implantation rates for all patient age groups. The data for all patients are shown below Table 37.6:

Dr. Jacques Stassart, Medical Director of Reproductive Medicine and Fertility Associates in Woodbury, Minnesota showed a statistically significant increase in their implantation rates. An increase in their pregnancy rate was seen, but it was not statistically significant. The data for all patients are shown below Table 37.7:

Dr. Sangita Jindal, Laboratory Director of The Institute for Reproductive Medicine and Health in Hartsdale, New York also had a similar increase in pregnancy and implantation rates. The data for all patients are shown below Table 37.8:

References

1. Schiewe M, Schmidt P, Bush M, Wildt D (1985) Toxicity potential of absorbed-retained ethylene oxide residues in cluture dishes on embryo development in vitro. J Anim Sci 60(6):1610–1618
2. Schiewe M, Schmidt P, Pontbriand D, Wildt D (1988) Toxicity potential of residual ethylene oxide on fresh or frozen embryos maintained in plastic straws. Gamete Res 19:31–39
3. Miller K, Fry K (2000) Failure of The American Association of Bioanalysis Culture Proficiency test to perform under certain culture conditions. Fertil Steril 74(Supp #3):S105–S106
4. Miller KF, Pursel VG (1987) Absorption of compounds in medium by the oil covering microdrop cultures. Gamete Res 17(1):57–61
5. AIA issues new guidelines for the design and construction of healthcare facilities. Healthc Hazard Manage Monit 2006;20(3):1–6
6. Wallace L (ed) (1985) Organic chemicals in indoor air: a review of human exposure studies and indoor air quality studies, Lewis Publishers, USA
7. Sterling D (ed) (1985) Volatile organic compounds in indoor air: an overview of sources, concentrations, and health effects, Lewis Publishers, USA
8. Harrison P (2007) Health impacts of indoor air pollution. Chem Ind 17:677–681
9. Wolfoff P, Nielsen G (2001) Organic compounds in indoor air and their relevance for perceived indoor air quality. Atmos Environ 35:4407–4417
10. Hall J, Gilligan A, Schimmel T, Cecchi M, Cohen J (1998) The origin, effects and control of air pollution in laboratories used for human embryo culture. Hum Reprod 13(S4):146–155
11. Cohen J, Gilligan A, Wiladsen S (1998) Culture and quality control embryos. Hum Reprod 13(S3):137–144
12. Cohen J, Gilligan A, Esposito W, Schimmel T, Dale B (1997) Ambient air and its potential effects on conception in vitro. Human reproduction, Oxford, England, 12(8):1742–1749
13. Compendium of methods for the determination of toxic organic compounds in ambient air, EPA; 1984/1988 April
14. Hirao Y, Yanagimachi R (1978) Detrimental effect of visible light on meiosis of mammalian eggs in vitro. J Exp Zool 206(3):365–369
15. Mayer J, Nehchinri F, Weedon V et al (1999) Prospective randomized crossover analysis of the impact on an incubator air filtration system (Coda, genX, Internation, Inc.) on IVF outcomes. Fertil Steril 72(Sup. 1):S42
16. Boone WR, Johnson JE, Locke AJ, Crane MMT, Price TM (1999) Control of air quality in an assisted reproductive technology laboratory. Fertil Steril 71(1):150–154
17. Worrilow K, Huynh H, Gwozdziewicz J, Schillings W, Peters A (2001) A retrospective analysis: The examination of a potential relationship between particulates and volatile organic compound levels in a clas 100 laboratory cleanroom and specific parapmeters of embryogenesis and rates of implantation. Fertil Steril 76(Supp 3):S15–S16
18. Worrilow K, Huynh H, Gwozdziewicz J, Schillings W, Peters A (2002) A retrospective analysis: Seasonal decline in implantation rates and its correlation with increased levels of volatile organic compounds (VOC). Fertil Steril 78(Supp 3):3S

Chapter 38
Preparation and Selection of Sperm for IVF and ICSI

Charles L. Bormann, Jose R. Alagretti, Eduardo L.A. da Motta, Paulo Serafini, and Gary D. Smith

Abstract Approximately 50% of all infertility problems are due to male factors. Some of the male factors preventing natural insemination or fertilization include ejaculatory problems, low sperm counts, abnormal sperm morphology, diminished sperm motility and function, and, often times, a combination of several of these factors. In vitro fertilization (IVF) was originally developed as a tool to overcome tubal defects in females and has since been widely utilized to achieve fertilization from men with a variety of abnormal sperm parameters. In cases in which sperm quality and quantity are severely compromised, injection of spermatozoon into the ooplasm of a mature oocyte is possible and is referred to as intracytoplasmic sperm injection (ICSI). Only a single sperm is required to perform ICSI, yet processing, isolation, and selection of a single healthy sperm from a subfertile man in an in vitro environment can be quite challenging. The objective of this chapter is to discuss the most commonly used methods of sperm separation and also to highlight the new methods currently being developed and tested for IVF and ICSI application. In addition, this chapter describes which separation process best suits the male factor in question and also the advantages and disadvantages associated with each method. Finally, this chapter describes the stringent morphological criteria necessary to select the best sperm for IVF and ICSI.

C.L. Bormann
Departments of Obstetrics and Gynecology and Urology, University of Michigan, Ann Arbor, MI, USA

J.R. Alagretti
Huntington Center for Reproductive medicine of Brazil, Sao Paulo, Brazil

E.L.A. da Motta
Huntington Center for Reproductive medicine of Brazil, Sao Paulo, Brazil

P. Serafini
Huntington Center for Reproductive medicine of Brazil, Sao Paulo, Brazil

G.D. Smith (✉)
Obstetrics and Gynecology, University of Michigan, 6410 Medical Science 1, 1301 E Catherine St, Ann Arbor, MI 48109-0617, USA
e-mail: smithgd@umich.edu

Keywords IVF • ICSI • Sperm separation • Sperm isolation • Sperm morphology • Sperm classification

38.1 Introduction

Approximately 10% of all couples have infertility problems, of which nearly half are related male factor [1]. In vitro fertilization (IVF) was originally developed as a treatment for tubal infertility; however, high rates of males with poor semen quality have led to the development of several preparation techniques to isolate motile sperm.

During natural insemination, semen is deposited in the vagina where potentially fertile spermatozoa are actively separated from immotile spermatozoa, debris, and seminal plasma by migration through the cervical mucus [2]. During this active separation, spermatozoa undergo maturational changes that enable them to fertilize oocytes. This process is known as capacitation [3, 4]. Factors within seminal plasma prevent spermatozoa from undergoing capacitation [5], and prolonged exposure to seminal plasma has been shown to inhibit sperm from undergoing the acrosome reaction [6] and to reduce their ability to fertilize oocytes [7]. Therefore, in a clinical setting where spermatozoa are being processed for IVF or ICSI, it is extremely important to separate spermatozoa from the seminal plasma as quickly as possible following ejaculation and liquefaction in order to reduce the inhibitory effects of seminal plasma. Several techniques have been developed to artificially isolate motile sperm from an ejaculate. The most commonly used techniques include simple washing and removal of seminal fluid, sperm migration or "swim-up," and density gradient centrifugation [8]. However, new technologies such as microfluidics are being used to isolate sperm for assisted reproductive purposes.

The goal of this chapter is to describe the most commonly used methods of sperm separation used in assisted reproduction and also to highlight the new methods currently being developed and tested for IVF and ICSI. In addition, this chapter describes which separation process best suits the male factor being treated and also the advantages and disadvantages

D.T. Carrell and C.M. Peterson (eds.), *Reproductive Endocrinology and Infertility: Integrating Modern Clinical and Laboratory Practice*,
DOI 10.1007/978-1-4419-1436-1_38, © Springer Science+Business Media, LLC 2010

associated with each separation technique. Finally, this chapter describes the best methods and stringent criteria necessary to choose viable sperm for IVF and ICSI.

38.2 Semen Collection

The most common method of obtaining a semen sample is through masturbation and ejaculation into a sterile nonsperm toxic cup. In cases in which ejaculation cannot be achieved via masturbation, whether due to religious or psychological reasons, a nontoxic condom can be used to collect the ejaculation during sexual intercourse. Coitus inter-ruptus is not recommended because of potential iatrogenic contamination and risk of incomplete sperm recovery. Following ejaculation, semen is maintained at body temperature and undergoes liquefaction within 30–60 min. When liquefaction is delayed or if the semen sample is very viscous, it is advisable to draw the sample through a 21-gauge needle to reduce viscosity [9].

In cases in which there is no ejaculation following orgasm, patients are asked to immediately urinate in a sterile cup, and the sample is analyzed for the presence of sperm. Presence of semen in the urine is an indicator of retrograde ejaculation. Men with this condition are prescribed stomach-acid buffering medications in order to neutralize the urine pH and thus provide a more hospitable environment for sperm during collection and processing.

In cases in which men cannot achieve an erection, emission, or ejaculation because of neurologic or psychogenic reasons, semen can still be collected via prostatic massage, electrical stimulation of the prostate or applied vibration to the penis. Samples collected from men with spinal cord injuries typically have high concentrations of sperm, poor motility, and red blood cell contamination of the ejaculate [9].

Spermatozoa may also be collected surgically from the epididymis or testicle in cases in which blockages prevent sperm transport. Most blockages are the result of a previous vasectomy, inflammation, tissue scarring or, a low percentage of cases, injury. In these cases, sperm are collected either by microsurgery or by percutaneous needle puncture. Depending on the skill of the physician, epididymal aspirates can be collected with minimal amounts of red blood cells or other cellular contaminants. Each sample aspirated is screened for the presence of spermatozoa. In some cases, enough sperm can be collected for use in IVF, intrauterine insemination (IUI), or freezing for future use.

In severe cases in which sperm cannot be located in ejaculates or aspirates, spermatozoa can be collected by way of testicular dissection or percutaneous needle biopsy. This method of collection is highly invasive and is generally the last resort in obtaining sperm for ICSI. Samples obtained by testicular dissection contain large amounts of red blood cells and testicular tissue and thus require additional steps to isolate a clean sample of spermatozoa.

As described earlier, there are many ways in which sperm are collected for IVF and ICSI. Each method produces a very different sample composition, some of which are rich in sperm or seminal plasma, those that are diluted in urine, and some containing high amounts of cellular debris and blood cells. Additionally, many of these alternative collection techniques (not including normal ejaculation) yield very small numbers of sperm in relation to high amounts of cellular debris, making processing and sperm isolation even more difficult.

38.3 Sperm Processing Techniques

38.3.1 Simple Washing and Dilution

The original method of sperm separation during the first cases of IVF involved diluting semen with culture media and isolation of spermatozoa by centrifugation at 200–300 × *g* [10]. Following centrifugation, the supernatant is removed, and the pellet is resuspended with additional culture media. This process is generally repeated two to three times to completely separate out seminal plasma. Main advantages of this technique are its simplicity and affordability.

Major disadvantages of using simple washing and dilution are that contaminants found in the original sample such as immotile sperm, cellular debris, epithelial cells and leukocytes remain in the washed sample. Cellular debris may produce reactive oxygen species (ROS) which impair functional competence of spermatozoa as well as cause DNA damage to spermatozoa [11]. In addition, it has been shown that increased levels of sperm DNA damage during IVF correlate with compromised embryo morphology at early cleavage stages [12], failure to advance to the blastocyst stage in vitro [13, 14], decreased pregnancy rates [15–17] and an increase in spontaneous abortions [18]. Repeated centrifugation has also been described to cause irreversible damage to spermatozoa that reduces motility and possibly even destroy the fertilization capacity of sperm (reviewed see: [19]). Because of limitations in separating spermatozoa from cellular debris and problems associated with repeated centrifugation, simple washing and dilution has been replaced in many instances with swim-up and density gradient separation techniques.

38.3.2 Swim-Up from Pellet

One of the oldest and most commonly used methods of sperm isolation is the swim-up procedure. This technique is used most commonly on normozoospermic males, was first described by Mahadevan and Baker in 1984, and is still widely used in IVF clinics worldwide [20]. The swim-up method is based on the active movement of motile sperm from a prewashed pellet of sperm into a layer of fresh medium above. The first step in swim-up involves repeat dilution and centrifugation (two to three times) of the semen sample to separate spermatozoa from seminal plasma. The speed of centrifugation should be low enough to prevent the final pellet from being too tightly compacted. This can be easily observed by tilting the test tube and visualizing whether or not the pellet tilts as well [9]. Each laboratory should determine their appropriate centrifugation speed to achieve this pellet formation. The pelleted spermatozoa can be both resuspended and overlaid with media, or the pellet can be uninterrupted and overlaid with media. If one chooses to disrupt the pellet, extreme care must be taken when overlaying media to prevent mixing and contamination with immotile sperm, debris and other cell types.

The efficiency of this technique is based on the surface of the cell pellet and the initial sperm motility in the ejaculate. Because there are many layers of sperm in the pellet, motile sperm situated in the bottom layers of the pellet are unlikely to ever reach the interface with the culture medium layer, thus limiting the yield of motile sperm.

To increase the surface area of the interface between the pellet and overlying culture media, the test tube can be tilted at 45° to facilitate migration of more sperm to the overlying culture media [9]. Resuspended or disrupted pellets can be placed in four-well dishes and overlaid with culture media to increase the surface area between the pellet and culture media [21].

The swim-up method using either the intact or disrupted sperm pellet is incubated at 37°C for 30–60 min in a buffered media to allow spermatozoa to migrate from the pellet to the culture medium. A visual change in turbidity of overlying culture media is an indication that migration has taken place. If the culture media appears still clear after 60 min, a longer period of time is allowed for motile sperm to swim from the pellet.

Following incubation, the upper layer of culture media is carefully aspirated without disrupting the pellet and is transferred to a clean test tube for further analysis. One advantage of this technique is that it isolates a population of sperm with greater than 90% motility without cellular debris. In addition, this swim-up technique isolates spermatozoa with increased swimming velocities and more normal morphology [22] and improves the rates of acrosome reaction and nuclear maturity [23]. The disadvantages of this technique are in the low overall recovery of motile spermatozoa due to the limited area of contact between the pellet and culture media. Another disadvantage is in the initial centrifugation and pelleting of sperm. Centrifugation and pelleting force spermatozoa in close contact with immotile spermatozoa, cellular debris and leukocytes, which are known to produce very high levels of ROS [24] and can inhibit subsequent fertilization ability.

38.3.3 Swim-Up from Nonpelleted Samples

The swim-up method can also be used directly on semen samples without need for the initial centrifugation step. Following liquefaction, semen samples can be allocated into four-well dishes or test tubes and overlaid with culture media. To reduce the chance of contaminating the upper layer of media with immotile sperm and cellular debris, it is possible to layer the semen under the culture media using a syringe [25]. Following incubation, the upper layer of culture media is carefully aspirated, transferred to a clean test tube and centrifuged at 300–600 × *g* for 4–10 min [9]. Next, the pelleted spermatozoa are suspended in media, analyzed and prepared for insemination.

The advantages of this method are the high populations of motile and morphologically normal sperm without contamination of nongerm cells and debris. In addition, this swim-up method does not require the initial centrifugation, which reduces the harmful effects from ROS. Some disadvantages of this method are the low yield of sperm from the original sample and the exposure to seminal fluid longer than the previously discussed other swim-up technique.

38.3.4 Density Gradient Centrifugation

The majority of all density gradients used to isolate spermatozoa are discontinuous and consist of two to three layers [19] although single layer gradients also work. The most commonly used materials for density gradients are colloidal silica with covalently bound silane molecules, which are nontoxic and approved for human in vivo use. Some of the major density separation products developed for clinical IVF and ICSI use are PureSperm® (NidaCon International AB, Göteborg, Sweden), Isolate® (Irvine Scientific, Santa Ana, CA, USA), IxaPrep (MediCult, Copenhagen, Denmark), and Enhance® (Conception Technologies, San Diego, CA, USA). These products are made isosmotic by the addition of polysucrose [9].

Density gradient medium is a colloid rather than a solution and has a low viscosity, which does not slow the sedimentation of spermatozoa [19]. During centrifugation, highly motile sperm migrate faster in the direction of the sedimentation gradient and are able to penetrate this interface faster than the low-motile or nonmotile spermatozoa [26]. This unimpeded density gradient separation produces a clean fraction of highly motile spermatozoa. The pellet is washed with culture media and centrifuged at 200 × *g* for 4–10 min [9]. This process is repeated two to three times to ensure the complete removal of contaminating density gradient medium.

There are many advantages in using a density gradient to process spermatozoa for IVF and ICSI. The entire ejaculate is used during the centrifugation process, resulting in a significantly higher yield of motile spermatozoa than can be obtained using other separation techniques. Thus this technique is ideal for patients with suboptimal semen parameters (e.g., oligozoospermia and asthenozoospermia). In addition, it has been shown that this separation technique produces a higher percentage of morphologically normal spermatozoa [27] with better DNA quality and chromatin packaging [28, 29] than other separation techniques. Another advantage of this technique is that it produces a relatively clean sample of spermatozoa, free of cellular debris and leukocyte contamination. This property significantly reduces ROS and problems associated with its contamination [26]. Disadvantages of this technique are that it is more expensive than the other techniques and that it requires repeat centrifugation.

38.3.5 Density Gradient and Swim-Up Combination

The advantages of both the density gradient and swim-up techniques can be achieved by combining the two sperm separation methods. Following liquefaction of semen, spermatozoa are separated as previously described using a discontinuous colloid gradient. The sperm pellet is resuspended in a buffered media, centrifuged and the supernatant is decanted to remove the contaminating density gradient medium. The pelleted spermatozoa can then be interrupted and overlaid with media, or the pellet can be maintained and overlaid with media and the swim-up separation takes place as described earlier. After density gradient separation, the swim-up is incubated at 37°C for 3–4 h in a buffered media to allow sufficient time for spermatozoa to migrate from the pellet to the culture medium. A visual change in turbidity of overlying culture media is the best indication that migration has taken place. Following incubation, the upper layer of culture media is carefully aspirated without disrupting the pellet and is transferred to a clean test tube for further analysis.

The greatest advantage in using this method is that it yields a clean sample of highly motile spermatozoa with extremely low levels of DNA fragmentation (unpublished data from our laboratory). Some of the disadvantages of this separation technique are that it is a bit more expensive, requires repeated centrifugation and a longer time for sperm swim-up in order to collect enough sperm for IVF.

38.3.6 Glass Wool Filtration

The two main ways to separate sperm using adherence and filtration are glass wool filtration and sephadex columns. These methods are based on the principal that dead or dying spermatozoa are extremely sticky and will attach to glass even in the presence of high concentrations of protein [25]. The initial step in glass wool filtration is an extensive rinsing of the glass wool to remove any loose wool fibers before filtration. The filter is produced by gently packing 30 mg of precleaned fibers into the barrel of a 3 ml disposable syringe [30]. The entire ejaculate is mixed with an equal volume of culture media, placed into 15-ml tubes (no more than 3 ml/tube) and centrifuged for 3 min. Following centrifugation, the pellet is resuspended with 1 ml of culture media and centrifuged again at 300 × *g* for 3 min. Following this centrifugation, one pellet is resuspended with 300 μl culture media, which is then used to resuspend all other remaining pellets. The washed spermatozoa (no more than 400 μl) are now gently layered on top of the prewet glass wool and filtered using gravity into a clean 15-ml tube. When the dripping stops, 100 μl of culture media is added to the filter for a final rinse and the filtrate is then analyzed and prepared for IVF and ICSI [9].

Glass wool filtration results in similar rates of sperm motility as the discontinuous density gradient with an average recovery of 50–70% progressively motile spermatozoa [31]. One major advantage of glass wool filtration is that it is more successful than a density gradient separation at separation of viable spermatozoa when there is a high percentage of asthenozoospermia or sperm with an abnormal hypo-osmotic (HOS) test [31]. Another advantage of this technique is that it uses the entire ejaculate, thus producing a high number of motile sperm, making this technique useful for patients with oligozoospermia and asthenozoospermia. This technique also separates sperm from urine in retrograde ejaculation cases [26]. Furthermore, it eliminates up to 90% of leukocytes present in semen and therefore greatly reduces ROS exposure of spermatozoa. Glass wool filtration also yields significantly more chromatin-condensed spermatozoa than swim-up or density gradient separation [32]. Disadvantages of this technique are that it is slightly more expensive due to the added expense of glass wool and that the final filtrate is not as clean as in other separation methods.

38.3.7 Sephadex Columns

Sephadex beads filter out dead and dying spermatozoa using the same separation principals as the glass wool technique. Here, sperm are diluted with an equal volume of culture media and centrifuged at 400 g for 6 min. The supernatant is removed and the sperm pellet is resuspended with enough culture media to bring the final concentration of sperm to 100×10^6 sperm/ml. Next, 1 ml of washed semen is gently placed in the filter column containing hydrated filtration beads and mixed [9]. After 15 min of filtration, the filtrate is centrifuged at $400 \times g$ for 6 min. Then, the pellet is resuspended with 1 ml of culture media, and sperm are analyzed and prepared for IVF or ICSI.

One advantage of this technique is the high yield of motile spermatozoa. Separation using sephadex beads yields significantly more sperm than with swim-up and migration-sedimentation [33]. This technique is ideal for patients with normal sperm motility and morphology but a lower than normal sperm count. Disadvantages are added expense of the Sephadex kits; the filtrate is not as clean as other techniques and potential risk of ROS due to the initial centrifugation wash process.

38.3.8 Microfluidics

Both sperm migration and gradient centrifugation result in the recovery of motile sperm. Nevertheless, these separation techniques are suboptimal for patients with severe oligozoospermia, as samples from many of these patients have large amounts of debris, and recovery rates from initial sperm samples have been reported to be as low as 0.8% for direct sperm migration [34, 35]. Therefore, separation of sperm using microfluidics is a possible alternative to traditional sperm isolation techniques. Development of a microfluidic device for sperm characterization was first developed by Kricka and colleagues (1993) using fabricated silicon and glass microfluidic devices [36]. In this study, sperm motility was assessed along the length of a network of branching microchannels (80 μm wide × 20 μm deep). The authors demonstrated that the amount of time it took for sperm to transverse the microchannel correlated with forward progression scores [37]. This method of sperm isolation provides a good measure of motility and forward progression, but does not give reliable information on sperm concentration or percent sperm motility.

Advancements in microfabrication (e.g., soft lithography) have made it possible to easily construct any desired [38, 39] micro-structures. Using these techniques, Cho and colleagues developed a novel gravity-driven pumping system to sort sperm samples [40]. The device, termed a microscale integrated sperm sorter (MISS), contains inlet/outlet ports, fluid reservoirs, gravity-driven power sources, and converging microchannels with laminar flow; all integrated components working together to facilitate sperm sorting [40]. The premise for this design was on the basis of a natural phenomenon of parallel laminar flow, characteristic of fluid movement at the microscale [41]. Laminar flow occurs when the Reynolds number (Re) is below 2,300. This number is a result of a calculation based on fluid density, velocity and viscosity and hydraulic diameter. As the Re approaches 2,300, the fluid becomes less steady and above this point the current becomes turbulent [42]. The orientation, geometry and size of the MISS reservoirs were designed to balance gravitational forces and surface tension forces and provide a pumping system, free of external energy, that generates steady flow rates over extended periods of time [40]. This device was designed so that converging streams of semen and media would flow in parallel, in a laminar fashion within a microchannel. The two parallel streams only mix by diffusion at the interface between streams, but motile sperm are able to swim across the contacting streamline and into the media for collection (Fig. 38.1). Nonmotile sperm, cellular debris, and seminal plasma do not cross this barrier and are shuttled into a waste reservoir.

Testing of this laminar flow sorting system was performed in two steps. First, 40 μl of unprocessed human semen was processed and second, semen samples were artificially filled with debris using a stock solution of round immature germ cells to simulate poor quality samples. For unprocessed semen, the device consistently produced a sorted fraction

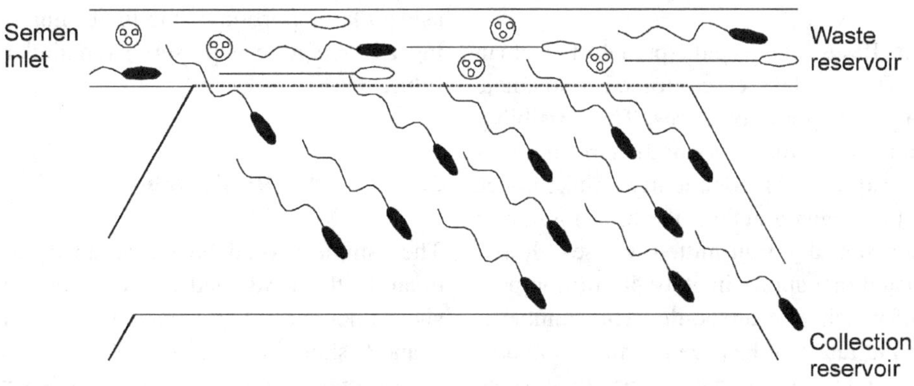

Fig. 38.1 Microfluid laminar flow collection of motile sperm

with increased motility (mean 98% motile) and improved strict sperm morphology (mean 22% normal forms) versus the initial specimen (mean 44 and 10%, respectively). For debris-filled samples, the device not only concentrated motile sperm (mean 98% motile) within the collected fraction, but also produced a round cell: sperm ratio of 1:33 when compared with a 10:1 ratio in the starting specimen [41].

A recent study by Schulte et al. demonstrated the beneficial effects on sperm parameters when using a microfluidics sperm sorter compared with other methods of sperm washing and separation [43]. In this experiment, a sperm chromatin dispersion (SCD) assay was used to assess DNA integrity, and sperm motility was used to measure sperm viability. Results from this study demonstrated a significant decrease in DNA fragmentation in sperm processed using microfluidics when compared with unprocessed sperm, as well as sperm isolated with serial centrifugation, density gradient centrifugation, and swim-up [43]. These results were further demonstrated on a similarly designed microfluidic platform made of quartz. In this study, a high percentage of highly motile sperm were separated within 5–10 min of processing and directly used for ICSI. A fertilization rate of nearly 50% was achieved but was not compared with other separation techniques [44].

Advantages of the microfluidic separation procedures are that it provides a simple, safe method of obtaining motile sperm of enriched normal morphology from both unprocessed normal semen and poor quality specimens containing significant debris. Additionally, this method greatly reduces the percentage of sperm with DNA fragmentation. The biggest disadvantage of this method of sperm separation is that it is not capable of processing an entire semen sample because of its small capacity. Secondly, it does not isolate every motile sperm. Additional modifications of the current system are underway, which may allow for large-scale processing of semen [41].

38.3.9 Viral Sperm Processing

By the end of the 1980s, the rapid spread of Human Immunodeficiency Virus (HIV) cases forced immediate changes in laboratory testing and practices. The possibility of sexual transmission and the discovery of the virus in seminal fluid [45, 46] forced the ART community to take notice and adapt practices to safeguard against the transmission of HIV [47] and other sexually transmitted viruses. It has recently been estimated that approximately 40 million people live with HIV, of which 94% are adults. This number is growing at a staggering rate as it has been further estimated that an additional four million people are newly infected annually. Improvements in antiretroviral therapies have greatly improved the quality and extended the lives of those infected with this disease and led to a 30% increase in the number of infected adults in reproductive age as well as those seeking infertility treatment [48].

Andrology laboratories should be well prepared for infected cases and thus operate under the strict laboratory guidelines outlined for class II biological security [49]. All procedures must be carried out with individual protection (nontalcum gloves, eye protection, and a facial mask). Recognizing that all biological samples should be handled with Universal Precaution, the routine processing of sperm from infected patients and noninfected patients in the same laboratory should be highly discouraged and ideally two separate laboratories should be maintained. Following processing, known contaminated samples should be stored in separate liquid nitrogen tanks as there is still some debate on vertical contamination during cryopreservation. Another option is to store samples in liquid nitrogen vapor.

One of the main goals in processing sperm from infected patients is to completely remove the virus from the sample. Cluster differentiation 4 (CD4) positive lymphocytes and macrophages, which are the primary receptors for HIV, are present in seminal liquid and must be removed during seminal preparation [50]. Therefore, independent of the procedure for which the sample will be prepared (IVF or ICSI); seminal preparation should always follow the same routine:

38.3.9.1 Previous Blood Test

It is necessary to establish a baseline CD4 count in order to determine any changes in a patient's health as well as to measure the viral load in blood.

38.3.9.2 Processing of the Sample

The semen sample should be processed using the combination of a discontinuous gradient and sperm swim-up as described earlier. The laboratory should be prepared to set aside a large portion of the final sample for viral RNA testing as well as cryopreserve remainder of the sample for future use.

38.3.9.3 RNA Viral Analysis

The sample should be measured using Real-time PCR to quantify the virus load in the sample. The HIV virus level should not exceed 50 copies/ml in the sample and Hepatitis B and C should not exceed 200 copies/ml.

It is important to recognize that detection of viral load, or lack there of, is directly related to sensitivity of the analysis.

Patient discussions and informed consent is absolute in attempting to process samples for viral load removal. One can expect that progress in this area will continue.

38.4 Postseparation Treatment of Spermatozoa

38.4.1 Sperm Motility-Stimulating Agents

One of the most obvious signs and useful measures of sperm viability is sperm motility. In cases where sperm are retrieved from the testis, spermatozoa have not undergone the maturation events acquired during migration through the epididymis and are often times immotile. Several chemicals enhance sperm motility including; relaxin, kallikrein, cysteine, taurine, prolactin, caffeine, adenosine, deoxyadenosine and pentoxifylline [51, 52]. Pentoxifylline is a methylxanthine derivative, and one of the most commonly used and widely studied compounds to stimulate movement in immobile sperm in both fresh [53–57] and cryopreserved spermatozoa [53, 56, 58, 59]. It also aids in the selection of viable sperm for ICSI. This nonspecific inhibitor of phosphodiesterase increases intracellular levels of cAMP by preventing its degredation. Elevated levels of cAMP stimulate motility, velocity and hyperactivity of spermatozoa. In addition, pentoxifylline has been shown to enhance the acrosome reaction [60] although premature induction of the acrosome reaction can be problematic [26]. Therefore, it is generally only recommended to use pentoxifylline on sperm prepared for ICSI and can especially be useful with testicular and epidiymal aspirated sperm.

Platelet-activating factor (PAF) can also be used to select viable sperm from males with asthenozoospermia. PAF factor has a positive effect on motility, capacitation, the acrosome reaction, and oocyte penetration [61, 62]. However, the mechanism by which PAF works is still not completely understood, and further studies are required to establish its importance in sperm function/processing.

38.4.2 Hypo-osmotic Swelling Test

In cases where chemical treatment of sperm is not possible or effective, another simple test exists to determine sperm viability. The Hypo-osmotic Swelling test is based of the semi-permeability of the intact and physiologically functional plasma membrane. Placement of viable spermatozoa into hypo-osmotic media causes an influx of water into the cell and expansion of the cell volume [63].

The HOS test can be performed immediately before ICSI. When setting up the ICSI plate, a small 5-μl drop of HOS media is placed next to two drops of culture media. The sperm suspension is then added to one of the drops of culture media. Individual spermatozoa are picked up with the ICSI pipette, placed in the HOS drop, and are immediately visualized for the presence of tail swelling or coiling. The tail swelling or coiling indicates the presence of an intact plasma membrane and cell viability. These cells are immediately removed from the HOS and transferred in the second wash drop to remove excess hypo-osmotic solution from the sperm and pipette. The spermatozoa are then transferred to a PVP drop and used normally for ICSI.

38.5 Selection Criteria

In IVF cases, sperm concentration, progressive motility and sperm morphology have all been demonstrated to be valuable predictors of fertilization and pregnancy rates [27, 64–70]. Liu and Baker studied the effect of sperm factors on over 1,000 IVF cases and ranked sperm morphology and zona binding as the most significant markers of fertilization. Additionally, Liu and Baker ranked normal intact acrosomes as correlating highly with fertilization rates [71]. Furthermore, Liu and Baker determined that sperm–ZP binding correlated with motility (as well as normal morphology and percentage acrosome-intact). On the basis of these results, the authors proposed that procedures that select for high numbers of sperm with normal morphology, forward progression, intact acrosomes and a high zona-binding capacity may improve the results of IVF [71].

It has further been shown that morphological abnormalities (particularly sperm head abnormalities) result in poor embryo quality and decreased pregnancy rates [72]. Grow et al. demonstrated that strict morphology could be used as a biomarker for fertilization [73]. In addition, Miller showed that sperm morphology could be related to blastocyst development [74] and Salumets et al. demonstrated that sperm morphology can be used to determine blastomere cleavage rates [75]. These results are not without debate as Host et al. was unable to find any correlation between sperm morphology and fertilization, embryo development and pregnancy rates when using Tygerberg and WHO analysis criteria [76, 77].

There is much debate as to whether sperm morphology can affect ICSI results. This question is difficult to answer because of the subjectivity of the ICSI technician selecting individual sperm to inject into oocytes, as it is probable that the most morphologically normal sperm will be selected and is likely not representative of the entire population of sperm.

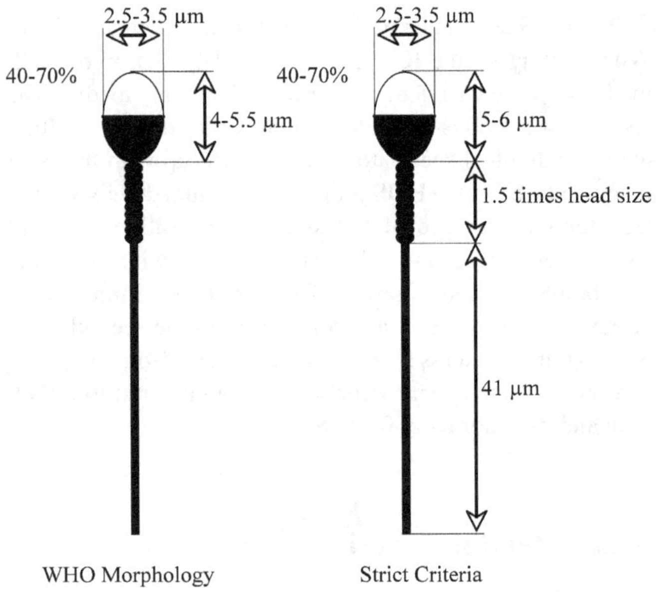

Fig. 38.2 Comparison of WHO and strict morphology criteria

It has been shown that sperm concentration, motility and morphology do not influence the outcome of ICSI [78–82]. Mansour et al., detected no differences in fertilization and pregnancy rates between patients with >95% teratozoospermia and those with <95% teratozoospermia [83]. In addition, Windt et al. found no differences in fertilization and pregnancy rates in ejaculated and testicular sperm that were classified as either good-prognosis or poor-prognosis spermatozoa [84]. Similarly, Yavetz et al. showed that head dimension, acrosome, and mid-piece abnormalities do not affect fertilization rates [85].

Despite reports demonstrating sperm morphology have no effect on fertilization and pregnancy rates, there are numerous reports that show strong correlations between sperm morphology and fertilization and subsequent development. Several groups have shown that in cases in which there is extremely high or complete teratozoospermia, there are no differences in embryo development; however, there is a significant decrease in pregnancy rates [86] and implantation potential, [69] and a higher rate of spontaneous abortion [87].

Owing to the subjective nature of selecting individual sperm for ICSI, it is important to classify each individual sperm used for ICSI instead of the population from which sperm are selected. Meticulous recording is necessary in determining the effect of various sperm abnormalities on subsequent fertilization and developmental outcomes. Levran et al. recorded the morphology of every sperm used for ICSI and found that fertilization was reduced when the following characteristics were present: short acrosome region, round head, and amorphous-head defect. In addition, no pregnancies were achieved when amorphous head defects were present. This study revealed that sperm head defects play a major role in decreased fertilization rates and poor embryo quality [32].

In a similarly designed study, De Vos et al. showed a decline in fertilization, implantation and pregnancy rates when morphologically abnormal sperm were used for ICSI [88]. De Vos et al. also showed that the lowest rates of fertilization are achieved when sperm with amorphous-head defects are used for ICSI [88]. Several other research groups have also shown that injection of sperm with macrocephalic heads results in low fertilization and pregnancy rates [89, 90]. Macrocephalic sperm have problems during meiosis I and II, resulting in failure of nuclear cleavage. For this reason, it has been suggested that sperm with this malformation should not be used in ICSI [89, 90]. Intracytoplasmic sperm injection with severely tapered sperm also decreases fertilization rates [91]. Spermatozoa with tapered heads are thought to have prolonged and incomplete decondensation patterns which may explain this decrease [91].

De Vos et al. showed that of fertilized oocytes, those injected with broken necks had reduced rates of embryo development and subsequent ability to establish pregnancy [88]. These results were in agreement with a study by Rawe et al., who also showed a negative effect on embryo development when sperm with head-tail junction alterations are used in ICSI [92]. Rawe et al. suggested that alterations in the neck region are caused by centriolar dysfunction [92]. The sperm centrosome provides the active division center for the embryo and plays a very important role in the first division of the embryo at syngamy. The functional, proximal sperm centriole is carried into the oocyte at fertilization, persists during sperm decondensation, and organizes the sperm aster and the first mitotic spindle [93]. Therefore, problems with centriolar function may result in insufficient sperm aster formation and problems during syngamy, cleavage and subsequent development.

38.5.1 PICSI™ Selection

To overcome the subjectivity of selecting the "best looking sperm" by an embryologist, a new noninvasive ICSI selection strategy has been developed to select only mature sperm. Previous research has shown a strong relationship between immature sperm and chromosomal disomies [94]. These findings suggest that selection of mature sperm may greatly reduce ICSI-related genetic disorders [94]. It has been demonstrated that sperm undergo a sperm plasma membrane remodeling during maturation [95], which facilitates the formation of hyaluronic acid (HA) sperm-binding site(s) for the zona pellucida [44, 96–100]. Immature sperm that have not undergone plasma membrane remodeling cannot bind to the zona pellucida or to immobilized HA [97, 101]. The presence of these binding sites allows for the selection of mature spermatozoa and is the scientific basis for the development of the PICSI™ plate (Biocoat, Inc).

The PICSI™ plate utilizes drops of hyaluronan (H), a major constituent of the cumulus matrix to bind mature sperm to the bottom of the plate. Once bound to the plate, the embryologist can simply pick-up the sperm using an ICSI pipette and proceed with normal ICSI. Using these principals for selection, Jacab et al. showed that HA-selected sperm had significantly reduced chromosomal disomy and sex chromosomal disomy frequencies when compared with unselected sperm [102]. In addition, Jacab demonstrated that there was no DNA fragmentation as assessed by DNA-nick translation and COMET assays in HA-selected sperm [102]. These results are especially encouraging as sperm shape and size can not be used to observe chromosomal abnormalities or DNA fragmentation.

In a recent study comparing the selection of sperm using PICSI™ and ICSI, Worrilow et al. demonstrated a statistically significant improvement in fertilization rates when using PICSI™ selected sperm [103]. In addition, the percentage of fragmentation was significantly less in embryos produced using PICSI™ selected sperm than in ICSI controls. Furthermore, positive beta hCG and clinical pregnancy rates for PICSI™ patients were higher than controls and the rate of miscarriage was significantly reduced in PICSI™ cases [103]. The results from this study further support the idea that selection of mature sperm with enhanced functional competence exerts a positive paternal influence on subsequent development.

38.6 Conclusions

Advancements in knowledge of male infertility reveal that there is not a single separation protocol that can be universally applied on all semen samples to achieve successful fertilization and development. Not only does the manner in which the semen is collected have to be considered when choosing a method for sperm preparation, but it is also important to consider the quality and quantity of spermatozoa as well as the way the sample is to be used. Some studies do not support the idea that sperm morphology can be used as a reliable marker for embryo development and pregnancy, while many others do. As more ICSI are being performed (greater than 70% in many ART clinics), so must the scrutiny with which we select sperm for these procedures increase. Advancements in microfluidics and in noninvasive methods to select HA-bound sperm have provided new methods of separation and isolation which can greatly reduce the chance of selecting sperm with DNA or chromosomal abnormalities. The integration of these new technologies will likely be useful. Additionally, discoveries of novel means of selecting the best sperm for fertilization, embryo development, pregnancy initiation, and birth of healthy children are required and they represent an exciting area of current and future research.

References

1. Mosher WD, Pratt WF (1991) Fecundity and infertility in the United States: incidence and trends. Fertil Steril 56:192–193
2. Mortimer D (1989) Sperm transfer in the human female reproductive tract. Oxford University Press, Oxford
3. Austin CR (1951) Observations on the penetration of the sperm in the mammalian egg. Aust J Sci Res (B) 4:581–596
4. Chang MC (1951) Fertilizing capacity of spermatozoa deposited into the fallopian tubes. Nature 168:697–698
5. Yanagimachi R (1994) Mammalian fertilization. In: Knobil E, Neill JD (eds) The physiology of reproduction, 2nd edn. Raven Press, New York
6. Rogers BJ, Perreault SD, Bentwood BJ, McCarville C, Hale RW, Soderdahl DW (1983) Variability in the human-hamster in vitro assay for fertility evaluation. Fertil Steril 39:204–211
7. Kanwar KC, Yanagimachi R, Lopata A (1979) Effects of human seminal plasma on fertilizing capacity of human spermatozoa. Fertil Steril 31:321–327
8. Trounson AO, Gardner DK (2000) Handbook of in vitro fertilization, 2nd edn. CRC Press, Boca Raton, FL
9. Nancy L, Bosset CJDJ (2007) Sperm preparation for IVF and ICSI. In: Gardner DK (ed) In vitro fertilization: a pratical approach. Informa Healthcare, New York
10. Jeulin C, Serres C, Jouannet P (1982) The effects of centrifugation, various synthetic media and temperature on the motility and vitality of human spermatozoa. Reprod Nutr Dev 22:81–91
11. Lopes S, Jurisicova A, Sun JG, Casper RF (1998) Reactive oxygen species: potential cause for DNA fragmentation in human spermatozoa. Hum Reprod 13:896–900
12. Virant-Klun I, Tomazevic T, Meden-Vrtovec H (2002) Sperm single-stranded DNA, detected by acridine orange staining, reduces fertilization and quality of ICSI-derived embryos. J Assist Reprod Genet 19:319–328
13. Benchaib M, Braun V, Lornage J et al (2003) Sperm DNA fragmentation decreases the pregnancy rate in an assisted reproductive technique. Hum Reprod 18:1023–1028
14. Seli E, Gardner DK, Schoolcraft WB, Moffatt O, Sakkas D (2004) Extent of nuclear DNA damage in ejaculated spermatozoa impacts on blastocyst development after in vitro fertilization. Fertil Steril 82:378–383
15. Bungum M, Humaidan P, Spano M, Jepson K, Bungum L, Giwercman A (2004) The predictive value of sperm chromatin structure assay (SCSA) parameters for the outcome of intrauterine insemination, IVF and ICSI. Hum Reprod 19:1401–1408
16. Henkel R, Hajimohammad M, Stalf T et al (2004) Influence of deoxyribonucleic acid damage on fertilization and pregnancy. Fertil Steril 81:965–972
17. Tesarik J, Greco E, Mendoza C (2004) Late, but not early, paternal effect on human embryo development is related to sperm DNA fragmentation. Hum Reprod 19:611–615
18. Carrell DT, Liu L, Peterson CM et al (2003) Sperm DNA fragmentation is increased in couples with unexplained recurrent pregnancy loss. Arch Androl 49:49–55

19. Mortimer D (2000) Sperm preparation methods. J Androl 21:357–366
20. Mahadevan M, Baker G (1984) Assessment and preparation of semen for in vitro fertilization. Springer, Berlin
21. Bongso A (1999) Handbook on blastocyst culture. National University of Singapore, Singapore
22. Oehninger S, Acosta R, Morshedi M, Philput C, Swanson RJ, Acosta AA (1990) Relationship between morphology and motion characteristics of human spermatozoa in semen and in the swim-up sperm fractions. J Androl 11:446–452
23. Erel CT, Senturk LM, Irez T et al (2000) Sperm-preparation techniques for men with normal and abnormal semen analysis. A comparison. J Reprod Med 45:917–922
24. Ford WC, McLaughlin EA, Prior SM, Rees JM, Wardle PG, Hull MG (1992) The yield, motility and performance in the hamster egg test of human spermatozoa prepared from cryopreserved semen by four different methods. Hum Reprod 7:654–659
25. Mortimer D, Mortimer ST (1992) Methods of sperm preparation for assisted reproduction. Ann Acad Med Singapore 21:517–524
26. Henkel RR, Schill WB (2003) Sperm preparation for ART. Reprod Biol Endocrinol 1:108
27. Hammadeh ME, Kuhnen A, Amer AS, Rosenbaum P, Schmidt W (2001) Comparison of sperm preparation methods: effect on chromatin and morphology recovery rates and their consequences on the clinical outcome after in vitro fertilization embryo transfer. Int J Androl 24:360–368
28. Morrell JM, Moffatt O, Sakkas D et al (2004) Reduced senescence and retained nuclear DNA integrity in human spermatozoa prepared by density gradient centrifugation. J Assist Reprod Genet 21:217–222
29. Tomlinson MJ, Moffatt O, Manicardi GC, Bizzaro D, Afnan M, Sakkas D (2001) Interrelationships between seminal parameters and sperm nuclear DNA damage before and after density gradient centrifugation: implications for assisted conception. Hum Reprod 16:2160–2165
30. Jeyendran RS, Van der Ven HH, Perez-Pelaez M, Al-Hassani S, Diedrich K (1987) Separation of viable spermatozoa by standardized glass woolcolumn. In Advances in Fertility and Sterility Series; In Vitro Fertilization, Vol 2, Ch 8, Ratman, Teoh, Ng (eds). Carnforth, Lancs, UK, Parthenon Publishing, p 49
31. Rhemrev J, Jeyendran RS, Vermeiden JP, Zaneveld LJ (1989) Human sperm selection by glass wool filtration and two-layer, discontinuous Percoll gradient centrifugation. Fertil Steril 51:685–690
32. Henkel RR, Franken DR, Lombard CJ, Schill W-B (1994) Selective capacity of glass wool filtration for chromatin condensed human spermatozoa: a possible therapeutic modality for male factor cases?. J Assist Reprod Genet 11:395–400
33. Gabriel LK, Vawda AI (1993) Preparation of human sperm for assisted conception: a comparative study. Arch Androl 30:1–6
34. Englert Y, Van den Bergh M, Rodesch C, Bertrand E, Biramane J, Legreve A (1992) Comparative auto-controlled study between swim-up and Percoll preparation of fresh semen samples for in-vitro fertilization. Hum Reprod 7:399–402
35. Smith S, Hosid S, Scott L (1995) Use of postseparation sperm parameters to determine the method of choice for sperm preparation for assisted reproductive technology. Fertil Steril 63: 591–597
36. Kricka LJ, Nozaki O, Heyner S, Garside WT, Wilding P (1993) Applications of a microfabricated device for evaluating sperm function. Clin Chem 39:1944–1947
37. Kricka LJ, Faro I, Heyner S et al (1997) Micromachined analytical devices: microchips for semen testing. J Pharm Biomed Anal 15:1443–1447
38. Anderson JR, Chiu DT, Jackman RJ et al (2000) Fabrication of topologically complex three-dimensional microfluidic systems in PDMS by rapid prototyping. Anal Chem 72:3158–3164
39. Unger MA, Chou HP, Thorsen T, Scherer A, Quake SR (2000) Monolithic microfabricated valves and pumps by multilayer soft lithography. Science 288:113–116
40. Cho BS, Schuster TG, Zhu X, Chang D, Smith GD, Takayama S (2003) Passively driven integrated microfluidic system for separation of motile sperm. Anal Chem 75:1671–1675
41. Schuster TG, Cho B, Keller LM, Takayama S, Smith GD (2003) Isolation of motile spermatozoa from semen samples using microfluidics. Reprod Biomed Online 7:75–81
42. Figeys D, Pinto D (2000) Lab-on-a-chip: a revolution in biological and medical sciences. Anal Chem 72A:330–335
43. Schulte RT, Chunga YK, Ohl DA, Takayama S, Smith GD (2007) Microfluidic sperm sorting device provides a novel method for selecting motile sperm with higher DNA integrity. Fertil Steril 88(Suppl 1):S76
44. Shibata D, Ando H, Iwase A, Harata T, Kikkawa F, Naruse K (2007) Analysis of sperm motility and fertilization rates after the separation by microfluidic sperm sorter made of quartz. Fertil Steril 88(Suppl 1):S110
45. Ho DD, Schooley RT, Rota TR et al (1984) HTLV-III in the semen and blood of a healthy homosexual man. Science 226:451–453
46. Zagury D, Bernard J, Leibowitch J et al (1984) HTLV-III in cells cultured from semen of two patients with AIDS. Science 226:449–451
47. Tyler JP, Dobler KJ, Driscoll GL, Stewart GJ (1986) The impact of AIDS on artificial insemination by donor. Clin Reprod Fertil 4:305–317
48. Chu MC, Pena JE, Thornton MH 2nd, Sauer MV (2005) Assessing the treatment efficacy of IVF with intracytoplasmic sperm injection in human immunodeficiency virus-1 (HIV-1) serodiscordant couples. Reprod Biomed Online 10:130–134
49. U.S. Public Health Service (2001) Updated U.S. public health service guidlines for the management of occupational exposure to HBV, HCV, and HIV and recommendations for postexposure prophylaxis. MMWR Recomm Rep 50(RR11):1–42
50. Sauer MV (2005) Sperm washing techniques address the fertility needs of HIV-seropositive men: a clinical review. Reprod Biomed Online 10:135–140
51. Hammitt DG, Bedia E, Rogers PR, Syrop CH, Donovan JF, Williamson RA (1989) Comparison of motility stimulants for cryopreserved human semen. Fertil Steril 52:495–502
52. Lindemann CB, Kanous KS (1989) Regulation of mammalian sperm motility. Arch Androl 23:1–22
53. Nassar A, Morshedi M, Mahony M, Srisombut C, Lin MH, Oehninger S (1999) Pentoxifylline stimulates various sperm motion parameters and cervical mucus penetrability in patients with asthenozoospermia. Andrologia 31:9–15
54. Paul M, Sumpter JP, Lindsay KS (1995) Action of pentoxifylline directly on semen. Hum Reprod 10:354–359
55. Rees JM, Ford WC, Hull MG (1990) Effect of caffeine and of pentoxifylline on the motility and metabolism of human spermatozoa. J Reprod Fertil 90:147–156
56. Sharma RK, Agarwal A (1997) Influence of artificial stimulation on unprocessed and Percoll-washed cryopreserved sperm. Arch Androl 38:173–179
57. Yovich JM, Edirisinghe WR, Cummins JM, Yovich JL (1990) Influence of pentoxifylline in severe male factor infertility. Fertil Steril 53:715–722
58. Gradil CM, Ball BA (2000) The use of pentoxifylline to improve motility of cryopreserved equine spermatozoa. Theriogenology 54:1041–1047
59. Stanic P, Sonicki Z, Suchanek E (2002) Effect of pentoxifylline on motility and membrane integrity of cryopreserved human spermatozoa. Int J Androl 25:186–190
60. Tesarik J, Mendoza C, Carreras A (1992) Effects of phosphodiesterase inhibitors caffeine and pentoxifylline on spontaneous and stimulus-induced acrosome reactions in human sperm. Fertil Steril 58:1185–1190

61. Krausz C, Gervasi G, Forti G, Baldi E (1994) Effect of platelet-activating factor on motility and acrosome reaction of human spermatozoa. Hum Reprod 9:471–476
62. Sengoku K, Tamate K, Takaoka Y, Ishikawa M (1993) Effects of platelet activating factor on human sperm function in vitro. Hum Reprod 8:1443–1447
63. Organisation WH (1999) WHO laboratory manual for the examination of human semen and sperm-cervical mucus interaction, 4th edn. Cambridge University Press, Cambridge
64. Coetzee K, Kruge TF, Lombard CJ (1998) Predictive value of normal sperm morphology: a structured literature review. Hum Reprod Update 4:73–82
65. Kruger TF, Acosta AA, Simmons KF, Swanson RJ, Matta JF, Oehninger S (1988) Predictive value of abnormal sperm morphology in in vitro fertilization. Fertil Steril 49:112–117
66. Kruger TF, Menkveld R, Stander FS et al (1986) Sperm morphologic features as a prognostic factor in in vitro fertilization. Fertil Steril 46:1118–1123
67. Ombelet W, Fourie FL, Vandeput H et al (1994) Teratozoospermia and in-vitro fertilization: a randomized prospective study. Hum Reprod 9:1479–1484
68. Sofikitis NV, Miyagawa I, Zavos PM, Toda T, Iino A, Terakawa N (1994) Confocal scanning laser microscopy of morphometric human sperm parameters: correlation with acrosin profiles and fertilizing capacity. Fertil Steril 62:376–386
69. Tasdemir I, Tasdemir M, Tavukcuoglu S, Kahraman S, Biberoglu K (1997) Effect of abnormal sperm head morphology on the outcome of intracytoplasmic sperm injection in humans. Hum Reprod 12:1214–1217
70. Vawda AI, Gunby J, Younglai EV (1996) Semen parameters as predictors of in-vitro fertilization: the importance of strict criteria sperm morphology. Hum Reprod 11:1445–1450
71. Liu DY, Baker HW (1992) Morphology of spermatozoa bound to the zona pellucida of human oocytes that failed to fertilize in vitro. J Reprod Fertil 94:71–84
72. Parinaud J, Mieusset R, Vieitez G, Labal B, Richoilley G (1993) Influence of sperm parameters on embryo quality. Fertil Steril 60:888–892
73. Grow DR, Oehninger S, Seltman HJ et al (1994) Sperm morphology as diagnosed by strict criteria: probing the impact of teratozoospermia on fertilization rate and pregnancy outcome in a large in vitro fertilization population. Fertil Steril 62:559–567
74. Miller JE, Smith TT (2001) The effect of intracytoplasmic sperm injection and semen parameters on blastocyst development in vitro. Hum Reprod 16:918–924
75. Salumets A, Suikkari AM, Mols T, Soderstrom-Anttila V, Tuuri T (2002) Influence of oocytes and spermatozoa on early embryonic development. Fertil Steril 78:1082–1087
76. Host E, Ernst E, Lindenberg S, Smidt-Jensen S (2001) Morphology of spermatozoa used in IVF and ICSI from oligozoospermic men. Reprod Biomed Online 3:212–215
77. Host E, Lindenberg S, Ernst E, Christensen F (1999) Sperm morphology and IVF: embryo quality in relation to sperm morphology following the WHO and Kruger's strict criteria. Acta Obstet Gynecol Scand 78:526–529
78. Hammadeh ME, al-Hasani S, Stieber M et al (1996) The effect of chromatin condensation (aniline blue staining) and morphology (strict criteria) of human spermatozoa on fertilization, cleavage and pregnancy rates in an intracytoplasmic sperm injection programme. Hum Reprod 11:2468–2471
79. Kupker W, Schulze W, Diedrich K (1998) Ultrastructure of gametes and intracytoplasmic sperm injection: the significance of sperm morphology. Hum Reprod 13(Suppl 1):99–106
80. Nagy ZP, Liu J, Joris H et al (1995) The result of intracytoplasmic sperm injection is not related to any of the three basic sperm parameters. Hum Reprod 10:1123–1129
81. Nagy ZP, Verheyen G, Tournaye H, Van Steirteghem AC (1998) Special applications of intracytoplasmic sperm injection: the influence of sperm count, motility, morphology, source and sperm antibody on the outcome of ICSI. Hum Reprod 13(Suppl 1):143–154
82. Sallam HN, Sallam A, Agamia AF (1998) The correlation between eight sperm parameters assessed objectively and the fertilization rate in IVF and ICSI. Fertil Steril 70:371
83. Mansour RT, Aboulghar MA, Serour GI, Amin YM, Ramzi AM (1995) The effect of sperm parameters on the outcome of intracytoplasmic sperm injection. Fertil Steril 64:982–986
84. Windt ML, Kruger TF (2004) The role of sperm cell morphology in intracytoplasmic sperm injection. In: Kruger TF, Franken DR (eds) Atlas of human sperm morphology evaluation. Taylor and Francis, Boca Raton, FL
85. Yavetz H, Yogev L, Kleiman S et al (2001) Morphology of testicular spermatozoa obtained by testicular sperm extraction in obstructive and nonobstructive azoospermic men and its relation to fertilization success in the in vitro fertilization-intracytoplasmic sperm injection system. J Androl 22:376–381
86. Moomjy M, Sills ES, Rosenwaks Z, Palermo GD (1998) Implications of complete fertilization failure after intracytoplasmic sperm injection for subsequent fertilization and reproductive outcome. Hum Reprod 13:2212–2216
87. O'Neil J, Lundquist L, Ritter J, Chantilis SJ, Carr BR, Byrd W (1998) Should strict morphology be used to indicate the need for intracytoplasmic sperm injection? Fetil Steril 70(Suppl 1):442
88. De Vos A, Van De Velde H, Joris H, Verheyen G, Devroey P, Van Steirteghem A (2003) Influence of individual sperm morphology on fertilization, embryo morphology, and pregnancy outcome of intracytoplasmic sperm injection. Fertil Steril 79:7
89. Devillard F, Metzler-Guillemain C, Pelletier R et al (2002) Polyploidy in large-headed sperm: FISH study of three cases. Hum Reprod 17:1292–1298
90. Viville S, Mollard R, Bach ML, Falquet C, Gerlinger P, Warter S (2000) Do morphological anomalies reflect chromosomal aneuploidies? case report. Hum Reprod 15:2563–2566
91. Osawa Y, Sueoka K, Iwata S et al (1999) Assessment of the dominant abnormal form is useful for predicting the outcome of intracytoplasmic sperm injection in the case of severe teratozoospermia. J Assist Reprod Genet 16:436–442
92. Rawe VY, Terada Y, Nakamura S, Chillik CF, Olmedo SB, Chemes HE (2002) A pathology of the sperm centriole responsible for defective sperm aster formation, syngamy and cleavage. Hum Reprod 17:2344–2349
93. Sathananthan AH, Ratnam S, Ng SC, Tarin JJ, Gianaroli L, Trounson A (1996) The sperm centriole: its inheritance, replication, and perpetuation in early human embryos. Hum Reprod 11:345–356
94. Kovanci E, Kovacs T, Moretti E et al (2001) FISH assessment of aneuploidy frequencies in mature and immature human spermatozoa classified by the absence or presence of cytoplasmic retention. Hum Reprod 16:1209–1217
95. Huszar G, Sbracia M, Vigue L, Miller DJ, Shur BD (1997) Sperm plasma membrane remodeling during spermiogenetic maturation in men: relationship among plasma membrane beta 1, 4-galactosyltransferase, cytoplasmic creatine phosphokinase, and creatine phosphokinase isoform ratios. Biol Reprod 56:1020–1024
96. Bharadwaj A, Ghosh I, Sengupta A et al (2002) Stage-specific expression of proprotein form of hyaluronan binding protein 1 (HABP1) during spermatogenesis in rat. Mol Reprod Dev 62:223–232
97. Huszar G, Ozenci CC, Cayli S, Zavaczki Z, Hansch E, Vigue L (2003) Hyaluronic acid binding by human sperm indicates cellular maturity, viability, and unreacted acrosomal status. Fertil Steril 79(Suppl 3):1616–1624
98. Huszar G, Willetts M, Corrales M (1990) Hyaluronic acid (Sperm Select) improves retention of sperm motility and velocity in normospermic and oligospermic specimens. Fertil Steril 54:1127–1134

99. Kornovski BS, McCoshen J, Kredentser J, Turley E (1994) The regulation of sperm motility by a novel hyaluronan receptor. Fertil Steril 61:935–940
100. Ranganathan S, Ganguly AK, Datta K (1994) Evidence for presence of hyaluronan binding protein on spermatozoa and its possible involvement in sperm function. Mol Reprod Dev 38:69–76
101. Huszar G, Vigue L, Oehninger S (1994) Creatine kinase immunocytochemistry of human sperm-hemizona complexes: selective binding of sperm with mature creatine kinase-staining pattern. Fertil Steril 61:136–142
102. Jakab A, Sakkas D, Delpiano E et al (2005) Intracytoplasmic sperm injection: a novel selection method for sperm with normal frequency of chromosomal aneuploidies. Fertil Steril 84:1665–1673
103. Worrilow KC, Huynh HT, Bower JB, Anderson AR, Schillings W, Crain JL (2007) PICSI™ vs ICSI: Statistically significant improvement in clinical outcomes in 240 in vitro fertilization (IVF) patients. Fertil Steril 88(Suppl 1):S37

Chapter 39
The Genetic and Epigenetic Contributions of Sperm to Early Embryogenesis

Denny Sakkas, Maria Lalioti, Hasan M. El-Fakahany, and Emre Seli

Abstract During fertilization, the sperm delivers a haploid set of chromosomes to the zygote. Genetic alterations, such as numerical or structural chromosome defects, can affect the ability of the embryo to undergo normal development. Similarly, epigenetic defects, such as abnormal methylation of gene promoters, may affect gene expression during embryogenesis and affect the viability or health of the developing embryo. This chapter explores the genetic and epigenetic contributions of sperm to normal embryogenesis.

Keywords Aneuploidy • DNA damage • DNA methylation • Embryogenesis • Epigenetics

39.1 Introduction

There is mounting evidence suggesting that the influence of the paternal genome on reproduction goes beyond that which can be appreciated by simple quantitative and morphologic evaluation of spermatozoa. This paternal influence spans from the gross nuclear contribution of a spermatozoon possessing the wrong chromosomal make up to that of a more subtle contribution as perceived in relation to the incorrect epigenetic state of the spermatozoal chromatin. Animal models have largely revealed the existence of this paternal influence; however, the increasing use of compromised spermatozoa via treatment modes, such as intracytoplasmic sperm injection (ICSI) in the human, have led to the belief and apprehension that such traits are more likely to be observed. Simple circumvention of fertilization using ICSI may increase the chances of deleterious effects arising from imperfect spermatozoa, and other reproductive parameters, such as embryo development, implantation, pregnancy loss, and live birth rate, may be affected. Therefore, it is necessary to identify molecular and cellular mechanisms that cause impaired spermatozoal function in order to develop personalized diagnostic and therapeutic interventions. In this chapter, we summarize the evidence pointing to this paternal effect and discuss whether our treatment options should be modified in certain patients. Invariably these treatment options largely revolve around the use of ICSI, as it is the power of this technique that allows us to push the limits of treatment of the male.

D. Sakkas (✉), M. Lalioti, H.M. El-Fakahany, and E. Seli
Department of Obstetrics, Gynecology and Reproductive Sciences, Yale University School of Medicine, New Haven, CT, USA

39.2 Aneuploidy of Paternal Origin

39.2.1 Incidence of Aneuploidy in Human

A small percentage of aneuploid fetuses survive and aneuploidy has important clinical implications as the leading cause of pregnancy loss and the most common cause of mental retardation. The detected incidence of aneuploidy in humans varies depending on the developmental time point examined. Approximately, 0.3% of newborns are aneuploid [1] with the most common abnormalities being trisomy 21 and sex-chromosome trisomies (47,XXX, 47,XXY, and 47,XYY). Among stillbirths (fetal deaths occurring between 20 weeks of gestation and term), the incidence of aneuploidy increases tenfold to approximately 4%, with the types of abnormality being similar to those identified among newborns. The incidence of aneuploidy among clinically recognized spontaneous pregnancy losses (between 6–8 weeks and 20 weeks of gestation) is estimated to be 35%. Unlike livebirths or stillbirths, various aneuploidies are detected in spontaneous abortions, including trisomies for almost all chromosomes. Analysis of preimplantation embryos generated by ART has revealed high aneuploidy rates [2]. These results are consistent with cytogenetic analyses of human gametes. An approximately 2% aneuploidy rate is reported in human spermatozoa [3], while in oocytes obtained for assisted reproductive technologies, it is much higher at 20–25% [4–6].

D.T. Carrell and C.M. Peterson (eds.), *Reproductive Endocrinology and Infertility: Integrating Modern Clinical and Laboratory Practice*,
DOI 10.1007/978-1-4419-1436-1_39, © Springer Science+Business Media, LLC 2010

39.2.2 Paternal Origin of Aneuploidy in Human

Sperm chromosomal analysis was initially investigated using the zona-free hamster egg penetration test, a costly, labor-intensive method that requires sperm-fertilizing ability [7]. Introduction of fluorescent in situ hybridization (FISH) has now made the cytogenetic analysis of a larger number of spermatozoa in a shorter period of time more feasible. Based on FISH studies, paternal errors account for 5–10% of autosomal trisomies, while maternal MI errors are the predominant etiology [1]. Paternal effect on sex chromosome trisomies is higher since 100% of 47,XYY, and nearly 50% of 47,XXY are paternal in origin [1, 8]. Seventy to eighty percent of 45,X have single maternally derived X chromosome and the paternal chromosome (X or Y) is lost either in meiosis or in an early stage of embryo development [9].

39.2.3 Incidence of Sperm Chromosome Aneuploidy and Implications on Reproduction

Hansen et al. [10] reported compiled data from the registries in Western Australia, involving 301 infants conceived with ICSI, 837 infants conceived with IVF, and 4,000 naturally conceived controls between 1993 and 1997. They found the incidence of major birth defects to be more than twofold higher for ICSI and IVF groups (8.6 and 9.0%, respectively) compared to normal controls (4.2%). Their data show an increased incidence of chromosomal abnormalities in the ICSI group (1.0% for all infants and 1.6% for singletons only) compared to IVF (0.7% for all infants and 0.6% for singletons only; the difference not statistically significant) and normal controls (0.2% for all infants and 0.2% for singletons only; $p<0.05$).

While some other studies failed to show an increase in major birth defects in children conceived with IVF and/or ICSI [11, 12], these were criticized for methodologic problems such as inadequate sample sizes, lack of appropriate data for comparison, use of different criteria to define major birth defects in infants conceived with ART and those conceived naturally [13].

The largest studies have arisen from registries established in Europe, especially from the Belgian groups. Van Steirteghem et al. summarized data from seven studies reporting karyotype analyses performed for prenatal diagnosis in a total of 2,139 pregnancies conceived with ICSI [14]. In comparison with the general population, they calculated a slight but significant increase in de novo sex chromosomal aneuploidy (0.6% vs. 0.2%), and structural autosomal abnormalities (0.7% vs. 0.04%), and an increased number of inherited (mostly from the father) structural aberrations.

Possible causes of elevated chromosome aneuploidy following ICSI include the technique itself or an increased risk from the sperm used for ICSI. Carrell et al. [15] found the mean aneuploidy rate for five chromosome (X ,Y, 13, 18, 21) to be 1.2% for fertile controls, 1.4% for general population, 2.6% for men with moderately diminished semen quality (count, motility, or morphology were diminished, but greater than 50% of normal value), 4.0% for men with severe terato-asthenooligozoospermia (count, motility, and morphology were all less than 50% of normal value), and 15.9% for men with rare ultrastructural defects. Their findings are consistent with previous reports and suggest that the incidence of chromosome aneuploidy in spermatozoa correlates with the severity of sperm defects.

The same group found the sperm chromosome aneuploidy rate to be higher in partners of women with recurrent pregnancy loss (2.77%) compared to the general population (1.48%) or fertile controls (1.19%) [16]. This is consistent with a previous report by Rubio et al. [17].

In summary, available evidence suggests a relationship between abnormal semen parameters and an increased incidence of sperm chromosomal aneuploidy. This increase may contribute to the higher rate of sex chromosomal aneuploidy reported in fetuses conceived with ICSI. Moreover, there may be a relationship between recurrent pregnancy loss and elevated sperm chromosomal aneuploidy. However, the relevance of these findings, beyond their use in counseling is currently unclear, because even in men with increased sperm chromosomal aneuploidy, only less than 5% of spermatozoa seem to have aneuploid chromosome content.

At present, we are unable to offer our patients a selection technique whereby spermatozoa with normal chromosome number can be used for fertilization. Very recently, Jakab et al. reported a new method based on the hyaluronic acid binding ability of spermatozoa [18]. Using this method, they were able to simulate ICSI techniques and select a spermatozoa population with a four- to fivefold decreased frequency of disomy or diploidy compared to unselected spermatozoa. While further validation is necessary, their findings are encouraging in providing a test that allows selection of spermatozoa prior to ICSI.

39.2.4 Klinefelter Syndrome as a Cause of Sperm Chromosome Aneuploidy

Klinefelter syndrome is the most common chromosomal disorder associated with male infertility, reported to occur in 1 in 500 newborn males. In approximately 95% of cases, it is characterized by a 47,XXY chromosome complement. The 47,XXY karyotype has a high incidence among infertile men, detected in 11% of men with azoospermia and in 0.7% of men with oligozoospermia.

The clinical presentation of Klinefelter syndrome includes small, firm testes, eunuchoid habitus, gynecomastia, elevated serum FSH levels, and azoospermia. While azoospemia is the usual finding among Klinefelter syndrome that carry a 47,XXY karyotype, oligozoospermia has been described in men with mosaicism. Moreover, rare cases of fertility have been reported among oligozoospermic Klinefelter syndrome patients.

Testicular histology in men with Klinefelter syndrome is characterized by the absence of spermatogenesis and hyalinization of seminiferous tubules. Those with mosaicism are less affected initially and the majority have normal size testes and spermatogenesis at puberty. However, their ability to reproduce is temporary as their reproductive function deteriorates rapidly and their seminiferous tubules become hyalinized shortly after puberty.

The ability of the germ cells from a 47,XXY male to proceed through meiosis and to generate XX or XY hyperhaploid gametes is not known. The presence of more than one X chromosome in a male germ cell is believed to be detrimental, although this notion has been challenged by FISH studies of spermatozoa in mosaic Kleinefelter's patients with 47,XXY, 46XY karyotype [19, 20]. An increased frequency of hyperhaploid 24,XY in these patients argues that such cells may indeed possess a meiotic capacity.

39.3 Y Chromosome Microdeletions

The human Y chromosome consists of a short and a long arm, termed Yp and Yq, respectively. The areas of sequence identity to the X chromosome that allows pairing and recombination during meiosis, called pseudoautosomal pairing regions (PARs), are located at the distal portions of Yp and Yq.

Y chromosome microdeletions are the second most frequent genetic cause of male infertility after Kleinefelter syndrome. Because the absence of meiotic recombination within most regions of the human Y chromosome impedes linkage analysis, mapping has been based on naturally occurring deletions. Initially, an interval map dividing the Y chromosome into seven segments was reported [21], and this was further delineated into 43 subintervals [22], resulting in the most commonly used map of the human Y chromosome. Almost 30 years ago, Tiepolo and Zuffardi were first to report microscopically detectable deletions in the distal potion of Yq in six azoospermic men [23]. Their findings suggested the presence of genes regulating spermatogenesis in the distal potion of Yq later referred to as the azoospermia factor (*AZF*). Further studies of men with nonobstructive severe oligozoospermia or azoospermia [24, 25] suggested the existence of a multitude of loci within Yq that may be associated with infertility, and lead to the characterization of three separate, nonoverlapping regions required for spermatogenesis referred to as *AZFa*, *AZFb*, and *AZFc* [25]. A fourth *AZF* subregion, positioned between *AZFb* and *AZFc* has also been proposed and named *AZFd* [26].

Studies of Y chromosome deletions have also demonstrated that although the genes within the nonrecombining portion play an important role in male fertility, their loss is not exclusively linked with azoospermia [27]. Indeed, microdeletions within the AZF regions have been associated with a multitude of clinical findings including Sertoli-cell-only syndrome, spermatogenic arrest, and morphological abnormalities of postmeiotic germ cells.

Naturally occurring infertility-associated deletions may be restricted to any one of the *AZF* regions or they may extend beyond a given region to encompass multiple subregions of *AZF*. In a series of reviews by Simoni and colleagues, four clinically relevant Y chromosome microdeletions found in men with oligo- or azoospermia: *AZFa*, *AZFb*, *AZFbc*, and *AZFc* [28]. The most frequently deleted region is *AZFc* (approximately 60% of cases), followed by deletions of the *AZFb* and *AZFbc* or *AZFabc* regions (35%), while isolated *AZFa* deletions are rare (5%) [29].

39.3.1 Phenotypes Associated with Y Chromosome Microdeletions

Deletions removing the entire *AZFa*, or *AZFb* regions (complete deletions) are associated with Sertoli cell only syndrome and spermatogenic arrest, respectively [30]. Partial deletions of *AZFa* or *AZFb* regions, or complete or partial deletions of *AZFc* region are associated with a variable phenotype ranging from oligozoospermia to Sertoli cell only syndrome. The broad range of phenotypes observed is not surprising in that several potentially functional genes or gene families lie in each *AZF* region. These include *USP9Y* (ubiquitin-specific protease 9, Y chromosome; initially identified as *DFFRY*, Drosophila fat facets related Y), and *DBY* (dead box on the Y) single genes in *AZFa*, *RBM* (RNA-binding motif) gene family in *AZFb*, and *DAZ* (deleted in azoospermia) gene family in *AZFc* [31]. Another explanation for the variable phenotype is the progressive regression of the germinal epithelium reported in patients with *AZFc* microdeletions [32, 33].

39.3.2 Y Chromosome Microdeletions in Fertile and Infertile Man

The pathogenic role of Y chromosome microdeletions in male infertility has been questioned by reports of naturally transmitted deletions removing the entire *AZFc* region [25, 34–36]. Sperm analysis was available in only two cases. Two fathers, one with reduced and the other with unknown sperm count, were able to father a single child [25, 34], whereas the father of four infertile sons was azoospermic many years later, after the natural conception of his sons [35].

Most studies investigating Y chromosome microdeletions used "proven fertile men" as controls rather than "normozoospermic men". Krausz and McElreavey summarized the results of 26 studies reported between 1995 and 2001 and calculated that only 12 of 2,295 proven fertile men, and none of 392 normospermic men had Y chromosome microdeletions [37]. In their elegant discussion, they pointed to the fact that the fertility potential of a man also depends on his partner's fertility potential, and that fertility is not a synonym of normozoospermia [37]. Indeed, the 12 fertile men with Y chromosome microdeletions reported in two studies [26, 34] could have been oligozoospermic. In summary, Y chromosome microdeletions have been found almost exclusively in patients with less than 1 million spermatozoa per milliliter, and are extremely rare (approximately 0.7%) among men with sperm concentrations greater than 5 million spermatozoa per milliliter [29], arguing for an important role for Y chromosome microdeletions in spermatogenic failure.

The incidence of Y chromosome microdeletions reported in infertile men varies between 1% [38] and 55% [39]. This variability may be caused by several factors including patient selection criteria, lack of rigorous testing of negative results, and ethnic variances among study populations [29].

39.3.3 Y Chromosome Microdeletions and ART Outcome

The introduction of ICSI combined with sperm retrieval techniques, such as testicular sperm extraction (TESE), now allows men with Y chromosome microdeletions to reproduce. Mulhall et al. [40] compared eight azoospermic men with *AZFc* deletions with 28 controls with normal Y chromosomes. All patients were treated with TESE and subsequent ICSI. While fertilization rates seemed to be lower in the *AZFc* deletion group compared to controls (36% vs. 45%), there was no statistically significant difference. Pregnancy rates did not differ between the two groups.

In a subsequent study, Van Golde et al. retrospectively compared the success rate of 19 ICSI treatments in eight couples with *AZFc* microdeletions to a control group of 239 ICSI treatments in 107 couples [41]. Ejaculated spermatozoa was used in both study groups. Although they found significantly lower fertilization rates (55% vs. 71%, $p<0.01$) and embryo scores in couples with *AZFc* microdeletions, overall pregnancy rates did not differ.

Oates et al. evaluated 713 men with nonobstructive azospermia or severe oligospermia and identified 42 (5.9%) with microdeletions, strictly confined to the *AZFc* region [42]. They were classified into four subgroups based upon spermatogenic capability: severe oligospermia (16 men); azoospermia with sperm detected on TESE or quantitative histological analysis (14 men); azoospermia with no sperm detected on TESE or quantitative histological analysis (seven men); azoospermia but no TESE or quantitative histological analysis was performed, leaving unanswered the question of whether testicular sperm might be present (five men). A total of 48 cycles of ICSI were performed in 26 of these couples. The overall fertilization rate was 47%, and the overall term pregnancy rate was 27%. The fertilization and term pregnancy rates for those cycles in which ejaculated sperm served as the gamete source were 64 and 47%, respectively. Fertilization rate and term pregnancy rate for the group who had used testicular sperm were 36 and 14%, respectively. Comparing fertilization rates from the ejaculated sperm group with the testicular sperm group revealed a statistically significant difference ($P<0.0001$).

Choi et al. [43] also reported their experience with 17 men with different types of Y chromosome microdeletions. Consistent with previous reports, they were unable to obtain spermatozoa with TESE in men with complete deletion of *AZFa* or *AZFb* or *AZFbc* regions. Spermatozoa was obtained from men with *AZFc* deficiencies and one with partial *AZFb* deficiency. Patients with Y chromosome microdeletions were studied in two groups depending on whether TESE or ejaculated spermatozoa was used. They were compared to matched controls. Although there was a tendency toward decreased fertilization and pregnancy rates, the differences were not statistically significant.

Overall, studies of ART outcome in patients with *AZFc* deletions suggest a tendency toward decreased fertilization rates, but not a significant change in overall pregnancy and delivery rates compared to matched controls [40–43]. Men with ejaculated spermatozoa seem to do significantly better than those who need TESE [42, 43].

39.3.4 Indications for Y Chromosome Microdeletion Testing in a Clinical Setting and the Need for Standardization

As summarized above, clinically relevant deletions are found in patients with azoospermia or a sperm concentration of less than one million spermatozoa per milliliter, and very rarely, in patients with sperm concentration between 1 and 5 million spermatozoa per milliliter [28]. Although the incidence of microdeletions is higher when patients are selected by testicular histology (e.g., Sertoli cell only syndrome), no absolute criteria exist for the selection of patients for molecular analysis. In general, Y chromosome testing is not indicated for patients with chromosomal abnormalities, obstructive azoospermia, or hypogonadotropic hypogonadism [28].

Patients with azoospermia or severe oligospermia who may be candidates for TESE combined with ICSI, should be offered Y chromosome testing because TESE should not be offered in cases of complete *AZFa* or *AZFb* or *AZFbc* deletions [28]. In addition, microdeletions of the *AZFc* region are transmitted to the male offspring if ART is performed [42, 44]. Therefore, information obtained from Y chromosome testing may be used in genetic counseling of patients contemplating ART [28].

With the aim of offering an additional diagnostic tool for male infertility, many laboratories across the world started offering polymerase chain reaction (PCR)-based deletion analysis using in-house methods. This occurred in the absence of a consensus on methodology. The European Academy of Andrology (EAA) and European Molecular Genetics Quality Network (EMQN) supported studies evaluating methodology used in different laboratories. These studies formed the basis of the 1999 Laboratory guidelines for molecular diagnosis of Y-chromosomal microdeletions [45]. Recently, a best practice meeting was held in Florence, Italy in October, 2003, and its conclusions was published [28].

39.4 Epigenetic Factors

Epigenetics refers to the covalent modifications of DNA and core histones that regulate gene activity without altering DNA sequence. To date, the best-characterized DNA modification associated with the modulation of gene activity is methylation of cytosine residues within CpG dinucleotides. CpG methylation, especially within the promoter region of genes, is associated with repression of transcription and provides a means to control gene expression. DNA methylation has been implicated in the regulation of a number of functions including allele-specific gene expression (also called genomic imprinting), X-chromosome inactivation, and heritable transcriptional silencing of parasitic sequence elements [46]. Human disorders associated with epigenetic abnormalities include rare imprinting diseases, molar pregnancies, and childhood cancers.

Germ cell development and early embryo development are critical times when epigenetic patterns are initiated or maintained. Striking modulations in methylation during gametogenesis and embryogenesis occur for imprinted genes that are expressed from only the maternal or the paternal genome. DNA methylation is the best-studied epigenetic mark that distinguishes the maternal and paternal alleles of imprinted genes. Most imprinted genes contain sequences that are differentially methylated in the gametes, and in most cases, the two parental alleles have different levels of DNA methylation. As a heritable, reversible, epigenetic mark, DNA methylation of imprinted genes can be stably propagated after DNA replication and can maintain monoallelic gene expression throughout life.

39.5 DNA Methylation in Gametes and Embryos

Early primordial germ cells (PGCs) are believed to carry somatic epigenetic patterns that are erased prior to and soon after their entry into the future gonads. In the mouse, erasure of DNA methylation in PGCs occurs at about the time these cells enter the gonad [47, 48] and results in a transformation from monoallelic to biallelic expression of imprinted genes [48]. Following the nearly genome-wide demethylation in PGCs, sex- and sequence-specific methylation patterns are re-established in the male and female gametes [49]. Although there is a second phase of genomic demethylation that occurs in the preimplantation embryo, some sequences, notably imprinted genes and some repeat sequences, retain their methylation status acquired at gamete stage. It is postulated that the gamete methylation that is retained during the wave of preimplantation demethylation is important for subsequent postimplantation embryo development.

Methylation at CpG dinucleotides in mammals is catalyzed by DNA (cytosine-5)-methyltransferase (DNMT) enzymes. DNMT1 is the predominant mammalian DNMT, although DNMT2, DNMT3a, DNMT3b, and DNMT3L have been characterized. To date, DNMT1, DNMT3a, and DNMT3b are the only known catalytically active DNMTs [50]. The expression of these three enzymes in both germlines are tightly regulated [51]. Due to embryonic lethality of mice homozygous for targeted deletions in *Dnmt1* [52] and *Dnmt3b* [53], determining the role of these enzymes during spermatogenesis will require germ cell-specific knockout or knockdown studies. *Dnmt3a*-deficient mice are underdeveloped, and die 3–4 weeks after birth. These mice show defects in spermatogenesis [53].

In the mouse and the rat, disruption of DNA methylation in male germ cells by chronic administration of cytosine analogs 5-azacytidine and 5-aza-2′-deoxycytidine has severe consequences for both germ cells and progeny outcome [54–56]. Adverse effects include decreased sperm counts, decreased fertility, and increased preimplantation loss. These findings argue for an important role for epigenetic mechanisms in the control of gamete and embryo development.

39.5.1 Implications of Altered Gamete and Early Embryo DNA Methylation

39.5.1.1 Gestational Trophoblastic Disease

The inability to establish appropriate maternal epigenetic marks on imprinted genes in the human germline has been associated with hydatiform moles. One group of molar pregnancies, termed complete hydatiform moles, is classically described as carrying two paternal haploid genomes. Interestingly, recent studies report complete hydatiform moles arising from normal fertilization events (uniting a maternal and a paternal haploid genome) where the maternal alleles carry paternal imprints or the paternal epigenotype [57–59]. Hayward et al. failed to detect mutations in the known DNMTs that might account for the failure of methylation in the female germline [60]. Their findings suggest that maternal imprinting during oogenesis may involve additional factors.

39.5.1.2 Imprinting Diseases

Animal studies suggest that epigenetic marks, especially DNA methylation, are unstable and can be altered by culture conditions [61, 62]. Assisted reproductive technologies rely on manipulation and culture of gametes and embryos at times when epigenetic programs are being acquired and modified. An initial study found no evidence of altered methylation at 15q11-13, the locus linked to the pathogenesis of the imprinting disorders Angelman and Prader-Willi syndromes, in samples from 92 children conceived using ICSI [63].

A number of studies have now reported the association of two imprinting disorders with assisted reproductive technologies; Beckwith–Wiedemann syndrome [64–67] and Angelman syndrome [68, 69].

Angelman syndrome has an incidence of approximately 1 in 15,000 children, and is characterized by mental retardation, ataxia, epilepsy, hypotonia, and absence of speech. It results from a loss of function of the maternal allele or duplication of the paternal allele within a region of 15q11-13 that spans the gene *UBE3A*. In 5% of affected children, the syndrome is due to loss of methylation within the *SNRPN* imprinting region, which then assumes a hypomethylated, paternal profile. Cox et al. [68] reported two children and Ostavik et al. [69] reported a third child with Angelman syndrome who were conceived using ICSI. In all three cases, a loss of methylation on the maternal *SNRPN* allele was found.

Beckwith–Wiedemann syndrome is characterized by prenatal or postnatal overgrowth, macroglossia, abdominal wall defects, neonatal hypoglycemia, hemihypertrophy, ear abnormalities, and an increased risk of embryonal tumors. Analysis of Beckwith–Wiedemann syndrome registries from three centers has shown the proportion of individuals with Beckwith–Wiedemann syndrome conceived using IVF to be 3/65, 6/149, and 6/149 syndrome [64–66]. These data, when combined, suggest that 4% of individuals with Beckwith–Wiedemann syndrome are conceived with IVF, a figure greater than that expected in relation to the use of IVF in these centers. Further interpretation of these results has been limited because of a reliance by these studies on case records of questionnaire data to determine the method of conception, a lack of use of appropriate controls, and a statistical significance that was either borderline [65, 66] or not mentioned [64]. More recently, Halliday et al. reported the first case–control study in an Australian population [67]. Among 1,316,500 live births in Victoria between 1983 and 2003, they identified 37 cases of Beckwith–Wiedemann syndrome. For each Beckwith–Wiedemann syndrome case, they randomly selected four live-born controls. IVF was the method of conception in four Beckwith–Wiedemann syndrome cases and in one control. Their results indicated that if a child has Beckwith–Wiedemann syndrome, the odds that the child was conceived using IVF was 18 times greater than that for a child without Beckwith–Wiedemann syndrome. The calculated risk of Beckwith–Wiedemann syndrome in the IVF population was 1/4,000, or nine times greater than the general population. Although this study has shortcomings including a large confidence interval, its results are concerning.

Beckwith–Wiedemann syndrome is linked to a loss of function of the maternal allele at 11p15 [70]. Two epigenetic DNA methylation defects have been associated with Beckwith–Wiedemann syndrome. The most common one involves loss of methylation at the maternal *KVDMR1/LIT1* (46% of cases) population [67], and the other a gain of methylation at *H19 DMD* on the maternal allele such that it assumes a paternal (methylated) profile (7% of cases). The rest is due to uniparental disomy of chromosome 11 (16%) and to an unidentified mutation (31%) [67].

A total of 15 cases with Beckwith–Wiedemann syndrome were evaluated for methylation defects in the four studies. Of those, 14 showed hypomethylation of maternal *KVDMR1/LIT1*. The preponderance of Beckwith–Wiedemann syndrome cases conceived by IVF that show hypomethylation of maternal *KVDMR1/LIT1* suggests that collection or in vitro culture conditions may disturb the methylation in the oocyte or the embryo, predisposing the maternal allele to demethylation. While the spermatozoon does not seem to be the source of altered methylation in the case of Beckwith–Wiedemann and Angelman syndromes, the same mechanisms may be effective in causing altered methylation of spermatozoal genes.

39.5.2 Imprinting in Spermatozoa of Men with Abnormal Semen Parameters

An initial study by Manning et al., using PCR-based techniques to analyze DNA extracted from spermatozoa of men with normal semen analysis ($n=30$) and from men with medium ($n=30$, 5–20 million spermatozoa/mL) and high-grade semen pathology ($n=30$, <5 million spermatozoa/mL) undergoing ICSI, failed to detect a difference in methylation status [71]. More recently, Marques et al. studied two oppositely imprinted genes in spermatozoan DNA from normozoospermic and oligozoospermic patients. In the mesodermal-specific transcript gene (MEST), bisulfite genomic sequencing showed that maternal imprinting was correctly erased in all 123 patients. However, methylation of the H19 gene did not change in any of 27 normozoospermic individuals (0%) compared with methylation changes in eight moderate (17%, $p=0.026$) and 15 severe (30%, $p=0.002$) oligozoospermic patients. Their findings suggest an association between abnormal genomic imprinting and hypospermatogenesis, and that spermatozoa from oligozoospermic patients carry a raised risk of transmitting imprinting errors [72]. Hartmann et al. [73] also analyzed imprinting in disruptive spermatogenesis. They explored the methylation pattern of SNRPN (paternally expressed) and H19 gene in different germ cell types obtained by testicular biopsies of a few infertile patients. They demonstrated correct genetic imprints for SNRPN and H19 in spermatogonia, primary spermatocytes and spermatids selected from seminiferous tubules exhibiting spermatogenic arrest. The conflicting results of these two reports clearly indicate that this area is still lacking in clear information.

Testicular sperm extraction and intracytoplasmic sperm injection (TESE-ICSI) is a frequently used therapeutic option in azoospermic males. Manning et al. used a heminested methylation-specific polymerase chain reaction for the target region 15q11-13 to analyze imprinting at the single-cell level in cells from different stages of spermatogenesis. They analyzed spermatozoa, elongated spermatids, and round spermatids and found completed establishment of the correct paternal imprint in these three developmental stages. However, the high rate of amplification failure in round spermatids in this study is a factor of uncertainty [74].

39.6 Conclusions

The rapid acceptance and success of ICSI to treat many types of male infertility has seen it surpass the concurrent need to diagnostically scrutinize the male infertility patient. A general outline for diagnostic screening of males is given in Fig. 39.1. Although it is impossible to deny treatment, it seems apparent from the current evidence that some vigilance is still needed prior to proceeding with treatment, especially in males with extremely poor sperm parameters.

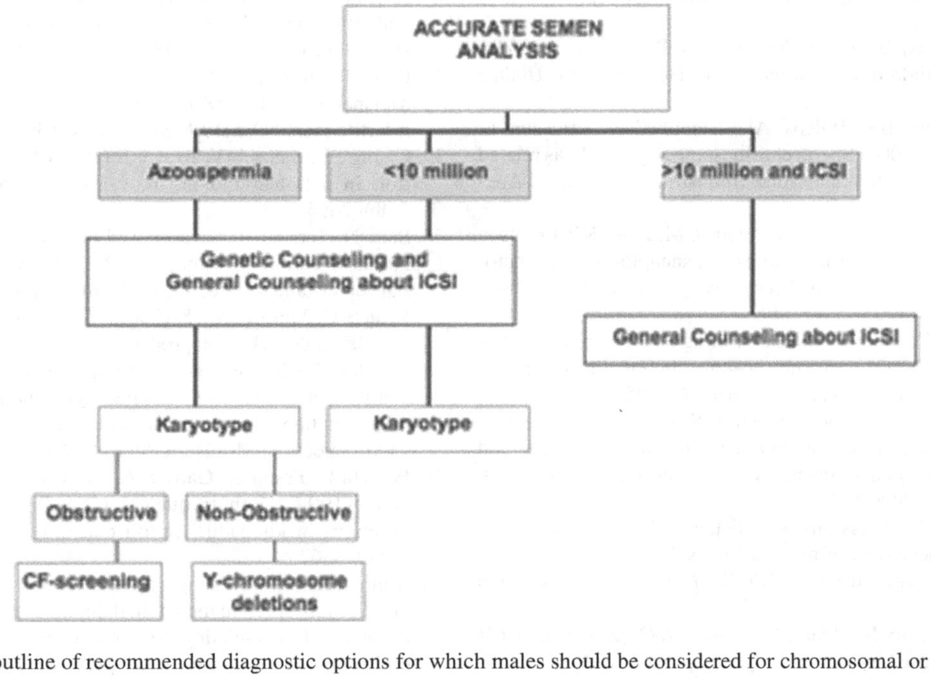

Fig. 39.1 A general outline of recommended diagnostic options for which males should be considered for chromosomal or genetic screening

References

1. Hassold T, Abruzzo M, Adkins K, Griffin D, Merrill M, Millie E et al (1996) Human aneuploidy: incidence, origin, and etiology. Environ Mol Mutagen 28(3):167–175
2. Gianaroli L, Magli MC, Ferraretti AP, Tabanelli C, Trombetta C, Boudjema E (2002) The role of preimplantation diagnosis for aneuploidies. Reprod Biomed Online 4(Suppl 3):31–36
3. Hassold TJ (1998) Nondisjunction in the human male. Curr Topics Dev Biol 37:383–406
4. Jacobs PA (1992) The chromosome complement of human gametes. Oxf Rev Reprod Biol 14:42–72
5. Marquez C, Cohen J, Munne S (1998) Chromosome identification in human oocytes and polar bodies by spectraal karyotyping. Cytogenet Cell Genet 51:254–258
6. Fragouli E, Wells D, Thornhill A, Serhal P, Faed MJ, Harper JC et al (2006) Comparative genomic hybridization analysis of human oocytes and polar bodies. Hum Reprod 21(9):2319–2328
7. Kamiguchi Y, Mikamo K (1986) An improved, efficient method for analyzing human sperm chromosomes using zona-free hamster ova. Am J Hum Genet 38:724–740
8. MacDonald M, Hassold T, Harvey J, Wang LH, Morton NE, Jacobs P (1994) The origin of 47,XXY and 47,XXX aneuploidy. Heterogenous mechanisms and the role of aberrant recombination. Hum Mol Genet 3:1365–1371
9. Jacobs P, Dalton P, James R, Mosse K, Power M, Obinson D et al (1997) Turner syndrome: a cytogenetic and molecular study. Ann Hum Genet 61:471–483
10. Hansen M, Kurinczuk JJ, Bower C, Webb S (2002) The risk of major birth defects after intracytoplasmic sperm injection and in vitro fertilization. N Engl J Med 346(10):725–730
11. Van Steirteghem A (1998) Outcome of assisted reproductive technology. N Engl J Med 338:194–195
12. Bonduelle M, Camus M, De Vos A, Staessen C, Tournaye H, Van Assche E et al (1999) Seven years of intracytoplasmic sperm injection and follow-up of 1987 subsequent children. Hum Reprod 14(Suppl 1):243–264
13. Kurinczuk JJ, Bower C (1997) Birth defects in infants conceived by intracytoplasmic sperm injection: an alternative interpretation. Br Med J 315:1260–1265
14. Van Steirteghem A, Bonduelle M, Devroey P, Liebaers I (2002) Follow-up of children born after ICSI. Hum Reprod Update 8:111–116
15. Carrell DT, Emery BR, Wilcox AL, Campbell B, Erickson L, Hatasaka HH et al (2004) Sperm chromosome aneuploidy as related to male factor infertility and some ultrastructure defects. Arch Androl 50:181–185
16. Carrell DT, Wilcox AL, Lowy L, Peterson CM, Jones KP, Erickson L et al (2003) Elevated sperm chromosome aneuploidy and apoptosis in patients with unexplained recurrent pregnancy loss. Obstet Gynecol 101:1229–1235
17. Rubio C, Simon C, Blanco V, Vidal F, Minguez Y, Egozcue J et al (1999) Implications of sperm chromosome abnormalities in recurrent miscarriage. J Assist Reprod Genet 16:253–258
18. Jakab A, Sakkas D, Delpiano E, Cayli S, Kovanci E, Ward D et al (2005) Intracytoplasmic sperm injection: a novel selection method for sperm with normal frequency of chromosomal aneuploidies. Fertil Steril 84(6):1665–1673
19. Cozzi J, Chevret E, Rousseaux S, Pelletier R, Benitz V, Jalbert H et al (1994) Achievement of meiosis in XXY germ cells: study of 543 sperm karyotypes from an XY/XXY mosaic patient. Hum Genet 93(1):32–34
20. Chevret E, Rousseaux S, Monteil M, Usson Y, Cozzi J, Pelletier R et al (1996) Increased incidence of hyperhaploid 24, XY spermatozoa detected by three-colour FISH in a 46, XY/47, XXY male. Hum Genet 97(2):171–175
21. Vergnaud G, Page DC, Simmler MC, Brown L, Rouyer F, Noel B et al (1986) A deletion map of the human Y chromosome based on DNA hybridization. Am J Hum Genet 38:109–124
22. Vollrath D, Foote S, Hilton A, Brown LG, Beer-Romero P, Bogan JS et al (1992) The human Y chromosome: a 43-interval map based on naturally occuring deletions. Science 258:52–59
23. Tiepolo L, Zuffardi O (1976) Localization of factors controlling spermatogenesis in the nonfluorescent portion of the human Y chromosome long arm. Hum Genet 34:119–124
24. Vogt P, Chandley AC, Hargreave TB, Keil R, Ma K, Sharkey A (1992) Microdeletions in interval 6 of the Y chromosome of males with idiopathic sterility point to disruption of AZF, a human spermatogenesis gene. Hum Genet 89:491–496
25. Vogt P, Edelman A, Kirsch S, Henegariu O, Hirschmann P, Kiesewetter F et al (1996) Human Y chromosome azoospermia factors (AZF) mapped to different subregions in Yq11. Hum Mol Genet 5:933–943
26. Kent-First M, Muallem A, Shultz J, Pryor J, Roberts K, Nolten W et al (1999) Defining regions of the Y-chromosome responsible for male infertility and identification of a fourth AZF region (AZF-d) by Y chromosome microdeletion detection. Mol Reprod Dev 53:27–41
27. Reijo R, Alagappan RK, Patrizio P, Page DC (1996) Severe oligozoospermia resulting from deletions of azoospermia factor gene on Y chromosome. Lancet 347:1290–1293
28. Simoni M, Bakker E, Krausz C (2004) EAA/EMQN best practice guidelines for molecular diagnosis of y-chromosomal microdeletions. State of the art 2004. Int J Androl 27:240–249
29. Krausz C, Forti G, McElreavey K (2003) The Y chromosome and male fertility and infertility. Int J Androl 26(2):70–75
30. Krausz C, Quintana-Murci L, McElreavey K (2000) Prognostic value of Y deletion analysis: what is the clinical prognostic value of Y chromosome microdeletion analysis? Hum Reprod 15(7): 1431–1434
31. Kent-First M (2000) The Y chromosome and its role in testis differentiation and spermatogenesis. Semin Reprod Med 18:67–80
32. Warchol JB, Jankowska A, Stecewicz D, Ciesielski M, Wasko R (2000) Analysis of the seminiferous tubules of patients with deletion of DAZ gene. Arch Perinatal Med 6:10–16
33. Colegero AE, Garofalo MR, Barone N, Palma AD, Vicari E, Romeo R et al (2001) Spontaneous regression over time of the germinal epithelium in a Y chromosome-microdeleted patient: case report. Hum Reprod 16:1845–1848
34. Pryor JL, Kent-First M, Muallem A, Van Bergen AH, Nolten WE, Meisner L et al (1997) Microdeletions in the Y chromosome of infertile men. N Engl J Med 336:534–539
35. Chang PL, Sauer MV, Brown S (1999) Y chromosome microdeletion in a father and his four infertile sons. Hum Reprod 14: 2689–2694
36. Saut N, Terriou P, Navarro A, Levy N, Mitchell MJ (2000) The human Y chromosome genes BPY2, CDY1, and DAZ are not essential for sustained fertility. Mol Hum Reprod 6:789–793
37. Krausz C, McElreavey K (2001) Y chromosome microdeletions in 'fertile' males. Hum Reprod 16(6):1306–1307
38. van der Ven K, Montag M, Peschka B, Leygraaf J, Schwanitz G, Haidl G et al (1997) Combined cytogenetic and Y chromosome microdeletion screening in males undergoing intracytoplasmic sperm injection. Mol Hum Reprod 3:699–704
39. Foresta C, Ferlin A, Garolla A, Moro E, Pistorello M, Barbaux S et al (1998) High frequency of well-defined Y chromosome deletions in idiopathic Sertoli cell only syndrome. Hum Reprod 13:302–307
40. Mulhall JP, Reijo R, Alagappan R, Brown L, Page D, Carson R et al (1997) Azoospermic men with deletion of the DAZ gene cluster are capable of completing spermatogenesis: fertilization, normal embryonic development and pregnancy occur when retrieved testicular spermatozoa are used for intracytoplasmic sperm injection. Hum Reprod 12(3):503–508

41. van Golde RJ, Wetzels AM, de Graaf R, Tuerlings JH, Braat DD, Kremer JA (2001) Decreased fertilization rate and embryo quality after ICSI in oligozoospermic men with microdeletions in the azoospermia factor c region of the Y chromosome. Hum Reprod 16(2):289–292
42. Oates RD, Silber S, Brown LG, Page DC (2002) Clinical characterization of 42 oligospermic or azoospermic men with microdeletion of the AZFc region of the Y chromosome, and of 18 children conceived via ICSI. Hum Reprod 17(11):2813–2824
43. Choi JM, Chung P, Veeck L, Mielnik A, Palermo GD, Schlegel PN (2004) AZF microdeletions of the Y chromosome and in vitro fertilization outcome. Fertil Steril 81(2):337–341
44. Page DC, Silber S, Brown LG (1999) Men with infertility caused by AZFc deletion can produce sons by intracytoplasmic sperm injection, but are likely to transmit the deletion and infertility. Hum Reprod 14:1722–1726
45. Simoni M, Bakker E, Eurlings MC, Matthijs G, Moro E, Muller CR et al (1999) Laboratory guidelines for molecular diagnosis of Y-chromosomal microdeletions. Int J Androl 22(5):292–299
46. Bestor TH (2000) The DNA methyltransferases of mammals. Hum Mol Genet 9:2395–2402
47. Szabo PE, Mann JR (1995) Biallelic expression of imprinted genes in the mouse germ line: implications for erasure, establishment, and mechanisms of genomic imprinting. Genes Dev 9:1857–1868
48. Szabo PE, Hubner K, Scholer H, Mann JR (2002) Allele-specific expression of imprinted genes in mouse migratory primordial germ cells. Mech Dev 115:157–160
49. Reik W, Dean W, Walter J (2001) Epigenetic reprogramming in mammalian development. Science 293(5532):1089–1093
50. Kelly TLJ, Trasler JM (2004) Reproductive epigenetics. Clin Genet 65:247–260
51. La Salle S, Mertineit C, Taketo T, Moens PB, Bestor TH, Trasler JM (2004) Windows for sex-specific methylation marked by DNA methyltransferase expression profiles in mouse germ cells. Dev Biol 268(2):403–415
52. Li E, Bestor TH, Jaenisch R (1992) Targeted mutation of the DNA methyltransferase gene results in embryonic lethality. Cell 69:915–926
53. Okano M, Bell DW, Haber DA, Li E (1999) DNA methyltransferases Dnmt3a and Dnmt3b are essential for de novo methylation and mammalian development. Cell 99:247–257
54. Doerksen T, Trasler JM (1996) Developmental exposure of male germ cells to 5-azacytidine results in abnormal preimplantation development in rats. Biol Reprod 55:1155–1162
55. Doerksen T, Benoit G, Trasler JM (2000) Deoxyribonucleic acidhypomethylation of male germ cells by mitotic and meiotic exposure to 5-azacytidine is associated with altered testicular histology. Endocrinology 141:3235–3244
56. Kelly TL, Li E, Trasler JM (2003) 5-aza-2′-deoxycytidine induces alterations in murine spermatogenesis and pregnancy outcome. J Androl 24:822–830
57. Helwani MN, Seoud M, Zahed L, Zaatari G, Khalil A, Slim RA (1999) A familial case of recurrent hydatiform molar pregnancies with biparental genomic contribution. Hum Genet 105:112–115
58. Moglabey YB, Kircheisen R, Seoud M, El Mogharbel N, Van De Veyver I, Slim R (1999) Genetic mapping of a maternal locus responsible for familial hydatiform moles. Hum Mol Genet 8:667–671
59. Fisher RA, Khatoon R, Paradinas FJ, Roberts AP, Newlands AS (2000) Repetitive complete hydatiform mole can be biparental in origin and either male or female. Hum Reprod 15:594–598
60. Hayward BE, De Vos M, Judson H, Hodge D, Huntriss J, Picton HM et al (2003) Lack of involvement of known DNA methyltransferases in familial hydatidiform mole implies the involvement of other factors in establishment of imprinting in the human female germline. BMC Genet 4:2
61. Doherty A, Mann M, Tremblay K, Bartolomei M, Schultz R (2000) Differential effects of culture on imprinted H19 expression in the preimplantation mouse embryo. Biol Reprod 62(6):1526–1535
62. Young L, Fernandes K, McEvoy T, Butterwith S, Gutierrez C, Carolan C et al (2001) Epigenetic change in IGF2R is associated with fetal overgrowth after sheep embryo culture. Nat Genet 27: 153–154
63. Manning M, Lissens W, Bonduelle M, Camus M, De Rijcke M, Liebaers I et al (2000) Study of DNA-methylation patterns at chromosome 15q11–q13 in children born after ICSI reveals no imprinting defects. Mol Hum Reprod 6(11):1049–1053
64. DeBaun MR, Niemitz EL, Feinberg AP (2003) Association of in vitro fertilization with Beckwith-Wiedemann syndrome and epigenetic alterations of LIT1 and H19. Am J Hum Genet 72(1): 156–160
65. Gicquel C, Gaston V, Mandelbaum J, Siffroi JP, Flahault A, Le Bouc Y (2003) In vitro fertilization may increase the risk of Beckwith-Wiedemann syndrome related to the abnormal imprinting of the KCN1OT gene. Am J Hum Genet 72(5):1338–1341
66. Maher ER, Brueton LA, Bowdin SC, Luharia A, Cooper W, Cole TR et al (2003) Beckwith-Wiedemann syndrome and assisted reproduction technology (ART). J Med Genet 40(1):62–64
67. Halliday J, Oke K, Breheny S, Algar E, Amor DJ (2004) Beckwith-Wiedemann syndrome and IVF: a case-control study. Am J Hum Genet 75(3):526–528
68. Cox GF, Burger J, Lip V, Mau UA, Sperling K, Wu BL et al (2002) Intracytoplasmic sperm injection may increase the risk of imprinting defects. Am J Hum Genet 71(1):162–164
69. Orstavik KH, Eiklid K, van der Hagen CB, Spetalen S, Kierulf K, Skjeldal O et al (2003) Another case of imprinting defect in a girl with Angelman syndrome who was conceived by intracytoplasmic semen injection. Am J Hum Genet 72(1):218–219
70. Weksberg R, Smith AC, Squire J, Sadowski P (2003) Beckwith-Wiedemann syndrome demonstrates a role for epigenetic control of normal development. [Review] [98 refs]. Hum Mol Genet 12(1): 61–68
71. Manning M, Lissens W, Liebaers I, Van Steirteghem A, Weidner W (2001) Imprinting analysis in spermatozoa prepared for intracytoplasmic sperm injection (ICSI). Int J Androl 24(2):87–94
72. Marques CJ, Carvalho F, Sousa M, Barros A (2004) Genomic imprinting in disruptive spermatogenesis. Lancet 363(9422): 1700–1702
73. Hartmann S, Bergmann M, Bohle RM, Weidner W, Steger K (2006) Genetic imprinting during impaired spermatogenesis. Mol Hum Reprod 12(6):407–411
74. Manning M, Lissens W, Weidner W, Liebaers I (2001) DNA methylation analysis in immature testicular sperm cells at different developmental stages. Urol Int 67(2):151–155

Chapter 40
Micromanipulation of Human Oocytes and Embryos: Applications of Intracytoplasmic Sperm Injection and Assisted Hatching in Infertility Treatment

Kenneth I. Aston and Klaus E. Weimer

Abstract Embryo micromanipulation methods, including intracytoplasmic sperm injection and assisted hatching, have become powerful tools in infertility treatment. These techniques have enabled the treatment of couples who would not otherwise be able to conceive using conventional IVF and have greatly improved the probability of success in many cases. While micromanipulation methods have revolutionized infertility treatment and a great deal of progress has been made since the inception of these techniques, continued research will further advance the technology and help clinicians in determining the best indications for the application of these techniques. This chapter discusses the current state of the technology as well as future directions for continued research.

Keywords IVF • Human oocytes • Micromanipulation • Human embryos • ICSI • Assisted hatching

40.1 Introduction

The use of micromanipulation to improve fertilization outcomes and implantation potential is an adaptation of techniques commonly used to improve the genetic quality of economically important animals in the field of animal husbandry. Early applications of micromanipulation in domesticated species were usually confined to increasing the number of embryos available for embryo transfer in genetically valuable animals. Specifically, embryos obtained at later stage by uterine lavage were either split in two or used for nuclear transplantation [1, 2].

The adaptation of these techniques to clinical human embryology was undertaken to attempt to improve fertilization outcomes in cases with suboptimal semen parameters. The first human pregnancy resulting from microsurgical fertilization was reported by Malter and Cohen in 1989 [3]. The methodology described by these investigators was called "partial zona dissection" (PZD) and was a means of introducing a small gap in the zona pellucida (ZP) with a fine needle through the perivitelline space of oocytes shortly after retrieval. This small gap allowed motile spermatozoa to freely circumvent the barrier of the zona. This technique worked best in cases where sperm numbers were so low that fertilization by conventional means would have been highly unlikely. The second microsurgical method applied to male factor cases is called subzonal sperm injection (SUZI, or SZI). The technique is performed by aspirating several sperm into a sharp, beveled microneedle. The loaded needle is then placed into the perivitelline space of an oocyte and the sperm are deposited in this space [4]. Partial zona dissection and SUZI were the first microsurgical techniques, whereby patients with poor semen parameters could become biological parents with the use of in vitro fertilization (IVF). It provided a viable alternative to the use of donor sperm. However, the successful application of these techniques was technically challenging with consistent results requiring great care and skill. Nonetheless, these techniques were landmark because they successfully introduced the concept of gamete micromanipulation in a clinical human embryology setting.

The common aspect between PZD and SZI is that there was no direct contact of the microneedle with the oolemma of the oocyte. Early experiments involving direct injection of the spermatozoa in the oocyte cytoplasm demonstrated that sperm nuclear decondensation can occur without the requirement of sperm and egg membrane fusion [5]. This process of direct spermatozoal injection, referred to as intracytoplasmic sperm injection (ICSI) was utilized in the successful production of live rabbits in 1987 [6]. In 1992, Palermo et al. [7] reported the first human pregnancies and healthy births following ICSI. Since this time, the use of ICSI has replaced various methods of microsurgical fertilization. To review the ICSI technique, a

K.I. Aston (✉)
Department of Urology, University of Utah School of Medicine, Salt Lake City, UT, USA
e-mail: kiaston@utah.edu

K.E. Weimer
Northwest Center for Reproductive Sciences, Kirkland, WA, USA
e-mail: kwiemer@nwreprosci.com

D.T. Carrell and C.M. Peterson (eds.), *Reproductive Endocrinology and Infertility: Integrating Modern Clinical and Laboratory Practice*,
DOI 10.1007/978-1-4419-1436-1_40,

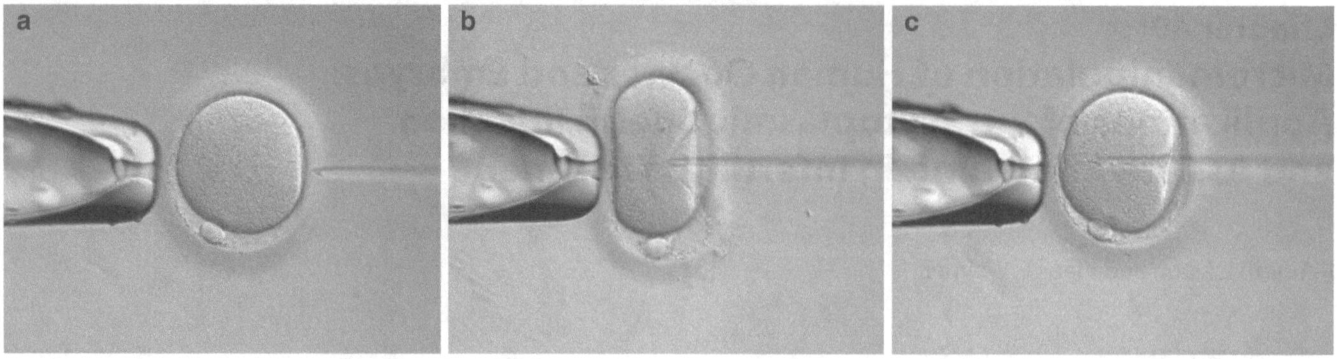

Fig. 40.1 The basic ICSI procedure using a beveled pipette. (**a**) Polar body is positioned at 6 or 12 o'clock. (**b**) Following penetration of the zona, the oolemma is distended and gently aspirated to facilitate controlled breakage of the membrane. (**c**) Following oolemma penetration the spermatozoa (*visible near the end of the pipette*) is deposited deep within the ooplasm

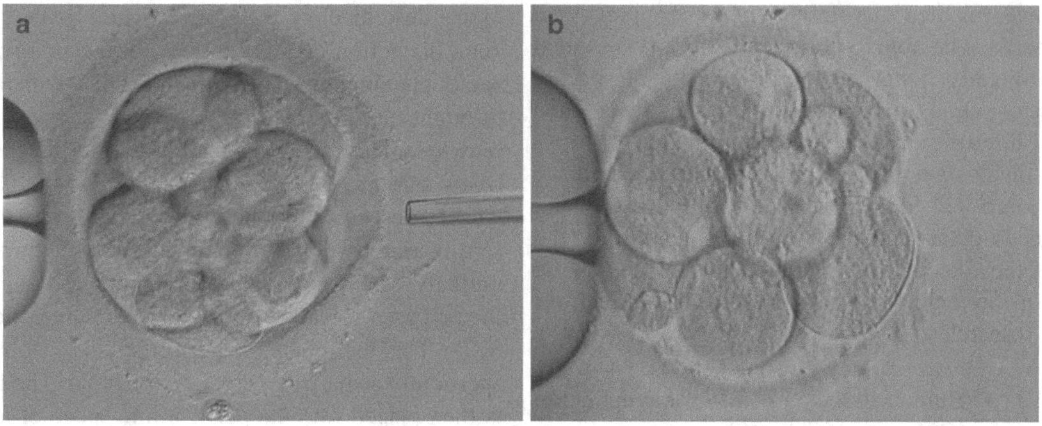

Fig. 40.2 Embryos following AH. Embryos hatched using (**a**) acid Tyrode's and (**b**) laser (laser photo courtesy of Dr. Denny Sakkas, Yale University). Hatching is generally performed in an area of the embryo adjacent to an area of empty perivitelline space or extracellular fragments. A widened region of perivitelline space corresponding to the junction between blastomeres. Note the differences in the holes created by the two methods

microneedle containing an immobilized sperm is used to deliver the sperm deep within the ooplasm following controlled breakage of the oolemma (Fig. 40.1). Today, ICSI offers fertilization rates that equal or surpass rates obtained using conventional insemination techniques with sperm possessing normal parameters.

Following IVF, the culture of human embryos can often result in less than ideal morphological attributes. Specifically, embryos can develop at inconsistent rates and often contain blastomeres of unequal size and orientation as well as poor cell-to-cell adhesion (compaction) in relation to other blastomeres. In addition, blastomeres can begin to undergo fragmentation or extrude cellular material, which can result in the presence of fragments within the embryo. It is possible that these fragments can interfere with the subsequent development of the embryo prior to hatching. Other dimorphic features noted in developing embryos include vacuoles, grainy and/or loose cytoplasm and contracted cytoplasm. These morphological aspects and others have been noted in many embryos despite the improvements made to culture media formulations. In some cases, these deficiencies result in failure of the embryo to properly hatch from the zona and subsequently implant.

Assisted embryo hatching (AH) is another micromanipulation technique utilized in human embryology in an effort to improve implantation rates following IVF. The technique involves thinning or breeching the zona pellucida to facilitate embryonic hatching (Fig. 40.2). It was fist demonstrated to improve implantation rates in 1990 by Cohen et al. and has since become a common micromanipulation technique in human IVF [8].

40.2 Intracytoplasmic Sperm Injection

Intracytoplasmic sperm injection is an alternative to standard microdrop insemination that allows the production of viable embryos even in cases of severe male factor infertility. The procedure involves the direct injection of a single spermatozoon into a mature oocyte (Fig. 40.1). Intracytoplasmic sperm injection is generally indicated in cases of low sperm motility, abnormal morphology, low sperm count, and repeated fertilization failure after conventional IVF. The criteria for utilizing ICSI over microdrop insemination vary from lab to lab. Since the first successful ICSI pregnancies in human ART in 1992, ICSI has become commonplace in human infertility centers. In 2005, ICSI was used in approximately 62% of all IVF cases in SART reporting labs in the United States, and some labs use ICSI exclusively in all IVF cases [9]. Similarly, statistics from European labs reporting to ESHRE for 2004 indicated 59% of all IVF cases used ICSI [10]. While ICSI associated with non-male factor infertility generally results in pregnancy rates equivalent to conventional IVF, no data supports the exclusive use of ICSI in all IVF cycles, and the overuse of ICSI raises concerns about potential consequences of unnecessary interventions.

40.3 ICSI Methods

The basic techniques for ICSI are quite straightforward. In general, cumulus cells are removed from mature oocytes by pipetting in an enzymatic solution often containing hyaluronidase. Following cumulus cell removal, oocytes are secured by aspiration with a small internal diameter, polished pipette with the polar body in either the 6 o'clock or 12 o'clock position and the sperm injection occurring at the 3 o'clock or 9 o'clock position; depending on the orientation of the holding pipette. With the oocyte held in place, an immobilized mature spermatocyte is subsequently injected into the oocyte cytoplasm. Variations of the ICSI procedure include incomplete removal of cumulus cells, the utilization of different tools for sperm injection, artificial activation of ICSI embryos, deviation in polar body location during the sperm injection process, variations in sperm cell selection methods, and the injection of various stages of sperm cells.

40.3.1 Cumulus Cells and ICSI

While the exact role of cumulus cells in oocyte growth and maturation and early embryo development have not been fully elucidated [11], it has been demonstrated that coculture with cumulus cells results in improved embryonic development [12, 13]. Recently, a prospective study by Ebner et al. demonstrated that the incomplete removal of cumulus cells prior to ICSI results in improved preimplantation development in some cases [14]. To date, data regarding the importance of cumulus cells on embryo development following ICSI is limited, but it appears that they may aid in ICSI embryo development as they do following conventional IVF. It may be possible that the cumulus cells might be altering the media composition by either adding factor(s) or removing compounds from the media.

40.3.2 ICSI Tools

While the basic methodology for ICSI is essentially the same among embryology labs, there are several choices for injection tools. A beveled glass pipette is most commonly used for sperm injection, however other options include laser assisted ICSI, the piezo-driven pipette as well and a recently developed rotationally oscillating drill (Ros-Drill). The piezo-driven pipette relies on the rapid expansion of a piezoelectric material when acted upon by an electrical pulse. Rapid longitudinal oscillation of the piezo-driven pipette facilitates zona penetration and reduces oocyte deformation [15]. Piezo-assisted ICSI has been shown to result in improved fertilization and cleavage rates when compared with the standard injection system [15], but data is limited. Laser-assisted ICSI, which employs a laser beam to penetrate the zona prior to sperm injection, has also been successfully utilized on a limited basis [16, 17]. The use of this technique has been primarily limited to oocytes with very thin or fragile zona pellucidae. The Ros-Drill creates rotational oscillations to facilitate penetration of the zona and oolemma [18]. Relatively good fertilization rates have been reported using this technology in mice [18], but there are no data reporting its efficacy in human ICSI.

40.3.3 Artificial Activation Following ICSI

While ICSI generally results in higher fertilization rates than conventional IVF, complete fertilization failure following ICSI occurs in approximately 1–3% of cases [19–21]. In many cases, complete fertilization failure following ICSI is the result of failed oocyte activation [22, 23]. Activational failure following ICSI is commonly associated with globozoospermia because of the absence of an acrosome [24]. Failure of the sperm to activate the oocyte following ICSI can be overcome by a variety of artificial oocyte activation methods.

Typical oocyte activation following fertilization by conventional IVF or ICSI is characterized by a series of repetitive calcium release and resequestration events [25]. These calcium transients are required for cell cycle resumption and subsequent development of the early embryo [26]. In the absence of calcium transients, activation and normal fertilization fail to occur.

Several methods have been employed to overcome activation failure by artificially inducing calcium transients within the embryo. Oocyte activation by applying an electrical stimulus to the embryo creates transient pores in the oolemma through which extracellular calcium can pass creating an artificial rise in intracellular calcium concentration. This method has been shown to be effective in overcoming failed activation following ICSI as demonstrated by the pregnancy and birth of healthy twins following the procedure [27].

Other methods for artificial oocyte activation used successfully in human IVF include treatment with calcium ionophore [24, 28, 29], or strontium chloride [30, 31], and a modified ICSI procedure [32, 33] involving repeated ooplasm aspiration and expulsion during the ICSI procedure. Each of these methods has resulted in the birth of healthy babies following fertilization failure in a previous ICSI cycle. A follow-up on the physical and mental development of five babies born following strontium chloride activation at 1 year of age indicated these babies were developing normally [31].

To date, no large-scale studies have been undertaken to assess the utility and safety of artificial oocyte activation following ICSI. The information available from a handful of case reports and smaller studies so far indicates that artificial activation is both a safe and effective intervention in some cases of failed fertilization.

40.3.4 Sperm Selection

Sperm morphology has long been known to be an important predictor of successful fertilization following conventional IVF; however, early reports indicated that sperm morphology was not an important predictor of ICSI success [34, 35]. It has, in fact, been demonstrated that ICSI with morphologically abnormal and immotile sperm can result in a successful outcome [36]. Recently, a growing body of information indicates sperm morphology is an important consideration in ICSI cases [37, 38].

Sperm selection for conventional ICSI generally occurs at 400× magnification. Ideally, morphologically normal, motile sperm are utilized. If no motile sperm are available, viable sperm can be selected utilizing the hyper-osmotic swelling test (HOS) or pentoxifylline treatment.

While gross morphologically abnormal sperm can be avoided using 400× magnification, fine structural anomalies may be missed using this technique. Some groups have recently shown improved fertilization and ICSI pregnancy rates by selecting sperm based on normal morphology evaluated using digitally enhanced high magnification [39, 40]. A recently developed technique known as motile sperm organellar morphology examination (MSOME) utilizes Nomarski optics coupled with a high power (100×) objective and a CCD camera to produce a digital image at over 6,000× magnification for fine morphological analysis of sperm.

Evaluation of six sub cellular sperm organelles (acrosome, postacrosomal lamina, neck, mitochondria tail, and nucleus) in sperm populations in early retrospective studies utilizing MSOME found an association between sperm morphology and fertilization rates but not pregnancy rates [38]. The study did reveal a positive association between nuclear morphology and pregnancy rate following ICSI [38].

These findings have recently given rise to a technique known as intracytoplasmic morphologically selected sperm injection (IMSI), involving the use of MSOME for the selection of morphologically normal sperm for ICSI. An early prospective IMSI study compared pregnancy rates following conventional ICSI and IMSI in couples with at least two previous failed ICSI cycles and found that sperm selection based on nuclear morphology resulted in significantly higher pregnancy rates when compared with conventional ICSI (66.0% versus 30.0%) [41].

A more recent study by the same group compared outcomes of two IMSI groups: one consisting of patients for whom no morphologically normal nuclei were found and the other of patients for whom sperm with morphologically normal nuclei were utilized for ICSI. The results were significantly higher implantation and pregnancy rates (25.0% and 52.6% versus 12.9% and 18.4%) and significantly lower miscarriage rates (10.0% versus 57.1%) in the normal nuclei group when compared with the abnormal nuclei group [42].

A recent randomized prospective study by a different group obtained similar results using IMSI [40]. In this study, 446 couples were treated either with ICSI or IMSI. In agreement with previous studies, higher clinical pregnancy rates were achieved using the IMSI protocol compared with conventional ICSI (39.2% versus 26.5%) [40]. The authors further concluded that the group that benefited most from IMSI in terms of increased pregnancy rates and decreased miscarriage rates was the group of patients with two or more previous failed IVF attempts. In this subgroup, pregnancy rates were 29.8% following IMSI when compared with 12.9% following ICSI, and miscarriage rates were 17.4% and 37.5% respectively [40].

While the technology is relatively new, and the data are limited, early indications based on a few studies indicate IMSI may be a useful sperm selection technique particularly for specific groups of patients such as those with few morphologically normal sperm or previous failed IVF cycles.

40.3.5 ICSI with Nonejaculated Sperm

Standard ICSI involves the injection of mature spermatocytes to overcome low sperm concentration or motility; however, ICSI is also a viable treatment option for some cases in which no ejaculated sperm can be found. In addition to ejaculated spermatozoa, epididymal and testicular spermatozoa have also been used for ICSI with pregnancy rates comparable to rates following ICSI with ejaculated sperm [43–46].

Early work evaluating postfertilization dynamics following ICSI with ejaculated versus testicular spermatozoa reported no difference in the timing of pronuclear formation between the two groups despite the differing levels of maturity and nuclear compaction between ejaculated and testicular sperm [47].

Fertilization, blastocyst development, and pregnancy rates were evaluated following ICSI using ejaculated spermatozoa, epididymal and testicular spermatozoa from obstructive azoospermic patients, and testicular spermatozoa from nonobstructive azoospermic patients [48]. In this study, fertilization and blastocyst formation rates as well as the incidence of expanded and hatching blastocysts were lower in nonobstructive azoospermic patients. In addition, implantation rates were higher in embryos derived from ejaculated sperm; however, clinical pregnancy rates were not different between groups [48].

A recent study evaluated pregnancy and miscarriage rates following ICSI with ejaculated sperm from oligozoospermic and normospermic men ($n=421$) compared with sperm obtained by percutaneous epididymal aspiration (PESA; $n=69$) and testicular sperm extraction (TESE; $n=47$). This group reported no significant differences in pregnancy or miscarriage rates between the three groups [43].

Recently, Kanto et al. compared fertilization and pregnancy rates following ICSI using sperm obtained by TESE from obstructive azoospermic (OA) versus nonobstructive azoospermic (NOA) men. In contrast to the study by Balaban et al. cited previously [48], this group found no significant differences in fertilization rates between groups, but there was agreement between the two studies that pregnancy rates were not dependent upon the type of azoospermia [44].

Sperm can be recovered by TESE in about 60% or more of nonobstructive azoospermia cases, making ICSI an invaluable tool for such treatment [49]. In cases in which no sperm are recoverable by TESE, the use of haploid round spermatids for ICSI (round spermatid injection [ROSI] or round spermatid nuclear injection [ROSNI]) has been suggested as a potential option for fertility treatment. The idea was originally proposed and tested by Ogura et al. by injecting round spermatid nuclei into hamster oocytes [50]. These experiments demonstrated the capacity of spermatid nuclei to form pronuclei and undergo DNA synthesis. This work was closely followed by another report by the same group, in which homologous electro-fusion of mouse and hamster round spermatids with mature oocytes was utilized to introduce spermatid nuclei into oocytes [51]. In these early experiments, it was observed that a limited number of oocytes were activated, and some developed to the 2-cell stage, however the male pronuclei remained small in most cases [51]. After 1 year the group reported the birth of mice derived from round spermatid nuclei by the same process although only about 1.7% of 2-cell embryos transferred developed to term [52].

The successes demonstrated in mice inspired attempts at ROSNI in humans. The safety and effectiveness of ROSNI has been a topic of considerable debate over the past few years. While ROSNI has been demonstrated to be successful in a few cases [53, 54], fertilization and pregnancy rates are extremely low, and a number of concerns have been raised about the safety of ROSNI.

In one study of 143 oocytes from 14 couples injected with round spermatids, only 36% of oocytes were fertilized successfully, and 7.7% developed beyond the 1-cell stage [55]. Furthermore, no pregnancies were established from the transfer of 11 embryos, and the authors found chromosomal abnormalities in seven of 23 arrested oocytes analyzed by FISH with probes for chromosomes 13, 18, 21, X and Y [55].

In another relatively large study involving 58 couples and over 1,000 oocytes injected by ROSI, only 202 (19.7%) developed 2PN embryos, 126 (12.3%) developed 1 PN embryos, and a total of 16 embryos developed to blastocyst [56]. Twelve embryos were transferred and no pregnancies resulted [56]. Likewise, Yamanaka et al. transferred 24 embryos derived from round spermatids to nine women and failed to achieve pregnancies [57].

In addition to the exceedingly low efficiency of ROSNI, several safety concerns have been raised regarding the practice. Round spermatids are the earliest haploid stage spermatogenic cells and as such are epigenetically very different from mature spermatozoa. At the round spermatid stage, DNA is packaged with histones and remains transcriptionally active. In later stages, beginning with the elongating spermatid stage, transcription is markedly suppressed, and histones are replaced by transition proteins which are subsequently replaced by protamines to achieve a highly compacted and transcriptionally inactive chromatin state [58].

Two groups have demonstrated in the mouse that gene expression in early ROSI embryos is altered when compared with controls raising additional concerns about the safety of the procedure [59, 60].

Elongating spermatid injection (ELSI) has been proposed as an alternative to ROSNI, and this method results in somewhat improved fertilization and pregnancy rates when compared with ROSNI [54, 61, 62], however similar questions regarding safety of this procedure have been raised. Zech et al. reported that of four pregnancies achieved by ELSI, two resulted in major congenital malformations [63]. While in this case causality was not demonstrated directly, the report does illustrate a potential concern.

Given the extremely low efficiencies of ELSI and ROSNI as well as the questions regarding the safety of these procedures, the injection of round and elongating spermatids in ICSI programs is not currently a clinically viable option.

40.4 Indications for the Use of ICSI

A major area of research regarding ICSI involves designating the proper conditions under which its use is indicated. The use of ICSI has risen dramatically in the past few years. Initially the use of ICSI was indicated exclusively for male factor infertility in cases where insufficient progressively motile sperm were available to ensure a reasonable fertilization rate following conventional IVF. Today, the criteria for utilizing ICSI vary widely from lab to lab. Some labs utilize ICSI exclusively, regardless of the source of infertility, because of the relatively high fertilization rates achieved using ICSI and the low incidence of fertilization failure, while other labs use a more conservative approach and apply ICSI only in cases of male factor infertility or previous failed cycles.

Advocates in favor of the exclusive use of ICSI argue that overall, higher fertilization rates are achieved by ICSI than standard IVF, and ICSI offspring are consistently healthy and normal. Conversely, those who advocate the use of ICSI only when conditions warrant it argue that while ICSI is necessary in some cases, ICSI eliminates the competitive selection process of sperm that occurs during natural fertilization and conventional IVF, potentially giving rise unnecessarily to problems in ICSI offspring. In addition, ICSI can affect the developmental rate of embryos.

Intracytoplasmic sperm injection is indicated in cases of obstructive or non-obstructive azoospermia in which immature testicular or epididymal spermatozoa are utilized as well as other cases of male factor infertility such as low motility, abnormal morphology, and low sperm concentration [64]. Cases in which previous IVF attempts have resulted in fertilization failure are generally treated with ICSI as well as cases where sperm concentration is less than 5×10^6/ml in the original sample [65]. A progressively motile sperm concentration of <500,000/ml with <4% normal strict morphology is also generally treated by ICSI [65], while increased oocyte immaturity at retrieval seems to be a contraindication for ICSI [66]. Other cases such as postcancer treatment [67] or a limited number of oocytes [64] also often warrant the use of ICSI.

Sperm function assays (reviewed in chapter by Alukal and Lamb) may be used to help select patients in need of ICSI therapy. One diagnostic tool that has been demonstrated to be effective in assessing the need for ICSI is the sperm penetration assay (SPA) [68]. The assay measures the ability of capacitated sperm to penetrate zona-free hamster eggs in vitro. A prospective study was designed to evaluate the utility of various semen parameters in predicting fertilization rates following conventional IVF [68]. In the study, Freeman et al. found the SPA to be a more sensitive assay for the prediction of IVF fertilization rates than standard semen analysis parameters including concentration and motility [68]. While very low sperm concentrations and progressive motility scores were somewhat predictive of fertilization ability, SPA scores and fertilization rates for previous cycles were by far the most predictive parameters of those assessed [68].

The lack of universal standards or general criteria for the use of ICSI as well as the broad spectrum of criteria used by various IVF labs for deciding whether or not to use ICSI for a particular case strongly illustrates the need for further research.

40.5 ICSI Efficiency

A major impetus for the dramatic and continuing increase in the utilization of ICSI in fertility treatment is the high fertilization rate generally achieved by ICSI. Total fertilization failure rarely occurs with ICSI but is often unpredictable with conventional IVF. In addition to consistently high fertilization rates, embryo development and pregnancy rates are generally comparable following IVF and ICSI. A number of reports have demonstrated fertilization rates equal to or higher following ICSI when compared with conventional IVF [64, 69, 70]. Reports of differences in embryo development rates and embryo quality following IVF versus ICSI are conflicting.

A recent study evaluating embryonic development in sibling oocytes produced by IVF and ICSI found no differences in cleavage rates or embryo quality between the two groups when considering cases with a previous IVF fertilization rate of <40% [70]. However, this study did find ICSI resulted in improved embryo quality in cases of moderate male factor infertility [70]. In another sibling oocyte study in patients with borderline semen, embryo quality was better in ICSI embryos, however no differences were observed in pregnancy rates of transferred embryos [69]. Other studies have reported improved cleavage rates [71] and blastocyst rates [72] following ICSI. Conversely, reports of reduced development to blastocyst [66, 73–76], increased embryo fragmentation [77], and increased incidence of arrested embryos [76] associated with ICSI are numerous. These differences likely reflect differences in patient populations or ICSI protocols as well as differences in skill levels in ICSI technicians [72].

With regard to pregnancy rates, there is a general agreement that when good quality embryos are transferred, embryos derived by ICSI and conventional IVF are equally likely to establish pregnancy [64, 69, 75, 77, 78].

40.6 ICSI Safety

The primary concern with the overuse of ICSI in clinical practice is the potential for the more invasive procedure resulting in unnecessary fetal harm. While the general safety of the ICSI procedure has been well established, there are studies that indicate an increased risk for fetal abnormalities associated with IVF and ICSI. Since ICSI is a relatively new technology, with fewer than two decades of clinical practice in human fertility treatment, long-term follow-up studies evaluating the health and development of ICSI-derived offspring have not been performed. Nevertheless, a number of epidemiological studies and short-term follow-ups have been done, and the results have confirmed that while there are slightly different incidences of some types of fetal abnormalities following ICSI, the risks are quite low and comparable to standard IVF. Continued research with ever-increasing numbers will prove valuable in the future.

Assessment of risks associated with ART procedures in general, as well as ICSI specifically, have been made in a number of settings, and the conclusions of these assessments vary. A major confounder in the assessment of risks associated with IVF or ICSI is the large number of multiple-birth gestations associated with ART. Of infants born through ART procedures in the United States in 2005, 49% were twins or higher order multiples [9], and in Europe about 37.5% of ART infants were born as twins or triplets [10]. Interestingly, a number of reports have indicated ICSI might contribute to the increased incidence of monozygotic twins observed in ART cases, however results to date are inconclusive [79]. Multiple-birth gestations are inherently much more risky that singletons, so in many cases, it is difficult to determine whether the risks are associated with multiple-births in general or are specifically attributable to the ART procedure [80]. In addition, many of the studies that have addressed risks associated with ART have not specifically evaluated the effect of ICSI compared with conventional IVF.

A recent systematic review evaluated 59 studies that measured the neurological development of children born following IVF and ICSI [81]. After selecting experimentally sound studies, On the basis of the data available from experimentally sound studies, the authors concluded that there are no consistent neurological differences in IVF and ICSI children when compared with naturally conceived children in terms of neuromotor development, behavior, speech and language, or overall cognition (Middleburg 101) [81]. Comparison of neurological development between IVF and ICSI children likewise did not reveal specific risks associated with ICSI. The authors did stress however that the children assessed were of preschool age or younger, and longer-term follow-up studies will be necessary to make an accurate assessment of potential risks associated with ART procedures [81].

Evaluation of data on major birth defects in infants born between 1993 and 1997 in Western Australia found a minor but significant increase in malformations associated with ART; however, incidences of malformations did not differ between ICSI and conventional IVF infants [82]. In agreement with this study, a meta-analysis evaluating the risk of birth defects associated with ICSI compared with other ART procedures found no significantly increased risks in ICSI cases for any of the birth defects evaluated [83].

While the majority of published reports indicate congenital risks are associated with ART procedures in general, and not specifically with ICSI, there are reports of ICSI-dependent risk factors. Comparison of neonatal outcomes following the transfer of cryopreserved ICSI or IVF embryos found a two-fold increase (6.4% versus 3.1%) in major malformations following ICSI when compared with IVF [84]. A cohort study evaluating the health of 5-year-old naturally conceived, IVF and ICSI children found the only significant difference in IVF when compared with ICSI children was an increase in uro-genital malformations in ICSI children–particularly boys [85]. This finding had been reported previously [86] and may be related to paternal genetics rather than the ICSI procedure.

While a number of reports indicate potentially increased incidences of congenital malformations and developmental problems associated with ART, there is a general agreement that these risks are independent of the type of ART procedure used [64]. Nevertheless, despite the encouraging reports regarding the safety of ICSI thus far, continued research and follow-up is imperative.

40.7 Assisted Hatching

Following fertilization and prior to implantation, the early embryo must emerge from the zona pellucida. In vivo, the process of embryo hatching occurs as a result of increased pressure on the zona exerted by the growing/expanding blastocyst [87] and is facilitated by the zona thinning activity of serine proteases produced by either embryonic or uterine cells [88, 89].

It has been postulated that one reason for reduced implantation rates following IVF and ICSI is a failure of the embryo to properly hatch from the zona because of zona hardening as a result of advanced maternal age, ovarian stimulation protocols, in vitro culture conditions, or cryopreservation. Assisted hatching, generally performed on day-two or day-three embryos, was developed as a means of facilitating blastocyst hatching in an attempt to improve implantation rates [8]. Since the first successful application of the technique in 1990 [8], AH has become a routine practice in many fertility centers. Over the years, a number of AH methods have been employed. Research is ongoing to determine the most effective methods for AH as well as the indications for its use.

40.8 Methods

The earliest reports of assisted hatching employed mechanical disruption of the zona using a glass micropipette to create an artificial opening in a process referred to as partial zona dissection (PZD) [8]. Partial zona dissection is performed by piercing the zona with a microneedle, exiting the zona with the microneedle at a distance approximately one-fifth the circumference of the embryo from the entry point, and subsequently rubbing the impaled section on the holding pipette to create a slit in the zona [90].

This method was followed by the use of acid Tyrode's (AT) to digest a portion of the zona creating either a thinned region or a hole through the zona (Fig. 40.2a). The basic procedure using AT involves blowing the solution over the surface of the zona to create a 30–35 μm depression adjacent to an area of empty perivitelline space or extracellular fragments [90]. A variation of this involves completely transversing the zona using care to cease applying AT in order to avoid damage to blastomeres. This method is used to reduce the overall thickness of the zona pellucida. Following the procedure, embryos are subsequently washed thoroughly to remove residual acidic solution.

More recently, diode lasers have been employed for AH (Fig. 40.2b). Laser AH simply involves applying two to three pulses of laser light for a duration of a few milliseconds to create a thinned region or hole in the zona [91]. The size of the hole created by laser AH varies from 10 to 30 μm.

Several groups have evaluated the affect of total zona removal on pregnancy and implantation rates and have shown improvements in pregnancy rates in some patients [92, 93]. A small observational study suggested that total zona removal of vitrified embryos was more effective than partial hatching using AT on the basis of pregnancy, implantation, and delivery rates [92].

Other methods for AH that have been used with much less frequency include piezo micromanipulation and pronase treatment. The piezo method involves generalized thinning of approximately one-third of the surface of the zona as well as the creation of a 20μm hole in the zona [94]. Assisted hatching by pronase is accomplished by bathing blastocysts in 0.2% pronase to thin the entire zona [95]. Both of these methods were demonstrated in prospective randomized trials to result in improved pregnancy and implantation rates when compared with untreated controls [94, 95].

A number of studies–both prospective and retrospective have evaluated the affect of the AH method on embryo development and pregnancy rates [90, 91, 96–99]. Results of these studies vary, probably as a result of different patient groups selected for study or differences in technician efficiencies using different AH methods.

Two studies comparing different laser AH techniques report similar results. Both groups found that thinning a region of the zona with a laser resulted in higher pregnancy rates compared with producing a hole in the zona [91, 96]; however, both studies were retrospective, and continued research is necessary.

Studies comparing the results of laser AH with other methods have reached conflicting conclusions. Again, these differences might reflect differences in patient etiology in each study as well as application of these methodologies.

An early prospective study comparing AT and laser AH on embryos from women 38 years of age and older reported significantly improved pregnancy and delivery rates following laser AH when compared with AT [97]. A more recent sibling oocyte study of a small number of patients who underwent AH either by laser or AT in conjunction with blastomere biopsy reported equivalent rates of blastocyst development and similar blastocyst quality in the two groups, however results beyond in vitro development were not reported [99].

A prospective randomized study comparing laser AH with mechanical PZD representing 319 patients 39 years of age or older reported the use of laser AH, significantly increased implantation rates as well as nonsignificant increases in clinical pregnancies and viable pregnancy (pregnancies progressing beyond the first trimester) rates were observed as compared to rates using mechanical PZD [98]. Similarly, a recently published retrospective study comparing AT and laser AH with PZD suggested both AT and laser AH are superior to PZD in terms of clinical pregnancy rates and viable pregnancy rates [90]. Conversely, a retrospective study comparing AT, laser, pronase and PZD reported similar pregnancy and abortion rates between groups [100].

The advantage of laser AH over other methods is the relative technical ease, precision, speed, and hands-off nature of the procedure. The main drawback to laser AH is the significant cost associated with a system. In addition, it is plausible that the transient heat produced by the laser beam might harm or injure the blastomeres that are closely associated with the zona breach. Continued research comparing AH outcomes in carefully controlled prospective studies will be valuable in determining the impact of the AH method on developmental efficiency.

The advantage of using AT for AH is that this method easily allows the removal of fragments as well as lysed blastomeres. This is especially important since several studies have indicated that the removal of lysed cells from fresh [101] and frozen-thawed [102] day 3 embryos is beneficial. The main disadvantage of using AT is the ability to consistently apply this technique. This technique has proven to be very difficult to replicate in many centers since the ability to apply the solution consistently is very difficult. It is quite possible that embryologists are making the holes either too large or small. In addition, this acid solution might be deleterious to the associated blastomeres. Further research in this area is necessary.

40.8.1 Indications

Research regarding the indications for AH and which cases benefit most from this procedure is ongoing, however, with little exception, there is general consensus that routine AH is not advantageous [103, 104]. Cases in which AH may be advantageous include embryos with thickened or hardened zonas [105, 106], women of advanced age [93, 105, 107, 108], cryopreserved embryos [109], and in cases of previous IVF failure [93, 104, 110, 111].

Cohen et al. demonstrated in a prospective randomized trial that embryos with zonas thicker than 15 µm benefited most from AH, while negative affects of AH were observed in embryos with zonas less than 13 µm thick [105]. Another study showed that AH of embryos that were determined during ICSI procedures to have a difficult-to-penetrate oolemma resulted in significantly improved pregnancy rates when compared with nonhatched controls [106].

In the study cited earlier, Cohen et al. also found that when selective AH based on increased zona thickness was performed, the benefit of AH was most pronounced in women 39 years of age and older [105]. In agreement with these results, two other studies found embryos from women of advanced maternal age implanted at a higher rate following AH [93, 111]. Other reports, however, have not found maternal age to be an important indicator for AH [108].

Few studies have evaluated the affect of AH on implantation rates of cryopreserved embryos; however, existing studies suggest it may beneficial [92, 109, 112]. Two different groups found post-thaw AH resulted in improved pregnancy and implantation rates, while the same benefits were not observed following AH of fresh embryos [109, 112]. Another study compared the affect of AH using AT compared with complete zona removal with laser and pipetting and found that complete zona removal resulted in improved pregnancy, implantation, and delivery rates [92].

Considering previous failed IVF cycles as an indicator for AH, the majority of studies indicate AH yields improved efficiencies [93, 110, 111], however, there is not complete consensus [109]. Selective AH for patients with at least three previous failed IVF cycles was demonstrated to yield improved clinical pregnancy and implantation rates when compared with unhatched controls, while the rate of miscarriage was similar for both groups [111]. When complete zona removal was performed on embryos from a group of women over the age of 40 and/or women with at least two previous failed IVF cycles, significantly higher pregnancy rates were reported [93]. Recently, a retrospective study found significant improvement in pregnancy and implantation rates in women following AH after a single failed IVF cycle [110], while another study found no benefit to AH based on maternal age [109].

40.8.2 Outcome

As discussed earlier, AH has been demonstrated to be beneficial in improving pregnancy, implantation, and delivery rates in some cases. Careful consideration must be given in determining which cases would benefit from AH, as it is certainly not beneficial in all cases, and in fact may result in reduced pregnancy rates under some circumstances. As with ICSI techniques, AH has been inconclusively implicated in increasing MZ twinning rates associated with ART, further emphasizing the need for selective use of the technique [79].

40.9 Conclusions

The primary aim of both ICSI and AH is to improve the efficiency of in vitro embryo production and embryo implantation, thereby expanding the population of patients who can benefit from ART techniques without providing undue harm. In order to achieve this goal, care must be given in determining under what circumstances these techniques are necessary and beneficial. Continued research focusing on ICSI and AH indications as well as improved methodologies will be of great benefit to the ART community as well as to those who benefit from infertility treatment.

References

1. Willadsen SM (1979) A method for culture of micromanipulated sheep embryos and its use to produce monozygotic twins. Nature 277:298–300
2. Willadsen SM (1986) Nuclear transplantation in sheep embryos. Nature 320:63–65
3. Malter HE, Cohen J (1989) Partial zona dissection of the human oocyte: a nontraumatic method using micromanipulation to assist zona pellucida penetration. Fertil Steril 51:139–148
4. Cohen J, Alikani M, Malter HE, Adler A, Talansky BE, Rosenwaks Z (1991) Partial zona dissection or subzonal sperm insertion: microsurgical fertilization alternatives based on evaluation of sperm and embryo morphology. Fertil Steril 56:696–706
5. Uehara T, Yanagimachi R (1976) Microsurgical injection of spermatozoa into hamster eggs with subsequent transformation of sperm nuclei into male pronuclei. Biol Reprod 15:467–470
6. Iritani A (1988) Current status of biotechnological studies in mammalian reproduction. Fertil Steril 50:543–551
7. Palermo G, Joris H, Devroey P, Van Steirteghem AC (1992) Pregnancies after intracytoplasmic injection of single spermatozoon into an oocyte. Lancet 340:17–18
8. Cohen J, Elsner C, Kort H et al (1990) Impairment of the hatching process following IVF in the human and improvement of implantation by assisting hatching using micromanipulation. Hum Reprod 5:7–13

9. Wright VC, Chang J, Jeng G, Macaluso M (2008) Assisted reproductive technology surveillance – United States, 2005. MMWR Surveill Summ 57:1–23
10. Andersen AN, Goossens V, Ferraretti AP et al (2008) Assisted reproductive technology in Europe, 2004: results generated from European registers by ESHRE. Hum Reprod 23:756–771
11. Gilchrist RB, Lane M, Thompson JG (2008) Oocyte-secreted factors: regulators of cumulus cell function and oocyte quality. Hum Reprod Update 14:159–177
12. Carrell DT, Peterson CM, Jones KP et al (1999) A simplified coculture system using homologous, attached cumulus tissue results in improved human embryo morphology and pregnancy rates during in vitro fertilization. J Assist Reprod Genet 16:344–349
13. Quinn P, Margalit R (1996) Beneficial effects of coculture with cumulus cells on blastocyst formation in a prospective trial with supernumerary human embryos. J Assist Reprod Genet 13:9–14
14. Ebner T, Moser M, Sommergruber M, Shebl O, Tews G (2006) Incomplete denudation of oocytes prior to ICSI enhances embryo quality and blastocyst development. Hum Reprod 21:2972–2977
15. Takeuchi S, Minoura H, Shibahara T, Shen X, Futamura N, Toyoda N (2001) Comparison of piezo-assisted micromanipulation with conventional micromanipulation for intracytoplasmic sperm injection into human oocytes. Gynecol Obstet Invest 52:158–162
16. Nagy ZP, Oliveira SA, Abdelmassih V, Abdelmassih R (2002) Novel use of laser to assist ICSI for patients with fragile oocytes: a case report. Reprod Biomed Online 4:27–31
17. Abdelmassih S, Cardoso J, Abdelmassih V, Dias JA, Abdelmassih R, Nagy ZP (2002) Laser-assisted ICSI: a novel approach to obtain higher oocyte survival and embryo quality rates. Hum Reprod 17:2694–2699
18. Ergenc AF, Li MW, Toner M, Biggers JD, Lloyd KC, Olgac N (2008) Rotationally oscillating drill (Ros-Drill(c)) for mouse icsi without using mercury. Mol Reprod Dev 75(12):1744–1751
19. Liu J, Nagy Z, Joris H, Tournaye H, Devroey P, Van Steirteghem A (1995) Successful fertilization and establishment of pregnancies after intracytoplasmic sperm injection in patients with globozoospermia. Hum Reprod 10:626–629
20. Esfandiari N, Javed MH, Gotlieb L, Casper RF (2005) Complete failed fertilization after intracytoplasmic sperm injection–analysis of 10 years' data. Int J Fertil Womens Med 50:187–192
21. Mahutte NG, Arici A (2003) Failed fertilization: is it predictable? Curr Opin Obstet Gynecol 15:211–218
22. Kovacic B, Vlaisavljevic V (2000) Configuration of maternal and paternal chromatin and pertaining microtubules in human oocytes failing to fertilize after intracytoplasmic sperm injection. Mol Reprod Dev 55:197–204
23. Sousa M, Tesarik J (1994) Ultrastructural analysis of fertilization failure after intracytoplasmic sperm injection. Hum Reprod 9:2374–2380
24. Tejera A, Molla M, Muriel L, Remohi J, Pellicer A, De Pablo JL (2008) Successful pregnancy and childbirth after intracytoplasmic sperm injection with calcium ionophore oocyte activation in a globozoospermic patient. Fertil Steril 90(4):1202.e1–1202.e5
25. Tesarik J, Sousa M, Testart J (1994) Human oocyte activation after intracytoplasmic sperm injection. Hum Reprod 9:511–518
26. Horner VL, Wolfner MF (2008) Transitioning from egg to embryo: triggers and mechanisms of egg activation. Dev Dyn 237: 527–544
27. Yanagida K, Katayose H, Yazawa H et al (1999) Successful fertilization and pregnancy following ICSI and electrical oocyte activation. Hum Reprod 14:1307–1311
28. Rybouchkin AV, Van der Straeten F, Quatacker J, De Sutter P, Dhont M (1997) Fertilization and pregnancy after assisted oocyte activation and intracytoplasmic sperm injection in a case of round-headed sperm associated with deficient oocyte activation capacity. Fertil Steril 68:1144–1147
29. Nasr-Esfahani MH, Razavi S, Javdan Z, Tavalaee M (2008) Artificial oocyte activation in severe teratozoospermia undergoing intracytoplasmic sperm injection. Fertil Steril 90(6):2231–2237
30. Yanagida K, Morozumi K, Katayose H, Hayashi S, Sato A (2006) Successful pregnancy after ICSI with strontium oocyte activation in low rates of fertilization. Reprod Biomed Online 13:801–806
31. Kyono K, Kumagai S, Nishinaka C et al (2008) Birth and follow-up of babies born following ICSI using SrCl2 oocyte activation. Reprod Biomed Online 17:53–58
32. Ebner T, Moser M, Sommergruber M, Jesacher K, Tews G (2004) Complete oocyte activation failure after ICSI can be overcome by a modified injection technique. Hum Reprod 19:1837–1841
33. Tesarik J, Rienzi L, Ubaldi F, Mendoza C, Greco E (2002) Use of a modified intracytoplasmic sperm injection technique to overcome sperm-borne and oocyte-borne oocyte activation failures. Fertil Steril 78:619–624
34. Svalander P, Jakobsson AH, Forsberg AS, Bengtsson AC, Wikland M (1996) The outcome of intracytoplasmic sperm injection is unrelated to 'strict criteria' sperm morphology. Hum Reprod 11: 1019–1022
35. Check M, Check JH, Summers-Chase D, Swenson K, Yuan W (2003) An evaluation of the efficacy of in vitro fertilization with intracytoplasmic sperm injection for sperm with low hypoosmotic swelling test scores and poor morphology. J Assist Reprod Genet 20:182–185
36. Nagy ZP, Liu J, Joris H et al (1995) The result of intracytoplasmic sperm injection is not related to any of the three basic sperm parameters. Hum Reprod 10:1123–1129
37. De Vos A, Van De Velde H, Joris H, Verheyen G, Devroey P, Van Steirteghem A (2003) Influence of individual sperm morphology on fertilization, embryo morphology, and pregnancy outcome of intracytoplasmic sperm injection. Fertil Steril 79:42–48
38. Bartoov B, Berkovitz A, Eltes F, Kogosowski A, Menezo Y, Barak Y (2002) Real-time fine morphology of motile human sperm cells is associated with IVF-ICSI outcome. J Androl 23:1–8
39. Berkovitz A, Eltes F, Lederman H et al (2006) How to improve IVF-ICSI outcome by sperm selection. Reprod Biomed Online 12:634–638
40. Antinori M, Licata E, Dani G et al (2008) Intracytoplasmic morphologically selected sperm injection: a prospective randomized trial. Reprod Biomed Online 16:835–841
41. Bartoov B, Berkovitz A, Eltes F et al (2003) Pregnancy rates are higher with intracytoplasmic morphologically selected sperm injection than with conventional intracytoplasmic injection. Fertil Steril 80:1413–1419
42. Berkovitz A, Eltes F, Yaari S et al (2005) The morphological normalcy of the sperm nucleus and pregnancy rate of intracytoplasmic injection with morphologically selected sperm. Hum Reprod 20:185–190
43. Naru T, Sulaiman MN, Kidwai A et al (2008) Intracytoplasmic sperm injection outcome using ejaculated sperm and retrieved sperm in azoospermic men. Urol J 5:106–110
44. Kanto S, Sugawara J, Masuda H, Sasano H, Arai Y, Kyono K (2008) Fresh motile testicular sperm retrieved from nonobstructive azoospermic patients has the same potential to achieve fertilization and pregnancy via ICSI as sperm retrieved from obstructive azoospermic patients. Fertil Steril 90(5):2010.e5–2010.e7
45. Moghadam KK, Nett R, Robins JC et al (2005) The motility of epididymal or testicular spermatozoa does not directly affect IVF/ICSI pregnancy outcomes. J Androl 26:619–623
46. Schwarzer JU, Fiedler K, Hertwig I et al (2003) Male factors determining the outcome of intracytoplasmic sperm injection with epididymal and testicular spermatozoa. Andrologia 35:220–226
47. Nagy ZP, Janssenswillen C, Janssens R et al (1998) Timing of oocyte activation, pronucleus formation and cleavage in humans after intracytoplasmic sperm injection (ICSI) with testicular sper-

matozoa and after ICSI or in-vitro fertilization on sibling oocytes with ejaculated spermatozoa. Hum Reprod 13:1606–1612
48. Balaban B, Urman B, Isiklar A et al (2001) Blastocyst transfer following intracytoplasmic injection of ejaculated, epididymal or testicular spermatozoa. Hum Reprod 16:125–129
49. Raman JD, Schlegel PN (2003) Testicular sperm extraction with intracytoplasmic sperm injection is successful for the treatment of nonobstructive azoospermia associated with cryptorchidism. J Urol 170:1287–1290
50. Ogura A, Yanagimachi R (1993) Round spermatid nuclei injected into hamster oocytes from pronuclei and participate in syngamy. Biol Reprod 48:219–225
51. Ogura A, Yanagimachi R, Usui N (1993) Behaviour of hamster and mouse round spermatid nuclei incorporated into mature oocytes by electrofusion. Zygote 1:1–8
52. Ogura A, Matsuda J, Yanagimachi R (1994) Birth of normal young after electrofusion of mouse oocytes with round spermatids. Proc Natl Acad Sci USA 91:7460–7462
53. Gianaroli L, Selman HA, Magli MC, Colpi G, Fortini D, Ferraretti AP (1999) Birth of a healthy infant after conception with round spermatids isolated from cryopreserved testicular tissue. Fertil Steril 72:539–541
54. Vanderzwalmen P, Zech H, Birkenfeld A et al (1997) Intracytoplasmic injection of spermatids retrieved from testicular tissue: influence of testicular pathology, type of selected spermatids and oocyte activation. Hum Reprod 12:1203–1213
55. Benkhalifa M, Kahraman S, Biricik A et al (2004) Cytogenetic abnormalities and the failure of development after round spermatid injections. Fertil Steril 81:1283–1288
56. Urman B, Alatas C, Aksoy S et al (2002) Transfer at the blastocyst stage of embryos derived from testicular round spermatid injection. Hum Reprod 17:741–743
57. Yamanaka K, Sofikitis NV, Miyagawa I et al (1997) Ooplasmic round spermatid nuclear injection procedures as an experimental treatment for nonobstructive azoospermia. J Assist Reprod Genet 14:55–62
58. Oliva R (2006) Protamines and male infertility. Hum Reprod Update 12:417–435
59. Ziyyat A, Lefevre A (2001) Differential gene expression in pre-implantation embryos from mouse oocytes injected with round spermatids or spermatozoa. Hum Reprod 16:1449–1456
60. Hayashi S, Yang J, Christenson L, Yanagimachi R, Hecht NB (2003) Mouse preimplantation embryos developed from oocytes injected with round spermatids or spermatozoa have similar but distinct patterns of early messenger RNA expression. Biol Reprod 69:1170–1176
61. Tesarik J, Cruz-Navarro N, Moreno E, Canete MT, Mendoza C (2000) Birth of healthy twins after fertilization with in vitro cultured spermatids from a patient with massive in vivo apoptosis of postmeiotic germ cells. Fertil Steril 74:1044–1046
62. Araki Y, Motoyama M, Yoshida A, Kim SY, Sung H, Araki S (1997) Intracytoplasmic injection with late spermatids: a successful procedure in achieving childbirth for couples in which the male partner suffers from azoospermia due to deficient spermatogenesis. Fertil Steril 67:559–561
63. Zech H, Vanderzwalmen P, Prapas Y, Lejeune B, Duba E, Schoysman R (2000) Congenital malformations after intracytoplasmic injection of spermatids. Hum Reprod 15:969–971
64. Neri QV, Takeuchi T, Palermo GD (2008) An update of assisted reproductive technologies results in the United States. Ann N Y Acad Sci 1127:41–48
65. Gosden LV, Yin H (2006) Micromanipulation in assisted reproductive technology: intracytoplasmic sperm injection, assisted hatching, and preimplantation genetic diagnosis. Clin Obstet Gynecol 49:73–84
66. Taylor TH, Wright G, Jones-Colon S, Mitchell-Leef D, Kort HI, Nagy ZP (2008) Comparison of ICSI and conventional IVF in patients with increased oocyte immaturity. Reprod Biomed Online 17:46–52
67. Zorn B, Virant-Klun I, Stanovnik M, Drobnic S, Meden-Vrtovec H (2006) Intracytoplasmic sperm injection by testicular sperm in patients with aspermia or azoospermia after cancer treatment. Int J Androl 29:521–527
68. Freeman MR, Archibong AE, Mrotek JJ, Whitworth CM, Weitzman GA, Hill GA (2001) Male partner screening before in vitro fertilization: preselecting patients who require intracytoplasmic sperm injection with the sperm penetration assay. Fertil Steril 76:1113–1118
69. van der Westerlaken L, Naaktgeboren N, Verburg H, Dieben S, Helmerhorst FM (2006) Conventional in vitro fertilization versus intracytoplasmic sperm injection in patients with borderline semen: a randomized study using sibling oocytes. Fertil Steril 85:395–400
70. Yoeli R, Orvieto R, Ashkenazi J, Shelef M, Ben-Rafael Z, Bar-Hava I (2008) Comparison of embryo quality between intracytoplasmic sperm injection and in vitro fertilization in sibling oocytes. J Assist Reprod Genet 25:23–28
71. Van Landuyt L, De Vos A, Joris H, Verheyen G, Devroey P, Van Steirteghem A (2005) Blastocyst formation in in vitro fertilization versus intracytoplasmic sperm injection cycles: influence of the fertilization procedure. Fertil Steril 83:1397–1403
72. Dumoulin JC, Coonen E, Bras M et al (2000) Comparison of in-vitro development of embryos originating from either conventional in-vitro fertilization or intracytoplasmic sperm injection. Hum Reprod 15:402–409
73. Shoukir Y, Chardonnens D, Campana A, Sakkas D (1998) Blastocyst development from supernumerary embryos after intracytoplasmic sperm injection: a paternal influence? Hum Reprod 13:1632–1637
74. Griffiths TA, Murdoch AP, Herbert M (2000) Embryonic development in vitro is compromised by the ICSI procedure. Hum Reprod 15:1592–1596
75. Menezo Y, Barak Y (2000) Comparison between day-2 embryos obtained either from ICSI or resulting from short insemination IVF: influence of maternal age. Hum Reprod 15:1776–1780
76. Miller JE, Smith TT (2001) The effect of intracytoplasmic sperm injection and semen parameters on blastocyst development in vitro. Hum Reprod 16:918–924
77. Frattarelli JL, Leondires MP, Miller BT, Segars JH (2000) Intracytoplasmic sperm injection increases embryo fragmentation without affecting clinical outcome. J Assist Reprod Genet 17:207–212
78. Westphal LM, Hinckley MD, Behr B, Milki AA (2003) Effect of ICSI on subsequent blastocyst development and pregnancy rates. J Assist Reprod Genet 20:113–116
79. Aston K, Peterson C, Carrell DT (2008) Monozygotic twinning associated with assisted reproductive technologies: a review. Reproduction 136(4):377–386
80. Alukal JP, Lamb DJ (2008) Intracytoplasmic sperm injection (ICSI) – what are the risks? Urol Clin North Am 35:277–288 ix–x
81. Middelburg KJ, Heineman MJ, Bos AF, Hadders-Algra M (2008) Neuromotor, cognitive, language and behavioural outcome in children born following IVF or ICSI – a systematic review. Hum Reprod Update 14:219–231
82. Hansen M, Kurinczuk JJ, Bower C, Webb S (2002) The risk of major birth defects after intracytoplasmic sperm injection and in vitro fertilization. N Engl J Med 346:725–730
83. Lie RT, Lyngstadaas A, Orstavik KH, Bakketeig LS, Jacobsen G, Tanbo T (2005) Birth defects in children conceived by ICSI compared with children conceived by other IVF-methods; a meta-analysis. Int J Epidemiol 34:696–701
84. Belva F, Henriet S, Van den Abbeel E et al (2008) Neonatal outcome of 937 children born after transfer of cryopreserved embryos obtained by ICSI and IVF and comparison with outcome data of fresh ICSI and IVF cycles. Hum Reprod 23(10):2227–2238
85. Bonduelle M, Wennerholm UB, Loft A et al (2005) A multi-centre cohort study of the physical health of 5-year-old children conceived

after intracytoplasmic sperm injection, in vitro fertilization and natural conception. Hum Reprod 20:413–419
86. Wennerholm UB, Bergh C, Hamberger L et al (2000) Incidence of congenital malformations in children born after ICSI. Hum Reprod 15:944–948
87. Sathananthan H, Menezes J, Gunasheela S (2003) Mechanics of human blastocyst hatching in vitro. Reprod Biomed Online 7:228–234
88. O'Sullivan CM, Liu SY, Karpinka JB, Rancourt DE (2002) Embryonic hatching enzyme strypsin/ISP1 is expressed with ISP2 in endometrial glands during implantation. Mol Reprod Dev 62:328–334
89. Cohen J (1991) Assisted hatching of human embryos. J In Vitro Fert Embryo Transf 8:179–190
90. Feng HL, Hershlag A, Scholl GM, Cohen MA (2008) A retroprospective study comparing three different assisted hatching techniques. Fertil Steril 91(Suppl. 4):1323–1325
91. Ghobara TS, Cahill DJ, Ford WC et al (2006) Effects of assisted hatching method and age on implantation rates of IVF and ICSI. Reprod Biomed Online 13:261–267
92. Hiraoka K, Fuchiwaki M, Horiuchi T, Murakami T, Kinutani M, Kinutani K (2007) Zona pellucida removal and vitrified blastocyst transfer outcome: a preliminary study. Reprod Biomed Online 15:68–75
93. Mansour RT, Rhodes CA, Aboulghar MA, Serour GI, Kamal A (2000) Transfer of zona-free embryos improves outcome in poor prognosis patients: a prospective randomized controlled study. Hum Reprod 15:1061–1064
94. Nakayama T, Fujiwara H, Yamada S, Tastumi K, Honda T, Fujii S (1999) Clinical application of a new assisted hatching method using a piezo-micromanipulator for morphologically low-quality embryos in poor-prognosis infertile patients. Fertil Steril 71:1014–1018
95. Isik AZ, Vicdan K, Kaba A, Dagli G (2000) Comparison of zona manipulated and zona intact blastocyst transfers: a prospective randomized trial. J Assist Reprod Genet 17:135–139
96. Mantoudis E, Podsiadly BT, Gorgy A, Venkat G, Craft IL (2001) A comparison between quarter, partial and total laser assisted hatching in selected infertility patients. Hum Reprod 16:2182–2186
97. Hsieh YY, Huang CC, Cheng TC, Chang CC, Tsai HD, Lee MS (2002) Laser-assisted hatching of embryos is better than the chemical method for enhancing the pregnancy rate in women with advanced age. Fertil Steril 78:179–182
98. Makrakis E, Angeli I, Agapitou K, Pappas K, Dafereras A, Pantos K (2006) Laser versus mechanical assisted hatching: a prospective study of clinical outcomes. Fertil Steril 86:1596–1600
99. Jones AE, Wright G, Kort HI, Straub RJ, Nagy ZP (2006) Comparison of laser-assisted hatching and acidified Tyrode's hatching by evaluation of blastocyst development rates in sibling embryos: a prospective randomized trial. Fertil Steril 85: 487–491
100. Balaban B, Urman B, Alatas C, Mercan R, Mumcu A, Isiklar A (2002) A comparison of four different techniques of assisted hatching. Hum Reprod 17:1239–1243
101. Keltz MD, Skorupski JC, Bradley K, Stein D (2006) Predictors of embryo fragmentation and outcome after fragment removal in in vitro fertilization. Fertil Steril 86:321–324
102. Eftekhari-Yazdi P, Valojerdi MR, Ashtiani SK, Eslaminejad MB, Karimian L (2006) Effect of fragment removal on blastocyst formation and quality of human embryos. Reprod Biomed Online 13:823–832
103. Hellebaut S, De Sutter P, Dozortsev D, Onghena A, Qian C, Dhont M (1996) Does assisted hatching improve implantation rates after in vitro fertilization or intracytoplasmic sperm injection in all patients? A prospective randomized study. J Assist Reprod Genet 13:19–22
104. Practice Committee of the Society for Assisted Reproductive Technology, Practice Committee of the American Society for Reproductive Medicine (2006) The role of assisted hatching in in vitro fertilization: a review of the literature. A committee opinion. Fertil Steril 85:544–546
105. Cohen J, Alikani M, Trowbridge J, Rosenwaks Z (1992) Implantation enhancement by selective assisted hatching using zona drilling of human embryos with poor prognosis. Hum Reprod 7:685–691
106. Ebner T, Moser M, Yaman C et al (2002) Prospective hatching of embryos developed from oocytes exhibiting difficult oolemma penetration during ICSI. Hum Reprod 17:1317–1320
107. Edi-Osagie E, Hooper L, Seif MW (2003) The impact of assisted hatching on live birth rates and outcomes of assisted conception: a systematic review. Hum Reprod 18:1828–1835
108. Lanzendorf SE, Nehchiri F, Mayer JF, Oehninger S, Muasher SJ (1998) A prospective, randomized, double-blind study for the evaluation of assisted hatching in patients with advanced maternal age. Hum Reprod 13:409–413
109. Valojerdi MR, Eftekhari-Yazdi P, Karimian L, Ashtiani SK (2008) Effect of laser zona pellucida opening on clinical outcome of assisted reproduction technology in patients with advanced female age, recurrent implantation failure, or frozen-thawed embryos. Fertil Steril 90:84–91
110. Dayal MB, Dubey A, Frankfurter D, Peak D, Gindoff PR (2007) Second cycle: to hatch or not to hatch? Fertil Steril 88:718–720
111. Magli MC, Gianaroli L, Ferraretti AP, Fortini D, Aicardi G, Montanaro N (1998) Rescue of implantation potential in embryos with poor prognosis by assisted zona hatching. Hum Reprod 13:1331–1335
112. Ge HS, Zhou W, Zhang W, Lin JJ (2008) Impact of assisted hatching on fresh and frozen-thawed embryo transfer cycles: a prospective, randomized study. Reprod Biomed Online 16:589–596

Chapter 41
Embryo Culture Techniques

Katharine V. Jackson and Catherine Racowsky

Abstract Many variables must be considered when choosing a clinical culture system. Although animal studies provide a strong evidence-based profile as to the composition of viable clinical systems, the true test of efficacy in a clinical setting is to test the system within one's own laboratory by randomizing sibling oocytes or embryos to the test system or the standard system currently in use. Using this methodology, clinical results can be maximized while minimizing the potential impact on patients.

Keywords Culture • Media • Air quality • Embryo density • Gas phase • Temperature • Light • Culture techniques

41.1 Introduction

There are many variables to consider when culturing human embryos in vitro. In a perfect culture system, all aspects of the in vivo microenvironment of eggs and embryos would be duplicated in vitro. This is a challenging endeavor, however, because our knowledge of the environments within the fallopian tube and uterus continues to evolve. Furthermore, standard embryo culture technology still relies on the use of static systems, thereby failing to capture the subtle nuances of the dynamic in vivo environment. In spite of these limitations, the fact that human embryos are able to produce live babies after culture in a wide variety of in vitro culture systems demonstrates their remarkable plasticity to adapt to the stresses imposed by these less than perfect systems.

Perhaps, the most fascinating and essential element to the proper practice of embryology is the ability to identify the individual and collective influences that in vitro culture conditions impose, and to adapt culture systems to minimize these effects. These conditions include, but are not limited to, the quality of the air in the IVF laboratory; the quality and composition of the gas in the incubator chambers; the type of culture dishes used; the selection of media used for gamete manipulation, embryo growth, and embryo transfer; and the specific technologies used to handle zygotes and embryos. In this chapter, we will explore each of these components after considering the historical development of embryo culture techniques and the more recent advancements in clinical IVF laboratory technologies.

41.2 Historical Perspective on Development of Embryo Culture Techniques

The embryo culture technologies used in clinical IVF today have their foundation in landmark studies undertaken with animal species over a century ago. These studies encompassed investigations with gametes, the fertilization process, and the resulting embryos, in addition to explorations of the reproductive cycle itself. Indeed, it was the confluence of research in these areas that enabled the development of culture systems capable of supporting fertilization and the formation of viable preimplantation embryos first in animal species, and then in the human (see Fig. 41.1).

The first reported attempt to achieve in vitro fertilization took place over 125 years ago when Viennese professor SL Schenk reported inseminating rabbit and guinea pig eggs in vitro and observing cleavage [1]. However, it was only with improved understanding of the adult estrus cycle and increased efficiency with embryo transfer techniques that the possibility of documenting successful in vitro embryo culture could be realized. In 1890, in extraordinary studies of the time, Walter Heape first reported the birth of live pups from the transfer of embryos from a donor female rabbit into a pregnant recipient [2]. These landmark studies revealed that the process of embryo development and implantation relied on complex processes that revolved around both the embryo and the adult reproductive processes.

K.V. Jackson (✉) and C. Racowsky
Department of Obstetrics, Gynecology and Reproductive Biology, Brigham and Women's Hospital, Harvard Medical School, Boston, MA, USA
e-mail: cracowsky@partners.org

D.T. Carrell and C.M. Peterson (eds.), *Reproductive Endocrinology and Infertility: Integrating Modern Clinical and Laboratory Practice*,
DOI 10.1007/978-1-4419-1436-1_41,

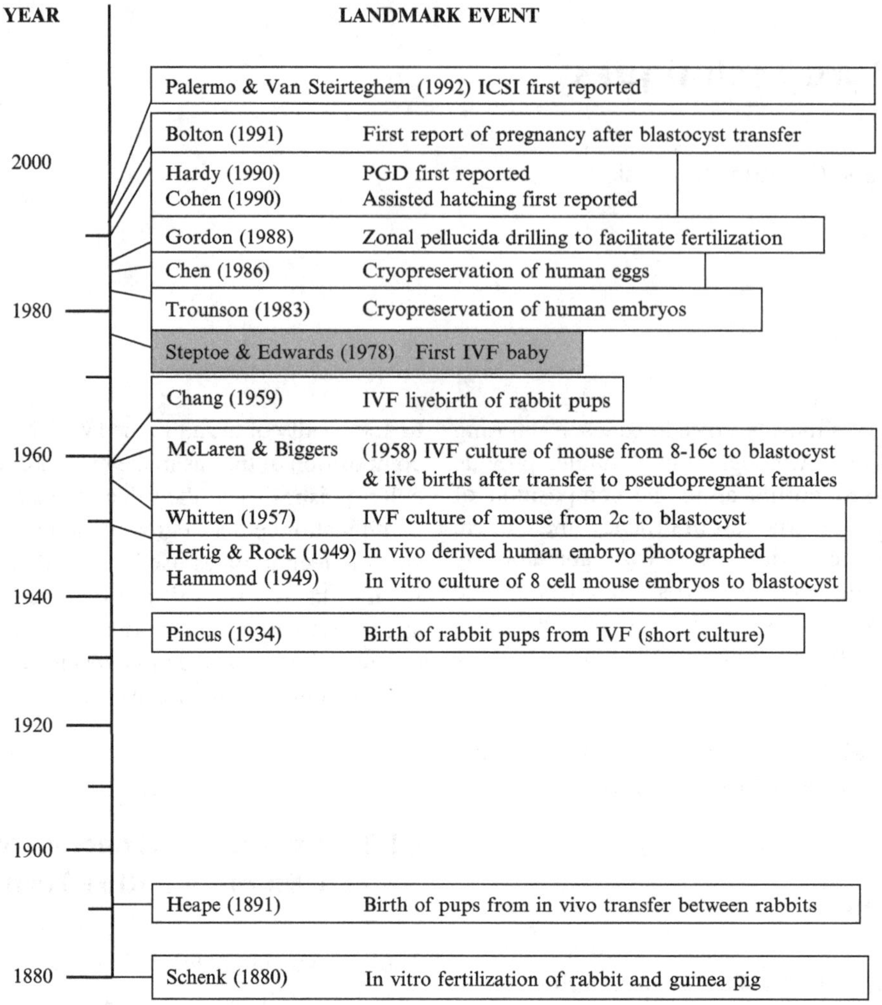

Fig. 41.1 Timeline of landmark events involved in the history of in vitro fertilization and embryo culture

It took another 50 years before the first successful in vitro fertilization and birth in an animal species was reported. In this 1934 study, Pincus reported the birth of seven rabbit pups resulting from "ova subjected to experiment manipulation in vitro" [3]. Since the in vitro exposure period consisted of only a 20 min incubation of eggs with sperm prior to their transfer into a pseudopregnant doe, there remains doubt as to whether or not this was indeed the first documented case of IVF in a mammalian species. Nevertheless, at the time this was considered a milestone in the field and sparked investigations to improve the formulation of embryo culture media.

In the late 1940s, Hammond reported the use of a simple salt solution for the culture of 8-cell mouse embryos through several cleavage divisions [4]. This formulation, which contained 6 mM glucose and 8–9% egg white, was able to support development to the blastocyst stage – quite extraordinary results indicating that simple salts, glucose, and protein can support early embryo development in culture. Whitten further refined this media to include calcium lactate instead of calcium chloride. In 1957, using this revised formulation, he was able to show that mouse embryos isolated as early as the 2-cell stage could remain in culture and form blastocysts, thus implicating that energy source changes affect embryo development [5]. The ability of in vitro culture systems to support live births was further demonstrated by McLaren and Biggers with the successful development and birth of mice cultured as early embryos [6], and then indisputably proven in 1959, when Chang reported the successful in vitro fertilization, embryo transfer into foster mothers, and birth of live rabbit pups [7].

While studies on animal culture systems were being refined, important research in human embryos was taking place. In rather provocative experiments, pathologist Arthur Hertig and obstetrician John Rock asked women scheduled for hysterectomy to document their menstrual cycles and sexual activities leading to the surgery. They then isolated concepti from the extracted reproductive tissue and correlated their developmental stage to morphology [8]. The studies were remarkable at two levels. First, they marked the first time that human embryos were ever observed and documented. Additionally, and perhaps more important for the field of embryology, it was the first time that an interdisciplinary union was established that successfully combined clinical and scientific expertise.

It took almost 30 years before Steptoe and Edwards, another interdisciplinary team, achieved the first successful birth of a human baby using in vitro fertilization [9]. Although Robert Edwards achieved fertilization of human ova in vitro as early as 1969 [10], it was not until he teamed up with Patrick Steptoe, an obstetrician who pioneered laparoscopic egg retrievals, that successful fertilization and embryo transfer were combined. Their first attempts were in patients stimulated with hMG and hCG [11], from whom they obtained oocytes which fertilized in vitro, grew into blastocysts and were transferred. However, the first IVF success was achieved following egg retrieval timed to the LH surge in a natural cycle, combined with culturing the embryo to the 8-cell stage. Of note, Leslie Brown was only the second patient to undergo this revised treatment regimen, resulting in the retrieval of a single ovum and the transfer of an 8 cell embryo into her uterus two and a half days later. After a 38-week gestation, Louise Brown, a 2,700 g infant was born on July 25, 1978, and the world of reproductive physiology was forever changed.

41.3 Advances in IVF Technologies

With the advent of this new treatment option, many reproductive clinics opened their doors in the late 1970s and early 1980s and further development of infertility treatments was undertaken. In the 10 years spanning 1982 and 1992, an unprecedented number of milestones in human reproductive physiology were passed. As early as 1983, techniques for cryopreserving embryos had been determined and the establishment of a pregnancy reported [12]. Three years later, Chen reported the successful cryopreservation of a human ovum that was subsequently thawed, fertilized, transferred, and resulted in a pregnancy [13]. Considering that we are still struggling with improving the efficacy of egg freezing more than 20 years later, this early success is quite remarkable.

By the late 1980s, advancements in the micromanipulation of human eggs and embryos were being made. In 1988, Gordon reported that it was possible to increase fertilization efficiency in human by inserting sperm under the zona pellucida [14]. Palermo and Van Steirteghem took this process one step further and revolutionized the field of male factor infertility when they described the successful fertilization of an oocyte by inserting the sperm directly into the cytoplasm [15]. In their first series using intracytoplasmic sperm injection (ICSI), they were able to attain a 66% fertilization rate ($n=47$ eggs) and a 26.7% implantation rate per embryo transferred! In 1990, Jacques Cohen demonstrated that implantation rates could be more than doubled when a hole was made in the zona pellucida of the embryo (6% vs. 25%, $P<0.023$) [16], a practice now commonly known as assisted hatching.

Even though the culture of human zygotes to the blastocyst stage was achieved as early as 1970 [11], it was not until the early 1990s that pregnancies were reported from their transfer, albeit with low pregnancy rates (10% viable pregnancy per ET) [17]. As advances were made in media development, the efficiency of blastocyst culture improved, and success rates of up to 66% per egg retrieval have now been reported [18]. This ability to let embryos grow 5 days in culture has impacted the industry in two ways. First, the approach allows those embryos that are the most robust to thrive, thus aiding in the selection process for transfer. In addition, opening the window of culture by two days allows sufficient time to perform preimplantation genetic diagnosis on day 3 embryos (i.e., removal and genetic analysis of one or two cells) followed by subsequent transfer of genetically normal embryos on day 4 or 5 [19]. The application of this technology will only be limited by the capabilities of the molecular biology assays developed.

The field of reproductive physiology has come a long way in a relatively short period of time. In just over 125 years, investigators have made great strides in the following key areas: (1) Determination and control of the physiology of estrous in adult females; (2) Development of techniques for the recovery, incubation, and fertilization of ova; (3) Establishment of methods to assist in the fertilization and implantation process; (4) Improvements in culture media such that embryo development can be supported through 5–6 days of in vitro; (5) Refinement of cryopreservation protocols such that we can now freeze oocytes, cleavage stage embryos, and blastocysts; and (6) The identification of methods for genetically screening embryos, and for diagnosing those that carry genetic mutations. In addition, the unique partnership between clinicians and scientists established long ago, and still so critical for the success of an IVF program, has continued to grow and flourish.

41.4 Culture Methods

The methods used to support gamete handling, fertilization, and embryo development encompass those at the macro-environmental level (i.e., the laboratory, the incubator, the hoods, and the microscopes), to those at the micro-environmental level (i.e., the dishes and the culture media). Variables common to all these environmental parameters prevail (such as air quality, temperature, and light) which must be critically controlled in order to optimize the overall culture system. In addition, there are many ways to culture embryos, thus variables such as dish pre-equilibration times, insemination concentration and timing, embryo density, number of direct observations and media renewal during culture can all affect the final outcome. In addition, peak observation intervals must be established so that assessment is timed to capture developmental mile-markers as the population mode dictates. The interplay of all these variables must be considered; thus the only way to determine the best culture methods is to optimize the all-encompassing system in the setting in which they will be used.

41.4.1 Air Quality

The quality of the laboratory air can impact IVF outcomes [20]. While little is known about the actual components that effect these changes, Cohen et al. have postulated that four different categories of pollutants are involved: volatile organic compounds (VOC's); small inorganic molecules such as N_2O, SO_2, and CO; substances derived from building materials (i.e., adhesives and floor tiles); and other polluting compounds (i.e., pesticides, aerosols, etc.). The use of clean-room technology has been shown to improve pregnancy rates [21, 22]. However, even after using centralized prefilter, carbon, and HEPA (high efficiency particulate air) filtration systems, the polished room air may still contain amounts of pollutants that exceed those of outside air [20]. In an effort to overcome such potential problems, two types of incubator filters, HEPA and VOC, have been developed for use in addition to clean-room technology. In one study involving human embryos, use of VOC filters increased blastocyst formation rates compared with use of HEPA filtration (29% vs. 23%, $P<0.02$) [22]. This finding is in agreement with another study that demonstrated increased pregnancy rates when carbon-based filters were placed in the incubators (41–45.3%, $P<0.04$) [23]. Thus, the toxicity of VOC's may be reduced by the use of in-incubator VOC filters.

In an effort to reduce these agents in our own laboratory, strict attention has been paid to using the lowest VOC-emitting products for all construction materials. We also use an inorganic agent that is water-based (Multiclean) for cleaning all equipment and facility surfaces rather than 70% ethanol, and we utilize special laboratory chairs that have non-out-gassing upholstery.

41.4.2 Temperature

The recognized industry standard regarding temperature for embryo culture is 37°C. However, it is almost impossible to maintain this temperature consistently when performing all laboratory interventions of a typical IVF cycle. Even in the most experienced hands, the temperature of microdrop cultures under oil experience minor cooling fluctuations when eggs or embryos are being observed, or during opening and closing of incubators.

Several studies have examined the impact of temperature on oocyte cytoarchitecture and embryo development when oocytes and embryos are subject to conditions similar to those experienced during IVF culture. As early as 1978, Hirao and Yanagimachi demonstrated that sperm fusion, cortical granule exocytosis, and the formation of pronuclei occurred more slowly in hamster eggs following insemination at 25°C, as compared with 37°C [24]. Additionally, they observed multiple "subnuclei" in the eggs that had been cooled and postulated that this was due to meiotic spindle malfunction. This observation was confirmed by Wang et al. in 2001, who used polarized light microscopy to image viable human oocytes and found that the ability of the human to recover spindle integrity is affected by the degree of cooling [25]. In fact, all oocytes cooled to 33°C and then rewarmed to 37°C were able to reform their spindles within 40 min, whereas only 2/5 of those cooled to 28°C and 0/5 of those cooled down to 25°C were capable of spindle reformation. It is noteworthy, however, that these experimental conditions are much more pronounced than those that eggs and embryos would likely experience in a clinical setting. Furthermore, and somewhat surprisingly, slight fluctuations around 37°C may actually be beneficial to IVF outcomes as evidenced by the results of Higdon et al. who recently reported a 19% increase in the clinical pregnancy rate when the incubator environment was <37°C as opposed to >37°C [22].

Most laboratories set their equipment to run at 37°C, but ambient air temperature can affect how temperature is maintained when embryos are outside an incubator. Cooling rates on stage warmers have been shown to double (1.6°C/m vs. 3.3°C/m), when ambient air temperatures drop from 22–24°C (71.6–75.2°F) to 18°C (64.4°F) [26]. Microscope stage warmers and incubator chambers also differ in their ability to hold the temperatures constant at 37°C. In a comparison between microscope stages with a surface of solid glass vs. black matte (with a 15 mm viewing hole in the middle), the rate of cooling was double (1.2°C/m vs. 2.4°C/m) when a viewing hole was present [27]. It was also found that recovery time varies according to the type of incubator used; water-jacketed incubators took more than 4 times longer to bring dish temperatures back to 37°C (after dish exposure to 35°C) than did MINC incubators, which rely on direct surface contact [27, 28]. On the basis of these findings, we recommend that laboratories set their thermostats to 71°C and above, use solid-viewing surface microscope stages, and limit the number of times water-jacketed incubators are opened.

41.4.3 Light

Handling of gametes and embryos in the IVF laboratory subjects them to light effects they would never encounter in vivo. Therefore, the effects of fluorescent and incandescent illumination on egg and embryo development must be considered, and the least detrimental type of illumination must be used. Cool white fluorescent light uses less energy and emits less heat than incandescent lighting, however, the light spectrum profile includes emission at mostly the 540–560 nm wavelength [29]. In contrast, incandescent and warm white fluorescent light emit both 540–560 nm and 620–640 nm wavelengths. Early studies conducted on cool white fluorescent illumination found that zona-free hamster embryos exposed for 15 m at 25°C demonstrated a 16% reduction in development as compared to controls, although it is unclear if this difference was significant [30]. While these findings are concerning, their value in an ART setting may be limited by the fact that they were conducted at 25°C. This consideration is supported by a later study that showed impairment in cell proliferation in rabbit embryos was compounded when light and temperature effects were administered jointly [31].

It does appear, however, that cool white fluorescent light is detrimental to development. In a recent study by Takenaka et al., it was found that after a 15 min exposure of mouse embryos to either no light, warm, or cool fluorescent light, significantly less reactive oxygen species (ROS) formed and more fetuses were obtained from embryos not exposed to cool fluorescence [29]. They also found that hamster embryos were affected to a higher degree than mouse embryos. Since different light sources emit different energy spectrums, it appears that light wavelength may be causing these changes (Fig. 41.2). Indeed, these effects have been examined using hamster embryos, where it was found that blue ray illumination (≤492 nm) impaired development, and red ray illumination (≥622 nm) improved development as compared to visible light [32]. These findings are not surprising when one considers that studies using low intensity light therapy in patients (630–1,000 nm wavelength) have been shown to increase wound healing and energy metabolism [33].

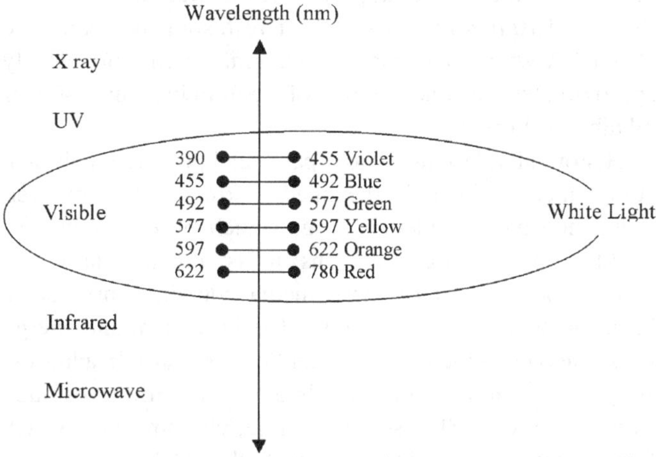

Fig. 41.2 Spectra of light waves and wavelengths of visible light

Consideration must also be given to possible detrimental effects of light intensity on gamete and embryo viability. While ambient laboratory light is typically 200–400 lux, the intensity of exposure from a microscope can vary from 2,300 to 5,000 lux and will vary among technicians [34]. Early studies in the rabbit and mouse demonstrated no effect on fertilization or development when eggs and embryos were exposed to light [35, 36]. These observations are supported by a more recent study that showed no effect on murine blastocyst formation rate or implantation rate from either light intensity or exposure time [37]. Contradictory to these findings, however, is a study conducted by Oh et al., who found that when 2-cell hamster embryos were exposed to three different light intensities (200, 500, and 900 lux) for 10 min, there was a trend toward increasing blastocyst development as light intensity was reduced, however, this effect was only significant at 200 lux as compared with 900 lux [32].

Taken together, available evidence suggests that there may be species-specific sensitivities to varying light intensities. Though it is unlikely that any of these experiments with animal models used lighting conditions that directly mimicked the IVF culture environment, they give us perspective on the correct use of light in a clinical IVF laboratory setting. When overhead lighting is generated by warm or incandescent lights and is kept at a subdued, yet comfortable level at or below 500 lux, it is not damaging to embryo development, thus the use of darkroom technology may not be necessary. Additionally, because wavelengths below 500 nm may be harmful to eggs and embryos, microscope filters should be used that exclude these wavelengths, with care given to the intensity of illumination and the amount of time eggs and embryos are viewed. Finally, it may be prudent for laboratories to purchase light lux meters and establish optimal light intensity levels using their own settings.

41.4.4 Incubator Gas Phase

Although the atmospheric level of oxygen at sea level is approximately 20.9%, physiological oxygen levels are lower, they vary in different parts of the reproductive tract, and they can fluctuate widely. In fact, oxygen concentrations differences of up to 4% have been reported in both human follicular fluid (range <1.5–5.5 % in 18–22 mm follicles) [38] and the uterus (range 0.9–4.6%) [39]. Therefore, the oxygen concentration that eggs and embryos are exposed to in vivo is 4–20 times lower than the 21% used in standard in vitro culture systems that employ a gas phase of 5–6% CO_2 in air.

Studies have investigated the relationship between oxygen tension and development. Van Blerkom et al. correlated the dissolved oxygen content of human follicular fluid at egg recovery to fertilization and embryo development in vitro [38].

They found that while fertilization rates did not correlate to the dissolved oxygen content (when comparing follicles with <1.5, 1.5–2.5, or 3–5.5% dissolved oxygen), significantly more embryos progressed to the 6–8 cell stage with increasing follicular fluid oxygen levels (42% vs. 66% vs. 79%, respectively, $P<0.001$). Several studies have compared in vitro culture of human embryos at 5% O_2 (i.e., a gas phase of 5% O_2+5% CO_2+90% N_2) vs. 20% O_2 (i.e. a gas phase of 5% CO_2 in air) [40, 41]. While these investigators showed no differences in fertilization rates, they also failed to demonstrate any differences in implantation or clinical pregnancy rates. However, in one of these studies, surplus embryos cultured to day 5 or 6, produced significantly more blastocysts when cultured in 5% O_2 as compared to 20% O_2 (30% vs. 23%, $P<0.01$) [40]. Animal studies confirm this finding. Using a mouse model, Rinaudo et al. found higher blastulation rates in low vs. atmospheric oxygen (69% vs. 81%, $P<0.05$) [42]. Of concern, however, differences in gene expression were also observed in this study; embryos cultured in 5% O_2 exhibited gene expression more closely resembling that of in vivo derived embryos. Additionally, there were fewer perturbations in the global pattern of gene expression in embryos cultured at 5% O_2 than those cultured at 20% O_2. Consequently, while oxygen tension may not affect common markers used for quality control in the IVF laboratory (i.e., fertilization or implantation rates), it may affect cleavage rates and result in molecular changes having long-range effects yet to be identified.

41.4.5 pH

In mammals, the pH shifts from an alkaline environment in the oviduct (7.60±0.01) to an acidic environment in the uterus (6.96±0.01) [43]. Since cellular processes are largely pH-dependent, this would imply that there are either stage-specific differences in the internal pH (pHi) during preimplantation development, or that eggs and embryos are able to regulate their pHi as they pass from the alkaline Fallopian tube into the more acidic uterus. The weight of experimental evidence supports the latter possibility. While little is known about the pHi of morulae and blastocysts, the pHi of human eggs has been measured and appears to remain constant during maturation and fertilization [44, 45]. The data regarding this absolute value for eggs are conflicting, however, which may be due to media differences. In one study of 111 samples incubated in Medicult Medium [44], the average pHi was found to be 7.4±0.1, while in a second study using KSOM, the pHi ranged from 6.98 to 7.04 pH ($n=22$), and only increased slightly in cleavage stage embryos to 7.12±0.01 ($n=199$) [45]. These studies also examined how eggs and embryos respond to acidosis and alkalosis and found that while both exhibited a robust recovery from alkalosis, eggs had lower rates of recovery from acidosis than did cleavage-stage embryos. Additionally, it was found eggs and embryos mainly rely on the presence of CO_2 and bicarbonate to maintain their pHi at 7.0–7.3 pH. Therefore, these regulation processes must be active during ovulation and migration through the alkaline environment of the oviduct, sperm penetration (which peaks at an extracellular pH of 7.5) [44], and entry into the acidic uterine environment. Due to these considerations, in a static laboratory environment, dogma dictates that pH's set at or near 7.3 may provide adequate conditions for insemination and embryo growth [46], because this is the midrange pH of those that are required for sperm penetration and embryonic pHi (i.e. 7.5–7.1). However, superior fertilization rates may be achieved when the insemination medium pH is set at 7.5 [44].

41.4.6 Media

The medium formulation used by most IVF laboratories in the early 1980s was HF10, a complex medium relatively high in glucose, and containing 20 amino acids and some vitamins. It was designed in 1963 as a media for the culture of diploid Chinese hamster and human cell lines [47] but was also found to support human in vitro fertilization and embryo cleavage. By the mid-1980s, IVF-specific formulations were being designed. The first such media was HTF, a media designed to mimic the concentrations of compounds in the human Fallopian tube [48]. Initially, 10–20% heated-inactivated maternal serum was used as the protein supplement, but now, (due to quality assurance issues and convenience) most laboratories use commercial protein products. These products include human serum albumin (HSA), packaged as a 10% protein solution in sterile saline; and synthetic serum substitute (SSS), a product packaged as a 6% protein solution in saline, containing 84% HSA and 16% alpha and beta globulins. These products are most often used at 10% v/v in culture media, resulting in a final protein concentration of 6 mg/ml (SSS) and 10 mg/ml (HSA). Of interest, some programs use 50% HSA v/v in their transfer medium, which more closely approximates the concentration of albumin in serum (40 mg/ml albumin) [49].

Historically, IVF laboratory personnel prepared their own culture media using published media formulations. However, as the industry expanded, it became much more effective (for quality control and cost reasons) to use commercially prepared products. All of these media contain simple salts, bicarbonate and/or HEPES for pH stabilization, and energy substrates (i.e., glucose, lactate and/or pyruvate). In addition, some also contain amino acids and other additives such as phenol red, EDTA, sodium citrate, vitamins and growth factors, antibiotics and hyaluronan (Table 41.1).

Table 41.1 Media Formulations. Products included in this table are representative of media products sold in the United States. Actual concentrations are included (mM, g/L or as indicated) if published. Symbols are as follows: "X" indicates the product is present, but concentration is not published, "ne" designates non essential amino acids, "e" designates essential amino acids

	Media for fertilization ± cleavage culture							Media for cleavage ± blastocyst culture							Media for blastocyst culture				
	Sage	Vitro Life	Irvine	Irvine	Many	Medicult	Cook	Sage	Vitro Life	Irvine	Life Global	Medicult	Cook	Sage	Vitro Life	Irvine	Life Global	Medicult	Cook
	Quinn's Advantage fertilization	GIVF	P1	HTF	HF10	Universal IVF	Sydney fertilization	Quinn's advantage cleavage	G1v5	EC medium	Global	Embryo Assist	Sydney cleavage	Advantage blastocyst	G2v5	Multiblast	Blastocyst	Blast Assist	Sydney blasto-cyst
Inorganic salt																			
Calcium chloride		X	2.01	1.84	0.285	X			X	1.70	X				X	1.70	X		
Cupric sulfate					9.5 nM														
Ferrous sulfate					0.003														
Magnesium chloride						X	X						X						X
Magnesium sulfate (anhyd)	X	X	0.20	0.18	0.591	X	X	X	X	0.20	X		X	X	X	0.20	X		X
Other						EBSS						EBSS						EBSS	
Orthophosphate 1 hydrate		X					X						X						X
Potassium chloride	X	X	4.69	4.22	3.630	X	X	X	X	2.50	X		X	X	X	2.50	X		X
Potassium phospate	X			0.33	0.580	X					X			X		0.35	X		
Sodium choride	X	X	101.6	91.44	121.0	X	X	X	X	102.7	X		X	X	X	101.50	X		X
Sodium dihydrogen		X																	
Sodium phosphate					1.030	X			X						X				
Zinc sulfate					0.000														
Energy source																			
Calcium lactate	X				1.170		X	X				X	X	X				X	X
Fructose		X																	
Glucose	X	X		2.50	5.810	X	X	X	X	0.50	X	X	X	X	X	3.00	X	X	X
Pyruvate (sodium)	X	X	0.33	0.30		X	X	X	X	0.33	X	X	X	X	X	0.20	X	X	X
Pyruvic acid					1.190														
Sodium lactate		X	21.40	19.30					X	20.77	X				X	20.00	X		
Antibiotics																			
Gentamycin	X	X	10 µg/ml	9 µg/ml	X		X	X	X	10 µg/ml	X		X	X	X	10 µg/ml	X		X
Penicillin					X	X						X						X	
Streptomycin						50 mg/L						50 mg/L						50 mg/L	
Other																			
Choline chloride					0.005									X					
EDTA	X	X					X	X	X	10 µm	X	X	X				X	X	
HEPES												X						X	

(continued)

Table 41.1 (continued)

	Media for fertilization ± cleavage culture							Media for cleavage ± blastocyst culture							Media for blastocyst culture					
	Sage	Vitro Life	Irvine	Irvine	Many	Medicult	Cook	Sage	Vitro Life	Irvine	Life Global	Medicult	Cook	Sage	Vitro Life	Irvine	Life Global	Medicult	Cook
	Quinn's Advantage fertilization	GIVF	P1	HTF	HF10	Universal IVF	Sydney fertilization	Quinn's advantage cleavage	G1v5	EC medium	Global	Embryo Assist	Sydney cleavage	Advantage blastocyst	G2v5	Multiblast	Blastocyst	Blast Assist	Sydney blastocyst
Heptahydrate		X																	
Hyaluronan									X						X				
Lipoic acid									X										
Pantothenate							X						X						X
Phenol red (sodium)	X		0.005 g/L	4.50	0.003	X		X		4.8 mg/L	X	X		X		4.8 mg/L	X	X	
Sodium bicarbonate	X		25.00	22.50	23.800	X	X	X	X	25.00	X	X	X	X	X	25.00	X	X	X
Sodium hydrogen carbonate		X																	
Sodium citrate	X	X	0.15 mg/L					X	X	0.15					X	1.00			
Taurine	X	X	0.05				X	X	X	0.05		X	X	X				X	X
Vitamins												X						X	
Biotin					X														
Folic acid					0.003									X					
Inositol														X					
Niacinamide					0.005														
Thiamine					0.003									X	X	0.05			
Vitamin B12					0.001														
Amino acids (L)	6 ne	9 ne	0	0	18ne 9e	0	8ne	6ne	8ne 1e	1ne	X	X	11ne 8e	14ne 9e	14ne 9e	11ne 9e	X	X	11ne 8e
Alanine		X			0.096		X		X				X		X	0.05			X
Alanyl glutamine	X	X			0.950		X	X	X	0.50			X	X	X	1.00			X
Arginine		X			1.150								X	X	X	0.30			X
Asparagine	X				0.108		X	X	X				X	X	X	0.05			X
Aspartic acid	X	X			0.095		X	X	X				X	X	X	0.05			X
Calcium pantothenate													X		X				X
Cysteine					0.190									X	X	0.05			
Cystine					0.190								X		X				X
Gluathione														X					
Glutamate		X					X		X										X
Glutamine		X			0.095											0.05			
Glycine	X	X			0.095		X	X	X					X	X	0.05			
Histidine (e)					0.141								X	X	X	0.10			X
Isoleucine(e)					0.019								X	X	X	0.20			X
Leucine (e)					0.095								X	X	X	0.20			X
Lysine (e)					0.191								X	X	X	0.20			X
Methionine (e)					0.029				X				X	X	X	0.05			X

myo-Inositol			0.003								
Pantothenic acid (hemical-cium)			0.003					X			
Phenyalanine (e)			0.029				X	X	X	0.10	X
Proline	X	X	0.095	X	X	X	X	X	X	0.05	X
Pyridoxine			0.001					X	X		
Riboflavin			0.001					X	X		
Serine	X	X	0.095	X	X	X	X	X	X	0.05	X
Thiotic acid			0.001								
Threonine (e)			0.029					X	X	0.20	
Thymidine			0.003					X			
Tryptophan (e)			0.003				X	X	X	0.02	X
Tyrosine			0.014				X	X	X	0.10	X
Valine (e)			0.028				X	X	X	0.20	X

Much research has been done to assess the impact of these various components on embryo development. Studies on glucose metabolism have unequivocally shown that high glucose concentrations (typically 2.5–5.5 mM) are needed in insemination media [50, 51]. Other studies on amino acid effects demonstrated superior rates of embryo development when nonessential amino acids and glutamine are present during cleavage to the 8-cell stage, whereas addition of both non-essential and essential amino acids favored development from the 8-cell stage to blastocyst [52]. On the other hand, penicillin and/or streptomycin may do more harm than good. At least one study in mice has shown lower fertilization rates (23% treated vs. 74% control) when using streptomycin at concentrations of 50 µg/ml or more [53]. In another study, the cleavage rate of human embryos was more than 1.5 times higher (94% vs. 58%, $P<0.01$) on day 3 when the embryos were grown in media without penicillin and streptomycin [54]. Currently, most culture media are supplemented with gentamicin in lieu of penicillin and streptomycin.

These findings, as well as others, have led to development of many different media formulations (Table 41.2), which undoubtedly are responsible, at least in part, for the improvement in implantation rates achieved in clinical IVF over the last decade or so. However, they have also sparked controversy as to which media system may be the best [55–60] and have led to debate as to whether sequential culture systems (i.e., systems using two different media, the first from days 1–3, the second from days 3–5) improve development when compared to single-media systems for the culture of gametes and embryos [61–63]. Sequential (two-step) culture systems are based on the original observation of Gardner et al. [64] that there is a changing energy substrate profile from the Fallopian tube to the uterine environment (lower glucose and higher lactate and pyruvate concentrations in the Fallopian tube, compared with the uterine environment). In contrast, the design of at least one of the monoculture (single-step) media has been based on rigorous experimental design using simplex optimization methodology [65].

Adding fuel to this controversy is the unknown effect different media formulations may have on gene imprinting. Concerning data in mouse indicate that the H19 gene, which is normally preferentially expressed from the maternal allele, was aberrantly expressed in embryos cultured in Whitten's media, but not KSOM-exposed embryos [66]. Additionally, some genes appeared to be unaffected, indicating that these molecular perturbations may be very subtle and difficult to quantify. Thus, it is critical that research continuing to target optimization of culture media formulations must appraise performance not only by implantation potential of the cultured embryos, but also by the assessment of potential down-stream adverse effects on the health of the offspring.

When considering which culture system may be superior, one must realize that media systems will perform differently

Table 41.2 Media manufacturers and media applications. Products included are representative of products sold in the United States

		Application			
Company	Media Name	Fertilization (Day 0)	Cleavage (Days 1–3)	Blastocyst culture (Days 3–6)	Web address
Sage	Quinn's Advantage Fertilization	x			www.coopersurgical.com
VitroLife	GIVF	x			www.vitrolife.com
Irvine	P1	x	x		www.irvinesci.com
Irvine	HTF	x	x		www.irvinesci.com
Medicult	Universal IVF	x			www.medicult.com
Cook	Sydney fertilization	x			www.cookmedical.com
Various Companies	HF10	x	x		
Sage	Quinn's advantage cleavage		x		
VitroLife	G1v5		x		
Irvine	ECM		x		
Medicult	EmbryoAssist		x		
Cook	Sydney Fertilization		x		
Lifeglobal	Global		x	x	www.lifeglobal.com
Sage	Quinn's advantage blastocyst			x	
VitroLife	G2v5			x	
Irvine	MultiBlast			x	
Medicult	BlastAssist			x	
Cook	Sydney blastocyst			x	
LifeGlobal	Blastocyst			x	

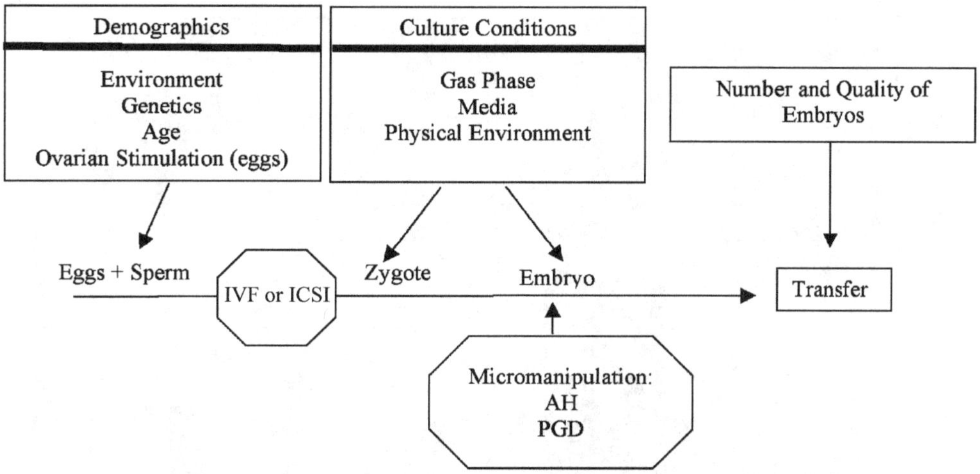

Fig. 41.3 Some of the variables that affect IVF outcomes

in different laboratories. This is an important consideration. Since atmospheric pressure, incubator quality control, and stimulation protocols (to name a few) can all affect performance, it is only reasonable that media formulations must be tested under the conditions in which they will be practiced (Fig. 41.3). Furthermore, one must realize that the culture system settled on by a laboratory does not have to subscribe to all the components of an entire vendor package (i.e., the complete media system marketed from egg collection to blastocyst culture) but rather, should reflect the optimum results obtained after careful testing of each product.

This systematic approach is one that we practice both to maximize results and to contain cost. For example, in one paradigm, we used Sage Quinn's Advantage Fertilization Media (SQAF) as our insemination media and VitroLife G1v3 (G3) as the day 1–3 cleavage medium. We arrived at this combination after several clinical trials in which we found this to be an efficacious and cost-effective media combination. However, we wished to test whether one medium was better for the culture of oocytes immediately after ICSI. Using a matched pair experimental design in which half the patient's oocytes were randomly allocated to each media after ICSI, we found advantages to using the G3 media (Fig. 41.4). Although there was no difference in the fertilization rates between G3 vs. SQAF (66.6% vs. 69.6%, $P=0.45$), 1.5 times more 8-cell embryos developed in eggs exposed to G3 media immediately after injection as compared to SQAF (1.38 ± 1.23 vs. 0.92 ± 1.01, $P<0.05$). On the basis of these results, we settled on the use of G3 media for post-ICSI culture, even though the manufacturing companies do not specifically indicate this combination of media.

41.4.7 Plating Considerations

Various plating techniques are used to culture embryos and they involve many combinations of variables. For instance, some embryologists prefer to overlay culture media with oil (i.e., a closed system) in order to improve the maintenance of osmolarity, pH, and temperature, whereas others prefer the use of systems without oil (open system). The two systems also differ in that the open system typically involves larger volumes of medium (ranging from 0.5 ml to 2 ml per dish) as compared with the closed system that usually involves microdrops of medium (ranging from 25 μl to 100 μl per drop). Plate design also varies (Fig. 41.5). Some of the more common plates used for human embryo culture include organ culture dishes, multi-well plates, and standard 30 mm or 60 mm tissue culture petri dishes. The basic difference in these plates is the size of the culture well. Organ culture dishes have a large central culture well (2 ml capacity) surrounded by a moat that can hold up to 7 ml of media and is often used for humidification and pre-wash of cells. Multi-well plates vary in capacity from 2 to 96 wells and can hold media droplets ranging from 0.10 to 1 ml depending on whether or not an oil overlay is used. The 60 mm plates have the largest capacity (8 ml) and, as with the 30 mm dishes, are typically used with microdrops of media in a closed system. A variation of the 60 mm plates has recently been developed that has pre-etched chambers for micro-drops (GPS embryo culture dishes, IVF Online); their efficacy is currently being evaluated.

Most of the studies involving direct comparisons of the open vs. closed culture systems have limitations due to

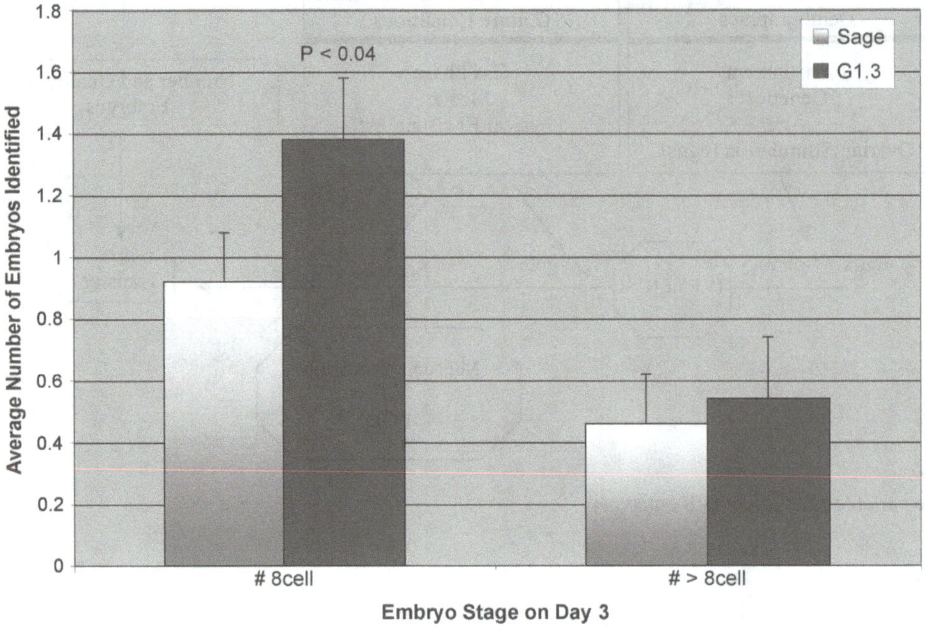

Fig. 41.4 Matched-pair comparison of Sage Quinn's Fertilization Media vs. VitroLife G1.3 for use as post-ICSI culture media. Data represent 39 patients for whom oocytes were randomized to one of the two media immediately post-ICSI. Results reported as average ± standard error

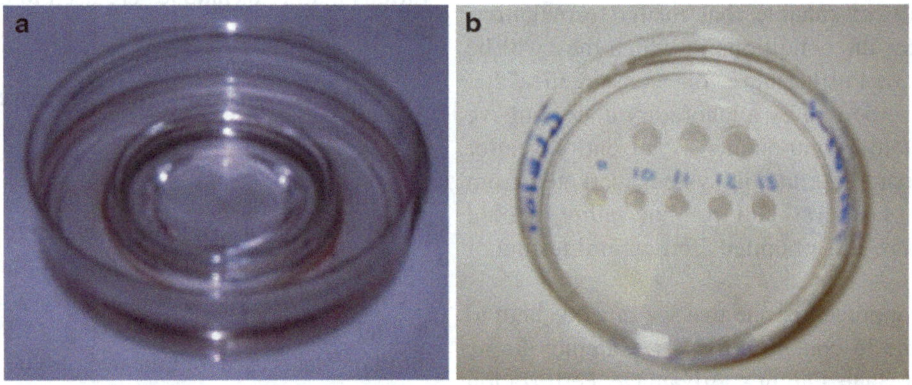

Fig. 41.5 Representative culture dishes used in clinical IVF: (a) standard Falcon organ culture dish (No. 3037) with outer ring for rinsing, and inner well for culturing cells; (b) closed microdrop system under oil in a Falcon culture dish (No.1007)

differences in plating volumes used; nevertheless, the weight of the evidence appears to favor use of a closed system for embryo culture. For instance, Sherbahn et al. compared blastocyst formation rates in mouse embryos cultured in groups (18 embryos/condition) using an open system (1 ml) vs. a closed system (30 µl drops) and found that significantly more blastocysts formed in the closed system as compared to the open system (14.6 vs. 10.2% $P<0.001$) [67]. A more recent clinical study by Petersen et al. supports these results. Although the published implantation and pregnancy rates appear to be reversed in the table, the results seem to show significantly higher implantation rates when embryos were cultured under oil (50 µl) as compared with when they were cultured without (1 ml) (25% vs. 3.8%, $P<0.05$) [68]. The results of these two studies are further supported by a bovine embryo study which demonstrated a significantly higher hatched blastocyst:blastocyst ratio when embryos were cultured in multiwell dishes containing 30–50 µl microdrops under oil as compared to those with 0.5 ml of media without oil (70.2% vs. 49.6% $P<0.05$) [69]. These findings are in direct opposition to those of Ozawa et al. [70], who found that pig embryos, when cultured in 5 ml of media without oil overlay, formed the same percentage of blastocysts compared with that using an oil overlay. Although this study controlled for both plate type and media volume, it used non-standard

IVF dishes and 5 ml of medium, thus the efficacy in a clinical IVF setting is unknown. Other studies have found no benefit to the use of oil unless there are toxic substances in the media [71]. Taken together, most of the available data, and all published clinical studies, support the use of an oil overlay for human embryo culture. It remains to be determined whether this overall benefit of an oil overlay is due to the accumulation of higher concentrations of autocrine factors in the microdrops, and/or to advantages accrued by the more stable environment imparted by the overlay itself.

There are two types of oil used for embryo culture: mineral and silicone oil. Mineral oil is comprised of mixtures of highly refined paraffinic liquid hydrocarbons [72], thus it is sometimes called paraffin oil. This can be confusing when one reviews the literature because some reports use both "mineral oil" and "paraffin oil" when making direct comparisons. In a strict sense, the two are the same; however, differences in the manufacturing process may lead to variations in performance. For instance, when mineral oil distributed by Sigma Aldrich was compared to that distributed by BDH, the BDH product was found to be embryotoxic as compared to the Sigma Aldrich product (0% vs. 11 % murine morula, $P<0.05$), and remained toxic even after washing with culture media [73]. In another study, when the same Sigma product was pre-washed and compared to OvOil ("light paraffin oil"; VitroLife, Inc), significantly fewer morulae and blastocysts formed as compared with those in OvOil (30.6% vs. 44.8%, $P<0.05$) [74]. Manufacturing considerations aside, it appears that mineral oil may be a better choice for use in embryo culture systems than silicone oil because of its hydrophobic properties. While both oil types absorb hydrocarbon compounds from the media, seven times more radiolabelled estrogen diffused from innoculated drops into pristine media drops when the drops were plated under silicone oil as compared to mineral oil [75]. Furthermore, twice as many blastocysts were formed when bovine eggs were inseminated and cultured under paraffin oil as compared to silicone oil (28.0 ± 6.0 vs. 14.0 ± 9.0, $P<0.001$) [76], a finding that was constant across two different lots of silicone oil.

Consideration should also be given to the potential adverse effects of lot-to-lot variation of oil. As with lot-to-lot variation of any product, these variations can be very subtle and difficult to track back, but can cause major problems in embryo culture performance. For instance, in one study, although two different lots of silicone oil produced comparable blastocyst formation rates (14% and 15% respectively) during fresh culture, none of the vitrified embryos from one lot survived the thaw process [76]. Lot variations in oil may be due to a myriad of variables. However, at least one study indicates that it may be attributable, at least in part, to variations in the peroxide value (POV), an indicator of oil oxidation associated with molecular oxygen [77]. In this study, one "bad" batch of oil was found to have 2.97 mEq/kg POV, whereas the control batch of oil that supported normal embryo development had 0 mEq/kg POV. This study is interesting in that it postulates that shelf-life and storage conditions can greatly effect oil performance. We have also observed this phenomenon. Using a mouse one-cell assay, mineral oil was tested the same week it was delivered or at various intervals up to 30 weeks of storage at room temperature in the dark (Fig. 41.6). While these storage criteria are well within the 1 year shelf-life per the manufacturer, we found significantly lower blastocyst formation rates as soon as 9 weeks after delivery. Therefore, we now limit the use of oil to within 6 weeks of the delivery date.

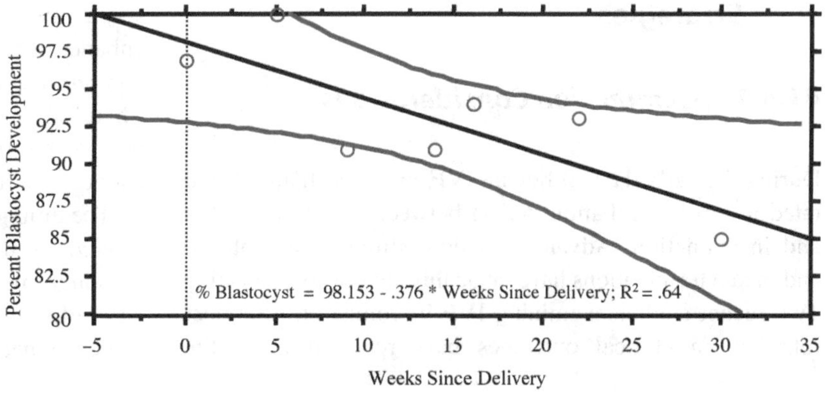

Fig. 41.6 Shelf life of oil. Fresh mouse embryos were cultured from the one cell stage through to blastocyst stage using HF10 in organ culture dishes with a 1 ml oil overlay. Data are reported as percent blastocyst development per 2-cell embryo (bivariate scattergram with regression line and 95% confidence bands as shown on the graph)

41.4.7.1 Dish Equilibration, Number of Observations and Media Renewal During Culture

Since temperature and pH affect embryo development, care needs to be taken to ensure complete equilibration of all media before use and during the culture period. However, few studies report the optimum equilibration time for culture solutions, perhaps because so many different culture systems are available. Nevertheless, of all the factors that come into play, it appears that pre-equilibration of dishes for 16–20 h in elevated CO_2 (typically 5–6%) with at least a 2 h pre-incubation at 37°C is required [78].

There are also very few studies, which address the effect on embryonic development of the number of times the embryos are taken out of the incubator. In one rather poorly described study, no differences in mouse blastulation rates were observed when embryos were examined at 24, 48, and 72 h intervals [79]. Thus, while frequent observation is not recommended, it appears not to harm embryos when done in an efficient manner. Indeed, it may be beneficial in order to derive cumulative developmental scores on embryos during culture (see Chap. 44).

It is unclear as to whether or not media renewal during the culture period is necessary. On the one hand, renewal has been shown to eliminate the build up of potentially harmful by products such as ammonia during culture [80]. On the other hand, it has been postulated that embryos condition media by autocrine secretion as they grow. In at least two studies, increased survival rates were obtained by renewal of the media [81, 82] and in another, changing media improved day 6 blastocyst rates, but only in serum-free media [83]. These data conflict with those from two other studies which found that media renewal either resulted in a decrease in the hatched blastocyst to blastocyst ratio [69] or had no effect [61]. Thus, it is likely that any benefit to culture media renewal is media-specific and dependent upon the duration of embryo culture.

41.5 Oocyte and Embryo Handling Strategies

41.5.1 Insemination Considerations

During the early days of human IVF, industry standards dictated a 2–6 h incubation period between oocyte collection and insemination. Advances in both stimulation protocols and media formulations have made this topic worth revisiting. Two recent studies examining IVF insemination time post-retrieval on clinical outcomes have reported conflicting results. In one study, pre-incubation of IVF eggs for increasing hourly intervals (range: 1 to ≥5 h) showed no effect on fertilization or ongoing pregnancy rates [84]. In contrast, another study showed that pre-incubation for less than 2.5 h or ≥5.5 h resulted in significantly lower fertilization rates than the hourly intervals between these two time points [85]. The findings for ICSI inseminations are also conflicted. While some have found that there is no advantage to pre-incubating the eggs prior to ICSI treatment [84–86], others have observed improved fertilization and embryo quality rates after pre-incubation for 2–4 h (180) or >3 h [87]. In fact, whether clinical outcome is impacted by the time interval between cumulus-corona removal and ICSI requires further resolution. Although the majority of IVF laboratories allow the lapse of 1 h between somatic cell removal and injection, at least one study has shown that this may not be necessary [86]. Given these contradictory findings, further research is clearly indicated. In the interim, it is recommended that each IVF laboratory assess their own data to identify the optimum times for insemination and ICSI in their own setting. In our laboratory, we perform IVF inseminations 4–6 h post-retrieval and ICSI injections at 4–5 h after retrieval, with allowance of a 1 h interval between cumulus-corona removal and injection.

The optimum concentration of sperm used must maximize the percentage of diploid zygotes formed, and minimize the incidence of polyspermic zygotes. In addition, consideration must be given to possible adverse effects of high numbers of sperm on embryo quality due to oxygen-free radical release. Numerous studies have attempted to identify the optimum sperm concentration. However, it is difficult to compare these studies, because many do not stipulate insemination conditions such as medium volume, or number of eggs inseminated [88–91]. Nevertheless, the weight of the evidence indicates that sperm concentrations ranging from 50,000 to 500,000/ml may be optimal for diploid rates, although polyspermy may increase with increasing concentrations [90, 91]. We therefore recommend that each laboratory perform trials within the same oocyte cohorts to identify the optimum sperm concentration to use within their own culture system. Furthermore, although increasing sperm numbers in cases of teratozoospermia appears to enhance fertilization rates, the quality of embryos appears compromised compared to those derived from ICSI [92]. Therefore, teratozoospermic patients having adequate numbers of motile sperm for standard insemination should be encouraged to utilize ICSI.

The timing of co-incubation of gametes should also be considered as it may affect fertilization and embryo quality. Although most clinics allow 16–18 h co-incubation of gametes before the oocytes are checked for fertilization, there is evidence that as little as a 1 h co-incubation may be all that is needed to maximize fertilization rates [93]. Furthermore, a prospective trial randomizing patients to different incubation times showed that cleavage rates may be superior in those embryos derived from reduced insemination time (55% vs. 40% embryos at the 4–5 cell stage on day 2, after 1 h vs. 16 h co-incubation, respectively; $P<0.005$) [93]. These findings were confirmed in another prospective randomized study [94], which also showed higher implantation (24.6% vs. 12.1%, $P<0.003$) and pregnancy rates (48.4% vs. 28.6%, $P<0.002$) for those embryos derived after short gamete co-incubation as compared to those from overnight incubations. Given these consistent findings, the efficacy of co-incubation of oocytes and sperm for 1–2 h should at least be tested by each laboratory when devising a standard insemination protocol.

41.5.2 Timing Fertilization Checks

The timing of formation of the pronuclei is dependent on the insemination method [95]. When sibling oocytes were subjected to either ICSI or IVF insemination, Nagy et al. observed that two pronuclei are visible as early as 6 h post ICSI and their visibility peaks between 10 and 12 h, with a slight decline by 18 h. In contrast, the pronuclei in IVF inseminated oocytes are delayed in their appearance, first being visible at approximately 8 h post insemination, with peak visibility at 18 h. Additionally, a 4-h time lag was noted with the start of the first cleavage division: ICSI embryos began cleaving at 20 h post ICSI whereas IVF embryos did so 24 h post insemination. Therefore, although current dogma is to perform the fertilization check between 16 and 18 h after routine insemination or ICSI, pronuclear formation is best visualized between 10 h and before 18 h for ICSI oocytes, and between 18 and 20 h for IVF oocytes. However, definitive windows for optimal visualization probably depend on the insemination medium, and should be established within each laboratory.

41.5.3 Embryo Density Issues

The number of oocytes and embryos cultured per drop must also be considered. While it is advantageous to use single embryo culture techniques in order to determine characteristics that support embryo developmental potential, data derived from animal experiments suggest that this may not be best for human eggs and embryos. However, most of the animal work has been performed in multi-ovulatory species wherein evolutionary mechanisms may favor inter-embryo co-operativity and may not be relevant to the mono-ovulatory human. Furthermore, comparison of results in the animal experiments is complicated by variances in media volume and grouping sizes.

In five of six animal studies, embryo development was improved with embryo co-culture; however, these improvements were affected by the number of embryos per drop and medium volume [82, 96–100]. Of concern when using group culture, however, is the effect that degenerating embryos may have on others in the group. Indeed, when degenerating embryos were added to group culture, the cell numbers in blastocysts were significantly reduced [99]. The results from human studies are a little less clear. In at least two studies, improved cleavage and pregnancy rates were seen when embryos were cultured in groups [101, 102]; yet in two others studies, no differences were seen in blastocyst formation rate or pregnancy rate when embryos were grown singly or in groups [103, 104]. Taken together, it appears that there may be no "right" way to culture human embryos with respect to embryo density. However, it may be prudent to use a single-embryo culture strategy when one considers possible detrimental effects of degenerating embryos on those that are viable, coupled with the advantages that may be gained by maintaining a unique embryo identity for selection purposes.

41.5.4 Embryo Transfer Day

In the early days of IVF, embryos were typically transferred on day 1 or day 2 due to concerns about the ability of the in vitro systems to sustain embryo development and the appreciation that a high proportion of human embryos undergo arrest in culture. With improvements in culture media in the early '90s, the opportunity to prolong the duration of culture led to the more common practice of transferring embryos on day 3. By the late '90s, the introduction of blastocyst culture media provided the opportunity for extending the culture for at least a further 48 h to perform transfers on day 5 or 6. These collective advancements in culture media development have led to one of the most heated controversies in ART: whether to transfer the embryos on day 3 or day 5 (Fig. 41.7).

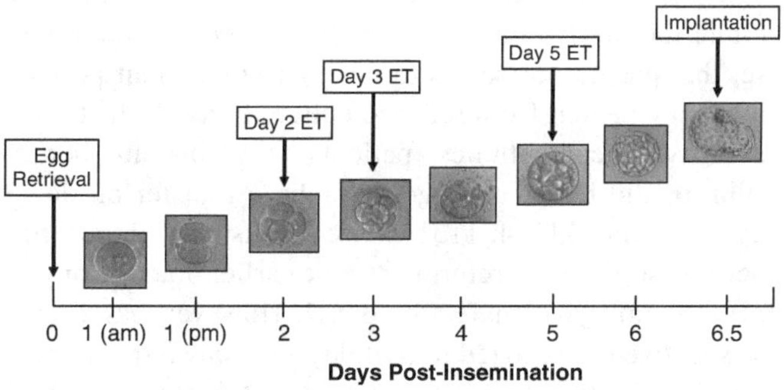

Fig. 41.7 Preimplantation developmental timeline in the human

There are several theoretical advantages to culturing embryos to the blastocyst stage and performing a day 5 or 6 transfer. They include: (1) improving synchronization of embryo development with uterine receptivity (cleavage stage embryos typically undergo development in the fallopian tube with traversal of the utero-tubal junction at the morula stage 4–5 days after fertilization); (2) providing the possibility of in vitro embryo selection (lesser quality embryos arrest and developmentally competent embryos cross developmental milestones to reach the blastocyst stage); (3) reducing the risk of multiple gestations by transferring fewer superior quality embryos [105, 106]; and (4) allowing sufficient time between blastomere biopsy and genetic analysis for fresh transfer to be performed in cases of preimplantation genetic diagnosis, as first described by Hardy et al. [18].

An early study showed that blastocyst transfer may be beneficial in good prognosis patients having ≥3, day three embryos with 8-cells [107]. This observation has been further substantiated in a study with egg donors following stratification of cycles according to those having ≥3 embryos with 7-cells [108]. Indeed, a recent Cochrane review evaluating the benefit of day 5 vs. day 3 transfer has provided further evidence indicating a significant increase in pregnancy and livebirth rates in favor of blastocyst transfer in good prognosis patients (36.0 % vs. 29.4% livebirth rate, OR 1.35 95% CI 1.05–1.74) [109]. However, there are disadvantages associated with blastocyst transfer. These include: (1) the risk of not having any blastocysts available for transfer [106, 109]; (2) a reduction in the number of embryos frozen [109, 110]; (3) an increased risk of monozygotic twinning [111]; and (4) an increased risk of the obstetrically more serious condition of monochorionic twinning [112]. Furthermore, animal data show that there may be increased induction of stress-activation proteins from pipetting [113], suggesting that increased embryo manipulation involved with prolonged culture should be held to a minimum. It is clear, therefore, that whether to transfer on day 3 or day 5 should be evaluated on case-by-case basis with patients being thoroughly counseled.

Despite advances in culture media developments, it is highly probable that any in vitro culture system does not mimic the in vivo environment. If one accepts this premise, the question arises as to whether any patient populations may benefit from reduced culture times. In fact, in at least two recent studies, patients with low number of embryos did better undergoing embryo transfer on day 2 instead of day 3 [114, 115]. These results may support further investigation of returning to the earlier practice of performing embryo transfers on day 2. However, based on a prospective randomized trial of day 1 vs. day 3 transfers, it seems unlikely that we will revert to transferring day 1 embryos [116].

41.5.5 Somatic Cell Co-culture

Given that even the most state-of-the-art culture systems are unlikely to mimic precisely the in vivo uterine environment, several studies have investigated possible benefit of co-culturing embryos with somatic cells. These somatic cells have involved either culture with cumulus or membrana granulosa cells or with frozen-thawed endometrial cells. In the granulosa cell studies, overall results showed beneficial effects on embryo quality [117–119], and implantation and pregnancy rates [120]. In fact, in poor prognosis patients, these positive effects can be dramatic as evidenced by a 14-fold increase in the percentage of good quality embryos in patients who went from a system without co-culture, to use of co-culture in a subsequent cycle [118]. Similar beneficial results have been obtained using endometrial co-culture systems [121, 122]. These benefits are dependent upon the day of luteal phase endometrial biopsy with biopsies performed 5 days or more post-LH surge (range 5–12 days) supporting superior embryo development than those performed less than 5 days post LH-surge [122]. When comparing these two co-culture approaches (granulosa vs. endometrial), it is clear that the granulosa cell approach is less labor-intensive, involves less intervention with the patient, and appears to provide similar benefits. However, no published studies have compared the two approaches head-to-head.

41.6 Developing Embryo Culture Techniques

In contrast to the dynamic properties that prevail in the in vivo environment provided by the Fallopian tube and uterine fluids, current embryo culture systems are static in nature. Efforts to compensate for this static property involve the introduction of nutrients in a temporal sequence that attempt to match metabolic and amino acid composition with specific developmental stages. Alternatively, systems using microperfusion of media across eggs and embryos are being developed to provide an in vivo-like dynamic environment in vitro. Such systems are being tested with animal embryos [123–126] and include various perfusion technologies. One promising study showed improved cleavage and blastocyst formation rates in mouse embryos cultured in microchannels vs. microdrops under oil [124]. However, further research is needed to refine the systems and to establish efficacy for use in the clinical IVF laboratory.

41.7 Conclusions

When determining the best clinical embryo culture system to use, multiple components must be considered. These include macro and micro-environmental issues as well as media, gamete and embryo handling, and culture duration choices. While it is important to test all these variables in one's own laboratory and adapt protocols to maximize clinical results, one must respect the fact that we may never fully mimic the in vivo environment. Furthermore, the standard measures of performance of a clinical IVF laboratory (i.e., fertilization, implantation, and live-birth rates) may not target the most critical outcome: that of neonate health and long-term downstream effects on health of the child and adult.

References

1. Schenk SL (1880) Des saugethieriei kumstlick befruchtet auBerh-all-des mutterthiesus. As cited by RE Hammer 1998. Int J Dev Biol 42:833–839. Mitt Embr Inst KK Univer Wien 1:107–118
2. Heape W (1890) Preliminary note on the transplantation and growth of mammalian ova within a uterine foster-mother. Proc R Soc Lond 48:457–458
3. Pincus G, Enzmann EV (1934) Can mammalian eggs undergo normal development in vitro? Proc Natl Acad Sci U S A 20:121–122
4. Hammond J (1949) Recovery and culture of tubal mouse ova. Nature 163:28–29
5. Whitten WK (1957) Culture of tubal ova. Nature 179:1081–1082
6. McLaren A, Biggers JD (1958) Successful development and birth of mice cultivated in vitro as early embryos. Nature182:877–878
7. Chang MC (1959) Fertilization of rabbit ova in vitro. Nature 84:466–467
8. Hertig AT, Rock J (1949) Two human ova of the pre-villous stage, having a developmental age of about 8 and 9 days respectively. Contrib Embryol 33(213–221):169–186
9. Steptoe PC, Edwards RG (1978) Birth after the reimplantation of a human embryo. Lancet 2:366
10. Edwards RG, Bavister BD, Steptoe PC (1969) Early stages of fertilization in vitro of human oocytes matured in vitro. Nature 221:632–635
11. Edwards RG (2005) An astonishing journey into reproductive genetics since the 1950's. Reprod Nutr Dev 45:299–306
12. Trounson A, Mohr L (1983) Human pregnancy following cryopreservation, thawing and transfer of an eight-cell embryo. Nature 305:707–709
13. Chen C (1986) Pregnancy after human oocyte cryopreservation. Lancet 350:186–187
14. Gordon JW (1988) Fertilization of human oocytes by sperm from infertile males after zona pellucida drilling. Fertil Steril 50(1):68–73
15. Palermo G, Joris H, Devroey P, Van Steirteghem AC (1992) Pregnancies after intracytoplasmic injection of single spermatozoon into an oocyte. Lancet 340:17–18
16. Cohen J, Elsner C, Kort H, Malter H, Massey J, Mayer MP, Weimer K (1990) Impairment of the hatching process following IVF in the human and improvement of implantation by assisting hatching using micromanipulation. Hum Reprod 5(1):7–13
17. Bolton VN, Wren ME, Parsons JH (1991) Pregnancies after in vitro fertilization and transfer of human blastocysts. Fertil Steril 55(4):830–832
18. Schoolcraft WB, Gardner DK, Lane M, Schlenker T, Hamilton F, Meldrum DR (1999) Blastocyst culture and transfer: analysis of results and parameters affecting outcome in two in vitro fertilization programs. Fertil Steril 172(4):604–609
19. Hardy K, Martin KL, Leese HJ, Winston RM, Handyside AH (1990) Human preimplantation development in vitro is not adversely affected by biopsy at the 8-cell stage. Hum Reprod 5(6):708–714
20. Cohen J, Gilligan EW, Schimmel T, Dale B (1997) Ambient air and its potential effects on conception in vitro. Hum Reprod 12(8): 1742–1749
21. Boone WR, Higdon HL III, Skelton WD (2007) How to design and implement an assisted reproductive technology (ART) cleanroom. Clin Emb 10(4):5–17
22. Higdon HL III, Blackhurst DW, Boone WR (2008) Incubator management in an assisted reproductive technology laboratory. Fertil Steril 89(3):703–710
23. Merton JS, Vermeulen ZL, Otter T, Mullaart E, De Ruigh L, Hasler JF (2007) Carbon-activated gas filtration during in vitro culture increased pregnancy rate following transfer of in vitro-produced bovine embryos. Theriogenology 67:1233–1238
24. Hirao Y, Yanagimanchi R (1978) Temperature dependence of sperm-egg fusion and post-fusion events in hamster fertilization. J Exp Zool 205:433–438
25. Wang WH, Meng L, Hackett RJ, Odenbourg R, Keefe DL (2001) Limited recovery of meiotic spindles in living human oocytes after cooling-rewarming observed using polarized light. Hum Reprod 16(11):2374–2378
26. Scott L (2004) Microanalysis of rapid temperature fluctuations in IVF culture systems. Clin Emb 7(4):1–6
27. Cooke S, Tyler JPP, Driscoll G (2002) Objective assessments of temperature maintenance using in vitro culture techniques. J Assist Reprod Genet 19(8):368–375
28. Fujiwara M, Takahashi K, Izuno M, Duan YR, Kazono M, Kimura F, Noda Y (2007) Effect of micro-environment maintenance on embyo culture after in-vitro fertilization: comparison of top-loading mini incubator and conventional front-load incubator. J Assist Reprod Genet 24:5–9
29. Takenaka M, Horiuchi T, Yanagimachi R (2007) Effects of light on development of mammalian zygotes. Proc Natl Acad Sci U S A 104:14289–14293
30. Hirao Y, Yanagimanchi R (1978) Detrimental effects of visible light on meiosis of mammalian eggs in vitro. J Exp Zool 206:365–370
31. Fischer B, Schumacher A, Hegel-Hartung C, Beier HM (1988) Potential risk of light and room temperature exposure to preimplantation embryos. Fertil Steril 50(6):938–944
32. Oh SJ, Gong SP, Lee ST, Lee EJ, Lim JM (2007) Light intensity and wavelength during embryo manipulation are important factors for maintaining viability of preimplantation embryos in vitro. Fertil Steril 88(S2):1150–1157
33. Desmet KD, Paz DA, Corry JJ, Eells JT, Wong-Riley MTT, Henry MM, Buchman EV, Connelly MP, Dovi JV, Liang HL, Henshel DS, Yeager RL, Millsap DS, Lim J, Gould LJ, Das R, Jett M, Hodgson BD, Margolis D, Whelan HT (2006) Clinical and Experimental Applications of NIR-LED Photobiomodulation. Photomed Laser Surg 24(2):121–128
34. Ottosen LDM, Hindkjaer J (2007) Light exposure of the ovum and perimplantation embryo during ART procedures. J Assist Reprod Genet 24:99–103
35. Bedford JM, Dobrenis A (1989) Light exposure of oocytes and pregnancy rates after their transfer in the rabbit. J Reprod Fertil 85(2):477–481
36. Jackson KV, Kiessling AA (1989) Fertilization and cleavage of mouse oocytes exposed to the conditions of human oocyte retrieval for in vitro fertilization. Fertil Steril 51(4):675–681
37. Barlow P, Puissant F, Van Der Zwalmn P, Vandromme J, Trigaux P, Leroy F (1992) In Vitro fertilization, development and implantation after exposure of mature mouse oocytes to visible light. Mol Reprod Dev 33:297–302
38. Van Blerkom J, Antczak M, Schrader R (1997) The developmental potential of the human oocyte is related to the dissolved oxygen content of follicular fluid: association with vascular endothelial growth factor levels and perifollicular blood flow characteristics. Hum Reprod 12:1047–1055

39. Ottosen LDM, Hindkjaer J, Husth M, Petersen DE, Kirk J, Ingerslev HJ (2006) Observations on intrauterine oxygen tension measured by fiber-optic micro sensors. Reprod Biomed Online 13(3):380–385
40. Dumoulin JCM, Meijers CJJ, Bras M, Coonen E, Geraedts JPM, Evers JLH (1999) Effect of oxygen concentraion on human in-vitro fertilization and embryo culture. Hum Reprod 14(2): 465–469
41. Bahceci M, Ciray HN, Karagnec L, Ulug U, Bener F (2005) Effect of oxygen concentration during the incubation of embryos of women undergoing ICSI and embryo transfer: a prospective randomized study. Reprod Biomed Online 11(4):438–443
42. Rinaudo PF, Giritharan G, Talbi S, Dobson AT, Schulz RM (2006) Effects of oxygen tension on gene expression in preimplantation mouse embryos. Fertil Steril 86(3):1252–1265
43. Hugentobler S, Morris DG, Kane MT, Sreenan JM (2004) In situ oviduct and uterine pH in cattle. Theriogenology 61(7–8): 1419–1427
44. Dale B, Menezo Y, Cohen J, DiMatteo L, Wilding M (1998) Intracellular pH regulation in the human oocyte. Hum Reprod 13(4):964–970
45. Phillips KP, Leveill MC, Claman P, Baltz JM (2000) Intracellular pH regulation in human preimplantation embryos. Hum Reprod 15(4):896–904
46. Pool TB (2004) Optimizing pH in Clinical Embryology. Clin Emb 7(3):1–17
47. Ham RG (1963) An improved nutrient solution for diploid chinese hamster and human cell lines. Exp Cell Res 29:515–526
48. Quinn P, Kerin JF, Warnes GM (1985) Improved pregnancy rate in human in vitro fertilization with the use of a medium based on the composition of human tubal fluid. Fertil Steril 44(4):493–498
49. Winkel P, Statland BE, Bokelund H (1974) Factors contributing to intra-individual variation of serum constituents: 5. Short term day-to-day and within-hour variation of serum constituents in healthy subjects. Clin Chem 20(12):1520–1527
50. Travis AJ, Tuntuncu L, Jorgez CJ, Ord TS, Jones BH, Kopf GS, Williams CJ (2004) Requirement for glucose beyond sperm capacititation during In vitro fertilization in the mouse. Biol Reprod 71:139–145
51. William AC, Ford WCL (2001) The role of glucose in supporting motility and capacitation in human spermatozoa. J Androl 22(4): 680–695
52. Lane M, Gardner DK (1997) Differential regulation of mouse embryo development and viability by amino acids. J Reprod Fertil 109(1):153–164
53. Lemeire K, Van Merris V, Cortvrindt R (2007) The antibiotic streptomycin assessed in a battery of in vitro tests for reproductive toxicology. Toxicol In Vitro 21(7):1348–1353
54. Magli MC, Gianaroli L, Fiorentino A, Ferraretti AP, Fortini D, Panzella S (1996) Improved cleavage rate of human embryos cultured in antibiotic-free medium. Hum Reprod 11(7):1520–1524
55. Aoki VW, Wilcox AL, Peterson CM, Parker-Jones K, Hatasaka HH, Gibson M, Huang I, Carrell DT (2005) Comparison of four media types during 3-day human IVF embryo culture. Reprod Biomed Online 10(5):600–606
56. Urman B, Yakin K, Ata B, Isiklar A, Balaban B (2007) Effect of hyaluronan-enriched transfer medium on implantation and pregnancy rates after day 3 and day 5 embryo transfers; a prospective randomized study. Fertil Steril: PMID17936283 90(3):604–612
57. Friedler S, Schachter M, Strassburger D, Ester K, Ron El R, Raziel A (2007) A randomized clinical trial comparing recombinant hyaluronan/recombinant albumin versus human tubal fluid for cleavage stage embryo transfer in patients with multiple IVF-embryo transfer failure. Hum Reprod 22(9):2444–2448
58. Cooke S, Quinn P, Kime L, Ayres C, Tyler JPP, Driscoll GL (2002) Improvement in early human embryo development using new formulation sequential stage-specific culture media. Fertil Steril 78(6):1254–1260
59. Van Langendonckt A, Demylle D, Wyns C, Nisolle M, Donnez J (2001) Comparison of G1.2/G2.2 and Sydney IVF cleavage/blastocyst sequential media for the culture of human embryos: a prospective, randomized, comparative study. Fertil Steril 76(5): 1023–1031
60. Hentemann M, Bertheussen K (2009) New media for culture to blastocyst. Fertil Steril: PMID18321494 91(3):878–883
61. Biggers JD, Racowsky C (2002) The development of fertilized human ova to the blastocyst stage in medium KSOMAA: is a two-step protocol necessary? Reprod Biomed Online 5(2): 133–140
62. Macklon NS, Pieters MHEC, Hassan MA, Jeucken PHM, Eijkemans MJC, Fauser BCJM (2002) A prospective randomized comparison of sequential versus monoculture systems for in-vitro human blastocyst development. Hum Reprod 17(10):2700–2705
63. Biggers JD, McGinnis LK, Lawitts JA (2005) One-step versus two-step culture of mouse preimplantation embryos: is there a difference? Hum Reprod 20:3376–3384
64. Gardner DK, Lane M, Calderon I, Leeton J (1996) Environment of the preimplantation human embryo in vivo: metabolite analysis of oviduct and uterine fluids and metabolism of cumulus cells. Fertil Steril 65:349–353
65. Biggers JD, Lawitts J (1991) Optimization of mouse embryo culture media using simplex methods. J Reprod Fertil 91(2):543–556
66. Doherty AS, Mann MRW, Tremblay KD, Bartolomei MS, Schultz RM (2000) Differential effects of culture on imprinted H19 expression in the preimplantation mouse embryo. Biol Reprod 62:1526–1535
67. Sherbahn R, Frasor J, Radwanska E, Binor Z, Wood-Molo M, Hibner M, Mack S, Rawlins RG (1996) Comparison of mouse embryo development in open and microdrop co-culture systems. Hum Reprod 11(10):2223–2229
68. Petersen CG, Mauri AL, Massaro FC, Oliveira JBA, Baruffi RLR, Franco Jr JG (2005) Human ICSI embryo: development and implantation in open and microdrop culture systems. ESHRE, 21st annual meeting, p 439
69. Fukui Y, Lee E, Araki N (1996) Effect of medium renewal during culture in two different culture systems on development to blastocysts from in vitro produced early bovine embryos. J Anim Sci 74:2752–2758
70. Ozawa M, Nagai T, Kaneko H, Noguchi J, Ohnuma K, Kikuchi K (2006) Successful pig embryonic development in vitro outside a CO2 gas-regulated incubator: effects of pH and osmolality. Theriogenology 65:860–869
71. Miller KF, Goldberg JM, Collins RL (1994) Covering embryo cultures with mineral oil alters embryo growth by acting as a sink for an embryotoxic substances. J Assist Reprod Genet 11(7):342–345
72. Expert Committee on Food Additives (1970) Toxicological evaluation of some extraction solvents and certain other substances. World Health Organ Tech Rep Ser:14th report
73. Lee S, Cho M, Kim E, Kim T, Lee C, Han J, Lim J (2004) Renovation of a drop embryo cultures system by using refined mineral oil and the effect of glucose and/or hemoglobin added to a serum-free medium. J Vet Med Sci 66(1):63–66
74. Tae JC, Kim EY, Lee WD, Park SP, Lim JH (2006) Sterile filtered paraffin oil supports in vitro developmental competence in bovine embryos comparable to co-culture. J Assist Reprod Genet 23(3):121–127
75. Miller KF, Pursel VG (1987) Absorption of compounds in medium by the oil covering microdrop cultures. Gamete Res 17:57–61
76. Van Soom A, Mahmoudzadeh AR, Christophe A, Ysebaert MT, de Kruit A (2001) Silicone oil used in microdrop culture can affect bovine embryonic development and freezability. Reprod Domest Anim 36:169–176

77. Otsuki J, Nagai Y, Chiba K (2007) Peroxidation of mineral oil used in droplet culture is detrimental to fertilization and embryo development. Fertil Steril 88(3):741–742
78. Bavister BD, Poole KA (2004) Duration and temperature of culture medium equilibration affect frequency of blastocyst development. Reprod Biomed Online 10(1):124–129
79. Zhu B, Walker SK, Maddocks S (2004) Optimisation of in vitro culture conditions in B6CBF1 mouse embryos. Reprod Nutr Dev 44:219–231
80. Lane M, Gardner DK (1994) Increase in postimplantation development of cultured mouse embryos by amino acids and induction of fetal retardation and encephaly by ammonium ions. J Reprod Fertil 102(2):305–312
81. Blum-Reckow B, Holtz W (1991) Transfer of porcine embryos after 3 days of in vitro culture. J Anim Sci 69(8):335–3342
82. Fujita T, Umeki H, Shimura H, Kugumiya K, Shiga K (2006) Effect of group culture and embryo-culture conditioned medium on development of bovine embryos. J Reprod and Dev 52(1):137–142
83. Carolan C, Lonergan P, Van Langendockt A, Mermilod P (1995) Factors affectiing bovine embryos development in synthetic oviduct fluid following oocyte maturation and fertilization in vitro. Theriogenology 43(6):115–1128
84. Jacobs M, Stolwijk AM, Wetzels AMM (2001) The effect of insemination/injection time on the results of IVF and ICSI. Hum Reprod 16(8):1708–1713
85. Ho JY-P, Chen M-J, Yi Y-C, Guu H-F, Ho ESC (2003) The effect of preincubation period of oocytes on nuclear maturity, fertilization rate, embryo quality, and pregnancy outcome in IVF and ICSI. J Assist Reprod Genet 20(9):358–364
86. Van de Velse H, De Vos A, Jris H, Nagy ZP, Van Steirteghem AC (1998) Effect of timing of oocyte denudation and micro-injection on survival, fertilization and embryo quality after intracytoplasmic sperm injecton. Hum Reprod 13(11):3160–3164
87. Rienzi L, Ubaldi F, Anniballo R, Cerulo G, Greco E (1998) Preincubation of human oocytes may improve fertilization and embryo quality after intracytoplasmic sperm injection. Hum Reprod 13(4):1014–1019
88. Abir R, Orvieto R, Raanani H, Fisch B, Schoenfeld A, Ginton D, Nitke S, Ben Rafael Z (2000) Can varying the number of spermatozoa used for insemination improve in vitro fertilization rates. J Assist Reprod Genet 17(7):397–399
89. Wolf DP, Byrd W, Dandekar P, Quigley MM (1984) Sperm concentration and the fertilization of human eggs in vitro. Biol Reprod 31:837–848
90. Dumoulin JCM, Bras M, Land JA, Pieters HEC, Enginsu ME, Geraedts JPM, Evers JLH (1992) Effect of number of inseminated spermatozoa on subsequent uman and mouse embryonic developmeny in vitro. Hum Reprod 7(7):1010–1013
91. Van der Ven HH, Al-Hasani S, Diedrich K, Hamerich U, Lehmann F, Krebs D (1985) Polyspermy in in vitro fertilization of human oocytes: frequency and possible causes. Ann N Y Acad Sci 442:88–95
92. Oehninger S, Kruger TF, Simon T, Jones D, Mayer J, Lanzendorf S, Toner JP, Muasher SJ (1996) A comparative analysis of embryo implantation potential in patients with severe teratozoospermia undergoing in-vitro fertilization with a high concentration or intracytoplasmic sperm injection. Hum Reprod 11:1086–1089
93. Gianaroli L, Fiorentino A, Magli MC, Ferraretti AP, Montanaro N (1996) Prolonged sperm-oocyte exposure and high sperm concentration affect human embryo viability and pregnancy rate. Hum Reprod 11(11):2507–2511
94. Kattera S, Chen C (2003) Short coincubation of gametes in in vitro fertilization improves implantation and pregnancy rates; a prospective, randomized, controlled study. Fertil Steril 80(4):1017–1021
95. Nagy ZP, Janssenswillen C, Janssens R, De Vos A, Staessen C, Van de Velde H, Van Steirteghem AC (1998) Timing of oocyte activation, pronucleus formation and cleavage in humans after intracytoplasmic sperm injection (ICSI) with testicular spermatozoa and after ICSI or in-vitro ferlilization on sibling oocytes with ejaculated spermatozoa. Hum Reprod 13(6):1606–1612
96. Palasz AT, Thundathil J (1998) The effect of volume of culture medium and embryo density on in vitro development of bovine embryos. Theriogenology 49(1):212
97. Canseco RS, Sparks AET, Pearson RE, Gwazdauskas FC (1992) Embryo density and medium volume effects on early murine embryo development. J Assist Reprod Genet 9(5):454–457
98. de Oliveira AT, Lopes RF, Rodrigues JL (2005) Gene expression and developmental competence of bovine embros produced in vitro under varying embryo density conditions. Theriognology 64(7):1559–1572
99. Salahuddin S, Ookutsu S, Goto K, Nakanishi Y, Nagata Y (1995) Effects of embryo density and co-culture of unfertilized oocytes on embryonic development of in-vitro fertilized mouse embryos. Hum Reprod 10(9):2382–2385
100. Fukuja Y, Kikuchi Y, Kondo H, Mizushima S (2000) Fertizability and developmental capacity of individually cultured bovine oocytes. Theriogenology 53:1553–1585
101. Moessner J, Dodson WC (1995) The quality of human embryo growth is improved when embryos are cultured in groups rather than separately. Fertil Steril 64(5):1034–1035
102. Almagor M, Bejar C, Kafka I, Yaffe H (1996) Pregnancy rates after communal growth of preimplantation human embryos in vitro. Fertil Steril 66(3):394–397
103. Rijnders PM, Jansen CAM (1999) Influence of group culture and culture volume on the formation of human blastocysts: a prospective randomized study. Hum Reprod 14(9):2333–2337
104. Spyropoulos I, Karamalegos C, Bolton VN (1999) A prospective randomixed study comparing the outcome of in vitro fertilization and embryo transfer following culture of human embryos individually or in groups before embryo transfer on day 2. Hum Reprod 14(1):76–79
105. Gardner DK, Vella P, Lane M et al (1998) Culture and transfer of human blastocysts increases implantation rates and reduces the need for multiple embryo transfers. Fertil Steril 69:84–88
106. Gardner DK, Schoolcraft WB, Wagley L, Schlenker T, Stevens J, Hesla J (1998) A prospective randomized trial of blastocyst culture and transfer in in-vitro fertilization. Hum Reprod 13:3434–3440
107. Racowsky C, Jackson KV, Cekleniak NA, Fox JH, Hornstein MD, Ginsburg ES (2000) The number of eight cell embyros is a key determinant for selecting day 3 or day 5 transfer. Fertil Steril 73:558–564
108. de los Santos MJ, Mercader MJ, Galan A, Albert C, Romero JL, Pellicer A (2003) Implantation rates after two, three, or five days of embryo culture. Placenta 24(b):S13–S19
109. Blake DA, Farquhar CM, Johnson N, Proctor M (2007) Cleavage stage versus blastocyst stage transfer in assisted conception. Cochrane Database Syst Rev 4:CD002118
110. Papanikolaou E, Camus M, Kolibianakis E et al (2006) In vitro fertilization with single blastocyst-stage versus single cleavage-stage embryos. N Engl J Med 354:1139–1146
111. Behr B, Fisch JD, Racowsky C, Miller K, Poole TB, Milki AA (2000) Blastocyst-ET and monozygotic twinning. J Assist Reprod Genet 17:349–351
112. Skiadas CC, Missmer SA, Benson CB, Gee RE, Racowsky C (2008) Risk factors associated with pregnancies containing a monochorionic pair following assisted reproductive technologies. Hum Reprod: PMID:18378561 23(6):1366–1371
113. Xie Y, Wang F, Puscheck EE, Rappolee DA (2007) Pipetting causes shear stress and elevation of phosphorylated stress-activated protein kinase/jun kinase in preimplantation embryos. Mol Reprod Dev 74:1287–1294
114. Shen S, Rosen MP, Dobson AT, Fujumoto VY, McCulloch CE, Cedars MI (2006) Day 2 transfer improves pregnancy outcome in

in vitro fertilization cycles with few available embryos. Fertil Steril 86(1):44–50
115. Bahceci M, Ulug U, Ciray HN, Akman MA, Erden HF (2006) Efficiency of changing the embryo transfer time from day 3 to day 2 among women with poor ovarian response: a prospective randomized trial. Fertil Steril 86(1):81–85
116. Jaroudi K, Al-Hassan S, Sieck U, Al-Sufyan H, Al-Kabra NM, Coskun S (2004) Zygote transfer on day 1 versus cleavage stage embryo transfer on day 3: a prospective randomized trial. Hum Reprod 19(3):645–648
117. Mansour RT, Aboulghar MA, Serour GI, Abbass AM (1994) Co-culture of human pronucleate oocytes with their cumulus cells. Hum Reprod 9(9):1727–1729
118. Dirnfeld M, Goldman S, Gonen Y, Koifman M, Calderon I, Abramovici H (1997) A simplified coculture system with luteinized granulosa cells improves enbryo quality and implantation rates, a controlled study. Fertil Steril 67:120–122
119. Fabbri R, Porcu E, Marsella T, Primavera MR, Cecconi S, Nottola SA, Motta PM, Venturoli S, Flamigni C (2000) Human embryo development and pregnancies in an homologous granulosa cell coculture system. J Assist Reprod Genet 17(1):1–12
120. Parikh FR, Nadkarni SG, Naik NJ, Naik DJ, Uttamchandani SA (2006) Cumulus coculture and cumulus-aided embryo transfer increases pregnancy rates in patients undergoing in vitro fertilization. Fertil Steril 86(4):839–847
121. Spandorfer SD, Pascal P, Parks J, Clarke R, Veeck L, Davis OK, Rosenwaks Z (2004) Autologous endometrial co-culture in patients with IVF failure: outcome of the first 1030 cases. J Reprod Med 49(6):463–467
122. Spandorfer SD, Barmat LI, Navarro J, Hung-Ching L, Veeck L, Rosenwaks Z (2002) Importance of the biopsy day in autologous endometrial co-cultures for patients with multiple implantation failures. Fertil Steril 77:1209–1213
123. Thompson JG (2006) Culture without the petri-dish. Theriogenology 67(1):16–20
124. Raty S, Walters EM, Davis J, Zeringue H, Beebe DJ, Rodriguez-Zas S, Wheeler MB (2004) Embryonic development in the mouse is enhanced via microchannel culture. Lab Chip 4: 186–190
125. Suh RS, Zhu X, Phadke N, Ohl DA, Takayama S, Smith GD (2006) IVF within microfluidic channels requires lower total numbers and lower concentrations of sperm. Hum Reprod 21(2): 477–483
126. Walters EM, Clark SG, Beebe DJ, Wheeler MB (2004) Mammalian embryo culture in a microfluidic device. Methods Mol Biol 254: 375–382

Chapter 42
In-Vitro Maturation of Human Oocytes

Ezgi Demirtas, Hananel Holzer, Weon-Young SON, Ri-Cheng Chain, and Seang Lin Tan

Abstract Since the birth of the first in-vitro fertilization (IVF) baby in 1978 [1], assisted reproductive technologies (ART) have helped thousands of couples to have children through the use of ovarian stimulation [2]. IVF was first performed in a natural cycle without any hormonal stimulation, and the oocyte retrieval was performed laparoscopically. However, natural cycle IVF was soon replaced by ovarian stimulation with clomiphene and gonadotropins to increase the number of oocytes available for retrieval. Although the opportunity to transfer multiple embryos and to select the highest-quality embryo(s) for transfer has improved the pregnancy rates remarkably, hormonal ovarian stimulation presents inherent risks, the most important of which is ovarian hyperstimulation syndrome (OHSS), a potentially life-threatening condition. Women with polycystic ovaries (PCO) and/or polycystic ovary syndrome (PCOS) undergoing ovarian stimulation are at increased risk of OHSS [3]. Severe OHSS affects 1–2% of all women undergoing controlled ovarian stimulation and up to 6–11% of women with PCO or PCOS [4, 5]. Although various strategies have been undertaken to reduce the risk of OHSS, the only way to eliminate it is to avoid ovarian stimulation altogether [6]. Hormonal ovarian stimulation has other disadvantages; it is an expensive treatment, especially due to the high cost of commercial gonadotropins. Patients must also be meticulously monitored by ultrasound examinations and serum estradiol measurements, which also increase the cost of treatment. In addition, it may not be preferred by women because of the inconvenience of daily injections and side effects such as bloating, breast tenderness, mood swings, and nausea. All of these factors can be major deterrents not only to women who are using their own oocytes but also to potential oocyte donors, who may decline undergoing the procedure due to its inherent risks [7]. In-vitro maturation (IVM) of immature oocytes obtained in an unstimulated cycle seems to provide a good alternative for these women, as it eliminates the risk of OHSS, simplifies monitoring, reduces the cost of treatment, and results in fair pregnancy outcomes particularly in young age groups.

Keywords Oocyte • Ovarian stimulation • OHSS • IVM • PCOS

42.1 History and Development of IVM of Human Oocytes

In 1983, Veeck et al. reported two pregnancies resulting from in-vitro matured oocytes [8]. These morphologically immature oocytes were recovered from human menopausal gonadotropin (HMG) and/or follicle stimulating hormone (FSH) and human chorionic gonadotropin (hCG) primed cycles in an in-vitro fertilization (IVF) program. This was followed by the report of Cha et al. in 1991 announcing a pregnancy in an oocyte recipient resulting from the fertilization of in-vitro matured oocytes obtained from unstimulated ovaries of another woman on cycle day 13 by direct aspiration during a gynecologic surgery [9].

The work leading to the eventual success of the IVM of human oocytes began in the 1930s, with Pincus, Enzman, and Saunders, who studied the in-vivo and in-vitro maturation of mammalian including human oocytes [10, 11]. They observed that when oocytes were removed from the follicles they spontaneously resumed meiosis and progressed to the metaphase-II (M-II) stage in the culture, as they do in vivo. In 1965, Edwards described the kinetics of oocyte maturation in vitro both in animals and in humans [12, 13]. He used the Tissue Culture Medium 199 (TCM-199) supplemented with fetal calf serum to culture the immature human oocytes, and showed that meiosis was resumed in 80% of immature oocytes independent of cycle day and without gonadotropin support. Most human oocytes examined after 43 h in culture were in M-II and had extruded the first polar body. Soon after, Edwards

E. Demirtas (✉), H. Holzer, W.-Y. SON, Ri.-C. Chain, and S.L. Tan
Department of Obstetrics and Gynecology, McGill University, Royal Victoria Hospital Women's Pavilion, Montreal, QC, Canada
e-mail: ezgidemirtas@yahoo.com

D.T. Carrell and C.M. Peterson (eds.), *Reproductive Endocrinology and Infertility: Integrating Modern Clinical and Laboratory Practice*,
DOI 10.1007/978-1-4419-1436-1_42,

demonstrated that in-vitro matured human oocytes could be fertilized [14]; after insemination, 18 of the 34 oocytes that had matured in vitro had spermatozoa in the zona pellucida and spermatozoa in the perivitelline space or pronuclei, indicating that most were undergoing fertilization.

Following the first report of IVM pregnancy obtained using in-vitro matured oocytes retrieved from the unstimulated ovaries in 1991 [9], the first pregnancy in a woman with anovulatory infertility using her own immature oocytes recovered in an unstimulated cycle without FSH/HMG or hCG priming was reported by Trounson et al. in 1994 [15]. The following year, same group reported another pregnancy in a woman with PCOS through the use of IVM combined with intracytoplasmic sperm injection (ICSI), assisted hatching, and blastocyst culture [16]. Other pregnancies were reported through the use of in-vitro matured oocytes recovered from unstimulated ovaries without hCG priming [17], and from ovaries stimulated by HMG but without hCG priming [18, 19] in 1990s. The first series of IVM treatments without FSH/HMG or hCG priming achieved a pregnancy rate of 27.1% and an implantation of 6.9% in 94 cycles in 64 women with PCOS where the average number of embryos transferred was 6.3 [20]. Indeed, the success rates of IVM remained low throughout most of the 1990s until the introduction of hCG priming prior to oocyte retrieval [21]. Chian et al. reported an implantation rate of 32% and a clinical pregnancy rate of 40% in their series of 25 women with PCOS who underwent oocyte retrieval 36 h following the administration of 10,000 IU of hCG. Since then, hCG priming has widely been adopted by many centers but it has not become a universal practice as it has in conventional IVF/ICSI cycles with ovarian stimulation.

Today, all centers report lower IVM pregnancy and live-birth rates compared with conventional IVF/ICSI cycles with hormonal ovarian stimulation. A case-control study of 107 IVM and 107 IVF cycles comparing the two methods in women with PCOS reported that the numbers of mature oocytes and embryos obtained in IVF cycles were significantly higher than that in IVM cycles, and implantation rate of IVF-derived embryos was also higher (17.1% vs. 9.5%) [5]. Furthermore, the final number of matured oocytes obtained in IVM cycles is relatively low compared with that in conventional stimulated cycles. In addition to lower oocyte numbers, the lower success rates in IVM might also be attributed to the asynchrony in the cytoplasmic and nuclear maturation of the oocyte, as well as the asynchrony in the endometrium. Therefore, investigators currently work on various strategies to improve IVM outcomes. While some investigators try to improve the in-vitro culture methods, others modify the clinical management of the treatment cycles to improve the quality and the number of the oocytes obtained and the endometrial synchrony.

42.2 Oocyte Maturation

42.2.1 Maturation In Vivo

Human oocytes stay arrested in prophase-I of meiosis during fetal life [22]. Prophase-I is characterized by the presence of an intact nuclear envelope, germinal vesicle. The oocytes in primordial follicles remain in prophase-I until the reproductive age, when they begin to grow in cohorts. Oocyte maturation is defined as the reinitiation and completion of the first meiotic division through prophase-I to metaphase-II. Pituitary gonadotropins are required for in-vivo maturation of oocytes. FSH is required for early growth of the follicles and is also necessary for the induction of the LH receptors in pre-ovulatory follicles. Luteinizing hormone initiates the resumption of meiosis in vivo in preovulatory oocytes.

Oocyte maturation is commonly referred to have two parts: nuclear maturation and cytoplasmic maturation. Nuclear maturation refers to the series of nuclear events starting with breakdown of the germinal vesicle in the prophase-I stage oocyte, followed by chromatin condensation, formation of meiotic spindle, separation of homolog chromosomes, polar body extrusion, and meiotic re-arrest at M-II stage until fertilization occurs [23]. While nuclear maturation is in progress, "cellular machinery" supplies the necessary molecules, controls, and regulates the series of nuclear events in the oocyte. The cellular machinery conducts mRNA and protein synthesis, modification and storage of the necessary molecules, and the timely reactivation of these molecules. Cytoplasmic maturation refers to this cellular machinery and is as important as the successful nuclear maturation for the developmentally competent mature oocyte and the embryo that will be obtained by its fertilization. Metabolism of an oocyte is best characterized by active transcription and translation in the cytoplasm during the preovulatory period. Developmental competence of the mature oocyte and the pre-embryo is dependent on mRNA and the protein accumulated in the cytoplasm during the follicular growth, since transcription ceases at the time of ovulation [24].

Cumulus cells play important roles in oocyte maturation in vivo. Human and other mammalian oocytes are surrounded by cumulus cells, which respond to gonadotropins and secrete various substances. Oocyte and cumulus cells are coupled by gap junctions, and cumulus cells control oocyte maturation through many potential factors. In-vivo maturation of oocytes is an induced process and is triggered by the LH surge; however, because there are no LH receptors on oocytes, LH probably induces germinal vesicle breakdown by an indirect action through the cumulus cells. The pattern of protein synthesis is also different between oocytes with and without cumulus cells indicating that gonadotropins modulate the protein synthesis pattern through cumulus cells [25].

42.2.2 Maturation In Vitro

It has been known for more than 70 years that immature oocytes can mature spontaneously when removed from the follicle. In-vivo maturation, on the other hand, is an induced process mediated by growth factors. It was suggested that untimely removal of the oocyte from its dynamic environment interrupts its in-vivo "capacitation" [26]. The deficiencies occurring during the maturation process will result in developmentally incompetent embryos and lower implantation rates. Therefore, the developmental competence of in-vitro matured oocytes is profoundly affected by culture conditions. Most deficiencies during maturation are associated with cellular machinery rather than the nuclear reprogramming. Despite insufficiencies in cytoplasmic maturation, oocytes frequently reach the mature stage. Nevertheless, incompetence of cellular machinery during oocyte maturation frequently causes a failure in embryonic development following fertilization. It was suggested that insufficient cytoplasmic maturation of the oocyte might fail to promote male pronuclear formation and might therefore increase chromosomal abnormalities after fertilization [27], and these abnormalities may result in an incompetent embryo in cleavage or peri-implantation stages. Some investigators suggested inhibiting or delaying spontaneous nuclear maturation in vitro following oocyte retrieval to give oocyte a chance to complete its capacitation. As an example, increasing cyclic AMP of the environment by adding phosphodiesterase type 3 inhibitor in media reversibly arrests the nuclear development of human oocytes [28].

Aspirated immature oocytes are cultured in maturation medium with surrounding cumulus cells. IVM media include basic energy substrates and molecules that establish the required osmolarity and pH; and are often supplemented with patients' serum or human serum albumin. Although gonadotropins are not required for in-vitro maturation, FSH and LH are added in most IVM media based on their physiologic role in vivo. Indeed, it has been shown that supplementing IVM medium with FSH does not significantly increase the ability of oocytes to reach M-II [29]. Nevertheless, oocytes exposed to FSH during culture have significantly higher fertilization [30] and cleavage rates [31, 32]. The actions of endocrine, paracrine, and autocrine factors controlling oocyte maturation in vivo and in vitro are mediated by cumulus cells. Culture medium supplemented with FSH and LH stimulates estrogen and progesterone secretions from the cumulus cells. Therefore, it is possible that the gonadotropins added in the culture medium may play a role in oocyte maturation through estrogen and progesterone [33]. It is believed that there are also oocyte-secreted factors that help regulate normal cumulus cell function during oocyte maturation [26]. As the dynamic relations of oocyte-cumulus cells are further clarified, modifications in in-vitro oocyte culture systems are likely to improve the IVM outcomes.

42.3 IVM in Practice

42.3.1 Anovulatory Women

Implantation and pregnancy rates in IVM cycles have a strong correlation with the number of immature oocytes retrieved [34, 35]. The number of oocytes retrieved can be predicted by the antral follicle count (AFC), ovarian volume, and peak ovarian stromal velocity measured by doppler ultrasound during the early follicular phase. Additionally, AFC is the most important independent ultrasonographic predictor of the number of immature oocytes recovered [35]. Therefore, the majority of IVM pregnancies in the literature have been in women with PCOS (Table 42.1), while pregnancy rates in women with normal ovaries appear to be lower [36]. In a prospective observational study, the clinical pregnancy rate per cycle in relation to AFC was reported as 6% when the follicle count was less than 20; 15% when the follicle count was 20–29, and 44% when the follicle count was higher than 29 [34]. In another comparison, IVM pregnancy and live birth rates were found to be less (26.2 and 15.9%) than that of IVF with ovarian stimulation (38.3 and 26.2%), even though the difference was not statistically significant [5]. The implantation rate of IVF-derived embryos was reported to be significantly higher than that for IVM (17.1% vs. 9.5%) in the same study [5]. On the other hand, 11.2% of the IVF cases had moderate or severe OHSS while there was no OHSS in IVM group [5]. The women who have the best chance for pregnancy by IVM are those with high AFC and they are also most prone to the OHSS. Therefore, women with PCO/PCOS having high numbers of antral follicles are the prime candidates for IVM treatment.

The ESHRE/ASRM-Sponsored PCOS Consensus Workshop Group has recently published a consensus report

Table 42.1 Summary of the published outcomes of IVM cycles in women with PCO/PCOS

Authors (year)	No. of cycles	Indication	No. of ET cycles at cleavage stage	Gn priming	Maturation rate (%)	Fertilization rate (%)	Implantation rate (%)	Pregnancy rate/ET (%)	Miscarriage rate (%)
Chian et al. (1999) [21]	25	PCOS	25	HCG	84	87	32	40	20
Cha et al. (2000) [20]	94	PCOS	85	None	75.1	67.9	6.9	27.1	26.1
Chian et al. (2000) [59]	11	PCOS	11	None	69.1	83.9	24.8	27.3	0
	13		13	HCG	84.3	90.7	16.6	38.5	40
Mikkelsen and Lindenberg (2001) [73]	12	PCOS	9	None	44.0	69.0	0	0	57.1
	24		21	FSH	59.0	70.0	21.6	33.3	
Child et al. (2002) [5]	107	PCO/PCOS	107	HCG	76.0	78.0	9.5	26.2	26.1
Lin et al. (2003) [74]	3533	PCOS	35	FSH+HCG	76.5	75.8	9.5	31.4	13.0
			33	HCG	71.9	69.5	11.3	36.4	
Chian (2004) [89]	254	PCO/PCOS	NA	HCG	78.8	69.2	11.1	24.0	NA
Soderstrom-Anttila et al. (2005) [40]	PCO: 13	PCO: 13	9 (IVF)	None	60.6	35.0	13.3	22.2	0
	7	7	5 (ICSI)		49.2	72.4	0	0	-
	PCOS: 18	PCOS: 18	17 (IVF)		54.3	82.5	34.5	52.9	33.3
	10	10	9 (ICSI)		53.2	70.0	12.5	22.2	50.0
Cha et al. (2005) [85]	203	PCOS	187	None	NA	NA	5.5	21.9	36.8
Torre et al. (2007) [90]	138	PCOS	NA	HCG	61.7	62	10.9	24.5[a]	42.3
Son et al. (2007) [78]	415	PCO/PCOS	415	HCG	74.0	80.1	9.7	28.4	NA
	106		106 (blastocyst)	HCG	78.2	80.5	26.8	51.9	21.8
Wei et al. (2007) [91]	3634	PCOS	36	FSH+HCG	70.4	67.7	6.2	16.7	16.7
			34	Metformin +FSH +HCG	76.7	70.0	15.3	38.2	23.1

[a]Per oocyte retrieval. ET = embryo transfer, Gn = gonadotropin, NA = not available

on infertility treatment related to PCOS [37, 38]. IVF was recommended as the third-line treatment in the PCOS Consensus Workshop report following clomiphene citrate as the first-line treatment for ovulation induction and exogenous gonadotropins and/or laparoscopic ovarian surgery as the second-line. In-vitro maturation was not mentioned as a treatment option in this report. A new treatment algorithm including IVM on infertility treatment for women with PCOS is proposed by the authors of this chapter in accordance with the recommendations of the ESHRE/ASRM-Sponsored PCOS Consensus Workshop Group consensus report (Fig. 42.1). IVM may be offered as a treatment option prior to conventional IVF with ovarian stimulation for the women with anovulatory infertility should the previous steps not result in a pregnancy.

42.3.2 Ovulatory Women

Although women with PCO(S) seem to be better candidates for IVM, encouraging treatment outcomes were achieved by IVM in ovulatory women with normal ovaries as well. The disadvantage of women with regular cycles for IVM is their relatively lower AFCs. Since the AFC is lower in these women, the numbers of oocytes retrieved and embryos generated are also less. This is reflected in the outcomes of the treatment cycles as lower implantation and pregnancy rates compared with IVM cycles conducted in women with PCO/PCOS (Table 42.2). However, Barnes et al. had reported that the immature oocytes recovered from regularly cycling women matured and fertilized at significantly higher rates than those from anovulatory women and women with irregular cycles, and the embryos from women with regularly ovulatory cycles had a significantly higher mean embryo development ratio [39]. However, the data were lacking implantation and pregnancy rates. A possible explanation for the better performance of in-vitro matured oocytes from women with regular cycles is that the putative unfavorable effects of intraovarian endocrine abnormalities on oocyte quality in women with PCOS on oocyte quality would be circumvented [40], [22]. Even though the data on IVM outcome in regularly cycling ovulatory women are limited, this method has been increasingly used for couples who had infertility due to causes other than anovulation, such as tubal factor or male factor. In the largest series to date in women with normal ovaries and regular cycles who underwent IVM, the implantation and the clinical pregnancy rates reported were as high as 22.6 and 31%, respectively, when IVF was undertaken as the fertilization method in comparison with ICSI [40]. To start an IVM cycle in regularly cycling women, the minimum recommended AFC on ultrasound examination in early follicular phase was recommended to be 10 [41].

42.3.3 Poor Responders

Poor responders require prolonged stimulation and higher doses of gonadotropins, and have a higher risk of cancelation. Oocyte donation offers the best pregnancy chance to these women and no single approach benefits those who prefer to use their own oocytes [42–44]. IVM has been employed in limited number of poor responders. Child et al. reported eight women with a previous poor response to ovarian stimulation treated by IVM [45]. An average of 2.3 immature oocytes was recovered following hCG priming in an unstimulated cycle and an average of 1.7 matured in vitro. Out of six women underwent embryo transfer one conceived and delivered.

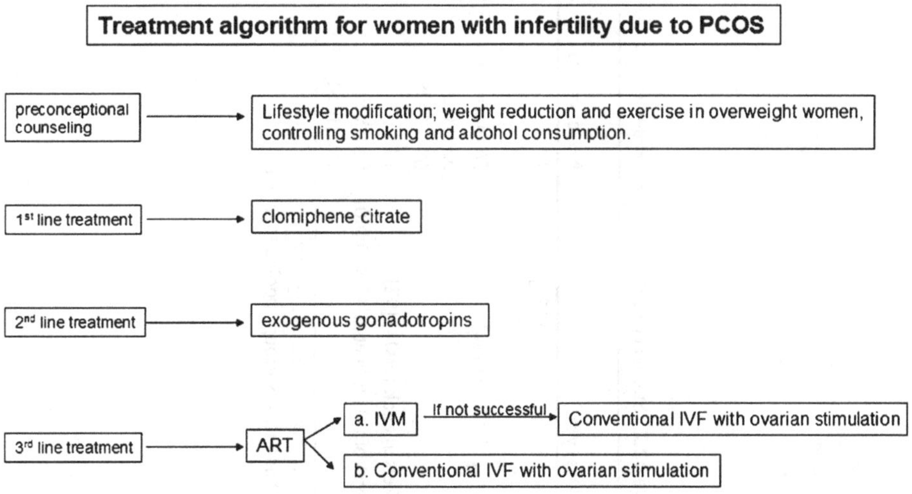

Fig. 42.1 Treatment algorithm for women with infertility due to PCOS

Table 42.2 Summary of the published outcomes of IVM cycles in women with regular cycles

Authors (year)	No. of cycles	No. of ET cycles at cleavage stage	Gn priming	Mean no. of oocytes retrieved	Maturation rate (%)	Fertilization rate (%)	Implantation rate (%)	Pregnancy rate/ ET (%)	Miscarriage rate (%)
Mikkelsen et al. (1999) [71]	10	9	None	37	76	62	18.8	33	20[a]
	10	9	FSH	40	85	65	11.8	22	
Child et al. (2001) [34]	56 (normal)	50	HCG	5.1 ± 3.7	79.5	67.7	1.5	4	50
	53 (PCO)	52	HCG	10 ± 5.1	75.0[b]	71.6[b]	8.9	23.1	25
	68 (PCOS)	67	HCG	11.3 ± 9.0			9.6	29.9	50
Mikkelsen et al. (2001) [92]	132	83	None	3.9	60.1	72.9	NA	18	NA
Soderstrom-Anttila et al. (2005) [40]	91 (IVF)	58 (IVF)	None	6.3 ± 3.4	66.9	35.9	22.6	31	33.3
	100 (ICSI)	86 (ICSI)		6.5 ± 3.6	54.5	67.1	15	21	16.7

[a]The two groups pooled together
[b]PCO and PCOS groups pooled together

42.3.4 IVM as a Rescue

IVF cycles are occasionally abandoned after a few days of FSH administration due to either high risk of ovarian stimulation or poor ovarian response. In both situations, it was proposed not to cancel the cycle but to proceed with earlier oocyte retrieval even if the follicular growth did not meet the retrieval criteria. Lim et al. suggested to administer full dose of hCG earlier, when the leading follicle reached 12–14 mm when a high risk of OHSS is anticipated to proceed with oocyte retrieval, IVM, ICSI, and embryo transfer in hyper-responders [46]. In their series of 123 cycles switched to IVM after ovarian stimulation started, mature oocyte retrieval rate was found to be 18.9% which was higher than expected in IVM cycles, and the overall pregnancy rate was 36.6% per embryo transfer [47]. Although 10,000 IU of hCG was administered, no case of OHSS was reported.

Similar rationale was adapted for women who showed poor ovarian response to ovarian stimulation, as well [48]. First, oocyte retrievals were performed without hCG priming, and 31.6% of pregnancy rate was obtained in 19 women who did not have a dominant follicle larger than 10 mm despite gonadotropin administration of more than 7 days [49]. In the second group, oocyte retrieval was performed 36 h after the administration of hCG, 10,000 IU, in 55 cycles [49]. Mature oocyte rate at retrieval was 14.7%; implantation and clinical pregnancy rates were reported as 15.8 and 40.4% [49]. The drawback of these studies in poor responders is that there were not any other criteria for the definition of poor response in these reports, except failure in growing a dominant follicle in response to ovarian stimulation. Indeed, the mean numbers of oocytes recovered in groups with and without hCG priming were 11.7 and 9.0, respectively. High numbers of oocytes recovered may indicate a selection bias and in fact at least some of these women might not be really having a poor ovarian reserve.

42.3.5 IVM for Fertility Preservation

One of the most important long-term effects of cancer treatments in young women is premature ovarian failure and infertility. With improving survival rates following cancer treatments and encouraging results of fertility preservation techniques, increasing number of young women are seeking methods to preserve their fertility. In fact, indications of fertility preservation are not limited to cancer. Any threat for a decrease in ovarian reserve can be an indication for fertility preservation, such as autoimmune diseases [36], endometriosis [37], genetic conditions like Turner's syndrome [38], and even natural aging itself. However, timeline for women diagnosed with cancer is much more limited for fertility preservation compared with women with other conditions. For women who have sufficient time before cancer treatment and no contraindication for hormonal ovarian stimulation, embryo or oocyte cryopreservation following controlled ovarian stimulation appears to be the most suitable approach. Indeed, ASCO and ASRM have endorsed IVF and embryo cryopreservation as the only method for female fertility preservation [53]. However, when estrogen-sensitive tumors and/or time constraints are involved, IVM may be a better option, as ovarian stimulation is not required and the time required for IVM is much less than an ovarian stimulation cycle [54]. In-vitro maturation and cryopreservation of oocytes retrieved from unstimulated ovaries seem to be a promising method for fertility preservation, as this technique avoids hormonal stimulation and is not associated with considerable delay in cancer treatment.

In a clinical trial at McGill Reproductive Center including 38 infertile women, oocyte cryopreservation by vitrification resulted in a mean survival rate of 81% post-thawing, a fertilization rate of 76% following ICSI, a clinical pregnancy rate of 45%, and a live birth rate of 40% with 22 healthy babies born [55]. Although pregnancy rates appear to be lower compared with in-vivo matured and vitrified oocytes, in a pilot study a live birth rate of 20% per cycle has been achieved with first four live births from vitrified IVM oocytes [55, 56].

Oocyte retrieval for fertility preservation can be performed at any day of the cycle in anovulatory women for fertility preservation. It is performed in the follicular phase in ovulatory patients for fertility preservation, based on the clinical practice of IVM in infertile couples. Although it is not routinely used, immature oocyte retrieval in the luteal phase has also revealed promising in-vitro maturation results [57, 58]. Immature oocytes recovered in the luteal phase can mature in vitro, can be fertilized, and can produce good-quality embryos. However, feasibility of this approach will only be ascertained when the implantation potential of these oocytes and embryos is tested.

42.4 Gonadotropin Priming in IVM Cycles

42.4.1 HCG Priming

The reason behind hCG priming before oocyte retrieval is to promote the initiation of oocyte maturation in vivo and to improve the developmental competence of oocytes by increasing their ability to mature, thus shortening the time required for maturation in vitro. Most of the studies published to date have reported hCG priming prior to oocyte retrieval as being advantageous in terms of treatment outcomes. However, it has not been adopted as a universal approach as it is in conventional IVF/ICSI cycles with ovarian stimulation.

A year after the first report announcing an IVM pregnancy rate of 40% in women with PCOS, in which oocyte retrieval was performed after hCG-priming [21], Chian et al. conducted a randomized controlled trial where oocyte retrieval was performed 36 h following the administration of 10,000 IU of hCG in 13 cycles, without hCG priming in 11 cycles [59]. The ratio of oocytes achieving maturation at 48 h was significantly higher in the hCG-primed group than in the non-hCG primed group (84.3% vs. 69.1%) and, more importantly, the number of oocytes that matured within 24 h was much higher in the hCG-primed group than in the non-hCG primed group (78.2% vs. 4.9%). They concluded that oocyte maturation was hastened in hCG-primed cycles [59]. This finding was supported by Son et al. [60], and it was suggested that the morphology of the oocyte cumulus complexes (OCC) was also affected by the hCG administration prior to oocyte retrieval [60, 61]. Most of the oocytes obtained in cycles where hCG 10,000 IU is administered prior to retrieval display a dispersed OCC morphology (Fig. 42.2a), while the majority of OCCs retrieved in cycles without hCG priming display compact or sparse appearance (Figs. 42.2b, c, d). The appearance of the dispersed OCC morphology resembles that of OCCs recovered in conventional IVF/ICSI with ovarian stimulation and hCG administration. This morphology may help identify immature oocytes in the aspirate under the stereomicroscope without using a filtration method; and, more importantly, there is a chance of recovering mature oocytes when oocyte retrieval is performed following hCG priming. It was reported that the presence of dispersed cumulus cells at retrieval was positively correlated with the rates of maturation and blastocyst development, and expression of LH receptor in cumulus cells was also correlated with the OCC morphology [61]. The mechanism of hCG action on small follicles remains unclear; however, it was shown that granulosa cells in small follicles in anovulatory women with PCOS responded LH prematurely [62]. This finding may be important to explain the mechanism of anovulation in PCOS and may help explain how hCG priming hastens oocyte maturation in vitro. The morphology of OCCs was further examined according to the presence of hormonal priming: without hCG or HMG priming; following low dose HMG priming; and following hCG priming [60]. Oocyte-cumulus complexes with dispersed cumulus cell morphology were observed only in the hCG-primed group and, interestingly,

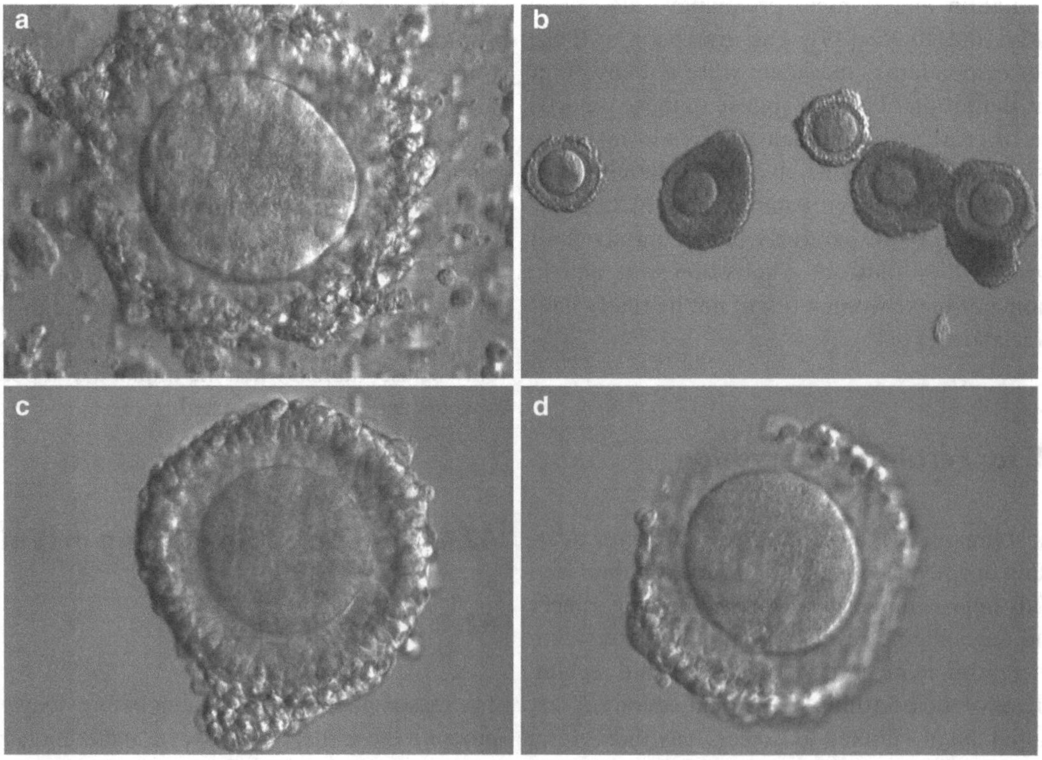

Fig. 42.2 Morphologic appearances of the oocyte cumulus complexes in IVM cycles at retrieval. (**a**) An oocyte with the appearance of dispersed cumulus cell morphology, retrieved following hCG priming (original magnification × 400). (**b**) Oocytes-cumulus complexes retrieved from a cycles without hCG priming (original magnification × 200). (**c**) An oocyte with compact cumulus cell morphology (original magnification × 400). (**d**)An oocyte with sparce cumulus morphology

11% of the oocytes showing dispersed cumulus cell morphology were mature at the time of retrieval [60]. Although there was no difference in the total maturation, fertilization, and cleavage rates, the pregnancy rate was found to be higher in the group that displayed dispersed OCC morphology following day-3 embryo transfer. Furthermore, the blastocyst development rate of the residual embryos was higher in the group with dispersed OCC morphology [60].

In an attempt to find the optimal dose of hCG prior to oocyte retrieval, a prospective randomized controlled trial demonstrated no improvement in oocyte maturation rates with 20,000 IU of hCG compared with 10,000 IU [63].

42.4.1.1 Timing of Oocyte Retrieval

The two important factors in timing of the oocyte retrieval in IVM cycles are the endometrial thickness and the leading follicle size. The literature has conflicting reports on the optimum size of the leading follicle before oocyte retrieval. Some reports suggest that the large follicles may compromise the developmental potential of the oocytes in the remaining small antral follicles [64]. However, other reports suggest that the developmental competence of oocytes retrieved from small antral follicles was not adversely affected by a growing dominant follicle in unstimulated cycles [65, 66]. In a recent study, it was shown that IVM cycles with in-vivo matured oocytes resulted in a higher clinical pregnancy rate compared with those with no mature oocytes at retrieval; the pregnancy rate was reported as 40% in IVM cycles with at least one mature oocyte at retrieval, compared with a pregnancy rate of 23% in cycles without any mature oocytes [67]. Retrieval of an in-vivo matured oocyte is more likely to occur in cycles where follicles are allowed to grow to 10–12 mm before oocyte retrieval in women with ovulatory cycles [67] (Fig. 42.3).

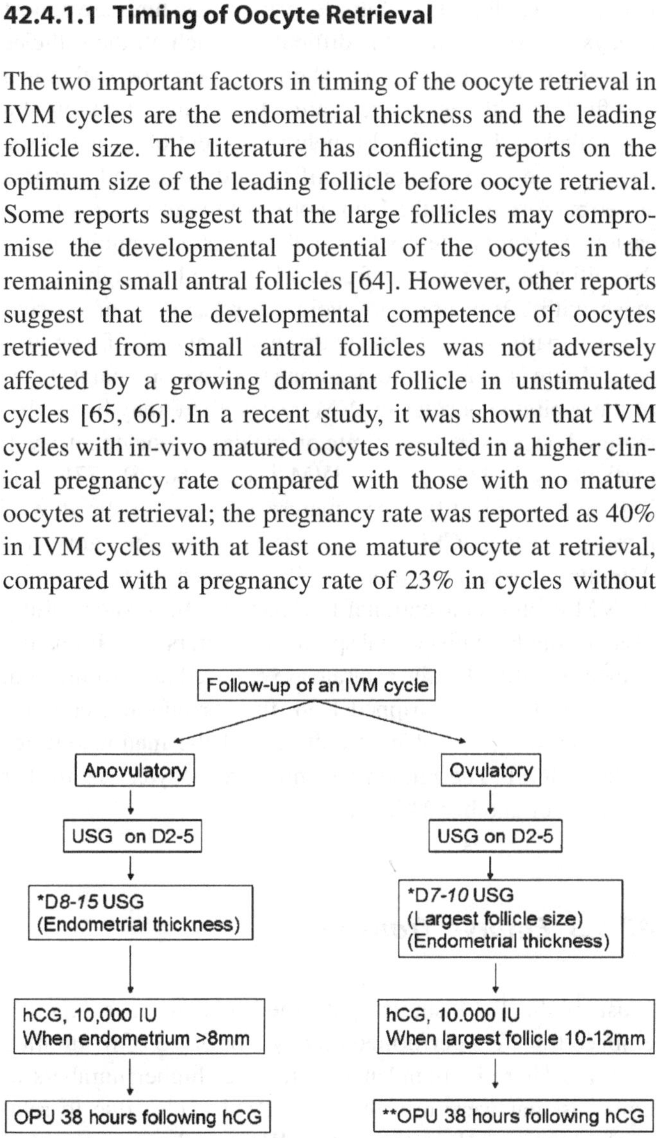

Fig. 42.3 Follow-up of an IVM cycle. *Dominant follicle size is an important factor in timing of oocyte retrieval in ovulatory cycles. **If the dominant follicle is larger than 13–14 mm on the day of hCG the oocyte retrieval is recommended to be performed earlier than 38 h due to the risk of ovulation

Time interval between hCG administration and oocyte retrieval in hCG-primed IVM cycles is another factor that is likely to play a role in retrieving mature oocytes in IVM cycles. In hCG primed IVM cycles, oocyte retrieval is most frequently performed 36 h after the hCG administration. However, when the intervals of 35 h vs. 38 h between hCG administration and oocyte retrieval were compared, the 38 h group yielded a significantly higher number of mature oocytes and maturation rate after 24 h in culture was higher in 38 h group [68]. Clinical pregnancy rates in the 38 h and 35 h groups were also significantly different in favor of 38 h group, 40.9% vs. 25%, respectively [68].

42.4.2 FSH Pretreatment

In 1998, Wynn et al. reported that pretreatment with a truncated course of 600 IU of FSH over 5 days increased the number of oocytes recovered at the retrieval and promoted the numbers of human oocytes reaching M-II by in-vitro maturation [69]. However, the following studies did not support this finding in regularly cycling women. Suikkari et al. proposed administration of low dose FSH starting from the previous luteal phase until the leading follicle reaches 10 mm in regularly cycling women and on the ninth day of progesterone administration in women with irregular cycles [70]. They found that the numbers of oocytes recovered, in-vitro maturation, and fertilization rates were comparable in both groups [70]. The possible effect of FSH priming in IVM cycles was later examined by Mikkelsen et al. in a prospective randomized study including 20 women with regular cycles, and there was no significant difference in number of oocytes obtained, maturation and cleavage rates between the two groups that underwent oocyte retrieval with and without FSH priming [71]. The same group examined the influence of withholding FSH for 2 days vs. 3 days before oocyte retrieval in a further study, and did not find any difference in the implantation rates between the two groups either [72].

On the other hand, studies imply that there may be a positive effect of FSH priming in women with anovulatory cycles. In a prospective randomized trial, Mikkelsen et al. reported a clinical pregnancy rate of 29% in 24 women who received 150 IU of FSH daily followed by FSH deprivation for 2 or 3 days [73]. The 12 women in the control group did not receive any FSH, and there was no pregnancy in this group. On the other hand, Lin et al. examined the possible effect of FSH priming in hCG primed cycles, however, did not find any additional benefit of FSH stimulation in women with PCOS [74].

Even though the study outcomes are conflicting, there may be potential benefits of FSH priming; easier oocyte retrieval due to larger follicle sizes, it may improve the maturational competence of the oocytes, and higher estradiol levels may improve endometrial lining. Interestingly, in an attempt to improve the thin endometrial lining in hCG-primed IVM cycles, low-dose FSH pretreatment was shown to be superior to micronized 17β estradiol in terms of implantation and pregnancy rates [75].

42.5 Overview of an IVM Cycle

42.5.1 Monitoring of the Cycle

Women with PCO and/or PCOS carrying the highest risk of OHSS and the best chance for pregnancy due to the higher AFC are the prime candidates for IVM, regardless of their ovulatory status. However, the follow-up of anovulatory and ovulatory women differs due to the development of a dominant follicle in ovulatory patients (Fig. 42.3).

The treatment cycle is initiated by progesterone administration to induce a withdrawal bleeding in anovulatory women. The first ultrasound examination is performed in early follicular phase, on cycle day 2–5 of the period, to rule out the presence of any ovarian cysts. A second ultrasound examination is performed to measure the endometrial thickness and to plan immature oocyte retrieval. An endometrial thickness of 6–8 mm before oocyte retrieval is preferable. If the endometrial thickness is not sufficient further ultrasound examination(s) is required. The time interval for the second and, if required, the third ultrasound examination and also for the oocyte retrieval is flexible for women with anovulatory cycles, since they do not have a growing follicle that limits the timeline for the oocyte retrieval. hCG administration is not a universal approach in IVM cycles; however, it is frequently undertaken and is administered at a dosage of 10,000 IU s.c., 36–38 h prior to oocyte retrieval [68, 76]. Women with regular cycles will develop a dominant follicle; therefore, a second examination is performed on cycle day 7–9, before the dominant follicle reaches preovulatory stage. The preferred diameter of the dominant follicle is 10–12 mm on the day of hCG [67].

42.5.2 Oocyte Retrieval and Identification

As in stimulated cycles, transvaginal ultrasound-guided follicular aspiration is used for oocyte retrieval, but several modifications are made. Depending on the accessibility of the ovaries, oocyte retrieval may be performed under general/spinal/epidural anesthesia or with intravenous sedation and local infiltration of injectable anesthetics. However, due to the multiple ovarian punctures often needed in immature oocyte retrieval, it is likely to be more painful than the oocyte retrieval in stimulated IVF cycles. The aspiration tubes are prepared with approximately 2-ml heparinized saline in the warming blocks before the retrieval. A fine-bore aspiration needle, preferably 19–21 G, is used for immature oocyte retrieval from small follicles and aspiration pressure is reduced to 75–80 mm Hg. Aspiration of small follicles requires good visibility of the these follicles on the ultrasound screen, and a high resolution is preferred if the ovaries are close to the vaginal vault. Still, it is difficult to aspirate follicles smaller than 4 mm and the needle is frequently removed and realigned with the small follicles. Multiple ovarian punctures are almost always necessary since it is difficult to reach all the follicles from the same puncture site. The needle may be withdrawn and flushed with heparinized saline following aspiration of a few follicles; this might also help to prevent blockage of the needle. The oocytes are identified and evaluated under a stereomicroscope in the laboratory. Although it is relatively easier to identify the oocytes with dispersed cumulus cells, the follicular aspirates are frequently filtered through a nylon mesh with 70 μm pores to avoid the possibility of missing oocytes particularly those with small amount of cumulus cells. There is an asynchrony among the developmental stages of the aspirated oocytes in IVM cycles; there may be in-vivo matured oocytes in the aspirate on the day of oocyte retrieval, particularly in hCG-primed IVM cycles [60, 61, 77]. It is important to identify these mature oocytes on the day of retrieval so that ICSI can be undertaken on the same day. Although most centers prefer ICSI as the fertilization method in IVM cycles, conventional IVF has also been successfully used in couples with normal sperm parameters [40]. Immature oocytes identified in the aspirate are cultured in IVM medium for 48 h. They are stripped from the surrounding cumulus cells following 18–24 h of culture and the mature oocytes undergo ICSI. The remaining immature oocytes are further cultured for another 24 h.

42.5.3 Embryo Transfer

Most of the IVM studies published to date have reported embryo transfers performed on day 2 or day 3 of maturation in vitro. There is a tendency to transfer higher numbers of embryos that were transferred in IVM cycles due to relatively lower implantation rates. When a large number of embryos are generated in IVM cycles, alternative approaches such as extended culture to blastocyst stage or a double transfer could be employed. It was reported that the blastocyst formation rate was 41.6% in cycles where seven or more fertilized eggs were obtained and the number of good-quality embryos on day 3 of fertilization was three or higher [78]. A double transfer is performed by transferring a cleavage stage embryo on day 2 or 3 and a blastocyst on day 5 or 6 [79].

42.5.4 Endometrial Preparation and Luteal Support

In conventional IVF/ICSI cycles with ovarian stimulation, the amount of estrogen produced by the ovaries is sufficient for endometrial preparation in the vast majority of women. However, in IVM cycles, the endometrium must be prepared by exogenous estrogen because the follicles are aspirated when they are smaller. The administration of estrogen usually starts on the day of oocyte retrieval [15, 34, 39, 40, 71, 74, 77, 80]. The recommended dose of estrogen depends on endometrial thickness on the day of oocyte retrieval and the dose is adjusted according to the thickness of the endometrial lining, and it varies between 2 and 12 mg (estradiol valerate) daily. Administration of estradiol starting from early follicular phase for a better endometrial lining may suppress follicular growth and compromised subsequent oocyte maturation in vitro (75, 81). The day on which progesterone administration should be started depends on the day of oocyte maturation. If at least one mature oocyte is identified on the day of oocyte retrieval, it is recommended that progesterone administration be started on the same day. If the first mature oocytes are obtained following IVM in culture, then it is recommended that progesterone administration should start on the day the matured oocytes are observed. Oral, vaginal, or intramuscular progesterone preparates may be used. Barnes et al. suggested that embryo and uterine synchrony were potentially enhanced by luteinization of the dominant follicle at the time of immature oocyte recovery [16]; however, in their randomized controlled study, Buckett et al. did not find any significant difference in endometrial thickness, uterine artery pulsatility index, or absent subendometrial blood flow between the groups that underwent immature oocyte retrieval with or without hCG priming, however, more embryos were generated by the hCG-primed group [82]. The administration of hCG prior to oocyte retrieval may be promoting the initiation of maturation of oocytes in vivo, thus improving the developmental potential of the embryos derived from them rather than improving the endometrium.

42.6 Outcome of IVM Cycles

The outcomes of IVM cycles in women with PCO(S) and with regular cycles are summarized in Tables 42.1 and 42.2. Women with PCO/PCOS have higher implantation and clinical pregnancy rates than women with normal ovaries. There is a higher rate of clinical miscarriage after IVM when compared with IVF and ICSI [83]. This appears to be related to polycystic ovary syndrome rather than to the IVM procedure. Early data concerning IVM pregnancies have generally been reassuring [82, 84, 85]. Recent studies also support these reports. Babies born to date following IVM treatment have shown no increased risk of congenital abnormalities or adverse perinatal outcomes over those already reported for IVF and ICSI [86]. The obstetric and perinatal outcomes of pregnancies following IVM are comparable with established ART data, and may even be associated with fewer low birth weight babies according to a study comparing the neonatal outcomes of 55 IVM, 217 IVF, and 160 ICSI babies [86]. From a total of 150 babies born following IVM, six major congenital anomalies have been reported [83]; omphalocele (1); cleft palate (2); ventriculo-septal defect (2) and 45XO/46XY mosaic (1). This rate is similar to that reported following other assisted reproductive technologies [60] and slightly higher than those in spontaneously conceived controls. A comparative study also shows a similar odds ratio when IVM is compared with IVF and with ICSI [83]. The odds ratio of any congenital abnormality following conception with IVF was reported to be 1.01; with IVM, 1.19; and with ICSI, 1.41. However, further data collection and matched studies are needed to obtain more detailed information.

42.7 Conclusions: Evidence-Based Guidelines

In-vitro maturation offers a more patient-friendly treatment option for the couples in need of assisted reproductive technologies compared with conventional IVF with ovarian stimulation. It is less expensive, avoids the risk of OHSS and other immediate side effects of hormonal stimulation, as well as the future concerns about the stimulation drugs.

Review of literature reveals that the best treatment outcomes in IVM cycles are obtained in women with high AFC regardless of the ovulatory status [21, 74, 78]. Therefore, women with high AFC are the prime candidates for IVM. IVM may be offered to these couples as a treatment option prior to conventional IVF with ovarian stimulation (Fig. 42.1).

HCG priming in unstimulated cycles hastens maturation in vitro of oocytes and offers better pregnancy chances [59, 60].

The current knowledge demonstrates that fertilization, cleavage, and pregnancy outcomes of in-vivo matured oocytes are superior to in-vitro matured oocytes [67]. Therefore, there is a benefit in recovering at least one mature oocyte even in unstimulated cycles for IVM. The dominant follicle size is the most important factor for the retrieval of a mature oocyte in ovulatory cycles. Current literature is lacking the studies determining the optimal size of the leading follicle for hCG administration. However, retrieval of in-vivo matured oocytes is more likely in cycles where follicles are allowed to grow to 10–12 mm before the administration of hCG in ovulatory cycles. A treatment guideline is drawn for IVM with respect to ovulatory status (Fig. 42.3).

Successful implantation requires a receptive endometrium as well as competent embryos. Inadequate exposure to estrogen in IVM cycles may lead to implantation failure [88]. Although the literature for FSH/HMG priming in IVM cycles is controversial, FSH/HMG priming may offer a potential benefit for a receptive endometrium. The duration and the target treatment group for FSH/HMG priming in IVM cycles remain to be further investigated.

References

1. Steptoe PC, Edwards RG (1978) Birth after the reimplantation of a human embryo. Lancet 2:366
2. Tan SL, Royston P, Campbell S, et al. (1992) Cumulative conception and livebirth rates after in-vitro fertilisation. Lancet 339:1390–4
3. MacDougall MJ, Tan SL, Jacobs HS (1992) In-vitro fertilization and the ovarian hyperstimulation syndrome. Hum Reprod 7:597–600
4. MacDougall MJ, Tan SL, Balen A, Jacobs HS (1993) A controlled study comparing patients with and without polycystic ovaries undergoing in-vitro fertilization. Hum Reprod 8:233–7
5. Child TJ, Phillips SJ, Abdul-Jalil AK, Gulekli B, Tan SL (2002) A comparison of in vitro maturation and in vitro fertilization for women with polycystic ovaries. Obstet Gynecol 100:665–70
6. Buckett W, Chian RC, Tan SL (2005) Can we eliminate severe ovarian hyperstimulation syndrome? Not completely. Hum Reprod 20:2367; author reply -8
7. Murray C, Golombok S (2000) Oocyte and semen donation: a survey of UK licensed centres. Hum Reprod 15:2133–9
8. Veeck LL, Wortham JW, Jr., Witmyer J, et al. (1983) Maturation and fertilization of morphologically immature human oocytes in a program of in vitro fertilization. Fertil Steril 39:594–602
9. Cha KY, Koo JJ, Ko JJ, Choi DH, Han SY, Yoon TK (1991) Pregnancy after in vitro fertilization of human follicular oocytes collected from nonstimulated cycles, their culture in vitro and their transfer in a donor oocyte program. Fertil Steril 55:109–13
10. Pincus G, Enzmann EV (1935) The comparative behaviours mammalian eggs in vitro and in vivo.II The activation of tubal eggs in the rabbit. Journal of Experimental Medicine 62:665–75
11. Pincus G, Saunders B (1939) The comparative behavior of mammalian eggs in vivo and in vitro. VI The maturation of human ovarian ova. Anat Rec 75:537–45
12. Edwards RG (1965) Maturation in vitro of human ovarian oocytes. Lancet 2:926–9
13. Edwards RG (1965) Maturation in vitro of mouse, sheep, cow, pig, rhesus monkey and human ovarian oocytes. Nature 208:349–51
14. Edwards RG, Bavister BD, Steptoe PC (1969) Early stages of fertilization in vitro of human oocytes matured in vitro. Nature 221:632–5
15. Trounson A, Wood C, Kausche A (1994) In vitro maturation and the fertilization and developmental competence of oocytes recovered from untreated polycystic ovarian patients. Fertil Steril 62: 353–62
16. Barnes FL, Crombie A, Gardner DK, et al. (1995) Blastocyst development and birth after in-vitro maturation of human primary oocytes, intracytoplasmic sperm injection and assisted hatching. Hum Reprod 10:3243–7
17. Nagy ZP, Cecile J, Liu J, Loccufier A, Devroey P, Van Steirteghem A (1996) Pregnancy and birth after intracytoplasmic sperm injection of in vitro matured germinal-vesicle stage oocytes: case report. Fertil Steril 65:1047–50
18. Liu J, Katz E, Garcia JE, Compton G, Baramki TA (1997) Successful in vitro maturation of human oocytes not exposed to human chorionic gonadotropin during ovulation induction, resulting in pregnancy. Fertil Steril 67:566–8
19. Jaroudi KA, Hollanders JM, Sieck UV, Roca GL, El-Nour AM, Coskun S (1997) Pregnancy after transfer of embryos which were generated from in-vitro matured oocytes. Hum Reprod 12:857–9
20. Cha KY, Han SY, Chung HM, et al. (2000) Pregnancies and deliveries after in vitro maturation culture followed by in vitro fertilization and embryo transfer without stimulation in women with polycystic ovary syndrome. Fertil Steril 73:978–83
21. Chian RC, Gulekli B, Buckett WM, Tan SL (1999) Priming with human chorionic gonadotropin before retrieval of immature oocytes in women with infertility due to the polycystic ovary syndrome. N Engl J Med 341:1624, 6
22. Cha KY, Chian RC (1998) Maturation in vitro of immature human oocytes for clinical use. Hum Reprod Update 4:103–20
23. Swain JE, Smith GD. Mechanism of oocyte maturation. In: Tan SL, Chian RC, Buckett WM, eds. (2007) In-vitro Maturation of Human Oocytes Basic science to clinical application London: informa Healthcare; 83–102
24. Telford NA, Watson AJ, Schultz GA (1990) Transition from maternal to embryonic control in early mammalian development: a comparison of several species. Mol Reprod Dev 26:90–100
25. Chian RC, Sirard MA (1995) Effects of cumulus cells and follicle-stimulating hormone during in vitro maturation on parthenogenetic activation of bovine oocytes. Mol Reprod Dev 42:425–31
26. Gilchrist RB, Thompson JG (2007) Oocyte maturation: emerging concepts and technologies to improve developmental potential in vitro. Theriogenology 67:6–15
27. Thibault C, Gerard M, Menezo Y (1975) Preovulatory and ovulatory mechanisms in oocyte maturation. J Reprod Fertil 45: 605–10
28. Nogueira D, Albano C, Adriaenssens T, et al. (2003) Human oocytes reversibly arrested in prophase I by phosphodiesterase type 3 inhibitor in vitro. Biol Reprod 69:1042–52
29. Durinzi KL, Wentz AC, Saniga EM, Johnson DE, Lanzendorf SE (1997) Follicle stimulating hormone effects on immature human oocytes: in vitro maturation and hormone production. J Assist Reprod Genet 14:199–204
30. Schroeder AC, Downs SM, Eppig JJ (1988) Factors affecting the developmental capacity of mouse oocytes undergoing maturation in vitro. Ann N Y Acad Sci 541:197–204
31. Jinno M, Sandow BA, Hodgen GD (1989) Enhancement of the developmental potential of mouse oocytes matured in vitro by gonadotropins and ethylenediaminetetraacetic acid (EDTA). J In Vitro Fert Embryo Transf 6:36–40
32. Morgan PM, Warikoo PK, Bavister BD (1991) In vitro maturation of ovarian oocytes from unstimulated rhesus monkeys: assessment of cytoplasmic maturity by embryonic development after in vitro fertilization. Biol Reprod 45:89–93
33. Chian RC, Ao A, Clarke HJ, Tulandi T, Tan SL (1999) Production of steroids from human cumulus cells treated with different concentrations of gonadotropins during culture in vitro. Fertil Steril 71:61–6

34. Child TJ, Abdul-Jalil AK, Gulekli B, Tan SL (2001) In vitro maturation and fertilization of oocytes from unstimulated normal ovaries, polycystic ovaries, and women with polycystic ovary syndrome. Fertil Steril 76:936–42
35. Tan SL, Child TJ, Gulekli B (2002) In vitro maturation and fertilization of oocytes from unstimulated ovaries: predicting the number of immature oocytes retrieved by early follicular phase ultrasonography. Am J Obstet Gynecol 186:684–9
36. Mikkelsen AL, Smith S, Lindenberg S (2000) Impact of oestradiol and inhibin A concentrations on pregnancy rate in in-vitro oocyte maturation. Hum Reprod 15:1685–90
37. Consensus on infertility treatment related to polycystic ovary syndrome. Hum Reprod 2008;23:462–77
38. Consensus on infertility treatment related to polycystic ovary syndrome. Fertil Steril 2008;89:505–22
39. Barnes FL, Kausche A, Tiglias J, Wood C, Wilton L, Trounson A (1996) Production of embryos from in vitro-matured primary human oocytes. Fertil Steril 65:1151–6
40. Soderstrom-Anttila V, Makinen S, Tuuri T, Suikkari AM (2005) Favourable pregnancy results with insemination of in vitro matured oocytes from unstimulated patients. Hum Reprod 20: 1534–40
41. Suikkari AM, Soderstrom-Anttila V (2007) In-vitro maturation of eggs: is it really useful? Best Pract Res Clin Obstet Gynaecol 21: 145–55
42. Nikolettos N, Al-Hasani S, Felberbaum R, et al. (2001) Gonadotropin-releasing hormone antagonist protocol: a novel method of ovarian stimulation in poor responders. Eur J Obstet Gynecol Reprod Biol 97:202–7
43. Lashen H, Ledger W, Lopez-Bernal A, Barlow D (1999) Poor responders to ovulation induction: is proceeding to in-vitro fertilization worthwhile? Hum Reprod 14:964–9
44. Surrey ES, Schoolcraft WB (2000) Evaluating strategies for improving ovarian response of the poor responder undergoing assisted reproductive techniques. Fertil Steril 73:667–76
45. Child TJ, Gulekli B, Chian RC, Abdul-Jalil AK, Tan SL (2000) In-Vitro Maturation (IVM) of Oocytes from Unstimulated Normal Ovaries of Women with a Previous Poor Response to IVF. Fertil Steril 74:S45
46. Lim KS, Son WY, Yoon HG, Lim JH (2002) IVM/F-ET in stimulated cycles for the prevention of OHSS. Fertil Steril 78:S10
47. Lim KS, Yoon SH, Lim JH. IVM as an alternative for over-responders. In: Tan SL, Chian RC, Buckett WM, eds. (2007) In-vitro maturation of human oocytes Basic science to clinical application. London: informa Healthcare; 345–52
48. Liu J, Lu G, Qian Y, Mao Y, Ding W (2003) Pregnancies and births achieved from in vitro matured oocytes retrieved from poor responders undergoing stimulation in in vitro fertilization cycles. Fertil Steril 80:447–9
49. Liu J, Lim JH, Chian RC. IVM as an alternative for poor responders. In: Tan SL, Chian RC, Buckett WM, eds. (2007) In-vitro maturation of human oocytes, basic science to clinical applicaton. London: Informa UK Ltd; 333–44
50. Elizur SE, Chian RC, Pineau CA, et al. Fertility preservation treatment for young women with autoimmune diseases facing treatment with gonadotoxic agents. Rheumatology (Oxford) 2008
51. Elizur SE, Chian RC, Holzer HE, Gidoni Y, Tulandi T, Tan SL. Cryopreservation of oocytes in a young woman with severe and symptomatic endometriosis: A new indication for fertility preservation. Fertil Steril 2007
52. Huang JY, Tulandi T, Holzer H, Tan SL, Chian RC (2008) Combining ovarian tissue cryobanking with retrieval of immature oocytes followed by in vitro maturation and vitrification: an additional strategy of fertility preservation. Fertil Steril 89:567–72
53. Lee SJ, Schover LR, Partridge AH, et al. (2006) American Society of Clinical Oncology recommendations on fertility preservation in cancer patients. J Clin Oncol 24:2917–31
54. Rao GD, Chian RC, Son WS, Gilbert L, Tan SL (2004) Fertility preservation in women undergoing cancer treatment. Lancet 363: 1829–30
55. Chian RC, Huang JY, Gilbert L, et al. Obstetric outcomes following vitrification of in vitro and in vivo matured oocytes. Fertil Steril 2008
56. Chian RC, Gilbert L, Huang JY, et al. Live birth after vitrification of in vitro matured human oocytes. Fertil Steril 2008
57. Oktay K, Demirtas E, Son WY, Lostritto K, Chian RC, Tan SL (2008) In vitro maturation of germinal vesicle oocytes recovered after premature luteinizing hormone surge: description of a novel approach to fertility preservation. Fertil Steril 89:228 e19–22
58. Demirtas E, Elizur S, Holzer H, et al. (2008) Immature oocyte retrieval in the luteal phaseto preserve fertility in cancer patients. RBM Online 17:520–3
59. Chian RC, Buckett WM, Tulandi T, Tan SL (2000) Prospective randomized study of human chorionic gonadotrophin priming before immature oocyte retrieval from unstimulated women with polycystic ovarian syndrome. Hum Reprod 15:165–70
60. Son WY, Yoon SH, Lim JH (2006) Effect of gonadotrophin priming on in-vitro maturation of oocytes collected from women at risk of OHSS. Reprod Biomed Online 13:340–8
61. Yang SH, Son WY, Yoon SH, Ko Y, Lim JH (2005) Correlation between in vitro maturation and expression of LH receptor in cumulus cells of the oocytes collected from PCOS patients in HCG-primed IVM cycles. Hum Reprod 20:2097–103
62. Willis DS, Watson H, Mason HD, Galea R, Brincat M, Franks S (1998) Premature response to luteinizing hormone of granulosa cells from anovulatory women with polycystic ovary syndrome: relevance to mechanism of anovulation. J Clin Endocrinol Metab 83:3984–91
63. Gulekli B, Buckett WM, Chian RC, Child TJ, Abdul-Jalil AK, Tan SL (2004) Randomized, controlled trial of priming with 10, 000 IU versus 20, 000 IU of human chorionic gonadotropin in women with polycystic ovary syndrome who are undergoing in vitro maturation. Fertil Steril 82:1458–9
64. Cobo AC, Requena A, Neuspiller F, et al. (1999) Maturation in vitro of human oocytes from unstimulated cycles: selection of the optimal day for ovum retrieval based on follicular size. Hum Reprod 14:1864–8
65. Smith LC, Olivera-Angel M, Groome NP, Bhatia B, Price CA (1996) Oocyte quality in small antral follicles in the presence or absence of a large dominant follicle in cattle. J Reprod Fertil 106: 193–9
66. Chian RC, Chung JT, Downey BR, Tan SL (2002) Maturational and developmental competence of immature oocytes retrieved from bovine ovaries at different phases of folliculogenesis. Reprod Biomed Online 4:127–32
67. Son WY, Chung JT, Demirtas E, et al. (2008) Comparison of in-vitro maturation cycles with and without in-vivo matured oocytes retrieved. Reprod Biomed Online 17:59–67
68. Son WY, Chung JT, Chian RC, et al. (2008) A 38 h interval between hCG priming and oocyte retrieval increases in vivo and in vitro oocyte maturation rate in programmed IVM cycles. Hum Reprod 23:2010–6
69. Wynn P, Picton HM, Krapez JA, Rutherford AJ, Balen AH, Gosden RG (1998) Pretreatment with follicle stimulating hormone promotes the numbers of human oocytes reaching metaphase II by in-vitro maturation. Hum Reprod 13:3132–8
70. Suikkari AM, Tulppala M, Tuuri T, Hovatta O, Barnes F (2000) Luteal phase start of low-dose FSH priming of follicles results in an efficient recovery, maturation and fertilization of immature human oocytes. Hum Reprod 15:747–51
71. Mikkelsen AL, Smith SD, Lindenberg S (1999) In-vitro maturation of human oocytes from regularly menstruating women may be successful without follicle stimulating hormone priming. Hum Reprod 14:1847–51

72. Mikkelsen AL, Host E, Blaabjerg J, Lindenberg S (2003) Time interval between FSH priming and aspiration of immature human oocytes for in-vitro maturation: a prospective randomized study. Reprod Biomed Online 6:416–20
73. Mikkelsen AL, Lindenberg S (2001) Benefit of FSH priming of women with PCOS to the in vitro maturation procedure and the outcome: a randomized prospective study. Reproduction 122:587–92
74. Lin YH, Hwang JL, Huang LW, et al. (2003)Combination of FSH priming and hCG priming for in-vitro maturation of human oocytes. Hum Reprod 18:1632–6
75. Elizur SE, Son WY, Yap R, Tan SL (2008) Low-dose humanmenopausal gonadotropin (hMG) is superior to micronized 17 beta estradiol in in-vitromaturation (IVM) cycles with thin endometrial lining. Fertil Steril in press
76. Chian RC (2004) In-vitro maturation of immature oocytes for infertile women with PCOS. Reprod Biomed Online 8:547–52
77. Son WY, Lee SY, Lim JH (2005) Fertilization, cleavage and blastocyst development according to the maturation timing of oocytes in in vitro maturation cycles. Hum Reprod 20:3204–7
78. Son WY, Lee SY, Yoon SH, Lim JH (2007) Pregnancies and deliveries after transfer of human blastocysts derived from in vitro matured oocytes in in vitro maturation cycles. Fertil Steril 87:1491–3
79. Phillips SJ, Dean NL, Buckett WM, Tan SL (2003) Consecutive transfer of day 3 embryos and of day 5–6 blastocysts increases overall pregnancy rates associated with blastocyst culture. J Assist Reprod Genet 20:461–4
80. Le Du A, Kadoch IJ, Bourcigaux N, et al. (2005)In vitro oocyte maturation for the treatment of infertility associated with polycystic ovarian syndrome: the French experience. Hum Reprod 20:420–4
81. Russell JB, Knezevich KM, Fabian KF, Dickson JA (1997) Unstimulated immature oocyte retrieval: early versus midfollicular endometrial priming. Fertil Steril 67:616–20
82. Buckett WM, Chian RC, Tan SL (2004) Human chorionic gonadotropin for in vitro oocyte maturation: does it improve the endometrium or implantation? J Reprod Med 49:93–8
83. Buckett WM, Chian RC, Dean NL, Sylvestre C, Holzer HE, Tan SL. Pregnancy loss in pregnancies conceived after in vitro oocyte maturation, conventional in vitro fertilization, and intracytoplasmic sperm injection. Fertil Steril 2007
84. Mikkelsen AL, Ravn SH, Lindenberg S (2003) Evaluation of newborns delevered after in vitro maturation. Hum Reprod 18:xviii
85. Cha KY, Chung HM, Lee DR, et al. (2005)Obstetric outcome of patients with polycystic ovary syndrome treated by in vitro maturation and in vitro fertilization-embryo transfer. Fertil Steril 83: 1461–5
86. Buckett WM, Chian RC, Holzer H, Dean N, Usher R, Tan SL (2007) Obstetric outcomes and congenital abnormalities after in vitro maturation, in vitro fertilization, and intracytoplasmic sperm injection. Obstet Gynecol 110:885–91
87. Hansen M, Kurinczuk JJ, Bower C, Webb S (2002) The risk of major birth defects after intracytoplasmic sperm injection and in vitro fertilization. N Engl J Med 346:725–30
88. Devroey P, Bourgain C, Macklon NS, Fauser BC (2004) Reproductive biology and IVF: ovarian stimulation and endometrial receptivity. Trends Endocrinol Metab 15:84–90
89. Chian RC, Buckett WM, Tan SL (2004) In-vitro maturation of human oocytes. Reprod Biomed Online 8:148–66
90. Torre A, Achour-Frydman N, Feyereisen E, Fanchin R, Frydman R. How do we improve implantation rate following in-vitro maturation of oocytes. In: Tan SL, Chian RC, Buckett WM, eds. In-vitro maturation of human oocytes Basic science to clinical application. London: Informa Healthcare; 2007:319–31
91. Wei Z, Cao Y, Cong L, Zhou P, Zhang Z, Li J. Effect of metformin pretreatment on pregnancy outcome of in vitro matured oocytes retrieved from women with polycystic ovary syndrome. Fertil Steril 2007
92. Mikkelsen AL, Andersson AM, Skakkebaek NE, Lindenberg S (2001) Basal concentrations of oestradiol may predict the outcome of in-vitro maturation in regularly menstruating women. Hum Reprod 16:862–7

Chapter 43
Integrating Preimplantation Genetic Diagnosis into the ART Laboratory

Kenneth C. Drury

Abstract Technology has become the driving force in the field of assisted reproductive infertility medicine. The ability to conduct in vitro fertilization, embryo micromanipulation, and cryopreservation allows the clinical embryologist to obtain an ever increasing ability to observe and test the viability of the human embryo in the laboratory. At the same time, molecular genetics and molecular biology have developed to the point of allowing the laboratory to detect and determine various aspects of the embryonic genome and knowledge of the detailed structure of human chromosomes. These technological abilities are now used not only to identify single gene mutations linked to specific diseases, but identify chromosomal abnormalities residing in the in vitro cultured human embryo as well. Selection of mutation-free and chromosomally normal embryos is now a reality that brings new hope to couples at risk for giving birth to affected offspring. There are also mounting indications that these technologies are also able to benefit couples facing other infertility issues such as failure to conceive during ART procedures. Ethical issues, concerning the use of these new technologies, have arisen from a number of quarters where it is troubling to think of, no less accept, the possible outcomes derived from their applications. One long sought after outcome, being requested by prospective parents, is to select the gender of the desired offspring for purely non-medical motives. Infertility programs throughout the United States and the world are now capable of utilizing these advanced technologies to make gender selection a reality for interested couples, as well as, enhance the ability to treat a variety of problems relating to infertility. Reproductive genetic programs may want to consider early on how they wish to utilize these technical abilities within their individual programs. There should be serious consideration of the pros and cons of developing these highly technical, time consuming and expensive procedures within a given facility. This chapter is designed to consider and help answer those questions.

K.C. Drury (✉)
Department of Obstetrics and Gynecology, Division of Reproductive Endocrinology and Infertility, University of Florida College of Medicine, Gainsville, FL100294 32610, USA
e-mail: drurykufl.edu

Keywords Assisted reproductive technology • Preimplantation genetic diagnosis • Preimplantation aneuploidy screening • Fluorescence in situ hybridization • Embryo biopsy • Chromosome • Embryo • Blastomere • Genetic disease • Egg • Sperm • Polar body • Blastocyst • Micromanipulation

43.1 Introduction

The use of new technology for infertility treatment is being introduced into assisted reproductive technology (ART) laboratories at an ever increasing rate [1–8]. Expanding novel embryo culture systems and the use of ever more complex culture media, are now being employed to enhance embryo viability and pregnancy potential [9–15]. The use of egg, sperm, and embryo micromanipulation procedures, utilizing advanced high technology equipment, has given rise to the possibility of handling and manipulating these in vitro specimens with unprecedented skill [16, 17]. As a result, breakthroughs in the treatment of infertility, affecting both female and male, are now standard in the great majority of infertility centers throughout the United States and around the world [18].

Another area utilizing ART technology is also rapidly advancing in its ability to diagnose in vitro cultured human embryos for deleterious genomic single gene mutations as well as chromosomal abnormalities [19, 20]. This was unheard of just 15 years ago. The very first article reporting the screening of human embryos for a genetic mutation (cystic fibrosis) was published in 1992 [21, 22]. Thus began the field of preimplantation genetic diagnosis (PGD).

Genetic tests now available for embryo PGD have increased nearly 100-fold [23, 24] to include not only those genetic diseases responsible for perinatal mortality but also those linked to later life morbidities/mortalities such as heart disease, breast cancer, and Alzheimer's disease [25–27]. Other more controversial uses of this technology have evolved to include HLA compatibility testing of in vitro embryos. These embryos can then be chosen for intra-uterine

D.T. Carrell and C.M. Peterson (eds.), *Reproductive Endocrinology and Infertility: Integrating Modern Clinical and Laboratory Practice*, 647
DOI 10.1007/978-1-4419-1436-1_43, © Springer Science+Business Media, LLC 2010

transfer and potentially produce placental stem cells from the resulting offspring that can be donated to a HLA compatible, but disease-affected sibling for rejection-free treatment. This procedure is sometimes referred to as "savior sibling PGD" [28–30].

The identification of chromosomal abnormalities, through the use of FISH, has also led to the prospects of averting pregnancy miscarriages, aneuploid live births, and sex chromosome anomalies. Of course, the ease and accuracy of determining gender of the preimplantation embryo, opens the door for gender selection by patients regardless of medical conditions, thus giving rise to additional ethical issues [31–33].

Even in the midst of these surrounding controversies vying for media attention, the technology available for employing preimplantation genetic (PGD) and chromosomal (PGD-AS) screening, is now within the means of most ART laboratories and infertility practices. If your program is determined to provide these specialized services to patients, how do you prepare and go about integrating this technology into your ART laboratory?

43.2 Rationale for PGD

A question that any infertility program may want to address is "Why do we want to provide this technology to our patients and how will it benefit them?" Of course, preimplantation genetic and chromosomal diagnosis can address many and varied infertility and pregnancy concerns. Prior familial diagnosed genetic abnormalities may be at the root of pregnancy abnormalities leading to the prospect of early pregnancy termination. The failure to conceive, or continue a detected pregnancy, may very well reside in a previously unknown chromosomal translocation event residing in either partner. Age-related chromosomal abnormalities, especially in the female, are the most prevalent causes of failure to conceive and carry a normal baby to term [34–36]. There may also be a case to be made for the failure to conceive through multiple-assisted reproductive procedures as a sign of potential chromosomal abnormalities [37, 38].

Any of the above mentioned concerns may very well propel your program to adopt and implement preimplantation embryo genetic/chromosomal diagnostic procedures.

43.3 PGD vs. PGD-AS

What is the difference between preimplantation genetic diagnosis (PGD) and preimplantation aneuploidy screening (PGD-AS)? It is important to understand the underlying technical demands that each of these procedures impose. PGD essentially identifies mutations within the genomic sequence of DNA which control the expression of genes or other regulatory elements necessary to develop, build, and maintain a healthy body. Every individual (on average) carries 6–8 potentially serious/lethal gene mutations in his or her DNA, which, under the right (wrong) circumstances, can be expressed and cause debilitating outcomes [39]. Cystic Fibrosis (CF) is a disease brought about by a mutation in a gene which regulates chloride channel transport [40]. This usually exhibits its expression or outcome in causing the failure of an individual's lungs to effectively and efficiently exchange carbon dioxide for oxygen and transport it to tissues within the body. It may also express itself in the failure of a male's vas deferens to fuse and transport sperm from the testis to the seminal vesicles, thus being a cause of male infertility [41]. There are now known to be over 1,000 site-specific mutations that govern the expression of this gene [40].

The ability to accurately determine the status of any specific gene mutation within a single cell is daunting at best. Prior to being able to detect and analyze sequences of nucleotides within a gene from a single cell (in this case, a single blastomere taken from an in vitro derived embryo), amplification of the genomic DNA (whole genome amplification – WGA) must take place over a million fold. This is accomplished through the use of the polymerization chain reaction (PCR) procedures [44] that create sufficient quantities of identical DNA strands for molecular diagnosis [42, 43]. This particular procedure is extremely sensitive to temperature control and environmental conditions. The most serious concern during this process is the inadvertent contamination of the test sample by extraneous DNA, which may then lead to an error in the diagnosis. Another difficultly leading to potential errors, originates from the PCR reaction itself, and is known as "allele dropout" [45]. This error or failure in the amplification of certain strands of DNA in the sample, may result in a false negative reading that will adversely affect the outcome of the diagnosis [46].

Needless to say, single gene analysis requires a great deal of specific expertise, equipment, and a separately maintained enclosed environment. Most "stand alone" infertility programs do not have the necessary patient-based volume for any specific disease to sustain this level and complexity of genetic diagnosis.

In comparison to PGD, PGD-AS screens for the presence or absence (or significant rearrangement) of whole chromosomes within a single cell [47]. PGD-AS relies on a technology known as fluorescence in situ hybridization (FISH), which does not require the amplification of genomic DNA [48]. As a result, multi-colored fluorescently-tagged commercially-available complementary DNA probe mixtures (Vysis, Rainbow) are used to link (hybridize) to chromosome-specific DNA sequence sites. These signals, observed with a fluorescence microscope, will then identify and enumerate specific chromosomes present within a particular cell. This information can then be used to classify the corresponding embryo as chromosomally normal (euploidy) or altered in a manner unsuitable (polyploidy, aneuploidy) for transfer. The major drawback to the use of FISH technology in the diagnosis of chromosomal fitness of an embryo, is the fact that only approximately a third of the 46 chromosomes (23 pairs) normally present can be identified and assessed [49]. This is due to the fact that chromosomes reside in an unstructured configuration (interphase) for most of the cell cycle and cannot be identified as individual entities (metaphase structures) as in a standard karyotype analysis. At least one FISH probe is now available for every chromosome, although only a restricted number can be simultaneously applied to a single interphase nucleus. This is because of the limited number of fluorochromes available and the risk of misdiagnosis due to overlapping signals.

Those chromosomes that are able to be screened, have been chosen primarily due to their occurrence in chromosomal defective live births or miscarriages [50–53]. These tend to include the sex chromosomes X & Y as well as 21, 18, 13, and 22. So, even though not all chromosomes can be assessed through FISH procedures, those accounting for the most prevalent chromosomal abnormalities in live-born offspring can be evaluated.

From this standpoint then, what will it take in terms of personnel, equipment, laboratory space, and program commitment to establish PGD and PGD-AS for patient treatment in your program?

43.4 Requirements for In-House PGD

For those programs interested in establishing in-house PGD capabilities, there are a number of general considerations to take into account. Some of these must take into account the community served, patient base size, personnel capabilities, existing laboratory facilities and technical expertise.

43.4.1 What Kind of Program Requires In-House PGD?

In-house PGD is probably best served through a larger-based infertility practice conducting on the order of 500 patient cycles + per year and residing in a metropolitan area of at least one million or greater inhabitants. This will allow a well-functioning and successful practice to invest the resources and personnel required to initiate, conduct, and maintain PGD.

43.4.1.1 Program Management and Personnel

In all likelihood, your present technical staff (those residing in the laboratory) will not have sufficient knowledge or experience to immediately undertake analysis of single embryonic cells, using PCR or FISH for patient diagnosis, requiring either PGD or PGD-AS.

In order to obtain and retain the required and necessary staff to prepare, conduct, and analyze results obtained from PGD, the medical management must firstly be absolutely committed to the demands and requirements of this technically intensive undertaking. Less than unanimous support and commitment to maintain all facets of preimplantation genetic analysis of in vitro embryos will result in failure, loss of patient confidence, and invested capital.

43.4.2 IVF Laboratory Micromanipulation Technology

The great majority of reproductive ART laboratories in the United States already have the technical expertise and skills to conduct essential micromanipulation procedures for those treatments requiring ICSI, assisted hatching, embryo defragmentation, and (with some additional training), embryo biopsy. All of these skills have to be carried out at the highest level of competence in order for biopsied embryos to retain viability and develop into healthy blastocysts during extended in vitro culture [54, 55].

There are various egg and embryo stages in which biopsy may be performed and cellular components obtained for genetic/chromosomal analysis. Each of these procedures demands various technical skills that will be required, at one time or another, in a PGD program. Below are the main stages of zygote and embryo development that can provide informative diagnosis.

43.4.2.1 Egg Polar Body (1st and 2nd) Biopsy

The mature egg (arrested at 2nd metaphase of meiosis), obtained during the egg retrieval procedure, has extruded the 1st polar body, consisting of a diploid complement of chromosomes. This egg now awaits in vitro fertilization by the addition of sperm, at which time, a 2nd (haploid) polar body is released by the egg. Both of these miniature cells (polar bodies) can be removed during separate procedures and utilized for DNA or chromosome analysis [56, 57].

Use of polar bodies during analysis can only provide genetic information pertaining to the egg, and therefore, any paternal abnormal contributions to the resulting embryo remain undetected. Timing of these respective biopsies is also critical due to the instability of polar bodies, which tend to degrade within hours.

43.4.2.2 Day 3 Eight-Cell Embryo Blastomere Biopsy

The eight-cell embryo provides a convenient and useful embryonic developmental stage from which to sample a single cell to determine the inheritance of either a single gene mutation or chromosomal abnormality. It also incorporates the paternal as well as maternal genetic components to give a more complete analysis of the potential offspring. Even though this eight-cell stage presents a number of difficulties and uncertainties pertaining to resulting outcomes obtained when using either PGD or PGD-AS, it has historically been the stage of choice for the majority of diagnostic procedures presented in the literature [58, 59].

43.4.2.3 Day 5 Blastocyst Embryo Trophectoderm Biopsy

The blastocyst stage embryo does not normally develop prior to the 5th day of in vitro culture. Utilizing biopsied material taken from this stage of development, presents an advantage and a number of disadvantages. The advantage is that more than one cell can be obtained during the biopsy procedure and used during testing to give confirmation and added confidence to the test results [60–63]. On the other hand, the embryo has now differentiated cellularly to contain both trophectoderm (placental destined) and inner-cell mass (destined for fetal development) cells. Present day biopsy procedures sample only trophectoderm cells to use for subsequent analysis and these cells may harbor characteristics that do not always pertain to the ICM or fetal-destined cells.

In any case, each of the cell types (polar bodies, blastomeres, and trophectoderm), obtained through the above biopsy procedures, require strict individual manipulation and processing in order to maintain a verifiable link to the respective biopsied embryo. Obtaining reliable results and making the proper diagnosis does not benefit your patient if they are assigned to the wrong embryo.

43.5 Referral PGD

Since the majority of ART laboratories already possess the requisite micromanipulation equipment in order to perform embryo biopsy procedures, (and there are embryo biopsy workshops available to acquire the required expertise), it may very well be advisable to process the biopsied cell(s) in-house and send it to be analyzed at a commercial PGD reference laboratory. This can usually be accomplished within a time frame that accommodates fresh blastocyst transfer. This strategy alleviates the most arduous aspects of making PGD available to your patients (see Appendix A).

Although both PGD and PGD-AS can be processed in this manner, it is highly recommended that single gene mutation PGD be referred to an experienced laboratory with expert skills in this area of genetic diagnosis. The technology is rapidly changing and the investment for developing whole genome amplification for use with comparative genome hybridization (CGH), fluorescent real-time PCR, and DNA micro-array technology is cost and expertise prohibitive [64–67]. Developing effective, accurate, and reproducible genetic tests, which utilize single cells, requires skills that few reproductive biologists possess.

As a result of the drawbacks likely to be encountered when establishing full karyotypic and gene-specific mutation analysis programs, this review will concentrate only on those requirements necessary to conduct FISH-based screening tests of chromosomal abnormalities – PGD-AS.

43.6 Setting up PGD-AS

There are a number of critical issues involved in preparing the ART laboratory for PGD-AS. Each of these issues must be approached differently using various resources and strategies. Many will be practice and facility-specific. Do not hesitate to seek experienced advice in order to prevent costly startup mistakes [70, 71].

43.6.1 How to Obtain a Blastomere for Analysis

Prior to being able to obtain a diagnosis and assigning it to an embryo, a well identified and intact specimen must be secured and processed. Each step of the protocol is critical from start to finish and mental concentration is just as important as technique. Here are some of the primary steps involved in the preparation of cell nuclei for FISH analysis [68, 69, 72].

43.6.1.1 Embryo Selection

It may seem intuitive that if there is an embryo available, you might as well biopsy it and process the cell for analysis. It is not that straightforward in many cases. Timing of development and embryo morphology can greatly impact the ability to carry out all subsequent procedures and impact the cost of doing so [73, 74].

It is recommended then that when considering a day three biopsy, that the embryo be judged in the morning hours of that day for both developmental and morphological features. Only those embryos that have attained a 6–10 cell status and a top 2–3 morphological classification (depending on the formula used) should be considered for biopsy. The ideal situation is to work with a 7–8 cell pre-biopsy grade 1 (best) embryo, removing only one cell for analysis. There may be acceptable reasons why more than a single cell is required to be removed during any particular biopsy. However, routinely removing two cells for purely diagnostic considerations is discouraged. As a result of employing the above-mentioned criteria for embryo selection, it has been found that developmental timeliness, good morphological parameters, and chromosomal euploidy are linked to produce high pregnancy potential [74].

43.6.1.2 Which Blastomere?

Is one blastomere just like any other within an eight-cell stage embryo? This is indeed a provocative question, which touches on many (developmental) issues other than just biopsy selection. However, there are reasons to think that the choice of a particular blastomere could have an impact on outcome [75–79].

It is often observed that even normally developing embryos divide asynchronously during early division stages. In these cases, the embryo may result as a mix of division stage blastomeres, resulting in some cells being anatomically larger than others; so which to choose? Some of these cells may display a visual nucleus, while others may not. Some may house multiple nuclei or micro-inclusions. Fragmentation present within the zona pellucida may have derived as the result of instability of a single blastomere. These are all considerations worthy of thought during the selection process of the biopsy procedure. In many cases, just choosing the blastomere most available will suit your biopsy technique. It has not been demonstrated that any selection process of a specific blastomere determines the effectiveness of PGD-AS. However, on the other hand, it has not been demonstrated not to. In the future, it may well be possible to identify each individual blastomere by positional characteristics within the eight-cell stage embryo. This may make it possible to always biopsy the same positional cell or to biopsy cells in a sequential manner and determine which are destined to develop as either trophectoderm (placental) or inner-cell mass (fetal) cells during differentiation to the blastocyst or implantation stage.

43.6.1.3 Embryo Biopsy

There are presently numerous and various techniques available for the successful and effective removal of polar bodies, single blastomeres, or trophectoderm cells for chromosomal analysis using PGD-AS.

Recently introduced technology, making use of a far infra-red (48 μm), non-contact laser system, has enhanced the biopsy process by making it less stressful on the embryo as well as the embryologist [80–83]. Less micromanipulation hardware is required and it allows a more precise entry through the zonal barrier in order to carry out the biopsy procedure. It is recommended then that a laser be added to the micromanipulation armamentarium.

43.6.2 Blastomere Fixation and Techniques

Blastomere preparation and nuclei fixation (required for the preparation of chromatin for hybridization) is probably the most critical and important procedure involved in the entire PGD-AS process. Not to make too much of a fine point, but fixation is the most important of all the other most important procedures to consider. Unfortunately, however, not all fixation outcomes resulting from this procedure are within the control of the technologist. This is not a comforting thought as the diagnostic outcome may very likely depend on the integrity and quality of the spread nucleus itself. Just as chromosomes undergo rearrangements from fully expanded to highly condensed states during the cell cycle, the nuclear plasm also changes consistency during this process and can affect the extent and characteristics of overall spreading and chromatin configuration once fixed for hybridization. Of course, if the particular cell chosen was in the process of degenerating (apoptotic degradation), then the nuclei may also behave in an abnormal manner. Uneven thickness of the spread nucleus can cause signal reading confusion post-hybridization, whereas, extended spreading can distort signal presentation and skew interpretation of the number and characterization of those signals present in the sample. These difficulties cannot be entirely avoided by any particular spreading technique.

On the other hand, various spreading techniques have been established and used successfully to allow for the adherence of an intact nucleus to the hybridization slide. The most cited and utilized spreading technique for single cells is a modified Tarkowsky's method using Carnoy's (3:1 methanol–acetic acid) solution [84, 85]. The use of a synthetic detergent (Tween-20) to assist spreading the nuclei has also been reported recently [86].

An especially useful "hybrid" version of both the above-mentioned techniques [87] has been employed with success. The benefit of using the hybrid-fix method is that the cell can be positioned exactly where required on the slide and allowed to dry without the need for constant monitoring to observe the "instant" of drying required before applying cold Carnoy's 3:1 solution. This procedure is also much less dependent on the environmental humidity factor and aids in the efficient processing of multiple cells and slides within a given time frame. However, the use of freshly made solutions is always a must.

Embryo blastomeres are much smaller and fragile than whole embryos. As a result, manipulation requires more agility, concentration, and practice in order to master these skills and become successful. Use of high-grade dissection scopes and proper manipulation tools are essential.

43.6.2.1 Identification and Mapping Fixed Nuclei

How does one confirm the placement of a nucleus on the hybridization slide so that it can be located once again during chromosomal analysis following hybridization? This is a multi-stepped process that begins with a clean (acid washed) microscope slide. The placement of a single cell or multiple cells on a single slide utilizes the same basic strategy. Inscribe the underside of a slide, using a diamond point pen and place a 2–3 mm diameter circle. Fix the nuclei within this circled area (as indicated above). Following fixation and drying, place the slide on the fluorescence microscope equipped with a stage micrometer. Locate the nuclei at low magnification and increase to 600×, using a 60× non-oil objective. Using the micrometer, document the two-dimensional stage coordinates of the centered nuclei. Correctly positioned coordinates are the key to locating the hybridized nuclei during the analysis phase. Remember, locating nuclei without a detailed map is like locating a hubcap in the middle of the Pacific Ocean.

43.6.3 Extended Culture and Tracking Individual Embryos

Directly following each embryo biopsy, strict identification, handling, and culture of singular embryos is imperative. The extended culture system should be able to sustain healthy embryo development upto at least the 5 or 6-day blastocyst stage.

Each individual embryologist has to be fully informed as to the culture system in use and whether or not biopsied embryos have been rearranged during the extended culture period.

43.6.4 Paperwork

Proper documentation of each procedure conducted, every culture medium and solution used, and each individual person conducting a specific activity is absolutely essential. Clear and frequent communication between embryologist, geneticist, nurse coordinator, and physician is critical. There are no designated procedures or formats in place to cover each program's unique structure. Therefore, a great deal of thought and reflection has to be incorporated into each facet of the PGD-AS program.

43.6.5 Chromosomal Diagnosis Using FISH

Chromosome detection, using FISH technology, is a powerful tool able to analyze single cells for both chromosomal abnormalities and single gene detection. FISH has been used experimentally and clinically since the mid 1980s [88–92] and is now the basis for aneuploidy screening of human oocytes and embryos [93].

43.6.5.1 What is Fluorescence In Situ Hybridization?

FISH is based on the competitive association of DNA–DNA complementary sequences taking place upon the reannealing of denatured strands of chromosomal DNA. This was first studied as DNA–DNA competitive duplex hybridization reactions (Cot curves), which were able to demonstrate the complexity of sequence distribution within the genome prior to the development of PCR DNA amplification, which allowed the identification of unique nucleotide sequences [94–96].

FISH makes use of amplified and fluorescently tagged DNA molecules, designed to seek out specific sequences residing only on specific chromosomes. The hybridized fluorescent tag can then be visualized using a microscope housing the appropriate wavelength filter devises. The identity and enumeration of that chromosome can then be determined [48, 90].

43.6.5.2 Quality Control Issues

Since the clinical use of this technology depends highly on the reaction's specificity and sensitivity, it is imperative that every aspect of the test be well quality controlled. Temperature is the driving force of the hybridization reaction, and therefore, every step must be validated and monitored for accurate temperature control.

It is surprising that not all temperature control units used for hybridization accurately reflect the programmed temperature output. Closely monitored devises are shown to be quite variable as to their ability to attain and sustain the programmed temperature settings. This can certainly impact conditions required to promote highly specific probe hybridization. This may subsequently render the interpretation of outcomes impossible.

43.6.5.3 Choosing Hybridizing Probes

Fluorescently tagged FISH probes are conveniently available commercially for many (but not all) chromosomes [97, 98]. Except for the highest volume programs, only preselected and packaged groups of probes are available from commercial vendors. However, these encompass those probes that detect chromosomes contributing to the most often detected abnormal outcomes (miscarriages and affected live births) about which patients are most concerned.

The most often tested chromosomes are: 7, 13, 15, 16, 17, 18, 21, 22, X, & Y.

43.6.5.4 Choosing and Maintaining Filters

The pre-labeled commercial FISH probes used (with their individual wavelength characteristics) will determine which filter sets are required to efficiently detect the emitted wavelength following excitation of the probe [99–101].

It is normally recommended that single wavelength filters be available for each specific probe color used. This enables the viewer to determine the specificity and position for each emitted wavelength. Dual and triple band pass filters can also be useful to combine signal detection within a single view. With each additional band pass capture, signal strength is compromised due to the decreased filtered light. Thus, a quad filter set is usually of no additional benefit.

Unless a "no burn out" filter is purchased, another essential quality control parameter is the monitoring of filter "burn out." Filter function and sensitivity should remain high for a number of years. However, filters should be checked yearly to see if the centers have been bleached. Bleaching will reduce signal strength until errors gradually creep into the interpretation of hybridization results. This may go unnoticed over time due to the gradual nature of the effect.

43.6.5.5 Hybridization Protocols

Current FISH protocols are based primarily on the use of fluorescently tagged DNA probes. This alleviates the use of additional reactions, such as combining biotinylated signals to the hybridized probe in order to detect the probe. It also helps to maintain the sensitivity of the test system. Standard protocols are now based on the combined denaturation of probes and target DNA simultaneously. This is known as co-denaturation and eliminates the need for two denaturation steps.

Conventional FISH

It is highly recommended that the newer program (just commencing FISH in their program) follow the stated recommendations and written protocols for hybridization supplied by the provider of the DNA probes. Most of the times, these can be obtained from the company website, and they can always be requested.

Basically, following the identification and scoring of the nuclei on a glass slide, probe sets are applied and covered with small cover-slips, which are then sealed. The probes and sample are co-denatured at 75°C for 5 min, followed by hybridization at 37°C for 5–16 h. Following hybridization, the slides are soaked in solutions prepared to wash unbound or nonspecifically bound probe from the sample. The slides are left to dry, and then prepared for analysis.

A counter stain/anti-fade solution is applied to the sample area and again a cover slip is positioned. The slide is carefully placed on the microscope stage and coordinates applied. Using a 40–60× (non-oil) objective, the background stained nuclei with colored signals is identified.

Microwave FISH

Due to the length of time taken for specific probes to interact and bind sufficiently to produce a clear and readable signal, a more rapid protocol has been developed to accelerate the process [102–104]. The new protocol makes use of microwave energy and speeds the interaction of probe and sample, thereby, enhancing the hybridizing reaction (Fig. 43.1). In this manner, the entire hybridization reaction can take as little as 5 min. When using mixed probes, such as those constructed to identify multiple or amplified sequences (centromeric) along with those identifying single copy stretches of sequences, then the procedure will extend to 1 h.

This shorter hybridization protocol has been found quite useful when applied to multi-round FISH (see below).

Multi-Round FISH

Multiple rounds of hybridization cycles, utilizing various probe sets, have been employed in order to increase the overall number of chromosomes that can be identified from a single cell [105]. This can boost the number of chromosomes analyzed to 12–13, following three rounds of hybridization.

Clinically though, three rounds of processing may actually jeopardize the ability to accurately assess or determine the true complement of chromosomes. This is due to the loss of variable amounts of chromatin/DNA during the extended processing taking place during these extra hybridization and washing steps.

43.6.5.6 Equipment and Image Capture Software

It is often unclear where to start when trying to choose the most appropriate equipment for a specific process as well as

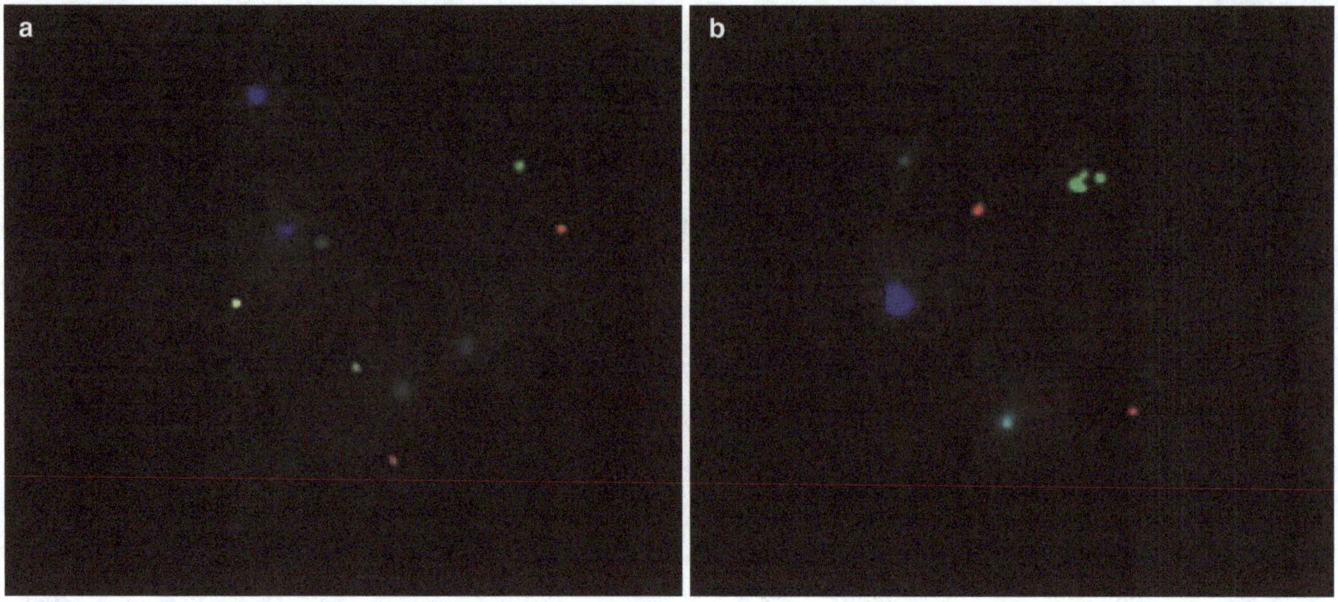

Fig. 43.1 (**a**) 1st round microwave 5 chromosome [13, 16, 18, 21, 22] FISH-diagnosed as normal. (**b**) 2nd round microwave 4 chromosome (X,Y,15,17) FISH-diagnosed as normal

purchasing it at a reasonable cost, while trying to fulfill the technical requirements of the new procedure. Luckily, in this case, the required pieces of equipment that are not already present in the ART laboratory will be minimal. However, that is not to say that they will not be expensive.

A good quality fluorescent microscope is the key and is at the heart of successful FISH chromosomal analysis. Two manufacturers that consistently provide microscopes of this quality are Nikon, Inc and Olympus. Both have some unique features that can be recommended. However, if your capital expense permits, it is recommended that a z-stacking stage accessory be included in your selection [106]. This accessory permits the identification of signals that may be otherwise slightly out of focus due to the inadequate focal depth of field provided by your 100× objective. As far as objectives are concerned, a high-grade 60× nonoil objective can be quite useful when performing your initial identification and assessment of probe signals. If reducing the magnification during this period is necessary, then oil will not interfere with readjustments. Final diagnosis is usually performed using the 100× oil objective.

As mentioned in the above section on quality control (43.6.5.2), the choice of hybridization equipment should be scrutinized closely in order to determine if the temperature profile accuracy meets requirements. Hybridization thermocontrol ovens are available and they are quite "handy." However, 37°C humidified CO_2 incubators (without the CO_2) are equally effective.

Image capture software and computer storage space is essential for accurate diagnosis and documentation of your results. Even though there are others available, it is recommended that the image capture programs of Applied Image (AI) be investigated [107]. These programs are now PC managed and network capable as well as validated in many laboratories.

Standard lab equipment is easily acquired: water bath heaters, pipettes, microscope slides, coplin jars, household microwaves, etc. can be purchased from most laboratory supply houses or kitchen store sections.

43.6.5.7 The Analysis

Control hybridizations are a basic feature of the clinical diagnosis; both positive and negative. Control slides prepared for CGH (Vysis, Downers Grove, IL USA) [108] make good positive controls since they provide not only interphase nuclei but also meta-phase stage (condensed) chromosomes plus most other stages. This slide can verify that not only did the probes hybridize during that particular processing run, but that they were specific for the chromosomes they were intended to detect. The negative slide will allow you to observe background noise, especially following multiple rounds of FISH.

Ideally, there will be two individuals trained and proficient in the process of analyzing FISH results. Mastering the technical procedures is demanding, but becoming highly proficient in the ability to accurately analyze and determine outcome takes considerable experience. A worthwhile exercise to accumulate reference material is to maintain a photo-book document, which will allow the review of many examples and variations of probe presentations. It is certainly recommended that knowledge of chromosomal arrangements during the cell cycle be well studied and appreciated. Single chromosomes may display doublet signals, which, if misinterpreted, can lead to the selection of an abnormal embryo. The learning curve is slow, so you must do this on a weekly basis to maintain the experience that you gain during these exercises.

There are a number of somewhat superficial rules to follow when in doubt: (a) determine whether the space in between doublet signals is greater or less than two signal diameters [109]. Greater will indicate two represented chromosomes, while less will signify the separation of chromatids of one chromosome. (b) Determine if there are connections between the two signals. These connections signal the attachment of chromatids. A possibly more convincing method is to observe all the signals for tell-tale signs of "doublets." Observing doublets will indicate that chromosomes are in a stage of the cell cycle (S phase), where chromatids separate.

Strong signals, proper filters, and clear objectives work together to enhance the chances of error-free FISH diagnosis. Experience and mental concentration is what your personnel have to bring to the process.

43.6.6 Laboratory Space

Every ART facility enters into a program such as PGD-AS with a laboratory "space" profile. It is rare that the first option of a program is to construct a separate PGD facility. If this should be the case, then you may want to proceed on to the next chapter. If, on the other hand, your program already maintains as much laboratory space as it is likely to obtain, then reallocation and reorganization is probably in order. It is not so much that a PGD laboratory has to be spacious, but it does have to utilize the space it has in particular ways.

Due to the nature of the fixatives used to prepare nuclei for hybridization, it is recommended that a site for this function be separate entirely from any aspect of the egg and embryo culture environment. If the cell fixative space is separate and small, then the presence of adequate ventilation and controlled humidity is required.

The hybridization process as well as the slide viewing operation for signal interpretation, requires relatively little overall space. However, this immediate space must have the capability of controlling illumination, and again, if small, clean fresh ventilation.

43.6.7 What's the Setup Cost?

The answer to the question of setup cost is highly variable. It may depend on any number of situations and circumstances; maybe even on the going rate of the Euro and the Yen. On the other hand, the primary expenditures encountered will be for big item equipment, and of course, qualified personnel (see below).

Not including the requisite micromanipulation station employed for embryo/polar body biopsy (or a standard dissection scope used primarily for initial cell fixation), there are basically only two big ticket items to be purchased.

First, a high-quality fluorescent microscope with a full complement of objectives (plus 60× non-oil) and possible z-stack option capability (as mentioned above) will cost in the neighborhood of $35,000. Second, a computer/image capture and processing system, along with the necessary filter accessories, will be in the neighborhood of $45,000. If you wish to purchase the convenience of a small bench-top hybridization heat controller, then add another $3,000 to $5,000.

As with all major purchases of indispensable equipment, there will be service contracts in the range of $12,000 to $15,000 over a three to five year period.

43.6.8 Qualified Personnel

Within the context of ART, and especially, within the subcontext of PGD, assessing the quality and qualifications of a particular individual is at best, difficult. As might be expected, there are few actual qualifications attached to this position, other than having good dexterity and some "learning" about genetics in general and chromosomes in particular. One does not take a graduate course to study clinical embryo preimplantation genetic diagnosis (yet). Therefore, individuals who are acknowledged to be qualified within this field have already spent years in the clinical or animal reproductive laboratory performing these intricate operations and diagnostic procedures in order to understand early embryo development and the genetic/chromosomal implications.

As a result, salary structure for such an individual can be, and is, quite variable. A nominal range may vary from $50,000 to $200,000, depending on the facility and region of the country.

43.7 Personnel Training

As mentioned previously, there is no official academic training opportunities currently available pertaining to the acquisition of PGD or PGD-AS diagnostic knowledge or skills for human ART programs. Many of those individuals currently active within this field have been trained in aspects of molecular biology, molecular cytogenetics, human genetics, animal genetics, or clinical ART. Most of the national board certified molecular geneticists (MD or PhD) do not recognize the validity of basing a diagnosis on results obtained from a single cell, which may or may not be representative of the tissue in question. So, the question remains, how will a clinical ART program train or obtain qualified testing personnel?

43.7.1 In-House Training

There is a strong likelihood that an existing PGD program or commercial business, which functions as a referral lab to other ART programs, will not be a ready source of training for competing programs. Therefore, in-house training may be one option for the ART laboratory. However, there is, at present, scarce information available to the clinical technologist that would serve as a step-by-step instruction source, enabling the development of a dependable and consistently reliable FISH-based embryo diagnosis operation.

43.7.2 Workshop Training

Various organizations, both here and abroad, make PGD-AS workshops available to those interested in establishing their own in-house program. These workshops can range from a pre-congress 1-day session, to the more extensive 3- to 5-day hands-on experience. Some may even offer a personalized training program for your own staff, with individual attention to setting up in a specific environment. Each may serve a particular need during the development of your facility.

43.7.3 Certification: State, National, and Federal

Institutional or individual certification requirements for the operation of a program designed to provide a genetic or chromosomal diagnosis for human in vitro cultured eggs and/or embryos (at whatever stage of development) is, at present, nonexistent. This, however, is likely to change over time. The College of American Pathologists (CAP), in coordination with the Society of Assisted Reproductive Technology (SART), has developed an IVF laboratory inspection service to meet the requirements of the federal government mandate to oversee laboratory function. They are not the only organization to be so "deemed," but they are the most utilized within the ART community. Although they do not currently have specific requirements for a facility performing clinical FISH diagnosis, they will include such facilities as an extension of the IVF lab and require similar quality control parameters to be maintained. They also require that the laboratory director attain national certification (High Complexity Laboratory Director – HCLD) in the specialties of Embryology and/or Andrology, which is currently only available through the agency of the American Board of Bioanalysis (ABB) [110, 111].

There are no local or State requirements imposed in order to perform PGD or PGD-AS on human embryos in particular. Remember, the diagnosis that is obtained is not applied to the patient, only the embryo, therefore, medical certification or licensing does not apply. Of course, the program operating such a service must be in compliance with Federal, State, and local medical licensing and certification standards. Therefore, the (titled) laboratory director is under the obligation to hold the requisite formal educational degree and certification.

43.8 Is There A Cost Breakeven Point?

Breakeven points are in the eye of the beholder (or the lease holder). Salaries, equipment, supplies, and consumables are often a function of locale and leverage. The breakdown that is presented here is very approximate, based on 2008 pricing, and is only meant to give a very rough estimate of potential scenarios. Salaries, of course, will be a major factor over time. Capital equipment (plus equipment warrantees) will constitute the greatest upfront expense. Supplies and consumables will vary to a degree as the patient base increases (or decreases). Dollar amounts are presented as the least to be expected. Salary expense is based on acquiring two skilled technologists ($100,000 per year each); however, as specified in (43.6.8), there can be a wide variation in this category. Initial equipment costs will run to at least $100,000. Yearly supplies (post setup) will likely be in the area of $5,000. Consumables (fluorescent probes, etc.) will be factored in as a function of the number of patients treated. An average expected setup cost would be in the vicinity of $250,000. Taking into account that the cost of equipment can be amortized over time (say 5 years), then $150,000 per year, over 5 years would present a breakeven point of 50 patient cycles per year, at a charge of $3,000 per cycle. Of course, if amortization is reduced to 3 years, then either the number of patients or the cost per cycles must increase. A charge of $3,000 per cycle is not competitive in today's market but is attainable. The breakeven numbers are not as interesting as the profit line, and in this respect, a sustainable patient base of at least 75–100 cycles per year is a near requirement to maintain a clear profit for the PGD program.

43.8.1 Who Pays for LeftOver Embryo Rediagnosis?

The question of who pays for the rediagnosis of abnormal embryos, whether obtained by PGD or PGD-AS, is really a question of whether or not your program performs rediagnosis on rejected embryos at all.

The question of rediagnosis has a number of important implications. First, this is an important quality control parameter, which can be used to verify the initial diagnosis and calculate potential error rates. Second, the problem of mosaicism residing within an embryo was only really appreciated through the rediagnosis of leftover embryos, so that important information can be obtained through this aspect of diagnostic QC. Having this information can also be the basis for counseling patients about the potential of false positive and false negative outcomes, which may impact the overall outcome of any particular cycle. Third, the rejected embryos make up an excellent source of practice material that can play a large role in the overall expertise maintained within the program.

Of course, there is the problem of who will absorb the cost of performing these follow-up tests. There are presently no mandatory regulations that stipulate this type of quality control be performed and it is often overlooked when using this technology in the clinical setting. However, this type of quality control, if employed, should be factored into the overall cost of doing business.

43.9 Ethical Considerations

There have always been questions concerning the ethics of producing human embryos in vitro no matter how they may be used. There were objections voiced from the medical establishment when IVF was first suggested for clinical application [112]. Today, clinical uses of in vitro-derived human embryos are available around the world, but this has not quelled the concerns over the proper treatment of these embryos from an ethical standpoint [113–116]. Each clinical program should understand and be ready to respond to the hesitations and concerns that may arise within this context.

43.9.1 Examples of Ethical Dilemmas

Current abilities to manipulate and potentially transform in vitro embryos within the ART laboratory gives rise to many speculations that are sometimes valid but many times uninform and even malicious. Two of the more interesting ethical dilemmas arising from the use of these technologies are: (a) HLA determination of preimplantation embryos so that stem cells issuing from term placental tissue can be used to treat a needy sibling [117], (b) determining the sex of embryos for patient-driven, non-medical selection [118, 119].

43.10 Government Involvement

Governments outside of the United States have taken steps to regulate, and even curtail particular uses of human embryos for clinical and research purposes [120–123]. Within the United States, few regulations mandate how a program should utilize the embryos they produce and leave it up to litigation to solve questions of misuse or negligence. There are currently no recognized "Code of Conduct or Ethics," covering activities within the ART laboratory and none have been proposed here in the United States. There are though, professional societies, which have produced position papers outlining expected member program practices [124] and the Food and Drug Administration (FDA) has issued specific requirements on the handling, storage, and use of donor tissue material to include eggs, sperm and embryos [125].

43.11 Genetics and Public Policy

With the clinical uses of PGD and PGD-AS (as well as newer technologies on the horizon) becoming firmly established as an adjunct to infertility practice, questions concerning their ethical uses have become more pressing, especially to the general public. Every clinical program utilizing these "life changing" procedures, should give ethical questions serious review and consideration. A good source of information on how the public relates to these issues can be viewed on the website of the Genetics and Public Policy Center, a Johns Hopkins effort funded by The Pew Charitable Trusts. (http://www.dnapolicy.org/science.assist.php) [126, 127].

43.12 Practice Controversy and Philosophical Polarization

Controversy within the clinical and scientific communities concerning the use and efficacy of the currently available technology used for embryo genetic and chromosomal diagnosis is becoming more and more polarized. Research supporting the use of FISH PGD-AS as a method to increase pregnancy rates (especially in the older population) and reduce miscarriage events in chronic pregnancy losses, is being called into question [128, 129]. There have been recent reports that the substandard use of current technology is unable to adequately address or solve any of these conditions [130].

Neither side can claim definitive proof of their respective positions at the present time. However, as indicated previously, the technical difficulties involved and expertise required in order to adequately carry out these procedures are considerable and to denounce their use is certainly premature. Patients should be aware of the potential benefits as well as specific drawbacks pertaining to their particular case when utilizing this technology. Genetic and chromosomal analysis of human embryos holds great promise in the future and newer technologies will address many of the current problems and difficulties observed in today's clinical practices [67].

43.13 Summary and Conclusions

Careful consideration is paramount when considering the establishment of an in-house ART laboratory program, utilizing any of the several technologies presently available to perform genetic and/or chromosomal analysis of in vitro grown human embryos. The potential benefits, available to those patients requiring or wishing to make use of this technology, are considerable. The commitment of a program wishing to make this technology available to their patients, is also considerable. Technologists must have superior skills and training, capital must be available to acquire specialized equipment, and a patient base must be present to support the effort.

Newer technology will eventually "leap-frog" and replace the current systems of chromosomal and genetic diagnosis. However, current technology, utilizing FISH as its diagnostic tool, will maintain its place in the ART laboratory for some years to come, finding a niche in patient treatment options.

Acknowledgments I am happy to acknowledge the cytogenetic and embryonic expertise of Larissa Kovalinskaia Ali, B.S., M.S., TS (ABB). She is a constant resource. I also wish to thank Frank Barnes, PhD, HCLD (ABB) for very informative discussions we have shared, based on PGD. It is also with great pleasure that I recognize my good friend and colleague Yaser Al-Katanani, PhD, HCLD (ABB) for his skills and insights in growing and biopsing embryos that develop into healthy children.

43.14 Appendix A

Recommended vender sites for PGD/PGS analysis of prepared embryo specimens. Request current testing and pricing.

1. Genesis Genetics: Preimplantation Genetic Diagnosis (PGD)
http://www.genesisgenetics.org/
2. Genetics & IVF Institute PGD
http://www.givf.com/pgd/whatispgd.cfm
3. Reproductive Genetics Institute
http://www.reproductivegenetics.com/
4. Reprogenetics provides PGD analysis to IVF centers,
http://www.reprogenetics.com/
5. Shady Grove Center for Preimplantation Genetics Diagnosis
http://www.pgdcenter.com/pgd_program/

References

1. Wilson M, Hartke K, Kiehl M, Rodgers J, Brabec C, Lyles R (2002) Integration of blastocyst transfer for all patients. Fertil Steril 77(4):693–696
2. Oktay K, Cil AP, Bang H (2006) Efficiency of oocyte cryopreservation: a meta-analysis. Fertil Steril 86(1):70–80
3. Mirkin S, Gimeno TG, Bovea C, Stadtmauer L, Gibbons WE, Oehninger S (2003) Factors associated with an optimal pregnancy outcome in an oocyte donation program. J Assist Reprod Genet 20(10):400–408
4. Schoolcraft WB, Gardner DK, Lane M, Schlenker T, Hamilton F, Meldrum DR (1999) Blastocyst culture and transfer: analysis of results and parameters affecting outcome in two in vitro fertilization programs. Fertil Steril 72(4):604–609
5. Veeck LL, Bodine R, Clarke RN, Berrios R, Libraro J, Moschini RM, Zaninovic N, Rosenwaks Z (2004) High pregnancy rates can be achieved after freezing and thawing human blastocysts. Fertil Steril 82(5):1418–1427
6. Wilson M, Hartke K, Kiehl M, Rodgers J, Brabec C, Lyles R (2004) Transfer of blastocysts and morulae on day 5. Fertil Steril 82(2):327–333
7. Kahraman S, Tasdemir M, Tasdemir I, Vicdan K, Ozgur S, Polat G, Islk AZ, Biberoğlu K, Vanderzwalmen P, Nijs M, Schoysman R (1996) Pregnancies achieved with testicular and ejaculated spermatozoa in combination with intracytoplasmic sperm injection in men with totally or initially immotile spermatozoa in the ejaculate. Hum Reprod 11(6):1343–1346
8. Palermo GD, Schlegel PN, Colombero LT, Zaninovic N, Moy F, Rosenwaks Z (1996) Aggressive sperm immobilization prior to intracytoplasmic sperm injection with immature spermatozoa improves fertilization and pregnancy rates. Hum Reprod 11(5):1023–1029
9. Johnson JE, Higdon HL 3rd, Boone WR (2008) Effect of human granulosa cell co-culture using standard culture media on the maturation and fertilization potential of immature human oocytes. Fertil Steril 90(5):1674–1679
10. Mercader A, Garcia-Velasco JA, Escudero E, Remohí J, Pellicer A, Simón C (2003) Clinical experience and perinatal outcome of blastocyst transfer after coculture of human embryos with human endometrial epithelial cells: a 5-year follow-up study. Fertil Steril 80(5):1162–1168
11. Spandorfer SD, Barmat L, Navarro J, Burmeister L, Veeck L, Clarke R, Liu HC, Rosenwaks Z (2002) Autologous endometrial coculture in patients with a previous history of poor quality embryos. J Assist Reprod Genet 19(7):309–312
12. d'Estaing SG, Lornage J, Hadj S, Boulieu D, Salle B, Guérin JF (2001) Comparison of two blastocyst culture systems: coculture on Vero cells and sequential media. Fertil Steril 76(5):1032–1035
13. Quea G, Romero K, Garcia-Velasco JA (2007) Extended embryo culture to increase implantation rate. Reprod Biomed Online 14(3):375–383. Review
14. Lane M, Gardner DK (2007) Embryo culture medium: which is the best? Best Pract Res Clin Obstet Gynaecol 21(1):83–100. Epub 2006 Nov 7. Review

15. Orasanu B, Jackson KV, Hornstein MD, Racowsky C (2006) Effects of culture medium on HCG concentrations and their value in predicting successful IVF outcome. Reprod Biomed Online 12(5): 590–598
16. Takeuchi T, Neri QV, Palermo GD (2005) Construction and fertilization of reconstituted human oocytes. Reprod Biomed Online 11(3):309–318
17. Nagy ZP (2004) Haploidization to produce human embryos: a new frontier for micromanipulation. Reprod Biomed Online 8(5): 492–495
18. Balen AH, Rutherford AJ (2007) Management of infertility. BMJ 335:608–611
19. Verlinsky Y, Handyside A, Grifo J, Munné S, Cohen J, Liebers I, Levinson G, Arnheim N, Hughes M, Delhanty J, et al (1994) Preimplantation diagnosis of genetic and chromosomal disorders. J Assist Reprod Genet 11(5):236–243. Review
20. Kanavakis E, Traeger-Synodinos E (2002) Preimplantation genetic diagnosis in clinical practice. J Med Genet 39:6–11
21. Handyside AH, Lesko JG, Tarín JJ, Winston RM, Hughes MR (1992) Birth of a normal girl after in vitro fertilization and Preimplantation diagnostic testing for cystic fibrosis. N Engl J Med 327(13):905–909
22. Ao A, Ray P, Harper J, Lesko J, Paraschos T, Atkinson G, Soussis I, Taylor D, Handyside A, Hughes M, Winston RM (1996) Clinical experience with preimplantation genetic diagnosis of cystic fibrosis(delta F508). Prenat Diagn 16(2):137–142
23. Thornhill AR, Snow K (2002) Molecular diagnostics in preimplantation genetic diagnosis. J Mol Diagn 4(1):11–29
24. Molina B, Dayal MD, MPH Shevetha M Zarek, MD (2008) Preimplantation genetic diagnosis. http://emedicine.medscape.com/article/273415-overview (free sign up)
25. Verlinsky Y, Rechitsky S, Verlinsky O, Masciangelo C, Lederer K, Kuliev A (2002) Preimplantation diagnosis for early-onset Alzheimer disease caused by V717L mutation. JAMA 287(8):1018–1021
26. Rechitsky S, Verlinsky O, Chistokhina A, Sharapova T, Ozen S, Masciangelo C, Kuliev A, Verlinsky Y (2002) Preimplantation genetic diagnosis for cancer predisposition. Reprod Biomed Online 5(2):148–155
27. Offit K, Sagi M, Hurley K (2006) Preimplantation genetic diagnosis for cancer syndromes: a new challenge for preventive medicine. JAMA 296(22):2727
28. Rechitsky S, Kuliev A, Tur-Kaspa I, Morris R, Verlinsky Y (2004) Preimplantation genetic diagnosis with HLA matching. Reprod Biomed Online 9(2):210–221
29. Verlinsky Y, Rechitsky S, Sharapova T, Morris R, Taranissi M, Kuliev A (2004) Preimplantation HLA testing. JAMA 291(17): 2079–2085
30. Verlinsky Y, Rechitsky S, Schoolcraft W, Strom C, Kuliev A (2001) Preimplantation diagnosis for Fanconi anemia combined with HLA matching. JAMA 285(24):3130–3133
31. Robertson JA (2003) Extending preimplantation genetic diagnosis: the ethical debate. Ethical issues in new uses of preimplantation genetic diagnosis. Hum Reprod 18(3):465–471
32. Heyd D (2003) Male or female, we will create them: the ethics of sex selection for non-medical reasons. Ethical Perspect 10(3–4):204–214
33. Pembrey M (2002) Social sex selection by preimplantation genetic diagnosis. Reprod Biomed Online 4(2):157–159
34. Keefe DL, Liu L, Marquard K (2007) Telomeres and aging-related meiotic dysfunction in women. Cell Mol Life Sci 64(2):139–143. Review
35. Pellestor F, Andréo B, Arnal F, Humeau C, Demaille J (2003) Maternal aging and chromosomal abnormalities: new data drawn from in vitro unfertilized human oocytes. Hum Genet 112(2): 195–203. Epub 2002 Oct 29
36. Lim AS, Tsakok MF (1997) Age-related decline in fertility: a link to degenerative oocytes? Fertil Steril 68(2):265–271
37. Rubio C, Rodrigo L, Pérez-Cano I, Mercader A, Mateu E, Buendía P, Remohí J, Simón C, Pellicer A (2005) FISH screening of aneuploidies in preimplantation embryos to improve IVF outcome. Reprod Biomed Online 11(4):497–506
38. Patrizio P, Bianchi V, Lalioti MD, Gerasimova T, Sakkas D (2007) High rate of biological loss in assisted reproduction: it is in the seed, not in the soil. Reprod Biomed Online 14(1):92–95
39. The Merck Manual of Medical Information – Home Edition Section 1. Fundamentals Chapter 2 Genetics Robert S. Porter, MD, Editor http://endoflifecare.tripod.com/huntdiseasefaqs/id16.html
40. Zielenski J, Tsui LC (1995) Cystic fibrosis: genotypic and phenotypic variations. Ann Rev Genet 29:777–807 see also: The genetics of cystic fibrosis http://www.cysticfibrosismedicine.com/CFdocs/CFText/gene.htm
41. Augarten A, Yahav Y, Kerem B, Halle D, Laufer J, Szeinberg A, Dor J, Mashiach S, Gazit E, Madgar I (1994) Congenital bilateral absence of vas deferens in the absence of cystic fibrosis. Lancet 344:1473–1474
42. Cheung VG, Nelson FS (1996) Whole genome amplification using a degenerate oligonucleotide primer allows hundreds of genotypes to be performed on less than one nanogram of genomic DNA. Proc Natl Acad Sci USA 93:14676–14679
43. Mullis K (1990) The unusual origin of the polymerase chain reaction. Sci Am 262(4):56–61, 64–65
44. Mullis K, Faloona F, Scharf S, Saiki R, Horn G, Erlich H (1992) Specific enzymatic amplification of DNA in vitro: the polymerase chain reaction. Biotechnology 24:17–27
45. Piyamongkol W, BermuÂdez MG, Harper JC, Wells D (2003) Detailed investigation of factors influencing amplification efficiency and allele drop-out in single cell PCR: implications for preimplantation genetic diagnosis. Mol Hum Reprod 9(7):411–420
46. Drury KC, Liu MC, Lilleberg S, Kipersztok S, Williams RS (2001) Results on single cell PCR for Huntington's gene and WAVE product analysis for preimplantation genetic diagnosis. Mol Cell Endocrinol 183(Suppl 1):S1–S4
47. Grifo JA, Ward DC, Boyle A (1990) In situ hybridization of blastomeres from embryo biopsy. In: Verlinsky Y, Kuliev A (eds) Preimplantation genetics: proceedings of the first international symposium on preimplantation genetics. September 14–19, Chicago, IL, pp 147–154
48. Scriven PN, Ogilvie CM (2007) Fluorescence in situ hybridization on single cells. (Sex determination and chromosome rearrangements). Meth Mol Med 132:19–30
49. Wilton L (2002) Preimplantation genetic diagnosis for aneuploidy screening in early human embryos: a review. Prenat Diagn 22: 512–518
50. Boue A, Boue J, Gropp A (1985) Cytogenetics of pregnancy wastage. Adv Hum Genet 14:1–57
51. Munne S, Magli C, Bahce M, Fung J, Legator M, Morrison L, Cohert J, Gianaroli L (1998) Preimplantation diagnosis of the aneuploidies most commonly found in spontaneous abortions and live births: XY, 13, 14, 15, 16, 18, 21, 22. Prenat Diagn 18:1459–1466
52. Lathi RB, Westphal LM, Milki AA (2008) Aneuploidy in the miscarriages of infertile women and the potential benefit of preimplanation genetic diagnosis. Fertil Steril 89(2) 353–357
53. Ljunger E, Cnattingius S, Lundin C, Anneren G (2005) Chromosomal anomalies in first-trimester miscarriages. Acta Obstet Gynecol Scand 84:1103–1107
54. Munné S, Gianaroli L, Tur-Kaspa I, Magli C, Sandalinas M, Grifo J, Cram D, Kahraman S, Verlinsky Y, Simpson JL (2007) Substandard application of preimplantation genetic screening may interfere with its clinical success. Fertil Steril 88(4):781–784
55. Cieslak-Janzen J, Tur-Kaspa I, Ilkevitch Y, Bernal A, Morris R, Verlinsky Y (2006) Multiple micromanipulations for preimplantation genetic diagnosis do not affect embryo development to the blastocyst stage. Fertil Steril 85(6):1826–1829

56. Verlinsky Y, Cieslak J, Ivakhnenko V, Evsikov S, Wolf G, White M, Lifchez A, Kaplan B, Moise J, Valle J, Ginsberg N, Strom C, Kuliev A (2001) Chromosomal abnormalities in the first and second polar body. Mol Cell Endocrinol 183(Suppl 1):S47–S49
57. Verlinsky Y, Cieslak J, Freidine M, Ivakhnenko V, Wolf G, Kovalinskaya L, White M, Lifchez A, Kaplan B, Moise J, Valle J, Ginsberg N, Strom C, Kuliev A (1996) Polar body diagnosis of common aneuploidies by FISH. J Assist Reprod Genet 13(2):157–162
58. Sandalinas M, Sadowy S, Alikani M, Calderon G, Cohen J, Munné S (2001) Developmental ability of chromosomally abnormal human embryos to develop to the blastocyst stage. Hum Reprod 16(9): 1954–1958
59. Magli MC, Jones GM, Gras L, Gianaroli L, Korman I, Trounson AO (2000) Chromosome mosaicism in day 3 aneuploid embryos that develop to morphologically normal blastocysts in vitro. Hum Reprod 15(8):1781–1786
60. Ruangvutilert P, Delhanty JD, Serhal P, Simopoulou M, Rodeck CH, Harper JC (2000) FISH analysis on day 5 post-insemination of human arrested and blastocyst stage embryos. Prenat Diagn 20(7):552–560
61. Veiga A, Gil Y, Boada M, Carrera M, Vidal F, Boiso I, Ménézo Y, Barri PN (1999) Confirmation of diagnosis in preimplantation genetic diagnosis (PGD) through blastocyst culture: preliminary experience. Prenat Diagn 19(13):1242–1247
62. Bielanska M, Jin S, Bernier M, Tan SL, Ao A (2005) Diploid-aneuploid mosaicism in human embryos cultured to the blastocyst stage. Fertil Steril 84(2):336–342
63. McArthur SJ, Leigh D, Marshall JT, de Boer KA, Jansen RP (2005) Pregnancies and live births after trophectoderm biopsy and preimplantation genetic testing of human blastocysts. Fertil Steril 84(6):1628–1636
64. Wells D (2004) Advances in preimplantation genetic diagnosis Eur J Obstet Gynecol Reprod Biol 115(1):S97–S101
65. Hu DG, Webb G, Hussey N (2004) Aneuploidy detection in single cells using DNA array-based comparative genomic hybridization. Mol Hum Reprod 10(4):283–289
66. Fiegler H, Geigl JB, Langer S, Rigler D, Porter K, Unger K, Carter NP, Speicher MR (2007) High resolution array-CGH analysis of single cells. Nucleic Acids Res 35(3):e15. Epub 2006 Dec 18
67. Treff NR, Su J, Mavrianos J, Bergh PA, Miller KA, Scott RT (2007) Accurate 23 chromosome aneuploidy screening in human blastomeres using single nucleotide polymorphism (SNP) microarrays . Fertil Steril 88:S1
68. Viville S, Messaddeq N, Flori E, Gerlinger P (1998) Preparing for preimplantation genetic diagnosis in France. Hum Reprod 13(4): 1022–1029
69. Staessen C, Van Assche E, Joris H, Bonduelle M, Vandervorst M, Liebaers I, Van Steirteghem A (1999) Clinical experience of sex determination by fluorescent in-situ hybridization for preimplantation genetic diagnosis. Mol Hum Reprod 5(4):382–389
70. Liu J, Tsai YL, Zheng XZ, Yazigi RA, Baramki TA, Compton G, Katz E (1998) Feasibility study of repeated fluorescent in-situ hybridization in the same human blastomeres for preimplantation genetic diagnosis. Mol Hum Reprod 4(10):972–977
71. Munné S (2002) Preimplantation genetic diagnosis of numerical and structural chromosome abnormalities. Reprod Biomed Online 4(2):183–196. Review
72. Pickering S, Polidoropoulos N, Caller J et al (2003) Strategies and outcomes of the first 100 cycles of preimplanation genetic diagnosis at the Guy's and St. Thomas' Center. Fertil Steril 79:81–90
73. Munné S, Tomkin G, Cohen J (2009) Selection of embryos by morphology is less effective than by a combination of aneuploidy testing and morphology observations. Fertil Steril 91(3): 943–945
74. Munné S, Chen S, Colls P, Garrisi J, Zheng X, Cekleniak N, Lenzi M, Hughes P, Fischer J, Garrisi M, Tomkin G, Cohen J (2007) Maternal age, morphology, development and chromosome abnormalities in over 6000 cleavage-stage embryos. Reprod Biomed Online 14(5):628–634
75. Edwards RG, Hansis C (2005) Initial differentiation of blastomeres in 4-cell human embryos and its significance for early embryogenesis and implantation. Reprod Biomed Online 11(2):206–218. Review
76. Edwards RG (2005) Genetics of polarity in mammalian embryos. Reprod Biomed Online 11(1):104–114. Review
77. Edwards RG (2000) The role of embryonic polarities in preimplantation growth and implantation of mammalian embryos. Hum Reprod 15(Suppl 6):1–8. Review
78. Edwards RG, Beard HK (1997) Oocyte polarity and cell determination in early mammalian embryos. Mol Hum Reprod 3(10): 863–905. Review
79. Scott LA (2000) Oocyte and embryo polarity. Semin Reprod Med 18(2):171–183. Review
80. Chatzimeletiou K, Morrison EE, Panagiotidis Y, Prapas N, Prapas Y, Rutherford AJ, Grudzinskas G, Handyside AH (2005) Comparison of effects of zona drilling by non-contact infrared laser or acid Tyrode's on the development of human biopsied embryos as revealed by blastomere viability, cytoskeletal analysis and molecular cytogenetics. Reprod Biomed Online 11(6):697–710
81. Han TS, Sagoskin AW, Graham JR, Tucker MJ, Liebermann J (2003) Laser-assisted human embryo biopsy on the third day of development for preimplantation genetic diagnosis: two successful case reports. Fertil Steril 80(2):453–455
82. Wang WH, Kaskar K, Gill J, Desplinter T (2007) A simplified technique for embryo biopsy for preimplantation genetic diagnosis. Fertil Steril 2008 90(2):438–442
83. Jones AE, Wright G, Kort HI, Straub RJ, Nagy ZP (2006) Comparison of laser-assisted hatching and acidified Tyrode's hatching by evaluation of blastocyst development rates in sibling embryos: a prospective randomized trial. Fertil Steril 85(2):487–491
84. Tarkowski AK (1966) An air-drying method of chromosome preparations from mouse eggs. Cytogenetics 5:394–400
85. Tarkowski AK (1971) Development of single blastomeres. In: Daniel JC (ed) Methods in mammalian embryology. Freeman, San Francisco, pp 172–185
86. Coonen E, Dumoulin JC, Ramaekers FC, Hopman AH (1994) Optimal preparation of preimplantation embryo interphase nuclei for analysis by fluorescence in-situ hybridization. Hum Reprod 9(3):533–537
87. Dozortsev DI, McGinnis KT (2001) An improved fixation technique for fluorescence in situ hybridization for preimplantation genetic diagnosis. Fertil Steril 76(1):186–188
88. Pinkel D, Straume T, Gray JW (1986) Cytogenetic analysis using quantitative, high-sensitivity, fluorescence hybridization. Proc Natl Acad Sci USA 83:2934–2938
89. Levsky JM, Singer RH (2003) Fluorescence in situ hybridization: past, present and future. J Cell Sci 116(14):2833–2838
90. Lichter P, Cremer T, Tang CC, Watkins PC, Manuelidis L, Ward DC (1988) Rapid detection of human chromosome 21 aberrations by in situ hybridization. PNAS 85(24):9664–9668
91. Tiiask BJ (1991) Fluorescence in situ hybridization: applications in cytogenetics and gene mapping. Trends Genet 7(5):149–154
92. Kuo WL, Tenjin H, Segraves R, Pinkel D, Golbus MS, Gray J (1991) Detection of aneuploidy involving chromosomes 13, 18, or 21, by fluorescence in situ hybridization (FISH) to interphase and metaphase amniocytes. Am J Hum Genet 49(1):112–119
93. Thornhill AR, deDie-Smulders CE, Geraedts JP, Harper JC, Harton GL, Lavery SA, Moutou C, Robinson MD, Schmutzler AG, Scriven PN, Sermon KD, Wilton L (2005) ESHRE PGD Consortium. ESHRE PGD Consortium Best practice guidelines for clinical preimplantation genetic diagnosis (PGD) and preimplantation genetic screening (PGS). Hum Reprod 20(1):35–48

94. Britten RJ, Davidson EH (1976) Studies on nucleic acid reassociation kinetics: Empirical equations describing DNA reassociation. Proc Natl Acad Sci USA 73(2):415–419
95. Wetmur JG, Davidson N (1968) Kinetics of renaturation of DNA. J Mol Biol 31(3):349–370
96. Smith MJ, Britten RJ, Davidson EH (1975) Studies on nucleic acid reassociation kinetics: reactivity of single-stranded tails in DNA–DNA renaturation. Proc Natl Acad Sci USA 72(12): 4805–4809
97. Website for the Vysis® AneuVysion Multicolor DNA Probe Kit http://www.aneuvysion.com/
98. Rainbow Scientific DNA FISH probes from Cytocell, Ltd. http://www.rainbowscientific.com/cytocell.html
99. Baart EB, Martini E, Van Opstal D (2004) Screening for aneuploidies of ten different chromosomes in two rounds of FISH: a short and reliable protocol. Prenat Diagn 24(12):955–961
100. FISH multiband combination filter sets: http://www.semrock.com/Catalog/BrightlineCatalog_Microscopy.htm#FISH_MB
101. Chroma Filter Set Ordering Guide. http://www.chroma.com/images/0708_ChromaPricelist.pdf
102. Durm M, Haar FM, Hausmann M, Ludwig H, Cremer C (1997) Optimized Fast-FISH with alpha-satellite probes: acceleration by microwave activation. Braz J Med Biol Res 30(1):15–23
103. Drury KC, Kovalinskaia L, Clark P, Williams RS (1997) Ultra-rapid (6 minute) FISH using microwave technology. Second international symposium on preimplantation genetics. Chicago, IL
104. Kovalinskaia L, Li S, Al-Katanani Y, Williams RS, Drury KC (2006) Rapid 2-Round FISH Aneuploidy Screening For 9 Chromosomes (X,Y, 13,15,16,17,18,21,22) Using Microwave Technology. Clin Embryol 9:1 pp 13–21
105. Abdelhadi I, Colls P, Sandalinas M, Escudero T, Munné S (2003) Preimplantation genetic diagnosis of numerical abnormalities for 13 chromosomes. Reprod Biomed Online 6(2): 226–231
106. Z-Stack multi-layer FISH capture. http://www.genetix.com/xhtml/technique03.aspx?tpid=54&tid=9
107. AI Cytovision Image Capture System. http://www.genetix.com/xhtml/downloads.aspx?pid=34&pcid=4
108. Vysis http://www.aneuvysion.com/
109. Munné S, Weier HU (1996) Simultaneous enumeration of chromosomes 13, 18, 21, X, and Y in interphase cells for preimplantation genetic diagnosis of aneuploidy. Cytogenet Cell Genet 75(4): 263–270
110. Hill DL, Li M (2004) What regulations for preimplantation genetic diagnosis? J Assist Reprod Genet 21(1):11–13
111. San Diego LJ (1997) Federal regulations: compliance and implications. Clin Lab Sci 10(6):339–346. Review
112. ABB Certification Standard for High-complexity Clinical Laboratory Director (HCLD). http://www.aab.org/hcld.htm
113. Henig RM. Second Best (The story of Landrum Shettles, MD). The New York Times Magazine, 28 December 2003
114. Scott R (2006) Choosing between possible lives: legal and ethical issues in preimplantation genetic diagnosis. Oxf J Leg Stud 26(1): 153–178
115. Roberts JC (2002) Customizing conception: a survey of preimplantation genetic diagnosis and the resulting social, ethical, and legal dilemmas. Duke Law Technol Rev 23:E1
116. Thomas C (2006) Preimplantation genetic diagnosis: development and regulation. Med Law 25(2):365–378
117. Klipstein S (2005) Preimplantation genetic diagnosis: technological promise and ethical perils. Fertil Steril 83(5):1347–1353. Review
118. Edwards RG (2004) Ethics of PGD: thoughts on the consequences of typing HLA in embryos. Reprod Biomed Online 9(2):222–224
119. Dahl E (2003) Ethical issues in new uses of preimplantation genetic diagnosis: should parents be allowed to use preimplantation genetic diagnosis to choose the sexual orientation of their children? Hum Reprod 18(7):1368–1369. Review
120. Pennings G (2002) Personal desires of patients and social obligations of geneticists: applying preimplantation genetic diagnosis for non-medical sex selection. Prenat Diagn 22(12):1123–1129. Review
121. Sutton A (1996) The British law on assisted reproduction: a liberal law by comparison with many other European laws. Ethics Med 12(2):41–45
122. Great Britain (1990) Human fertilisation and embryology act 1990. Bull Med Ethics 63:13–21
123. Krebs D (1996) Rules and ethics concerning assisted procreation established by the government in Germany. J Assist Reprod Genet 13(3):193–195
124. Walters L (1987) Ethics and new reproductive technologies: an international review of committee statements. Hastings Cent Rep 17(3):S3–S9. Review
125. Practice Committee of the Society for Assisted Reproductive Technology; Practice Committee of the American Society for Reproductive Medicine (2007) Preimplantation genetic testing: a Practice Committee opinion. Fertil Steril 88(6):1497–1504. Epub 2007 Oct 17. Review
126. Practice Committee of the American Society for Reproductive Medicine; Practice Committee of the Society for Assisted Reproductive Technology (2006) Guidelines for Gamete and Embryo Donation. Fertil Steril 86(Suppl 5):S38–S50
127. Baruch S, Kaufman D, Hudson KL (2007) Genetic testing of embryos: practices and perspectives of US in vitro fertilization clinics. Fertil Steril 10 [Epub ahead of print]
128. Kalfoglou A, Scott J, Hudson K (2005) PGD patients' and providers' attitudes about the use and regulation of PGD. Reprod BioMed Online 11:486–496. (also see: http://www.dnapolicy.org/pub.reports.php?action=detail&report_id=9#)
129. Mastenbroek S, Twisk M, van Echten-Arends J, Sikkema-Raddatz B, Korevaar JC, Verhoeve HR, Vogel NE, Arts EG, de Vries JW, Bossuyt PM, Buys CH, Heineman MJ, Repping S, van der Veen F (2007) In vitro fertilization with preimplantation genetic screening. N Engl J Med 357(1):9–17. Epub 2007 Jul 4
130. Staessen C, Platteau P, Van Assche E, Michiels A, Tournaye H, Camus M, Devroey P, Liebaers I, Van Steirteghem A (2004) Comparison of blastocyst transfer with or without preimplantation genetic diagnosis for aneuploidy screening in couples with advanced maternal age: a prospective randomized controlled trial. Hum Reprod 19(12):2849–2858. Epub 2004 Oct 7

Chapter 44
Evaluation and Selection of Preimplantation Embryos for Transfer

Lynette Scott

Abstract Proper selection of embryos with the highest implantation potential is essential for successful IVF. Traditionally, embryo morphology has been the major selection criterion used in selecting embryos for transfer. This chapter discusses new techniques for evaluating embryo competence throughout the culture period.

Keywords Blastocyst • Embryo morphology • Embryo scoring • Nucleoli • Polar body • Pronuclei • Sequential scoring system

44.1 Introduction

The practice of embryology has been, and currently is, a science of meticulous observation, documentation and empiric correlations, not too dissimilar to the classical studies in biology, anatomy and physiology in the early parts of the last two centuries. To date, there have been few easily integrated, clinically applicable, systems other than morphology and cell-cycle timing, to distinguish and differentiate oocytes and embryos from each other. However, it is clear that as we observe record and correlate more and more physical and morphological features with outcomemeasures and couple these observed features to biological, metabolic and molecular functions, and live outcome-data, we are becoming more efficient in selecting viable oocytes and embryos in clinical human in vitro fertilization (IVF) and assisted reproductive technologies (ART). Over the last few years, new innovative techniques for gamete and embryo selection have begun to emerge, but they are still too expensive and have not been fully validated for incorporation into a clinical, real life ART laboratory.

In nonhuman laboratory- and agricultural-assisted reproduction, ovulation induction, in vitro maturation, fertilization, and embryo culture and development, the overall efficiency and end points of experiments and investigations are scored differently to those in human ART. Research in nonhuman fields is not focused on the *inability* to reproduce but on the *manipulation of reproductive capacity*. Genetics, diet, lifestyle, and major clinical issues, which would negate subjects from being considered in laboratory trials and investigations in the non-human field, are not considered in human fertility treatment because in ART, we *treat the inability to perform reproduction* and attempt to *overcome this inability to conceive* and ultimately deliver a healthy infant. Female age, male reproductive potential, and previous male and female fertility profile are the major, and often the only, or rate limiting, issues considered in human ART. Research in the nonhuman reproductive field is directed and controlled, whereas research in the human ART field is empiric and based on observation and outcome data, where the subjects of study are also the subjects of treatment, and are often very poor controls for outcome data and any studies at hand.

With these considerations in mind, the key morphological features that are used for embryo selection also need to be tailored to fit the fertility profiles of both partners, and decisions made accordingly. Gamete and embryo selection needs to be dynamic since embryos are not static and more than one point in an embryos development should be used to decide the embryo for transfer [1]. Using a sequential embryo selection technique (SES), a profile of the developing embryo can be drawn/profiled, and if morphology is coupled to biology [2, 3], this profile can then help in selecting embryos with the maximum potential for implantation. The key element in developing a scoring system that can be used in a repeatable manner is timing; when are observations made? If observations are made relevant to hCG or to insemination, then data can be compared. If it is random, the results will reflect this with wide variations and little correlation.

This chapter presents the key scoring techniques, couple these to biology, and show how SES can be implemented at each stage of embryo scoring/selection.

44.2 Gamete Scoring

Gamete selection is not possible in any standard-insemination case. In these cases all oocytes are "selected" for insemination

L. Scott (✉)
Fertility Centers of New England, Reading, MA, USA

D.T. Carrell and C.M. Peterson (eds.), *Reproductive Endocrinology and Infertility: Integrating Modern Clinical and Laboratory Practice*,
DOI 10.1007/978-1-4419-1436-1_44,

and sperm are selected by gross separation/preparation techniques. The resulting fertilized oocytes are the result of the "fittest are fertilized". In ICSI cases, which only account for about 40% of all ART cases performed, the only morphological features that are generally considered are: is the oocyte mature/MII (have a visible polar body)? Are sperm motile and the correct shape? If there are very few sperm, anything that is moving is used. Within the constraints of delivering care, what an oocyte or sperm looks like will not dictate its use. The aim in ART is an embryo to score rather than gamete selection or more accurately, nonselection. Thus, data on oocyte and sperm morphology correlated to outcome data is lacking in the literature since the goal to create an embryo for transfer overrides all other observational techniques and parameters. Furthermore, there have been few techniques or parameters of gamete selection presented that have proven to be clinically relevant.

During maturation, the oocyte is dynamic and undergoes many physical changes, which include shrinking and expanding and finally the formation/extrusion of the first polar body PB1), which results in an oocyte that has a definite pole (defined by the first PB1) and which in the human (unlike the mouse) is spherical within the ZP. It is three dimensional, and everything that is scored or "seen" has to be related to this three dimensional aspect, regardless of the poles or orientation of the PB1.

On recording oocyte, morphology certain parameters have pointed to competence. There has been little definitive correlation of the overall morphology of the oocyte and outcome. Some reports point to the cytoplasmic appearance as being important, while others indicate little correlation [4–7]. Oocyte variance could result for patient and population variations or the stimulation protocols. No one parameter has been shown to affect implantation rates in a definitive manner.

The first polar body has been used as an indicator of oocyte competence. The LH surge or hCG injection triggers the final maturation events within the follicle, leading to the completion of the first meiotic division with extrusion of the first polar body, which is complete by about 40 h after hCG. The first polar body results from a very asymmetric cell division, resulting in a small polar body and large oocyte, ensuring only a fraction of cytoplasm is lost to the oocyte with the extrusion of half the DNA complement.

Most of the key signaling events that occur rapidly in the oocyte are controlled by protein kinases. The extrusion of the first polar body, formation of the spindle and condensation of chromosomes onto the spindle and finally its migration to the periphery of the oocyte are signaled and controlled by the *c-Mos-MAPK* pathway [8, 9]. After extrusion of the first polar body, the *c-Mos-MAPK* are involved in its degradation [9, 10] which is time-dependent and is complete by about 20 h in the human [11].

The first polar body morphology can give some insights to the events of meiotic spindle formation and the correct sequence of certain signaling events in the oocyte. Abnormally sized polar bodies will indicate a disruption in the spindle migration, which may indicate an aneuploid oocyte. Early fragmentation of the polar body may also indicate a disruption of the *c-Mos-MAPK* pathway, which again has implications for oocyte quality. This could be through the spindle and nondisjunction events or timing of cellular processes related to cell cycle control. Some studies have indeed linked the fragmentation of first polar bodies to decreased in vitro developmental competence and reduced implantation rates in human IVF [12–14]. These studies showed lowered fertilization rates, lowered development rates to the blastocyst stage and decreased implantation rates when the embryos were transferred. During ICSI cases, the state of the polar body can easily be recorded and embryos resulting from oocytes with abnormal or fragmenting polar bodies can be avoided. During IVF cycles, this presents a problem in that the cumulus mass is generally not removed. (see Fig. 44.1 for examples of PB morphology)

Some new microscopic techniques are available for viable sperm selection, using ultramicroscopic techniques [15], where head morphology becomes vital. However, these have not been validated in controlled clinical settings. The Hyaluran Binding Assay and "Sperm Chromatin Condensation Assay" have not proven efficacious when tested in controlled trials. Thus, sperm selection is still not done (standard insemination) and if it is (ICSI), it is by gross morphology and motility.

At the oocyte level, new technologies are available that may prove to be efficacious in the selection of viable oocytes with differential developmental are available. These include the appearance and shape of the metaphase spindle [16, 17], the birefringence, shape and thickness of the zona pellucida [18, 19], and oocyte respiration rates [20].

Zona: The zona pellucida (ZP) is an integral part of the oocyte since it is laid down by the developing oocyte during oogenesis. ZP material can be detected within the oocyte as early as in primordial follicles, and as the oocyte matures to primary and secondary stages, it moves to the oocyte periphery and then forms the ZP. Flaws in the ZP would suggest a flaw in the oocyte. [21]. The ZP is a trilaminate structure with aspects of a polarized structure, allowing visualization by polarized light microscopy. Variations in zona structure may affect sperm binding and this has been shown to correlate with abnormal embryo development [22, 23]. Polarized light microscopy highlights two different abnormalities in the zona: Birefringence of the layers: the outside layer should be polarized, the inner layer scattered and the middle layer partially polarized.

The second measurable aspect of the ZP is the regularity of zona, which can be quantified with birefringence. Oocytes in which ZP displays breaks or the irregularity of birefringence has proved to have lowered postfertilization potential [18, 24].

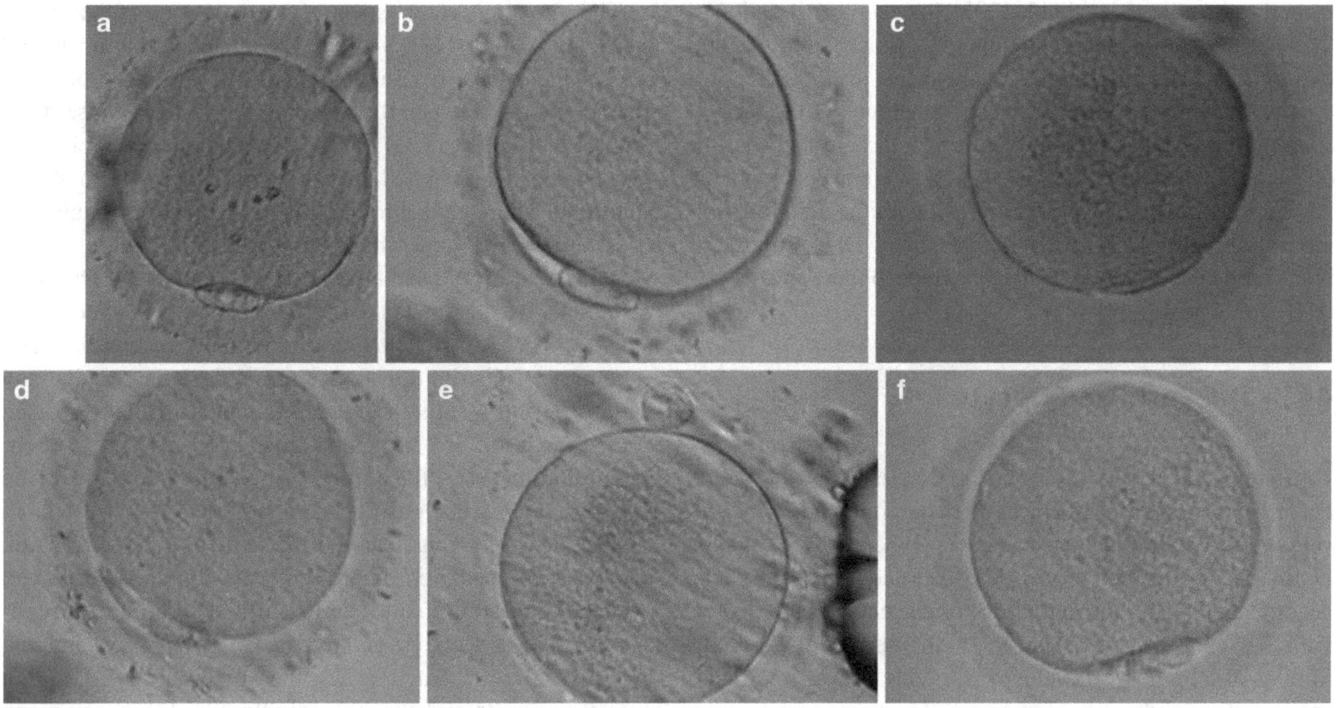

Fig. 44.1 Polar body morphologies: Panel a, b are normal; panel c the PB is flat and ill-defined; panel d, the PB has divided and is too large; panel e the PB is detached and could indicate an aged or abnormal oocyte; panel F the PB has not fully extruded which may indicate it is newly formed or abnormal

This system, or the use of polarized light microscopy to illuminate aspects of oocyte morphology, is an emerging technique, has not been fully validated in a clinical setting and requires the investment and introduction of new technology into the laboratory, which may limit its use in the short term. At present, it does not supercede the current morphology scoring and is not likely to result in rejection of oocytes until very strong pregnancy outcome data are available.

44.2.1 The Spindle

Ovulated or mature oocytes are arrested in the second meiotic division at metaphase II. The metaphase II spindle is bipolar with microtubules running from pole to pole with the chromosomes attached to it on the equatorial plane. The spindle is comprised of long microtubules, which run pole to pole and pass through the metaphase plate and short microtubules, which are associated with the chromosomes through their kinetechores. The whole structure is not static and turns over rapidly with assembly and disassembly of the tubulin molecules at each end [25]. Further, temperature drops to below 35 °C will also result in depolymerization and loss of structure.

The polarity of the spindle can be used to visualize with polarized light microscopy. Using this technique both the position of the spindle and its shape, is it bipolar or is there a disruption in shape, can be deduced. Spindles that are not bipolar have been associated with aneuploidy and aging [26]. Most spindles are in the hemisphere of the polar bodies, but rarely under them since there is movement away from the PB with time and with aging [27–29]. However, the data are not vast and due to the sensitive working environment, and the need to manipulate the oocytes in order to visualize the spindle, this has resulted in fairly limited use for clinical application. The largest application here will be in countries where limited numbers of oocytes can be used in fertilization or in egg cryo-banking.

44.2.2 Oocyte Respiration

Oocyte and embryo metabolism and respiration profiles have been suggested as means of differential selection for years. Very few studies have been conducted on human oocytes; however with new noninvasive technologies, this may become a means of oocyte selection [20]. Oocyte respiration has been shown to differ between oocytes and between cohorts and be correlated with already known fertility parameters such as age, FSH levels, and certain disease profiles, such as endometriosis and PCOS. It was also shown to correlate with oocyte health and ability to mature, but no outcome data either for fertilization or embryo development from these studies is available [20]. However, certification of the instrumentation and validation in a clinical setting is still required, and at present this is years away.

The drawback to each of these techniques is the lack of sound clinical data and controlled trials and the fact that the oocyte is not the whole story in embryo and fetal development. Although the oocyte is a powerful cell with the ability to correct some sperm dysfunction, such as minor DNA fragmentation, it still cannot overcome the fundamental flaws in sperm.

44.3 The Fertilized Oocyte

Fertilization is a very dynamic process, and as the sperm enters, there are waves of calcium release, mitochondrial activation, and dynamic cellular changes (see chapter by Sutovsky). During the fertilization process, the male and female pronuclei become visible and move/rotate into the center of the oocyte, with the concomitant extrusion of the second polar body. Timing of all embryo development events is systematic thus scoring also needs to be systematic. The time from hCG or fertilization of the events described will also be given.

After formation of the male pronucleus, there is further movement of the cytoplasm, to bring the nuclei together in a central position. As this occurs, there is continual movement of streaming of the nuclei and cytoplasm that can be observed on time-lapse video photography and appears as the halo in single observations [30, 31]. The presence of a halo in the pronuclear embryo at 16–18 h after insemination (56–58 h post hCG) is an indicator that redistribution of mitochondria is occurring, the cytoplasm is competent and is moving.

The one cell-fertilized oocyte has a number of features that have been strongly correlated with development competence in vitro, after transfer in vivo and with the aneuploidy status of the embryo. The main parameters that are scored at 16–18 h post insemination (56–58 h post hCG) are the number, position and size of the pronuclei, the number, alignment and size of the nucleolar precursor bodies (NPB's) within the pronuclei, and the appearance of the cytoplasm, or "halo".

There should be two nuclei of approximately the same size and centrally located. Nuclei that are not closely aligned will result in lack of alignment of male and female chromatin, lack of crossing over and the potential formation of a two-cell embryo in which the nuclear material in one cell is purely female and in the other male in origin, since the first cleavage plane is through the pronuclear axis, which is on the metaphase plate. Nuclei which are not centrally located will also result in abnormal first mitotic cleavage for the same reasons, resulting in a two-cell embryo with uneven cell size (see day 2 scoring). Nuclei of very different sizes have been shown to result in embryos that are aneuploid in the vast majority of cases [32].

The most important aspect of day 1 scoring is the spatial distribution of the NPB's within the nuclei, the numbers and size of the NPB's per nucleus, and the symmetry of these characteristics between the nuclei at 16–18 h post insemination (56–58 h post hCG). Using these parameters, fertilized oocytes can be assigned to two main groups, normal and abnormal. There are a number of scoring system, but all look at essentially the same characteristics and all assign normal vs. abnormal on the same parameters (Fig. 44.2). The most commonly used formats are the Tesarik and the Z-Score systems [2, 31, 33, 34]. Both require equality of numbers and symmetry of distribution for a normal designation, and any variation from results in lowered potential of that fertilized oocyte, both in vitro and after transfer [33, 35–39]. A more recent finding is that the numbers of NPB's should ideally be five to seven per nucleus [20] (Fig. 44.3).

The basis of pronuclear scoring relates to the chromatin, condensation of the chromatin onto the spindle and the cell cycle. An important feature of pronuclear scoring is the concept that both the oocyte and the nuclei are spherical and that the spindle is not flat. Further, the nuclei and NPB's align onto the spindle and that the spindle may lie in any plane between them, with chromatin condensing into chromosomes and attaching to the spindle. To score the NPBs requires mental rotation of the nuclei in order to look at the NPBs relative to a 2D plane between the nuclei. Scoring the numbers and alignment of the NPBs relates to the function of these organelles and the way they relate to the ability of the embryo to develop [2, 3].

As an oocyte develops from a primordial oocyte to a mature MII stage, they are growing and actively forming new protein, which is accomplished by the nucleoli. During the final stages of maturation, growth stops and the nucleoli disassemble into component parts, only reforming when the embryo begins growing again. All proteins in any cell are constructed on the nucleoli. Nucleoli are also the sites of ribosomal RNA (rRNA) production, and the production of some growth factors and developmental regulatory proteins [40]. The nucleoli develop on DNA at sites where the genes for rDNA are located, which are referred to as the nucleolar organizing regions (NORS) [41]. The NORs are clustered on the DNA on heterochromatin adjacent to rDNA genes. There are only five NOR-bearing chromosomes: 13, 14, 15, 21 and 22; the heterochromatic chromosomes [42]. Interestingly, these are also the chromosomes most likely to be abnormal during aneuploidy screening and pronuclear scoring has been correlated with aneuploidy [43].

Structurally, there are three functional components in nucleoli: the dense fibrillar component (DFC) that is required for transcription, the fibrillar component (FC) that is surrounded by the DFC and that stores inactive transcription factors and is the centre of the nucleolus and the granular or cytoplasmic component (GC) [23, 41]. During oocyte development, when

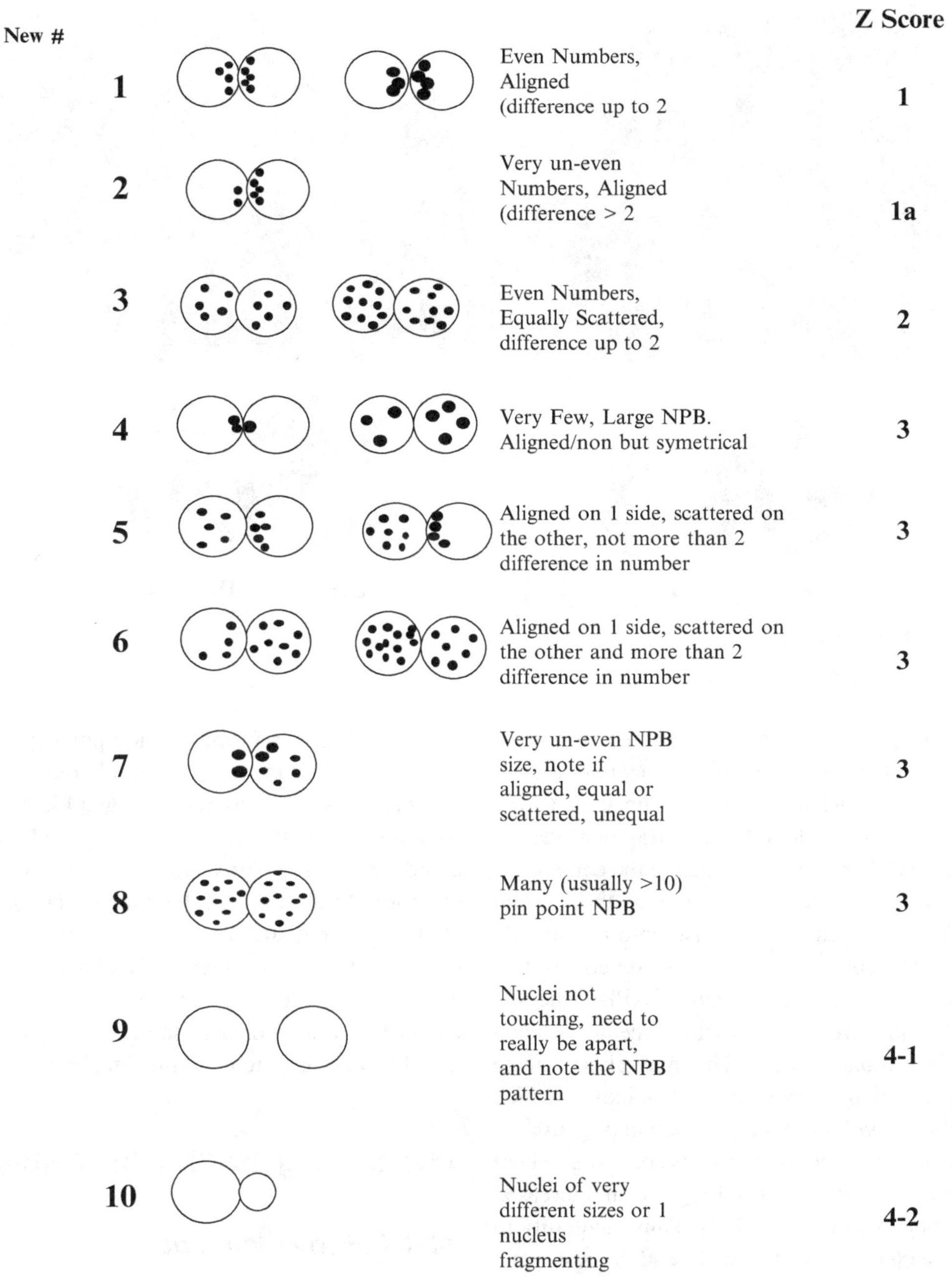

Fig. 44.2 Pronuclear score: The "new" designation describes a numerical system for each form of pronuclear pattern that can be seen. The pictures show how the NPBs can be visualized. The Z score relates to the system most commonly used, and how the observed patterns are scored. Use of an embryo is ideally 1, 3, 2, 4. Type 5 (Z-3) result in lowered but adequate positive pregnancy tests but few live offspring. Type 8 are the next best embryos after 1–4, but have lowered pregnancy rates. Types 9 and 10 are mainly abnormal and should not be used in transfer

the nucleoli disassemble, only the FC region remains; this is what is visible in the nuclei as the chromatin condenses and what is "scored" during pronuclear scoring. NPB's are the FC region on chromosomes 13, 14, 15, 21 and 22, the five heterochromatic chromosomes. In essence, what is being indirectly seen during scoring is the condensation of chromatin from these five chromosomes onto the spindle.

All human cells, including embryos and sperm, have between two and seven nucleoli per cell. During any mitotic cell division they dissociate into their component parts and the mitotic daughter cells show synchrony between the nuclei in terms of nucleoli content and patterns, with any asynchrony being attributed to abnormal chromosomal function [41].In abnormal cell division or growth, such as in tumors and other

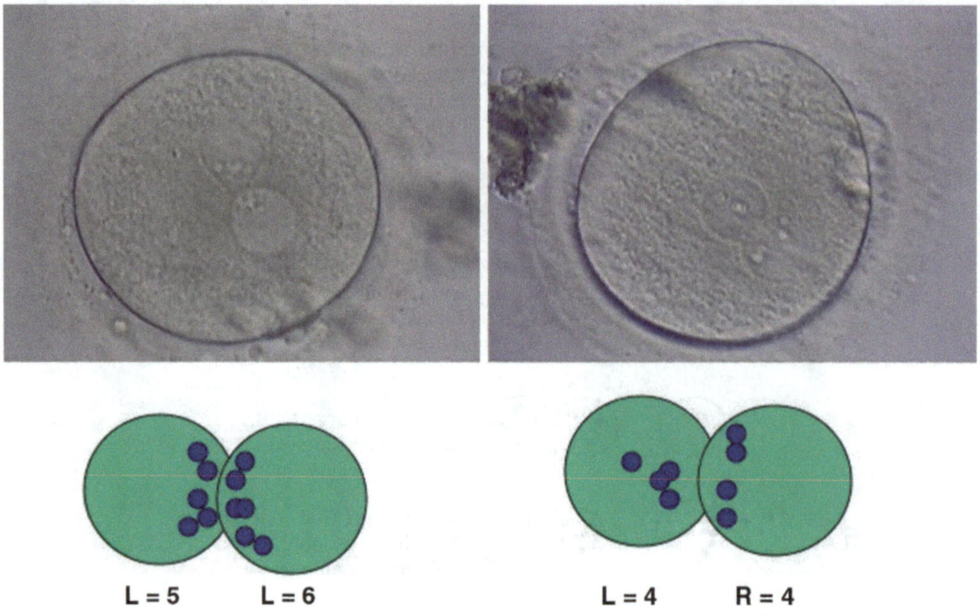

Fig. 44.3 Ratio of NPB's per pronucleus

cancerous tissue, there are more than the expected number of NORs or NORs of differing, abnormal or unequal sizes in mitotic daughter cells. Nucleoli are also connected to the process of aging, where the nucleoli begin to fragment, resulting in an increased number of dense bodies in the cells [44].

When chromatin begins to condense onto the mitotic spindle, the NPBs will appear to condense onto the spindle and be visible. In PN scoring, the lack of symmetry in this condensation is seen as unequal alignment of NPBs, unequal numbers of NPBs and different sizes which means delayed or fast condensation in one nucleus. This may also indicate abnormal or asynchronous karyo- and cyto-kinesis, which may result in embryos with little developmental potential.

Nucleoli are also connected to the process of aging, where the nucleoli begin to fragment, resulting in an increased number of dense bodies in the cells [44]. Thus inequality in NPB's between nuclei in oocytes will lead to abnormal development and increased number may indicate fragmentation and aging.

Strong correlations have been shown between PN score and aneuploidy with the incidence of chromosomally normal embryos being highest with equal sized nuclei and equal numbers of NPB that are aligned [43, 45–47].

Another aspect of pronuclear embryos that has been used as an indication of developmental competence is the appearance of a halo, or clearing in the cytoplasm on the periphery of the embryo [31, 48]. There are a number of theories as to what the streaming or halo represents. In low order animals, there is a similar streaming or cytoplasmic movement that sets up many of the fundamental axes that the embryo uses through development as well as localizing certain organelles into defined areas in the embryo [49–52]. Recent work indicates that axis formation and polarity in the mammalian embryo is a key to developmental competence and that this can begin as early as the oocyte [49, 51, 53, 54]. If this streaming is indicative of polarity and axis formation, it could be an easily observable parameter to use in embryo selection. In the human, the halo effect could also be attributed to the redistribution of mitochondria, with polarized mitochondria on the periphery and a dense core in the center of the embryo around the nuclei [55, 56]. Polarized mitochondria are localized in the periphery of the oocyte such that they can react to calcium signaling during sperm entry.

44.4 Scoring the Cleaving Embryo

44.4.1 Early Cleavage

The scoring term "early cleavage" (EC), designates fertilized oocytes that have nuclear membrane break down and the first mitotic division, at a set time after fertilization and hCG [31, 57–59]. EC is generally performed between 22 and 26 h post-insemination. The literature varies in timing and also in results, which could be a consequence of the lack of consensus as to when this parameter should be scored. [57, 60–62]. Variations in timing of as much as 4 h could lead to very different results. The timing of observation is crucial since entry into the first mitotic division is very rapid with fast breakdown of the nuclear membranes and then cleavage to the two cell stage. Embryos that undergo early cleavage (two-cell by at least 25 h post insemination) certainly are on a correct time clock and also tend to have better scores on day 2 and on day 3 and also result in higher implantation rates [60]. EC can be an added parameter in sequential embryo selection, especially when there are multiple embryos. Its use with fewer embryos may not be as great and may merely add another time point at which the embryos need to be removed from the incubator.

44.4.2 Day 2 Scoring

The completion of fertilization occurs with the first mitotic cell division, forming the two-cell embryo. This division is slightly unequal (as with the two polar bodies), is not random and the resulting cells are elliptical, not ovoid. The first mitotic division is an active one with the blastomeres moving and pulsing and rotating and finally arranging themselves into the two-cell embryo, which is not like animal models where it is a clean division with no rotation. After this division, the blastomeres do not rotate as much and settle into fixed positions. However, the second and third divisions, which happen in rapid succession, resulting in a four-cell embryo are also dynamic with pulsing and blastomere movement and some rotation. Due to the very dynamic nature of these first mitotic divisions, and the fact that embryos are on a time clock that starts with the LH surge/hCG injection [63, 64], day 2 scoring needs to be timed very carefully. The subsequent divisions have a degree of asynchrony, probably to allow spatial orientation in the embryo, which is also correlated with increased developmental potential [65].

The position of the meiotic spindle in the oocyte will affect this fist cleavage division. If it is off center, the oocyte may cleave down a plane that would result in a two-cell embryo with very different cell sizes. This becomes important when considering cell linage and the abnormal cytokinesis in this event will lead to blastocysts with allocation of cellular constituents that are abnormal [1, 54, 66–68]. If unequal cleavage was not due to aberrant positioning of the spindle, any cytokinesis resulting in two cells of grossly different sizes would suggest abnormal cellular processes resulting in an embryo with little developmental potential [69].

Day 2 scoring is probably the most important scoring point for embryos. When coupled to day1 pronuclear scoring, it allows for the selection of embryos that have originated from gametes that are most likely normal. Day 2 scoring considers three main parameters. At a set point, generally 42–44 h after insemination, the number of blastomeres are counted, the state of nucleation within these blastomeres scored and the relative sizes of each blastomeres recorded.

Ideally, an embryo should be at the four-cell stage by 42–44 h post-insemination. Embryos with uneven numbers of blastomeres (three and five) are generally abnormal unless the three-cell embryo progresses very rapidly to a four-cell stage. Five cell and greater embryos are cleaving too fast or originate from multinucleated embryos at the two-cell stage (see below). Embryos that are at the two-cell stage are necessarily developing slower than the four-cell embryos. It has been shown that embryos that are at the four-cell stage have greater developmental potential than those at the two-cell [33].

Multinucleation can arise through various mechanisms. In embryos, it could be true multinucleation or it could be nuclear fragmentation, many small nuclei. At the two-four cell stage, multinucleation arises through an abnormal mitotic event at the end of the fertilization process. This could be a duplication of the microtubule-organizing center (MTOC), which is known to occur in cells placed in culture [70]. It could indicate that spindle integrity and the mitotic process in the oocyte have been disrupted. It can also arise when karyokinesis occurs without cytokynesis. Whatever the cause, two and four-cell embryos with multinucleation have a lowered implantation rate [40, 71] and an increased incidence of aneuploidy [72, 73]. However, if only one cell is affected, they can give rise to normal offspring [74].

Polyspermic oocytes will often spontaneously cleave from the one cell stage to three and four-cell embryos. This is due to three (or more) centriole positions being set up and thus greater than one cleavage plane. Applying this to multinucleated blastomeres, what can occur is multiple planes of cleavage. This will result in embryos with greater than the expected number of blastomeres and within these, there may be no chromatin or fragments of chromatin, resulting in aneuploidy and decreased developmental potential.

The third aspect of day 2 scoring is the evenness of cell size. This relates directly to cleavage planes and spindles (see above). Allocation of cellular components is also affected, as is continued development. It is a very easy parameter to score and correlates directly with implantation potential [1]. (See Fig. 44.4–44.6 for day 2 scoring parameters)

Finally, without day 2 scoring, there is no information on the timing of development from the one-cell fertilized oocyte to the six to eight cell stage. Cell cycles are fundamental to gene expression and the events that occur in a sequential manner in the developing embryo. If an embryo's cell cycle is not on the basic rhythm, the resulting blastocyst will be abnormal and fail to implant. Figure 44.7 presents two embryos where cleavage was delayed and which resulted in adequate day 3 embryos, but which were grossly abnormal. Without the information from day 2, these could conceivably be used in either transfer or cryopreservation, on the basis of their day 3 morphology.

44.4.3 Day 3 Scoring

In embryos from the two to eight cell stage, there can only be three sizes of cells and no more than two sizes in any one embryo, which correspond to the cell stages [65]. The orientation of these in a three dimensional space is also important

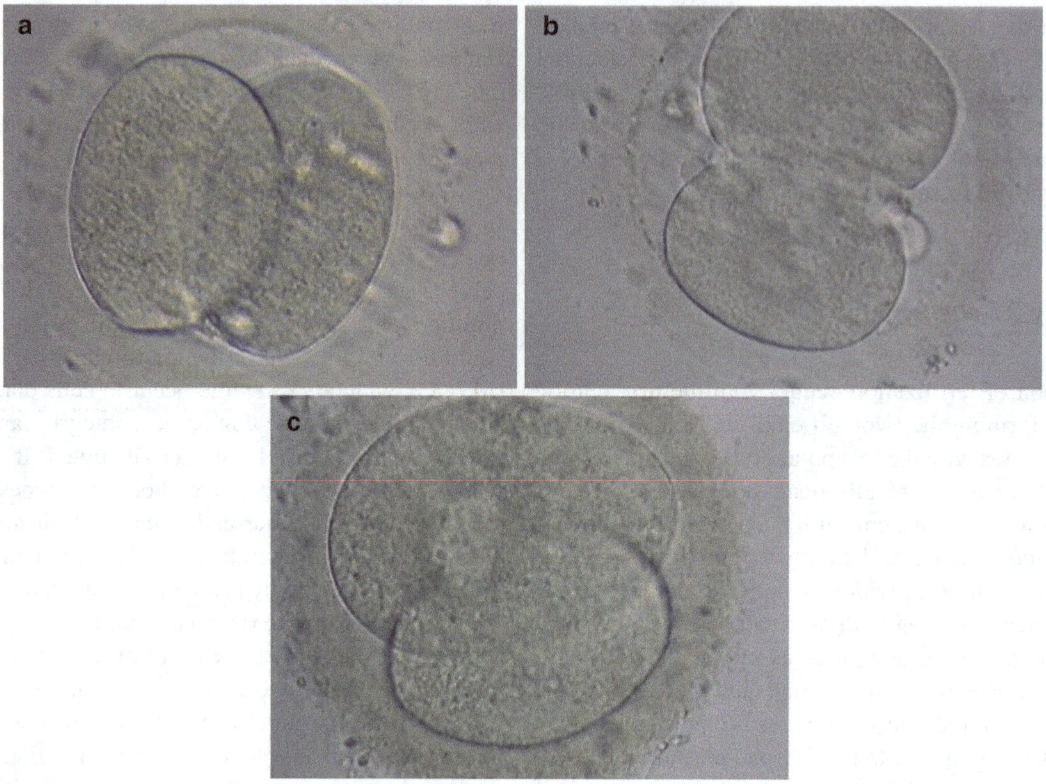

Fig. 44.4 Day 2, 2-cell morphology. Panel a, even sized, one nucleus per blastomeres; panel b, even size but multinucleated; panel c, Uneven sized blastomeres (30% difference)

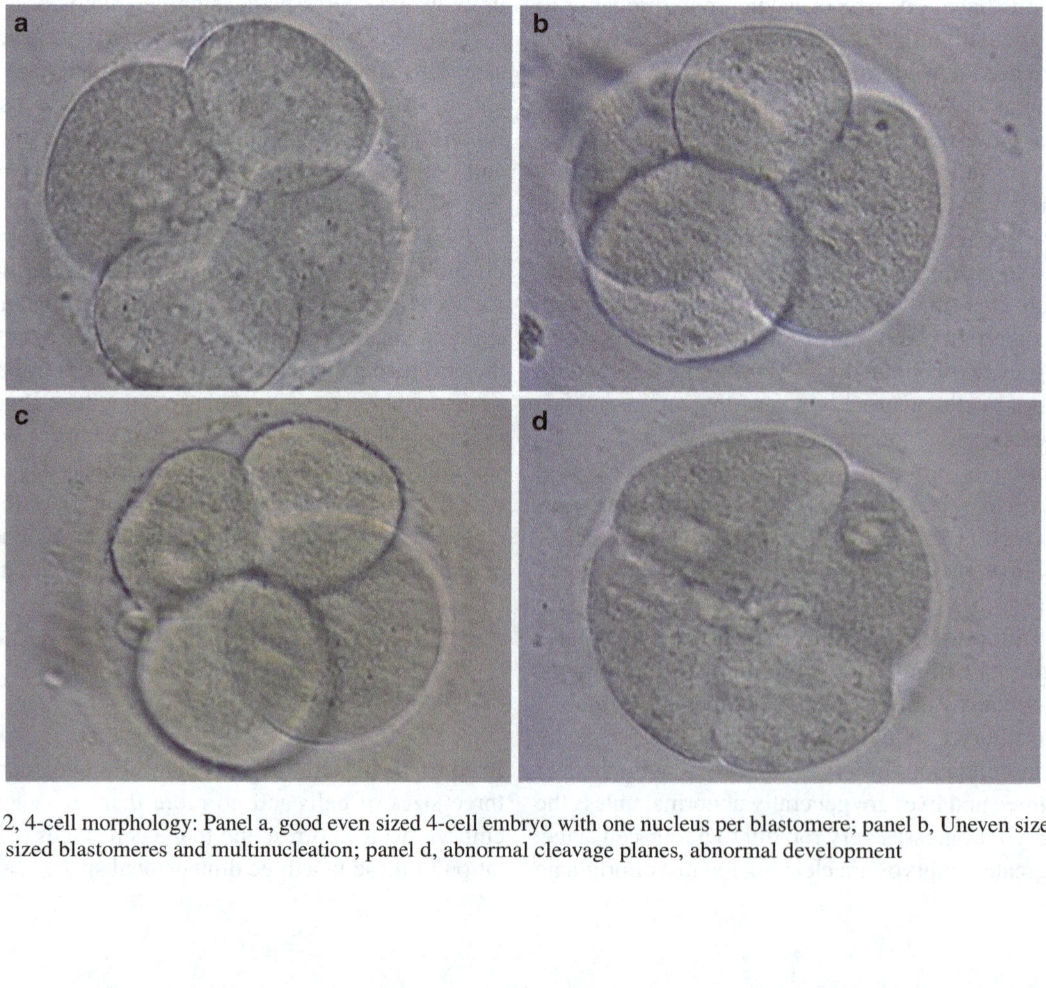

Fig. 44.5 Day 2, 4-cell morphology: Panel a, good even sized 4-cell embryo with one nucleus per blastomere; panel b, Uneven sized blastomeres,; panel c Uneven sized blastomeres and multinucleation; panel d, abnormal cleavage planes, abnormal development

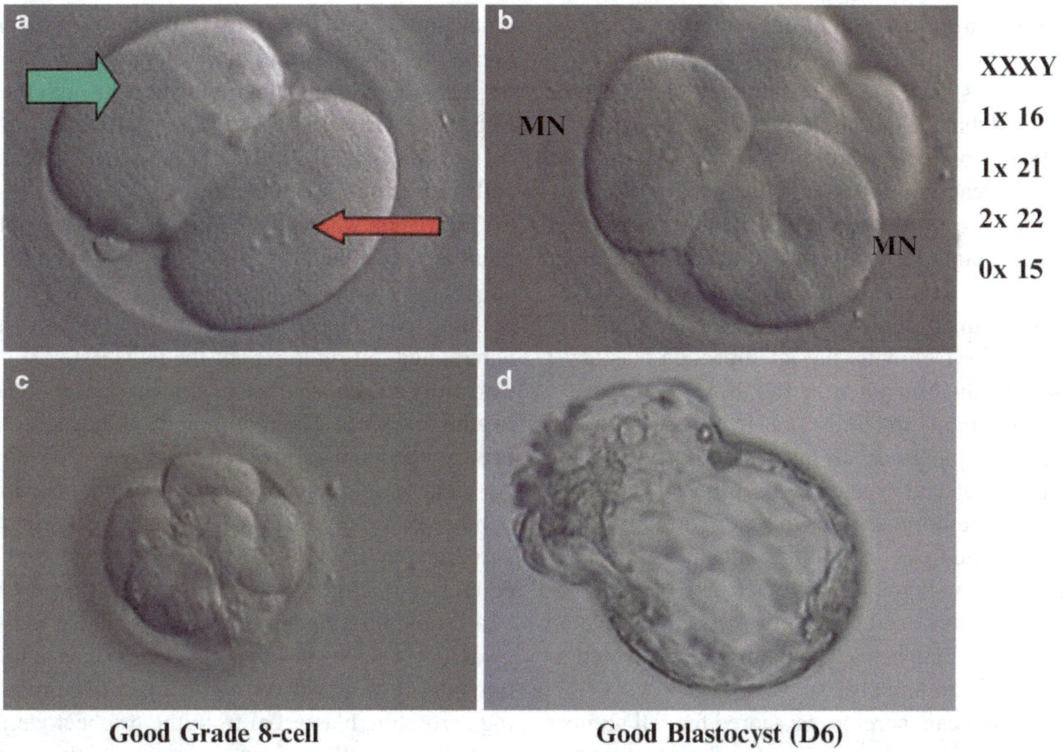

Fig. 44.6 The progression of multinucleated 2-cell embryo, through the 4-cell stage, showing continued multi-nucleation, the formation of an adequate 8-cell embryo prior to biopsy and finally a hatching Day 6 blastocyst. The FISH results from this embryo indicate a highly abnormal embryo, complex abnormal, which was predicted from Day 2 scoring

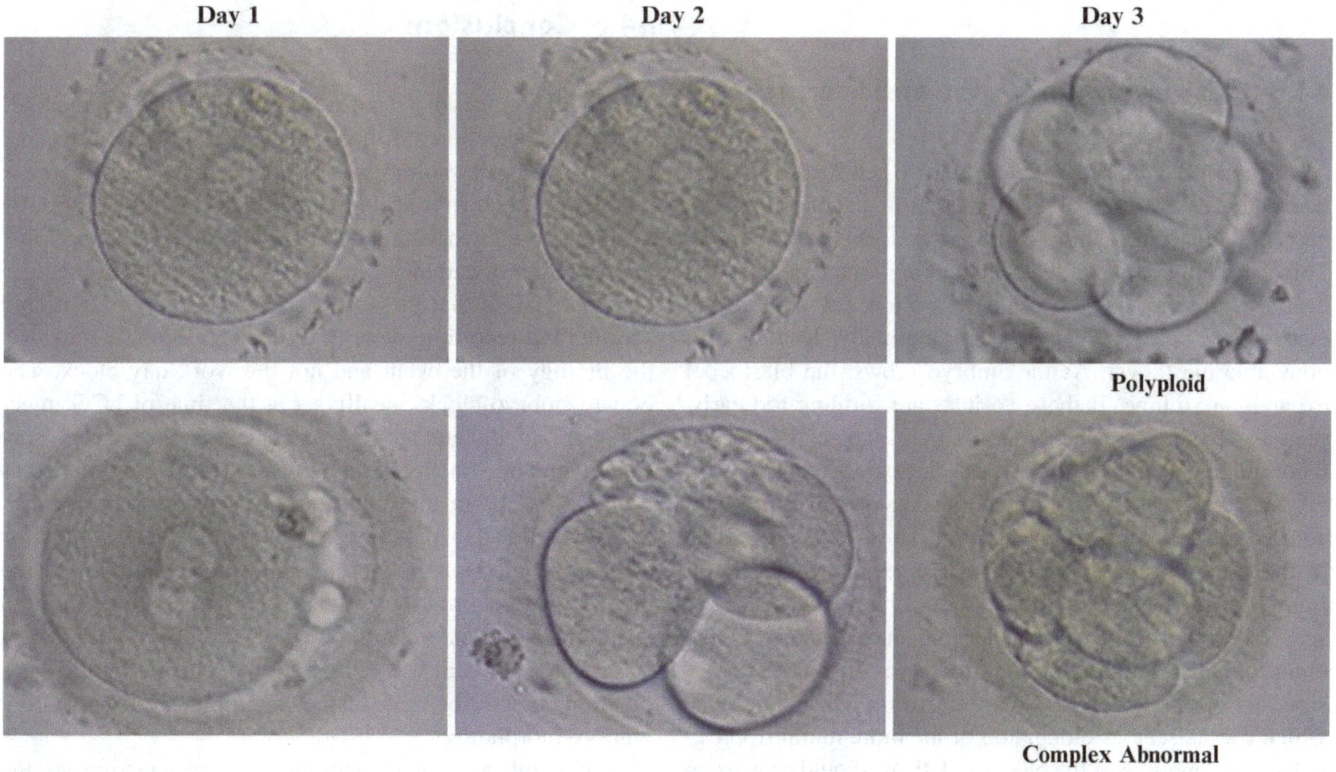

Fig. 44.7 Development of 2 embryos from day to day 3. The upper panel shows an embryo that failed to cleave on time from Day 1 to Day 2 but then went though rapid cleavage to an 8-cell stage (or spontaneously cleaved from a 1 cell to 8-cell, due initial karyokinesis without cytokinesis). The lower panels show an embryo that cleaved to an even celled 3-cell embryo and then into an adequate 6-cell embryo. The formation of 3-cell embryos is abnormal. The FISH results on both embryos indicated that both were highly abnormal, and which could be predicted from Day 2 scoring

for the directional development of the embryo and fetus [49, 53, 75].

All of these points have been realized in scoring systems that variously show that the morphology of cleaving embryos, [76–81] the degree of fragmentation [77, 82, 83], and the degree of multinucleation impacts on implantation [84, 85].

Since embryos are on time clocks, the rate of development is also important. The embryo initiates key developmental events related to this clock and not according to the cell number [63]. This is shown clinically where the rate of development of embryos in vitro has an impact on blastocyst formation and implantation potential [86, 87].

As the embryo begins to compact at the eight to 16 cell stage and form tight junctions, an inside and outside, or the first differentiation of cell types, occurs. There need to be sufficient cells in the embryo for this to occur correctly. Early compaction could lead to an embryo that allocates all its cells to the outside, which will go on to form a trophoblastic vesicle with no inner cell mass and therefore no ability to develop a fetus [64]. Early compaction can only be observed if embryos are scored sequentially.

Cleaving embryos can therefore be scored for cell number at a set point after hCG, the equality of cell size, the three dimensional distribution of the cells, the degree of fragmentation and multinucleation (see below), and the degree to which they are beginning to compact.

44.5 Blastocysts Formation and Scoring

As the embryo compacts at the eight to 16 cell stage, refractile bodies that are found in all blastomers from the one-cell stage onward begin to fuse in specific areas to form the blastocoel. This is initially between the cells making up the outside and inside of the morula [88]. If there are too few cells in the embryo, this process cannot occur normally, leading to a nonviable blastocyst. As the embryo grows, the blastocoel expands in volume. If these vesicles are forming too early, seen as a paving like vacuole formation in the early morula, it could indicate a disruption of the embryonic clock.

Once the blastocoel is formed, the outside cells are totally committed to become trophectoderm. These cells proliferate in the early blastocyst but not in the expanded blastocyst [89]. In early blastocysts, there should be a ring of evenly spaced, evenly sized cells all around the periphery of the embryo, indicating that proliferation is occurring. At expansion, the trophectoderm cells transform into giant-cells, which can be seen as elongation of the more mural trophectoderm. At one side of the blastocoel, there should be a group of evenly sized cells, protruding into the cavity, the inner cell mass (ICM). In the region of the ICM, the trophectoderm cells, or polar trophectoderm, remain mitotically active with a net flow of cells from this region to the opposite side, or mural area [90]. The junction between the polar and mural trophectoderm can be distinguished through the processes or finger like projections, that extend from the migrating polar cells to the ICM [89, 91]. These should breakdown as the cells move into the mural area.

The region where the ICM is located is the polar region, the point at which the polar body should still be located, and the site that defines the embryonic-abembryonic [54, 75], the first defining axis of gastrulation in the fetus [92, 93] and the dorso-ventral and left right axes of the fetus [94, 95]. As the blastocyst fully expands, it increases in size and the inner ICM begins to flatten. The morphology of blastocysts in vitro has been studied and various scoring systems developed [96–98]. An ideal blastocyst should have a blastocoel with an adequate number of evenly spaced equal sized cells in the trophectoderm, and an obvious ICM that is compact and comprised of equal sized cells by approximately 154 h post hCG or 112–114 h post-insemination. Overly expanded blastocyst should be avoided as they have been shown to have a lower implantation rates [86]. Blastocysts with finger like projections stretching across the blastocoel from the trophectoderm to the ICM [51] show a failure of full migration of the polar cells to the mural region, which could lead to developmental anomalies.

44.6 Conclusions

Within the confines of a clinical ART practice, the best methods of embryo selection are those that do as little harm to, and rely on the basic biology of the oocyte and embryo. These techniques are easily accomplished with the tools currently available to the working laboratory, and merely require time and accurate documentation. Oocytes and embryos need to be separated so that they can be followed individually and scoring and recording done in a timely fashion, dictated by the biology of the event and not the work day clock. The oocyte/embryo clock, ideally set at the time of hCG injection, should dictate all scoring and recording. This may require an adjustment of timing of procedures in practice as a whole or just in the time that key scoring is performed. Whatever the day of embryo transfer is, there should be sequential selection and not a single static evaluation of the embryo. This should start in the ovary and continue through until embryo transfer. Each oocyte and embryo needs to be scored at each point with elimination occurring on the basis of the parameter being assessed, regardless of the resulting embryo morphology.

Taking into account the various points of selection and the biology behind each criteria, the embryo should dictate and not the day of development, for transfer. Assuming a sequential selection system, an embryo that does not pass a scoring

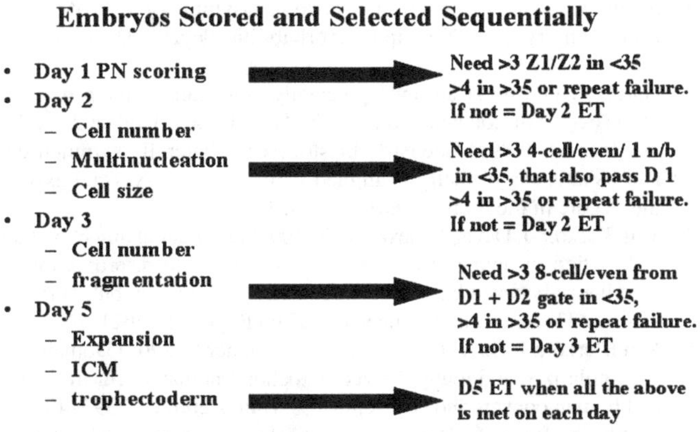

Fig. 44.8 Sequential embryo scoring and selection of transfer day based on embryo morphology

"gate" should be deselected, regardless of the morphology on subsequent days. In this manner, the fittest embryos on each day can be determined and selected for transfer of cryopreservation. If, within a cohort, only two or three embryos pass the first scoring point, a day 2 transfer can be performed. The same situation pertains on day 2, as allowing selection of embryos on day 3 from a poor day-2 cohort will not increase the like hood of success. Figure 44.8 provides a guideline for embryo selection and transfer day, on the basis of strict sequential selection.

References

1. Scott L, Finn A, O'Leary T, McLellan S, Hill J (2007) Morphologic parameters of early cleavage-stage embryos that correlate with fetal development and delivery: prospective and applied data for increased pregnancy rates. Hum Reprod 22:230–240
2. Scott L (2003) In: Van Blerkom J, Gregory L (eds) Morphological correlates of oocyte and embryo competence-identification. Kluwer Press, London
3. Scott L (2003) The biological basis of non-invasive strategies for selection of human oocytes and embryos. Hum Reprod Update 9:237–249
4. Van Blerkom J (1990) Occurrence and developmental consequences of aberrant cellular organization in meiotically mature human oocytes after exogenous ovarian hyperstimulation. J Electron Microsc Tech 16:324–346
5. Van Blerkom J (1994) Intrinsic factors affecting the outcome of laboratory assisted conception in the human. In: Van Blerkom J (ed) The biological basis of early reproductive failure in the human: applications to medically-assisted conception. OUP, Oxford, UK, pp 283–325
6. Van Blerkom J (1996) The influence of intrinsic and extrinsic factors on the developmental potential and chromosome normality of the human oocyte. J Soc Gynecol Invest 3:3–11
7. Van Blerkom J, Henry G (1992) Oocyte dysmorphism and aneuploidy in meiotically-mature human oocytes after ovulation stimulation. Hum Reprod 7:379–390
8. Araki K, Naito K, Haraguchi S et al (1996) Meiotic abnormalities of c-mos knockout mouse oocytes: activation after the first meiosis or entrance into third meiotic metaphase. Biol Reprod 55:1315–1324
9. Verlhac M, Kubiak J, Clarke H, Maro B (1994) Microtubule and chromatin behavior follow MAP kinase activity but not MPF activity during meiosis in mouse oocytes. Development 120:1017–1025
10. Choi T, Fukasawa K, Zhou R et al (1996) The MOS/mitogen-activated protein kinase (MAPK) pathway regulates the size and degradation of the first polar body in maturing mouse oocytes. Proc Natl Acad Sci USA 93:7032–7035
11. Ortiz M, Lucero P, Croxatto H (1983) Post ovulatory aging of human ova: spontaneous division of the first polar body. Gamete Res 7:269–276
12. Ebner T, Moser M, Sommergruber M, Tews G (2003) Selection based on morphological assessment. Hum Reprod Update 9: 251–262
13. Ebner T, Moser M, Yaman C, Feichtinger O, Hartl J, Tews G (1999) Elective transfer of embryos selected on the basis of first polar body morphology is associated with increased rates of implantation and pregnancy. Fertil Steril 72:599–603
14. Ebner T, Yaman C, Moser M, Sommergruber M, Feichtinger O, Tews G (2000) Prognostic value of first polar body morphology on fertilization rate and embryo quality in intracytoplasmic sperm injection. Hum Reprod 15:427–430
15. Bartoov B, Berkovitz A, Eltes F et al (2003) Pregnancy rates are higher with intracytoplasmic morphologically selected sperm injection than with conventional intracytoplasmic injection. Fertil Steril 80:1413–1419
16. Montag M, Schimming T, van der Ven H (2006) Spindle imaging in human oocytes: the impact of the meiotic cell cycle. Reprod Biomed Online 10:192–198
17. Rienzi L, Ubaldi F, Iacobelli M, Minasi M, Romano S, Greco E (2005) Meiotic spindle visualization in living human oocytes. Reprod Biomed Online 10:192–198
18. Montag M, Schimming T, Köster M et al (2008) Oocyte zona birefringence intensity is associated with embryonic implantation potential in ICSI cycles. Reprod Biomed Online 16:239–244
19. Nottola S, Makabe S, Stallone T, Familiari G, Correr S, Macchiarelli G (2005) Surface morphology of the zona pellucida surrounding human blastocysts obtained after in vitro fertilization. Arch Histol Cytol 68:133–141
20. Scott L, Berntsen J, Davies D, Gundersen J, Hill J, Ramsing N (2008) Human oocyte respiration-rate measurement- potential to improve oocyte and embryo selection? RBMOnline 17:461–469
21. Bousquet D, Léveillé M, Roberts K, Chapdelaine A, Bleau D (2005) The cellular origin of the zona pellucida antigen in the human and hamster. J Exp Zool 215:215–218
22. Familiari G, Relucenti M, Heyn R, Micara G, Correr S (2006) Three-dimensional structure of the zona pellucida at ovulation. Microsc Res Tech 69:415–426
23. Schwartz P, Hinney B, Nayudu P, Michelmann H (2003) Oocyte-sperm interaction in the course of IVF: a scanning electron microscopy analysis. Reprod Biomed Online 7:192–198
24. Shen Y, Stalf T, Mehnert C, Eichenlaub-Ritter U, Tinneberg H (2005) High magnitude of light retardation by the zona pellucida is associated with conception cycles. Hum Reprod 20:1596–1606
25. Gorbsky G, Simerly C, Schatten G, Borisy G (1990) Microtubules in the metaphase-arrested mouse oocyte turn over rapidly. Proc Natl Acad Sci USA 87:6049–6053
26. Battaglia D, Goodwin P, Klein N, Soules M (1996) Influence of maternal age on meiotic spindle assembly in oocytes from cycling women. Hum Reprod 11:2217–2222
27. Garello C, Baker H, Rai J et al (1999) Pronuclear orientation, polar body placement, and embryo quality after intracytoplasmic sperm injection and in-vitro fertilization: further evidence for polarity in human oocytes? Hum Reprod 14:2588–2595
28. Hardarson T, Lundin K, Hamberger L (2000) The position of the metaphase II spindle cannot be predicted by the location of the first polar body in the human oocyte. Hum Reprod 15:1372–1376

29. Silva CP, Kommineni K, Oldenbourg R, Keefe D (1999) The first polar body does not predict accurately the location of the metaphase II meiotic spindle in mammalian oocytes. Fertil Steril 71:719–721
30. Hardarson T, Lofman C, Coull G, Sjogren A, Hamberger L, Edwards R (2002) Internalization of cellular fragments in a human embryo: time-lapse recordings. Reprod BioMed Online 5:36–38
31. Scott LA, Smith S (1998) The successful use of pronuclear embryo transfers the day following oocyte retrieval. Hum Reprod 13: 1003–1013
32. Sadowy S, Tomkin G, Munne S (1998) Impaired development of zygotes with uneven pronuclear size. Zygote 63:137–141
33. Scott LA, Alvero R, Leondires M, Miller BT (2000) The morphology of human pronuclear embryos is positively related to blastocyst development and implantation. Hum Reprod 15(11):2394–2403
34. Tesarik J, Greco E (1999) The probability of abnormal preimplantation development can be predicted by a single static observation on pronuclear stage morphology. Hum Reprod 14(5):1318–1323
35. Borini A, Cattoli M, Sereni E, Sciajno R, Flamigni C (2005) Predictive factors for embryo implantation potential. Reprod Biomed Online 10:653–668
36. Chen C, Kattera S (2006) Comparison of pronuclear zygote morphology and early cleavage status of zygotes as additional criteria in the selection of day 3 embryos: a randomized study. Fertil Steril 85:347–352
37. Ludwig M, Schopper B, Katalinic A, Strum R, Al-Hasani S, Diedrich K (2000) Clinical use of a pronuclear stage score following intracytoplasmic sperm injection: impact on pregnancy rates under the conditions of the German embryo protection law. Hum Reprod 15(2):325–329
38. Senn A, Urner F, Chanson A, Primi M, Wirthner D, Germond M (2005) Morphological scoring of human pronuclear zygotes for prediction of pregnancy outcome. Hum Reprod 21:234–239
39. Zollner U, Steck T (2003) Pronuclear scoring. Time for international standardization. J Reprod Med 48:365–369
40. Pedersen T (1998) Growth factors in the nucleolus? J Cell Biol 143:279–281
41. Goessens G (1984) Nucleolar structure. Int Rev Cytol 87:107–158
42. Dimitri P, Corradini N, Rossi F, Vernì F (2005) The paradox of functional heterochromatin. Bioessays 27:29–41
43. Gianaroli L, Magli MC, Ferraretti AP, Fortini D, Grieco N (2003) Pronuclear morphology and chromosomal abnormalities as scoring criteria for embryo selection. Fertil Steril 80(2):341–349
44. Guarente L (1997) Link between aging and the nucleolus. Genes Dev 11:2449–2455
45. Edirisinghe W, Jemmott R, Smith C, Allen J (2005) Association of pronuclear Z scores with rates of aneuploidy in in vitro-fertilised embryos. Fertil Dev 17:529–534
46. Gamiz P, Rubio C, de los Santos M, Mercader A, Simone C (2003) The effect of pronuclear morphology on early development and chromosomal abnormalities in cleavage stage embryos. Hum Reprod 18:2413–2419
47. Kahraman S, Bahce M, Samli H et al (2000) Healthy births and ongoing pregnancies obtained by preimplantation genetic diagnosis in patients with advanced maternal age and recurrent implantation failure. Hum Reprod 15:2003–2007
48. Payne D, Flaherty SP, Barry MF, Mathews CD (1997) Preliminary observations on polar body extrusion and pronuclear formation in human oocytes using time-lapse video cinematography. Hum Reprod 12:532–541
49. Edwards RG, Beard HK (1997) Oocyte polarity and cell determination in early mammalian embryos. Mol Hum Reprod 3(10):863–905
50. Kloc M, Etkin LD (1995) Two distinct pathways for the localisation of RNA at the vegetal cortex in *Xenopus* oocytes. Development 121:287–297
51. Scott L, Alvero R, Leondires M, Miller B (2000) The morphology of human pronuclear embryos is positively related to blastocyst development and implantation. Hum Reprod 15(11):2394–2403
52. Seydoux G, Fire A (1994) Soma-germline asymmetry in the distribution of embryonic RNA's in Caenorhabditis elegans. Development 120:2823–2834
53. Gardner RL (1996) Can developmentally significant spatial patterning of the egg be discounted in mammals? Hum Reprod Update 2:3–27
54. Gardner RL (1997) The early blastocyst is bilaterally symmetrical and its axis of symmetry is aligned with the animal-vegetal axis of the zygote in the mouse. Development 124:289–301
55. Van Blerkom J, Davis P, Alexander S (2000) Differential mitochondrial distribution in human pronuclear embryos leads to disproportionate inheritance between blastomeres: relationship to microtubular organization, ATP content and competence. Hum Reprod 15:2621–2633
56. Van Blerkom J, Davis P, Mathwig V, Alexander S (2002) Domains of high-polarized and low-polarized mitochondria may occur in mouse and human oocytes and early embryos. Hum Reprod 17:393–406
57. Lundin K, Bergh C, Hardarson T (2001) Early embryo cleavage is a strong indicator of embryo quality in human IVF. Hum Reprod 16:2652–2657
58. Sakkas D, Percival G, D'Arcy Y, Sharif K, Afnan M (2002) Assessment of early cleaving human embryos at the 2-cell stage before transfer improves embryo selection. Fertil Steril 76:1150–1156
59. Shoukir Y, Campana A, Farley T, Sakkas D (1997) Early cleavage of in-vitro fertilized human embryos to the 2-cell stage: a novel indicator of embryo quality and viability. Hum Reprod 12:1531–1536
60. Lawler C, Baker H, Edgar D (2007) Relationships between timing of syngamy, female age and implantation potential in human in vitro-fertilised oocytes. Reprod Fertil Dev 19:482–487
61. Salumets A, Hydén-Granskog C, Mäkinen S, Suikkari A, Tiitinen A, Tuuri T (2003) Early cleavage predicts the viability of human embryos in elective single embryo transfer procedures. Hum Reprod 18:821–825
62. Van Montfoort A, Dumoulin J, Kester A, Evers J (2004) Early cleavage is a valuable addition to existing embryo selection parameters: a study using single embryo transfers. Hum Reprod 19:2103–2106
63. Johnson M, Day M (2000) Egg timers: how is developmental time measured in the early vertebrate embryo? BioEssays 22:57–63
64. Johnson M, Ziomek C (1981) The foundation of two distinct cell linages within the mouse morula. Cell 24:71–80
65. Roux C, Joanne C, Agnani G, Fromm M, Clavequin MC, Bresson JL (1995) Morphometric parameters of living human in-vitro fertilized embryos: importance of the asynchronous division process. Hum Reprod 10:1201–1207
66. Antczak M, Van Blerkom J (1997) Oocyte influences on early development: the regulatory proteins leptin and STAT3 are polarized in mouse and human oocytes and differentially distributed within the cells of the preimplantation stage embryo. Mol Hum Reprod 3(12):1067–1086
67. Gardner R, Davies T (2006) An investigation of the origin and significance of bilateral symmetry of the pronuclear zygote in the mouse. Hum Reprod 21:492–502
68. Hansis C, Edwards R (2003) Cell differentiation in the preimplantation human embryo. Reprod Biomed Online 6:215–220
69. Ciray H, Karagenc L, Ulug U, Bener F, Bahceci M (2005) Use of both early cleavage and day 2 mononucleation to predict embryos with high implantation potential in intracytoplasmic sperm injection cycles. Fertil Steril 84:1411–1416
70. Sorimachi K, Naora H, Akimoto K, Niwa A, Naora H (1998) Multinucleation and preservation of nucleolar integrity of macrophages. Cell Biol Int 22:352–357
71. Moriwaki T, Suganuma N, Hayakawa M et al (2004) Embryo evaluation by analysing blastomere nuclei. Hum Reprod 19(1):152–156
72. Kligman I, Benadiva C, Alikani M, Munne S (1996) The presence of multinucleated blastomeres in human embryos is correlated with chromosomal abnormalities. Hum Reprod 11:1492–1498
73. Staessen C, Van Steirteghem A (1998) The genetic constitution of multinuclear blastomeres and their derivative daughter blastomeres. Hum Reprod 13:1625–1631

74. Balakier H, Cadesky K (1997) The frequency and developmental capability of human embryos containing multinucleated blastomeres. Hum Reprod 12:800–804
75. Gardner R (2001) Specification of embryonic axes begins before cleavage in normal mouse development. Development 128: 839–847
76. Dawson KJ, Conaghan J, Ostera GR, Winston RML, Hardy K (1995) Delaying transfer to the thrid day post-insemination, to select non-arrested embryos, increases development to the fetal heart stage. Hum Reprod 10:177–182
77. Desai N, Goldstein J, Rowland D, Goldfarb J (2000) Morphological evaluation of human embryos and derivation of an embryo quality scoring system specific for day 3 embryos: preliminary study. Hum Reprod 15:2190–2196
78. Rijnders PM, Jansen CAM (1998) The predictive value of day 3 embryo morphology regarding blastocyst formation, pregnancy and implantation rate after day 5 transfer following in-vitro fertilization or intracytoplasmic sperm injection. Hum Reprod 13:2869–2873
79. Steer CV, Mills CL, Tan SL, Campbell S, Edwards RG (1992) The cumulative embryo score: a predictive embryo scoring technique to select the optimal number of embryos to transfer in an in-vitro fertilization and embryo transfer programme. Hum Reprod 7:117–119
80. Tan SL, Royston P, Cambell S (1992) Cumulative conception and live birth rates after in-vitro fertilization. Lancet 339:1390–1394
81. Van Royen E, Mangelschots K, De Neubourg D, Laureys I (2001) Calculating the implantation potential of day 3 embryos in women younger than 38 years of age: a new model. Hum Reprod 16:326–332
82. Alikani M, Calderon G, Tomkin G, Garrisi G, Kokot M, Cohen J (2000) Cleavage anomalies in early human embryos and survival after prolonged culture in-vitro. Hum Reprod 15:2634–2643
83. Van Blerkom J, Davis P, Alexander S (2001) A microscopic and biochemical study of fragmentation phenotypes in stage-appropriate human embryos. Hum Reprod 16:719–729
84. Hardarson T, Hanson C, Sjogren A, Lundin K (2001) Human embryos with unevenly sized blastomeres have lower pregnancy and implantation rates: indications for aneuploidy and multinucleation. Hum Reprod 16:313–318
85. Pickering S, Taylor A, Johnson M, Braude P (1995) An analysis of multinucleated blastomere formation in human embryos. Hum Reprod 10:1912–1922
86. Racowsky C, Jackson K, Cekleniak N, Fox J, Hornstein M, Ginsburg E (2000) The number of eight-cell embryos is a key determinant for selecting day 3 or day 5 transfer. Fertil Steril 73:558–564
87. Shapiro B, Harris D, Richter K (2000) Predictive value of 72-hour blastomere cell number on blastocyst development and success of subsequent transfer based on the degree of blastocyst development. Fertil Steril 73:582–586
88. Calcaro PG, Brown EH (1969) An ultrastructural and cytological study of preimplantation development of the mouse. J Exp Zool 171:253–283
89. Gardner R (2000) Flow of cells from polar to mural trophectoderm is polarized in the mouse blastocyst. Hum Reprod 15:694–701
90. Gardner RL, Nichols J (1991) An investigation of the fate of cells transplanted orthotopically between morulae/nascent blastocysts in the mouse. Hum Reprod 6:25–35
91. Flemming TP, Warren PD, Chisholm TC, Johnson MH (1984) Trophectodermal processes regulate the expression of totipotency within the inner cell mass of the mouse expanding blastocyst. J Embryol Exp Morphol 84:63–90
92. Smith LJ (1980) Embryonic axis orientation in the mouse and its correlation with blastocysts' relationships to the uterus. Part 1. Relationship. J Embryol Exp Morphol 55:257–277
93. Smith LJ (1985) Embryonic axis orientation in the mouse and its correlation with blastocysts' relationship to the uterus. Part II relationships from 41/2 to 91/2 days. J Embryol Exp Morphol 89:15–35
94. Yost H (1995) Vertebrate left-right development. Cell 82:689–692
95. Yost H (2001) Establishment of left-right asymmetry. Academic Press, London
96. Balaban B, Urman B, Isklar A et al (2001) The effects of pronuclear morphology on embryo quality parameters and blastocyst transfer outcome. Hum Reprod 16:2357–2361
97. Dokras A, Sargent IL, Barlow DH (1993) Human blastocyst grading: an indicator of developmental potential. Hum Reprod 8:2119–2127
98. Gardner DK, Lane M, Stevens J, Schlenker T, Schoolcraft WB (2000) Blastocyst score affects implantation and pregnancy: towards a single blastocyst transfer. Fertil Steril 73:1155–1158

Chapter 45
Embryo Transfer in IVF: Evidence-Based Clinical Practice

Lindsay Mains and Bradley J. Van Voorhis

Abstract Since the first pregnancy using in vitro fertilization (IVF) was achieved nearly 30 years ago, many aspects of this procedure have undergone significant progress. In contrast, the technique of embryo transfer (ET) has remained relatively unchanged. A simple yet critical element in the final step of IVF, embryo transfer, has received little attention until recently. As poor implantation rates have increasingly hindered the growing success of IVF, the procedure of embryo transfer is now under great scrutiny. While poor embryo quality or suboptimal uterine receptivity may be responsible for implantation failures, the transfer technique itself is now also recognized as an important determinant of IVF success. Optimizing the technique of embryo transfer should take several factors into consideration.

In general, the procedure starts by placing a speculum in the vagina to visualize the cervix, which is cleansed with saline solution or culture media. Additional mucus in the cervical canal can be aspirated using a sterile syringe. A transfer catheter is loaded with the embryos and handed to the clinician after confirmation of the patient's identity. The catheter is inserted through the cervical canal and advanced into the uterine cavity where the embryos are deposited. The catheter is then withdrawn and handed to the embryologist who inspects it for retained embryos.

The ultimate goal of a successful embryo transfer is to deliver the embryos atraumatically to a location in the uterus where implantation is maximized. Potential reasons for a failed transfer include disruption of the endometrium by the catheter, induction of uterine contractions, deposition of the embryos in a suboptimal location, or damage to the embryos during the process. Numerous technical aspects of this procedure have been studied to minimize these complications and determine their effect on pregnancy outcome. Though much of the published data that evaluate these factors are conflicting or are confounded by variables in the IVF process that are difficult to hold constant, several aspects of the procedure warrant consideration.

Keywords Embryo transfer • Embryo culture medium • Antibiotics • Ultrasound guidance • Transfer catheter

L. Mains
Department of Obstetrics and Gynecology,
University of Iowa, Iowa City, IA, USA

B.J. Van Voorhis (✉)
Department of Obstetrics and Gynecology,
University of Iowa Hospitals and Clinics, Iowa City, IA, USA
e-mail: brad-van-voorhis@uiowa.edu

45.1 Ease of Transfer

An abundance of literature suggests that the overall "ease" of the embryo transfer is strongly correlated to pregnancy outcome [1–5]. Despite the apparent simplicity of this procedure, difficult transfers often occur and have been shown to significantly lower pregnancy and implantation rates compared to easy transfers [2]. The "difficulty" of a transfer is somewhat subjective but is often used to describe transfers that are time consuming, require a firmer catheter, cause discomfort, or involve additional instrumentation such as a tenaculum. One mechanism by which difficult or traumatic transfers can hinder implantation is thought to be through the stimulation of uterine contractions [6, 7]. Contractions may be initiated by fundal contact or cervical manipulation associated with the release of prostaglandins and oxytocin [6, 8]. Presence of blood on the catheter, often an indication of a difficult transfer, is also associated with decreased pregnancy rates and a higher incidence of retained embryos [4, 9]. Despite its subjectivity, "ease of transfer" is generally accepted as an important factor in successful implantation.

The most common reasons for a difficult transfer are cervical stenosis or a large degree of ante/retroversion or ante/retroflexion of the uterus [10, 11]. Several methods have been suggested and evaluated as ways to minimize the difficulty of a transfer, including trial transfer, ultrasound guidance, and use of a soft catheter.

D.T. Carrell and C.M. Peterson (eds.), *Reproductive Endocrinology and Infertility: Integrating Modern Clinical and Laboratory Practice*,
DOI 10.1007/978-1-4419-1436-1_45,

45.2 Trial Transfers

Trial transfers, or mock transfers, can be done at any point prior to the actual transfer, but the two most common times are prior to starting an ovarian stimulation and immediately before the actual embryo transfer. Some in vitro fertilization (IVF) centers will perform trial transfers at both of these points. During the trial transfer prior to stimulation, a catheter is often advanced to the uterine fundus in order to measure the full length of the uterine cavity and cervical canal. Any notes regarding the type of speculum required, type of catheter used, need for a tenaculum, and the direction and curve of the catheter can be recorded for future reference. This sounding may be done blindly, since the uterine fundus is identified by feel, though abdominal ultrasound may be used if any difficulty is encountered.

Findings from this trial transfer may lead a clinician to take additional precautions prior to the actual transfer. For example, in cases of severely flexed uteri, which require a tenaculum on the cervix for traction, a cervical stitch cut long can be placed at the time of oocyte retrieval and then used for relatively atraumatic traction at embryo transfer. If the trial reveals a cervix too stenotic to permit passage of the catheter, cervical dilatation can be planned well before the embryo transfer. Dilatation at the start of stimulation allows sufficient time for the endometrium to recover from any trauma, inflammation, or bacterial contamination before embryo transfer. In cases of cervical stenosis, lower pregnancy rates are associated with cervical dilatation done within 5 days of transfer [4, 12]; however, dilatation several weeks out appears to improve pregnancy rates [13, 14].

A trial transfer can also be done at the time of embryo transfer. Often done under ultrasound guidance, the catheter should only be advanced to the internal os so as not to disrupt the endometrial lining. If this is easily accomplished, the catheter can be removed and the transfer catheter loaded with the embryos can then be inserted. Alternatively, the other sheath from this trial catheter can be left in place, either routinely or with difficult cases, while the soft inner catheter is loaded with the embryos and advanced through the sheath to the correct placement. This method, sometimes referred to as the "afterloading" technique, may also decrease mucus contamination of the catheter [15].

In an RCT of 335 patients, examining the effect of an early trial transfer on outcome, pregnancy and implantation rates were improved in the trial transfer group. This group also had no difficult embryo transfers while 50 (29.8%) patients had difficult transfers when no trial transfer was done [2]. However, reported implantations rates were low, and no further prospective randomized trials have been published. The value of a trial transfer has been challenged as the length and position of the uterus can change before the actual transfer. For example, a retroverted uterus at trial transfer can often be anteverted at actual transfer when large stimulated ovaries are in the posterior cul-de-sac [16]. Some authors have therefore suggested performing a trial transfer at the time of oocyte retrieval. Though this could theoretically alter endometrial receptivity, a retrospective study of 289 women showed no difference in ongoing pregnancy rates when the trial was done prior to starting ovulation induction compared to at retrieval (47.6 and 48.4%) [17].

45.3 Ultrasound Guidance Versus Clinical Touch

Ultrasound guidance (UG) is another method used to facilitate nontraumatic insertion of the catheter, as well as ensure correct location in the uterine cavity. Touching the fundus can easily be avoided with ultrasound, and one can be certain that the catheter is beyond the internal os in cases of an elongated cervical canal. Ultrasound can be especially helpful in uteri distorted by fibroids or those with previous caesarean section scars in which the catheter can get hung up or misdirected. Direct visualization of the catheter at the cervicouterine angle can facilitate its insertion, allowing the physician to place an appropriate curve on the catheter, which can be particularly helpful in severely flexed uteri. The full bladder required for abdominal ultrasound also helps to straighten the cervicouterine angle and facilitate entry of the catheter, particularly for the strongly anteverted uterus [18–20]. Ultrasound at transfer can be useful to assess the degree of intraperitoneal ascites and ovarian enlargement prior to proceeding with a transfer in cases at risk for ovarian hyperstimulation syndrome. Sonographic guidance can be extremely instructive at training facilities because it provides reassurance and feedback to clinicians in training. Patients also seem to take great comfort in visualizing this final step of an often long and difficult process.

Disadvantages with ultrasound may include the need for a second operator, a longer procedure time, and the inconvenience of filling the patient's bladder [21]. Some have suggested that moving the catheter to identify its location, a motion that is not necessary in transfers performed by "clinical touch," could potentially disrupt the endometrium [22]. However, this movement is usually unnecessary with the echogenic catheters that are now available.

Many clinicians still use the "clinical touch" method. The potential disadvantages of this method are inadvertent contact with the fundus and inaccurate assessment of the catheter position. Clinicians using this method must rely on tactile assessment or patient discomfort to indicate fundal contact [6]. However, discomfort is often indicative of uterine contractility which may lead to expulsion of the embryos, a possible explanation for their association with lower pregnancy rates [7]. In one study on 121 transfers done by clinical touch and then visualized by transvaginal ultrasound, abutment of the catheter tip with the fundus occurred in 17.4% and the tubal ostia in 7.4% [23]. Some advocates of this method will transfer the embryos at a fixed distance from the external os (~6 cm), though this would certainly not take into account variation in cervical length or uterine size [6].

Since first described by Strickler et al. in 1985 [24], numerous studies evaluating the effect of ultrasound guidance in embryo transfer on pregnancy rates have been published. A 2007 Cochrane review of 13 randomized controlled trials comparing ultrasound versus "clinical touch" concluded that ultrasound did increase live birth and ongoing clinical pregnancy rates (452/1,376 vs. 353/1,338, OR 1.40, 95% CI 1.18–1.66, $P<0.0001$) [25]. Three other recent meta-analyses of randomized controlled trials have shown similar findings [18, 26, 27]. However, the quality of most of the studies to date have been limited due to inadequate randomization, low power, and nonstandardized reporting of outcomes. Several recent studies with improved methodology have shown little or no benefit with ultrasound, including an RCT of 300 women and a single clinician [28] and another RCT of 387 oocyte donor cycles [22, 29]. Ultrasound has also been associated with fewer ectopic pregnancies in several RCTs, [22, 29, 30] though other studies have shown no effect [22, 28, 31]. Other clinical investigators have tried to extend the method by using 3D/4D ultrasound [32, 33] or vaginal ultrasound [34] with encouraging results.

Occasionally, intrauterine fluid is detected on ultrasound at the time of embryo transfer, particularly in patients with a hydrosalpinx or caesarean section scar. In the case of a hydrosalpinx, cryopreservation of the embryos for future transfer after removal or proximal obstruction of the hydrosalpinx is likely beneficial [35]. Though aspiration of this fluid is an option, it is unlikely to be of any benefit due to the likelihood of reaccumulation [36, 37]. It is not clear if aspiration provides any benefit when this fluid originates from a caesarean section scar.

45.4 Preparing the Patient

Analgesia or anesthesia for transcervical embryo transfer is not necessary in most cases. However, some centers advocate the routine or occasional use of a benzodiazepine, such as diazepam. Use of other medications has been suggested as a way to reduce uterine contractility, such as progesterone, b-mimetics, antiprostaglandins, and nitric oxide. Limited data exists regarding the benefit of such measures. To date, only progesterone has shown any uterus-relaxing effect [38].

Historically, the position of the uterus dictated the position of the patient during transfer to bring the uterine fundus into a dependent level. The knee-chest position was used for an anteverted uterus, and the dorsal position for the retroverted uterus. Today, we generally place all patients in the dorsal lithotomy position regardless of uterine position as this does not appear to affect pregnancy rates [39]. As the procedure is not necessarily a sterile one, it may be done in clinic or in an operating room.

Pelvic infection is an uncommon complication of IVF despite the invasive nature of oocyte retrieval and embryo transfer [40]. However, subclinical infection of the endometrium from the transfer procedure has been implicated as a possible cause for failure to implant. Positive cultures from the cervix or catheter have been associated with diminished pregnancy rates [41, 42]. In a study of 110 women, cultures were positive from cervical mucus in 71% of patients, and the catheter tip in 49% of patients. These patients had a clinical pregnancy rate of 29.6% compared to 57.1% in patients with negative cultures [41]. Cleaning the cervical mucus with saline may reduce bacterial contamination to some extent. Vaginal antiseptics are not recommended at embryo transfer due to potential toxicity to the embryos. Use of antibiotics prior to ET has been suggested but has not been shown to increase pregnancy rates [43]. Due to the lack of proven benefit as well as the potential to disrupt normal cervical flora and result in an inflammatory response, antibiotics are currently not recommended for embryo transfer. Systemic antimicrobials at the time of retrieval as well as an antimicrobial in the culture media are routinely used, however. Antibiotics at the time of retrieval are associated with a reduction in positive cultures of catheter tips at transfer with significantly higher implantation and pregnancy rates [44].

Cervical mucus can be responsible for plugging the tip of the catheter which may interfere with delivery of the embryos inside the uterine cavity. Embryos may also adhere to the mucus around the catheter and be inadvertently displaced during catheter withdrawal. Cervical mucus can be removed with a sterile cotton ball or gauze soaked in saline or transfer medium. Additional mucus from the cervical canal can be aspirated using a sterile syringe attached to a transfer catheter. Use of a cytobrush to remove endocervical mucus has also been described [45]. Removal of cervical mucus was associated with increased clinical pregnancy rates in one prospective controlled trial [46], but this effect was not significant in another RCT [47]. Vigorous flushing of the cervix has also yielded mixed results [48, 49].

45.5 Preparing the Catheter

A variety of embryo transfer catheters are commercially available today. The ideal ET catheter is soft enough to avoid trauma to the endocervix or endometruim but malleable enough to be directed into the uterine cavity along its natural contour. Firm catheters may facilitate placement, particularly in difficult transfers, but can be associated with more bleeding, trauma, and stimulation of uterine contractions. With the widespread use of ultrasound for embryo transfer, several echogenic catheters are now available, in which the tip or the entire catheter are easily visualized on ultrasound.

Several studies have compared different types of transfer catheters, but the issue of catheter type is still a controversial one. In general, "soft" catheters, such as the Cook (Cook Ob/Gyn, Inc. Bloomington, IN) and the Wallace catheters (Marlow Technologies, Willoughby, OH), are preferred to "firm" ones such as the TDT (metal obturator) (Laboratoire CCD, Paris, France), Frydman (Laboratoire CCD), Tomcat (Kendell Health Care, Hampshire, MA), Tefcat (Kendell Health Care), and Rocket ET catheters (Rocket Medical, Watford, UK) because they are less likely to induce cervical and endometrial lacerations [3, 50, 51]. In two recent meta-analyses of randomized controlled trials, the use of soft catheters was associated with a higher pregnancy rate than firm catheters [52, 53]. Ultrasound monitoring during IUI demonstrated disrupted endometrium in 50% of patients when a Tomcat catheter was used compared to 12.5% with a Wallace catheter [54]. Hysteroscopic studies also suggest that there is less trauma after mock transfer when soft catheters are used [55]. The pregnancy rates among various soft catheters have not been shown to be significantly different [56–60].

While a difficult transfer may require a firm catheter, the rigid outer sheath of a soft catheter can also be bent to align the catheter to the uterine axis. Though cannulation of the cervix to negotiate a difficult internal os has not been shown to decrease pregnancy rates, [61] this outer sheath should be used minimally and, if possible, stopped short of the internal os to avoid any release of prostaglandins.

Typically, a column of fluid totaling about 20 μl surrounds the embryo in the catheter with most of this fluid proximal to the embryo to increase the chance of embryo expulsion. Transfer volumes >60 μl may result in expulsion of the embryos into the vagina, [62] while volumes <10 μl may also negatively affect implantation rates [63]. The embryo-containing medium is often bracketed by air. The use of air bubbles in the catheter has not been shown to affect pregnancy or implantation rates [64], nor in the extrusion of fluid within [2]. Nevertheless, the air fluid interface is easily visualized on ultrasound and is therefore a useful tool in an ultrasound-guided transfer.

Commercial media are primarily made up of various concentrations of ions, amino acids, and carbohydrates. The concentration of protein and the viscosity of the transfer medium have not been shown to affect outcome [65, 66]. A fibrin sealant added to the medium has been studied in two RCTs, one study showing a nonsignificant improvement in pregnancy rate and the second showing a benefit in older patients [67, 68]. Recently, hyaluronan, a glycosaminoglycan found throughout the female reproductive tract, has been used in transfer medium as several of its properties suggest a beneficial effect on early embryo development and implantation. In a recent RCT of 1,282 patients, use of hyaluronan-enriched transfer medium (HETM, EmbryoGlue; Vitrolife, Englewood, CO, USA) significantly improved clinical pregnancy rates (54.6% vs. 48.5%, OR 1.28) and implantation rates (32% vs. 25%, OR 1.43) [69]. However, no significant benefit in pregnancy or implantation rates was shown in another RCT of 815 patients [70]. A recent RCT of 101 patients with >4 previous transfer failures showed increased ongoing pregnancy rates (31.3% vs. 4.0%, $p=0.0005$) with hyaluronan, suggesting that it may provide benefit in a select group of patients [71].

45.6 Depositing the Embryos

Traditionally, the tip of the catheter has been placed 5–10 mm from the uterine fundus [72]. However, several recent studies suggest that transfer further from the fundus, may be more ideal. In an RCT performed in patients undergoing UGET, a higher pregnancy rate (60% vs. 39.3%) was achieved when the distance was 15–20 mm as compared to 10 mm [73]. Other studies that have shown that embryos deposited less than 5 mm from the fundus have a decreased pregnancy rate and an increased ectopic pregnancy rate [6, 23, 74–76]. Some have suggested that the desired location should take into account the length of the cavity rather than be a fixed reference point, such as the distance from the fundus [77]. In a prospective cohort study, clinical pregnancy rates increased with ET directed at the lower to middle uterine segment. Another RCT showed that clinical pregnancy or implantation rates were similar in the upper and lower uterus, but significantly improved closer to the mid-portion of the uterus [78].

After injection of the embryos, pressure on the plunger of the syringe should be maintained until the catheter is completely withdrawn from the uterus. Furthermore, the outer sheath should be completely retracted and removed simultaneously with the inner catheter to avoid a "plunger" effect. Withdrawing the catheter slowly will also minimize negative pressure. Some authors suggest waiting before removing the catheter so that the uterus can become stabilized, whereas others report good results with immediate withdrawal. In a randomized controlled trial of 100 women, a 30 s delay before catheter withdrawal did not significantly increase pregnancy rates (60.8% and 69.4%) [79].

The time interval from loading the ET catheter to depositing the embryos in the uterus should be minimized, as embryos may be vulnerable to exposure to the environmental temperature, light, or other agents in the catheter. A longer time interval has been shown to lower pregnancy and implantation rates with an interval of more than 120 s carrying a poor prognosis [80]. However, the significance of this factor is unclear, as another study, limited to good quality embryos, showed no effect of the duration of the procedure on the outcome, with transfers lasting up to 7.5 min [81].

45.7 After the Procedure

Following the transfer, the catheter should be handed to the embryologist to be flushed and inspected for retained embryos. Any retained embryos should be properly reloaded for transfer into the uterus. This event can often cause concern for patients. However, they should be reassured that the effect of retained embryos in the transfer catheter on pregnancy outcome is likely minimal. While one study reported lower pregnancy rates (3% vs. 20.3%) when retained embryos were identified and retransferred, [4] two more recent studies did not show a difference [9, 82].

Historically, patients have been placed on bed rest for varied amounts of time following the transfer, as decreased physical activity was thought to improve embryo retention within the uterine cavity. Patients were routinely rested strictly flat on their backs for 24 h. Embryo transfer subsequently became an outpatient procedure, as prolonged bed rest was shown not to improve pregnancy rates [83–85]. Even brief bed rest (30 min) has since been shown to offer no benefit over immediate ambulation (47.0% vs. 51.0%, OR 0.85, 0.39–1.85) in a randomized controlled trial of 164 patients [86]. Following the air–fluid interface on ultrasound showed that standing immediately after transfer was associated with no movement in 94% of cases, less than 1 cm of movement in 4%, and more than 4 cm of movement in 2% [23]. Intercourse during the peritransfer period also does not appear to influence pregnancy rates [87].

45.8 Alternative Methods

Transmyometrial embryo transfer is an alternative method to the conventional transcervical ET and may be useful in patients with severe cervical stenosis or history of several failed IVF cycles in which transfers were extremely difficult. Alternatively called the "Towako method," Kato et al. presented their four-year experience with this method on 1,298 cases with a 44.9% pregnancy rate in transfers with ICSI embryos. The procedure is performed using an endovaginal US probe. A special needle (K-TTET-18-32-5; William A. Cook, Queensland, Australia) with its stylet attached to the vaginal probe needle holder is inserted transmyometrially and sonographically guided into the endometrial cavity. The stylet is removed, and a transfer catheter, loaded with embryos, is passed through the needle [88]. Due to increased pain, this method should be reserved for extremely difficult transfers by conventional techniques. An alternative method for such cases would be laparoscopic zygote intrafallopian tube transfer, or ZIFT.

45.9 Number of Embryos to Transfer

Multiple births are now the greatest challenge facing infertility specialists in the United States. The dramatic rise in the birthrates of twins, triplets, and higher order multiples over the past two and a half decades is largely attributable to the growth of IVF. According to 2004 data from the CDC, 32% of pregnancies conceived by IVF procedures were multiple gestations, affecting 50% of the infants born through IVF. The rate for triplets and higher-order multiples was 6%, approximately 42 times higher than the general U.S. population [89]. With an increased awareness of the morbidity and mortality associated with multiple pregnancies, an effort has been made to reduce the contribution of ART to the multiple gestation rate in the U.S. The Society for Assisted Reproductive Technology (SART), in conjunction with the American Society for Reproductive Medicine, has published guidelines that recommended limiting the number of embryos for women with a good prognosis [90, 91] (Table 45.1). During the 5 years following the initial publication of these guidelines in 1998, the ratio of triplet and quadruplet+ births per 1,000 total births conceived by ART decreased by 45% and 61% respectively [92, 93].

The rate of twin births per 1,000 total U.S. births, however, increased by 12% over this time [92, 93]. Although much of the focus of maternal, fetal, and neonatal complications has been placed on triplets or other higher order multiple gestations, twin gestations are also associated with significantly increased morbidity and mortality [94, 95].

Table 45.1 Recommended limits on the numbers of embryos to transfer

Cleavage-state embryos				
Prognosis	Age <35	Age 35–37	Age 38–40	Age >40
Favorable	1–2	2	3	5
All others	2	3	4	5
Blastocysts				
Prognosis	Age <35	Age 35–37	Age 38–40	Age >40
Favorable	1	2	2	3
All others	2	2	3	3

Favorable = First cycle of IVF, good embryo quality, excess embryos available for cryopreservation, or previous successful IVF cycle

ASRM Practice Committee. Guidelines on number of embryos transferred. Fertil Steril 2006

Twins have been found to have an increased incidence of low birth weight, premature delivery, stillbirth, cerebral palsy, and perinatal mortality, compared to singletons [94, 96]. IVF twins have also been found to have a higher frequency of NICU admissions, surgical interventions, and special needs than IVF singletons [94]. The mother of a twin gestation is also at increased risk for hypertension of pregnancy, placental abruption, postpartum hemorrhage, delivery by caesarean section, and maternal mortality [94, 95].

Twin pregnancies place a huge financial burden on our health care system. The estimated charges associated with a twin delivery are close to $40,000 compared to $10,000 for a singleton delivery [97, 98]. These costs do not include the cost associated with infertility treatment, outpatient obstetric management, maternal admissions before delivery, and loss of work from hospitalizations or home bed rest. Other less studied outcomes are the difficulties that families face when dealing with multiple births, which can pose significant parenting, marital, and social challenges [95, 99–101].

In the early years of IVF, poor implantation rates necessitated transfer of multiple embryos to achieve an acceptable pregnancy rate. Even today, there is substantial pressure on IVF programs as well as patients to maximize success rates by transferring more embryos. However, recent advancements have improved pregnancy and implantation rates, allowing us to limit the number of embryos to transfer while maintaining pregnancy rates. Improved IVF success rates are now steering many practitioners toward single embryo transfer in good prognosis couples in an effort to lower the twin gestation rate. Furthermore, the most recent SART/ASRM guidelines regarding embryo number for transfer reflect their support of this strategy (Table 45.1) [91]. However, implementation of this practice in the U.S. has been difficult due to concerns about a reduced pregnancy rate and patient dissatisfaction.

Addressing the effect of single embryo transfers on pregnancy rates, several prospective randomized trials have compared transfer of a single embryo with transfer of two embryos, primarily in Scandinavian centers. These trials demonstrated that transferring in a single day two or three embryos resulted in a lower pregnancy rate than transferring two embryos (Table 45.2) [102–106]. However, the difference in pregnancy rates was generally small, and cumulative pregnancy rates were often equivalent when single cryopreserved embryo transfers were taken into account. Thus, a similar pregnancy rate can be achieved by transferring one embryo in the fresh cycle and one additional embryo in the frozen cycle, as compared to placing two embryos in the fresh cycle. This strategy leads to marked reductions in twinning rates, from 30% to 50% with two embryos to less than 5% with single embryo transfer (Table 45.2) [102–106].

Transferring a single blastocyst can result in even higher pregnancy rates due to the improved ability to select a healthy embryo with a high implantation rate [107]. A prospective randomized trial reported a 61% pregnancy rate with transfer of a single blastocyst compared to a 76% pregnancy rate with transfer of two blastocysts, a nonsignificant difference. However, no twins occurred with transfer of one blastocyst versus a 47% twinning rate after transfer of two [105]. Several observational trials have also shown that elective transfer of a single blastocyst can result in ongoing pregnancy rates between 40% and 76% (Table 45.3) [108–110].

Table 45.2 Single versus double embryo transfer: prospective, randomized trials

			SET (Ongoing PR)		DET (Ongoing)		Cumulative PR	
Author	Country	Day of ET	Delivery rate	Twin rate	Delivery rate	Twin rate	SET	DET
Martikainen	Finland	2	22/74 (30%)	5%	28/70 (40%)	39%*	47%	59%
Gerris	Belgium	2 or 3	10/26 (38%)	5%	20/27 (74%)*	30%*		
Thurin	Sweden Norway Denmark	2	91/330 (28%)	1%	142/331 (43%)*	34%*	39%	43%
Gardner	USA	5	14/23 (61%)	0	19/25 (76%)	47%*		
Lukassen	Netherlands	3	14/54 (26%)	0	19/53 (36%)	37%*	41%	36%

*$p \leq 0.05$

Table 45.3 Observational trials of single blastocyst transfers

		SET		DET		Cumulative PR	
Author	Country	Pregnancy rate	Twin rate	Pregnancy rate	Twin rate	SET	DET
Henman	Australia	50/121 (41%)	2%	152/285 (53%)	44%*	65%	64%
Criniti	USA	31/41 (76%)	3%	52/66 (79%)	62%*	83%	83%
Ryan	USA	51/77 (66%)	2%	116/183 (63%)	41%*	80%	N/A

*$p \leq 0.05$

Admittedly, patients having a single embryo transfer are likely a select group with a good prognosis for pregnancy.

Given this information, our program has adopted a policy that mandates good prognosis patients to have only a single blastocyst transferred [110]. Specifically, women less than the age of 38 who have never failed a previous IVF cycle, and who have a good or excellent embryo to transfer [111], will have only a single blastocyst transferred. We have found that educating patients about the risks of multiple gestations and our rationale for limiting embryo number prior to the start of their cycle, increases their receptiveness to this policy. Studies have shown that 30% of IVF patients consider twins the most ideal outcome, and this desire was associated with a lack of knowledge about the adverse outcomes associated with a twin gestation [112–117]. Important components of this program are patient education, high blastocyst implantation rates, and a successful cryopreservation program, allowing for the successful transfer of any additional blastocysts at a later time. Cumulative pregnancy rates (fresh and frozen cycles from one retrieval) have exceeded 80% in our program for women who qualify for single blastocyst transfer [110].

National data from Scandinavian countries that have emphasized single embryo transfer for many years has demonstrated markedly reduced multiple birth rates while maintaining pregnancy rates from IVF. In 2003, Swedish law required single embryo transfer for all women up to the age of 38 in the first two IVF treatment cycles when one good quality embryo was available, resulting in single embryo transfers in greater than 70% of women this age. While multiple birth rates dropped from nearly 25 to 5%, national delivery rates per cycle were maintained. Single embryo transfer is now the norm in Sweden and is widely accepted by both patients and physicians [118, 119]. This type of national data is encouraging for a wider application of single embryo transfer in the United States. However, physician endorsement of this policy will be necessary.

45.10 Blastocyst Versus Cleavage Stage Embryo Transfer

Prolonged culture of embryos to the blastocyst stage offers several theoretical advantages. Embryos that develop to the blastocyst stage have been shown to have a lower rate of aneuploidy [120]. In addition, temporal synchronization between the blastocyst embryo and the endometrium is improved and better simulates in vivo conditions. On the other hand, prolonged culture extends the time that the embryo is in an unnatural environment. Blastocyst formation rates have ranged from 28% to nearly 50% in various series [121], which necessitates increasing the number of embryos for culture to ensure survival of a blastocyst for transfer [91]. Occasionally, patients with few embryos will have nothing for transfer after prolonged cultured to the blastocyst stage. Thus, many programs restrict blastocyst transfer to patients with a good prognosis, as determined by ovarian stimulation or embryo formation.

A meta-analysis of trials comparing day 2 and day 3 embryo transfers with blastocyst transfers found no significantly different live birth rates (OR 1.03, 95% CI 0.74–1.44), despite a higher implantation rate with blastocyst embryos (33% vs. 26%) [122]. This was likely the result of a higher number of women randomized to extended culture having no blastocysts to transfer. A recent prospective randomized study of good prognosis patients found a higher embryo implantation rate and a higher live birth rate when a single blastocyst was transferred, compared to a single cleavage stage embryo [107]. Thus, good prognosis couples of a younger age and with more embryos may benefit from blastocyst transfer, particularly if a single embryo is to be transferred. Of concern is the finding in some studies that blastocyst transfers result in a higher rate of monozygotic twinning [123–125]. Because of the higher implantation rates and the risk of monozygotic twinning, practitioners should be particularly cautious about transferring multiple blastocysts.

45.11 Summary: Evidence-based guidelines

1. "Difficult" transfers are associated with lower pregnancy rates with IVF.
2. Ultrasound guidance will result in easier transfers with improved outcomes.
3. Soft catheters should be used when feasible.
4. Single embryo transfers reduce the rate of twin gestations.

Recommendations based on expert opinion

1. Trial transfers allow better preparation for difficult transfers.
2. Cervical mucus should be removed to potentially decrease bacterial contamination and mucus plugging of the catheter.
3. Embryos should be deposited 1–2 cm from the uterine fundus.
4. Negative pressure should be minimized during withdrawal of the catheter.
5. The procedure should be done in a minimum amount of time.
6. IVF patients should be counseled on the obstetrical risks associated with multiple gestations.

References

1. Englert Y, Puissant F, Camus M, Van Hoeck J, Leroy F (1986) Clinical study on embryo transfer after human in vitro fertilization. J In Vitro Fert Embryo Transf 3:243
2. Mansour R, Aboulghar M, Serour G (1990) Dummy embryo transfer: a technique that minimizes the problems of embryo transfer and improves the pregnancy rate in human in vitro fertilization. Fertil Steril 54:678–681
3. Wood EG, Batzer FR, Go KJ, Gutmann JN, Corson SL (2000) Ultrasound-guided soft catheter embryo transfers will improve pregnancy rates in in-vitro fertilization. Hum Reprod 15: 107–112
4. Visser DS, Fourie FL, Kruger HF (1993) Multiple attempts at embryo transfer: effects on pregnancy outcome in an in vitro fertilization and embryo transfer program. J Assist Reprod Genet 10:37–43
5. Tomas C, Tikkinen K, Tuomivaaara L, Tapanqinen JS, Martikainen H (2002) The Degree of difficulty of embryo transfer is an independent factor for predicting pregnancy. Hum Reprod 17:2632
6. Lesny P, Killick SR, Tetlow RL, Robinson J, Maguiness SD (1998) Embryo transfer-can we learn anything new from the observation of junctional zone contractions. Hum Reprod 13(6):1540–1546
7. Fanchin R, Righini C, Olivennes F, Taylor S, de Ziegler D, Frydman R (1998) Uterine contractions at the time of embryo transfer alter pregnancy rates after in vitro fertilization. Hum Reprod 13:1968–1974
8. Dorn C, Reinsberg J, Schlebusch H, Prietl G, van der Ven H, Krebs D (1999) Serum oxytocin concentration during embryo transfer procedure. Eur J Obstet Gynecol Reprod Biol 87(1):77–80
9. Goudas VT, Hammitt DG, Damario MA, Session DR, Singh AP, Dumesic DA (1998) Blood on the embryo transfer catheter is associate with decreased rates of embryo implantation and clinical pregnancy with the use of invitro fertilization-embryo transfer. Fertil Steril 70(5):878–882
10. Lass A, Abusheikha N, Brinsden P, Kovacs GT (1999) The effect of a difficult embryo transfer on the outcome of IVF. Hum Reprod 14:2417
11. Garzo VG (2006) Embryo transfer technique. Clin Obstet Gynecol 49(1):117–122
12. Groutz A, Lessing JB, Wolf Y, Azem F, Yovel I, Amit A (1997) Comparison of transmyometrial and trasncervical embryo transfer in patients with previously failed in vitro fertilization-embryo transfer cycles and/or cervical stenosis. Fertil Steril 67(6):1073–1076
13. Yanushpolsky EH, Ginsburg ES, Fox JH, Stewart EA (2000) Transcervical placement of a Malecot catheter after hysteroscopic evaluation provides for easier entry into the endometrial cavity for women with histories of difficult intrauterine inseminations and/or embryo transfers: a prospective case series. Fertil Steril 73(2):402–405
14. Glatstein IZ, Pang SC, McShane PM (1997) Successful pregnancies with the use of laminaria tents before embryo transfer for refractory cervical stenosis. Fertil Steril 67(6):1172–1174
15. Neithardt AB, Segars JH, Hennessy S, James AN, McKeeby JL (2005) Embryo afterloading: a refinement in embryo transfer technique that may increase clinical pregnancy. Fertil Steril 83(3):710–714
16. Henne MB, Milki AA (2004) Uterine position at real embryo transfer compared with mock embryo transfer. Hum Reprod 19:570
17. Katariya KO, Bates GW, Robinson RD, Arthur NJ, Propst AM (2007) Does the timing of mock embryo transfer affect in vitro fertilization implantation and pregnancy rates? Fertil Steril 88(5):1462–1464
18. Sundrstrom P, Wramsby H, Person PH, Liedhom P (1984) Filled bladder simplifies human embryo transfer. Br J Obstet Gynecol 91:506–507
19. Lewin A, Schenker JG, Avrech O, Shapira S, Safran A, Friedler S (1997) The role of uterine straightening by passive bladder distension before embryo transfer in IVF cycles. J Assist Reprod Genet 14:32–34
20. Oorusso F, Depalo R, Bettocchi S, Vacca M, Vimercati A, Selvaggi L (2005) Outcome of in vitro fertilization after transabdominal ultrasound-assisted embryo transfer with a full or empty bladder. Fert Steril 84(4):1046–1048
21. Martins A, Baruffi R, Mauri A, Petersen C, Oliveira J, Contart P, Pontes A, Franco J Jr (2004) Ultrasound guidance is not necessary during easy embryo transfers. J Assist Reprod Genet 21(12):421–425
22. Garcia-Velasco J, Isaza V, Martinez-Salazar J, Landazabal A, Requena A, Remohi J, Pellicer A, Simon C (2002) Transabdominal ultrasound guided embryo transfer does not increase pregnancy rates in ooctye recipients. Fertil Steril 78(3):534–539
23. Woolcott R, Stanger J (1997) Potentially important variables identified by transvaginal ultrasound-guided embryo transfer. Hum Reprod 12(5):963–966
24. Strickler RC, Christianson C, Crane JP, Curato A, Knight AB, Yang V (1985) Ultrasound guidance for human embryo transfer. Fertil Steril 43:54–61
25. Brown JA, Buckingham K, Abou-Setta A, Buckett W (2007) Ultrasound versus "clinical touch" for catheter guidance during embryo transfer in women. Cochrane Database of Syst Rev (1) http://www.cochrane.org/reviews/en/ab006107.htmlAccessed 24 Jan, 2007
26. Buckett WM (2003) A meta-analysis of ultrasound-guided versus clinical touch embryo transfer. Fertil Steril 80:1037–1041
27. Abou-Setta AM, Mansour RT, Al-Inany HG, Aboulghar MM, Aboulghar MA, Serour GI (2007) Among women undergoing embryo transfer, is the probability of pregnancy and live birth improved with ultrasound guidance over clinical touch alone? A systemic review and meta-analysis of prospective randomized trials. Fertil Steril 88(2):333–341
28. Kosmas IP, Janssens R, De Munch L, Al Turki A, Van Der Elst J, Tournaye H, Devroey P (2007) Ultrasound-guided embryo transfer does not offer any benefit in clinical outcome: a randomized controlled trial. Hum Reprod 22(5):1327–1334
29. Tang OS, Ng EH, So WW, Ho PC (2001) Ultrasound-guided embryo transfer: a prospective randomized controlled trial. Hum Reprod 16:2310–2315
30. Sallam HN, Sadek S (2003) Ultrasound-guided embryo transfer: a meta-analysis of randomized controlled trials. Fertil Steril 80(4):1042–1046
31. Matorras R, Urguijo E, Mendoza R, Corcostegui B, Exposito A, Rodriguez-Escudero FJ (2002) Ultrasound-guided embryo transfer improves pregnancy rates and increases the frequency of easy transfers. Hum Reprod 17(7):1762–1766
32. Gergely R, DeUgarte CM, Danzer H, Surrey M, Hill D, DeCherney AH (2005) Three dimensional/four dimensional ultrasound-guided embryo transfer using the maximal implantation potential point. Fertil Steril 84(2):500–503
33. Baba K, Ishihara O, Hayashi N, Saitoh M, Taya J, Kinoshita K (2000) Three-dimensional ultrasound in embryo transfer. Ultrasound Obstet Gynecol 16:372–373
34. Johnson NP, Mak W, Sowter MC (2004) Surgical treatment for tubal disease in women due to undergo in vitro fertilization. Cochrane Database Syst Rev (3):CD002125
35. Anderson RE, Nugent NL, Gregg AT, Nunn SL, Behr BR (2002) Transvaginal ultrasound-guided embryo transfer improves outcome in patients with previous failed in vitro fertilization cycles. Fertil Steril 77:769–775

36. Hinckley MD, Milki AA (2003) Rapid reaccumulation of hydrometra after drainage at embryo transfer in patients with hydrosalpinx. Fertil Steril 80:1268–1271
37. Hofmann GE, Warikoo P, Jacobs W (2003) Ultrasound detection of pyometra at the time of embryo transfer after ovum retrieval for in vitro fertilization. Fertil Steril 80:637–638
38. Fanchin R, Righini C, Ziegler D, Olivennes F, Ledee N, Frydman R (2001) Effects of vaginal progesterone administration on uterine contractility at the time of embryo transfer. Fertil Steril 75(6):1136–1140
39. Egbase PE, Al-Sharhan M, Grudzinskas JG (2000) Influence of position and length of uterus on implantation and clinical pregnancy rates in IVF and embryo transfer treatment cycles. Hum Reprod 15(9):1943–1946
40. Sowerby E, Parsons J (2004) Prevention of iatrogenic pelvic infection during in vitro fertilization – current practice in the UK. Hum Fertil 7:135–140
41. Egbase PE, al-Sharhan M, al-Othman S, al-Mutawa M, Udo EE, Grudzinskas J (1996) Incidence of microbial growth from the tip of the embryo transfer catheter after embryo transfer in relation to clinical pregnancy rate following in-vitro fertilization and embryo transfer. Hum Reprod 11(8):1687–1689
42. Moore DE, Soules MR, Klein NA, Fujimoto VY, Agnew KJ, Eschenbach DA (2000) Bacteria in the transfer catheter tip influence the live-birth rate after in vitro fertilization. Fertil Steril 74(6):1118–1124
43. Brook N, Khalaf Y, Coomarasamy A, Edgeworth J, Braude P (2006) A randomized controlled trial of prophylactic antibiotics (co-amoxiclav) prior to embryo transfer. Hum Reprod 21(11):2911–2915
44. Egbase PE, Edo E, Al-Sharhan M, Grudzinskas P (1999) Prophylactic antibiotics and endocervical microbial inoculation of the endometrium at embryo transfer. Lancet 354(9179): 651–652
45. Michael E, Ahmady A (2005) The use of a cytobursh in cervical canal preparation for embryo transfer procedures. Fertil Steril 84:S357
46. Eskandar MA, Abou-setta AM, El-Amin M, Almushait MA, Sobande AA (2007) Removal of cervical mucus prior to embryo transfer improves pregnancy rates in women undergoing assisted reproduction. Reprod Biomed Online 14(3):308–313
47. Visschers BA, Bots RS, Peeters MF, Mol BW, van Dessel JH (2007) Removal of cervical mucus: effect on pregnancy rates in IVF/ICSI. Reprod Biomed Online 15(3):310–315
48. McNamee P, Huang T, Carwile A (1998) Significant increase in pregnancy rates achieved by vigorous irrigation of endocervical mucus prior to embryo transfer with a Wallace catheter in an IVF-ET program. Fertil Steril 70(S1):S228
49. Glass KB, Green CA, Fluker MR et al (2000) Multicenter randomized trial of cervical irrigation at the time of embryo transfer. Fertil Steril 74(S1):S31
50. McDonald JA, Norman RJ (2002) A randomized controlled trial of a soft double lumen embryo transfer catheter versus a firm single lumen catheter: significant improvements in pregnancy rates. Hum Reprod 17(6):1502–1506
51. Sallam HN, Agameya AF, Rahman AF et al (2003) Impact of technical difficulties, choice of catheter, and the presence of blood on the success of embryo transfer: experience from a single provider. J Assist Reprod Genet 20:135–142
52. Abou-Setta AM, Al-Inany HG, Mansour RT, Serour GI, Aboulghar MA (2005) Soft versus firm embryo transfer catheters for assisted reproduction: a systematic review and meta-analysis. Hum Reprod 20(11):3114–3121
53. Buckett W (2006) A review and meta-analysis of prospective trials comparing different catheters used for embryo transfer. Fertil Steril 85(3):728–734
54. Lavie O, Margalioth EJ, Geva-Eldar T, Ben-Chetrit A (1997) Ultrasonographic endometrial changes after intrauterine insemination: a comparison of two catheters. Fertil Steril 68:731–734
55. Marconi G, Vilela M, Bello J et al (2003) Endometrial lesions caused by catheters used for embryo transfers: a preliminary report. Fertil Steril 80:363–367
56. Al-Shawaf T, Dave R, Harper J et al (1993) Transfer of embryos into the uterus: how much do technical factors affect pregnancy rates? J Assist Reprod Genet 10:31–36
57. Ghazzawi IM, Al-Hasani S, Karaki R, Souso S (1999) Transfer technique and catheter choice influence the incidence of transcervical embryo expulsion and the outcome of IVF. Hum Reprod 14:677–682
58. Urman B, Aksoy S, Slatas C et al (2000) Comparing two embryo transfer catheters. Use of a trial transfer to determine the catheter applied. J reprod Med 45:135–138
59. Burke LM, Davenport AT, Russell GB, Deaton JL (2000) Predictors of success after embryo transfer; experience from a single provider. Am J Obstet Gynecol 182:1001–1004
60. Saldeen P, Abou-Etta A, Bergh T, Sundstrom P, Holte J (2008) A prospective randomized controlled trial comparing two embryo transfer catheters in an ART program. Fertil Steril 90(3):599–603
61. Silberstein t, Weitzen S, Franfurter D, Trimarchi FR, Keefe DL, Plosker SM (2004) Cannulation of a resistant internal os with the malleable outer sheath of a coaxial soft embryo transfer catheter does not affect in vitro fertilization-embryo transfer outcome. Fertil Steril 82:1402–1406
62. Poindexter AN, Thompson DJ, Gibbons WE, Findley WE, Dodson MG, Young RL (1986) Residual embryos in failed embryo transfer. Fertil Steril 46(2):262–267
63. Ebner T, Yaman C, Moser M, Sommergruber M, Polz W, Tews G (2001) The ineffective loading process of the embryo transfer catheter alters implantation and pregnancy rates. Fertil Steril 76(3):630–632
64. Moreno V, Balasch J, Vidal E et al (2004) Air in the transfer catheter does not affect the success of embryo transfer. Fertil Steril 81:1366–1370
65. Khan I, Staessen C, Devroey P, Van Steirteghem AC (1991) Human serum albumin versus serum: a comparative study on embryo transfer medium. Fertil Steril 56:98–101
66. Menezo Y, Arnal F, Humeau C, Ducret L, Nicollet B (1989) Increased viscosity in transfer medium does not improve the pregnancy rates after embryo transfer. Fertil Steril 52:680–682
67. Feichtinger W, Strohmer H, Radner KH, Goldin M (1992) The use of fibrin sealant for ET: development and clinical studies. Hum Reprod 7:890–893
68. Ben-Rafael Z, Ashkenazi J, Shelef M et al (1995) The use of fibrin sealant in in vitro fertilization and embryo transfer. Int J Fertil Menopausal Stud 40:303–306
69. Urman B, Yakin K, Ata B, Isiklar A, Balaban B (2008) Effect of hyaluronan-enriched transfer medium on omplantation and pregnancy rates after day 3 and day 5 transfers: a prospective randomized study. Fertil Steril 90(3):604–612
70. Karimian L, Rezazadeh VM, Baghestani AR, Moeini A (2004) A prospective randomized comparison of two commercial embryo transfer medium in IVF/ICSI cycles. Hum Reprod 19(Supp 1):i52
71. Friedler S, Schacter M, Strassburger D, Esther K, Ron El R, Raziel A (2007) A randomized clinical trial comparing recombinant hyaluronan/recombinant albumin versus human tubal fluid for cleavage stage embryo transfer in patients with multiple IVF-embryo transfer failure. Hum Reprod 22(9):2444–2448
72. Jones HW (1998) In vitro fertilization. In Behrman SJ, Kistner RW, Patton GW (eds) Progress in Infertility, 3rd edn. Little, Brown and Co., Boston, pp 543–561
73. Coroleu B, Barri PN, Carreras O et al (2002) The influence of the depth of the embryo replacement into the uterine cavity on implantation

rates after IVF: a controlled, ultrasound-guided study. Hum Reprod 17:341–346
74. Pope CD, Cook EK, Arny M et al (2004) Influence of embryo transfer depth on in vitro-fertilization and embryo transfer outcomes. Fertil Steril 81:51–58
75. Yovich JL, Turner SR, Murphy AJ (1985) Embryo transfer technique as a cause of extopic pregnancies in in vitro fertilization. Fertil Steril 44:318–321
76. Nazari A, Askari HA, Check JH, O'Shaughnessy A (1993) Embryo transfer technique as a cause of ectopic pregnancy in in vitro fertilization. Fertil Steril 60:919–921
77. Frankfurter D, Trimarchi JB, Silva CP, Keefe DL (2004) Middle to lower uterine segment embryo transfer improves implanation and pregnancy rates compared with fundal embryo transfer. Fertil Steril 81:1273–1277
78. Franco JG Jr, Martins AM, Baruffi RL et al (2004) Best site for ET: the upper or lower half of endometrial cavity? Hum Reprod 19:1785–1790
79. Martinez F, Coroleu B, Parriego M, Carreras O, Belil I, Parera N, Hereter L, Buxaderas R, Barri P (2001) Ultrasound-guided embryo transfer: immediate withdrawal of the catheter versus a 30 s wait. Hum Reprod 16(5):871–874
80. Matorras R, Mendosa R, Exposito A, Rodriguez-Escudero FJ (2004) Influence of the time interval between embryo catheter loading and discharging on the success of IVF. Hum Reprod 19:2027–2030
81. Ciray HN, Tosum S, Hacifazlioglu O, Mesut A, Bahceci M (2007) Prolonged duration of transfer does not affect outcome in cycles with good embryo quality. Fertil Steril 87(5):1218–1221
82. Nabi A, Awonuga A, Birch H, Barlow S, Stewart B (1997) Multiple attempts at embryo transfer: does this affect in-vitro fertilization treatment outcome? Hum Reprod 12(6):1188–1190
83. Sharif K, Afnan M, Lashen H et al (1998) Is bed rest following et necessary? Fertil Steril 69:478–481
84. Botta G, Grudzinskas G (1997) Is a prolonged bed rest following embryo transfer useful? Hum Reprod 12:2489–2492
85. Amarin ZO, Obeidat BR (2004) Bed rest versus free mobilization following ET: a prospective randomized study. BJOG 111:1273–1276
86. Purcell KJ, Schembri M, Telles TL, Fujimoto VY, Cedars MI (2007) Bed rest after embryo transfer: a randomized controlled trial. Fertil Steril 87(6):322–326
87. Tremellen KP, Valbuena D, Landeras J et al (2000) The effect of intercourse on pregnancy rates during assisted human reproduction. Hum Reprod 15:2653–2658
88. Kato O, Takatsuka R, Asch RH (1993) Transvaginal-transmyometrial embryo transfer: the Towako method; experiences of 104 cases. Fertil Steril 59(1):51–53
89. CDC (2006) 2004 Assisted reproductive technology success rates. In: Center for Disease Control and Prevention (ed) US Department of Health and Human Services, Atlanta, GA
90. American Society for Reproductive Medicine (1998) Guidelines on number of embryos transferred. A practice committee report. American society for Reproductive Medicine, Birmingham, AL
91. The Practice Committee of the Society for Assisted Reproductive Technology and the Practice Committee of the American Society for Reproductive Medicine (2006) Guidelines on number of embryos transferred. Fertil Steril 86(Suppl 4):S51–S52
92. Dickey R (2007) The relative contribution of assisted reproductive technologies and ovulation induction to multiple births in the United States 5 years after the Soceity for Assisted reproductive Technology/American Society for Reproductive Medicine recommendation to limit the number of embryos transferred. Fertil Steril 88(6):15541561
93. Jain T, Missmer SA, Hornstein MD (2004) Trends in embryo-transfer practice and in outcomes of the use of assisted reproductive technology in the United States. N Engl J Med 350:1639–1645
94. Pinborg A, Loft A, Schmidt L, Anderson AN (2003) Morbidity in a Danish national cohort of 472 IVF/ICSI twins, 1132 non-IVF-ICSI twins and 634 IVF/ICSI singletons: health-related and social implications for the children and their families. Hum Reprod 18:1234–1243
95. Pinborg A (2005) IVF/ICSI twin pregnancies: risks and prevention. Hum Reprod Update 11:575–593
96. Scher AI, Petterson B, Blair E, Ellenberg JH, Grether JK, Haan E et al (2002) The risk of mortality or cerebral palsy in twins: a collaborative population-based study. Pediatr Res 52:671–681
97. Callahan TL, Hall JE, Ettner SL, Christiansen CL, Greene MF, Crowley WF (1994) The economic impact of multiple-gestation pregnancies and the contribution of assisted-reproduction techniques to their incidence. N Engl J Med 331:244–249
98. Hidlebaugh DA, Thompson IE, Berger MJ (1997) Cost of assisted reproductive technologies for a health maintenance organization. J Reprod Med 42:570–574
99. Glazebrook C, Sheard C, Cox S, Oates M, Ndukwe G (2004) Parenting stress in first-time mothers of twins and triplets conceived after in vitro fertilization. Fertil Steril 81:505–511
100. Olivennes F, Golombok S, Ramogida C, Rust J et al (2005) Behavioral and cognitive development as well as family functioning of twins conceived by assisted reproduction: findings from a large population study. Fertil Steril 84:725–733
101. Ellison MA, Hotamisligil S, Lee H, Rich-Edwards JW, Pang SC, Hall JE (2005) Psychosocial risks associated with multiple births resulting from assisted reproduction. Fertil Steril 83: 1422–1428
102. Martikainen H, Orava M, Lakkakorpi J, Tuomivaara L (2004) Day 2 elective single embryo transfer in clinical practice: better outcome in ICSI cycles. Hum Reprod 19(6):1364–1366
103. Gerris J, De Neubourg D, Mangelschots K, Van Royen E, Vercruyssen M, Barudy-Vasquez J, Valkenburg M, Ryckaert G (2002) Elective single day 3 embryo transfer halves the twinning rate without decrease in ongoing pregnancy rate of an IVF/ICSI programme. Hum Reprod 17:2626–2631
104. Thurin A, Hausken J, Hillensjö T, Jablonowska B, Pinborg A, Strandell A et al (2004) Elective single-embryo transfer versus double-embryo transfer in in vitro fertilization. N Engl J Med 351:2392–2402
105. Gardner DK, Surrey E, Minjarez D, Leitz A, Stevens J, Schoolcraft WB (2004) Single blastocyst transfer: a prospective randomized trial. Fertil Steril 81:551–555
106. Lukassen HG, Braat DD, Wetzels AM et al (2005) Two cycles with single embryo transfer versus one cycle with double embryo transfer: a randomized controlled trial. Hum Reprod 20: 702–708
107. Papanikolaou EG, Camus M, Kolibianakis EM, Van Landuyt L, Van Steirteghem A, Devroey P (2006) In vitro fertilization with single blastocyst-stage versus single cleavage-stage embryos. N Engl J Med 354:1139–1146
108. Henman M, Catt JW, Wood T, Bowman MC, de Boer KA, Jansen RP (2005) Elective transfer of single fresh blastocysts and later transfer of cryostored blastocysts reduce the twin pregnancy rate and can improve the in vitro fertilization live birth rate in younger women. Fertil Steril 84(6):1620–1627
109. Criniti A, Thyer A, Chow G, Lin P, Klein N, Soules M (2005) Elective single blastocyst transfer reduces twin rates without compromising pregnancy rates. Fertil Steril 84(6):1613–1619
110. Ryan GL, Sparks AE, Sipe CS, Syrop CH, Dokras A, Van Voorhis BJ (2007) A mandatory single blastocyst transfer policy with educational campaign in a United States IVF program reduces multiple gestation rates without sacrificing pregnancy rates. Fertil Steril 88(2):354–360
111. Gardner DK, Schoolcraft WB (1999) In-vitro culture of human blastocysts. In: Jansen R, Mortimer D (eds) Towards reproductive

certainty: fertility and genetics beyond 1999. Parthenon, Carnforth, pp 378–388
112. Coetzee K, Stewart B, Peek J (2007) Acceptance of single-embryo transfer by patients. Fertil Steril 87(1):207–209
113. Murray S, Shetty A, Rattray A, Taylor V, Bhattacharya S (2004) A randomized comparison of alternative methods of information provision on the acceptability of elective single embryo transfer. Hum Reprod 19:911–916
114. Pinborg A, Loft A, Schmidt L, Andersen AN (2003) Attitudes of IVF/ICSI-twin mothers towards twins and single embryo transfer. Hum Reprod 18:621–627
115. Child TJ, Henderson AM, Tan SL (2004) The desire for multiple pregnancy in male and female infertility patients. Hum Reprod 19:558–561
116. Ryan GL, Zhang SH, Dokras A, Syrop CH, Van Voorhis BJ (2004) The desire of infertile patients for multiple births. Fertil Steril 81:500–504
117. Newton CR, McGride J, Feyles V, Tekpetey F, Power S (2007) Factors affecting patients' attitudes' toward single- and multiple-embryo transfer. Fertil Steril 87(2):269–278
118. Karlstrom P, Berg C (2007) Reducing the number of embryos transferred in Sweden-impact on delivery and multiple birth rates. Hum Reprod 22(8):2202–2207
119. Bergh C, Söderström-Anttila V, Selbing A, Aittomaki K, Hazekamp J, Loft A, Nygren KG, Wennerholm UB (2007) Attitudes towards and management of single embryo transfer among Nordic IVF doctors. Acta Obstet Gynecol 86:1222–1230
120. Li M, DeUgarte CM, Surrey M, Danzer H, DeCherney A, Hill DL (2005) Fluorescence in situ hybridization reanalysis of day-6 human blastocysts diagnosed with aneuploidy on day 3. Fertil Steril 84(5):1395–1400
121. Langley MJ, Marek DM, Gardner DK, Doody KM, Doody KJ (2001) Extended embryo culture in human assisted reproductive treatments. Hum Reprod 16(5):902–908
122. Blake D, Proctor M, Johnson N, Olive D (2005) Cleavage stage versus blastocyst stage embryo transfer in assisted conception (review). Cochrane Database Syst Rev (2):CD002118
123. Milki AA, Jun SH, Hinckley MD, Behr B, Giudice LC, Westphal LM (2003) Incidence of monozygotic twinning with blastocyst compared to cleavage-stage transfer. Fertil Steril 79:503–506
124. Sheiner E, Har-Vardi I, Potashnik G (2001) The potential association between blastocyst transfer and monozygotic twinning. Fertil Steril 75:217–218
125. Kissin DM, Schieve LA, Reynolds MA (2006) Multiple-birth risk associated with IVF and extended embryo culture: USA, 2001. Hum Reprod 20:2215–2223

Chapter 46
Cryopreservation of Human Oocytes and Embryos

Barry Behr and Yimin Shu

Abstract With the advent of assisted reproductive technology, controled ovarian hyperstimulation (COH) is usually carried out to stimulate the growth of multiple follicles and produce multiple oocytes. Accordingly, multiple embryos are transferred to the uterus to increase the chances of success. However, multiple embryos can also increase the likelihood of multiple pregnancies, which are accompanied by a whole series of complications affecting both mother and child. There has been a trend toward transferring fewer embryos during the last decade. According to Center for Disease Control and Prevention (CDC), the average number of embryos transferred to women under 35 has dropped from 4.0 in 1995 to 2.8 in 2001 in the United States (N Engl J Med 350:1639–1645, 2004). In Europe, IVF centers in many countries have reduced the number of replaced embryos to two or even one (Ann N Y Acad Sci 1034:110–116, 2004). It is, therefore, very important to have a reliable technique to effectively cryopreserve the supernumerary embryos after transfer. The first pregnancy following the transfer of a frozen-thawed human embryo was reported by Trounson et al. in 1983 (Nature 305:707–709, 1983). Since then, embryo cryopreservation has become a very important part of the clinical use of in vitro fertilization. To date, human embryos have been successfully cryopreserved at the pronuclear, cleavage, and blastocyst stages of development. Moreover, recent advances in cryopreservation techniques have expanded the female fertility preservation from embryo to oocyte and ovarian tissue.

Keywords Cryopreservation • Vitrification • Cryoinjury • Cryoprotectant • Embryo storage

B. Behr (✉)
Department of Obstetrics & Gynecology, Stanford University, 900 Welch Road, Suite 14, Palo Alto, CA, USA
e-mail: behr@stanford.edu

Y. Shu
Senior Embryologist-Research Stanford Ferlility and Reproductive Medicine Center, Palo Alto, CA, USA

46.1 Basics of Cryopreservation

Cryopreservation involves a series of complex and dynamic physiochemical processes of temperature and water transport between a cell and the surrounding medium. The basic goal of cryopreservation, including slow freezing and vitrification, is to achieve intracellular vitrification while avoiding intracellular ice formation and membrane and organelle damage. Understanding these processes and their interactions with the cell biology is essential to develop successful cryopreservation methodologies.

46.1.1 Cryoprotectant Agents

Cryopreservation of oocytes and embryos routinely involves the use of cryoprotectants. A cryoprotectant is a substance that is used to protect biological tissue from cryopreservation damage. Cryoprotectants are typically categorized into two groups, permeating and nonpermeating cryoprotectants. Permeating cryoprotectants, such as 1, 2-Propanediol (PROH), Glycerol, Ethylene Glycol (EG), and Dimethyl Sulfoxide (DMSO), usually possess low molecular weight and, therefore, penetrate the cell membrane and displace the water molecules out of the cell. Effective working concentrations of permeating cryoprotectants are usually in the order of 1–4 mol/l. Polyvinyl pyrrolidone, sucrose, glucose, and other sugars are cryoprotectants that do not have to penetrate the cellular membrane. They are usually effective at low concentrations (0.01–0.2 mol/l). The cryoprotectants act as "antifreeze" in several different ways. Freezing point depression due to colligative properties of permeating cryoprotectants prevents the formation of destructive intracellular ice crystals. The mixture of nonpermeating cryoprotectants and permeating cryoprotectants aids in cellular dehydration during the cryopreservation process. In addition, the use of nonpermeating macromolecules produces an osmotic counterforce to restrict water movement across the membranes and prevent excessive swelling of the cells during the removal of cryoprotectant [1, 2].

DOI 10.1007/978-1-4419-1436-1_46,

While cryoprotectants are used to control or prevent ice formation in many preservation protocols, they themselves tend to be damaging. Cryoprotectants are toxic to embryos at high concentrations and long exposure times. In addition, the toxicity of cryoprotectant agents (CPAs) generally increases with temperature. For mammalian tissues, glycerol is generally the least toxic of the conventional CPAs, which can be ordered by toxicity as: propylene glycol>DMSO>ethylene glycol>glycerol [3]. It has been proposed that the intrinsic toxicity of cryoprotectants is largely due to their hydrophobicity, and the potential ability to denature DNA and proteins. To overcome cryoprotectant toxicity, a mixture of several cryoprotectants is usually used at lower individual concentrations.

In general, cryopreservation methods fall into two categories: equilibrium (slow freezing) and nonequilibrium (rapid cooling), according to the cooling rates and CPAs used [4]. Two major methods are used in the cryopreservation of human oocytes and embryos: controlled slow freezing and vitrification. Slow freezing attempts to maintain a delicate balance between cryoprotectants and the aqueous embryo compartment, whereas the strategy of the vitrification method is a rapid solidification of liquid without ice crystal formation.

46.1.2 Slow Freezing

The principle behind conventional slow freezing procedures is to induce ice formation extracellularly, thereby raising the solute concentration. The cryopreservation procedure can be divided into the following phases: prefreeze, freezing, storage, thawing, and postthaw [5]. The prefreeze phase gives the cells a brief equilibration period to uptake the cryoprotectants (Fig. 46.1). When the cells are transferred from isotonic solution to hyperosmotic solutions with permeating cryoprotectants, they shrink immediately as water leaves in response to the difference of osmotic pressure between intracellular and extracellular solutions. As the cryoprotectant permeates, water enters the cells to maintain intracellular osmotic equilibrium. Shrinkage stops when equilibrium is reached between the efflux of water and the influx of cryoprotectants. After that, the cryoprotectant enters the cells at a rate dependent on its permeability characteristics. Equilibration is complete when no further osmotic and chemical gradients with regard to the cryoprotectants as well as water exist. Optimal equilibration prior to slow cooling should be long enough for permeating cryoprotectants to enter the cells while minimizing the toxic effect of cryoprotectants.

The optimal cooling rate is determined by a number of biophysical factors and is cell-type-specific. A cooling rate of −1°C to −3°C/min is satisfactory for most animal cell cultures. Oocytes and embryos have lower surface-to-volume ratio and larger size as compared to somatic cells. Accordingly, a slower cooling rate is required to allow enough time for cell dehydration. After being loaded into plastic straws or vials, oocytes or embryos are cooled at a rate of −1°C to −2°C/min from room temperature to a temperature slightly below the melting point of the solution, which is approximately −5°C to −7°C. At this point, manual seeding is performed to initiate the extracellular ice formation in a controlled manner and avoid supercooling by touching the straw or vial with liquid nitrogen prechilled forceps or spatulas. The oocytes and embryos are again allowed to equilibrate for 5–10 min, and the temperature is lowered at a rate of −0.3°C to −0.5°C/min until below −30°C. Osmotic imbalance caused by the increasing extracellular solute concentrations following extracellular ice formation drives water out of the cells. As ice crystals grow, the extracellular solution becomes more concentrated and the cells are exposed to an increasingly hypertonic environment. The cooling process continues until the intracellular cryoprotectant concentration is high enough to allow vitrification, preventing intracellular ice formation when the cell is plunged into liquid nitrogen. The frozen oocytes and embryos are then stored in the liquid nitrogen tank for future use.

Thawing is the reverse of the freezing process and involves the removal of the frozen straws or vials from liquid nitrogen, removal of cryoprotectant from the frozen cells by stepwise dilution and warming the thawed cells to 37°C. The optimal thawing protocol depends on the specific freezing protocol and cryoprotectants used. If the cooling is terminated at a high subzero temperature of −30 to −40°C, a moderately rapid warming (200–350°C/min) is required to maximize the

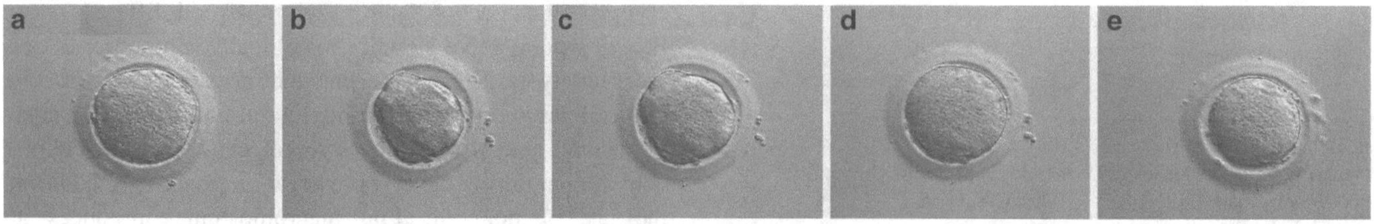

Fig. 46.1 The morphological appearance of immature metaphase I (MI) human oocytes during the prefreeze phase at room temperature, (**a**) MI oocyte in isotonic culture medium, (**b**) a rapidly shrunken oocyte after 50 s of exposure to 1.5 M 1,2-propandiel (PROH); (**c**) shrinkage stops when equilibrium is reached between the efflux of water and the influx of cryoprotectants. (**d**) an oocyte returning to normal volume as the PROH penetrates the oocyte after 10 min exposure to 1.5 M PROH; (**e**) The oocyte shrinks considerably due to the presence of nonpermeating cryoprotectant sucrose (1.5 M PROH + 0.2 M Sucrose)

survival rate. Embryos cooled slowly to temperatures below −60°C prior to being plunged into liquid nitrogen requires a rather slow warming rate of about 25°C/min or less. Due to the fact that oocytes and embryos are more permeable to water than cryoprotectants, the frozen cells will swell or burst if they are placed directly to a medium without cryoprotectants after thawing. To control the degree of swelling during the removal of cryoprotectants, a high concentration of sucrose is used as an osmotic buffer to counteract the high concentration of cryoprotectants in the cell [6].

46.1.3 Cryodamage

The process of cryopreservation has profound effects on cells, many of which result in sublethal damage to the cells and a subsequent reduction of function. There are several mechanisms underlying cryodamage during the freezing and thawing process.

46.1.3.1 Cold Shock

Cold shock, or direct chilling injury, is a form of injury following exposure of cells to temperatures lower than normal growth temperatures, but not freezing temperatures. Its severity increases with both an increase in cooling rate and the absolute temperature of the exposure. The main damage caused by chilling is to the membranes. Direct chilling injury induces temperature-induced phase transitions of phospholipids from the liquid crystalline- to the gel-phase, which results in separation of membrane proteins and lipid, change membrane permeability, and cause a decline in the activity of membrane bound enzymes. Chilling injury also affects the oocyte meiotic spindles, microtubules, and microfilaments [7–9]. Mammalian oocytes and embryos at different developmental stages have varying degrees of sensitivity to chilling. In bovine, resistance to chilling increased with advancing stage from 8-cell to morula to blastocyst [10]. For a given developmental stage, survival declines with increasing length of exposure to a given low temperature. Lipid phase transition in human oocytes at different developmental stages takes place at higher temperatures than that in zygotes, which explains the increased sensitivity of oocytes to cooling and cryoinjury and indicates the necessity to adjust the cryopreservation protocols in order to minimize cryoinjury [11].

46.1.3.2 Osmotic Stress

The water inside a living cell can be roughly divided into two parts, osmotically active freezable water (bulk water) and osmotically inactive, unfreezable water (bound water). Bulk water can be removed by exposure to a hypertonic environment. Bound water consists of about 10% of cellular water and is tightly hydrogen-bonded to the hydrophilic surfaces of proteins, nucleic acids, or the polar end-groups of membrane lipids. Removal of bulk water does not cause dehydration damage, but excessive loss of bound water results in the loss of structural support to proteins and lipids [12]. Oocytes and embryos are dehydrated before and during the cooling process through the addition of cryoprotectants and rehydrated by the removal of cryoprotectants during the thawing process. This volumetric shrinkage and swelling are capable of causing damage or even cell death. It is therefore of critical importance to maintain a delicate balance between the removal of bulk water that could potentially form ice crystals and the removal of bound water.

46.1.3.3 Ice Crystal Formation and Solution Effects

Survival of frozen cells after thawing depends largely upon the cooling rates. The optimal cooling rate should be slow enough to allow cells time to dehydrate and fast enough to prevent excessive dehydration damage (Fig. 46.2). If cells are cooled too rapidly, the water cannot leave fast enough to prevent

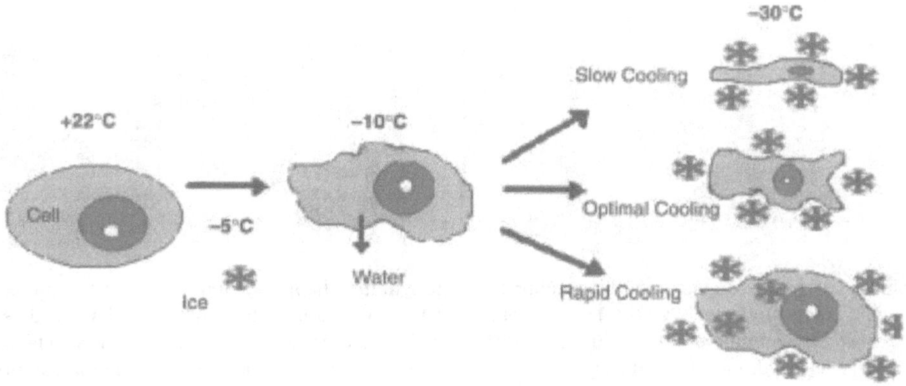

Fig. 46.2 Schematic of physical events in cells during slow freezing. Reproduced from [128]

extensive supercooling, which eventually leads to lethal intracellular ice formation [4]. If the cooling is too slow, too much extracellular ice crystal formation can cause cellular damage due to mechanical forces on cell membrane. Prolonged exposure of cells to a highly concentrated solution could also lead to cell injury termed as solution effects [13]. High concentrations of electrolytes affect ionic interactions, including those that help stabilize the native state of enzymes.

Although the above stresses induced by the freezing process can lead to cell injury, the warming rate is of critical importance as well. If the thawing rate is too slow, small ice crystal formed from the small amount of intracellular water could recrystallize to larger damaging crystals [4]. However, if the thawing rate is too rapid when the freezing has been slow, the abrupt entrance of water to the cell due to insufficient egress of excess cryoprotectants from the cell may cause its death [14].

46.1.4 Vitrification

Vitrification is a cryopreservation strategy in which cells are converted into a glass-like amorphous solid which is free of any crystalline structure. As a nonequilibrium cryopreservation method, vitrification is achieved by the combination of high concentration of cryoprotectants and an extremely high cooling rate. Compared to slow freezing, vitrification is simpler and more convenient without the requirement of expensive equipment (i.e., controlled rate freezer). Vitrification is also able to eliminate the ice crystal formation in the intra- and extracellular spaces. Although controlled slow freezing remains the main method of cryopreservation in most IVF laboratories, vitrification technique has entered more and more the mainstream of human assisted reproductive technology.

Although the freezing temperature of water is close to 0°C, pure water requires very small amount of volume and incredibly fast cooling rate to achieve vitrification. It has been shown that vitrification of small droplets of water would require a cooling rate of about 3,000,000°C/s [15], which is not practical for clinical use. At very high cooling rates (up to 7.2×10^{5}°C/min), human spermatozoa can be successfully vitrified without cryoprotectants [16]. Fortunately, the addition of high concentration of cryoprotectants substantially decreases the critical cooling rate to achieve successful vitrification. The total concentration of cryoprotectant ranges from 5 to 8 M in the vitrification protocols currently used in the cryopreservation of human oocyte and embryos. A maximized cooling rate could be achieved by the use of minimized volume of vitrification medium and direct contact between the solution and liquid nitrogen [17]. Cryoprotectants are not always needed in vitrification. Although high survival rate of vitrified human oocytes and embryos have been obtained by using open carrier systems, such as Electron Microscopic Grids [18], Cryoloops [19], Open Pulled Straws (OPS) [20], and hemistraw system [21], direct contact between oocytes or embryos and liquid nitrogen raises the concern of contamination from nitrogen-born bacteria and/or viruses. An aseptic alternative device such as closed pulled straw has been tried; however, their efficacy needs further evaluation [22, 23].

Compared to slow freezing, vitrification involves a very high cooling rate and passages rapidly through the dangerous temperature zone between +15°C and −5°C, significantly decreasing chilling injury to the oocytes and embryos [24]. However, not all cell injuries are avoided by vitrification. High concentration of cryoprotectants is an obstacle to vitrification. More severe osmotic stress and toxic effects are potentially imposed upon the cells during vitrification/warming than slow freezing/thawing (Fig. 46.3.). A stepwise addition of cryoprotectants can help reduce the toxic and osmotic damage induced by cryoprotectants at high concentrations [25].

46.2 Cryopreservation of Human Embryos

Embryo cryopreservation has several advantages in the practice of human in vitro fertilization. Transfer of the frozen-thawed embryos following a fresh IVF cycle offers a patient a chance to have one or more additional children without additional ovarian stimulation and oocyte retrieval, which can help reduce costs and increase the cumulative pregnancy rate. For patients with severe ovarian hyperstimulation syndrome

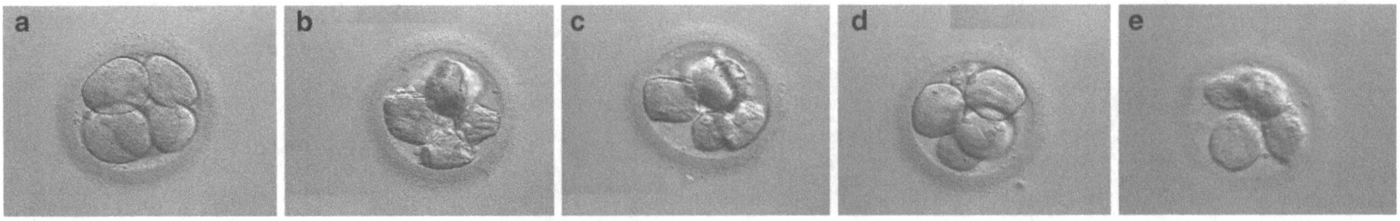

Fig. 46.3 Embryo morphological changes during a two-step equilibration in a vitrification solution containing ethylene glycol (EG) and dimethyl sulfoxide (DMSO). (**a**) a 5-cell stage embryo before vitrification, (**b**) the embryo undergoes a sudden dehydration immediately after exposure to equilibration solution with 7.5% EG+7.5% DMSO, (**c**) partial rehydration happens within 2 min as cryoprotectants enter the embryo, (**d**) equilibration stops when an balanced is reached between the efflux of water and the influx of cryoprotectants, (**e**) the embryo undergoes further dehydration in vitrification solution with 15% EG+15% DMSO

(OHSS), the postponement of a fresh embryo transfer and cryopreservation of all embryos can help prevent the patient's situation from deteriorating [26]. Embryo cryopreservation also provides the opportunity to delay the embryo transfer to a later time for patients whose health would not be conducive with pregnancy. Moreover, in the last decade, there has been a trend towards reducing the number of embroys transferred in both the United States and Europe [27, 28], resulting more surplus embroys for cryopreservation. The ability to successfully cryopreserve human embryos is therefore of critical importance in reducing the number of embryos transferred and decreasing therefore multiple pregnancy rates [29].

46.2.1 Cryopreservation of Cleavage Stage Embryos

Although glycerol and DMSO contributed to the first pregnancy following transfer of a frozen-thawed 8-cell stage embryo [30], slow freezing/rapid thawing protocols using PROH and sucrose as cryoprotectants have been the standard protocols of pronuclear and early cleavage stage embryos for years [31–34]. Freezing of human embryos at the pronuclear stage is more acceptable to some patients with ethical problems, primary due to the fact that the cryopreservation occurs before syngamy. Cryopreservation of cleavage stage embryo allows the selection of better embryos for transfer in fresh cycles, resulting in high pregnancy and embryo implantation rates [35].

Poor quality embryos do not survive well and are usually not chosen for cryopreservation. A multicell embryo (2–8 cell stage) is defined as surviving when ≥50% blastomeres remain intact. With the development of cryopreservation techniques, 70–80% of day 2 and day 3 human embryos can successfully survive the freezing and thawing process currently, among which 5–20% of transferred embryos implant [36–38]. Embryo quality prior to cryopreservation has a profound effect on the clinical outcome of frozen embryo transfer. For day 2 frozen embryos, intact 4-cell embryos have a significantly higher implantation rate (16.9%) than 2-cell embryos (7.2%) [34].

In general, pregnancy rates after transfer of frozen–thawed embryos are lower than fresh embryo transfers [39]. However, cryopreservation per se does not seem to affect subsequent embryo development in vivo following embryo transfer, as supported by the fact that fully intact thawed embryos have been shown to have similar implantation rate as fresh embryos with equivalent cell number [34, 40]. The impact of cryopreservation on the embryo implantation potential is manifested only when there is blastomere lysis, [34]. Blastomere loss is a common occurrence in cryopreserved embryos. As shown by Edge (2000) [34], 44.5% (2,480/5,572) of day 2 frozen embryos showed blastomere loss after thawing. Fully intact thawed embryos were more than twice as likely to implant compared with those that had lost one or more of their blastomeres [41]. A quantitative analysis performed by Edgar et al. [42] showed a highly significant association between blastomere loss and reduction in implantation potential even in embryos with ≥50% blastomeres surviving. There was very little chance to achieve pregnancy (1%) by transfer of thawed embryos with less than 50% blastomere survived [34].

Precise mechanisms of blastomere loss on thawed embryo development are still investigational. The presence of necrotic blastomeres may disrupt cell signaling communication and morphological restructuring of embryonic cells, resulting in impaired preimplantation development and reduced cell numbers in resultant blastocysts [43, 44]. To eliminate the potentially toxic effect of dead blastomere on further embryonic development, removal of the necrotic blastomeres has been performed and proven to effectively improve the implantation rate of partially damaged thawed embryos [45, 46]. It has been suggested that necrotic blastomere removal be applied routinely for all partially damaged embryos when appropriate [47].

Resumption of mitotic division (i.e., further cleavage) after in vitro culture of frozen-thawed early-cleaved embryos has reported to be effective in aiding the selection of viable embryos for transfer by several studies [45, 48]. Significantly, higher implantation rates were obtained after the transfer of embryos that had resumed cell division compared to those without further cleavage. Guerif et al. reported that the implantation rate per transferred embryo was significantly higher for cleaved embryos compared with uncleaved embryos (19.7% and 3%, respectively) [49]. A similar trend was observed by Tang et al. [38], who reported a reduced rate of embryo implantation (13.4% versus 2.8%) for those embryos with and without blastomere division in single embryo transfers. These data strongly support that priority should be given to thawed embryos with further cleavage and suggest leaving postthaw embryos in culture to allow for subsequent cell division.

Limited data is available regarding the application of vitrification in the cryopreservation of pronuclear and cleavage stage human embryos [50–52]. This is probably because acceptable rates of embryo survival and pregnancy have been achieved by using the slow freezing method. By using single pronucleate (1PN) and three pronucleate (3PN) zygotes, Liebermann et al. [53] demonstrated that vitrification did not impact the developmental potential of human pronuclear stage embryos. Similar rates of embryo cleavage, cavitation, and blastocyst formation were obtained between vitrified groups and the unvitrified control groups. Desai et al. reported the largest number of pregnancies obtained from vitrified 6–8 cell stage human embryos [54]. In her study, 85% (201/236) of the vitrified embryos survived warming. The clinical pregnancy rate was 44% (34/77) and implantation rate was 20% (40/201). Although the existing data support that vitrification yields satisfactory survival rate, direct comparison between slow freezing and vitrification of cleavage stage embryos is still lacking.

46.2.2 Blastocyst Cryopreservation

Since the advent of sequential culture media, the utility of blastocyst culture has gained popularity in human assisted reproductive technology programs. Accordingly, the need to cryopreserve supernumerary blastocysts is increasing. The main characteristic of the blastocyst is its fluid-filled cavity, the blastocoele. For cleavage stage embryos, a large proportion of water content is present inside the totipotent blastomeres (2–8 cell stage); the osmolarity-induced changes during the cryopreservation process are manifested at the cellular level. However, the in vitro derived human blastocyst contains a large number (60 ~ 100) of two structurally and functionally differentiated cell populations (inner cell mass (ICM) and trophectoderm (TE)) [55]. These cells are small in size and volume, and it is the blastocoele that contains the largest amount of water of a blastocyst [56]. Blastocysts, therefore, behave differently from cleavage stage embryos, as not only the volumetric changes of the blastomere but more importantly changes of blastocoele size together constitute the integrated whole of osmotic behavior of blastocysts during the cryopreservation process.

Different from the cleavage stage embryo, the viability of cryopreserved blastocyst is less easy to define by detecting the further cleavage of survived blastomeres even under inverted microscope [57]. Prolonged culture of thawed blastocysts provides a chance to evaluate blastocoele reexpansion, which is a relatively fast event that can happen within 1–2 h postthaw [58]. Blastocoele re-expansion has been shown to be predictive of blastocyst viability [59, 60]. Although the precise mechanism remains unclear, trophectoderm epithelium has proven to play a key role in the reestablishment of the blastocoelic cavity [59]. Tranfers of a single thawed blastocyst with more than 50% blastocoele re-expansion resulted in significantly higher rate of clinical pregnancy compared to early or un-reexpanded blastocysts [59, 62]. Studies in human and bovine showing that reexpanded blastocysts had higher glucose consumption than those without re-expansion verify the accuracy of fast re-expansion as a good morphological marker in selection of good embryos [63, 64].

The most commonly used freezing protocol for human blastocyst is the Menezo 2-step slow freezing/rapid thawing protocol as previously described by Menezo et al. [65, 66]. For example, in our protocol, freezing and thawing solutions consist of the cryoprotectants in a HEPES-buffered human tubal fluid medium (mHTF) (CooperSurgical, Inc, Trumbull, CT) supplemented with 20% Serum Protein Substitute (SPS). Equilibration with the freezing solutions is carried out at room temperature. Blastocysts are first exposed to a 5% glycerol solution for 10 min and then to 9% glycerol + 0.2 mol/l sucrose solution for another 10 min. They are then loaded into cryostraws (Cryo Bio System, IMV Technologies, Paris, France) and placed in a programmable freezer (CL-8000, Cryologic, Mulgrave, Victoria, Australia). The straws are cooled from −6.5°C at which point a 1 min pre-seeding hold is maintained before manual seeding is performed. An additional 9 min hold at −6.5°C is provided for further equilibration. Cooling resumes at a rate of −0.3°C/min to −35°C before the cryostraws are plunged and stored in liquid nitrogen.

For blastocyst thawing, cryoprotectants are removed at room temperature by stepwise dilution. Cryostraws are removed from liquid nitrogen and exposed in air for 30 s before being warmed in a water bath at 30°C for 45 s. Blastocysts are then expelled from the cryostraws into a 0.5 mol/l sucrose solution and left for 10 min, followed by 0.2 mol/l sucrose solution for another 10 min. The thawed blastocysts are then washed in mHTF with 20% SPS without sucrose, after that blastocysts are transferred to Quinn's Advantage Blastocyst Medium with 20% SPS and further cultured at 37°C with 5% CO_2, 5% O_2, and 90% N_2 for 2–4 h until transfer. Blastocysts undergo multiple changes in blastocoele size in response to external osmotic stress during the freezing–thawing process, as illustrated in Figs. 46.4 and 46.5.

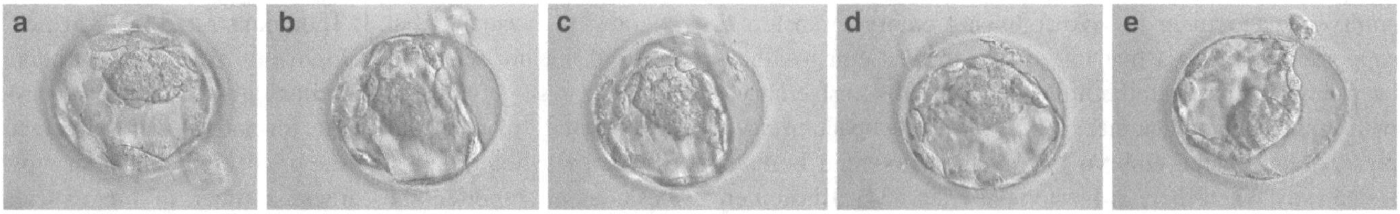

Fig. 46.4 Morphological changes of a human blastocyst during the 2-step equilibration prior to slow cooling. (**a, b**) a blastocyst floats and starts to shrink within a few seconds in 5% glycerol, (**c**) the blastocyst shranks rapidly to between 60% of their isotonic volume and maximum shrinkage occurs within 3 min, (**d**) the blastocyst undergoes slow re-expansion and regains 80% of its initial blastocoele volume, (**e**) the blastocyst undergoes further shrinkage within a few seconds of exposure to 9% glycerol + 0.2 mol/l sucrose and remained shrunken

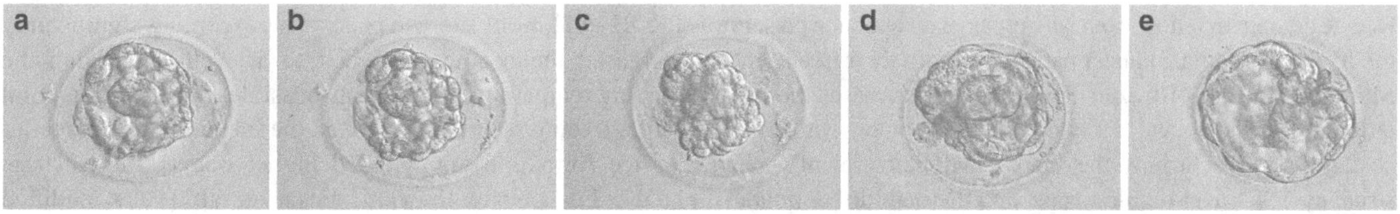

Fig. 46.5 Blastocoele re-expansion of a thawed blastocyst. (**a**) a thawed blastocyst expelled from the frozen straw immediately after the thaw, (**b**) the thawed blastocyst shrinks slowly after being transferred into thawing media containing 0.5 mol/l sucrose, (**c**) the blastocyst continues to shrink in thawing solution with 0.2 mol/l sucrose, (**d**) the thawed blastocyst starts to re-expand within 1 h incubation in isotonic blastocyst medium without sucrose, (**e**) the thawed blastocyst shows 90% blastocoele re-expansion after 2 h in vitro culture

Slow freezing has been widely used in the cryopreservation of human blastocysts; however, inconsistent results were obtained, with pregnancy rates of 0–59.2% [60, 67–69]. Suboptimal culture conditions might have influenced the freezability of blastocysts. Very poor clinical outcome was achieved following the replacement of frozen/thawed blastocysts cultured in a single medium [70]. The availability of a number of successful sequential culture systems has led to the production of high quality blastocysts and acceptable pregnancy rates. Moreover, a decrease of the number of junctional contacts between the trophoblastic cells of in vitro produced blastocysts has been observed through ultrastructure observation, leading to poor postthaw survival and decreased rate of re-expansion as compared to in vivo produced counterparts with similar morphology [71–73].

Frozen blastocyst transfer provides a very good model to investigate the synchronization of endometrium and embryonic development. As demonstrated by Shapiro et al. [75], transferred embryos reaching blastocyst stage on day 5 are approximately twice as likely to implant compared to those for which expansion and transfer are delayed until day 6, implying the importance of developmental rate in the establishment of a successful pregnancy in a fresh transfer cycle. However, several studies have shown that day 6 and day 5 frozen blastocysts have similar survival rates and implantation potential [69, 76]. The fact that cryopreservation rescues developmentally retarded blastocyst frozen on day 6 indicates the critical role of endometrial receptivity in the reduced success rates of later developing embryos [77, 78].

Since the first pregnancy following transfer of a vitrified human blastocyst reported in 2000 [79], successful pregnancies and live births have been obtained by using different carrier methods: Cryoloops [80], Electron Microscopy Grids [81], plastic micropipettes [82], Cryotops [76], and cut standard straws (CSS) [22]. A decreased rate of blastocyst survival after vitrification has been noted when the volume of the blastocoelic cavity is increased, with morula and early blastocysts surviving better than expanded and hatching blastocysts [56]. This is probably due to the insufficient permeation of cryoprotectant into the blastocoele, with residual water in the blastocoelic cavity increasing the potential for ice crystal formation during the vitrification process. Artificial shrinkage of the blastocoele by using a micro-needle or a laser pulse prior to the cooling steps of vitrification has been proven to significantly improve the blastocyst survival and implantation rates [56, 83]. Although slow freezing is still the main stream of blastocyst cryopreservation, direct comparison between slow freezing and vitrification has demonstrated that vitrification was superior or at least equal to slow freezing [76, 84]. Considering the tremendous economic advantage of vitrification over slow freezing, it is conceivable that vitrification will be more widely used in human blastocyst cryopreservation.

46.3 Cryopreservation of Human Oocytes

Oocyte cryopreservation offers potential benefits for several categories of infertile and fertile women. While embryo cryopreservation is routine and well-established, it is suitable only for women with a male partner and may not be acceptable to some patients due to ethical, moral, and religious reasons. Oocyte cryopreservation bypasses these issues and potentially offers the patients an alternative to embryo cryopreservation. Women in the Western hemisphere have been delaying initiation of childbearing to later in life. In 2002, the rate of first birth increased by 28% for women 35–39 years of age and 44% for women aged 40–45 when compared with 1990 [83]. However, female fertility declines with the advancing age, with poor oocyte quality being the main cause. A woman over 35 has more difficulty in conceiving and some of them have to seek oocyte donation. Oocyte cryopreservation preserves a woman's future ability to have a child at a later date without losing the chance to use their own oocytes. In 2001, over 625,000 women in the United States were diagnosed with some form of invasive cancer [86, 87]. Approximately 8%, or 50,000 of these women were under the age of 40 [88]. While progress in cancer therapy has increased the 5-year relative survival rate for all cancers combined from 56% to 64% in women [89], the risk of loss of ovarian function is a well-known side effect of antineoplastic treatment.

Oocyte cryopreservation potentially provides an option to preserve the fertility of female cancer patients prior to their treatments. Moreover, the use of frozen donor oocytes decreases the limitations of fresh oocyte donation, such as donor availability, cost, need to synchronize the donor's and the recipient's menstrual cycles, travel requirements, and the inability to quarantine oocytes [90].

The first pregnancy after human oocyte cryopreservation was reported in 1986 by using DMSO as the cryoprotectant supplemented with sucrose [91]. Despite considerable efforts hat had been made to improve the outcome of oocyte cryopreservation, only a few more pregnancies were obtained in the following 10 years [92, 93]. On the basis of the assumption that oocytes were similar to embryos, oocytes were cryopreserved in a similar way as cleavage stage embryos at the early stage of oocyte cryopreservation. Unfortunately, slow freezing/rapid thawing protocol derived from embryos was not applicable to oocytes, as manifested by the low rates of survival, fertilization, and poor embryonic development. An appreciation of the specific biophysical characteristics of oocytes is helpful to understand why oocytes were so difficult to be successfully cryopreserved. First of all, the oocyte is a large single cell with a small surface:volume ratio, which can slow water and cryoprotectant efflux and influx and increase the likelihood of intracellular ice formation [94]. Secondly, the meiotic spindle apparatus is highly sensitive to chilling injury and easily damaged by intracellular ice crystal formation during the freezing and thawing process. It has been reported that even transient cooling to room temperature for 10 min could cause irrevisible disruption of the meiotic spindle in the human oocytes [95]. Thirdly, oocytes are less permeable to water and cryoprotectants as compared to zygotes and early cleavage stage embryos. Lastly, the cryopreservation process initiates parthenogenetic activation and the hardening of the zona pellucida, which can adversely affect the normal fertilization process [96].

For these reasons, several modifications have been made to the slow freezing protocols derived from embryos in recent years. Eighty percent of the frozen oocytes (37/46) were successfully recovered by using PROH as cryoprotectant [97]. The addition of high concentrations of sucrose in the freezing solution not only ensures high rates of oocyte survival, but also improves oocyte quality. According to Fabbri et al. [98], the survival rate of cumulus-free oocytes was improved from 30% to 60% and 81% when the concentration of sucrose was increased from 0.1 mol/l to 0.2 and 0.3 mol/l respectively. More frozen-thawed oocytes displayed normal meiotic spindle configuration and chromosome organization under a protocol adopting 0.3 mol/l sucrose (69.7%) as compared to using 0.1 mol/l sucrose (50.8%) [99]. Reducing or eliminating sodium in the freezing medium has also exerted beneficial effects on the survival of immature and mature human oocytes [100]. Fabbri et al. [98] showed that a longer preincubation (from 10.5 to 15 min) in 1.5 mol/l PROH + 0.2 mol/l sucrose prior to slow cooling significantly increased the oocyte survival rate as well. Increasing the seeding temperature as close as possible to the melting point of the freeing solution decreased the incidence of intracellular ice formation and yielded higher oocyte survival rate [101]. For oocyte thawing, Fosas et al. [102] modified Fabbri's protocol by shortening the exposure time in the rehydration solutions at room temperature from 30 to 12.5 min. They reported a survival rate of 90% and obtained four pregnancies out of seven transfers. Three to four hours postthaw incubation is necessary for meiotic spindle restoration and is reported to facilitate normal fertilization and subsequent embryonic development [100]. Microinjection of small amount of trehalose provides another alternative to protect human oocytes against freezing damage [103]. These modifications as well as the introduction of ICSI have increased the efficiency of oocyte freezing and resulted in many healthy live births.

As an alternative method to slow freezing, vitrification involves the use of very high concentrations of cryoprotectants and rapid cooling rate. The rapid cooling rate used to achieve vitrification allows less time for ice formation. In contrast to slow freezing in which the meiotic spindle was inevitably damaged and a 3–4 h postthaw incubation was required for the reconstruction of the cryo-damaged spindle [104], vitrification performed at 37°C had negligible impact on the meiotic spindle [105]. The first birth following transfer of embryos obtained from vitrified human oocytes was reported by Kuleshova et al. [106]. Successful pregnancies and live births have been achieved by vitrification of human oocytes using different carrier systems: OPS [20], Cryotops [107, 108]; Cryoleaves [109*]. Oocyte vitrification protocols vary significantly in the literature with different type and concentration of the cryoprotectants being used. The most commonly used mixture of cryoprotectants for human oocyte vitrification are EG and DMSO. Liebermann's experience indicated that an EG + DMSO mixture can be an effective cryoprotectant strategy for human oocyte vitrification [110]. In his large series of 1,120 human oocytes vitrified with cryoloop, more than 80% of the vitrified oocytes survived after warming. By using and Cryotop technique, Antinori et al. vitrified mature oocytes in a mixture of 15% EG, 15% DMSO, and 0.5 mol/l sucrose and achieved a survival rate as high as 99.4% (328/330), with the pregnancy and implantation rates of 32.5% and 13.2% being obtained respectively [107]. These results are encouraging; however, it should be noted that high concentrations of cryoprotectants are cytotoxic. Maximizing the cooling rate by minimizing the volume of vitrification solution containing oocytes is one of the most promising strategies to reduce the concentration of cryoprotectants, leading to less cryoprotectant toxicity to the oocytes. High oocyte survival rate (91%, 58/64) has been achieved by employing tiny drops as small as 0.1 μl in volume [108]. To eliminate the risk of contamination during oocyte storage in liquid nitrogen, further studies are needed to assure the efficacy of open vs. closed carrier systems.

Similar to embryos, membrane permeability of oocytes decreases as maturation proceeds. Immature oocytes at GV and metaphase I stages have been shown to have a higher permeability than mature oocytes for a given cryoprotectant [111], making it more difficult to cryopreserve mature oocytes. Due to the lack of understanding of the mechanism regulating oocyte maturation and the limited number of births from in vitro matured human oocytes, most published reports focused on the cryopreservation of mature oocytes. The difficulty of cryopreserving mature oocytes also lies in the presence of meiotic spindle, which is essential for correct alignment and segregation of chromosomes. Oocyte quality is another factor affecting the recovery rate, with high quality oocytes surviving better than poor ones. The presence of cumulus cells during freezing process is helpful to increase the cell surface/volume ratio of oocytes. However, results from different groups show some divergence, probably due to different freezing/thawing protocols of investigation [112]. The removal of cumulus cells before vitrification has been shown to enhance the survival rate of both mature and immature oocytes, however, the developmental competence of immature oocytes was impaired [113, 114].

Live births have been obtained from cryopreserved human oocytes by using either slow freezing or vitrification method. It is estimated that there have been 300 to 600 children born from cryopreserved human oocytes worldwide during the last two decades [115]. A major concern about oocyte cryopreservation is the potential damage of meiotic spindle and its effect on the safety of the offspring. In a recent survey performed by Borini et al. [116], two malformations were found out of 105 babies born after frozen oocytes, with one infant being affected by choanae atresia and the other by Rubinstein–Taydi Syndrome. However, the fathers of those two babies were affected by severe male factor. A prospective follow-up with adequate numbers of patients for a sufficient length of time will be valuable to help evaluate the long-term safety and development of the children born after oocyte cryopreservation. Due to the limited number of births, oocyte cryopreservation is still considered to be an experimental procedure and advised to be performed under institutional review board (IRB) research protocol by American Society for Reproductive Medicine (ASRM).

46.4 Storage of Cryopreserved Oocytes and Embryos

Advances in assisted reproductive technologies (ART) over the last two decades have led to better cyropreservation techniques and the wider use of cryopreserved human embryos. As of April 11, 2002, nearly 400,000 embryos were stored in the United States, the majority of which (88.2%) were targeted for patient use [117]. Among these embryos, 99% were stored in the IVF clinics, with the other 1% being stored in offsite facility. Patients consenting to the frozen storage of oocytes or embryos quite rightly expect the IVF clinics or offsite facilities to do everything reasonably possible to keep them in optimum conditions [118]. Both the process of cryopreservation and the cryofacility are loaded with risk, from patient/sample processing, through to the eventual utilization or disposal of specimens. The IVF clinics and offsite storage facilities must ensure that there is a system to manage risks associated with cryopreservation, which include, but are not limited to, staff injury, premature warming of cells and tissues, and transmission of infection [118].

Attention should be paid to the safety aspects involved in cryopreservation and storage. It is a matter of good laboratory practice to wear gloves and eye protection when handling liquid nitrogen. A continued supply of liquid nitrogen must be ensured to maintain ultralow temperature for the safekeeping of cryopreserved specimens. Alarms linked to external warning systems such as autodialers or fire alarm panels to deal with out of hours emergencies should also be in place. Cross-contamination within a liquid nitrogen storage tank is another concern of frozen oocyte and embryo storage. Human immunodeficiency virus (HIV), hepatitis B (HBV) and C (HCV) viruses, and possibly other viruses can survive in liquid nitrogen, making it possible for cross contamination of samples to occur in liquid nitrogen storage tanks [119]. While there is no direct evidence of cross-contamination of gametes and embryos stored in the same tank, there is however, evidence of the presence of HCV virus in different ejaculates of the same semen donor [120]. It is therefore of critical importance to screen all patients for HIV, HBV, HCV prior to sperm, oocyte and embryo cryopreservation. Cryopreserved samples must also be maintained in quarantine while test results are still pending. Ideally, separate storage tanks for HIV-, HBV-, and HCV-infected specimens are advised [119]. Both oocytes and embryos can be associated with a number of potentially pathogenic agents when stored in open containers or are introduced through leakage due to faulty seals or container breakage [121, 122]. To reduce the risks of cross contamination of samples in liquid nitrogen storage, specimen containers must be guaranteed by the manufacturer to withstand freezing temperatures and thawing cycles.

Another strategy to minimize the potential for transmission is the use of nitrogen vapor instead of liquid nitrogen itself. Vapor storage has been proposed to minimize or eliminate the possibility of cross-contamination [123, 124]. A major concern of the vapor storage is the risk of loss of cell viability. Human sperm survive satisfactorily with good recovery in the vapor of liquid nitrogen [125]. Similar rates of embryo survival and blastocyst formation were obtained between 1-cell mouse embryos stored in liquid nitrogen and nitrogen vapor [124]. Although no published data is available on human embryos, nitrogen vapor storage does not compromise the viability of vitrified human oocytes [126].

46.5 Conclusions

Recent advances in the understanding of oocytes and embryos have contributed significantly to the improvement of the efficiency of human oocyte and embryo cryopreservation. However, it should be noted that attempts to cryopreserve human oocytes, embryos and ovarian tissues have been based mostly on empirical approaches [127]. As a well-established technique with reasonable outcomes, embryo cryopreservation has been accepted as an integral part of human assisted reproductive technology. Although encouraging results have been recently obtained in oocyte cryopreservation by using vitrification techniques, there is still much to learn and understand today. As an alternative method to oocyte and embryo cryopreservation, ovarian tissue cryopreservation is an experimental technology and its efficacy remains to be determined. Due to the complex nature of the cryopreservation process, membrane permeability coefficients to water and cryoprotectants vary among cell types and developmental stages. To optimize the oocyte and embryo cryopreservation protocols, further studies need be performed to elucidate the biochemical and biophysical events by theoretical analysis.

References

1. Leibo SP (1984) A one-step method for direct nonsurgical transfer of frozen-thawed bovine embryos. Theriogenology 21:767–790
2. Kasai M, Komi JH, Takakamo A, Tsudera H, Sakurai T, Machida T (1990) A simple method for mouse embryo cryopreservation in a low toxicity vitrification solution, without appreciable loss of viability. J Reprod Fertil 89:91–97
3. Baudot A, Alger L, Boutron P (2000) Glass-forming tendency in the system water-dimethyl sulfoxide. Cryobiology 40:151–158
4. Mazur P (1990) Equilibrium, quasi-equilibrium, and nonequilibrium freezing of mammalian embryos. Cell Biophys 17:53–92
5. Schneider U (1986) Cryobiological principles of embryo freezing. J In Vitro Fert Embryo Transf 3:3–9
6. Leibo SP (1983) A one-step in situ dilution method for frozen-thawed bovine embryos. Cryo Letters 4:387–400
7. Albertini DF, Eppig JJ (1995) Unusual cytoskeletal and chromatin configurations in mouse oocytes that are atypical in meiotic progression. Dev Genet 16:13–19
8. Zenzes MT, Bielecki R, Casper RF, Leibo SP (2001) Effects of chilling to 0 degrees C on the morphology of meiotic spindles in human metaphase II oocytes. Fertil Steril 75:769–777
9. Songsasen N, Yu IJ, Ratterree MS, VandeVoort CA, Leibo SP (2002) Effect of chilling on the organization of tubulin and chromosomes in rhesus monkey oocytes. Fertil Steril 77:818–825
10. Balasubramanian S, Rho G (2006) Effect of chilling on the development of in vitro produced bovine embryos at various cleavage stages. J Assist Reprod Genet 23:55–61
11. Ghetler Y, Yavin S, Shalgi R, Arav A (2005) The effect of chilling on membrane lipid phase transition in human oocytes and zygotes. Hum Reprod 20:3385–3389
12. Wright DL, Eroglu A, Toner M, Toth TL (2004) Use of sugars in cryopreserving human oocytes. Reprod Biomed Online 9:179–186
13. Mazur P, Leibo SP, Chu EHY (1972) A two-factor hypothesis of fleezing injury. Exp Cell Res 71:345–355
14. Mazur P (1984) Freezing of live cells: mechanisms and implications. Am J Physiol 247:C125–C142
15. Lepault J, Booy FP, Dubochet J (1983) Electron microscopy of frozen biological suspensions. J Microsc 129(Pt 1):89–102
16. Isachenko V, Montag M, Isachenko E, Dessole S, Nawroth F, van der Ven H (2006) Aseptic vitrification of human germinal vesicle oocytes using dimethyl sulfoxide as a cryoprotectant. Fertil Steril 85:741–747
17. Vajta G, Nagy ZP (2006) Are programmable freezers still needed in the embryo laboratory? Review on vitrification. Reprod Biomed Online 12:779–796
18. Hong SW, Chung HM, Lim JM, Ko JJ, Yoon TK, Yee B, Cha KY (1999) Improved human oocyte development after vitrification: a comparison of thawing methods. Fertil Steril 72:142–146
19. Yeoman RR, Gerami-Naini B, Mitalipov S, Nusser KD, Widmann-Browning AA, Wolf DP (2001) Cryoloop vitrification yields superior survival of Rhesus monkey blastocysts. Hum Reprod 16:1965–1969
20. Selman H, Angelini A, Barnocchi N, Brusco GF, Pacchiarotti A, Aragona C (2006) Ongoing pregnancies after vitrification of human oocytes using a combined solution of ethylene glycol and dimethyl sulfoxide. Fertil Steril 86:997–1000
21. Liebermann J, Tucker MJ (2002) Effect of carrier system on the yield of human oocytes and embryos as assessed by survival and developmental potential after vitrification. Reproduction 124:483–489
22. Isachenko V, Katkov II, Yakovenko S, Lulat AG, Ulug M, Arvas A, Isachenko E (2007) Vitrification of human laser treated blastocysts within cut standard straws (CSS): novel aseptic packaging and reduced concentrations of cryoprotectants. Cryobiology 54:305–309
23. Chen SU, Lien YR, Cheng YY, Chen HF, Ho HN, Yang YS (2001) Vitrification of mouse oocytes using closed pulled straws (CPS) achieves a high survival and preserves good patterns of meiotic spindles, compared with conventional straws, open pulled straws (OPS) and grids. Hum Reprod 16:2350–2356
24. Ambrosini G, Andrisani A, Porcu E, Rebellato E, Revelli A, Caserta D, Cosmi E, Marci R, Moscarini M (2006) Oocytes cryopreservation: state of art. Reprod Toxicol 22:250–262
25. Rall WF (1987) Factors affecting the survival of mouse embryos cryopreserved by vitrification. Cryobiology 24:387–402
26. Wada I, Matson PL, Troup SA, Morroll DR, Hunt L, Lieberman BA (1993) Does elective cryopreservation of all embryos from women at risk of ovarian hyperstimulation syndrome reduce the incidence of the condition? Br J Obstet Gynaecol 100:265–269
27. Jain T, Missmer SA, Homstein MD (2004) Trents in embryo-transfer practice and in outcomes of the use of assisted reprodnctive technology in the United States N Engl J Med 350: 1639–1645
28. Burlow DH, Beard HK, William AC (2004) Assisted reproductive technologies in europe encompass diverse and complex ethical viewprints issues to be considered in repoting research in human reproduction. Ann NY Acad Sci 1034: 110–111
29. Anderson AR, Wilkinson SS, Price S, Crain JL (2005) Reduction of high order multiples in frozen embryo transfers. Reprod Biomed Online 10:402–405
30. Trounson A, Mohr L (1983) Human pregnancy following cryopreservation, thawing and transfer of an eight-cell embryo. Nature 305:707–709

31. Lassalle B, Testart J, Renard JP (1985) Human embryo features that influence the success of cryopreservation with the use of 1, 2 propanediol. Fertil Steril 44:645–651
32. Testart J, Lassalle B, Belaisch-Allart J, Hazout A, Forman R, Rainhorn JD, Frydman R (1986) High pregnancy rate after early human embryo freezing. Fertil Steril 46:268–272
33. Mandelbaum J, Junca AM, Plachot M, Alnot MO, Salat-Baroux J, Alvarez S, Tibi C, Cohen J, Debache C, Tesquier L (1988) Cryopreservation of human embryos and oocytes. Hum Reprod 3:117–119
34. Edgar DH, Bourne H, Jericho H, McBain JC (2000) The developmental potential of cryopreserved human embryos. Mol Cell Endocrinol 169:69–72
35. Fauser BC, Bouchard P, Coelingh Bennink HJ, Collins JA, Devroey P, Evers JL, van Steirteghem A (2002) Alternative approaches in IVF. Hum Reprod Update 8:1–9
36. Balakier H, Cabaca O, Bouman D, Shewchuk AB, Laskin C, Squire JA (2000) Spontaneous blastomere fusion after freezing and thawing of early human embryos leads to polyploidy and chromosomal mosaicism. Hum Reprod 15:2404–2410
37. Hu Y, Maxson WS, Hoffman DI, Ory SJ, Eager S (1999) A comparison of post-thaw results between cryopreserved embryos derived from intracytoplasmic sperm injection and those from conventional IVF. Fertil Steril 72:1045–1048
38. Tang R, Catt J, Howlett D (2006) Towards defining parameters for a successful single embryo transfer in frozen cycles. Hum Reprod 21:1179–1183
39. Tucker MJ, Morton PC, Sweitzer CL, Wright G (1995) Cryopreservation of human embryos and oocytes. Curr Opin Obstet Gynecol 7:188–192
40. Archer J, Gook DA, Edgar DH (2003) Blastocyst formation and cell numbers in human frozen-thawed embryos following extended culture. Hum Reprod 18:1669–1673
41. El-Toukhy T, Khalaf Y, Al-Darazi K, Andritsos V, Taylor A, Braude P (2003) Effect of blastomere loss on the outcome of frozen embryo replacement cycles. Fertil Steril 79:1106–1111
42. Edgar DH, Archer J, Gook DA, Jericho H, Wilton L, Bourne H (2004) Survival and developmental potential of stored human early cleavage stage embryos. Eur J Obstet Gynecol Reprod Biol 115(Suppl 1):S8–S11
43. Hardarson T, Löfman C, Coull G, Sjögren A, Hamberger L, Edwards RG (2002) Internalization of cellular fragments in a human embryo: time-lapse recordings. Reprod Biomed Online 5:36–38
44. Houghton FD, Barr KJ, Walter G, Gabriel HD, Grümmer R, Traub O, Leese HJ, Winterhager E, Kidder GM (2002) Functional significance of gap junctional coupling in preimplantation development. Biol Reprod 66:1403–1412
45. Rienzi L, Nagy ZP, Ubaldi F, Iacobelli M, Anniballo R, Tesarik J, Greco E (2002) Laser-assisted removal of necrotic blastomeres from cryopreserved embryos that were partially damaged. Fertil Steril 77:1196–1201
46. Rienzi L, Ubaldi F, Iacobelli M, Minasi MG, Romano S, Ferrero S, Sapienza F, Baroni E, Tesarik J, Greco E (2005) Developmental potential of fully intact and partially damaged cryopreserved embryos after laser-assisted removal of necrotic blastomeres and post-thaw culture selection. Fertil Steril 84:888–894
47. Nagy ZP, Taylor T, Elliott T, Massey JB, Kort HI, Shapiro DB (2005) Removal of lysed blastomeres from frozen-thawed embryos improves implantation and pregnancy rates in frozen embryo transfer cycles. Fertil Steril 84:1606–1612
48. Van der Elst J, Van den Abbeel E, Vitrier S, Camus M, Devroey P, Van Steirteghem AC (1997) Selective transfer of cryopreserved human embryos with further cleavage after thawing increases delivery and implantation rates. Hum Reprod 12:1513–1521
49. Guerif F, Bidault R, Cadoret V, Couet ML, Lansac J, Royere D (2002) Parameters guiding selection of best embryos for transfer after cryopreservation: a reappraisal. Hum Reprod 17:1321–1326
50. Mukaida T, Wada S, Takahashi K et al (1998) Vitrification of human embryos based on the assessment of suitable conditions for X-cell mouse embryos. Hum Reprod 13:2874–2879
51. El-Danasouri I, Solman H (2001) Successful pregnancies and deliveries after a simple vitrilk;ition protcK-ol for day 3 human embryos. Fertil Steril 76:400–402
52. Rama Raju GA, Haranath GB, Krishna KM et al (2005) Vitrification of human 8-cell embryos, a modified protocol for better pregnancy rates. Reprod Biomed Online 11:434–437
53. Liebermann J, Tucker MJ, Graham JR, Han T, Davis A, Levy MJ (2002) Blastocyst development after vitrification of multipronuclear zygotes using the Flexipet denuding pipette. Reprod Biomed Online 4:146–150
54. Desai N, Blackmon H, Szeptycki J, Goldfarb J (2007) Cryoloop vitrification of human day 3 cleavage-stage embryos: post-vitrification development, pregnancy outcomes and live births. Reprod Biomed Online 14:208–213
55. Hardy K, Handyside AH, Winston RM (1989) The human blastocyst: cell number, death and allocation during late preimplantation development in vitro. Development 107:597–604
56. Vanderzwalmen P, Bertin G, Debauche Ch, Standaert V, van Roosendaal E, Vandervorst M, Bollen N, Zech H, Mukaida T, Takahashi K, Schoysman R (2002) Births after vitrification at morula and blastocyst stages: effect of artificial reduction of the blastocoelic cavity before vitrification. Hum Reprod 17: 744–751
57. Guerif F, Cadoret V, Poindron J, Lansac J, Royere D (2003) Overnight incubation improves selection of frozen-thawed blastocysts for transfer: preliminary study using supernumerary embryos. Theriogenology 60:1457–1466
58. Kosasa TS, McNamee PI, Morton C, Huang TT (2005) Pregnancy rates after transfer of cryopreserved blastocysts cultured in a sequential media. Am J Obstet Gynecol 192:2035–2040
59. Desai N, Goldfarb J (2005) Examination of frozen cycles with replacement of a single thawed blastocyst. Reprod Biomed Online 11:349–354
60. Veeck LL, Bodine R, Clarke RN, Berrios R, Libraro J, Moschini RM, Zaninovic N, Rosenwaks Z (2004) High pregnancy rates can be achieved after freezing and thawing human blastocysts. Fertil Steril 82:1418–1427
61. Offenberg H, Thomsen PD (2005) Functional challenge affects aquaporin mRNA abundance in mouse blastocysts. Mol Reprod Dev 71:422–430
62. Shu YM, Watt J, Gebhardt J, Applying J, Behr B (2009) The value of fast blastocoele re-expansion in the selection of a shows blastocyst for transfer. Fert Steril 91: 401–406
63. Gardner DK, Pawelczynski M, Trounson AO (1996) Nutrient uptake and utilization can be used to select viable day 7 bovine blastocysts after cryopreservation. Mol Reprod Dev 44:472–475
64. Gardner DK, Lane M, Stevens J, Schoolcraft WB (2003) Changing the start temperature and cooling rate in a slow-freezing protocol increases human blastocyst viability. Fertil Steril 79:407–410
65. Menezo Y, Nicollet B, Herbaut N, Andre D (1992) Freezing cocultured human blastocysts. Fertil Steril 58:977–980
66. Menezo Y, Veiga A (1997) Cryopreservation of blastocysts. In: Proceedings of the 10th World Congress on IVF and Assisted Reproduction, Vancouver, Canada, 24–28 May 1997. Monduzzi Editore, Bologna, Italy, pp 41–45
67. Troup SA, Matson PL, Critchlow JD, Morroll DR, Lieberman BA, Burslem RW (1991) Cryopreservation of human embryos at the pronucleate, early cleavage, or expanded blastocyst stages. Eur J Obstet Gynecol Reprod Biol 38:133–139
68. Pantos K, Stefanidis K, Pappas K, Kokkinopoulos P, Petroutsou G, Kokkali G, Stavrou D, Tzigounisv V (2001) Cryopreservation of embryos, blastocysts, and pregnancy rates of blastocysts derived from frozen-thawed embryos and frozen-thawed blastocysts. J Assist Reprod Genet 18:579–582

69. Behr B, Gebhardt J, Lyon J, Milki AA (2002) Factors relating to a successful cryopreserved blastocyst transfer program. Fertil Steril 77:697–699
70. Ménézo Y, Veiga A, Benkhalifa M (1998) Improved methods for blastocyst formation and culture. Hum Reprod 13(Suppl 4):256–265
71. Boni R, Tosti E, Roviello S, Dale B (1999) Intercellular communications in in vivo- and in vitro-produced bovine embryos. Biol Reprod 61:1050–1055
72. Leibo SP, Loskutoff NM (1993) Cryobiology of in vitro-derived bovine embryos. Theriogenology 39:81–94
73. Zhu SE, Zeng SM, Yu WL, Li SJ, Zhang ZC, Chen YF (2001) Vitrification of in vivo and in vitro produced ovine blastocysts. Anim Biotechnol 12:193–203
74. Fair T, Lonergan P, Dinnyes A, Cottell DC, Hyttel P, Ward FA, Boland MP (2001) Ultrastructure of bovine blastocysts following cryopreservation: effect of method of blastocyst production. Mol Reprod Dev 58:186–195
75. Shapiro BS, Richter KS, Harris DC, Daneshmand ST (2001) A comparison of day 5 and day 6 blastocyst transfers. Fertil Steril 75:1126–1130
76. Liebermann J, Tucker MJ (2006) Comparison of vitrification and conventional cryopreservation of day 5 and day 6 blastocysts during clinical application. Fertil Steril 86:20–26
77. Utsunomiya T, Ito H, Hirai K, Otsu E, Watanabe H, Mori T (2006) Developmentally retarded frozen blastocysts can be rescued by synchronizing culture prior to transfer. Reprod Biomed Online 12:622–629
78. Richter KS, Shipley SK, McVearry I, Tucker MJ, Widra EA (2006) Cryopreserved embryo transfers suggest that endometrial receptivity may contribute to reduced success rates of later developing embryos. Fertil Steril 86:862–866
79. Yokota Y, Sato S, Yokota M, Ishikawa Y, Makita M, Asada T, Araki Y (2000) Successful pregnancy following blastocyst vitrification. Hum Reprod 15:1802–1803
80. Mukaida T, Nakamura S, Tomiyama T, Wada S, Kasai M, Takahashi K (2001) Successful birth after transfer of vitrified human blastocysts with use of a cryoloop containerless technique. Fertil Steril 76:618–620
81. Son WY, Yoon SH, Yoon HJ, Lee SM, Lim JH (2003) Pregnancy outcome following transfer of human blastocysts vitrified on electron microscopy grids after induced collapse of the blastocoele. Hum Reprod 18:137–139
82. Cremades N, Sousa M, Silva J, Viana P, Sousa S, Oliveira C, Teixeira da Silva J, Barros A (2004) Experimental vitrification of human compacted morulae and early blastocysts using fine diameter plastic micropipettes. Hum Reprod 19:300–305
83. Hiraoka K, Hiraoka K, Kinutani M, Kinutani K (2004) Blastocoele collapse by micropipetting prior to vitrification gives excellent survival and pregnancy outcomes for human day 5 and 6 expanded blastocysts. Hum Reprod 19:2884–2888
84. Stehlik E, Stehlik J, Katayama KP, Kuwayama M, Jambor V, Brohammer R, Kato O (2005) Vitrification demonstrates significant improvement versus slow freezing of human blastocysts. Reprod Biomed Online 11:53–57
85. Martin JA, Hamilton BE, Ventura SJ, Menacker F, Park MM, Sutton PD (2002) Births: final data for 2001. Natl Vital Stat Rep 51:1–102
86. American Cancer Society (2001) Cancer facts and figures—2001. American Cancer Society, Atlanta, GA
87. National Cancer Institute (1999) SEER*Stat software, version 2.0, National Cancer Institute, SEER cancer incidence public-use database, 1973-1996, August 1998 submission. Bethesda, MD
88. Ries LAG, Percy CL, Bunin GR (1999) Introduction. In: Ries LAG, Smith MA, Gurney JG, Linet M, Tamra T, Young JL, Bunin GR (eds) Cancer incidence and survival among children and adolescents: United States SEER Program 1975-1995 [NIH Pub. No. 99-4649]. National Cancer Institute, Bethesda, MD, pp 1–15
89. Jemal A, Clegg LX, Ward E, Ries LA, Wu X, Jamison PM, Wingo PA, Howe HL, Anderson RN, Edwards BK (2004) Annual report to the nation on the status of cancer, 1975–2001, with a special feature regarding survival. Cancer 101:3–27
90. Jain JK, Paulson RJ (2006) Oocyte cryopreservation. Fertil Steril 86(Suppl 4):1037–1046
91. Chen C (1986) Pregnancy after human oocyte cryopreservation. Lancet 330:884–886
92. Al-Hasani S, Diedrich K, van der Ven H, Reinecke A, Hartje M, Krebs D (1987) Cryopreservation of human oocytes. Hum Reprod 2:695–700
93. van Uem JF, Siebzehnrübl ER, Schuh B, Koch R, Trotnow S, Lang N (1987) Birth after cryopreservation of unfertilized oocytes. Lancet 329:752–753
94. Shaw JM, Oranratnachai A, Trounson AO (2000) Fundamental cryobiology of mammalian oocytes and ovarian tissue. Theriogenology 53:59–72
95. Pickering SJ, Johnson MH (1987) The influence of cooling on the organization of the meiotic spindle of the mouse oocyte. Hum Reprod 2:207–216
96. Matson PL, Graefling J, Junk SM, Yovich JL, Edirisinghe WR (1997) Cryopreservation of oocytes and embryos: use of a mouse model to investigate effects upon zona hardness and formulate treatment strategies in an in-vitro fertilization programme. Hum Reprod 12:1550–1553
97. Gook DA, Schiewe MC, Osborn SM, Asch RH, Jansen RP, Johnston WI (1995) Intracytoplasmic sperm injection and embryo development of human oocytes cryopreserved using 1, 2-propanediol. Hum Reprod 10:2637–2641
98. Fabbri R, Porcu E, Marsella T, Rocchetta G, Venturoli S, Flamigni C (2001) Human oocyte cryopreservation: new perspectives regarding oocyte survival. Hum Reprod 16:411–416
99. Coticchio G, De Santis L, Rossi G, Borini A, Albertini D, Scaravelli G, Alecci C, Bianchi V, Nottola S, Cecconi S (2006) Sucrose concentration influences the rate of human oocytes with normal spindle and chromosome configurations after slow-cooling cryopreservation. Hum Reprod 21:1771–1776
100. Boldt J, Cline D, Mclaughlin D (2003) Human oocyte cryopreservation as an adjunct to IVF-embryo transfer cycles. Hum Reprod 18: 1250–1255
101. Trad FS, Toner M, Biggers JD (1999) Effects of cryoprotectants and ice-seeding temperature on intracellular freezing and survival of human oocytes. Hum Reprod 14:1569–1577
102. Fosas N, Marina F, Torres PJ, Jové I, Martín P, Pérez N, Arnedo N, Marina S (2003) The births of five Spanish babies from cryopreserved donated oocytes. Hum Reprod 18:1417–1421
103. Eroglu A, Toner M, Toth TL (2002) Beneficial effect of microinjected trehalose on the cryosurvival of human oocytes. Fertil Steril 77:152–158
104. Rienzi L, Martinez F, Ubaldi F, Minasi MG, Iacobelli M, Tesarik J, Greco E (2004) Polscope analysis of meiotic spindle changes in living metaphase II human oocytes during the freezing and thawing procedures. Hum Reprod 19:655–659
105. Larman MG, Minasi MG, Rienzi L, Gardner DK (2007) Maintenance of the meiotic spindle during vitrification in human and mouse oocytes. Reprod Biomed Online 15:692–700
106. Kuleshova L, Gianaroli L, Magli C, Ferraretti A, Trounson A (1999) Birth following vitrification of a small number of human oocytes: case report. Hum Reprod 14:3077–3079
107. Antinori M, Licata E, Dani G, Cerusico F, Versaci C, Antinori S (2007) Cryotop vitrification of human oocytes results in high survival rate and healthy deliveries. Reprod Biomed Online 14: 72–79
108. Kuwayama M, Vajita G, Kato O, Leibo SP (2005) Highly efficient vitrification method for cryopreservation of human oocytes. Reprod Biomed Online 11:300–308

109. Chian RC, Son WY, Huang JY, Cui SJ, Buckett WM, Tan SL (2005) High survival rates and pregnancies of human oocytes following vitrification: preliminary report. Fertil Steril 84(Suppl 1):S36
110. Liebermann J, Tucker MJ, Sills ES (2003) Cryoloop vitrification in assisted reproduction: analysis of survival rates in > 1000 human oocytes after ultra-rapid cooling with polymer augmented cryoprotectants. Clin Exp Obstet Gynecol 30:125–129
111. Valdez DM, Miyamoto A, Hara T, Seki S, Kasai M, Edashige K (2005) Water- and cryoprotectant-permeability of mature and immature oocytes in the medaka (Oryzias latipes). Cryobiology 50:93–102
112. Fabbri R (2006) Cryopreservation of human oocytes and ovarian tissue. Cell Tissue Bank 7:113–122
113. Chian RC, Kuwayama M, Tan L, Tan J, Kato O, Nagai T (2004) High survival rate of bovine oocytes matured in vitro following vitrification. J Reprod Dev 50:685–696
114. Bogliolo L, Ariu F, Fois S, Rosati I, Zedda MT, Leoni G, Succu S, Pau S, Ledda S (2007) Morphological and biochemical analysis of immature ovine oocytes vitrified with or without cumulus cells. Theriogenology 68:1138–1149
115. Maher B (2007) Little consensus on egg freezing. Nature 449(7165):958
116. Borini A, Cattoli M, Mazzone S, Trevisi MR, Nalon M, Iadarola I (2007) Survey of 105 babies born after slow-cooling oocyte cryopreservation. Fertil Steril 88(Suppl 1):S13–S14
117. Hoffman DI, Zellman GL, Fair CC, Mayer JF, Zeitz JG, Gibbons WE, Turner TG Jr, Society for Assisted Reproduction Technology (SART) and RAND (2003) Cryopreserved embryos in the United States and their availability for research. Fertil Steril 79: 1063–1069
118. Tomlinson M (2005) Managing risk associated with cryopreservation. Hum Reprod 20:1751–1756
119. Practice Committee of the American Society for Reproductive Medicine (2006) Guidelines for reducing the risk of viral transmission during fertility treatment. Fertil Steril 86(5 Suppl):S11–S17
120. McKee TA, Avery S, Majid A, Brinsden PR (1996) Risks for transmission of hepatitis C virus during artificial insemination. Fertil Steril 66:161–163
121. Russel PH, Lyaruu VH, Millar JD, Curry MR, Watson PF (1997) The potential transmission of infectious agents by semen packing during storage for artificial insemination. Anim Reprod Sci 47:337–342
122. Bielanski A, Nadin-Davis S, Sapp T, Lutze-Wallace C (2000) Viral contamination of embryos cryopreserved in liquid nitrogen. Cryobiology 40:110–116
123. Clarke GN (1999) Sperm cryopreservation: is there a significant risk of cross-contamination? Hum Reprod 14:2941–2943
124. Tomlinson M, Sakkas D (2000) Is a review of standard procedures for cryopreservation needed?: safe and effective cryopreservation-should sperm banks and fertility centres move toward storage in nitrogen vapour? Hum Reprod 15: 2460–2463
125. Saritha KR, Bongso A (2001) Comparative evaluation of fresh and washed human sperm cryopreserved in vapor and liquid phases of liquid nitrogen. J Androl 22:857–862
126. Cobo A, Pérez S, Santos MJ, Pellicer A, Remohí J (2007) Comparison between storage of vitrified oocytes by cryotop method in liquid nitrogen vs. vapour phase of liquid nitrogen tanks. Fert Steril 88(Suppl 1):S91
127. Fahy GM (2007) Theoretical considerations for oocyte cryopreservation by freezing. Reprod Biomed Online 14:709–714
128. Gao D, Critser JK (2000) Mechanisms of cryoinjury in living cells. ILAR J 41(4):187–196

Chapter 47
Preserving Fertility

Kutluk Oktay and Ozgur Oktem

Abstract Negative impact of modern cancer treatment methods on human reproduction has been recognized. In this chapter, we first summarize the facts about cancer and treatment-related adverse outcomes in female reproductive function, then discuss the needs, and outline the current strategies and the future directions of fertility preservation and ovarian cryopreservation and transplantation in adult and adolescent female patients whose fertility are jeopardized by the therapies required for the treatment of their primary illnesses.

Keywords Fertility preservation • Cancer • Gonadotoxic • Chemotherapy • Radiation • Cryopreservation

47.1 Facts About Cancer

Cancer is one of the biggest public health problems in the world. In 2008, approximately 1.5 million new cancer cases and 500,000 deaths from cancer were expected to occur in the US. Approximately 700,000 of these cases would be females. Cancers of the breast, lung and bronchus, and colon and rectum, leukemia and lymphomas, and cervical cancer are commonly diagnosed in females under the age 40. The probability of being diagnosed with an invasive cancer for women under the age 40 is 2%. This rate climbs up to 9% by the age 60 [1]. Leukemia is the leading cause of cancer death among females before age 20. Breast cancer ranks first at age 20–59 years, and leaves its place to lung cancer in women at age 60 years and older. Overall, cancer is the leading cause of death among women aged 40–79 years [1].

Childhood cancers are another important health issue as cancer is the second leading cause of death among children between ages 1 and 14 years in the United States. Most common types of childhood tumors are leukemia, tumors of the central nervous system, neuroblastoma, Wilms tumor and nonHodgkin lymphoma [1].

Advanced diagnostic modalities, improved surgical technique, combination chemotherapy, radiotherapy, and supportive care have led to an increase in the 5-year survival rates for many cancer types. For instance, the survival rate in adults increased from 50% in 1970s to 66% in 2003 when cancers of all sites and all races are considered [1]. The figures are more encouraging in children. The 5-year relative survival rate among children for all cancer sites combined improved from 58% for patients diagnosed in 1975–1977 to 80% for those diagnosed in 1996–2003 [1].

47.2 Cancer Therapy: Gonadal Cytotoxicity

Modern combination chemotherapy and radiotherapy regimens have a substantial negative impact on reproductive organs. Premature ovarian failure and other poor reproductive outcomes such as preterm births and abortions are major sequels subsequent to cancer therapies. Ovaries are endowed with a limited number of eggs, which are very sensitive to cytotoxic cancer drugs and radiation. Reproductive life span (ovarian reserve) is determined by the number of quiescent primordial follicles in the ovary. Germ cells differentiate into primordial follicles, and their number is established before birth even though this dogma has been recently challenged by two studies [2, 3]. Direct or indirect toxic insults to the oocyte, surrounding steroid-producing somatic cell layers (granulosa and theca cells) or both are associated with accelerated and premature depletion of germ cells in the gonads. This is the main mechanism underlying gonadal failure induced by chemotherapy and radiation [4]. Patient's age, the type, dose, and intensity of chemotherapy and/or radiotherapy are the main factors determining the magnitude of the damage in the ovary. Older patients have lower ovarian reserve when compared with younger ones; therefore they have higher risk for ovarian failure during or after chemotherapy or radiation. Sadly, as

K. Oktay (✉) and O. Oktem
Department of Obstetrics and Gynecology, New York Medical College-Westchester Medical Center, Valhalla, NY, USA

D.T. Carrell and C.M. Peterson (eds.), *Reproductive Endocrinology and Infertility: Integrating Modern Clinical and Laboratory Practice*,
DOI 10.1007/978-1-4419-1436-1_47, © Springer Science+Business Media, LLC 2010

noted in the adult survivors of childhood cancers, there are some other adverse *extragonadal* effects such as abnormalities in the regulation of growth and endocrine functions, and other poor reproductive outcomes that appear later in life such as preterm births and miscarriages.

Besides malignancies, treatment of certain precancerous and benign conditions such as myelodysplasia, aplastic anemia, and systemic lupus erythematosus may necessitate the administration of high dose chemotherapeutics with and without stem cell transplantation [5]. Therefore, preservation of gonadal function and fertility has become one of the major qualities of life issues for cancer survivors at reproductive ages. Accordingly, clinical guidelines, encouraging fertility preservation among all young cancer survivors with interest in fertility, have been recently issued by American Society of Clinical Oncology [6].

47.3 Chemotherapy Agents: Ovarian Toxicity

Gonadotoxic potentials of chemotherapeutics may differ depending upon their mechanisms of action. Data on their toxicity profile has accumulated from important sources; clinical trials and animal studies. In most of the clinical studies, status of menstrual function has been the main parameter to evaluate the magnitude of the impact of chemotherapy on human ovary. However, menstrual status may not be a reliable marker of gonadotoxicity or fertility as shown previously in patients who were still menstruating despite their critically elevated FSH levels and diminished ovarian reserve [7]. Moreover, the use of multiagent chemotherapy drugs in many regimens precludes assessment of individual gonadotoxicity of each drug in a given regimen.

Markers of ovarian reserve such as FSH, estradiol, and anti-Mullerian hormone (AMH) measurements [7] as well as antral follicle counts [8] can be used for a better assessment of ovarian reserve before and after chemotherapy. However, their predictive value in evaluating the impact of chemotherapy regimens remains to be determined. Unfortunately, neither of these markers is direct measures of ovarian reserve. More accurate information of gonadotoxicity on human ovary can only be obtained by real-time quantitative analysis of primordial follicle counts using histomorphological methods in ovarian samples. This necessitates an operation it cannot be done in clinical settings for ethical and practical reasons. Moreover, as new agents are introduced to adjuvant setting, their long-term impact on human ovary is extremely difficult to determine from short-term studies.

As another source of information on gonadotoxicity, a number of animal studies have been conducted mainly in rodents. Even though these models showed individual gonadotoxicity of certain cancer drugs such as cyclophosphamide and doxorubicin [9, 10] however, some discrepancies may exist between animal and human ovaries. Therefore by considering all these needs, we developed a human xenograft model [11]. That model enabled us to characterize the time course and the mechanism of action of gonadal damage induced by chemotherapy agents via quantitative histomorphometric analysis of primordial follicle counts and cell death assays.

A solid body of evidence consistently showed that chemotherapy agents of alkylating group appear to have more toxic effects in the gonads of both sexes, therefore are associated with the highest risk of infertility as shown in clinical and animal studies. Alkylating antineoplastic agents include nitrogen mustard family (cyclophosphamide, uramustine, chlorambucil and melphalan, mechlorethamine), alkyl sulfonates (busulfan), nitrosureas (carmustine, streptozocin), ethyleneimines and methylmelamines (hexamethylmelamine and thiotepa), triazenes (dacarbazine) and imidazotetrazines (temozolomide). Cyclophosphamide is one of the most commonly used and one of the most effective antineoplastic drugs in the treatment of many solid and hematologic malignancies as well as certain autoimmune diseases [4]. We recently characterized gonadotoxicity of cyclophosphamide in human ovary using a xenograft model [11]. Cyclophosphamide based regimens CEF, CMF, CAF, AC (combinations of cyclophosphamide with methotrexate, epirubicin, fluorouracil, doxorubicin) are commonly used in the adjuvant treatment of breast cancer. Cyclophosphamide and busulfan combination are administered at high doses for myeloablative conditioning prior to hematopoietic stem cell transplantation. CHOP (in combination with doxorubicin and vincristine) is another cyclophosphamide-based alkylating regimen commonly used in the treatment of leukemia and lymphomas. All these regimens are associated with higher risk of permanent and premature ovarian failure especially in patients at age 40 and older with diminished ovarian reserve even at smaller doses. Patients who receive these combinations at ages between 30 and 39 or younger than 30 possess lower risk for gonadal failure because of their higher ovarian reserve [6].

Data on ovarian toxicity associated with the use of other antineoplastic agents are scarcer. Cisplatin and Adriamycin posses intermediate risk for gonadotoxicity whereas administration of nonalkylating agents such as vincristine methotrexate, fluorouracil, Idarubicin or ABVD combination (doxorubicin/bleomycin/vinblastin/dacarbazine) may pose lower risk for ovarian failure because of less harmful nature of these agents [5, 6].

It should be emphasized that newer drugs with unknown toxicity profile such as, Taxanes, Oxaliplatin, Irinotecan, monoclonal antibodies (trastuzumab, bevacizumab, cetuximab), or tyrosine kinase inhibitors (erlotinib, imatinib), or less cytotoxic agents when used at higher doses, longer duration of use, or at more frequent intervals may be associated with higher risk for premature ovarian failure.

A recent study quantified the impact of chemotherapy on primordial follicle count in age-matched cancer patients undergoing ovarian freezing before and after chemotherapy administration by providing histological evidence for chemotherapy induced primordial follicle loss [12].

Another important point to be emphasized is that ovarian stromal cells may play a role in ovarian endocrine function and possibly in restoration of ovulatory function postchemotherapy [13]. Since the importance of stromal cells has been shown in other organs such as bone marrow, in which stromal cells previously exposed to cancer drugs suppress hematopoiesis from normal donor cells [14], studies that address whether chemotherapy induced damage in ovarian stromal cells has important in the restoration of ovarian stromal function are needed. We showed that in vitro, ovarian cortical pieces from individuals who were previously exposed to chemotherapy (chemotherapy group) produced significantly less estradiol when compared with those who were not (control group) [12].

47.4 Ovarian Damage Induced by Radiation

Ovarian damage and failure may develop during or after radiotherapy. Abdominal, pelvic, or spinal irradiation are associated with increased risk of developing acute ovarian failure, especially if both ovaries are within the treatment field [15, 16]. Ovarian damage may occur not only by direct exposure to radiation such as in the case of pelvic or low abdominal irradiation, but also scatter radiation may cause significant damage even if gonads are outside of the radiation. Direct actions of particles such as neutrons on DNA are predominant mechanism of damage, while indirect actions come from the interaction of radiation with other substances in the cell such as water leading to formation of free radicals and DNA damage. This mechanism is particularly true for sparsely ionizing radiation such as X-rays. Increased radiation doses are associated with a higher risk of gonadal failure. The extent of the damage could be more pronounced with single dose rather than fractionated dose [17]. The LD 50, the radiation dose required to kill 50% of oocytes of the human oocyte is <2 Gray (Gy).

As younger ovaries harbor higher number of primordial follicles, younger individuals are more resistant to permanent damage from irradiation than are older individuals [18, 19]. For instance, 6 Gy may be sufficient to produce irreversible ovarian damage in women older than 40 years of age when compared with 10–20 Gy doses needed to induce permanent ovarian failure in the majority of females treated during childhood [20, 21]. Perhaps, the most devastating damage in the ovary occurs in patients who receive a stem cell transplant with high dose total body irradiation (TBI). One study showed that almost all of the patients who had undergone a marrow transplant with TBI after age 10 years developed acute ovarian failure, whereas approximately 50% of girls who had received a transplant before age 10 years suffered acute loss of ovarian function [22]. TBI given as a single dose or fractionated (10–15 Gy), is often used in combination with gonadotoxic cyclophosphamide or melphalan. The use of cyclophosphamide in conjuction with radiation increases further the extent of the damage as exemplified by a study showing that all of 144 patients receiving TBI with cyclophosphamide for bone marrow transplantation (BMT) developed amenorrhea in the first 3 years. Return of menses occurred 3–7 years posttransplant only in nine patients; all were younger than age 25 [23].

47.5 Other Reproductive Harms Associated with Chemotherapy and Radiation

Increased survival rates associated with newer modern cancer therapies have given rise to a new population, *adult survivors of childhood cancer*. As a result of exposure to high cumulative doses of specific chemotherapeutic agents (e.g., alkylating agents, anthracyclines) and radiotherapy or both, many treatment-related adverse health outcomes have been identified in this newly described group of patients, ranging from metabolic and endocrine abnormalities to cognitive function deficits. There are some other long-term adverse outcomes in reproductive function, especially among survivors of childhood cancer after exposure to chemotherapy and radiotherapy, due to their extra gonadal effects. It appears that female sex is more commonly associated with higher treatment-related risks such as cognitive dysfunction after cranial irradiation, poor cardiovascular outcomes, obesity, radiation-associated differences in pubertal timing, development of primary hypothyroidism, breast cancer as a second malignant neoplasm and osteonecrosis [24]. The timing of menarche may be altered in survivors of childhood cancer, especially in those exposed to cranial and craniospinal radiotherapy when compared with those treated with chemotherapy alone. Therefore, those exposed to cranial and craniospinal radiotherapy, especially at a young age, should be monitored closely for abnormal timing of menarche [25].

Uterine function is also often compromised by radiation-induced damage to uterine vascular and muscular structures resulting in decreased uterine blood flow, reduced uterine volume, decreased endometrial thickness, and loss of distensibility. Whole body irradiation (20–30 Gy) during childhood has documented to cause mid-trimester miscarriages [26]. Unfortunately, women exposed to radiation postpubertally have larger uterus and greater likelihood of livebirth than those exposed prepubertally [27]. Sadly, women with ovarian failure secondary to whole body irradiation (20–30 Gy) have significantly reduced uterine size with no improvement in blood flow and endometrial thickness in response to exogenous sex hormones [28]. Another adverse effect of radiation therapy is lower birth weight in the offspring and a higher risk of miscarriage in childhood cancer survivors according to the report of the Childhood Cancer Survey Study [29]. Restricted fetal growth and early births may occur as late effects among the offspring of female childhood cancer survivors, especially in those who had received pelvic irradiation [30].

Amenorrhea occurring post exposure to radiation may be hypothalamic in origin rather than ovarian as seen in individuals receiving radiation at doses >30 Gy to the hypothalamic – pituitary unit [31].

47.6 Strategies to Preserve Reproductive Function

There are different fertility preservation options in female patients depending upon the patient's age, type of treatment, diagnosis, whether she has a partner, the time available and the potential that cancer has metastasized to her ovaries.

47.7 Ovarian Tissue Freezing

Animal studies of ovarian tissue cryopreservation and transplantation date back to the 1950s. But its application to human ovarian tissue is confined to last decade [32]. Studies related to several animal models such as sheep, mice, rat, and primate have documented feasibility of ovarian tissue freezing and transplantation [33]. Prepubertal children and adult patients who do not have time to undergo ovarian stimulation for oocyte or embryo cryopreservation should be considered ovarian cryopreservation. Primardial follicles are located in ovarian cortex and contain oocytes arrested in the diplotene stage of prophase of first meiotic division. Banking of ovarian tissue relies on the relative resistance of primordial follicles to cryo-toxicity/ischemia because of their relatively high surface/volume ratio, low metabolic rate, the absence of zona pellucida, and lack of metaphase spindles when compared with follicles at other developmental stages [34].

As our understanding about cryobiology and cryo damage improved along with the advent of effective modern cryoprotectants such as ethylene glycol, dimethyl sulfoxide (DMSO) and propanediol and new sophisticated automated cryopreservation machines, more encouraging results have been obtained in human. In order to determine the optimum way of freezing human ovarian tissue, several points need to be considered:

- *Patient age* is one of the most important factors determining the success of ovarian freezing and transplantation procedure. More than 60% of primordial follicles are lost after transplantation during ischemic period until revascularization is established according to animal autograft [35] and human xenograft studies [11]. An additional 7% appear to be lost during freezing and thawing. Since there is an age-related decline in primordial follicle counts [36], women older than 40 tend to have low follicle density; therefore, they may not be good candidates for the procedure. The losses are tolerated better in younger patients with higher ovarian reserve.
- *Size of the cortical pieces* is another important factor. Even though we still don't know the optimum size of the pieces for freezing and grafting, long term survival and follicle growth are achieved in 0.5×0.5–1 cm pieces. Excessive tissue slicing may damage the primordial follicle reserve in the tissue and, small cortical pieces may not be manageable for future transplantation. Because of these considerations, we have utilized ovarian cortical pieces with 0.5×1 cm long and 0.1–0.2 cm for cryopreservation.
- *Cryoprotectant* can be DMSO, propanediol or ethylene glycol. Glycerol is not as effective for ovarian tissue freezing and therefore should not be used [37]. At the present time, slow freezing technique appears to be the most suitable technique for ovarian tissue freezing, and vitrification has not yet produced reliable results.

47.8 Ovarian Transplantation

Two main approaches have been developed to autotransplant ovarian cortical pieces in humans. *Orthotopic* transplants involve grafting these strips near the infundibulopelvic ligament or possibly on a postmenopausal ovary. In the *heterotopic* transplant, tissues can be grafted subcutaneously at various locations including forearm and abdominal wall.

We reported the first case of autologous ovarian transplantation with cryopreserved tissue in 2000 [37]. The case was a 29 year old patient suffering from severe endometriosis and underwent orthotopic transplantation in which the grafts were sutured to a peritoneal pocket created in the left pelvic ovarian bursa. The grafts were stimulated with gonadotropins and ovulation was documented 15 weeks postgrafting. Endocrine function continued up to 9 months posttransplantation. Likewise, we also reported the first cases of embryo generation and spontaneous pregnancies following subcutaneous transplantation of frozen banked tissue in 2004 and 2006, respectively [13, 38]. In both cases, the grafts were transplanted heterotopically beneath the skin of abdomen. In the first case, ovarian tissue was cryopreserved from a 30-year-old woman with breast cancer before chemotherapy-induced menopause, and this tissue was transplanted beneath the skin of her abdomen 6 years later. Ovarian function returned in the patient 3 months after transplantation, as shown by follicle development and oestrogen production. The patient underwent eight oocyte retrievals percutaneously and 20 oocytes were retrieved. Of the eight oocytes suitable for in-vitro fertilization, one fertilized normally and developed into a four-cell embryo. The other patient was a Hodgkin lymphoma survivor who became menopausal for two and a half years following a HSCT. Interestingly, following a heterotopic ovarian transplantation, the patient spontaneously conceived within 4 months of transplantation, concurrently with follicular activity in the ovarian transplant under her abdominal skin. She eventually delivered a healthy girl who is now 2 years old. This case clearly illustrates that spontaneous pregnancies can occur even in those who appear to be in menopause for years, and even after unilateral oophorectomy for ovarian cryopreservation. It also brings up a new research question as to whether ovarian transplants could play a role in the recovery of the damaged ovary by triggering regeneration of oocytes postchemotherapy [13, 39].

Recently, live births following autologous ovarian transplantation to pelvis have been reported. Even though these results are encouraging, some argued that it is not possible to confirm if the patients have ovulated from their preexisting ovaries or from the transplanted tissues [40–42].

Overall, the experience with ovarian cryopreservation is still limited, the utilization rate of banked tissue is very low because the procedure itself is a relatively new technology and the patients are young and some are still undergoing cancer treatment and/or surveillance [43].

47.9 Embryo Cryopreservation

For patients with partners and sufficient amount of time before cancer treatment, in vitro fertilization (IVF) with embryo cryopreservation is the most established fertility preservation technique. It is not technically challenging and has been used for nearly two decades to store the unused embryos from IVF and embryo transfer cycles.

Low-temperature storage methods of embryos at the pronuclear, early cleavage stage, and more recently at the blastocyst stage, have been successfully established [44]. It is not within the scope of this chapter to review literature and provide detailed technical information on embryo freezing; rather, we mainly focus on the ovarian stimulation protocol with aromatase inhibitors recently developed by us for IVF and embryo or oocyte freezing as a means of fertility preservation in breast cancer patients.

An IVF cycle typically takes approximately 2 weeks to complete, and this time period may not be available to most cancer patients except breast cancer patients who have a 6 week period between surgery and initiation of adjuvant therapies. However, standard ovarian stimulation protocols are contraindicated in patients with breast cancer because of high estrogen levels. Since most of these tumors are estrogen sensitive, supraphysiologic estrogen levels (typically greater than 1,000 pg/mL compared to peak levels of 200–350 pg/mL in natural cycles) attained with gonadotropin stimulation during ovarian stimulation, in general, is not considered safe in women with breast cancer. We recently developed an ovarian stimulation protocol using aromatase inhibitors in combination with FSH for the purpose of preserving fertility via embryo or oocyte cryopreservation in breast cancer patients [45, 46]. Letrozole appears to be the best aromatase inhibitor drug for this purpose as it has a proven efficacy in the prevention of breast cancer recurrence and because, coincidentally, has ovulation-inducing properties [47]. When combined with gonadotropins letrozole cycles results in similar oocyte and embryo yield as IrF cycles [45].

47.10 Oocyte Freezing

Cryopreservation of oocyte is an emerging option suitable for young adolescents, women without partners, or women who do not wish to have their oocytes fertilized by sperm from a partner or anonymous donor. Since the first report of a live birth after successful oocyte cryopreservation in human in 1986 [49], several additional pregnancies and deliveries using a slow freeze, rapid thaw technique were reported [50, 51]. Unfortunately, it is still associated with lower pregnancy rates in contrast to more encouraging results with IVF and embryo freezing due to some technical challenges encountered during the freeze – thaw process and the in vitro maturation of immature oocytes. Mature oocytes are arrested at metaphase II and therefore more prone to cryodamage because the spindle apparatus is fully extended at metaphase II and prone to disassembly at lower temperature, with subsequent chromosome dispersion and aneuploidy [52, 53]. Large size, high water content, and relatively impermeable zona layer are other features of oocytes that also make them more vulnerable to ice crystal formation, rupture, and limited penetration of cryoprotectant solutions. We recently conducted meta-analysis to determine the efficiency of oocyte cryopreservation relative to IVF with unfrozen oocytes [54]. The success rates of IVF with slow-frozen oocytes are significantly lower when compared with the case of IVF with unfrozen oocytes. Although oocyte cryopreservation with the SF method appears to be justified for preserving fertility when a medical indication exists, its value for elective applications remains to be determined. Pregnancy rates with VF appear to have improved, but further studies will be needed to determine the efficiency and safety of this technique.

47.11 Ovarian Transposition (Oophoropexy) and Other Options

Administration of spinal radiation for the treatment of acute lymphoblastic leukemia and brain tumors appears to result in clinically significant ovarian damage in some young females [55]. Girls treated with whole abdominal and/or pelvic irradiation for Hodgkin disease, Wilms tumor, or other solid tumors (e.g., rhabdomyosarcoma, neuroblastoma) are at high risk of acute ovarian failure [56, 57]. Ovarian transposition performed prior to radiotherapy may rescue some ovarian function in the majority of young girls and adolescent females [58, 59]. If the patient is to undergo an abdominal surgery, ovaries can be transposed simultaneously, or if she is to be treated nonsurgically, laparoscopic transposition can be performed before the scheduled radiotherapy. The success with fertility preservation by ovarian transposition prior to radiotherapy varies between 16 and 90% [5]. This likelihood of success is affected by the degree of scatter radiation, vascular compromise, the age of the patient, dose of radiation, whether the ovaries were shielded, whether concomitant chemotherapy is used, and whether vaginal brachytherapy or pelvic external beam irradiation plus brachytherapy were used. In addition, this surgical procedure is not without complications; Fallopian tube infarction, chronic ovarian pain, ovarian cyst formation, and migration of ovaries back to their original position before radiotherapy have been reported, some of which may require additional gynaecological surgeries [60]. When ovaries are transposed to an abdominal position, spontaneous pregnancy may not be possible unless a second procedure is performed to relocate ovaries back to pelvis. In addition, should these patients need IVF in the future, oocyte retrieval may become technically more challenging. Therefore, candidates for ovarian transposition should be selected carefully, accounting for all the variables that may affect its success rates. It should also be borne in mind that, when gonadotoxic chemotherapy is used along with radiation, there is no strong rationale to perform this procedure.

Another option to decrease the dose of scattered radiation to the ovaries is intensity modulated radiotherapy (IMRT). IMRT is a new conformal radiotherapy that delivers radiation to tumor more precisely while sparing the surrounding tissues. Its ability of simultaneously creating multiple targets and multiple avoidance structures may guide oncologist to reduce the scattered dose to the ovary [61].

It has been hypothesized, largely based on the debated role of gonadal suppression in men in preserving testicular function against chemotherapy, and partially the misbelief that prepubertal girls are not affected by gonadotoxic cancer treatment, that ovarian suppression can be protective. Even though there are some animal studies with conflicting results of the protective effect of GnRH agonists against chemotherapy and radiotherapy [62, 63] and some anecdotal clinical trials done with a few patients with short term follow-ups and historical controls [64], there is neither a reliable clinical study nor molecular evidence showing that GnRH agonists protect the human ovaries from chemo and radiation [12, 65, 66].

Sphingosine-1-phosphate (S1P), a metabolite in ceramide signaling pathway has been shown to provide protection in mouse ovaries against chemotherapy and radiation. While we still do not know if this drug protects the germ cells in human ovaries from chemotherapy and radiation, there is one recent study that showed that S1P may decrease germ cell apoptosis in-vitro in human ovaries when cultured without serum [67].

47.12 Conclusion: Evidence-Based Guidelines

As a recently emerging field, fertility preservation is still investigational. When chosing a fertility preservation technique, details such as patient's age, type of treatment, diagnosis, whether she has a partner, the time available and the potential that cancer has metastasized to her ovaries have to be taken into account. Appropriate counseling and good communication with the oncologist is also vital to facilitate and perform the fertility preservation procedures safely and without delay.

Ovarian tissue freezing should be considered for prepubertal children and adult women patients who do not have a partner or time to undergo ovarian stimulation for oocyte or embryo cryopreservation.

Oocyte cryopreservation is an emerging option for young adolescents, women without partners, or women who do not wish to have their oocytes fertilized by sperm from a partner or anonymous donor.

IVF and embryo cryopreservation is the most established fertility preservation technique if the patient has a partner and sufficient amount of time before cancer treatment. Recently, aromatase inhibitors have been introduced for ovarian stimulation in breast cancer patients. While large-scale and long term prospective randomized studies are needed to validate the safety of this form of ovarian stimulation protocols in breast cancer patients, with 5-year follow-up [48], letrozole appears to be a safe alternative to conventional ovarian stimulation protocols, which are contraindicated because of endogenous estradiol rising to the levels several times higher than natural cycles.

References

1. Jemal A, Siegel R, Ward E et al (2008) Cancer statistics, 2008. CA Cancer J Clin 58:71–96
2. Johnson J, Bagley J, Skaznik-Wikiel M et al (2005) Oocyte generation in adult mammalian ovaries by putative germcells in bone marrow and peripheral blood. Cell 122:303–315
3. Johnson J, Canning J, Kaneko T et al (2004) Germline stem cells and follicular renewal in the postnatal mammalian ovary. Nature 428:145–150
4. Oktem O, Oktay K (2008) Preservation of menstrual function in adolescent and young females. Ann N Y Acad Sci 1135:237–243
5. Sonmezer M, Oktay K (2004) Fertility preservation in female patients. Hum Reprod Update 10:251–266
6. Lee SJ, Schover LR, Partridge AH et al (2006) American Society of Clinical Oncology recommendations on fertility preservation in cancer patients. J Clin Oncol 24:2917–2931
7. Oktay K, Oktem O, Reh A (2006) Measuring the impact of chemotherapy on fertility in women with breast cancer. J Clin Oncol 24:4044–4046
8. Scheffer GJ, Broekmans FJ, Looman CW et al (2003) The number of antral follicles in normal women with proven fertility is the best reflection of reproductive age. Hum Reprod 18:700–706
9. Plowchalk DR, Mattison DR (1991) Phosphoramide mustard is responsible for the ovarian toxicity of cyclophosphamide. Toxicol Appl Pharmacol 107:472–481
10. Morita Y, Perez GI, Paris F et al (2000) Oocyte apoptosis is suppressed by disruption of the acid sphingomyelinase gene or by sphingosine-1-phosphate therapy. Nat Med 10:1109–1114
11. Oktem O, Oktay K (2007) A novel ovarian xenografting model to characterize the impact of chemotherapy agents on human primordial follicle reserve. Cancer Res 67(21):10159–10162
12. Oktem O, Oktay K (2007) Quantitative assessment of the impact of chemotherapy on ovarian follicle reserve and stromal function. Cancer 110:2222–2229
13. Oktay K (2006) Spontaneous conceptions and live birth after heterotopic ovarian transplantation: is there a germline stem cell connection? Hum Reprod 21:1345–1348
14. Schwartz GN, Warren MK, Rothwell SW et al (1998) Post-chemotherapy and cytokine pretreated marrow stromal cell layers suppress hematopoiesis from normal donor CD341 cells. Bone Marrow Transplant 22:457–468
15. Stillman RJ, Schinfeld JS, Schiff I et al (1981) Ovarian failure in long term survivors of childhood malignancy. Am J Obstet Gynecol 139:62–66
16. Sklar C (2005) Maintenance of ovarian function and risk of premature menopause related to cancer treatment. J Natl Cancer Inst Monogr 34:25–27
17. Wallace WHB, Thompson AB, Kelsey TW (2003) Radiosensitivity of the human oocyte. Hum Reprod 18:117–121
18. Horning SJ, Hoppe RT, Kaplan HS, Rosenberg SA (1981) Female reproductive potential after treatment for Hodgkin's disease. N Engl J Med 304:1377–1382
19. Lushbaugh CC, Casarett GW (1976) The effects of gonadal irradiation in clinical radiation therapy: a review. Cancer 37:1111–1120
20. Thibaud E, Ramirez M, Brauner R et al (1992) Preservation of ovarian function by ovarian transposition performed before pelvic irradiation during childhood. J Pediatr 121:880–884
21. Sarafoglou K, Boulad F, Boulad F, Sklar C (1997) Gonadal function after bone marrow transplantation for acute leukemia during childhood. J Pediatr 130:210–216
22. Sklar C (1995) Growth and endocrine disturbances after bone marrow transplantation in childhood. Acta Paediatr 411(suppl):57–61
23. Sanders JE, Hawley J, Levy W et al (1996) Pregnancies following high-dose cyclophosphamide with or without high-dose busulfan or total-body irradiation and bone marrow transplantation. Blood 87:3045–3052
24. Armstrong GT, Sklar CA, Hudson MM, Robison LL (2007) Long-term health status among survivors of childhood cancer: does sex matter? J Clin Oncol 25:4477–4489
25. Chow EJ, Friedman DL, Yasui Y et al (2008) Timing of Menarche among survivors of childhood acute lymphoblastic leukemia: a report from the Childhood Cancer Survivor Study. Pediatr Blood Cancer 50:854–858
26. Wallace W, Shalet SM, Crowne EC, Morris-Jones PH, Gattamaneni HR (1989) Ovarian failure following abdominal irradiation in childhood: natural history and prognosis. Clin Oncol 1:75–79
27. Bath LE, Wallace WH, Critchley HO (2002) Late effects of the treatment of childhood cancer on the female reproductive system and the potential for fertility preservation. BJOG 1092:107–114
28. Critchley HO, Wallace WH, Shalet SM, Mamtora H, Higginson J, Anderson DC (1992) Abdominal irradiation in childhood: the potential for pregnancy. Brit J Obstet Gynaecol 99:392–394
29. Green DM, Whitton JA, Stovall M et al (2002) Pregnancy outcome of female survivors of childhood cancer: a report from the Childhood Cancer Survivor Study. Am J Obstet Gynecol 187: 1070–1080
30. Cohen SLB, SS BC et al (2006) Female survivors of childhood cancer: preterm birth and low birth weight among their children. J Natl Cancer Inst 98:1453–1461
31. Sklar CA, Constine LS (1995) Chronic neuroendocrinological sequelae of radiation therapy. Int J Radiat Oncol Biol Phys 31:1113–1121
32. Oktay K, Newton H, Aubard Y, Salha O, Gosden RG (1998) Cryopreservation of immature human oocytes and ovarian tissue: an emerging technology? Fertil Steril 69:1–7
33. Shamonki MI, Oktay K (2005) Oocyte and ovarian tissue cryopreservation: indications, techniques, and applications. Semin Reprod Med 23:266–276
34. Oktem O, Sonmezer M, Oktay K (2004) Ovarian tissue cryopreservation and other fertility preserving strategies. In: Gardner DK, Weismann A, Howles CM, Shoham Z (eds) Textbook of assisted reproductive techniques, 2nd edn. Taylor & Francis, Florida, pp 315–327
35. Baird DT, Webb R, Campbell BK, Harkness LM, Gosden RG (1999) Long-term ovarian function in sheep after ovariectomy and transplantation of autografts stored at −196°C. Endocrinology 140:462–471
36. Oktay K (2001) Ovarian cryopreservation and transplantation: preliminary findings and implications for cancer patients. Hum Reprod Update 7:526–534
37. Oktay K, Karlikaya G (2000) Ovarian function after transplantation of frozen, banked autologous ovarian tissue. N Engl J Med 342:1919
38. Oktay K, Buyuk E, Veeck L et al (2004) Embryo development after heterotopic transplantation of cryopreserved ovarian tissue. Lancet 363:837–840
39. Oktay K, Oktem O (2007) Regeneration of oocytes after chemotherapy: connecting the evidence from mouse to human. J Clin Oncol 25:3185–3187

40. Donnez J, Dolmans MM, Demylle D et al (2004) Livebirth after orthotopic transplantation of cryopreserved ovarian tissue. Lancet 364:1405–1410
41. Meirow D, Levron J, Eldar-Geva T et al (2005) Pregnancy after transplantation of cryopreserved ovarian tissue in a patient with ovarian failure after chemotherapy. N Engl J Med 353:318–321
42. Demeestere I, Simon P, Buxant F et al (2006) Ovarian function and spontaneous pregnancy after combined heterotopic and orthotopic cryopreserved ovarian tissue transplantation in a patient previously treated with bone marrow transplantation: case report. Hum Reprod 21:2010–2014
43. Oktay K, Oktem O Safety and utilization of ovarian cryopreservation for fertility preservation in cancer patients: long term experience. Fertil Steril (2008)
44. Borini A, Cattoli M, Bulletti C, Coticchio G (2008) Clinical efficiency of oocyte and embryo cryopreservation. Ann N Y Acad Sci 1127:49–58
45. Oktay K, Hourvitz A, Sahin G et al (2006) Letrozole reduces estrogen and gonadotropin exposure in women with breast cancer undergoing ovarian stimulation before chemotherapy. J Clin Endocrinol Metab 91:3885–3890
46. Oktay K, Buyuk E, Libertella N, Akar M, Rosenwaks Z (2005) Fertility preservation in breast cancer patients: a prospective controlled comparison of ovarian stimulation with tamoxifen and letrozole for embryo cryopreservation. J Clin Oncol 23:4347–4353
47. Fisher B, Costantino J, Redmond C et al (1989) A randomized clinical trial evaluating tamoxifen in the treatment of patients with node-negative breast cancer who have estrogen-receptor-positive tumors. New Engl J Med 320:479–484
48. Azin AA, Constantini-Fernando M, Oktay K (2008) Safety of fertility preseration by ovarian stunulation with letrozole and gonadotropins in patients with breast cancer: a prospective controlled study. J Clin Oncol 16:2612–2613
49. Chen C (1986) Pregnancy after human oocyte cryopreservation. Lancet 1:884–886
50. Van Uem JFHM, Siebzehnruebl ER, Schuh B et al (1987) Birth after cryopreservation of unfertilized oocytes. Lancet 1:752–753
51. Chen C (1988) Pregnancies after human oocyte cryopreservation. Ann N Y Acad Sci 541:541–549
52. Boiso I, Marti M, Santalo J, Ponsa M, Barri PN, Veiga A (2002) A confocalmicroscopy analysis of the spindle and chromosome configurations of human oocytes cryopreserved at the germinal vesicle and metaphase II stage. Hum Reprod 17:1885–1891
53. Cobo A, Rubio C, Gerli S, Ruiz A, Pellicer A, Remohi J (2001) Use of fluorescence in situ hybridization to assess the chromosomal status of embryos obtained from cryopreserved oocytes. Fertil Steril 75:354–360
54. Oktay K, Cil AP, Bang H (2006) Efficiency of oocyte cryopreservation: a meta-analysis. Fertil Steril 86:70–80
55. Hamre MR, Robison LL, Nesbit ME et al (1987) Effects of radiation on ovarian function in long-term survivors of childhood acute lymphoblastic leukemia: a report from the Childrens Cancer Study Group. J Clin Oncol 5(11):1759–1765
56. Wallace WH, Shalet SM, Hendry JH, Morris-Jones PH, Gattamaneni HR (1989) Ovarian failure following abdominal irradiation in childhood: the radiosensitivity of the human oocyte. Br J Radiol 62(743):995–998
57. Papadakis V, Vlachopapadopoulou E, Van Syckle K et al (1999) Gonadal function in young patients successfully treated for Hodgkin disease. Med Pediatr Oncol 32(5):366–372
58. Cowles RA, Gewanter RM, Kandel JJ (2007) Ovarian repositioning in pediatric cancer patients: Flexible techniques accommodate pelvic radiation fields. Pediatr Blood Cancer 49(3):339–341
59. Thibaud E, Ramirez M, Brauner R et al (1992) Preservation of ovarian function by ovarian transposition performed before pelvic irradiation during childhood. J Pediatr 121(6):880–884
60. Meirow D, Nugent D (2001) The effects of radiotherapy and chemotherapy on female reproduction. Hum Reprod update 7(6):535–543
61. Guerrore Urbano MT (2004) Clinical use of intensity-modulated radiotherapy: part II. Br J Radiol 77:177–182
62. Ataya K, Rao LV, Lawrence E, Kimmel R (1995) Luteinizing hormone-releasing hormone agonist inhibits cyclophosphamide-induced ovarian follicular depletion in rhesus monkeys. Biol Reprod 52(2):365–372
63. Ataya K, Pydyn E, Ramahi-Ataya A, Orton CG (1995) Is radiation-induced ovarian failure in rhesus monkeys preventable by luteinizing hormone-releasing hormone agonists?: preliminary observations. J Clin Endocrinol Metab 80(3):790–795
64. Blumenfeld Z, Avivi I, Linn S et al (1996) Prevention of irreversible chemotherapy-induced ovarian damage in young women with lymphoma by a gonadotrophin-releasing hormone agonist in parallel to chemotherapy. Hum reprod 11(8):1620–1626
65. Oktay K, Sonmezer M, Oktem O, Fox K, Emons G, Bang H (2007) Absence of conclusive evidence for the safety and efficacy of gonadotropin-releasing hormone analogue treatment in protecting against chemotherapy-induced gonadal injury. Oncologist 12(9): 1055–1066
66. Linch DC, Gosden RG, Tulandi T, Tan SL, Hancock SL (2000) Hodgkin's lymphoma: Choice of Therapy and Late Complications. Hematology Am Soc Hematol Educ Program 205–221
67. Oktem O, Oktay K (2007) Sphingosine-1-phosphate enhances human primordial follicle survival and blocks ovarian apoptosis in vitro. Fertil Steril 88:S270

Chapter 48
Ovarian Hyperstimulation Syndrome

Kenneth H.H. Wong

Abstract Ovarian hyperstimulation syndrome is a relevant and increasingly common complication of modern IVF therapy. The complications associated with ovarian hyperstimulation syndrome are serious and potentially life threatening. This chapter highlights the risk factors and appropriate methods to eliminate risk, along with current strategies of treating ovarian hyperstimulation syndrome.

Keywords Ovarian hyperstimulation syndrome • Polycystic ovary syndrome • hCG • GnRH agonist • Albumin • Dopamine agonist • Thromboprophylaxis • Pregnancy termination

48.1 Introduction

Ovarian hyperstimulation syndrome (OHSS) is a potential iatrogenic complication of ovarian stimulation in the treatment of infertility. This entity is increasingly being recognized due to the high number of women undergoing assisted reproductive techniques. The syndrome is typically associated with exogenous gonadotropins, but has also been associated with clomiphene-induced cycles as well as spontaneous pregnancies.

OHSS is a potentially lethal disease with hallmarks of extravascular exudate accumulation combined with profound intravascular depletion and hemoconcentration. These changes accompany ovarian enlargement, exaggerated ovarian steroidogenesis, and the potential for multiorgan failure, including renal, hepatic, and respiratory dysfunction.

48.2 Risk Factors

One of the most important factors in safeguarding against OHSS development is identifying the population at risk. Risk factors that are associated with OHSS development include:

K.H.H. Wong (✉)
Southern California Permanente Group, 9985 Sierra AveFontana, CA 92335, Loma Linda University, Center for Fertility and In Vitro Fertilization, 11370 Anderson Street, Loma Linda, California 92354, USA
e-mail: khhw@aol.com

1. Age: A younger age is associated with development of OHSS.
2. Polycystic Ovary Syndrome (PCOS): It is well established that OHSS develops more frequently in PCOS patients undergoing ovarian stimulation. In addition, there is a higher incidence of OHSS in women with an ultrasonographic phenotype of PCOS.
3. Parameters specific to infertility treatments: Exogenous hCG is pivotal in the development of OHSS. The use of GnRH-agonists rather than GnRH-antagonists has been associated with an increased incidence of OHSS.
4. Risk of OHSS also increases with elevated serum estradiol levels, large number of developing follicles or a large number of oocytes obtained at retrieval.
5. Pregnancy prolongs and increases the severity of the disease.

48.3 Classification

OHSS has been traditionally classified into three categories of mild, moderate, and severe. Mild OHSS is characterized by ovarian enlargement and chemical hyperstimulation, occurring in up to 1/3 of superovulation cycles. In addition to the clinical characteristics of mild OHSS, moderate OHSS features abdominal distention, bloating, nausea, vomiting, and/or diarrhea. Severe OHSS, which occurs in 0.1–2.0% of patients, comprises massive (>12 cm) ovarian enlargement, as well as ascites, hydrothorax, or pericardial effusion. Anasarca, renal dysfunction and hemoconcentration will also upgrade moderate to severe OHSS. In 1992, life-threatening OHSS was added to the classification having criteria of adult respiratory distress syndrome (ARDS), tense ascites, hydrothorax, pericardial effusion, oliguria, creatinine less than 1.6 mg/dL, creatinine clearance less than 50 mL/min, severe hemoconcentration (>55%), profound leucocytosis (WBC ≥ 25,000) and thromboembolic phenomena.

OHSS has also been classified by the time of onset. Early onset OHSS occurs 3–7 days after the administration of hCG. In contrast, late-onset OHSS is believed to be related to

D.T. Carrell and C.M. Peterson (eds.), *Reproductive Endocrinology and Infertility: Integrating Modern Clinical and Laboratory Practice*,
DOI 10.1007/978-1-4419-1436-1_48,

pregnancy-related hCG and occurs more than a week after the initial hCG administration.

48.4 Prevention of OHSS

Cycle cancelation and withholding of hCG administration whenever a high risk situation arises represent a well-established and occasionally unavoidable method of preventing OHSS. Other strategies for the prevention of OHSS in high risk situations include:

1. Lower dose of hCG: The traditional dose of ovulatory hCG is 10,000 IU. Lowering the dose (5,000 IU) may reduce the risk. 2,500 IU of hCG has also been used without compromising pregnancy rates.
2. Coasting: Withholding gonadotropins while maintaining GnRH analog until serum estradiol levels return to a safe level has been used successfully to diminish OHSS development. What constitutes an optimal strategy (number of days of coasting, level of estradiol to start, etc.) still needs further study.
3. LH for triggering: Recombinant LH may offer a replacement for hCG. The European rLH study group revealed that a dose of 15,000–30,000 IU of rLH resulted in a similar number of oocytes, embryos and pregnancies, as well as a reduction of OHSS when compared with 5,000 IU hCG.
4. GnRH agonist triggering: GnRH agonist administration can stimulate the release of LH. However, the clinical pregnancy rate appears to be lower than with the use of hCG. Recent evidence points to no reduction of pregnancy rates and a reduction in the development of OHSS.
5. Cryopreservation of embryos: Elective cryopreservation of all embryos for the postponement of transfer can decrease the risk of late OHSS from pregnancy. However, a Cochrane review did not draw sufficient evidence for the routine use of cryopreservation to prevent OHSS.
6. Albumin administration: Despite a Cochrane review showing a possible benefit of albumin, recent studies have revealed that human albumin administration at the time of hCG administration does not appear to prevent OHSS development.
7. Dopamine agonist: Dopamine agonists have been found to inactivate VEGF receptor-2 and prevent VEGF induced vascular permeability. Dopamine agonists have been used successfully in the prevention of OHSS. Further studies with larger numbers of patients are needed before dopamine agonists become routine prophylactic treatment for the prevention of OHSS.

48.5 Treatment

There is no specific treatment for OHSS. The therapy is mainly supportive until this mostly self-limited condition resolves.

48.5.1 Outpatient Management

Mild to moderate OHSS is initially treated with daily monitoring of weight and urine output, oral intake of electrolyte-supplemented drinks (sport drinks), and serial follow-up of hematocrit concentration, electrolytes and creatinine. Close observation is necessary since moderate OHSS may progress rapidly to the severe form.

48.5.2 In Patient Management

In severe and life-threatening forms of OHSS, hospital admission is warranted. The assessment of hemodynamic and respiratory status is the first step in the management of these patients. After a full physical examination with careful attention to look for deep venous thrombosis is performed, intravenous access needs to be established. Either peripheral intravenous catheters or central venous catheter must be placed. An advantage of central venous catheter placement is the possible measurements of the central venous pressure, especially helpful in the management of fluids. In addition, a urinary catheter may be helpful in monitoring of urinary output.

All patients will require blood tests to measure white blood count, hemoglobin concentration, hematocrit, serum electrolytes and liver enzymes. Additional tests may include creatinine clearance, prothrombin time and partial thromboplastin time, oxygen saturation and blood gasses. Imaging tests will include pelvic and abdominal ultrasounds, chest X-ray, and possible tests for ruling out pulmonary embolism. Many recommend the use of thromboprophylactic agents in severe OHSS.

The goals of medical treatment for OHSS are to maintain circulatory function and to mobilize the intra-abdominal fluid. Normal saline is the crystalloid of choice and potassium containing fluids should be avoided. Albumin can be given as a volume expander in cases with significant hypovolemia, hemoconcentration, hypoalbuminemia or severe ascites. Diuretics may be used to assess renal function, but premature or overzealous use may aggravate hypovolemia or hemoconcentration. Other volume expanders that have been in use include dextran and fresh frozen plasma, although the use of dextran in OHSS has been associated with the development of OHSS.

The usual treatment of hydrothorax in OHSS is observation, but in the progression of respiratory symptoms, thoracentesis may be performed. If ARDS develops, mechanical ventilation is required as well as lung-protective strategies. Steroid-pulse treatment has been utilized in life threatening OHSS with ARDS.

Ultra-sound guided (trans-abdominal or trans-vaginal) paracentesis may produce a dramatic improvement in renal function. The markedly increase size in ovarian size may make paracentesis difficult to perform. In severe cases of ascites, drainage of fluid two to three times a week may be required. A percutaneous placement of a pigtail catheter may be an attractive alternative to multiple paracentesis in this group.

Surgical intervention may be necessary in the presence of adnexal torsion, ovarian cyst rupture or ovarian cyst hemorrhage. In the case of torsion, early diagnosis and prompt surgical intervention is critical for a successful outcome in salvaging the involved ovary. In rare circumstances in which OHSS increases in severity despite all interventions, pregnancy termination should be considered.

48.6 Treatment/Evaluation Algorithm

Prevention
Identification of risk factors
Cycle cancelation/withhold hCG
Lower dose of hCG
Coasting
Cryopreservation of embryos
Possible future preventive measures:
Dopamine agonist
GnRH agonist trigger
Recombinant LH trigger

Evaluation
CBC
Serum electrolytes
BUN/Creatinine, creatinine clearance
Albumin
ALT, AST, alkaline phosphatase
PT, PTT, D-dimer
Ultrasound
Possible chest radiograph and/or abdominal CT

Treatment
Crystalloid
Volume expanders
Paracentesis
Possible surgical intervention
Therapeutic abortion

References

1. Navot D, Bergh PA, Laufer N (1996) The ovarian hyperstimulation syndrome. In: Adashi EY, Rock JA, Rosenwaks Z (eds) Reproductive endocrinology, surgery, and technology, vol 2, 1st edn. Lippincott-Raven, Philadelphia, pp 2215–2232
2. Avecillas JF, Falcone T, Arroliga AC (2004) Ovarian hyperstimulation syndrome. Crit Care Clin 20:679–695
3. Chen SU, Chen CD, Yang YS (2008) Ovarian hyperstimulation syndrome (OHSS): new strategies of prevention and treatment. J Formos Med Assoc 107:509–512

Chapter 49
Pregnancy Outcomes in Infertile Couples

Caroline Signore and Uma M. Reddy

Abstract The use of assisted reproductive technologies (ART) is increasing worldwide. Though most ART pregnancies are uncomplicated and result in the birth of healthy children, it should be noted that some ART pregnancies are at higher risk for adverse maternal and perinatal outcomes as compared to spontaneously conceived pregnancies. For many of these outcomes, it is not clear whether and to what extent observed complications are related to ART procedures themselves vs. the underlying condition(s) impairing fertility. Additional research is needed, keeping in mind specific methodological challenges.

It is abundantly clear, however, that complications arising from multiple gestations conceived with ART are the major contributor to the adverse outcomes seen among ART mothers and children. Continued emphasis on reducing morbidity and mortality by reducing the number of embryos transferred per cycle while maintaining reasonable pregnancy rates is imperative.

Recent data indicate that even singleton ART pregnancies are at higher risk of perinatal and possibly longer-term child health and developmental problems than naturally conceived singleton pregnancies. Couples seeking infertility treatment and ART should be carefully counseled about these risks.

Keywords Assisted reproductive technologies • Infertility • Adverse pregnancy outcomes • Multiple pregnancy • Congenital malformations • Perinatal morbidity

49.1 Introduction

Since the first delivery of an infant conceived by assisted reproductive technologies (ART) roughly 30 years ago, there has been continued growth in the use of these procedures to overcome infertility. In 2004, a total of 49,458 infants conceived with ART were live-born in the United States, accounting for 1% of all births [1], and these numbers appear to be steadily increasing. Currently, ART conceptions account for 2–3% of all births in several European countries [2]. While ART has made parenthood possible for thousands of infertile couples, these pregnancies may be at increased risk for adverse outcomes when compared to their spontaneously conceived counterparts. The goal of ART should be the birth of healthy babies rather than an increase in pregnancy rates alone. The increased incidence of multiple gestations among pregnancies conceived with ART is a well-known contributor to the increased risk of complicated pregnancies and adverse perinatal outcomes. However, evidence suggests that ART singletons also experience increased adverse outcomes.

49.2 Competing Risks

49.2.1 Multifetal Gestation

In the United States, more than 50% of infants born through ART in 2004 were multiple births; this contrasts with a 3% rate of multiple births in the general population [1]. The twin rate is approximately 15-fold higher among ART pregnancies than the baseline U.S. rate; for triplets and higher-order births, the rate is about 42-fold higher [1]. The increased rate of multiple gestation among ART conceptions is related both to the practice of transferring multiple embryos into the uterus to enhance pregnancy rates, and to an increased rate of embryo splitting associated with these procedures.

Multiple gestations are associated with increased risks to the mother and fetus, for example, from preeclampsia, cesarean delivery, preterm birth, low birthweight, sudden infant death syndrome, and cerebral palsy [3–10] (see Box 49.1). This risk of preterm delivery and resultant morbidity and mortality is especially pronounced among higher-order

C. Signore and U.M. Reddy (✉)
Department of Health and Human Services, Pregnancy and Perinatology Branch, Eunice Kennedy Shriver, National Institute of Child Health and Human Development, National Institutes of Health, Bethesda, MD 20892-7510, USA
e-mail: reddyu@mail.nih.gov

D.T. Carrell and C.M. Peterson (eds.), *Reproductive Endocrinology and Infertility: Integrating Modern Clinical and Laboratory Practice*,
DOI 10.1007/978-1-4419-1436-1_49, © Springer Science+Business Media, LLC 2010

multiples, with 45% of triplet pregnancies delivering before 32 weeks gestation [11]. However, the greater proportion of multiples among ART pregnancies are twins, and these account for the majority of perinatal morbidity and mortality associated with ART. Twins conceived via in-vitro fertilization (IVF) have an average gestational age at delivery 3 weeks earlier, and birthweight 800–1,000 g less than IVF singletons [12]. In a study of more than 8,600 ART births in the Danish National Birth Cohort, Pinborg and colleagues reported a tenfold increase in delivery before 37 weeks and a sevenfold increase in delivery before 32 completed weeks among ART twins compared with similarly conceived singletons. Stillbirth was twice as common among twins resulting from IVF with or without intracytoplasmic sperm injection (ICSI) than in singletons (13.1/1000 vs. 6.6/1000, $p=0.002$) [13].

49.2.1.1 Influence of Zygosity and Chorionicity

Additionally, ART has been associated with an increased risk of embryonic splitting leading to monozygotic, monochorionic twin gestation (1.5–4.5% of pregnancies in which zygosity was determined) compared to 0.45% among spontaneously conceived gestations [14–18]. The increased risk of perinatal morbidity and mortality among monozygotic and monochorionic twin pregnancies is well-documented [18, 19]. Of particular concern is the risk of twin-to-twin transfusion syndrome, which complicates approximately 10–15% of monochorionic twin pregnancies and is associated with discordant fetal growth, in utero fetal death, and central nervous system injury in surviving infants [20].

49.2.1.2 ART vs. Spontaneous Twins

While IVF twins have poorer outcomes than similarly conceived singletons, their rates of prematurity, low birthweight, perinatal mortality, congenital anomalies, and neurodevelopmental abnormalities are the same as seen in spontaneously conceived twins in most [21–25], but not all [26, 27], studies. A recent systematic review found a slightly increased risk of very preterm delivery among assisted conception compared to spontaneous twins (RR 1.07, 95% CI 1.02–1.13), but a 40% decrease in perinatal mortality [21].

49.2.1.3 Triplet and Higher-Order Pregnancy

Adverse pregnancy and long-term outcomes are substantially more common among triplet and higher-order pregnancies than among twins. While the average gestational age at delivery for dichorionic twins is 36.7 weeks, and for monochorionic/diamnionic twins is 35.6 weeks [28], triplets are delivered at 32.2 weeks, and quadruplets at 29.9 weeks, on average [29, 30]. Prematurity is a major risk factor for long-term handicap in surviving children. Twenty percent of triplet and 50% of quadruplet pregnancies result in at least one child with a major disability; cerebral palsy is 17 times more common among triplets than singletons [31]. Along with prematurity, an increased risk of intrauterine growth restriction among higher order multiples may underlie some of these poor outcomes [31, 32].

49.2.1.4 Spontaneous Reduction

Fetal number may be reduced by spontaneous death of one or more embryos or fetuses in a multiple pregnancy. In one study of 1,597 IVF/ICSI pregnancies, 12% of clinically documented twin pregnancies ended with delivery of a singleton [33]. These so-called "vanishing twin" pregnancies may be associated with increased perinatal risks for the surviving co-twin. Pinborg and associates [34] compared outcomes between 642 ART singletons who had survived the intrauterine demise of a co-twin and 5,237 ART singletons without vanish. When loss of the co-twin occurred before 22 weeks, the surviving fetus had higher risk of low birthweight <2,500 g (adjusted OR 1.7, 95% CI 1.2–2.2), very low birthweight <1,500 g (aOR 2.1, 95% CI 1.3–3.6), and very preterm birth <32 weeks (aOR 2.3, 95% CI 1.4–4.0). There were no significant increased risks of these outcomes in the subset with losses occurring before 8 weeks gestation, suggesting that obstetric risk increases the later in pregnancy the spontaneous reduction occurs.

49.2.1.5 Reducing Multiples

A number of strategies have been developed to minimize the risk of adverse outcomes arising from multifetal gestations in ART pregnancies.

Multifetal Pregnancy Reduction

Over the last decades, multifetal pregnancy reduction in which one or more fetuses are terminated (MFPR) has been employed as a means to reduce the perinatal and maternal risks of high-order (i.e., triplet or greater) pregnancies arising from ART. Patients with more than twins are faced with the options of continuing the pregnancy with all risks previously described, terminating the entire pregnancy, or reducing the number of fetuses in an effort to decrease the risk of maternal and perinatal morbidity and mortality. Multifetal pregnancy reduction (MFPR) decreases risks associated with preterm delivery, but often creates profound ethical dilemmas. Pregnancy loss is the main risk of MFPR. However, current data suggest that such complications have decreased as experience with the procedure has grown. The incremental risk of loss of the entire pregnancy secondary to MFPR is approximately 1% [35].

In general, the risk of loss after MFPR increases if the number of fetuses at the beginning of the procedure is more than three. While there is little difference between the loss rates observed when the final number of viable fetuses is two or one, the loss rate is higher in pregnancies reduced to triplets. Pregnancies that are reduced to twins appear to do as well as spontaneously conceived twin gestations, although there is an increased risk of fetal growth restriction in reduced multifetal pregnancies [36]. In a recent retrospective study of 389 twin ART pregnancies and 353 high-order ART pregnancies reduced to twins, Cheang and colleagues [37] demonstrated small, but significant decreases in gestational age and birthweight among reduced twins (35.2 vs. 35.8 weeks, and 2,137 vs. 2,305 g, respectively), though the rate of infant mortality was unchanged.

The perinatal benefit of MFPR compared to continuation of triplet and higher-order gestations can be documented because reduction prolongs the length of gestation of the surviving fetuses. This has been demonstrated for triplets, which have a 30–35% risk of birth under 32 weeks compared to twins which is 7–10%.

Reduced/Single Embryo Transfer

Complications of multifetal gestation can be avoided without the potential risks of selective fetal reduction by limiting the number of embryos transferred to the uterus during ART. Recently [38], the American Society for Reproductive Medicine (ASRM) and the Society of Assisted Reproductive Technology (SART) have issued guidelines for the number of embryos to be transferred during a single cycle of infertility treatment. As demonstrated in several Northern European Centers, elective single embryo transfer (SET) can reduce the rate of multiple pregnancies while maintaining acceptable pregnancy rates in appropriately selected patients [39]. Good-prognosis candidates for SET include women under age 35 who are undergoing their first cycle of IVF, and who have embryos of high morphologic quality in sufficient numbers to warrant cryopreservation of excess embryos [38]. Results of a randomized trial indicate that in women under age 36 with at least two high-quality embryos, transfer of a single fresh embryo – followed by transfer of a single thawed embryo in a subsequent cycle if necessary – resulted in similar live birth rates (38.8% vs. 42.9%), but a significant reduction in multiple gestation rates (0.8% vs. 33.1%, $p<0.001$) compared to the initial transfer of two fresh embryos [40].

Practice trends are changing. The proportion of IVF cycles in which three or more fresh embryos were transferred declined significantly in the United States between 1996 and 2002 (92 to 54%, $p<0.001$); however, the proportion of SET cycles remained small (2.5% in 2002) [41]. SET is more common in Europe, reaching 15.7% in 2003 [2]. In Belgium, where recent legislation restricts the number of embryos transferred, the rate of SET increased from 14 to 49% while the rate of twin gestations decreased from 19 to 3% [42].

49.2.2 Underlying Infertility

Another important factor to consider when assessing perinatal risks in ART pregnancies is the extent to which observed complications are due to the condition underlying the couple's infertility vs. the ART procedures themselves. Live birth rates from ART vary by diagnosis, so it is natural to assume that pregnancy outcomes may vary by cause of infertility. Often infertility is attributed to multiple etiologies or the etiology is classified as unknown (Fig. 49.1). This problem is further compounded by the lack of standardized definitions for the various etiologies and lack of a hierarchy to prioritize these etiologies.

A number of studies have shown increased risks of adverse outcomes among patients with subfertility or prolonged time to pregnancy [43–46]. Thomson and colleagues [46] reported increased risks of preeclampsia, placenta previa, placental abruption, and cesarean delivery among 1,437 subfertile women who delivered singleton infants after taking >1 year to conceive, compared to the general population ($n=21{,}688$), noting that there were no differences in adverse outcomes between subfertile women who had and had not received treatment. In a study conducted within the Danish National Birth Cohort [43], women who conceived spontaneously after >1 year of attempting pregnancy had higher risk of preterm birth (adjusted OR 1.36 95% CI 1.08–1.71). Women who report a history of delayed conception prior to achieving pregnancy experience a roughly threefold increase in perinatal mortality, whether the index pregnancy arose from infertility treatment (adjusted OR 2.7, 95% CI 1.5 4.7) or not (adjusted OR 3.3, 95% CI 1.6 6.8) [47].

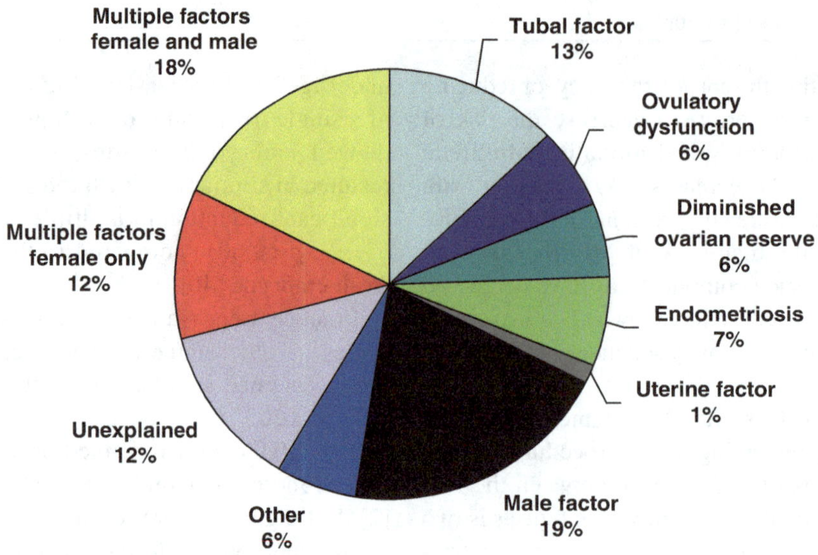

Fig. 49.1 Diagnoses among couples who had ART cycles using fresh nondonor eggs or embryos, 2003. *Source*: Wright VC, Chang J, Jeng G, Maculuso M (2006) Assisted reproductive technology surveillance-United States, 2003. MMWR Surveill Summ 55:1–22. Reprinted with permission from [104]

Box 49.1 Complications Associated with Multifetal Pregnancy

Fetus and Infant

Abortion
Perinatal mortality
Low birthweight

- Preterm birth
- Fetal growth restriction

Abnormal presentation
Placental vascular anastomoses
Hydramnios
Cord accidents

- Prolapse
- Vasa previa
- Cord entanglement

Congenital malformations
Cerebral palsy
Infant death

Maternal

Pregnancy induced hypertension/preeclampsia
Gestational diabetes
Anemia
Hyperemesis gravidarum
Placental abruption
Placenta previa
Postpartum hemorrhage
Cesarean delivery
Excess weight gain

49.3 Pregnancy Outcomes

49.3.1 Pregnancy Loss

Clinically recognized spontaneous pregnancy loss is not uncommon among naturally conceived pregnancies, occurring in 10–15% [48]. Care must be taken when evaluating abortion risk in ART pregnancies for a number of reasons. Pregnancies conceived with ART are under early and intense surveillance, so more early losses are ascertained. Additionally, couples undergoing ART are more likely to have conditions that predispose to pregnancy loss, such as higher maternal age, uterine abnormalities, or chromosomal aberrations. There are conflicting data as to whether spontaneous abortion is increased among ART pregnancies. A large study using US population-based data adjusted for maternal age and plurality showed no increase in spontaneous abortion in ART conceptions compared to baseline rates [49]. In another study, however, Wang and colleagues [50] compared 1,945 pregnancies conceived via ART with a historical prospective cohort of naturally conceived pregnancies diagnosed with urine hCG at 4 to 5 weeks of gestation ($N=549$). The spontaneous loss rate among ART pregnancies was 21% vs. 16% in the naturally conceived pregnancies (crude RR 1.33; 95% CI 1.08–1.65). Overall risk of spontaneous abortion was significantly higher in both the first and second trimesters (16.5% vs. 14.0%, $p<0.05$ and 4.5% vs. 2.0%, $p<0.05$, respectively). After adjusting for maternal age and history of previous spontaneous abortion, the relative risk was reduced to 1.20 (95% CI 1.03–1.46). The authors noted that among ART pregnancies, age ≥40 and history of three or more previous losses were independent predictors of spontaneous abortion [50]. Farr and colleagues analyzed 148,494 ART pregnancies from 1999 to 2002, including biochemical pregnancies, and documented a 29% overall risk of pregnancy loss. Women over age 42 had nearly three times the risk of pregnancy loss as women aged less than 33 years. At a gestational age of 6 weeks, women <33 years had a 10.2% conditional probability of subsequent pregnancy loss, while women >42 years had a 44.7% probability [51]. By 20 weeks gestation, the probability of later pregnancy loss among all ages was less than 2.0%. Pregnancy loss rates were higher for singleton compared to multiple gestations, and for thawed embryos compared to fresh [51].

49.3.2 Maternal Disease

Maternal complications of pregnancy are increased among women who conceive with ART. A recent meta-analysis of 15 studies controlled for maternal age and parity demonstrated that singleton IVF pregnancies are at significantly higher risk of preeclampsia (OR 1.55, 95% CI 1.23 1.95) and gestational diabetes (OR 2.00, 95% CI 1.36 2.99) [52]. It is likely that some portion of these increased risks is related to other maternal conditions and the underlying infertility [53]. The risks of preeclampsia and gestational diabetes increase with body mass index among obese and morbidly obese women with IVF pregnancies [54].

Women with assisted conceptions are at higher risk for cesarean delivery [21], both elective and emergent [52]. Using a prospectively collected database of 36,000 pregnancies, Shevell, et al. [55] found a 2.4-fold increased risk of placental abruption and a 6.0-fold increased risk of placenta previa among IVF singletons compared to controls.

Table 49.1 Potential adverse outcomes in singleton IVF pregnancies

	Absolute risk (%) ART pregnancies	OR (95% CI)[a]
Perinatal risks		
Preterm birth [52]	11.5%	2.0 (1.7–2.2)
Low birthweight (<2,500 g) [52]	9.5%,	1.8 (1.4–2.2)
Very low birthweight (<1,500 g) [52]	2.5%	2.7 (2.3–3.1)
Small for gestational age [52]	14.6%	1.6 (1.3–2.0)
NICU admissions [52]	17.8%	1.6 (1.3–2.0)
Stillbirth [52]	1.2%	2.6 (1.8–3.6)
Neonatal mortality [52]	0.6%	2.0 (1.2–3.4)
Cerebral palsy [22]	0.4%	2.8 (1.3–5.8)
Maternal risks		
Preeclampsia [52]	10.3%	1.6 (1.2–2.0)
Placenta previa [52]	2.4%	2.9 (1.5–5.4)
Placental abruption [55]	2.2%	2.4 (1.1–5.2)
Gestational diabetes [52]	6.8%	2.0 (1.4–3.0)
Cesarean delivery [52]	26.7%	2.1 (1.7–2.6)
Genetic risks		
Epigenetic/Imprinting disorders [95][b]	0.03%	17.8 (1.8–432.9)
Major birth defects [69]	4.3%	1.5 (1.3–1.8)
Chromosomal abnormalities (post ICSI) [79]		
De-novo sex chromosomal aneuploidy	0.6%	3.0
Structural autosomal abnormalities	0.4%	5.7

[a]ART singleton vs. spontaneously conceived singleton offspring
[b]Absolute risk and OR reported for Beckwith–Wiedemann syndrome
Reprinted with permission from [104]

49.3.3 Singleton Gestations

Although the majority of singleton pregnancies arising from ART are uncomplicated, recent meta-analyses have indicated increased risk of adverse perinatal outcomes in ART singletons compared to spontaneously conceived singletons (Table 49.1). A 2004 meta-analysis of 15 studies [52], which compared 12,283 in vitro fertilization (IVF) singleton pregnancies to 1.9 million spontaneous singletons, found increased odds of perinatal mortality (OR 2.2), preterm birth (OR 2.0), low and very low birthweight (ORs 1.8 and 2.7, respectively), and small for gestational age infants (OR 1.6). These findings were very similar to those reported in a systematic review by Helmerhorst and colleagues [21], who analyzed 25 controlled studies of assisted reproduction pregnancies and natural conceptions. Among assisted conceptions, there was an increased risk of very preterm delivery <32 weeks (OR 3.3), perinatal mortality (OR 1.7), cesarean delivery (OR 1.5), and small for gestational age (OR 1.4). Higher perinatal mortality in ART pregnancies results from the combined increased risks of neonatal death (most often related to prematurity) and antepartum fetal death [21, 52]. Farr et al. reported a conditional probability of pregnancy loss at 40 weeks gestation of 0.16% among ART conceptions [51]; the corresponding probability in a general obstetric population is 0.05–0.08% [56].

At this time, it is difficult to determine whether and how much ART procedures contribute to these increased risks. An important question is whether adverse outcomes are attributable to the cause of underlying infertility. A number of studies have shown that the risk of preterm birth, low birthweight, and small for gestational age infants is positively correlated with the time-to-pregnancy interval [44, 53, 57, 58]. Furthermore, women who receive ART treatment are older than those who conceive spontaneously, and increased age is an independent risk factor for many adverse outcomes.

49.3.4 Infant and Child Health Outcomes

Neonatal and childhood morbidity may be increased among ART-conceived singletons [25]. In a retrospective case–control study of 36 infants with grade III–IV intraventricular hemorrhage (IVH) and 69 controls matched for gestational age and birthweight, IVF conception was significantly associated with high-grade IVH (OR: 4.34; 95% CI: 1.42–13.3) [59]. Children conceived via ART may have higher utilization of health care resources than their spontaneously conceived counterparts. In a 5-year follow-up study of 540 ICSI, 437 IVF, and 538 naturally conceived children, children born after ART had significantly higher rates of childhood illness, surgical procedures, medical therapies, and hospital admissions [60].

Overall, studies of neurodevelopmental outcomes in children conceived with ART are reassuring [61]; however, the strength of this evidence is limited by small sample sizes and low statistical power, selection bias, inadequate or inappropriate comparison groups, and loss to follow-up. A recent population-based study with improved methodology, however, showed an increased risk of cerebral palsy (OR 3.7) and developmental delay (OR 4.0) among IVF children compared to controls [22]. Much of this increased risk could be attributed to the high proportion of multiple births among the IVF group. However, risk persisted in singletons, who demonstrated a 2.8-fold increased risk of cerebral palsy compared to controls [22]. Another recent registry-based study noted a significant 1.8-fold increased risk of cerebral palsy among singleton IVF children compared to spontaneously conceived children [62]. Using the Danish Medical Birth Register, Hvidtjorn and colleagues [63] recently demonstrated a 1.6-fold increased risk of cerebral palsy among IVF children, but found that adjustment for multiplicity and gestational age at delivery abolished the difference. The authors concluded that the large proportion of preterm births among ART twins and singletons poses an increased risk for cerebral palsy in these children [63]. Some authors have suggested that the increased risk of cerebral palsy among singleton ART births may be related to adverse effects of spontaneous reduction of what was originally a multiple conception [34, 64].

49.3.4.1 Congenital Anomalies

A large number of studies have investigated the risk of congenital malformations among ART conceptions. As is the case with other pregnancy complications, it is difficult to determine to what degree, if any, birth defects associated with assisted reproduction are related to the ART treatment vs. the underlying infertility. Current evidence is limited by methodological concerns, including small sample sizes and low statistical power, inconsistent ascertainment and definitions of anomalies, incomplete follow-up, and confounding by underlying parental factors, such as genetic defects, that may contribute to infertility and the incidence of malformations [64]. As in other studies of ART outcomes, it is particularly difficult to identify appropriate control populations for studies of congenital malformations among ART conceptions. There are no possible controls for infertile couples whose *only* means to achieve pregnancy are through the use of ART. A study design in which ART are used in a control group of fertile couples is not ethically justifiable.

Recent population-based studies suggest an increased relative risk of birth defects among ART infants compared to spontaneously conceived infants, though the absolute risk remains small [65, 66]. One meta-analysis of 16 studies involving 28,524 IVF infants and 2,520,988 spontaneously conceived controls and seven studies involving 7,234 ICSI infants and 978,078 controls showed a pooled odds ratio of 1.29 (95% CI 1.01–1.67) for major malformations [67]. Another meta-analysis [68] produced very similar results. Similarly, a large study based on the Finnish Registry of Congenital Malformations demonstrated an adjusted odds ratio for major malformations among IVF children of 1.3 (95% CI 1.1–1.6) [69]. When results were stratified by plurality and gender, the increase in risk was confined to singleton boys; female multiples had a decreased risk of major malformations (OR 0.5, 95% CI 0.2–0.9) [69]. Bonduelle and colleagues examined 2,889 infants born after ICSI and 2,995 infants born after IVF and found no difference in overall major malformation rates between the two groups [70].

There are few studies of sufficient size on which to base conclusions about the risk of specific malformations among ART-conceived children. A structural anomaly that has been studied often in ART children – particularly those from ICSI – is hypospadias [65, 69, 71, 72]. In a Swedish population-based study of children born after ICSI [71], the odds ratio for hypospadias was 3.0 (95% CI 1.09–6.50) compared to spontaneously conceived children. Pinborg et al. [13] reported a significantly increased risk of hypospadias among ICSI children compared to IVF (9.1% vs. 4.0%, $p=0.05$), but a recent meta-analysis of four studies comparing ICSI to IVF children found no such difference [73]. Because the numbers of affected children in these studies are small, and because of variability in the severity and diagnostic criteria for hypospadias, it is difficult to determine from the current evidence whether hypospadias is increased among children conceived through IVF with or without ICSI.

A number of other studies, subject to similar limitations, have reported associations between ART and other genitourinary anomalies [68, 69, 72, 74], neural tube defects [65, 72, 75], gastrointestinal defects [65], musculoskeletal defects [68, 72, 76], and cardiovascular defects [68, 76, 77].

49.3.4.2 Chromosomal and Other Genetic Abnormalities

Increased risks of numerical and structural chromosomal abnormalities have been reported among conceptions resulting from ICSI treatment of male factor infertility [78, 79]. In a study of 1,586 ICSI fetuses karyotyped via invasive prenatal testing, 3% were abnormal: 10 (0.6%) had de novo sex chromosome anomalies, 15 (0.9%) had de novo autosomal anomalies, and 22 (1.4%) had inherited anomalies; these defects were related to sperm concentration and motility [78]. De novo sex chromosomal aneuploidy and structural autosomal abnormalities were also observed more frequently in live-born ICSI children compared with a general neonatal population [79]. Infertile males have higher rates of chromosomal abnormalities including microdeletions of the long arm of the Y chromosome and translocations [80–83]. Interestingly, female partners of couples undergoing ART have also been noted to have an increased risk of chromosomal abnormalities [84]. Thus, it is not possible, at present, to clearly determine to what degree chromosomal anomalies among ICSI offspring are related to the treatment itself or to the underlying cause of infertility.

49.3.4.3 Disorders of Genetic Imprinting

Animal and in vitro studies demonstrate the potential for ART procedures to induce epigenetic effects. Genomic imprinting refers to heritable changes in gene function in which genes are expressed in a parent-of-origin-specific manner. A number of retrospective studies have suggested a link between ART and rare imprinting disorders such as Angelman Syndrome [85–87], Beckwith–Wiedemann Syndrome [88, 89], and Russell–Silver dwarfism [90], though two national follow-up studies of 6,052 Danish and 16,280 Swedish IVF children found rates of imprinting disorders similar to those expected in the general population [91].

Angelman syndrome (AS) is a severe developmental disorder characterized by profound mental retardation, ataxia, seizures, microcephaly, and characteristic behaviors including frequent laughing [92]. A link between AS and ICSI was first suggested in 2002, when Cox et al. reported two cases of a rare (1/300,000) subtype of AS with an imprinting defect, both of whom had been conceived with ICSI [85]. A follow-up report described a similar case [86], resulting in concern that the ICSI procedure could be involved in abnormal imprinting. Another imprinting disorder, Beckwith–Weidemann Syndrome (BWS) is an overgrowth condition characterized by gigantism, macroglossia, abdominal wall defects, and increased risk of embryonic tumors such as Wilms' tumor [93]. BWS was also linked with ART when three register-based studies described a higher-than expected prevalence of ART conception among children with BWS (RR 3–6) [88, 89, 94].

The imprinting-related incidence of these conditions is so uncommon (1 in 100,000 to 1 in 300,000) [90] that even a large increase in relative risk associated with ART would translate to a small number of affected children. In one case–control study of Beckwith–Weidemann syndrome, the odds of having been conceived by IVF were nearly 18-fold higher among affected children than control children; this translated into one case of Beckwith–Weidemann syndrome per 4,000 IVF births [95]. The existing evidence should be interpreted with caution, however, because these studies are small, and are often based on genetic disease registries, which are subject to bias. Couples of higher socioeconomic status are more likely to undergo ART and to participate in disease registries. Again, underlying infertility and its association with genetic or epigenetic disorders may be contributing to these observed effects [96, 97].

49.3.4.4 Other Risks

There are limited data examining the risk of early childhood cancer in ART offspring; most studies indicate no increased risk [98–102]. A recent report from the Netherlands [103], however, raises concern that the risk of retinoblastoma may be increased in children conceived with IVF. Moll and colleagues [103] identified five cases of retinoblastoma in IVF children in a 2-year period. Given that the baseline incidence of retinoblastoma in the Netherlands is one in 17,000 live births, the authors estimated a 4.9- to 7.2-fold increased risk of the disease associated with ART. Large prospective studies with long-term follow-up are needed to further investigate these risks.

49.4 Counseling

It is no longer sufficient to define successful treatment with ART as the establishment of pregnancy, or achieving a live birth. Rather, emphasis should be placed on the delivery of a healthy term or late preterm singleton infant. At a 2005 National Institute of Child Health and Human Development workshop on pregnancy outcomes after ART, expert panelists concluded that counseling for potential ART patients should be nondirective, and provided well in advance of any invasive procedures, in a relaxed and unrushed environment [104]. All treatment options should be discussed, and patients should be given time to consider the risks and ask questions. Attending clinicians are responsible for the content of counseling, but counseling processes may be varied to include group meetings, one-on-one sessions, or the use of trained physician extenders [104]. Couples should be informed not only of the risks of the treatment itself, or anticipated pregnancy rates, but also of the risks of potential perinatal complications for which well-documented outcome data exist [104].

49.4.1 Multiple Gestations

Because of the persistent excess of multiple gestations – especially twins, but also higher-order multiples – among ART patients, couples should be fully advised of the consequences of multiple births [105–109]. These discussions should take into account multiple- vs. single-embryo transfer, risks of adverse perinatal outcomes, and the possible costs or other effects of additional ART cycles. The risks of preterm birth should be quantified [105, 107]. Counseling should cover both immediate and long-term outcomes of multiple gestation for both mother and infant and the influence these outcomes may have on the family. Families raising twins and higher-order multiples may experience higher levels of physical, emotional, and financial stress [110]. Compared to mothers of IVF singletons at 1 year after delivery, mothers of IVF multiples are more than five times more likely to report severe parenting stress, and are 70% less likely to be in paid employment [111]. Informing couples of these risks and psychosocial consequences may influence their preference for specific treatment options (e.g., number of embryos transferred) [112].

49.4.2 Obstetric Complications

Couples should be made aware that even singleton pregnancies resulting from ART are at increased risk for obstetric complications, including preterm birth and small for gestational age infants, compared to spontaneously conceived gestations. The observed frequency of adverse outcomes should be described (see Table 49.1), and comparison with frequencies in spontaneous conceptions may be discussed. It is not possible, at this time, to quantify for patients the separate contributions of the ART procedures and the underlying fertility disorder to the excess risk, nor does sufficient evidence exist to allow a differential estimate of perinatal risks by specific treatment or etiology of infertility. Similarly, no specific data exist on which clinicians caring for women with ART pregnancies can base recommendations for any particular antenatal monitoring for or effective preventive measures against these outcomes, beyond current standard obstetrical practice.

49.4.3 Congenital Malformations and Chromosomal Abnormalities

Patients should be informed of the risks of congenital malformations and aneuploidy, and options for prenatal screening and diagnosis should be discussed. While it may be emphasized that the overall risk is small, certain clinical scenarios may warrant more extensive genetic counseling. Male partners with severe oligospermia or azospermia may transmit numerical sex chromosome aberrations or Y chromosomal microdeletions to their offspring [80, 81, 83]. In these patients, paternal karyotyping and Y deletion testing are recommended prior to attempting IVF with ICSI [81, 83, 105, 107]. Obstructive azoospermia or congenital bilateral absence of the vas deferentia in male factor infertility patients warrant referral for genetic counseling and testing for cystic fibrosis [81, 83, 105, 107].

49.4.4 Other Risks

Data suggesting associations between ART and long-term neurodevelopmental or behavioral disorders, childhood cancer, and epigenetic disorders are still preliminary and require further investigation.

References

1. Wright VC, Chang J, Jeng G, Chen M, Macaluso M (2007) Assisted reproductive technology surveillance – United States, 2004. MMWR Surveill Summ 56:1–22
2. Andersen AN, Goossens V, Gianaroli L, Felberbaum R, de Mouzon J, Nygren KG (2007) Assisted reproductive technology in Europe, 2003. Results generated from European registers by ESHRE. Hum Reprod 22:1513–1525
3. Doyle P (1996) The outcome of multiple pregnancy. Hum Reprod 11:110–117
4. Elster N (2000) Less is more: the risks of multiple births. The Institute for Science, Law, and Technology Working Group on Reproductive Technology. Fertil Steril 74:617–623
5. Graham GM III, Gaddipati S (2005) Diagnosis and management of obstetrical complications unique to multiple gestations. Semin Perinatol 29:282–295
6. Norwitz ER, Edusa V, Park JS (2005) Maternal physiology and complications of multiple pregnancy. Semin Perinatol 29:338–348
7. Pharoah PO (2006) Risk of cerebral palsy in multiple pregnancies. Clin Perinatol 33:301–313
8. Taylor MJ (2006) The management of multiple pregnancy. Early Hum Dev 82:365–370
9. Warner BB, Kiely JL, Donovan EF (2000) Multiple births and outcome. Clin Perinatol 27:347–361
10. Getahun D, Demissie K, Lu SE, Rhoads GG (2004) Sudden infant death syndrome among twin births: United States, 1995–1998. J Perinatol 24:544–551

11. Kaufman GE, Malone FD, Harvey-Wilkes KB, Chelmow D, Penzias AS, D'Alton ME (1998) Neonatal morbidity and mortality associated with triplet pregnancy. Obstet Gynecol 91:342–348
12. Pinborg A (2005) IVF/ICSI twin pregnancies: risks and prevention. Hum Reprod Update 11:575–593
13. Pinborg A, Loft A, Nyboe AA (2004) Neonatal outcome in a Danish national cohort of 8602 children born after in vitro fertilization or intracytoplasmic sperm injection: the role of twin pregnancy. Acta Obstet Gynecol Scand 83:1071–1078
14. Alikani M, Cekleniak NA, Walters E, Cohen J (2003) Monozygotic twinning following assisted conception: an analysis of 81 consecutive cases. Hum Reprod 18:1937–1943
15. Blickstein I (2005) Estimation of iatrogenic monozygotic twinning rate following assisted reproduction: pitfalls and caveats. Am J Obstet Gynecol 192:365–368
16. Derom C, Vlietinck R, Derom R, Van den Berghe H, Thiery M (1987) Increased monozygotic twinning rate after ovulation induction. Lancet 1:1236–1238
17. Schachter M, Raziel A, Friedler S, Strassburger D, Bern O, Ron-El R (2001) Monozygotic twinning after assisted reproductive techniques: a phenomenon independent of micromanipulation. Hum Reprod 16:1264–1269
18. Toledo MG (2005) Is there increased monozygotic twinning after assisted reproductive technology? Aust N Z J Obstet Gynaecol 45:360–364
19. Rao A, Sairam S, Shehata H (2004) Obstetric complications of twin pregnancies. Best Pract Res Clin Obstet Gynaecol 18:557–576
20. Wee LY, Fisk NM (2002) The twin-twin transfusion syndrome. Semin Neonatol 7:187–202
21. Helmerhorst FM, Perquin DA, Donker D, Keirse MJ (2004) Perinatal outcome of singletons and twins after assisted conception: a systematic review of controlled studies. BMJ 328:261
22. Stromberg B, Dahlquist G, Ericson A, Finnstrom O, Koster M, Stjernqvist K (2002) Neurological sequelae in children born after in-vitro fertilisation: a population-based study. Lancet 359:461–465
23. Pinborg A, Loft A, Rasmussen S et al (2004) Neonatal outcome in a Danish national cohort of 3438 IVF/ICSI and 10, 362 non-IVF/ICSI twins born between 1995 and 2000. Hum Reprod 19:435–441
24. Luke B, Brown MB, Nugent C, Gonzalez-Quintero VH, Witter FR, Newman RB (2004) Risk factors for adverse outcomes in spontaneous versus assisted conception twin pregnancies. Fertil Steril 81:315–319
25. Klemetti R, Sevon T, Gissler M, Hemminki E (2006) Health of children born as a result of in vitro fertilization. Pediatrics 118:1819–1827
26. Nassar AH, Usta IM, Rechdan JB, Harb TS, Adra AM, Abu-Musa AA (2003) Pregnancy outcome in spontaneous twins versus twins who were conceived through in vitro fertilization. Am J Obstet Gynecol 189:513–518
27. Smithers PR, Halliday J, Hale L, Talbot JM, Breheny S, Healy D (2003) High frequency of cesarean section, antepartum hemorrhage, placenta previa, and preterm delivery in in-vitro fertilization twin pregnancies. Fertil Steril 80:666–668
28. Hack KE, Derks JB, Elias SG et al (2008) Increased perinatal mortality and morbidity in monochorionic versus dichorionic twin pregnancies: clinical implications of a large Dutch cohort study. BJOG 115:58–67
29. Elliott JP (2005) High-order multiple gestations. Semin Perinatol 29:305–311
30. Martin JA, Hamilton BE, Sutton PD, Ventura SJ, Menacker F, Munson ML (2003) Births: final data for 2002. Natl Vital Stat Rep 52:1–113
31. (2004) ACOG Practice Bulletin #56: Multiple gestation: complicated twin, triplet, and high-order multifetal pregnancy. Obstet Gynecol 104:869–883
32. Garite TJ, Clark RH, Elliott JP, Thorp JA (2004) Twins and triplets: the effect of plurality and growth on neonatal outcome compared with singleton infants. Am J Obstet Gynecol 191:700–707
33. Tummers P, De SP, Dhont M (2003) Risk of spontaneous abortion in singleton and twin pregnancies after IVF/ICSI. Hum Reprod 18:1720–1723
34. Pinborg A, Lidegaard O, la Cour FN, Andersen AN (2005) Consequences of vanishing twins in IVF/ICSI pregnancies. Hum Reprod 20:2821–2829
35. Stone J, Eddleman K, Lynch L, Berkowitz RL (2002) A single center experience with 1000 consecutive cases of multifetal pregnancy reduction. Am J Obstet Gynecol 187:1163–1167
36. Depp R, Macones GA, Rosenn MF, Turzo E, Wapner RJ, Weinblatt VJ (1996) Multifetal pregnancy reduction: evaluation of fetal growth in the remaining twins. Am J Obstet Gynecol 174:1233–1238
37. Cheang CU, Huang LS, Lee TH, Liu CH, Shih YT, Lee MS (2007) A comparison of the outcomes between twin and reduced twin pregnancies produced through assisted reproduction. Fertil Steril 88:47–52
38. Society for Assisted Reproductive Technology (2006) Guidelines on number of embryos transferred. Fertil Steril 86:S51–S52
39. Gerris JM (2005) Single embryo transfer and IVF/ICSI outcome: a balanced appraisal. Hum Reprod Update 11:105–121
40. Thurin A, Hausken J, Hillensjo T et al (2004) Elective single-embryo transfer versus double-embryo transfer in in vitro fertilization. N Engl J Med 351:2392–2402
41. Reynolds MA, Schieve LA (2006) Trends in embryo transfer practices and multiple gestation for IVF procedures in the USA, 1996–2002. Hum Reprod 21:694–700
42. Gordts S, Campo R, Puttemans P et al (2005) Belgian legislation and the effect of elective single embryo transfer on IVF outcome. Reprod Biomed Online 10:436–441
43. Basso O, Baird DD (2003) Infertility and preterm delivery, birthweight, and Caesarean section: a study within the Danish National Birth Cohort. Hum Reprod 18:2478–2484
44. Henriksen TB, Baird DD, Olsen J, Hedegaard M, Secher NJ, Wilcox AJ (1997) Time to pregnancy and preterm delivery. Obstet Gynecol 89:594–599
45. Joffe M, Li Z (1994) Association of time to pregnancy and the outcome of pregnancy. Fertil Steril 62:71–75
46. Thomson F, Shanbhag S, Templeton A, Bhattacharya S (2005) Obstetric outcome in women with subfertility. BJOG 112:632–637
47. Draper ES, Kurinczuk JJ, Abrams KR, Clarke M (1999) Assessment of separate contributions to perinatal mortality of infertility history and treatment: a case-control analysis. Lancet 353:1746–1749
48. Wilcox AJ, Treloar AE, Sandler DP (1981) Spontaneous abortion over time: comparing occurrence in two cohorts of women a generation apart. Am J Epidemiol 114:548–553
49. Schieve LA, Tatham L, Peterson HB, Toner J, Jeng G (2003) Spontaneous abortion among pregnancies conceived using assisted reproductive technology in the United States. Obstet Gynecol 101:959–967
50. Wang JX, Norman RJ, Wilcox AJ (2004) Incidence of spontaneous abortion among pregnancies produced by assisted reproductive technology. Hum Reprod 19:272–277
51. Farr SL, Schieve LA, Jamieson DJ (2007) Pregnancy loss among pregnancies conceived through assisted reproductive technology, United States, 1999–2002. Am J Epidemiol 165:1380–1388
52. Jackson RA, Gibson KA, Wu YW, Croughan MS (2004) Perinatal outcomes in singletons following in vitro fertilization: a meta-analysis. Obstet Gynecol 103:551–563
53. Basso O, Weinberg CR, Baird DD, Wilcox AJ, Olsen J (2003) Subfecundity as a correlate of preeclampsia: a study within the Danish National Birth Cohort. Am J Epidemiol 157:195–202

54. Dokras A, Baredziak L, Blaine J, Syrop C, VanVoorhis BJ, Sparks A (2006) Obstetric outcomes after in vitro fertilization in obese and morbidly obese women. Obstet Gynecol 108:61–69
55. Shevell T, Malone FD, Vidaver J et al (2005) Assisted reproductive technology and pregnancy outcome. Obstet Gynecol 106:1039–1045
56. Smith GC (2001) Life-table analysis of the risk of perinatal death at term and post term in singleton pregnancies. Am J Obstet Gynecol 184:489–496
57. Ghazi HA, Spielberger C, Kallen B (1991) Delivery outcome after infertility – a registry study. Fertil Steril 55:726–732
58. Williams MA, Goldman MB, Mittendorf R, Monson RR (1991) Subfertility and the risk of low birth weight. Fertil Steril 56:668–671
59. Linder N, Haskin O, Levit O et al (2003) Risk factors for intraventricular hemorrhage in very low birth weight premature infants: a retrospective case-control study. Pediatrics 111:e590–e595
60. Bonduelle M, Wennerholm UB, Loft A et al (2005) A multi-centre cohort study of the physical health of 5-year-old children conceived after intracytoplasmic sperm injection, in vitro fertilization and natural conception. Hum Reprod 20:413–419
61. Olivennes F, Fanchin R, Ledee N, Righini C, Kadoch IJ, Frydman R (2002) Perinatal outcome and developmental studies on children born after IVF. Hum Reprod Update 8:117–128
62. Lidegaard O, Pinborg A, Andersen AN (2005) Imprinting diseases and IVF: Danish National IVF cohort study. Hum Reprod 20:950–954
63. Hvidtjorn D, Grove J, Schendel DE et al (2006) Cerebral palsy among children born after in vitro fertilization: the role of preterm delivery – a population-based, cohort study. Pediatrics 118:475–482
64. Sutcliffe AG, Ludwig M (2007) Outcome of assisted reproduction. Lancet 370:351–359
65. Ericson A, Kallen B (2001) Congenital malformations in infants born after IVF: a population-based study. Hum Reprod 16:504–509
66. Hansen M, Kurinczuk JJ, Bower C, Webb S (2002) The risk of major birth defects after intracytoplasmic sperm injection and in vitro fertilization. N Engl J Med 346:725–730
67. Rimm AA, Katayama AC, Diaz M, Katayama KP (2004) A meta-analysis of controlled studies comparing major malformation rates in IVF and ICSI infants with naturally conceived children. J Assist Reprod Genet 21:437–443
68. Hansen M, Bower C, Milne E, de Klerk KN, Kurinczuk JJ (2005) Assisted reproductive technologies and the risk of birth defects – a systematic review. Hum Reprod 20:328–338
69. Klemetti R, Gissler M, Sevon T, Koivurova S, Ritvanen A, Hemminki E (2005) Children born after assisted fertilization have an increased rate of major congenital anomalies. Fertil Steril 84:1300–1307
70. Bonduelle M, Liebaers I, Deketelaere V et al (2002) Neonatal data on a cohort of 2889 infants born after ICSI (1991–1999) and of 2995 infants born after IVF (1983–1999). Hum Reprod 17:671–694
71. Wennerholm UB, Bergh C, Hamberger L et al (2000) Incidence of congenital malformations in children born after ICSI. Hum Reprod 15:944–948
72. Zhu JL, Basso O, Obel C, Bille C, Olsen J (2006) Infertility, infertility treatment, and congenital malformations: Danish national birth cohort. BMJ 333:679
73. Lie RT, Lyngstadaas A, Orstavik KH, Bakketeig LS, Jacobsen G, Tanbo T (2005) Birth defects in children conceived by ICSI compared with children conceived by other IVF-methods; a meta-analysis. Int J Epidemiol 34:696–701
74. Wood HM, Trock BJ, Gearhart JP (2003) In vitro fertilization and the cloacal-bladder exstrophy-epispadias complex: is there an association? J Urol 169:1512–1515
75. (1990) Births in Great Britain resulting from assisted conception, 1978–87. MRC Working Party on Children Conceived by In Vitro Fertilisation. BMJ 300:1229–1233
76. Anthony S, Buitendijk SE, Dorrepaal CA, Lindner K, Braat DD, den Ouden AL (2002) Congenital malformations in 4224 children conceived after IVF. Hum Reprod 17:2089–2095
77. Koivurova S, Hartikainen AL, Gissler M, Hemminki E, Sovio U, Jarvelin MR (2002) Neonatal outcome and congenital malformations in children born after in-vitro fertilization. Hum Reprod 17:1391–1398
78. Bonduelle M, Van Assche E, Joris H et al (2002) Prenatal testing in ICSI pregnancies: incidence of chromosomal anomalies in 1586 karyotypes and relation to sperm parameters. Hum Reprod 17:2600–2614
79. Van Steirteghem AC, Bonduelle M, Devroey P, Liebaers I (2002) Follow-up of children born after ICSI. Hum Reprod Update 8:111–116
80. Calogero AE, Burrello N, De Palma A, Barone N, D'Agata R, Vicari E (2003) Sperm aneuploidy in infertile men. Reprod Biomed Online 6:310–317
81. Dohle GR, Halley DJ, Van Hemel JO et al (2002) Genetic risk factors in infertile men with severe oligozoospermia and azoospermia. Hum Reprod 17:13–16
82. Foresta C, Garolla A, Bartoloni L, Bettella A, Ferlin A (2005) Genetic abnormalities among severely oligospermic men who are candidates for intracytoplasmic sperm injection. J Clin Endocrinol Metab 90:152–156
83. Johnson MD (1998) Genetic risks of intracytoplasmic sperm injection in the treatment of male infertility: recommendations for genetic counseling and screening. Fertil Steril 70:397–411
84. Schreurs A, Legius E, Meuleman C, Fryns JP, D'Hooghe TM (2000) Increased frequency of chromosomal abnormalities in female partners of couples undergoing in vitro fertilization or intracytoplasmic sperm injection. Fertil Steril 74:94–96
85. Cox GF, Burger J, Lip V et al (2002) Intracytoplasmic sperm injection may increase the risk of imprinting defects. Am J Hum Genet 71:162–164
86. Orstavik KH (2003) Intracytoplasmic sperm injection and congenital syndromes because of imprinting defects. Tidsskr Nor Laegeforen 123:177
87. Sanchez-Albisua I, Borell-Kost S, Mau-Holzmann UA, Licht P, Krageloh-Mann I (2007) Increased frequency of severe major anomalies in children conceived by intracytoplasmic sperm injection. Dev Med Child Neurol 49:129–134
88. DeBaun MR, Niemitz EL, Feinberg AP (2003) Association of in vitro fertilization with Beckwith-Wiedemann syndrome and epigenetic alterations of LIT1 and H19. Am J Hum Genet 72:156–160
89. Gicquel C, Gaston V, Mandelbaum J, Siffroi JP, Flahault A, Le BY (2003) In vitro fertilization may increase the risk of Beckwith-Wiedemann syndrome related to the abnormal imprinting of the KCN1OT gene. Am J Hum Genet 72:1338–1341
90. Maher ER (2005) Imprinting and assisted reproductive technology. Hum Mol Genet 14(Spec No 1):R133–R138
91. Lidegaard O, Pinborg A, Andersen AN (2006) Imprinting disorders after assisted reproductive technologies. Curr Opin Obstet Gynecol 18:293–296
92. Lalande M, Calciano MA (2007) Molecular epigenetics of Angelman syndrome. Cell Mol Life Sci 64:947–960
93. Enklaar T, Zabel BU, Prawitt D (2006) Beckwith-Wiedemann syndrome: multiple molecular mechanisms. Expert Rev Mol Med 8:1–19
94. Maher ER, Brueton LA, Bowdin SC et al (2003) Beckwith-Wiedemann syndrome and assisted reproduction technology (ART). J Med Genet 40:62–64
95. Halliday J, Oke K, Breheny S, Algar E, Amor J (2004) Beckwith-Wiedemann syndrome and IVF: a case-control study. Am J Hum Genet 75:526–528
96. Edwards RG, Ludwig M (2003) Are major defects in children conceived in vitro due to innate problems in patients or to induced genetic damage? Reprod Biomed Online 7:131–138

97. Horsthemke B, Ludwig M (2005) Assisted reproduction: the epigenetic perspective. Hum Reprod Update 11:473–482
98. Bergh T, Ericson A, Hillensjo T, Nygren KG, Wennerholm UB (1999) Deliveries and children born after in-vitro fertilisation in Sweden 1982–95: a retrospective cohort study. Lancet 354:1579–1585
99. Bruinsma F, Venn A, Lancaster P, Speirs A, Healy D (2000) Incidence of cancer in children born after in-vitro fertilization. Hum Reprod 15:604–607
100. Doyle P, Bunch KJ, Beral V, Draper GJ (1998) Cancer incidence in children conceived with assisted reproduction technology. Lancet 352:452–453
101. Ericson A, Nygren KG, Olausson PO, Kallen B (2002) Hospital care utilization of infants born after IVF. Hum Reprod 17:929–932
102. Klip H, Burger CW, de Kraker J, van Leeuwen FE (2001) Risk of cancer in the offspring of women who underwent ovarian stimulation for IVF. Hum Reprod 16:2451–2458
103. Moll AC, Imhof SM, Cruysberg JR, Schouten-van Meeteren AY, Boers M, van Leeuwen FE (2003) Incidence of retinoblastoma in children born after in-vitro fertilisation. Lancet 361:309–310
104. Reddy UM, Wapner RJ, Rebar RW, Tasca RJ (2007) Infertility, assisted reproductive technology, and adverse pregnancy outcomes: executive summary of a National Institute of Child Health and Human Development workshop. Obstet Gynecol 109:967–977
105. (2005) ACOG Committee Opinion #324: Perinatal risks associated with assisted reproductive technology. Obstet Gynecol 106: 1143–1146
106. (2006) Elements to be considered in obtaining informed consent for ART. Fertil Steril 86:S272–S273
107. Allen VM, Wilson RD, Cheung A (2006) Pregnancy outcomes after assisted reproductive technology. J Obstet Gynaecol Can 28:220–250
108. Emery M, Beran MD, Darwiche J et al (2003) Results from a prospective, randomized, controlled study evaluating the acceptability and effects of routine pre-IVF counselling. Hum Reprod 18:2647–2653
109. Hock DL, Seifer DB, Kontopoulos E, Ananth CV (2002) Practice patterns among board-certified reproductive endocrinologists regarding high-order multiple gestations: a united states national survey. Obstet Gynecol 99:763–770
110. Practice Committee of the American Society for Reproductive Medicine (2006) Multiple pregnancy associated with infertility therapy. Fertil Steril 86:10
111. Glazebrook C, Sheard C, Cox S, Oates M, Ndukwe G (2004) Parenting stress in first-time mothers of twins and triplets conceived after in vitro fertilization. Fertil Steril 81:505–511
112. Grobman WA, Milad MP, Stout J, Klock SC (2001) Patient perceptions of multiple gestations: an assessment of knowledge and risk aversion. Am J Obstet Gynecol 185:920–924

Chapter 50
The Impact of Complementary Medicine on In Vitro Fertilization

Laurence C. Udoff and Grant Zhang

Abstract The high cost and limited success rates of In Vitro Fertilization (IVF) have driven many patients to pursue alternative or complementary medicine options. Though many options exist, only the Traditional Chinese Medicine of acupuncture as adjuvant treatment in IVF has received significant scientific scrutiny. Despite an extensive body of literature that includes numerous randomized clinical trials and a meta-analysis, definitive conclusions are lacking. Though results to date suggest a statistically significant improvement in pregnancy rates with adjuvant acupuncture, important issues remain to be addressed. These include the chance of a placebo effect, the possible impact of patient selection and baseline pregnancy rates, and the lack of biologically plausible mechanism. Larger, randomized placebo-controlled trials are underway to address these concerns.

Keywords Acupuncture • Alternative medicine • Complementary medicine

50.1 Introduction

Despite significant advances, pregnancy and delivery rates with In Vitro Fertilization (IVF) remain limited, particularly in older patients. Additionally, the expense of IVF is substantial, often costing more than $10,000 per attempt. These factors combine to drive patients to pursue complementary or alternative medicine (CAM) options. Anecdotal reports have suggested a rapidly growing trend of CAM usage by IVF patients in the United States [1]. Published studies from Europe and Australia have recorded estimates that range from 32–66% of infertility patients reporting the use of CAM for treatment [2–4]. It is most likely that physicians are unaware of CAM usage by their infertility patients, as a nationwide survey in the United States found that only 38.5% of patients utilizing CAM for a variety of reasons disclosed this information to their health care provider [4].

As defined by the National Center for Complementary and Alternative Medicine (NCCAM) [5], a component of the National Institutes of Health, CAM is a group of diverse medical and health care systems, practices, and products that are not presently considered to be part of conventional medicine. Complementary medicine is used together with conventional medicine, whereas alternative medicine is used in place of conventional therapy. NCCAM further categorizes these therapies into whole medical systems and four domains that include mind–body medicine, biologically based practices, manipulative and body-based practices, and energy therapies. Examples of whole medical systems include homeopathic, naturopathic, traditional Chinese medicine (TCM), and Ayurveda therapies. Mind–body medicine includes techniques, such as meditation, prayer, mental healing, and therapies that use creative outlets such as art, music, or dance. Biologically based practices utilize substances found in nature, such as herbs, foods, and vitamins, to treat disease and promote health. Manipulative and body-based practices use movement of one or more parts of the body, such as osteopathic manipulation and message. Energy medicine includes the use of biofield therapies, such as qi gong, Reiki and therapeutic touch, as well as the unconventional use of pulsed fields, magnetic fields, or alternating-current or direct-current fields.

Unfortunately, most of the diverse therapies noted above have received little scientific scrutiny, leaving the practitioner with no credible data on which to base recommendations. One notable exception would be the TCM of acupuncture as adjuvant therapy for patients undergoing IVF. A significant body of literature is available for review examining the effects of acupuncture on numerous IVF outcomes and includes several randomized clinical trials. Therefore, as a practical matter, this chapter will focus on the impact of acupuncture in IVF patients, and will provide

L.C. Udoff (✉)
Department of Obstetrics, Gynecology and Reproductive Sciences, University of Maryland School of Medicine, 405 W. Redwood Street, 3rd floor, Baltimore, MD, 21201, USA
e-mail: ludoff@umm.edu

G. Zhang
Center for Integrative Medicine, University of Maryland School of Medicine, Baltimore, MD, USA

D.T. Carrell and C.M. Peterson (eds.), *Reproductive Endocrinology and Infertility: Integrating Modern Clinical and Laboratory Practice*,
DOI 10.1007/978-1-4419-1436-1_50, © Springer Science+Business Media, LLC 2010

the reader with evidence-based conclusions that can be used in patient counseling.

Acupuncture has been utilized in China for centuries to regulate the female reproductive system. Traditional Chinese medicine views that everything is created and ruled by two principle energy forces called "yin and yang." Balance and free flow of these energies are critical to the health of our body and mind [6]. Too little (deficiency), too much (excess), or blockage of the free flow of the energy, are common examples of causes of illness. In considering conception and fertility, Kidney essence and Liver energy are particularly important [7, 8]. Generally speaking, acupuncture treatment is given by two forms: a fixed protocol, which composes predetermined acupuncture points and frequency of treatment and an individualized treatment, where points change with each patient, following a TCM diagnosis. Besides the choice of the acupuncture points, the way of manipulating the acupuncture needles, such as rotating the needles in a certain direction, or in conjunction with electro-stimulation, are also part of the treatment components. These manipulations are believed to enhance the effect of the needles in balancing the energy, or opening the energetic pathways.

Despite centuries of use, only recently have modern investigational methods been employed to evaluate the impact of acupuncture on infertility. These studies can be categorized as those that focus on possible mechanisms by which acupuncture may impact IVF outcomes (i.e., associated physiological and psychological changes associated with acupuncture), and studies whose primary endpoints are clinical outcomes, such as pregnancy rates or live births.

50.2 Physiological Changes: Beta-Endorphin

One of the best characterized physiological changes associated with acupuncture is the increase in circulating and local tissue beta-endorphin concentrations. Beta-endorphin is an endogenous opioid peptide derived from its precursor protein proopiomelanocortin, which is present in abundant amounts in neuronal cells of the arcuate nucleus of the hypothalamus, pituitary, medulla, and in peripheral tissues, including intestines and ovaries [9–11]. Proopiomelanocortin cleaves to form adrenocorticotropic hormone and beta-lipoprotein. Further cleavage of beta-lipoprotein yields neuropeptides, including beta-endorphin. Mayer et al. [13] first reported that acupuncture analgesia was induced through endorphin production and antagonized by the opioid receptor antagonist naloxone. Other studies similarly suggested that certain effects of acupuncture are mediated through the nervous system, within which beta-endorphin and other neuropeptides have been implicated [13–15]. Acupuncture was shown by Petti et al. [14] to cause a significant increase in beta-endorphin levels during treatment, which lasted for up to 24 h.

A change in the level of endorphins may affect reproductive physiology through the hypothalamic-pituitary-gonadal axis. The hypothalamic beta-endorphin center and the GnRH pulse generator, are both situated within the arcuate nucleus. Ching [17], Orstead [18], and Whisnat [19], respectively, showed that opioid peptides suppress GnRH release in rats, rabbits, and the ewe. A more recent review concluded that endogenous opioid peptides mediate the negative feedback action of progesterone on GnRH pulse frequency during the luteal phase of the ovine estrous cycle [19]. Investigations in humans have noted an increased opioid inhibition of LH secretion in hyperprolactinemic patients with pituitary microadenomas [20], and have demonstrated the role of opioid peptides in the initiation of the midcycle LH surge in normal cycling women [21].

Beta-endorphin and other neuropeptides have been identified in the ovaries of multiple species, including humans [9, 10, 22, 23]. It has been suggested that endogenous opioids like beta-endorphin are locally produced, since pro-opiomelanocortin mRNA has been identified in the ovary [10, 23], and follicular fluid beta-endorphin levels are several times higher than that found in plasma [25] and do not correlate with plasma levels. Gene expression and follicular fluid concentrations of POMC-related peptides have been found to change during the menstrual cycle. In rats, treatment with PMSG resulted in a profound increase in ovarian POMC-like mRNA [23]. In women, Petraglia [22] measured follicular fluid levels of POMC-related peptides in various menstrual phases, and demonstrated that beta-endorphin concentrations were significantly higher in the preovulatory days than in the other periods. Further investigations have suggested that intrafollicular beta-endorphin levels vary based on the size and maturity of the follicle. Aleem et al. noted that follicles greater than 1 cm in size contained higher levels of beta-endorphin than follicles less than 1 cm [25]. Facchinetti et al. [9] were not able to detect beta-endorphin in immature follicles, but noted that the highest concentrations were in follicles greater than 22 mm obtained after superovulation for IVF. Expanding the investigations in women undergoing superovulation for IVF, Facchinetti et al. [26] reported that beta-endorphin levels were higher in the follicular fluid from follicles that contained oocytes that were subsequently fertilized. Most recently, Gallinelli et al. [11] studied POMC gene expression in fertile and postmenopausal women. They reported that POMC mRNA from the ovarian parenchyma and germinative follicles of women of fertile age appeared higher than samples from postmenopausal women. Additionally, no POMC mRNA signals were noted in corpora lutea suggesting that POMC gene expression is localized in the human ovary. They concluded that the physiological role for the POMC gene (and products such as beta-endorphin) is unclear and warrants further investigation. At present, no study has examined the effect of acupuncture on beta-endorphin expression in the ovary.

50.2.1 Physiological Changes: Autonomic Nervous System and Regulation of Blood Flow

Another pathway by which acupuncture may impact reproductive function is through effects on the autonomic nervous system. Numerous studies in animals as well as human subjects have documented changes in sympathetic and parasympathetic activity in association with acupuncture [27–37]. Techniques employed include measuring changes in skin temperature, thermography, plethysmography, blood pressure, and muscle-sympathetic nerve activity. More recently, spectral analysis has been utilized to measure the low frequency and high frequency components of heart rate variability to reflect sympathetic and parasympathetic activity. Since the studies vary to such a high degree in methods employed, acupuncture points used, and organ system studied, one can not draw a simple conclusion regarding the impact of acupuncture on the autonomic nervous system. Some studies report an increase in sympathetic activity [27, 28, 37] while others have documented a sympathoinhibitory effect [29–36]. It is the latter that has led some to hypothesize that acupuncture could increase blood flow to the uterus and ovaries, which could result in beneficial changes in reproductive function at these sites. This hypothesis was investigated by Stener-Victorin et al. [38] who measured uterine artery blood flow impedance in ten infertile women with a high baseline pulsatility index ($PI \geq 3.0$). Patients had endogenous hormone activity suppressed by a GnRHa, and underwent EA twice a week for 4 weeks. The PI was significantly reduced after the eighth EA treatment and remained significantly lower up to 14 days later. In contrast, Paulus et al. [39], in a larger, randomized study of infertility patients undergoing IVF could find no acupuncture-associated changes in the uterine artery PI. However, a different acupuncture protocol and patient population (baseline normal uterine artery blood flow impedance) prevent a direct comparison between studies. Changes in ovarian blood flow in response to EA have been studied in anesthetized rats [40]. This report concluded that low-frequency EA stimulation increases ovarian blood flow as a reflex response via the ovarian sympathetic nerves. In related studies, the same group has recently shown, in rats with steroid-induced polycystic ovary syndrome, that EA produces a decline in ovarian concentrations of endothelin-I, a potent vasoconstrictor [41].

A basic assumption common to these studies is that an increase in blood flow to the uterus and/or ovary would improve reproductive function. However, based on available evidence, it would be difficult to predict whether an acupuncture mediated increase in uterine and/or ovarian blood flow would ultimately result in an improvement in IVF pregnancy rates. Regarding the uterus, multiple studies have investigated uterine artery blood flow and endometrial vascularity and its relationship to endometrial receptivity and pregnancy rates [42–47]. The studies vary widely regarding inclusion/exclusion criteria, the various forms of treatment utilized (e.g., IVF, intracytoplasmic sperm injection, frozen embryo transfer), the timing of the assessment of blood flow (e.g., at the start of ovarian stimulation, at the time of hCG administration, on the day of oocyte retrieval and on the day of embryo transfer), and the tools used to assess blood flow (color Doppler, intrauterine laser Doppler, 3D power Doppler). Results have been mixed. Some studies have concluded that an increase in uterine blood flow/endometrial vascularity is associated with higher pregnancy rates [42, 43, 46–50] while others did not find a significant correlation [42–44, 51–53]. Results from investigations focusing on uterine blood flow and the risk of miscarriage have also been contradictory with a study by Isaksson [54] showing no correlation and a study by Ng [43] concluding that a higher vascularization index in the endometrium is associated with a lower pregnancy loss rate. Regarding the ovary, early investigations showed that stromal peak systolic velocity prior to the beginning of ovarian stimulation in IVF cycles was associated with the number of oocytes retrieved [55, 56]. More recent studies have employed the technique of 3D power Doppler, which is thought to have methodological advantages over bidimensional pulsed Doppler [57, 58]. Conflicting results have been noted regarding the association and predictive value of 3D power Doppler measurements and IVF outcomes. In some studies, an increase in ovarian blood flow as measured by higher indices has been associated with a greater number of follicles and a higher number of retrieved oocytes as well as an improvement in pregnancy rates [57–60]. Other studies found no significant association between these measurements and IVF outcomes [61, 62]. Additionally, further statistical analysis in several of these studies [57, 58, 62] found these measurements to be poor predictors of IVF outcomes, including pregnancy rates.

50.2.2 Psychological Changes: Anxiety and Depression

Lastly, it has been postulated that acupuncture may improve IVF outcomes through a positive impact on psychological factors. It has been well-documented that infertility patients commonly have psychiatric diagnoses. Chen et al. [63] performed a structured psychological interview on 112 consecutive patients at an assisted reproduction clinic and reported that overall, 40.2% of patients met criteria for a psychiatric disorder. The most common disorder was generalized anxiety disorder (23.2%), followed by major depressive disorder (17%) and dysthymic disorder (9.8). It has also been well-documented in numerous studies that distress adversely affects IVF outcomes. In a review by Domar et al. [64], 21 studies on stress and IVF were identified, with 15 supporting the theory that distress adversely affects pregnancy rates, two noted a trend for this relationship, and three found no relationship between stress and IVF outcome and one study did not reach a conclusion. However, to date there is only one randomized controlled prospective trial to investigate whether the treatment of distress improves IVF outcomes. In this study performed in Turkey [65], 60 couples undergoing ART were randomized to receive routine care or to take part in a counseling services model. Couples in the experimental group had lower anxiety and depression scores, higher life satisfaction scores and a higher clinical pregnancy rate (43% treatment, 17% control). However, at present, it is unknown whether acupuncture, as a specific intervention, improves depression and/or anxiety in IVF patients. Data that are available include reports that IVF patients receiving acupuncture often report a relaxing effect [66] and studies have shown that acupuncture has a beneficial effect on depression and anxiety disorders [67–70]. However, recent reviews on this topic site insufficient evidence to reach a firm conclusion [71, 72].

50.3 Clinical Outcome Data: Non-IVF Studies

Though the extensive body of literature discussed above provides support for further research, recommendations regarding the use of acupuncture in IVF patients should be based on studies reporting results that are more directly related to the outcome of live births. The earliest such reports focused on the use of acupuncture to treat ovulatory disorders. In 1992, Gerhard and Postneck [73] studied the effect of auricular acupuncture on infertile women diagnosed with oligomenorrhea or luteal insufficiency. The results of this group were compared to a control group treated with hormone therapy. The groups were matched according to age, duration of infertility, body mass index, previous pregnancies, menstrual cycle, and tubal patency. Eleven pregnancies occurred out of 45 women treated with acupuncture compared to 15 pregnancies from the control group of 45 women treated with hormones. It was concluded that auricular acupuncture was a reasonable alternative to traditional ovulation induction therapy. In a smaller trial, Chen [74] treated 11 anovulatory patients with electroacupuncture (EA) and noted that 46% of menstrual cycles that followed were ovulatory. More recently, Stener-Victorin et al. [75] examined the use of EA for ovulation induction in 24 oligo-amenorrheic women with polycystic ovarian syndrome (PCOS). The percentage of ovulatory cycles in all subjects was shown to improve from 15 to 66% up to 3 months after treatment. Their result suggested that acupuncture could be considered as an alternative or adjunct to pharmacological ovulation induction in these selected patients with PCOS.

50.3.1 Clinical Outcome Data: IVF

More recently, the focus has been on the impact of acupuncture on IVF outcomes. Numerous studies are available for review but they vary significantly in regard to methodology (e.g., retrospective case–control studies, prospective randomized trials with no treatment control group, prospective randomized double-blind sham control trials) acupuncture protocol, infertility treatment (i.e., IVF with or without intracytoplasmic sperm injection (ICSI)), and subject selection (average prognosis patients, poor prognosis patients, good prognosis patients). To facilitate reaching a conclusion as to whether acupuncture improves success with IVF, studies will be grouped for discussion based on the quality of study design and presumed weight of their respective results.

Several studies have noted the impact of acupuncture on IVF, though it was recorded as a secondary outcome with the primary focus being acupuncture as perioperative analgesia for an oocyte retrieval. This could be a very significant distinction, as treatment aimed at pain relief may not be expected to necessarily alter fertility. The earliest of these reports was from Stener-Victorin et al. [76] who randomized 150 women to receive electro-acupuncture plus paracervical block or alfentanil (short acting opiate), plus paracervical block as anesthesia for an oocyte retrieval as part of an IVF cycle. They concluded that electro-acupuncture (EA) was as good as alfentanil in inducing adequate perioperative analgesia during oocyte retrieval. Additional analysis revealed a significantly higher implantation rate (27.2% vs. 16.3%), pregnancy rate (45.9% vs. 28.3%) and take-home baby rate (41% vs. 19.4%) per embryo transfer in patients receiving EA compared to patients receiving alfentanil. Interestingly, a larger ($n=286$) more recent study by the same group [77] confirmed the effectiveness of acupuncture as peri-operative analgesia during oocyte retrieval but did not show a difference in pregnancy rates between the acupuncture and alfentanil group. It was concluded that since this study was more adequately powered to test this hypothesis, acupuncture as applied for the purpose of peri-operative anesthesia does not improve pregnancy rates in IVF. This is in agreement with the conclusion reached by a recent Cochrane Database review, which found no difference in clinical pregnancy rates in women using alternative methods for pain relief during oocyte retrieval [78]. Two additional studies have been published since this review. One study randomized 200 patients to either a short duration electroacupuncture technique or standard care and found no significant difference between treatment and control groups (pregnancy rates 52.3, and 55.6%, respectively) [79]. The other study [80] randomized 94 women to auricular acupuncture with or without electrical stimulation or a placebo. Pregnancy rates per embryo transfer in the acupuncture groups were significantly higher than the placebo group (47% vs. 24.1%, respectively).

Many more investigations have had pregnancy rate and live birth rate with adjuvant acupuncture as the primary study endpoint. This would include a retrospective analysis by Magarelli et al. presented in abstract form in 2004 [81, 82]. This group utilized a case control study design to investigate the impact of acupuncture on over 50 IVF patients compared to a similar number of selected control patients. Treatments were administered pre- and post-embryo transfer with some patients also receiving treatment prior to the oocyte retrieval. Methods included electrostimulation as well as traditional/auricular acupuncture protocols. In both good prognosis and poor prognosis patients, it was concluded that the main impact of treatment was to increase the birth rate per cycle mainly through a reduction in the rate of miscarriages (23% more births/pregnancy with acupuncture). The following year, a similar conclusion was reached by Khorram and colleagues in an abstract presentation [83]. In this report, 238 conventional IVF cases were reviewed, in which 127 patients received acupuncture consisting of a minimum of two session given 5–7 days prior to and on the day of embryo transfer. The groups were similar in most variables recorded, except the acupuncture group had a significantly lower number of oocytes retrieved and fewer first trimester miscarriages. Two, more recent published reports, have also concluded through a retrospective analysis that acupuncture is not associated with an increase in pregnancy rates. Johnson [84] compared the results of 26 IVF cycles with adjuvant acupuncture (pre- and post-embryo transfer and variable prior) to a control group. The clinical pregnancy rate per cycle in the acupuncture group was 57.7%, which was not significantly different than the control group rate of 45.3%. Wang et al. [85] reviewed the experience of 32 patients undergoing IVF and acupuncture. A slightly different protocol was used, in which acupuncture sessions were limited to the follicular and luteal phases of the stimulation, omitting treatment on the day of embryo transfer. The ongoing pregnancy rate for acupuncture patients was 37.5% per transfer, which was not significantly different than the rate of 43.7% in matched controls.

The results of these retrospective studies would suggest that adjuvant acupuncture for IVF patients does not improve the chances of conceiving, though it may decrease the risk of miscarriage. However, these findings could be due to small sample sizes as well as inherent biases in study design. There are multiple confounding variables to consider when evaluating IVF outcomes including the age of the patient, ovarian reserve, number of prior treatment cycles, prior pregnancies, and infertility diagnosis. As these studies were retrospective reviews, patients were free to choose acupuncture or no treatment. It is possible that patients with a poorer prognosis would be more likely to choose acupuncture as a means of doing anything they can to improve their chances of success. Conversely, patients that believe they have a good prognosis may be less likely to try anything unproven that could jeopardize their chances. Unfortunately, most of these studies did not adequately control for these variables. To address this problem and other potential biases, the study design of choice would be a randomized clinical trial.

The first randomized clinical trial of acupuncture as adjuvant therapy in IVF was reported by Paulus et al. [39]. In this study, 160 IVF (or ICSI) patients with good quality embryos were randomly assigned to traditional and auricular acupuncture 25 min before and after embryo transfer or no treatment. Patient groups were similar with respect to age, number of previous cycles, number of transferred embryos (German law mandates no more than three), endometrial thickness, plasma estradiol on day of transfer, use of ICSI, clinical indications for treatment, and blood flow impedance in the uterine arteries (pulsatility index = PI). The clinical pregnancy rate in the acupuncture group was significantly greater than the group receiving no adjuvant treatment (42.5% vs. 26.3%). The authors concluded that acupuncture before and after embryo transfer produces a statistically significant increase in pregnancy rates, though a placebo-controlled trial would be needed to rule out the possibility that acupuncture produces only a psychological or psychosomatic effect. To this end, a year later, the same group reported in abstract form the results of a similar trial that included a placebo acupuncture needle [86]. Two hundred patients with good quality embryos were randomized to acupuncture or placebo needling (same acupuncture points but did not penetrate the skin). The clinical pregnancy rate in the acupuncture group was 43.0%, which was not significantly different than the rate of 37% recorded for the control group.

The results of these two trials highlight an ongoing debate regarding the use of sham control groups in acupuncture studies. Many experts in the field have called for all future trials to include a placebo control group [1, 87–89]. They site the possibility of a placebo effect leading to false conclusions regarding the true impact of acupuncture on IVF outcomes. Specifically, it has been noted that many people who receive sham acupuncture report a calming affect and some have hypothesized that a reduction in stress can impact IVF outcomes [1] Additionally, it has become the expected medical standard for a treatment to compare itself to a placebo before making any legitimate claims as to its efficacy (e.g., FDA approval standards). Placebo interventions are also required for adequate blinding, though in the specific setting of IVF, the motivating factors are so strong for success, it seems very unlikely there would be any difference in care given to intervention and nonintervention groups.

There is also a compelling argument that the need for a placebo or sham treatment group in this particular area of study is overstated. It has been asserted that a true, inert placebo for acupuncture is not available [90, 91]. For example, it has been hypothesized that there is a subset of patients that are very sensitive to touch/manipulation, so that even superficial needling produces an effect based on the principles of TCM. The issue of sham acupuncture was directly addressed in two recent trials. Kaptchuk et al. [90] randomized 270 patients with arm pain to acupuncture, sham acupuncture (Streitberger placebo needle), amitriptyline or inert pill. They concluded that sham acupuncture had greater effects than the placebo pill on self-reported pain and severity of symptoms, both subjective outcomes. However, this was not seen with objective measures such as arm strength and grip strength. Haake et al. [91] studied 1,162 patients with chronic low back pain, randomizing patients to acupuncture, sham acupuncture (superficial needling at nonacupuncture points), and conventional therapy. The response rate, based on responses to standardized pain/ability questionnaires (i.e., subjective measures) was 47.6% in the acupuncture group, 44.2% in the sham acupuncture group, and 27.4% in the conventional therapy group. The differences between acupuncture and conventional therapy and sham acupuncture and conventional therapy were statistically significant. The difference between acupuncture and sham acupuncture was not statistically significant. Several reports have addressed the issue of sham controls and subjective versus objective outcomes. Hrobjartsson and colleagues [92, 93] have shown in two separate systematic reviews that in trials with binary outcomes or when continuous outcomes were reported by observers (i.e., objective outcomes), there was no statistically significant effect of placebo interventions. However, a statistically significant effect was noted with patient-reported continuous outcomes (i.e., subjective outcome). Additionally, at a recent Cochrane Colloquium, Wood et al. [94] presented metaepidemiological data suggesting that failure to double-blind is associated with exaggerated treatment estimates, but only for trials with subjective outcomes. With these issues in mind, the most recent randomized clinical trials examining acupuncture and IVF will be discussed deemphasizing the distinction between placebo-controlled and no intervention trials.

In 2006, five randomized clinical trials investigating adjuvant acupuncture and IVF outcomes were reported. Two of these were reported in abstract form at the American Society for Reproductive Medicine annual meeting [95, 96] and three were published together in the same edition of Fertility and Sterility with accompanying editorials [97–99]. Two of these trials reported an increase in the clinical pregnancy rate with acupuncture [97, 99], whereas three of the trials reported no statistically significant difference [95, 96, 98].

One of the trials reporting no statistically significant impact of adjuvant acupuncture on IVF pregnancy rates was from Domar et al. [95] This study was a randomized, controlled, prospective, single-blind study 146, undergoing IVF at a major US center and utilizing the same acupuncture protocol as described by Paulus et al. [39] just before and after embryo transfer. Patients randomized to no treatment lay quietly for the same amount of time as the acupuncture patients. Acupuncture and no treatment groups did not differ significantly in age, mean number of embryos transferred, or clinical pregnancy rate (acupuncture 30.8%, no treatment 33.8%). This study also used standardized questionnaires to assess the mental status of patients and found acupuncture patients were more relaxed and more optimistic.

Another study that failed to find a significant difference in outcomes with patients utilizing adjuvant acupuncture was reported by Benson et al. [96] This was a prospective, single blind, randomized trial of 258 IVF patients at a large US fertility clinic that randomly assigned subjects to five separate treatment arms: needle acupuncture, laser acupuncture, sham laser acupuncture, relaxation, or no intervention. Acupuncture groups followed the Paulus [39] protocol of treatment just before and after embryo transfer. Although the clinical pregnancy rate in the traditional acupuncture group was the highest at 54.7% compared to 44% for no treatment with the other groups falling in between, statistical analysis revealed this to be a nonsignificant trend. The authors concluded that further study with larger patient groups is warranted, as this trial lacked the required statistical power.

Though studying more than twice the number of patients in acupuncture and control groups, Smith and colleagues from Australia [98] also reported no statistically significant difference in IVF outcomes with acupuncture. In this study, 228 subjects were randomized to traditional acupuncture or control with a placebo needle (nonpenetrating) placed in nonacupuncture points. The treatment schedule was a modification of the Paulus protocol [39] by adding a treatment session on day 9 of ovarian stimulation and adding acupuncture points based on TCM diagnosis. The study was adequately powered (power of 80%, two-sided testing at the 5% significance level) to detect a significant difference between groups based on the findings from Paulus et al. [39] The acupuncture group recorded a clinical pregnancy rate of 31% compared to 23% for control subjects, a difference that was not statistically significant. The authors concluded that acupuncture did not produce a significant impact on IVF pregnancy rates. However, they did note that a smaller effect could not be excluded and would require a larger study.

Appearing in the same journal issue as Smith et al. [98] and studying a similar number of subjects, Westergaard and colleagues [99] reached the opposite conclusion. In this investigation conducted at a Danish IVF center, patients were randomly assigned to treatment with traditional acupuncture on the day of embryo transfer only (Paulus protocol [39]), on that day and again 2 days later or no treatment. Clinical pregnancy rates in the group receiving acupuncture only on the day of embryo transfer were significantly higher than the no treatment group (39% vs. 24%). There was a trend toward a higher pregnancy rate in the group receiving the extra session (36% vs. 24%), though this was not statistically significant. Possible confounding variables were similar between groups, such as age, body mass index, duration of infertility, proportion of primary infertility patients, number of previous IVF attempts, and cause of infertility. Additionally, the distribution of various ovarian stimulation protocols was comparable between groups. It was recognized that the results could possibly be related to a placebo affect, as there was no sham control group. However, if this were the case, one would expect the group with the extra session to have the same or an enhanced affect. Also, this would be inconsistent with results from a subanalysis that showed only patients under age 38 showed a statistically significant improvement in clinical and ongoing pregnancy rates.

Addressing this issue by including a sham acupuncture control, Dieterle et al. [97] reported their results from a randomized, prospective study of 225 patients in a German infertility clinic. IVF patients were randomized to acupuncture based on the principles of TCM or sham acupuncture (needle insertion at nonrelevant points) performed immediately after the embryo transfer and again 3 days later. There was no statistically significant difference between the groups with regards to possible confounding variables, such as age, body mass index, duration/cause of infertility, and number of previous cycles. Clinical and ongoing pregnancy rates per transfer were significantly higher in the acupuncture group compared to control (33.6% vs. 15.6% and 33% vs. 15%, respectively). It was noted that the control group had a lower pregnancy rate than average based on data from the German IVF/ICSI register (24.6% for IVF and 22.6% for ICSI). This raised the possibility that the sham acupuncture protocol had an unexpected adverse effect. It was also noted that this trial had to adhere to the German Embryo Protection Law, which prohibits embryo selection and limits the number of embryos that can be transferred to three, which can impact pregnancy rates.

In an attempt to clarify this situation of conflicting study results, Manheimer et al. [100] recently reported the results of a meta-analysis of randomized controlled trials evaluating the impact of acupuncture on pregnancy rates and live birth rates from IVF. Studies were chosen to be included in the analysis if they met the following criteria: randomized, prospective clinical trial, evaluating acupuncture (i.e., insertion of needles into traditional meridian points) as a complement to the embryo transfer procedure with the objective of improving pregnancy rates, and extractable data on clinical and/or ongoing pregnancy rate and/or live birth rate. Articles could have appeared as a full article or as an abstract and could have had either a sham control or no intervention control group. Authors were contacted as needed to provide additional data to strengthen the analysis. Applying these standards, seven trials were identified [39, 86, 95–99], studying a total of 1,366 patients. Complementing the embryo transfer process with acupuncture was associated with a higher clinical pregnancy rate (odds ratio = 1.65, 95% CI, 1.27–2.14), ongoing pregnancy rate (odds ratio = 1.87, CI, 1.40–2.29), and live birth (odds ratio = 1.91, CI, 1.39–2.64). Further analysis found that for every ten patients receiving adjuvant acupuncture, one additional clinical pregnancy could be expected. Of note, a subgroup analysis revealed no statistically significant impact for acupuncture if analyzing only the three trials reporting control group pregnancy rates equal to or greater than European averages. It was concluded that further study would be needed to address this issue and better define the clinical situations that may benefit from acupuncture.

Since the meta-analysis by Manheimer et al., several other notable studies and meta-analyses have been published with differing conclusions. Craig et al. [101] reported the results of a multi-center, prospective and randomized trial of 107 IVF patients who received acupuncture before and after embryo transfer or no intervention. The clinical pregnancy rate in the control group was 69.6%, which was statistically higher than the rate of 43.8% calculated in the acupuncture group. Of note, all acupuncture occurred off-site in contrast to most of the previous trials reported. El-Toukhy [102] reported no impact of acupuncture on IVF clinical pregnancy rates (RR=1.23, 95% CI 0.96-1.58, P=0.1) after performing a meta-analysis of 8 randomized clinical trials in which sham acupuncture or no treatment was used in the control group. This study differed from the previous meta-analysis [100] by including data from the Craig et al. study and by including the group receiving laser acupuncture in the Benson et al. [96] trial. A systemic review and meta-analysis from China [103], reached the opposite conclusion, excluding the data from Craig et al. and Benson et al. and adding data from studies that were excluded in the other meta-analyses. Specifically, Ng et al. reported a significant improvement in the pregnancy rate for acupuncture treatment with an odds ratio [OR] 1.42, and 95% CI 1.17-1.72. Lastly, So and colleagues [104] from China, reported the results of a randomized double blind comparison of real and placebo acupuncture (sham acupuncture needles) and IVF treatment in 370 patients. The protocol involved treatment only on the day of embryo transfer (25 minutes before and after the procedure) and involved assessment of endometrial and subendometrial vascularity, serum cortisol levels and anxiety levels. No significant difference was found in live birth rates between the two groups, Both groups showed a similar treatment associated decline in endometrial vascularity, serum cortisol and anxiety levels. This led the authors to conclude that placebo acupuncture may not be inert.

50.4 Summary: Evidence-Based Guidelines

In conclusion, there is an extensive though not exhaustive body of literature regarding the impact of acupuncture on IVF. Studies have investigated physiological and psychological endpoints that could impact IVF outcomes as well as studying the impact of adjuvant acupuncture on pregnancy rates and live birth rates. Regarding physiological changes, it has been well established that treatment with acupuncture is associated with a significant increase in the endogenous neuropeptide beta-endorphin. Additionally, studies have suggested a role for beta-endorphin and other neuropeptides in regulation of the GnRH pulse generator, and locally, in the ovary. However, no studies have investigated the impact of acupuncture on beta-endorphin levels in patients undergoing IVF. Acupuncture has also been associated with changes in the autonomic nervous system that could lead to alterations in blood flow. Evaluating the impact of acupuncture on uterine blood flow in humans has led to conflicting results, whereas data from studies in animals have concluded that acupuncture causes an increase in ovarian blood flow. It is unknown how these changes would impact IVF success rates as, despite numerous studies, it is unclear whether measurements of blood flow to the uterus or ovaries are good predictors of success with IVF. Acupuncture has also been found to have a beneficial effect on patients with depression and anxiety disorders, issues commonly seen in infertility patients and that have been associated with poor IVF outcomes. However, more study is needed to determine whether acupuncture during IVF improves these conditions. Regarding pregnancy rates, a review of the literature finds more than 20 separate reports investigating the impact of adjuvant acupuncture on IVF outcomes. Though initial randomized clinical trials and a meta-analysis concluded that acupuncture improves IVF pregnancy rates, more recent reports have raised significant doubt regarding this conclusion. Studies have almost uniformly shown little risk of serious adverse events.

Prior to making definitive recommendations, several issues need to be addressed. It is possible that the few, relatively small, studies that concluded that acupuncture was associated with a significant improvement in pregnancy rates did so by chance (α error) [87]. This seems possible especially when the data is examined closer, revealing that if a few more pregnancies occurred in the control group (to reach pregnancy rates closer to the average for that region), the differences would no longer be statistically significant [39, 97, 99]. There is also the possibility that the impact of acupuncture is dependent on the baseline pregnancy rate. This issue was raised by the observation that trials with higher control group pregnancy rates failed to show a significant difference when acupuncture was added [100]. There have also been concerns voiced regarding a placebo effect in studies with no treatment controls and the concern that placebo acupuncture may not be inert. Additionally, the possibility of publication bias skewing results of the meta-analysis. Lastly, there is the lack of a biologically plausible mechanism by which a single acupuncture treatment before and after embryo transfer results in an improvement in live birth rates. This is especially important as it is well established with other disease states that TCM often requires multiple courses of treatment over time to have an impact. It is hoped that these issues will be addressed in future studies, as currently there is insufficient agreement amongst studies to conclude that adjuvant acupuncture improves IVF success rates, though there appears to be little risk of serious side-effects.

References

1. Domar A (2006) Acupuncture and infertility: we need to stick to good science. Fertil Steril 85:1359
2. Coulson C, Jenkins J (2005) Complementary and alternative medicine utilization in NHS and private clinic settings: a United Kingdom survey of 400 infertility patients. J Exp Clin Assist Reprod 2:5
3. Boivin J, Schmidt L (2007) Who uses complementary therapy? Predictors in an infertile population. In: Abstracts of the 23rd Annual Meeting of the ESHRE, Lyon, France, July 2007, (Abstract O-229)
4. Stankiewicz M, Smith C, Alvino H, Norman R (2007) The use of complimentary medicine and therapies by patients attending a reproductive medicine unit is South Australia: a prospective survery. Aust N Z J Obstet Gynaecol 47(2):145–149
5. National Center for Complimentary and Alternative Medicine, National Institutes of Health. http://www.Nccam.nih.gov
6. Eisenberg D, Davis R, Ettner S, Appel S, Wilkey S, Van Rompay M, Kessler R (1998) Trends in alternative medicine use in the United States, 1990–1997, results of a follow-up national survey. JAMA 280:1569–1575
7. Kaptchuk TJ (2000) The web that has no weaver. Understanding Chinese medicine. Contemporary Publishing Group, Chicago, IL
8. Maciocia G (1998) Obstetrics & gynecology in Chinese medicine. Churchill Livingstone. Philadelphia, Pennsylvania, USA
9. West Z (2001) Acupuncture in pregnancy and childbirth. Churchill Livingstone, New York
10. Facchinetti F, Storchi AR, Petraglia F, Volpe A, Genazzani AR (1988) Expression of proopiomelanocortin-related eptides in human follicular fluid. Peptides 9:1089–1092
11. Gallinelli A, Garuti G, Matteo ML, Genazzani AR, Facchinetti F (1995) Expression of proopiomelanocortin gene in human ovarian tissue. Hum Reprod 10:1085–1089

12. DeBold CD, Menefee JK, Nicholson WE, Orth DN (1988) Proopiomelanocortin gene is expressed in many normal human tissues and intumors not associated with ectopic adrenocorticotropin syndrome. Mol Endocrinol 2:862–870
13. Mayer DJ, Price DD, Rafil A (1977) Antagonism of acupuncture analgesia in man by the narcotic antagonist naloxone. Brain Res 121:368–372
14. Petti F, Bangrazi A, Liguori A, Reale G, Ippoliti F (1998) Effects of acupuncture on immune response related to opioid-like peptides. J Tradit Chin Med 18:55–63
15. Ulett GA, Han S, Han JS (1998) Electroacupuncture: mechanisms and clinical application. Biol Psychiatry 44:129–138
16. Ku Y, Chang Y (2001) Beta-endorphin and GABA-mediated depressor effect of specific electroacupuncture surpasses pressor response of emotional circuit. Peptides 22:1465–1470
17. Ching M (1983) Morphine suppresses the proestrous surge of GnRH in pituitary portal plasma of rats. Endocrinology 1120: 2209–2211
18. Orstead KM, Spics HG (1987) Inhibition of hypothalamic gonadotropin releasing hormone release by endogenous opioid peptides in the female rabbit. Neuroendocrinology 46:14–23
19. Whisnat S, Havern R, Goodman R (1991) Endogenous opioid suppression of luteinizing hormone pulse frequency and amplitude in the ewe: hypothalamic sites of action. Neruoendocrinology 54:587–593
20. Goodman R, Gibson M, Skinner D, Lehman M (2002) Neuroendocrine control of pulsatile GnRH secretion during the ovrarian cycle: evidence from the ewe. Reprod Suppl 59:41–56
21. Quigley ME, Sheeham KL, Casper RF, Yen SSC (1980) Evidence for an increased opioid inhibition of luteinizing hormone secretion in hyperprolactinemic patients with pituitary microadenoma. J Clin Endocrinol Metab 50:427–446
22. Rossmanith WG, Mortola JF, Yen SSC (1988) Role of endogenous opioid peptides in the initiation of the mid-cycle luteinizing hormone surge in normal cycling women. J Clin Endocrinol Metab 67:695–700
23. Petraglia F, DiMeo G, Storchi R, Segre A, Facchinette F, Szalay S et al (1987) Proopiomelanocortin-related peptides and methionine enkephalin in human follicular fluid: changes during the menstrual cycle. Am J Obstet Gynecol 157:142–146
24. Chen C, Chang C, Krieger D, Bardin C (1986) Expression and regulation of proopiomelanocortin-like gene in the ovary and placenta: comparison with the testis. Endocrinology 118:2382–2389
25. Aleem FA, Eltabbakh GH, Omar RA, Couthren AL (1987) Ovarian follicular fluid beta-endorphin levels in normal and polycystic ovaries. Am J Obstet Gynecol 156:1197–1200
26. Facchinetti F, Artini P, Monaco M, Volpe A, Genazzani A (1989) Oocyte fertilization in vitro is assoicated with high follicular immunoreactive beta-endorphin levels. J Endocrinol Invest 12: 693–698
27. Knardahl S, Elam M, Olausson B, Wallin BG (1998) Sympathetic nerve activity after acupuncture in humans. Pain 75:19–25
28. Tokumaru C, Chen J (1005) Effects of acupressure on gastric myoelectrical activity in healthy humans. Scand J Gastroenterol 40:319–325
29. Ernst M, Lee M (1985) Sympathetic vasomotor changes induced by manual and electrical acupuncture of the Hoku point visualized by thermography. Pain 21:25–33
30. Andersson S, Lundeberg T (1995) Acupuncture-from empiricism to science: functional background to acupuncture effects in pain and disease. Med Hypotheses 45:271–281
31. Haker E, Egekvist H, Bjerring P (2000) Effect of sensory stimulation (acupuncture) on sympathetic and parasympathetic activities in healthy subjects. J Auton Nerv Syst 79:52–59
32. Middlekauff H, Hui K, Yu J, Hamilton M, Fonarow G, Moriguchi J, Maclellan W, Hage A (2002) Acupuncture inhibits sympathetic activation during mental stress in advanced heart failure patients. J Card Fail 8:399–406
33. Loaiza L, Yamaguchi S, Ito M, Ohshima N (2002) Electro-acupuncture stimulation to muscle afferents in anesthetized rats modulates the blood flow to the knee joint through autonomic reflexes and nitric oxide. Auton Neurosci 97:103–109
34. Sakai S, Hori E, Umeno K, Kitabayashi N, Ono T, Nishijo H (2007) Specific acupuncture sensation correlates with EEGs and autonomic changes in human subjects. Auton Neurosci 133:158–169
35. Schneider A, Weiland C, Enck P, Joos S, Streitberger K, Maser-Gluth C, Zipfel S, Bagheri S, Herzog W, Friederich H (2007) Neruoendrocrinological effects of acupuncture treatment in patients with irritable bowel syndrome. Complement Ther Med 15: 255–263
36. Bäker M, Grossman P, Schneider J, Michalsen A, Knoblauch N, Tan L, Niggemeyer C, Linde K, Melchaart D, Dobos G (2008) Acupuncture in migraine: investigation of autonomic effects. Clin J Pain 24:106–115
37. Takagi K, Yamaguchi S, Ito M, Ohshima N (2005) Effects of electroacupuncture stimulation applied to limb and back on mesenteric microvascular hemodynamics. Jpn J Physiol 55:191–203
38. Stener-Victorin E, Waldenstrom U, Andersson SA, Wikland M (1996) Reduction of blood flow impedance in the uterine arteries of infertile women with electro-acupuncture. Hum Reprod 11: 1314–1317
39. Paulus WE, Zhang M, Strehler E, El-Danasouri I, Sterzik K (2002) Influence of acupuncture on the pregnancy rate in patients who undergo assisted reproduction therapy. Fert Steril 77:721–724
40. Stener-Victorin E, Kobayashi R, Kurosawa M (2003) Ovarian blood flow responses to electro-acupuncture stimulation at different frequencies and intensities in anaesthetized rats. Auton Neurosci 108(1–2):50–56
41. Stener-Victorin E, Kobayashi R, Watanabe O, Lundeberg T, Kurosawa M (2004) Effect of electro-acupuncture stimulation of different frequencies and intensities on ovarian blood flow in anaesthetized rats with steroid-induced polycystic ovaries. Reprod Biol Endocrinol 2:16
42. Schild R, Knobloch C, Dorn C, Fimmers R, van der Ven H, Hansmann M (2001) Endometrial receptivity in an in vitro fertilization program as assessed by spiral artery blood flow, endometrial thickness, endometrial volume, and uterine artery blood flow. Fertil Steril 75:361–366
43. Ng EHY, Chan CCW, Tang OS, Yeung WSB, Ho PC (2007) Endometrial and subendometrial vascularity is higher in pregnant patients with live birth following ART than in those who suffer a miscarriage. Hum Reprod 22:1134–1141
44. Aytoz A, Ubaldi F, Tournaye H, Nagy Z, Van Steirteghem A, Devroey P (1997) The predictive value of uterine artery blood flow measurements for uterine receptivity in an intracytoplasmic sperm injection program. Fertil Steril 68:935–937
45. Bloechle M, Schreiner T, Kuchler I, Schurenkamper P, Lisse K (1997) Colour Doppler assessment of ascendant uterine artery perfusion in an in-vitro fertilization-embryo transfer programme after pituitary desensitization and ovarian stimulation with human recombinant follicle stimulating hormone. Hum Reprod 12:1772–1777
46. Yang J, Wu M, Chen C, Jiang M, Ho H, Yang Y (1999) Association of endometrial blood flow as determined by a modified colour Doppler technique with subsequent outcome of in-vitro fertilization. Hum Reprod 14:1606–1610
47. Sher G, Fisch J (2000) Vaginal sildenafil (Viagra): a preliminary report of a novel method to improve uterine artery blood flow and endometrial development in patients undergoing IVF. Hum Reprod 15:806–809
48. Battaglia C, Artini P, Giulini S, Salvatori M, Maxia N, Petraglia F et al (1997) Color Doppler changes and thromboxane production

after ovarian stimulation with gonadotrophin-releasing hormone agonist. Hum Reprod 12:2477–2482
49. Kupesic S, Bekavac I, Bjelos D, Kurjak A (2001) Assessment of endometrial receptivity by transvaginal color Doppler and three-dimensional power Doppler ultrasonography in patients undergoing in vitro fertilization procedures. J Ultrasound Med 20: 125–134
50. Wu H, Chiang C, Huang H, Chao A, Wang H, Soong Y (2003) Detection of the subendometrial vascularization flow index by three-dimensional ultrasound may be useful for predicting the pregnancy rate for patients undergoing in vitro fertilization-embryo transfer. Fertil Steril 79:507–511
51. Zaidi J, Campbell S, Pittrof R, Tan S (1995) Endometrial thickness, morphology, vascular penetration and velocimetry in predicting implantation in an in vitro fertilization program. Ultrasound Obstet Gynecol 6:191–198
52. Applebaum M (1995) The uterine biophysical profile. Ultrasound Obset Gynecol 5:67–68
53. Yuval Y, Lipitz S, Dor J, Achiron R (1999) The relationship between endometrial thickness and blood flow and pregnancy rates in in-vitro fertilization. Hum Reprod 14:1067–1071
54. Isaksson R, Tiitinen A, Cacciatore B (2000) Uterine artery impedance to blood flow on the day of embryo transfer does not predict obstetric outcome. Ultrasound Obstet Gynecol 15:527–530
55. Zaidi J, Barber J, Kyei-Mensah A, Bekir J, Campbell S, Tan S (1996) Relationship of ovarian stromal blood flow at the baseline ultrasound scan to subsequent follicular response in an in vitro fertilization program. Obstet Gynecol 88:779–784
56. Engmann L, Sladkevicius P, Agrawal R, Bekir J, Campbell S, Tan S (1999) Value of ovarian stromal blood flow velocity measurement after pituitary suppression in the prediction of ovarian responsiveness and outcome of in vitro fertilization treatment. Fertil Steril 71:22–29
57. Mercé L, Santiago B, Barco M, Troyano J, Gay R, Sotos F, Villa A (2006) Assessment of the ovarian volume, number and volume of follicles and ovarian vascularity by three-dimensional ultrasonography and power doppler angiography on the HCH day to predict the outcome in IVF/ICSI cycles. Hum Reprod 21: 1218–1226
58. Mercé L, Barco M, Bau S, Troyano J (2007) Prediction of ovarian response and IVF/ICSI outcome by three-dimensional ultrasonography and power Doppler angiography. Eur J Obstet Gynecol Reprod Biol 132:93–100
59. Kupesic S, Kurjak A (2002) Predictors of IVF outcome by three-dimensional ultrasound. Hum Reprod 17:950–955
60. Kupsesic S, Kurjak A, Bjelos D, Vujisic S (2003) Three-dimensional ultrasonographic ovarian measurements and in vitro fertilization outcome are related to age. Fertil Steril 79:190–197
61. Jarvela I, Sladkevicius P, Kelly S, Ojha K, Campbell S, Nargund G (2003) Quantification of ovarian power Doppler signal with three-dimensional ultrasonography to predict response during in vitro fertilization. Obstet Gynecol 102:816–822
62. Ng E, Tang O, Chan C, Ho P (2006) Ovarian stromal vascularity is not predictive of ovarian response and pregnancy. Reprod Biomed Online 12:43–49
63. Chen T, Chang S, Tsai C, Juang K (2004) Prevalence of depressive, and anxiety disorders in an assisted reproductive technique clinic. Hum Reprod 19:2313–2318
64. Domar A (2005) Infertility and the mind/body connection. Female Patient 30:24–28
65. Terzioglu F (2001) Investigation into effectiveness of counseling on assisted reproductive techniques in Turkey. J Psychosom Obstet Gynaecol 22:133–141
66. Johnson D (2006) Acupuncture prior to and at embryo transfer in an assisted conception unit- a case series. Acupunct Med 24:23–28
67. He Q, Ahzng J, Tang Y (2007) A controlled study on treatment of mental depression by acupuncture plus TSM medication. J Tradit Chin Med 27(3):166–169
68. Allen JJB, Schnyer R, Hitt S (1998) The efficacy of acupuncture in the treatment of major depression in women. Psychol Sci 9(5): 397–401
69. Roschke J, Wolf C, Muller M et al (1998) The benefits from whole body acupuncture in major depression. J Affect Disord 57:73–81
70. Manber R, Schnyer RN, Allen JJ, Rush AJ, Blasey CM (2004) Acupuncture: a promising treatment for depression during pregnancy. J Affect Disord 83:89–95
71. Pilkington K, Kirkwood G, Rampes H, Cummings M, Richardson J (2007) Acupuncture for anxiety and anxiety disorders- a systematic literature review. Acupunct Med 25(1–2):1–10
72. Smith C, Hay P (2005) Acupuncture for depression. Cochrane Database Syst Rev 18(2):CD004046
73. Gerhard I, Postneck F (1992) Auricular acupuncture in the treatment of female infertility. Gynecol Endocrinol 6(3):171–181
74. Chen BY (1997) Acupuncture normalizes dysfunction of hypothalamic-pituitary-ovarian axis. Acupunct Electrother Res 22: 97–108
75. Stener-Victorin E, Waldenstrom U, Tagnfors U, Lundeberg T, Lundstedt G, Janson PO (2000) Effects of electro-acupuncture on anovulation in women with polycystic ovary syndrome. Acta Obstet Gynecol Scand 79:180–188
76. Stener-Victorin E, Waldenstrom U, Nisson L, Wikland M, Janson P (1999) A prospective randomized study of electro-acupuncture versus alfentanil as anaesthesia during oocytes aspiration in in-vitro fertilization. Hum Reprod 14:80–84
77. Stener-Victorin E, Urban W, Mattis W, Nilsson L, Hagglund L, Lundeberg T (2003) Electro-acupuncture as a preoperative analgesic method and its effects on implantation rate and neuropeptide Y concentrations in follicular fluid. Hum Reprod 18:1454–1460
78. Kwan I, Bhattacharya S, Knox F, McNeil A (2005) Conscious sedation and analgesia for oocytes retrieval during in vitro fertilization procedures. Cochrane Database Syst Rev 20(3):CD004829
79. Humaidan P, Stener-Victorin E (2004) Pain relief during oocytes retrieval with a new short duration electro-acupuncture technique-an alternative to conventional analgesic methods. Hum Reprod 19:1367–1372
80. Satro-Katzenshlager S, Wolfler M, Kozek-Langenecker A, Sator K, Sator P, Li B, Heinze G, Sator M (2006) Auricular electro-acupuncture as an additional perioperative analgesic method during oocytes aspiration in IVF treatment. Hum Reprod 21:2114–2120
81. Magarelli P, Cridennda D, Cohen M (2004) Acupuncture and good prognosis IVF patients: synergy. Fertil Steril 82:S80 (Abstract O-200)
82. Magarelli P, Cridennda D (2004) Acupuncture and IVF poor responders: a cure? Fertil Steril PCRS abstracts 81:S20 (Abstract P-10)
83. Khorram N, Horton S, Sahakian V (2005) The effect of acupuncture on outcome of in vitro fertilization. Fertil Steril 84:S364 (Abstract P-587)
84. Johnson D (2006) Acupuncture prior to and at embryo transfer in an assisted conception unit- a case series. Acupunct Med 24:23–28
85. Wang W, Check J, Liss J, Choe J (2007) A matched controlled study to evaluate the efficacy of acupuncture for improving pregnancy rates following in vitro fertilization-embryo transfer. Clin Exp Obstet Gynecol 34:137–138
86. Paulus W, Ahang M, Strehler E, Seybold B, Sterzik K (2003) Placebo-controlled trial of acupuncture effects in assisted reproduction therapy. Hum Reprod 18(xviii):18–19 (Abstract O-052)
87. Collins J (2006) The play of chance. Fertil Steril 85:1364
88. Myers E (2006) Acupuncture as adjunctive therapy in assisted reproduction: remaining uncertainties. Fertil Steril 85:1362

89. Dieterle S (2006) Invitation to an international multicenter study of the effect of acupuncture on the outcome of in vitro fertilization and intracytoplasmic sperm injection. Fertil Steril 85:1370
90. Kaptchuk TJ, Stason WB, Legedza DRB, AR SRN, Kerr CE et al (2006) Sham device v inert pill: randomised controlled trial of two placebo treatments. BMJ 332:391–397
91. Haake M, Muller JJ, Schade-Brittinger C, Basler H, Schafer H, Maier C et al (2007) German acupuncture trials for chronic low back pain. Arch Intern Med 167:1892–1898
92. Hrobjartsson A, Gotzsche PC (2001) Is the placebo powerless? An analysis of clinical trials comparing placebo with no treatment. N Engl J Med 344:1594–1602
93. Hrobjartsson A, Gotzsche PC (2004) Is the placebo powerless? Update of a systematic review with 52 new randomized trials comparing placebo with no treatment. J Int Med 256:91–100
94. Wood L, Egger M, Gluud LL, Schulz K, Altman D, Juni P et al (2006) The association of allocation concealment and blinding with estimated treatment effect varies according to type of outcome: a combined analysis of meta-epidemiological studies. In: 14th Cochrane Colloquium, Dublin, Ireland, October 23–26, 2006 (Abstract O-19)
95. Domar AD, Meshay I, Kelliher J, Alper M, Powers RD (2009) The impact of acupuncture on in vitro fertilization outcome. Fertil Steril 91(3):723–726
96. Benson MR, Elkind-Hirsch KE, Theall A, Fong K, Hogan RB, Scott RT (2006) Impact of acupuncture before and after embryo transfer on the outcome of in vitro fertilization cycles: a prospective single-blind randomized study. Fertil Steril 86:S135 (Abstract P-18)
97. Dieterle S, Ying G, Hatzmann W, Neuer A (2006) Effect of acupuncture on the outcome of in vitro fertilization and intracytoplasmic sperm injection: a randomized, prospective, controlled clinical study. Fertil Steril 85:1347–1351
98. Smith C, Coyle M, Norman RJ (2006) Influence of acupuncture stimulation on pregnancy rates for women undergoing embryo transfer. Fertil Steril 85:1352–1358
99. Westergaard LG, Mao Q, Krogslund M, Sandrini S, Lenz S, Grinsted J (2006) Acupuncture on the day of embryo transfer significantly improves the reproductive outcome in infertile women: a prospective, randomized trial. Fertil Steril 85:1341–1346
100. Manheimer E, Zhang G, Udoff L, Haramati A, Langenberg P, Berman B, Bouter L (2008) Effects of acupuncture on rates of pregnancy and live birth among women undergoing in vitro fertilization: systematic review and meta-analysis. BMJ 336: 545–549
101. Craig L, Criniti A, Hansen L, Marshall A, Soules M (2007) Acupuncture lowers pregnancy rates when performed before and after embryo transfer. Fertil Steril 88:S40 (Abstract O-106)
102. El-Toukhy T, Sunkara SK, Khairy M, Dyer R, Khalaf Y, Coomarasamy A (2008) A systematic review and meta-analysis of acupuncture in in-vitro fertilization. BJOG 115:1203–1213
103. Ng EHY, So WS, Gao J, Wong YY, Ho PC (2008) The role of acupuncture in the management of subfertility. Fertile Steril 90(1):1–12
104. So EWS, Ng EHY, Wong YY, Lau EYL, Yeung WSB, Ho PC (2009) A randomized double blind comparison of real and placebo acupuncture in IVF treatment. Hum Reprod 24(2):341–348

Part VI
Research in the REI Practice and Laboratories

Chapter 51
Designing a Clinical Research Infrastructure

Tonya Edvalson, Emily Hixson, and Michael Varner

Abstract The design, conduct, and supervision of clinical research trials in the early twenty-first century American medical setting are increasingly complex processes. With increasing awareness that clinical trial outcomes must focus on clinically significant, rather than surrogate, outcomes, the need for larger multi-site extramurally funded studies is becoming more apparent. The administration of such studies requires careful attention to research personnel administration, careful and thorough financial accounting, and appropriate timely approval mechanisms. Institutions committed to long-term sustainable research programs will need to develop research infrastructures capable of proactive administration. This chapter provides guidelines for infrastructure development as well as specific examples from the authors' institution.

Keywords Research • Grants • Contracts, research administration • Personnel

51.1 Introduction

Reproductive medicine, from before conception to the puerperium, is characterized by normal physiology and normal outcomes for both mother and her baby(ies). Even many of the clinical entities of interest to the readers of this book (infertility, polycystic ovary syndrome (PCOS), endometriosis, varicocele, etc.) occur infrequently enough that few clinical centers have sufficient clinical volumes to mount adequately powered single-center clinical trials of individuals or couples with well-characterized conditions. Likewise, the end points of clinical trials should ideally be clinically significant, and not surrogate outcomes. In addition, the study of infrequent outcomes can be complicated by the lack of sensitive and specific predictive tests remote from the clinical outcome of interest. For all these reasons, there is a growing trend toward multicenter clinical trial networks.

For example, the National Institute of Child Health and Human Development (NICHD) now has at least seven reproductive endocrinology/infertility (REI) multicenter clinical trials networks (Table 51.1). While the number of networks as well as their memberships will doubtless change over the years, it is already clear that these clinical trial networks are dominated by a relatively small number of institutions that have established clinical research infrastructures.

The authors of this contribution have developed such an infrastructure in an obstetrics and gynecology department, initially focusing on obstetric clinical trials but now expanded to cover the entire department. The authors have been recruited to fill key positions in the research infrastructure of the Department of Obstetrics and Gynecology at the University of Utah. It is the purpose of this contribution to provide some background and guidance to those individuals and clinical centers that might wish to design a clinical research infrastructure.

51.2 Patient Population

Because any clinical research infrastructure must be tailored to the population(s) that it will study, it is thus important to first consider the effect(s) of patient population(s) on infrastructure design. In particular, if a research infrastructure is being developed around an existing clinic/clinics that is/are already seeing a substantial number of women with specific REI diagnoses, the requirements are likely quite different from an infrastructure being created for population-based studies. In reality, many research programs will need and want to be able to recruit subjects from both groups.

T. Edvalson, E. Hixson, and M. Varner (✉)
Department of Obstetrics and Gynecology, University of Utah School of Medicine, 30 N. Medical Drive, 2B200, Salt Lake City, UT, 13126, USA
e-mail: Michael.varner@hsc.utah.edu

D.T. Carrell and C.M. Peterson (eds.), *Reproductive Endocrinology and Infertility: Integrating Modern Clinical and Laboratory Practice*,
DOI 10.1007/978-1-4419-1436-1_51, © Springer Science+Business Media, LLC 2010

Table 51.1 NICHD networks in reproductive endocrinology and infertility

Network	NICHD contact	Number of centers	Network focus
Contraceptive Clinical Trials Network (CCTN)	Trent MacKay MD, MPH	14	Phase I, II, and III trials of oral, injectable, implantable, or topical contraceptive drugs and contraceptive devices
Cooperative Contraceptive Research Centers	Diana Blithe, PhD	5	Basic or clinical research on new contraceptives
Cooperative Reproductive Science Research Centers (CRSRC) at minority institutions	Estella Parrott MD, MPH	3	Development of competitive research environments in reproductive science at minority institutions
Cooperative Research Program on Male Fertility Regulation	Louis DePaolo, PhD	8	Development of male contraceptives, including a combination of basic, applied, and clinical research
National Cooperative Program for Infertility Research (NCPIR)	Louis DePaolo, PhD	2	Genetic etiology of polycystic ovarian syndrome
Reproductive Medicine Network (RMN)	Tracy Rankin, PhD	8	Multicenter clinical trials in the areas of male and female infertility, reproductive diseases and disorders
Specialized Cooperative Centers Program in Reproduction Research (SCCPRR)	Louis DePaolo, PhD	14	Research focus groups were established in the areas of male reproduction, endometrial biology, ovarian physiology, and reproductive neuroendocrinology

51.2.1 Specialty- or Subspecialty-Based Recruitment

Many patients seen for diagnosis and/or treatment of the entities identified in Table 51.1 will likely be seen in REI subspecialty clinics. Recruitment of research subjects in this setting generally requires less infrastructure support because the subjects are already identified. However, recruitment by diagnosis in specialty clinics leaves open the questions of incidence (the number of new occurrences of a condition in a population over time) and prevalence (the measure of a condition in a population at a given moment in time). This may be because some proportion of subspecialty clinics in a community or region are not included in the population base or because some proportion of potential subjects are seen by other providers (general obstetrician-gynecologists, urologists, family physicians, etc.). In either case, the more extensively a research network is integrated with its community(ies), the more fully representative will be its patient population of the diagnosis and/or treatment entities it wishes to study.

The authors have a 17+ year experience with population-based recruitment as a result of their initial preparation for, and subsequent involvement with, the NICHD Maternal-Fetal Medicine Units (MFMU) Network. The Utah site in this Network consists of the five tertiary care perinatal centers in the northern Utah urban corridor (90% of the State's population) and thus allows research access to almost all women with significant pregnancy complications (recognizing that a proportion of such women will present to their local facilities and require immediate delivery rather than maternal transport). The authors worked for 5 years (1990–1995) to nurture the relationships with providers and health-care facilities that would be necessary for a fundable multicenter collaborative clinical trials network. The two areas of emphasis that proved most successful in our endeavors were collaborative research and collaborative education, both of which are frameworks on which to construct political and economic relationships that are either mutually neutral or mutually advantageous.

51.2.1.1 Collaborative Research

Initial collaborative research need not begin with randomized controlled trials. Rather, simple descriptive statistics, either prospectively or retrospectively acquired, can be valuable for establishing collaboration (and resultant mutual trust), providing useful community and/or institutional benchmarks, and establishing a basis for collaborative publications. Preparation and submission of collaborative publications can prove particularly valuable for documenting previous collaboration when funding applications are eventually submitted.

While telephones, mailings, and internet communications (websites, e-mails, etc.) are all vitally important communications media for the early twenty-first century, there remains no substitute for "face time" when developing relationships. We have found that regular "research road shows," in which the research administration visits both administrators (hospital and clinic) and providers, are truly invaluable for establishing and maintaining personal relationships based on trust, respect, and understanding. These relationships are even more important than research protocols for maintaining long-term research collaboration.

For a collaborative research relationship to be truly synergistic and sustainable, consideration needs to be given to the prospect of all partners being eligible to pursue funding opportunities. Said another way, "research colonialism" (in which one institution gets all the academic credit and indirect cost funding while some considerable proportion of the actual work is done elsewhere) is not a viable option. A "research commonwealth," in which all partners have opportunities to pursue funding opportunities according to their individual interests, strengths, and expertise, is – at least in the authors' opinion – the strategy most likely to be successful over extended time-periods.

51.2.1.2 Collaborative Education

The development of collaborative education programs (Grand Rounds that rotate amongst institutions, CME programs, "mini-residencies," etc.) is not directly related to research collaboration but, at least in the authors' experience, has proven very helpful for establishing, nurturing, and expanding the mutual trust, respect and multidirectional communication that is absolutely essential for any long-term research relationship. In the authors' specific situation, the development of collaborative research and education programs among providers and health-care facilities as well as the publication of collaborative research activities were both absolutely critical to the success of our initial (1996) and subsequent multicenter clinical trial network applications.

51.2.2 Population-Based Recruitment

Population-based recruitment largely obviates concerns about incidence and prevalence. However, they require long-term, extensive involvement with the entire community. Prospective population-based recruitment studies can generally only be accomplished after widespread engagement of providers, health-care facilities, and/or populations.

Population-based studies can sometimes also be augmented by collaboration with regional Health Departments. Health Departments are interested in community-wide outcomes and can provide valuable background data. Their surveillance systems may also provide valuable contacts for expanding clinical access.

Two examples of NIH-funded population-based recruitment studies with which the authors have specific experience are the Stillbirth Collaborative Research Network and the National Children's Study. In both cases, they were build on the foundations of collaborative research (and publications) and education described in the preceding section.

51.2.2.1 Collaborative Stillbirth Research Network

The Collaborative Stillbirth Research Network (CSRN) is an NICHD-funded multicenter geographic population-based study of the incidence of fetal deaths at 20 weeks gestation or greater. An extensive clinical protocol has been developed, and cases plus controls are now being recruited at five clinical sites (Brown University, Emory University, University of Texas Medical Branch–Galveston, University of Texas–San Antonio, University of Utah). The Utah clinical center is collecting cases and controls from women who are residents of Salt Lake County, Utah. This involves "real-time" identification and recruitment of cases in all hospitals in Salt Lake County ($n=8$) as well as those hospitals in immediately adjacent counties ($n=8$) where women who are Salt Lake County residents might seek obstetric services.

Based on relationships originally developed in preparation for the MFMU Network application, the Utah investigators were able to enlist the participation of all 16 hospitals and the majority of the obstetric care providers in Salt Lake County. This emphasizes the importance not only of establishing community relationships, but also of maintaining them over time.

51.2.2.2 National Children's Study

The National Children's Study (NCS) is a large, long-term longitudinal study of environmental and genetic influences on children's health and development. It expects to enroll a sufficient number of women of reproductive age, either preconceptionally or early in pregnancy, to result in 100,000 live births. Monitoring of the mother's exposures will continue throughout pregnancy to birth, and possibly beyond. The child will then be followed for a wide range of health and developmental outcomes and NCS-defined environmental exposures throughout childhood until at least 21 years of age. It will be conducted in 105 preassigned jurisdictions across the country that were selected to represent the population of the country as a whole. One of these jurisdictions is Salt Lake County. On behalf of Salt Lake County, the University of Utah is one of the seven selected NCS Vanguard Centers (for more information, see http://www.nationalchildrensstudy.gov).

Besides enlisting the support of health-care providers and facilities, the NCS Vanguard Centers are expanding the research infrastructure to involve employers, advocacy groups, neighborhoods, schools, faith groups, media, and health departments.

51.3 Protocols

51.3.1 *Single Site Versus Multi-site*

Recruitment of research participants from a single site (hospital, clinic, etc) offers obvious geographic advantages but has the potential of limiting enrollment, particularly when protocol entry criteria are restrictive. On the other hand, multi-site recruitment offers access to larger, and sometimes more diverse, patient populations but carries with it the challenges of parallel administrative functions, often between disparate institutions.

Multi-site recruitment may involve a single investigator functioning in more than one hospital or clinic or could involve multiple investigators and multiple hospitals or clinics. While the latter situation has the additional complexity of organizing multiple investigators (mercifully beyond the scope of this contribution), both situations require understandings between institutions. It has been our experience that misunderstandings are substantially less when contractual agreements are in place between the various organizations that outline both the research projects (equivalent IRB approvals, procurement and distribution of supplies and equipment, etc.) and personnel issues (job descriptions, supervision and evaluation, access requirements and/or restrictions, funding streams, etc.).

51.3.2 *Grants Versus Contracts*

Grant submissions generally require more investigator preliminary results but, once awarded, allow more flexibility in approach. While it remains vitally important to develop mechanisms by which resource utilization is accurately tracked and reported, actual research outcomes will be based on data collection and/or experimental outcomes.

In clinical trials, the double-edged option of capitated enrollment may also be present. If recruitment and protocol execution can be accomplished efficiently, then income can exceed expenses and the remaining funds may (sometimes requiring sponsor approval) be used to support the research infrastructure. On the other hand, when expenses exceed income, the institution either needs to change its procedures or limit/cease its participation. It is also vitally important that all appropriate administration be made aware of any capitated funding mechanisms (before the fact!), including provisions for covering any deficits that might develop. Such an awareness requires timely and accurate research accounting.

Contracts offer less opportunity for intellectual input and are generally specifically prescribed protocols. Research infrastructures based primarily on contracts require careful attention to the prescribed protocols and timelines. It is specifically important to be able to track, and be responsive to, reporting deadlines, as contracts can be rendered null and void if these deadlines are missed. Likewise, performance on previous contracts (at least for US government contracts) is a significant consideration in the evaluation of any subsequent contract submissions.

Contracts also have more stringent requirements for changes in personnel, equipment, and scope of work. This can be constraining but can also be advantageous, as any requested change from the original scope of work should require an appropriately funded supplement or amendment to the original contract.

51.4 Personnel

51.4.1 *Research*

Case reports and retrospective reviews are most commonly performed by individuals or groups of investigators and require little in the way of research infrastructure, although IRB approval (usually expedited) will generally be required.

While some prospective research, such as case series, can still be accomplished by individuals or groups of investigators, more sophisticated prospective research, particularly clinical trials, almost always require research personnel in addition to the investigator(s).

Most clinical trials require an initial screening procedure, a decision about eligibility, enrollment, then monitoring and data collection during and following the intervention. The key personnel decision, in our experience, for such studies is: "How much education and technical knowledge is required to conduct the study(ies) with acceptable precision?" The crux of this issue generally involves whether to utilize nurses (generally registered nurses (RNs)) or research assistants (generally, licensed practical nurses (LPNs), medical assistants (MAs), or individuals without specific health sciences degrees). The difference in hourly salaries between these two groups are substantial and can result in substantial cost-savings (as long as recruitment numbers and data quality remain high).

In our experience, the two steps in a clinical trial that are most vulnerable to suboptimum outcomes are screening for randomization and outcomes data collection. The level of educational requirements for these, as well as any interventions and interval assessments, can – and should – be tailored to the individual protocol in order to utilize available research personnel with optimal cost-efficiency.

Health status screening of potential research participants frequently requires an extensive understanding of clinical medicine that might not be intuitive to individuals with little or no clinical training or experience. For example, if a woman was being screened for a drug trial for which liver disease was an exclusion criterion and she reported to a research screener that she had had "liver failure in my pregnancy" (that was actually severe preeclampsia that completely resolved), an individual unfamiliar with preeclampsia might exclude her, whereas a more educated and/or experienced individual would recognize that preeclampsia is a self-limiting pregnancy complication that generally resolves completely and that the woman in question could be eligible for study participation. Because incorrect determinations of protocol eligibility are so critically important in clinical trials, we have generally utilized RNs for screening. However, exceptions to this policy can, do, and should, occur. For example, if a protocol is limited to women with asymptomatic bacteriuria and large numbers of women are to be screened for a straightforward biologic outcome prior to actual study recruitment, it could be cost-effective to utilize individuals with less training and experience for the specific process of obtaining permission to obtain a clean-catch urine sample.

The informed consent process (discussed in more detail in Sect. 6 below) also requires extensive understanding of the biologic basis of the proposed study, its inclusion and exclusion criteria, and potential side effects. We generally utilize RNs or physicians at this critically important step as well.

Biologic sample collections in clinical research characteristically follow prescribed protocols and do not generally require the same clinical acumen necessary for enrollment and randomization. Although many clinical research programs utilize RNs for these activities as well, we have enjoyed success – and some appreciable savings – using research assistants (RAs).

Although beyond the scope of this chapter, the majority of research-oriented health facilities will have data analysis personnel available (generally biostatisticians, bioinformaticists, or other quantitative health scientists). In the event that such expertise is not available locally, it is becoming increasingly accessible online.

51.4.2 Administrative

51.4.2.1 Human Resources

The previous several decades have seen a seemingly inexorable increase in administrative requirements for clinical research. Research personnel at all levels are required to have annual certification in Health Information Portability and Accountability Act (HIPAA) and some sort of research conduct certification (for example, CITI = Collaborative Institutional Training Initiative). Many institutions also have their own additional research certification/recertification programs. For example, the University of Utah has a Research Administration Training Series, or RATS (http://www.education.research.utah.edu/). For any research organization to be effective, sufficient human resources (HRs) personnel must be available to track these issues for all new and ongoing personnel. For our research enterprise, we now employ a full-time Research Administrator who supervises all research personnel, both within the University and in the other health-care networks in which we screen, recruit, and follow research subjects.

The extension of clinical research programs across multiple health-care systems is becoming more common. The coordination of HR activities (job expectations, performance review, etc) across health-care systems is becoming more complex, in part because of the increasing concerns by health-care administrations about research employees of another health-care system conducting research activities in their system. More and more health-care systems will no longer allow this practice and in those that still permit the practice, the certification process is becoming increasingly complex and time-consuming. In addition, HIPAA-related concerns about involvement of research personnel from outside the "covered entity" further compounds these problems.

Our research network extends across several health-care systems and we have found it easier to hire research personnel through the respective health-care systems. Their salaries are paid by their respective health-care systems via subcontracts with the University of Utah. The HR issues for these employees are managed collaboratively by their institutional supervisors and by the University Research Administrator under terms specified by the subcontracts.

51.4.2.2 Accounting

It has always been important to track research expenditures. This process was relatively straightforward in the setting of single investigator research, particularly bench research where personnel requirements are less and research supplies can be credited to a single account.

The process becomes more complex with clinical trial networks that involve multiple concurrent protocols and multiple institutions. For example, at the time of this writing, our Department is participating in seven federally funded clinical trial networks conducting a total of 14 different protocols that are being conducted in 12 hospitals (not all protocols are being conducted at all hospitals!).

The tracking of expenditures (supplies and personnel effort) and income (base and capitated) requires considerable accounting expertise and resources, the precise amounts of which will obviously vary from one situation to the next.

At present, our research accounting efforts require two full-time positions, a Research Accounting Manager and Financial Analyst.

51.4.2.3 Research Coordination

In addition to HR and accounting expertise, one individual should be designated as a Research Coordinator. His or her responsibility will be to decide, in conjunction with the Principal Investigators, which research personnel will work on specific protocols and where each protocol will, or will not, be conducted. This person can be either a senior research nurse or a physician.

51.4.2.4 Institutional Review Board Specialist

If a research enterprise is conducting more than a few protocols in more than a couple of institutions, the Institutional Review Board (IRB) requirements for new protocol submissions, annual reviews, adverse event reporting, etc. can rapidly become overwhelming. In our infrastructure, we employ a full-time IRB Specialist who tracks each protocol for renewals, amendments, and adverse event reporting. This is a particularly challenging position when a given protocol is conducted in multiple hospitals (we have several protocols that are being conducted in all eight hospitals in Salt Lake County that have obstetrics and gynecology services).

51.4.2.5 Others

Multicenter clinical trials often require data entry specialists. Our research program employs approximately three FTEs for these efforts (two full-time individuals plus part-time efforts by several research project coordinators). While it requires some additional expenditure, we have found that our data quality can be optimized with routine double data entry.

51.5 Finances

51.5.1 Infrastructure Support

The financial support necessary to support a research infrastructure can come from a variety of sources, such as clinical income, returned indirects, industry research, in-sourcing, and fundraising.

Income from patient visits, procedures, and surgeries is the primary source of revenue for almost all clinical departments. It is often left to departmental leadership to determine how to best use clinical income to support central functions. One option is to assess a tax on physicians' clinical income to fund a research infrastructure, in whole or in part. Not all physicians are involved directly with the research being conducted in their departments and may not want a portion of their income to go to a resource that does not directly benefit them. Department leadership will need to determine if a tax on clinical income is an acceptable method of funding, based on the culture of the department and institution.

Options are available to avoid a perceived disconnect between a clinical funding source and research infrastructure expenses, including returned indirects and industry-sponsored research.

Funding awards include a budget for the work that is to be done (direct costs), as well as a budget to cover the institutional costs of supporting research (facilities and administrative costs). Facilities and Administrative costs (F&A) are often known as indirect costs and are costs that are incurred for common or joint objectives and, therefore, cannot be identified readily and specifically with a particular sponsored project, an instructional activity, or any other institutional activity. Depending on the institution, some of these indirect costs may be available to support research infrastructure. For example, at the University of Utah, a small percentage of the indirect costs collected are returned to the departments that administer the grants. These returned indirects are budgeted at the department's discretion for research-related costs such as investigator start-up costs, seed grants, and research administrative support.

Industry-sponsored projects, as opposed to those funded by federal and nonprofit sponsors, may offer a means to supplement a research infrastructure budget. These sponsors most often used a fixed price budget in which a flat fee is paid for each milestone reached or participant enrolled. If the work can be done for less money than the sponsor is paying, the difference can be used to support other research endeavors, including a research infrastructure. The opposite, however, is also true – if the project costs more to do than the sponsor is willing to pay, the investigator must make up the difference. For this reason, it is risky to rely solely on industry research for steady revenue. It has been noted that the only way to make a small fortune from clinical research is to start with a large fortune. With a well-designed budget and closely monitored expenses, the risk of running out of funds can be reduced. Remaining funds from well-managed industry-sponsored projects can be a good supplement to infrastructure funding.

As a research infrastructure is formed and proficiency is built, the expertise gained is often sought after by other departments and institutions. This provides the opportunity for in-sourcing. An established research team can offer it services to others for a negotiated fee. These services can include budget development, proposal preparation, compliance management, clinical research services, financial reporting, study close-out, or any combination of these and others. Such an arrangement allows departments without research resources to benefit from existing expertise and provides financial support for the infrastructure.

Fundraising is also a viable option for securing the funds necessary to support a research infrastructure. This can take several forms, from an annual donation campaign to naming opportunities – such as the ABC Center for Women's Health Research Administration or the XYZ Nephrology Research Network. Most universities have public relations and development offices that can offer professional services to publicize a department's research and to create a plan to solicit financial support.

51.5.2 Protocol Expenses

As mentioned previously, the tracking of expenditures (supplies and personnel effort) and income (base and capitated) requires considerable accounting expertise and resources, the precise amounts of which will obviously vary from one situation to the next. We have found it imperative to track expenses and income separately for each protocol and currently track the hours expended during each pay period by every research employee. While requiring considerable effort, it is necessary in order to be able to assess which protocols are being conducted in a cost-effective fashion and which are not. In addition, research funding sources expect – and deserve – a precise accounting of how and where their funding was utilized.

51.5.3 Subcontracts

Whenever research activities extend across multiple healthcare systems, subcontracts are necessary to ensure that collective expectations are met regarding personnel, finances, equipment/supplies, and access to potential participants. A potentially important consideration with federal funding is the limitation of indirect expenses on subcontracts. In particular, indirect costs are only allowable on the first $25,000 of a subcontract. Beyond that amount, the indirect costs must be either returned to the funding agency or else approved for local use by that funding agency. We have found it mutually advantageous to request of the federal funding agency permission to utilize these funds for either research equipment or for other research projects related to the originally funded protocols. In this age of tight federal funding, this mechanism is often appealing to federal funding agencies, as it ensures that they do not have unutilized funds at the end of their funding cycle.

This limitation on indirect funding for subcontracts is understandably not always seen favorably by the institution(s) to whom subcontracts are disbursed. We have made concerted efforts to support our subcontractors' efforts to achieve research funding of their own, including the utilization of our grant preparation expertise. These efforts, besides being successful in procuring research funding, are of substantial benefit for developing and expanding relationships based on trust and respect.

51.5.4 Participant Remuneration

Research subjects can, and should, be appropriately compensated for their time and travel when participating in research studies. In the past, this has sometimes been conducted in a haphazard fashion, with the distribution of cash, gift certificates, move tickets, etc. by research personnel. Such activities are not advisable. We require each participant to complete a W-2 form (income from research participation in excess of $600/year is taxable), including a social security number, and then submit a requisition through our University Research Accounting office. This mechanism provides a trackable record of payment and receipt (e.g., a cashed check).

51.6 IRB/Compliance

Research participants have the right to protection and dignity when enrolling in a research study. Investigators and institutions have the obligation to design and conduct studies in such a way that this right is not infringed upon. A successful and ethical research infrastructure develops a process that acknowledges three levels of accountability and compliance: Institutional Accountability, Investigator Accountability, and Institutional Review Board (IRB) Accountability (1). For the purposes of this chapter, Investigator Accountability is discussed in terms of its ability to facilitate research compliance with local and federal policies and regulations.

Institutions and departments are best served by having experienced staff that understand the importance of human research protection from an ethical and regulatory perspective in addition to understanding the rights of the investigator. Such staff should have the ethical and regulatory background in order to proactively advise investigators in submission and ongoing monitoring of projects. Individuals in this role also require a working knowledge of federal-level agency interactions (e.g., Office of Human Research Protections and Food and Drug Administration, etc.) in order to facilitate discussions with local IRBs and monitor situations where an audit by any of these agencies, study sponsors, etc. is conducted.

51.6.1 Basic Ethical Principles

In the United States, research on human participants is subject to basic ethical principles as outlined in 1979 by The Belmont Report (2). The Belmont Report proposes three basic ethical principles (Respect for Persons, Beneficence, and Justice) that are relevant not only to the actual conduct of a research study, but to the "corporate mentality" of the research infrastructure as well. A strong research infrastructure will recognize these principles and advise investigators from initial study design through project completion.

51.6.2 Research Regulations

In addition to the framework set by The Belmont Report, adherence to the federal human subjects protection regulation must be understood by both investigators and research administrators/support personnel. The regulations discussed here are not all-inclusive and may be amended in the future. There may also be additional requirements based on specialized fields. However, these are the currently most important for research using human participants whether it be basic medical records research through drugs and devices. Depending on the type of study undertaken, any or all of these may apply.

51.6.2.1 Common Rule and Subparts

Human research participant protection regulations are primarily codified at 45 CFR 46 (3). Subpart A is currently adopted by 15 Federal agencies. Subpart A, commonly referred to as the "Common Rule" delineates the specific regulations for the overall protection of human subjects research. These regulations also consist of three additional subparts (B–D): Subpart B – Pregnant Women, Human Fetuses, and Neonates; Subpart C – Prisoners; and Subpart D – Children (4). These latter subparts have been adopted by all federal agencies. These regulations apply to all federally funded research. However, institutions can choose (and are most likely) to apply these regulations to all research studies, regardless of funding source. It is important for research administration to understand local policies.

Table 51.2 Selected FDA regulatory compliance documents

General/administrative:
21 CFR 11: Electronic records; electronic signatures
21 CFR 50: Protection of human subjects
21 CFR 54: Financial disclosure by clinical investigators
21 CFR 56: Institutional review boards
ICH-E6: Good clinical practice (consolidated guidance for investigators)
FDA information sheets: guidance for institutional review boards and clinical investigators
FDA compliance program guidance manual, chapter 48 – bioresearch monitoring: clinical investigators
Drugs:
21 CFR 312: Investigational new drug application
21 CFR 314: Applications for FDA approval to market a new drug
Devices[a]:
21 CFR 803: Medical device reporting
21 CFR 812: Investigational device exemptions
21 CFR 814: Premarket approval of medical devices

[a]Additional regulations apply to manufacturing and importation

51.6.2.2 Food and Drug Administration

Clinical studies that investigate and support applications for research and marketing permits for all products are subject to Food and Drug Administration (FDA) regulations (e.g., foods, drugs, dietary supplements that claim nutrient or health qualities, infant formulas, food and color additives, drugs for human use, biological products for human use, and electronic projects) (5).The FDA has multiple regulations and guidance documents of which all research administrators should be aware in ensuring compliance (see Table 51.2) (6).

51.6.2.3 HIPAA Privacy and Research

This set of regulations applies to the protection of individually identifiable information and is codified as 45 CFR 164 (3).

51.6.2.4 Informed Consent

The consent process is just that a process. Much focus and attention is given to the actual document. However, investigators and research administrators are obligated to make this process dynamic between the research staff and the participant. Revisiting The Belmont Report's principle of Respect for Persons emphasizes the importance of individuals acting as autonomous agents. Therefore, relaying the necessary information to make an informed decision can be done in many ways. The consent document is the means by which this process has been documented (7).

The federal requirements of informed consent are outlined in 45 CFR 46.116. Generally speaking, however, the consent must contain enough information that explains to the participant that he/she is being asked to volunteer in a research study. The voluntary nature of this study must include assurance that no penalties will be assessed as a result of nonparticipation. At a minimum, the participant must be provided with enough information about the procedures (including any alternatives to the research), the risks and benefits of these procedures, contact information for questions and to report injury/ concerns. Under no circumstances can a document include exculpatory language wherein the participant waives (or appears to waive) his/her legal rights or limit the liability of the institution or its agents.

Although the regulations specifically address certain requirements, there may be additional elements required at an institutional level. It is important that these be addressed and understood by all research staff. It is important that the original signed document be kept with research files until the study is complete (e.g., no more procedures, data collection, or potential for audit) and the documentation is destroyed.

Not all research studies will include direct access to participants and a signed consent document is not practicable (e.g., medical records review). The regulations allow for a waiver of informed consent in these instances. The investigator needs to demonstrate that the research involves no more than minimal risk to the participants; the waiver will not adversely affect the rights and welfare of participants; the research could not be practicably carried out without the waiver; and the participants will be provided with additional pertinent information (if appropriate) (4).

Since institutions vary with regard to their requirements, investigators and research administrators are cautioned to review local policies to ensure strictest compliance.

51.6.2.5 Review Process

Institutions will have a broad range of how the review process is conducted. The investigator and research administration should review local policies to ensure that they are met. The federal regulations have basic requirements regarding how each review is conducted. These are discussed in this section.

Initial Review

The initial review will likely be the most intensive process over the course of a project. A working knowledge of local policies and federal regulations should enable an investigator and research team to have a more positive experience. Research administration should be involved early in this process to allow for a more streamlined submission. The compliance coordinator within research administration should also be in contact with the grants/contracts manager to ensure that there will be an organized approach to begin the study. It is incredibly frustrating and much time is lost for all involved if these considerations are not made before IRB approval is obtained.

Continuing Review

Federal regulations require that research be reviewed no less than once a year. Review may be required by the IRB at greater intervals throughout the year based on the degree of risk in the study (8, 9). This must be closely monitored by the investigator and/or research administration since research must not proceed unless it has been approved by the IRB. Typically, researchers rely on the IRB for notices that the study will expire. However, the investigator is ultimately responsible for monitoring this date and submitting the continuing review documents per local policy.

51.7 Conclusions

The design, conduct, and supervision of clinical research trials in the early twenty-first century American medical setting are increasingly complex processes. With increasing awareness that clinical trial outcomes must focus on clinically significant, rather than surrogate, outcomes, the need for larger multi-site extramurally funded studies is becoming more apparent. The administration of such studies requires careful attention to research personnel administration, careful and thorough financial accounting and appropriate timely approval mechanisms. Institutions committed to long-term sustainable research programs will need to develop research infrastructures capable of proactive administration. This chapter provides guidelines for infrastructure development as well as specific examples from the authors' institution.

References

1. Bankert E, Amdur R (2006) Institutional review board management and function, 2nd edn. Jones and Bartlett, Sudbury, MD
2. http://ohsr.od.nih.gov/guidelines/belmont.html (1979)
3. US Department of Health and Human Services (2008) Office for Human Research Protections, Code of Regulations http://www.hhs.gov/ohrp.htm
4. 45CFR26.116(d). Accessed at http://www.hhs.gov/ohrp.htm
5. FDA (2008) 21CFR56.101(a). Accessed at http://www.fda.gov
6. FDA (2008) Accessed at http://www.fda.gov
7. 45CFR46.117. Accessed at http://www.hhs.gov/ohrp.htm
8. 21CFR56.109(f) (2008) Accessed at http://www.fda.gov
9. 45CFR46.110(e). Accessed at http://www.hhs.gov/ohrp.htm

Chapter 52
Integrating Research into a Clinical Practice

Douglas T. Carrell

Abstract While exposure to research techniques is a standard component of the training of most physicians and laboratory directors, the progressive migration of reproductive medicine clinics away from academic institutions and into private practice has decreased the exposure and involvement of many clinicians and laboratory technicians away from clinical or basic science research studies. This chapter explores the benefits of implementing research into reproductive endocrinology clinics and laboratories. Benefits may include the development of a broader clinical knowledge base, enhanced reasoning skills, and improved career satisfaction. The inclusion of research in a clinical practice can proceed in a prudent and measured manner consistent with the aims and assets of the practice. Simple initial tools include journal clubs and focused study, and the use of an invaluable tool, the quality assurance program. Clinicians can establish collaborative relationships with basic scientists by providing careful characterization, documentation, and organization of records for patients (phenotyping) and by providing relevant clinical insights. The benefits of participation in research studies are available to all clinical practices by the careful assessment of resources and sustained commitment to the endeavor.

Keywords Research • Quality assurance • Collaboration • Journal club • Phenotyping • Collaboration

52.1 Introduction

Most clinicians have participated in research at some point during their education and training. For many, their experience in research involved retrospective chart reviews to evaluate a clinical practice outcome. For others, the research may have involved a randomized evaluation of a novel drug therapy, or perhaps even a basic science study characterizing a specific pathological cell type. Regardless of the type of research performed, the researcher was introduced to basic practices of research, such as a thorough literature review, careful design, critical observation and data analysis, and integration of data into a cogent theory for further testing [1].

Most agree that research is important, and that the principles learned doing research are of benefit in clinical practice. Historically, reproductive endocrinology and infertility is a subspecialty in which most clinicians were actively involved in research, especially during doctoral or specialty training. However, in recent years, the treatment of infertile couples has tended to move away from large academic research institutions and into private practices, therefore, many within our industry have lost impetus and resources necessary for research [2–4]. Nevertheless, the potential benefits of being a clinician researcher exist independent of the practice structure [5–7]. This chapter will comment briefly on the reasons for integrating research into a clinical practice and focus on a few key ideas and methods for undertaking the integration of research into a busy clinical practice.

52.2 Benefits of Integrating Research into a Clinical Practice

In order for research to succeed in a clinical practice, it must be a priority. Several negative criteria can preclude making research a priority but can usually be narrowed down to two major factors, cost and time. The financial and time expenses, along with the potential emotional expense involved in performing research, are real and should not be ignored [5, 8]. However, the benefits of research are also real and may outweigh the negative factors. Therefore, a careful consideration of the benefits of research to an individual and practice is important. Some of the common benefits of active participation in research are listed in the following section. Individual clinics will undoubtedly have unique benefits in addition to those listed.

D.T. Carrell (✉)
Departments of Surgery (Urology), Obstetrics and Gynecology, and Physiology, University of Utah School of Medicine, Salt Lake City, UT, USA
e-mail: douglas.carrell@hsc.utah.edu

D.T. Carrell and C.M. Peterson (eds.), *Reproductive Endocrinology and Infertility: Integrating Modern Clinical and Laboratory Practice*,
DOI 10.1007/978-1-4419-1436-1_52, © Springer Science+Business Media, LLC 2010

52.2.1 An Improved Knowledge Base and Critical Thinking Skills

Perhaps, the greatest benefit of integrating research into a clinical practice is to improve your knowledge base and critical reasoning skills by evaluating evidence from the literature and from your own studies. This process, termed evidence-based practice, has been shown to improve clinical decision making ability [9, 10]. Evidence-based clinical practice has been emphasized as an essential means of improving patient care, and consists of obtaining and critically evaluating the evidence presented by other clinicians and researchers and integrating it with your clinical expertise and your patients' preferences in order to provide the most effective form of clinical practice [11]. Although many studies have consistently demonstrated improved patient outcomes when evidence-based medicine is practiced, a relatively small percentage of clinical practices have integrated evidence-based techniques [12]. One reason is the lack of experience and skill in acquiring and critically evaluating evidence.

Research, at its core, is the development of critical reasoning. From an initial observation to review of the relevant literature, critical analysis and reasoning are necessary. The formulation of a hypothesis and the design of a relevant study require logic and insight. Careful analysis of data and interpretation of the data to obtain correct conclusions are the heart of critical thinking and evidence-based medicine. Therefore, while participation in research is not essential to acquiring critical reasoning skills, it facilitates the process. It is likely that the development and continued nurturing of critical thinking skills among the staff of any practice is improved through participation in research projects, and may be useful in avoiding and identifying errors and developing better techniques and policies [13].

52.2.2 Improved Job Satisfaction

Most clinicians choose to become clinicians because of the rewards of assisting patients and enjoy providing patient care, but variety in daily routine is almost always beneficial to improving attitude. Research not only provides variety, but also helps illuminate daily routines from new angles. The spark of insight gleamed from a recent study, or the idea for a new study, can change a routine clinical consultation from mundane to exciting. Additionally, pride in the knowledge that you have contributed to better care of patients both within your practice and outside is a positive and rewarding experience.

52.2.3 Service to Patients and Community

Although several selfish reasons exist to do research, altruistic reasons also exist. Perhaps, the strongest altruistic reason to commit resources to research is the belief that we as clinicians have a debt to our patients to not only distill therapy, but to also improve therapies. Inherent in that belief is an understanding that we all have individual skills and assets to contribute. While the drive for profit or the constraints of resources may dim such an altruistic desire, altruistic motives should be encouraged and nurtured. Research to benefit the community has been considered an essential part of medical practice and should be an aim of all clinicians [5, 14, 15].

52.3 Tools to Implement Research into a Clinical Practice

52.3.1 Review the Literature

For most researchers, the study of relevant scientific or medical literature is the key stimulus in the development of questions that lead to research studies. Research is always built on the foundations set by prior studies, and nearly every study sets the stage for further studies. Most research reports specifically discuss further study options and questions, but reading and thinking should also stimulate novel questions and insights based on your personal experience and interests.

Relevant literature not only includes journals specific to your field, but should also include periodic review of broad based journals such as *Nature*, *Science*, or the *New England Journal of Medicine*, which may stimulate ideas for translating cutting edge techniques into your specific field. Several online resources are available to help in focusing study efforts, such as Pubmed, Scopus, Biowizard, and others [16, 17]. These services allow customized searches and immediate access to abstracts, and in some cases, full research reports. Additionally, some services perform regular searches of keywords and electronically send relevant reports to your email.

52.3.2 Discuss Ideas with Colleagues

Regular discussion of ideas and questions with a colleague is invaluable in broadening your scope and perspective regarding ideas and can stimulate practical ideas for study. Indeed, many agree that often more is learned at society meetings during casual hallway or dinner conversation than during formal sessions of the meeting.

One recent aid in stimulating conversation is online discussion forums, such as "Embryomail" and "Andrology". These online forums are available to share ideas, questions, and protocols and may help pinpoint areas of critical need in which you may have an interest and/or ability to contribute to the knowledge. Additionally, vendors of laboratory supplies, instruments, and medicines can be a resource for practical information and often distribute useful literature that may be of benefit in educating staff in both the specific topic and in the general skill of critical reading and interpretation of data. Vendor literature may describe a new tool that has not previously been applied to your field, but could yield immediate useful information.

52.3.3 Involve Staff in a Journal Club

Journal clubs vary in format and intensity, but can be beneficial to all clinicians [18]. Historically, journal clubs were generally established to review literature and keep clinicians abreast of advances reported in the one or two journals relevant a particular field. However, the explosion of studies reported in dozens of journals relevant to reproductive medicine makes the goal of keeping up with all literature nearly impossible. Therefore, some journal clubs have evolved into a tool for evaluating specific topics, rather than journals. Topic-based study may lead to study of topics for improved patient care, questions to explore through the clinic's quality assurance program, or areas of transitional research in which the clinic may design relevant clinical studies.

Journal clubs are invaluable in educating staff on the differences in well designed research and poorly designed studies, defects in interpreting data, the importance of validating studies, and in short, the importance of critical thinking skills. Indeed, one of the first lessons learned in journal clubs is that "not all studies are created equally." This lesson not only teaches the importance of critically evaluating studies, but may inspire the implementation of the same principles into daily responsibilities.

Implementation of a few key principles can improve the quality of any journal club [19]. Successful journal clubs are built on the foundation of an atmosphere of open dialogue, without belittling or criticism of questions and comments. Diversity in the make-up of the journal club is important in stimulating creativity and broad views, therefore, it may be of benefit to include nurses and laboratory technician in a common journal club, a tool which may also stimulate team unity. Consistency is paramount, and providing incentives, like food, may initially help in prioritization of the meeting in the mind of staff. The main objective of a journal club should be to stimulate questions, such as "Why do we it this way?" and "would this technique be a better way of doing it?" These are the foundations of clinical research.

52.3.4 Evaluate Your Situation and Utilize Your Assets

Just as it would be imprudent for a sedentary person to attempt to run a marathon without prior training, it is important that the researcher carefully evaluates available assets and priorities and plans research contributions with prudence. Assessment of assets includes personnel skills and work loads, available physical facilities, monetary issues, and the availability of reference and support agencies, such as biostatistical support, institutional review boards, and core laboratories that can assist [20].

It is important to realize that the most valuable research resource that most clinicians possess is a study population. Clinicians generally have populations of highly phenotyped patients that are key to basic and translational research studies. Therefore, a common and prudent approach is to begin the research process by enhancing the phenotyping (clinical characterization) documentation of patients and implementing an effective means to retrieve patients with desired phenotypes for future studies. Such improved documentation and data management procedures usually have direct clinic benefits in addition to facilitating research. In the laboratory, similar efforts may include coding of surplus tissue and banking the tissue for future studies. Tissue banking requires patient consent and Institutional Review Board (IRB) oversight (see Chap. 53), but is invaluable to future studies.

52.3.5 Delegate

Most clinicians are extremely busy and unable to devote large amounts of time to research. Effective delegation can maximize time usage from all staff to accomplish otherwise impossible projects. Additionally, delegation to staff can improve job satisfaction by increasing variety and team unity. However, delegation requires organization and accountability to be effective.

One technique our clinic has employed is to delegate responsibilities not only for certain research projects, but also for attendance of certain meeting presentations, ongoing literature reviews, journal clubs, databases, etc. An especially motivating tool is to send a clinical employee to a symposium or training course to learn a technique for which that person will be the "resident expert."

52.3.6 Use Your Quality Assurance Program

Current regulations require that laboratories and clinical practices implement quality assurance programs [21]. A quality assurance program is essentially a method to ask relevant questions about the efficacy of practice, measurement of outcomes, and evaluation of the data to revise and improve clinical care. It is readily apparent that the quality assurance process mirrors research methodology. More importantly, the quality assurance program lends itself as a tool for initiating clinical research studies [22]. For example, if routine monitoring of embryo transfer results demonstrates a consistent difference between the outcomes of two physicians, differences in techniques can be determined and studied. Such internal quality assurance may evolve into a useful clinical study of significant benefit.

52.3.7 Build on Small Successes

Nothing is more discouraging than failure, and success drives further success. Those two maxims should always be remembered while establishing a research program. When you have identified your assets, it is best to begin with simple, achievable projects. Then, minor successes should be lauded and built upon. Waiting to celebrate or extol an effort until a "major" paper is published may discourage personnel and impede the progress of the project.

52.3.8 Collaborate

Successful research programs are founded on the premise of collaboration. While important studies can be accomplished within a small clinical lab, refusal to collaborate limits the scope and quality of most studies. This is due to the fact that as a clinical researcher identifies a topic of interest and assesses their assets, the determination may be made that the clinic lacks the tools, patient volume and/or laboratory skills, to study the question at a high level of quality. Additionally, collaborative relationships may foster mentoring of the less experienced researcher [23]. The step to collaboration may require a higher level of commitment, and sometimes a leap of faith, but it is usually rewarded with a better outcome.

Two specific suggestions may be beneficial in facilitating collaboration. First, evaluate the research interests of faculty at local universities to identify possible areas of overlap. This can usually be done using online resources from the university, but can also be taken further by visiting with a faculty member or attending seminars to acquaint yourself with others. If local resources are not available, expand to national or international resources. These resources are usually available at society meetings or can be identified through online searches. As mentioned earlier, it is important to realize that as a clinician you are valuable to a basic scientist because you can provide patients/tissues that are properly phenotyped and/or valuable clinical insights.

A second suggestion is to consider increasing the power of your study by joining multi-center studies. Multi-center studies are often necessary to obtain statistical power, and are generally better trusted than small studies from one site. While national collaborative groups are available, such as the Reproductive Medicine Network or the Tyho Galilleo Research Group, most collaborations are formed during informal discussions. Such collaborations are generally rewarding in both the quality of research, and the relationships established.

52.3.9 Establish a Research-Oriented Team

Nothing will facilitate clinical research as much as instilling within the staff the importance of research, and maximizing their desire to participate. Within our clinical Andrology and IVF laboratories, we specifically attempt to instill a "spirit of research" by insisting that each employee be involved in at least one research study, including medical assistants and clerical staff. Each employee has skills of meaningful help to a study, and participation is expected. Several techniques can help, including, as discussed earlier, the consistent holding of journal clubs and attendance of national and regional meetings. However, the most beneficial tolls, in my opinion, are the establishment of the expectation of research participation and the rewarding of successes. Rewarding of successes usually involves acknowledgement of progress, and ultimately of publication, verbally in private or at group meetings, but may include celebratory lunches or other creative awards recognizing their efforts.

It is usually helpful to consider the potential research abilities and emphasize the expectation of research participation before hiring staff applicants. Discussing research during the interview process not only aids in selecting employees with useful skills, but also sets a tone of the importance of research prior to hiring. It may be helpful to specifically consider individuals with prior experience, such as clinical research coordinators or graduate level students. Personnel with experience in the process of working with IRB committees and data management may be of particular assistance.

52.3.10 Consistently Monitor Progress

Accountability is critical in any group project, and careful monitoring of research progress should be consistently performed. Group research reports are critical, either in a dedicated research meeting or as part of a general staff meeting. Additionally, a list of ongoing studies and responsible personnel should be placed in suitable work areas for constant reinforcement. Lastly, individual reminders and discussions are necessary to reinforce the importance of the project and resolve hurdles. The essential principle is that continued monitoring aids in adding emphasis of importance, in addition to helping with general logistical factors.

52.3.10.1 Make it Fun

The adage that everything is easier if you make it fun is certainly true for research. Making research fun requires creativity and customization. One method our laboratory has employed is to implement debates on controversial subjects. Such debates develop reasoning skills and familiarity with the available literature, but sometimes cross into the realm of entertainment as the debaters imitate internationally known proponents of a given position. Another idea we have implemented is to encourage the historical perspectives and human aspects of a given study and the researchers involved. Humanizing science can not only make it more interesting, but also help in understanding the reasons for some current situations. Lastly, for large, group-related aspects of research, such as the goal of recruiting a given number of participants to a study, it is suitable to plan a celebration for the achievement of the goal. Celebrations of publications and grants are common, but in establishing a research program in a nontraditional setting, such as a clinic, celebrating smaller accomplishments may be helpful in building inertia.

52.4 Conclusions

Developing a research program within a clinical setting is difficult and requires consistent emphasis. However, the benefits can be useful in improving staff morale and raising the quality of clinical performance. Creativity and consistency in implementing the principles discussed earlier can assist any clinic in developing a research program.

References

1. Kenton K, Brubaker L (2007) Research education in obstetrics and gynecology: how are we doing? Am J Obstet Gynecol 197(5): 532 e1–4
2. Sauer MV (2005) Surviving the shifting focus from basic research to clinical activities in reproductive endocrinology and infertility. Fertil Steril 84(3):573–575 discussion 83
3. Soules MR (2005) Assisted reproductive technology has been detrimental to academic reproductive endocrinology and infertility. Fertil Steril 84(3):570–572
4. Ebbert JO, Montori VM, Schultz HJ (2001) The journal club in postgraduate medical education: a systematic review. Med Teach 23(5):455–461
5. Macaulay AC (2007) Promoting participatory research by family physicians. Ann Fam Med 5(6):557–560
6. Marquez IC, Andrews C, Matthews DC, Clovis JB (2007) From clinician to researcher – a first-hand account. J Can Dent Assoc 73(3):247–251
7. Bailey CJ (2007) Practitioner to researcher: reflections on the journey. Nurse Res 14(4):18–26
8. Avins AL, Goldberg H (2007) Creating a culture of research. Contemp Clin Trials 28(4):557–562
9. Ernst E (2008) Science, clinical practice, and a synthesis of both. Am J Med 121(1):2
10. Clancy CM (2008) Clinical research training: scientific literacy for the twenty-first century. J Gen Intern Med 23(2):219–220
11. Oman KS, Duran C, Fink R (2008) Evidence-based policy and procedures: an algorithm for success. J Nurs Adm 38(1): 47–51
12. Coomarasamy A, Khan KS (2004) What is the evidence that postgraduate teaching in evidence based medicine changes anything? A systematic review. BMJ 329(7473):1017
13. Fritsche L, Greenhalgh T, Falck-Ytter Y, Neumayer HH, Kunz R (2002) Do short courses in evidence based medicine improve knowledge and skills? Validation of Berlin questionnaire and before and after study of courses in evidence based medicine. BMJ 325(7376):1338–1341
14. Harris J (2005) Scientific research is a moral duty. J Med Ethics 31(4):242–248
15. Brassington I (2007) John Harris' argument for a duty to research. Bioethics 21(3):160–168
16. Krupski TL, Dahm P, Fesperman SF, Schardt CM (2008) How to perform a literature search. J Urol 179(4):1264–1270
17. Vincent B, Vincent M, Ferreira CG (2006) Making PubMed searching simple: learning to retrieve medical literature through interactive problem solving. Oncologist 11(3):243–251
18. Linzer M, Brown JT, Frazier LM, DeLong ER, Siegel WC (1988) Impact of a medical journal club on house-staff reading habits, knowledge, and critical appraisal skills. A randomized control trial. JAMA 260(17):2537–2541
19. Swift G (2004) How to make journal clubs interesting. Adv Psychiatr Treat 10:67–72
20. Keenan AM, Redmond AC (2002) Integrating research into the clinic. What evidence based practice means to the practising podiatrist. J Am Podiatr Med Assoc 92(2):115–122
21. Hamlin WB (1999) Requirements for accreditation by the College of American Pathologists Laboratory Accreditation Program. Arch Pathol Lab Med 123(6):465–467
22. Doezema D, Hauswald M (2002) Quality improvement or research: a distinction without a difference? IRB 24(4):9–12
23. Blixen CE, Papp KK, Hull AL, Rudick RA, Bramstedt KA (2007) Developing a mentorship program for clinical researchers. J Contin Educ Health Prof 27(2):86–93

Chapter 53
Research Regulations: The Role of the Institutional Review Board

Benjamin R. Emery and Mark A. Munger

Abstract The successful assisted reproductive therapy (ART) clinic may wish to support the altruistic nature of medicine with the endeavor of advancing emerging technologies and patient care through clinically related research. Clinical research is quite common in academic medicine, but can also be of great benefit to private practitioners. Indeed, the private practice has a unique environment and viewpoint that may not be present in academic medicine. Additionally, human reproductive tissues that are unsuitable for ART use or no longer desired by the patient are often used for training personnel in the IVF laboratory or even for diagnostic testing. Therefore, it is likely that all ART clinics are affected by regulations regarding the oversight of human research and/or tissue storage. This chapter will give insight into establishing a reasonable method of procurement, storage, and tracking of such tissues. Because an ethics committee must oversee all research involving human subjects, a role most often filled by a local institutional review board (IRB), we will discuss how to work with and submit research proposals to the IRB. The maintenance and coding of stored tissues is also discussed, as it is also mandated under the Code of Federal Regulations.

Keywords Research regulation • Informed consent • Institutional review board • Tissue banking

53.1 Background

53.1.1 The Ethics Committee for Medical Research

53.1.1.1 Establishment of Federal Regulations

There are three main federal regulations covering biomedical research that relate to patient consent and ethical treatment of individuals within that setting. The Federal Food, Drug, and Cosmetic Act of 1938 (Public Law 75-717) covers the use of medical devises and therapeutic goods. The "Common Rule," of 1991 (U.S. Code of Federal Regulations 45CFR Part 46) provides for Institutional Review Boards (IRBs) and gives direction on what can take place as medical research. Lastly, the Health Insurance Portability and Accountability Act (HIPAA) of 1996 (Public Law 104-191, 45CFR Parts 160 and 164) addresses confidentiality of personal information in health care, including research.

These regulations provide a structure under which the tradeoff between good medical practice, the well-being of the patient, and continued medical advancement is weighed. The weight of this debate still falls on the shoulders of the ethics committee reviewing the procedures and ultimately the clinician treating the patient and contributing to the research. For this reason, this chapter will give details on how to work within the governmental regulations and support the advancement of science.

53.1.1.2 Definition/Description of an Ethics Committee (The IRB)

The U.S. Office of Human Research Protections (OHRP) is the federal oversight body for assurance of compliance to the Code of Federal Regulations (CFR) 45, part 46, which stipulates the review of all research conducted involving human subjects. This mandate is achieved, in part, by local medical/ethical review boards, which are referred to as institutional review boards (IRBs) by the OHRP. The IRB has become a common term at most universities and medical centers around the U.S. The functioning review board does not have to carry this title, but must maintain the required standards described in the CFR. The OHRP has a very useful website (http://www.hhs.gov/ohrp/) with FAQ pages and copies of the relevant CFRs.

The review board is structured to contain at least five members with a diverse outlook on biomedical research. The review board, whenever possible, should contain members of both sexes. The members are to be chosen based on their

B.R. Emery(✉)
Department of Urology, Andrology & IVF Laboratories, University of Utah School of Medicine, 675 S. Arapeen Dr., Ste 205, Salt Lake City, UT 84108, USA

M.A. Munger
Department of Pharmacology, University of Utah College of Pharmacy, Salt Lake City, UT, USA

D.T. Carrell and C.M. Peterson (eds.), *Reproductive Endocrinology and Infertility: Integrating Modern Clinical and Laboratory Practice*,
DOI 10.1007/978-1-4419-1436-1_53,

ability to address issues of diversity (including race, gender, and cultural background), their sensitivity to community attitudes, expertise, and experience in dealing with issues of local and national law and resources of the institution conducting the research.

The CFR also requires that the board be well balanced in its membership. All members cannot be from the same type of occupation. One member should be from the community at large without any relationship to the affiliated institution. One member should be a scientist and one member is needed who is not involved with biomedical research or scientific research in general. The review board is allowed to have pre-approved alternates to fill vacancies, invite competent professionals for expert opinion on protocols (these gests are not allowed to vote on the presented protocols), or invite the principal investigator to inform the review board in more detail. If any member of the board has a conflicting interest in the research, an approved alternate must replace them for review of the given protocol. Any one member may fill more than one of the diversity requirements, but the board must still consist of five members.

The charge of the review board is outlined in CFR 45 part 46.111 (Table 53.1). These guidelines help to ensure that the research being performed is first and foremost, safe for the participants and equitable to the local community. Additionally, guidelines require that the potential participant be well informed of the purpose, risks, benefits, and impact of the research on them, and the benefits gained by society as a whole.

Table 53.1 Charge of the Institutional Review Board (adapted from 45CFR46.111)

1. Risks to subjects are minimized: (a) By using procedures which are consistent with sound research design and which do not unnecessarily expose subjects to risk, and (b) whenever appropriate, by using procedures already being performed on the subjects for diagnostic or treatment purposes.
2. Risks to subjects are reasonable in relation to anticipated benefits, if any, to subjects, and the importance of the knowledge that may reasonably be expected to result. In evaluating risks and benefits, the IRB should consider only those risks and benefits that may result from the research (as distinguished from risks and benefits of therapies subjects would receive even if not participating in the research). The IRB should not consider possible long-range effects of applying knowledge gained in the research (for example, the possible effects of the research on public policy) as among those research risks that fall within the purview of its responsibility.
3. Selection of subjects is equitable. In making this assessment, the IRB should take into account the purposes of the research and the setting in which the research will be conducted and should be particularly cognizant of the special problems of research involving vulnerable populations, such as children, prisoners, pregnant women, mentally disabled persons, or economically or educationally disadvantaged persons.
4. Informed consent will be sought from each prospective subject or the subject's legally authorized representative, in accordance with, and to the extent required by CFR 46.116.
5. Informed consent will be appropriately documented, in accordance with, and to the extent required by CFR 46.117.
6. When appropriate, the research plan makes adequate provision for monitoring the data collected to ensure the safety of subjects.
7. When appropriate, there are adequate provisions to protect the privacy of subjects and to maintain the confidentiality of data.

53.2 Finding and Choosing an Institutional Review Board

Any academic institution that receives funds from the National Institutes of Health is required to operate an IRB for approval of medical research as mandated by CFR 45. Therefore, clinicians who are operating under the umbrella of a major university have an IRB functioning in-house. For those in private practice, or even adjunct to a university, finding a private not-for-profit review board may be a more feasible option. There are several national agencies operating in major metropolitan areas that are available.

A word of caution is warranted. Finding a reputable review board agency is paramount. The collapse or unprofessional behavior of a contracted oversight body will cause endless problems with not only re-establishing your protocols and patient consents, but is likely to effect the confidence of your patients and referral base. For this reason, it is suggested that investigators use an IRB from the registered list at the United States Department of Human Services, Office for Human Research Protections (OHRP). The OHRP maintains a searchable database at http://ohrp.cit.nih.gov/search/asearch.asp.

53.3 The Application Process

53.3.1 What to Expect in Submission

Upon locating and registering with an IRB, one must then start the application process. The typical review board will have a standardized format for submission. The submission forms will include detailed instructions for completing the paperwork and guidelines for determining the type of consent that should be proposed for the study procedure. The forms will ask for disclosure and description of:

1. The type of study (clinical drugs, medical devices, basic science studies, genetic analysis)
2. The type of participant (minors, women, minorities, mentally disabled, prisoners, at risk groups, age range, etc.)
3. Will exclusion/inclusion criteria be used (height/weight/diagnosis)

4. How many patients will be approached
5. What is the maximum and minimum number of enrollees
6. What is the scientific justification for the number of participants
7. How will the data be analyzed
8. Who will have access to the data and how will access be restricted
9. Who is responsible for maintaining the records of consent and participation and tissue procurement
10. What are the qualifications of those involved in the research protocols
11. What type of protocols will be used for sample procurement (patient interventions)
12. What type of protocols will be used for analysis
13. Where will the study and patient intervention occur
14. Who will inform the patients (potential enrollees or study participants) of the proposed research
15. Who will consent them for participation and do the investigators have any conflict of interest with the study protocol or outcome of the study itself
16. What is the clinical relevance of the study
17. A description of how the benefit of the study (either directly to the patient or to society) outweighs the risk to the patient (relative risk assessment)
18. How is the project funded (internal funding or extramural resources) and
19. Is there a financial burden or reimbursement for the study participant?

In addition to the line item description, the review committee will require a protocol summary. The summary will include a background, study objectives, study design and procedure. These items are in the format of a typical grant submission, but the details included maybe less than what is required for a typical grant.

To determine how much information is needed, one must try to put themselves in place of the review board members. The key is to be able to readily see the risk to benefit ratio, or relative risk, and discern what the expected outcomes are and how they benefit both the patient and society as a whole must be clear in the proposed document. In some cases, the intervention may be minor, and it is easy to see the patient benefit. Other research, especially when gametes and embryos are used (due to the politically and morally charged nature of research involving gametes, embryos, and embryonic stem cells), may be less obvious and need more background or justification to grasp the relative risk of the research. It is important to remember that many of those serving on the review board are not scientists, and it is unlikely someone on the board is familiar with the kind of work being proposed. The easier the protocol is to read and the less background work the reviewer has to do independently, the quicker the turnaround on the review will be. Saving time and resources is always of paramount concern. Most review boards will have a posted schedule. Timing your submission and returning your revisions in a timely fashion will also reduce downtime. Lastly, the submission will include a draft of the consent document. The specifics of this document are not addressed here, but are discussed in detail below.

After the initial submission to the review committee and review by either the full committee or expedited review, the protocols, and consents will be returned with revisions requested to clarify the study procedures, refinement of the consent documentation and procedures and possibly additional justification for conducting the study.

53.3.2 Informed Consent

53.3.2.1 Overview

The first issue of informed consent is to determine when consent is needed. The answer is always [1–3]. Unfortunately, obtaining consent is not always possible. One case in point, following good quality control and quality assurance practices may yield an interesting perspective and be worthy of dissemination to the medical community. Such retrospective chart reviews and data analysis protocols should be proposed to the IRB for review, but may pose little to no risk to the patient, therefore not requiring written consent. It is imperative to remember that this judgment of exemption should not be made by the investigational team, but proposed to the IRB for an impartial evaluation.

The exemption from consent is regulated under the FDA set forth in 45CFR 46.116(d); An IRB may approve a consent procedure which does not include, or which alters, some or all of the elements of informed consent set forth in this section, or waive the requirements to obtain informed consent provided the IRB finds and documents that:

1. The research involves no more than minimal risk to the subjects
2. The waiver or alteration will not adversely affect the rights and welfare of the subjects
3. The research could not practicably be carried out without the waiver or alteration; and
4. Whenever appropriate, the subjects will be provided with additional pertinent information after participation.

It is important for researchers in assisted reproductive technology (ART) to remember that any type of research using human gametes, embryos, or embryonic stem cells is held to a higher standard due to the moral stigma tied to reproductive tissues and embryos [4–6]. Additionally, the use of embryos or gametes retrieved from oocyte and sperm donors should be consented for use by both the intended parent and the donor [7]. Education of the patients and the community at large will likely increase the acceptance of such research protocols, allowing the important work of understanding early gametogenesis, the developmental processes, and realization of embryonic stem cell potential.

53.3.2.2 Consent Document

The content of the consent document is required to contain several key components, as directed by the Code of Federal Regulations, 45CFR.46.116 (Table 53.2). In addition to these items, the review board will look for readability of the document. The investigator should also be aware that the review board may also have exact phrases that must be present in the consent document for their approval, check with the IRB that is reviewing to find out more about such statements. In most cases, the content should be readable and understandable by a person with an eighth-grade education. In drafting the document, one may wish to use the Fry's Readability Scale to determine how complex the text is, many online tools are available through the use of an online internet browser [8]. The resource will indicate the grade level of the text. Unfortunately, using the readability scale only factors such as the length of the words and sentences can be considered. Using the readability scale will not:

1. Indicate how complex the ideas are
2. Whether or not the content is in a logical order
3. Whether the vocabulary is appropriate for the audience
4. Whether there is a gender, class or cultural bias
5. Whether the design is attractive and helps or hinders the reader, or
6. Whether the material appears in a form and type that is easy or hard to read.

Consideration of these six points and the Fry's Readability Scale allows the document to be better understood by all those who are to be consented. By no means will the consent document stand alone without discussion of the consent by the informing or consenting member of the medical team. The patient must be able to ask questions and have any portion of the document clarified by the presenter.

Lastly, the document must contain space for signature of the patient(s) consenting to the protocols contained therein, the consenting individual, and when the consenting individual is to be blinded from the enrollment, a witness to the patient's signature.

Table 53.2 Information to be included in the informed consent document (adapted from 45CFR.46.116)

1. A statement that the study involves research.
2. An explanation of the purpose of the research, an invitation to participate and explanation of why the participant was selected, and the expected duration of the participant's participation.
3. A description of procedures to be followed and identification of which procedures are investigational and which might be provided as standard care to the participant in another setting. Use of research methods such as randomization and placebo controls should be explained.
4. A description of any foreseeable risks or discomforts to the participant, an estimate of their likelihood, and a description of what steps will be taken to prevent or minimize them; as well as acknowledgment of potentially unforeseeable risks.
5. A description of any benefits to the participant or to others that may reasonably be expected from the research, and an estimate of their likelihood.
6. A disclosure of any appropriate alternative procedures or courses of treatment that might be advantageous to the participant.
7. A statement describing to what extent records will be kept confidential, including examples of who may have access to research records such as hospital personnel, the FDA, and drug sponsors.
8. For research involving more than minimal risk, an explanation and description of any compensation and any medical treatments that are available if participants are injured through participation; where further information can be obtained, and whom to contact in the event of research-related injury.
9. An explanation of whom to contact for answers to questions about the research and the research participant's rights (including the name and phone number of the Principal Investigator (PI)).
10. A statement that research is voluntary and that refusal to participate or a decision to withdraw at any time will involve no penalty or loss of benefits to which the participant is otherwise entitled.
11. A statement indicating that the participant is making a decision whether or not to participate, and that his/her signature indicates that he/she has decided to participate having read and discussed the information presented.

When appropriate, or when required by the IRB, one or more of the following elements of information will also be included in the consent document:

1. If the participant is or may become pregnant, a statement that the particular treatment or procedure may involve risks, foreseeable or currently unforeseeable, to the participant, or to the embryo or fetus.
2. A description of circumstances in which the participant's participation may be terminated by the investigator without the participant's consent.
3. Any costs to the participant that may result from participation in the research.
4. The possible consequences of a participant's decision to withdraw from the research and procedures for orderly termination of participation.
5. A statement that the PI will notify participants of any significant new findings developed during the course of the study that may affect them and influence their willingness to continue participation.
6. The approximate number of participants involved in the study.

There may also be additional stipulations from the IRB, when minors are to participate in the research protocol.

53.3.2.3 Who Should Consent the Patient and When?

The patient consent process begins with, as does consent for a medical procedure, a disclosure of the risks and benefits involved in the donation of time, personal medical information, and body tissue and/or fluids [9, 10]. It is often difficult to choose the right person to consent patients for medical research. The American Society of Reproductive Medicine (ASRM) guidelines stress that the primary caregiver should not obtain consent for embryo donation [5, 6]. The rationale behind the ASRM guideline lies in which patients may consent to research and they would not otherwise agree with if they feel their reproductive endocrinologist is depending on them to donate. Removing the primary caregiver from the consent process avoids this pressure on the patient and may also remove the caregiver from some conflict of interest. If the treating physician is not involved in the research, this may help to ensure that the consent of the patient is truly voluntary.

Another option is to have the laboratory director or a scientist involved in the research consent the patient. This is often a feasible option, but special attention should be paid to the abilities of the presenter. Whereas, the embryology team that often has experience in speaking with patients, likely competent in the basic science, may be a useful resource. Although, be cautious of researchers who are not part of the patient's clinical care or basic scientists who are not trained in patient interaction. A poorly conducted research consent is likely to cause undue stress to the patient who will be put off by the experience and lose faith in the treating clinics professionalism.

Whereas, the physician is often considered by the patient as a reliable source of information, and the most effective protocol may be to have the treating physician inform the patient of the research, then leave the signing of the consent to be witnessed by the support staff. The treating physician is then unaware of the consent status. This ensures that the patient is properly informed; the patient is assured that his or her well-being is foremost in the clinic and potential social, and scientific benefits are not lost.

The highly emotional nature of medical treatment in general, and specifically ART, also introduces constraint as to when it is a ppropriate to consent patients for donation. For the researcher, it is optimal to have consent prior to starting an in vitro fertilization (IVF) procedure, so gametes and embryos may be collected in a time-sensitive manner. The shortcoming of consenting at the onset of this extended procedure is that the attitude of the patient towards the embryos and collected gametes may change as they experience the collection of oocytes and the creation of their embryos. Consenting only once at the beginning of treatment may make the patients feel as if they made their decision without fully understanding the implications of donation, later regretting the consent and even perceiving they were unfairly treated or even coerced into participation. For this reason, consent may need to be reaffirmed during the treatment period.

53.4 Patient Privacy and Sample Storage

53.4.1 Sample and Medical Record Coding and Protected Health Information (PHI)

HIPPA does indeed cover samples retrieved from research participants and must be addressed during the consent procedure, as noted above. After samples have been donated to research, they must be tracked meticulously in order to preserve patient privacy and the fidelity of the research. Random number generator for sample coding is an excellent method for coding materials. This device can be found online through a basic internet searching tool or built into a secured database for sample storage and inventory control.

Coding samples is a necessity, but complete de-identification of material is not always the best option. There are contingencies that may require the investigator to track the samples back to the donor. The results may be of clinical significance or the investigator may need to contact the donor to validate results, ask for familial data, or verify the sample has been appropriately tested prior to using derived cell lines or products for clinical use with another patient; embryonic stem cells are of particular interest in this regard.

The principal investigator or research coordinator should maintain linked identifiers with limited access. An alternative to maintain the linked identifiers is to retrieve all pertinent data at the time of tissue collection, remove all PHI and link the coded data to the collected samples. This may be an option for much of the research performed. It is suggested that only the necessary information be collected for the research to proceed and then to disseminate only the pertinent information to collaborators, thus reducing the potential for breach of the federal mandate and loss of standing in the medical community and possibly the community at large.

These types of assurances are even more difficult to maintain in the current age of digital media storage and huge datasets that are only manageable through computerization. The review board often requires the use of secured servers maintained by certified professionals. The flipside is that these digital systems can afford increased ease of sample tracking. A well-designed sample storage database can save valuable time and resources. Turnkey systems are available for a premium price, but an in-house system designed through a simple database engine may very well be sufficient for most users.

53.5 Summary

The regulatory mandates put into place by the federal government are truly daunting when taken all at once. The consolation is that with proper preparation and close communication with your local review board, the regulations can be easily met. The patient will then be well cared for and, as has been the case, medical research will continue forward. Table 53.3 contains additional reading suggestions for those who wish to delve further into the inner workings of the review process and establishment of the current law.

Table 53.3 Practical references

Beauchamp, Tom L., and Childress, James F. *Principles of Biomedical Ethics*, 3d ed. New York: Oxford University Press, 1989.
Maloney, Dennis M. *Protection of Human Research Subjects: A Practical Guide to Federal Laws and Regulations*. New York: Plenum Press, 1984.
"The Common Rule" CFR45 part 46 (http://www.hhs.gov/ohrp/humansubjects/guidance/45cfr46.htm).

References

1. Maloney DM (1984) Protection of human research subjects: a practical guide to federal laws and regulations. Plenum, New York
2. Lo B, Chou V, Cedars MI et al (2004) Informed consent in human oocyte, embryo, and embryonic stem cell research. Fertil Steril 82(3):559–563
3. Levine RJ (1986) Ethics and regulation of clinical research. Urban and Schwarzenberg, Baltimore
4. Natinal Bioethics Advisory Commission (1999) Research involving human biological materials:ethical issues and policy guidance. In: Commission NBA (eds) Rockville, MD.
5. Ethics Committee of the American Society for Reproductive Medicine (2004) Donating spare embryos for embryonic stem-cell research. Fertil Steril 82(Suppl 1):S224–S227
6. American Society for Reproductive Medicine Ethics Committee (2002) Donating spare embryos for embryonic stem-cell research. Fertil Steril 78(5):957–960
7. Congressional Information Service (1978) Index to the code of federal regulations. In: Information Handling Services, Englewood, CO, v
8. Berland GK, Elliott MN, Morales LS et al (2001) Health information on the Internet: accessibility, quality, and readability in English and Spanish. JAMA 285(20):2612–2621
9. Shannon TA (1987) In vitro fertilization: ethical issues. Women Health 13(1–2):155–165
10. Robertson JA (1995) Ethical and legal issues in human embryo donation. Fertil Steril 64(5):885–894

Chapter 54
Technology Transfer and Its Role in the Practice of Reproductive Endocrinology and Infertility

Ashley J. Stevens

Abstract This chapter is very different from the other chapters in this book. Rather than addressing specific reproductive endocrinology and infertility diagnostic and therapeutic needs and situations, it is intended to help clinicians who come up with ideas that have the potential to improve the practice of reproductive endocrinology and infertility translate those ideas from bench to bedside.

Keywords Invention • commercialization • Technology transfer • Intellectual property • Patents • Copyrights • Trademarks • Trade secrets and mask works

54.1 Technology Transfer

Technology transfer means the transfer of a technology from one party to another. So, when for example Hewlett Packard or IBM establishes a factory in Singapore or Bangalore to manufacture a product developed in the US, it involves a transfer of technology, from one country to another, but generally the technology stays within the same company.

In the US, however, the term "technology transfer" has come to mean the transfer of a technology developed at an academic institution, often with federal or philanthropic funding, to a company which can secure the necessary private funds to develop the technology, secure any necessary regulatory or standards approvals to market the product and then manufacture and bring the product to market.

Academic institutions have developed offices and resources of varying degrees of sophistication to facilitate this process, which we will discuss later.

A.J. Stevens (✉)
Institute for Technology Entrepreneurship and Commercialization
School of Management and Technology Transfer, Boston University,
53 Bay State Road, Boston, MA, USA
e-mail: astevens@bu.edu

54.2 A Brief History of Technology Transfer in the United States

Until 1980, if an academic researcher made an invention with federal funding, the government owned the resultant patent rights. The government had a firm policy that it would not grant exclusive licenses to inventions it owned, but would only license them non-exclusively. This meant that there was little incentive for companies to make the investment necessary to develop academic technologies because once they had made the investment and proved the viability of the technology, their competitors could then obtain a license on the same terms without having to make the same high risk investment.

As a result, in 1978 the government owned 28,000 academic patents and had licensed fewer than 4% of them. Inventions reported to NSF and NIH were declining even though federal funding of research was booming. And perhaps worst of all, companies would talk of research being "tainted" if it had received federal funding because of their fear of the government being able to grant nonexclusive licenses if it owned the patent rights (or even jointly owned them by virtue of having provided part of the funding to develop the technology).

Also at this time, the US economy was perceived as being in trouble under the double burden of high interest rates and high oil prices, coupled with a loss of leadership of manufacturing efficiency to Europe and Japan.

Senators Robert Dole (R. KS) and Birch Bayh (D., IN) led a bipartisan effort to help restore the vitality all of the US economy by removing the barriers to widespread integration of academic innovation into the mainstream economy.

In 1980, Congress enacted the Bayh–Dole Act [1] which allowed US universities, teaching hospitals, research institutes and small businesses to have the automatic right to take title to inventions made with federal funding.

The Act imposed a few requirements on institutions:

- Institutions were required to share any income they receive with inventors
- Institutions may only use the remainder on research and education

D.T. Carrell and C.M. Peterson (eds.), *Reproductive Endocrinology and Infertility: Integrating Modern Clinical and Laboratory Practice*,
DOI 10.1007/978-1-4419-1436-1_54,

- Institutions were expected to file patents on inventions they elect to own
- Institutions were encouraged to collaborate with commercial concerns to promote the utilization of inventions arising from federal funding
- Institutions were expected to give licensing preference to small businesses
- Products sold in the US must be manufactured in the US
- The government retained a nonexclusive license to practice the patent throughout the world
- The government retained march-in rights to grant additional licenses in the public interest if the invention is not being exploited in the public good.

Little was visible for quite some time. Institutions established offices of technology transfer to seek patent protection on these inventions and license them to existing and new businesses for development and commercialization, but there did not seem to be much impact on the economy at large. The 1980s were still a difficult time for the US economy, with oil prices reaching record levels in 1982 that were only exceeded in inflation-adjusted terms in the summer of 2008, and with the US semiconductor industry sustaining heavy losses and loss of market share in DRAM memory chips.

As recently as April 1992, the cover story of Business Week trumpeted gloom and doom and called on the government to establish an industrial policy. It said: "The very phrase rattles the teeth. It implies bureaucracy. It suggests that government will pick winners and losers. Done badly, it would certainly hurt America. But with the Cold War over and the global economy taking shape, American needs to shore up its competitiveness. How? Certainly by investing in education and infrastructure. But that's not enough. We must recharge the knowledge base – the basic science and technology that are the foundation of an advanced industrial society. Perhaps we should call it a "growth policy."

Just six months later, Business Week was trumpeting an entirely different message. "Hot Spots" was the theme off the issue with the subtitle "America's New Growth Regions." Inside it was clear that the recharging of the knowledge base had already taken place. A map showed a series of clusters from Ceramic Corridor in Upstate New York to Laser Lane in Orlando, Florida to optics Valley in Tucson, Arizona and up to Boomtown Boise in Boise, Idaho. The map stated that 600,000 people held high-tech jobs in these places.

As notable as anything was the omission of the traditional high-tech clusters of Route 128 in Boston, Research Triangle in North Carolina, and Silicon Valley in California from the map.

The article correctly identified the ingredients for a high tech cluster that hold true today, starting with a major research university:

- A major research university
- Quality of life
- Build on local industry
- Cooperation between local university, business and government
- Technology transfer from the university
- Funding sources – state, venture capital, angels
- Incubators.

54.3 The Impact of Technology Transfer

Since 1991, the Association of University Technology Managers has published an annual survey which has quantified the magnitude of the US's technology transfer enterprise [2]: For instance, in 2006, institutions

- Managed 18,874 new invention disclosures
- Filed 15,908 total U.S. patent applications
- Had 3,255 U.S. patents issued
- Signed 4,963 new licenses
- Managed 12,672 licenses and options that are yielding active income.
- Had 697 new products introduced to the market in 2006 from active licensees;
- Introduced more than 4,350 new products into the market in the nine years from FY1998 to FY2006.
- Launched 553 new startup companies in 2006 and 5,724 since 1980.

Academic technology transfer generates new products in a broad range of sectors of society and industry, but has had a particular impact on two sectors:

- Healthcare, reflecting the large amount of federal funding for healthcare research
- The Internet, reflecting its academic origins.

A recent study [3] quantified the considerable contribution to improve public health through the discovery, patenting, licensing and successful development of over 130 small molecule and biological drugs, vaccines and in vivo diagnostics,

Some of the contributions of academic institutions to the development of the Internet are shown in Table 54.1.

Table 54.1 Components of the internet that originated in academic institutions

Component	Originating institution
World Wide Web	European Organization for Nuclear Research (CERN)
Mosaic (Internet Explorer)	University of Illinois Urbana Champaign
Eudora	University of Illinois Urbana Champaign
Yahoo	Stanford
Lycos	Carnegie Mellon
Akamai	MIT
Google	Stanford

It is not surprising therefore that some institutions have garnered enormous returns from technology transfer. The 2006 AUTM Licensing Activity Survey showed that overall, US academic institutions received almost $2 billion in licensing income. However, this income is highly concentrated in a small number of institutions who have had one big success, frequently a drug – the so-called "big hit".

54.4 Intellectual Property

Technology transfer starts with intellectual property. Intellectual property is a blanket term for a number of different mechanisms for protecting the results of intellectual activity. The most common of these, and the most important in life sciences research, is the patent system. Other important mechanisms are copyrights, trademarks, trade secrets and mask works.

It may seem antithetical to the spirit of science to try and sequester knowledge, and certainly a number of the critics of technology transfer make that argument. However, this view reflects a fundamental misunderstanding of the intention and purpose of the patent system, which has always been to provide incentives to inventors to fully disclose their inventions to the world so that others may build on them, in return for the inventor being given a period of exclusive use of their innovation, rather than holding the knowledge close to their chest and practicing it in secret. By properly utilizing the patent system, a scientist can publish his or her findings and advance the body of scientific knowledge, while reserving for him or herself the exclusive commercial use of those findings. Indeed, a recent study of publications in Nature Biotechnology found that almost 50% of articles in that journal between 1997 and 1999 had a counterpart issued US patent by 2006, a phenomenon the author termed the Paper-Patent-Pair [4].

That said, a minority of academic scientists make the effort to commercialize their scientific findings. A study of 3,342 science faculty at six universities over 17 years [5] found that almost 65% of faculty never disclose an invention, another 22% disclose an invention once or twice in their careers and fewer than 15% are prolific users of the commercialization process. The data are shown in Table 54.2.

Table 54.2 Faculty invention disclosure rates

Number of disclosures	%
Never disclose	64.2
Disclosed once	14.8
Disclosed twice	7.6
Disclosed three to five times	11.4
Disclosed eight or more times	2.0

Table 54.3 Relationship of faculty performance to industrial research support

Variable	No. of publications	Teaching time	No. of service activities	Publication-trends score
No industrial support	10.1	16.6	1.8	2.1
Industrial support	14.6	16.0	2.3	4.2
1–33%	16.8	17.7	2.8	5.0
34–66%	16.4	19.3	2.2	5.3
67–100%	12.1	15.8	2.1	2.5

Research has also shown that faculty who are involved with commercialization are better faculty, as measured by publication rate and participation on faculty committees than faculty who are not involved with industry [6]. The data are shown in Table 54.3. This relationship holds true until industrial support accounts for more than 2/3rd of total support for the lab.

54.5 Who Owns Your Invention?

Who owns your invention will have a lot to do with how it gets handled and how much you will benefit from it.

If you work for a company, you will have undoubtedly been required to sign an invention agreement when you joined the company, in which you agreed to assign any inventions you made to the company.

If you work for a university or an academic medical center (AMC) which is affiliated with a university, then you will have signed also an invention agreement, commonly known as a patent policy or patent policy agreement, in which you also agreed to assign ownership of your inventions to the University or AMC. Unlike a company agreement, where you will most likely have been given "$1 and other good and valuable consideration (such as keeping your job)" when you assigned your rights in the patent to the company but you will not share in the profits made from your inventions, the University patent policy agreement will probably include a detailed description of just how much of the university's income you will receive. As we noted earlier under the discussion of the Bayh–Dole Act, it is a legal requirement that the inventor share in the income. Theoretically, the university could have a separate policy for income from inventions that were not federally funded, but the majority of institutions have a single policy. Typical rates are from 25–35% though some institutions have tiered distributions which give a higher percentage of the early income to the inventors and lower percentages as income increases. There may be an additional percentage allocated to your own laboratory. If there is no lab share, there will undoubtedly be a share allocated to your department or college, and you should negotiate with the chair/chief/dean for somewhere between one third to one half of this department/college share to be allocated to your lab account.

There will be an office of technology transfer/licensing/industrial relations to whom you should submit the invention disclosure and which will manage the process for you, with your enthusiastic support.

If you work for a community hospital, a for-profit hospital, a nonprofit HMO, a group practice or in private practice, then it is likely that the total basis for your employment is clinical practice with no research component to it. In those circumstances, there will likely be no policies on inventorship and ownership, in which case you will be free to pursue (and pay for!) your inventions entirely by and for yourself.

54.6 The Invention

In the course of your clinical practice, you will frequently identify an unmet medical need, something that you would buy and use if it were available, but which you find is not available commercially. It may be a new diagnostic test, a new instrument, an improvement on an existing instrument, a new drug, a new use for an existing drug, a combination of two existing drugs, a new way of delivering or dosing an existing drug, and so forth.

One thing that is no longer worth patenting is a surgical procedure. In the early 1990s, Dr. Samuel Pallin filed a patent infringement suit against Dr. Jack Singer alleging infringement of U.S. Patent No. 5,080,111 on a patented surgical technique for use during cataract surgery [7]. The case caused widespread outrage both within the medical profession, among the public and in Congress. The 1996 Omnibus Appropriations bill, Public Law 104-208, contained a section, which limited the legal remedies available for infringement of patents on medical procedures. That said, if you identify a new surgical procedure that you think has merit, the way to extract value from it would be to develop and patent a new instrument or machine to carry out the procedure.

54.7 Obtaining a Patent

The basic criteria for obtaining a patent are that the invention must be:

- Novel
- Useful
- Nonobvious; and
- Adequately described.

54.7.1 Novelty

Novelty means that the invention has not been identically described in the literature anywhere in the world, or put on sale in the country in which patent protection is being sought. In the US or Canada, an inventor can publish his or her invention and still apply for a patent within a year, and in Japan within six months. In the rest of the world, a patent examiner somewhere must be the first person to learn about an invention for it to be patentable, so a US inventor who takes advantage of this one-year "grace period" will lose the opportunity for worldwide protection. Fortunately, the advent of provisional patent applications in the US has greatly facilitated the patent application process for academic inventors, by reducing substantially the time and effort needed to file an initial patent application.

54.7.2 Utility

Utility means that the inventor must disclose a use of his invention. He or she doesn't have to disclose all the uses and doesn't even have to disclose the most important use he or she knows of. These can be added at a later stage.

54.7.3 Nonobviousness

Nonobviousness means that the invention could not have been anticipated by putting together two existing inventions. In many academic inventions, these are some of the most difficult arguments made by the patent examiner to overcome. A patent examiner frequently combines references from widely different areas of science and claims that these make the invention obvious.

This has always been one of the most difficult patent examiner objections to overcome, and the examiners' hands were strengthened by a 2007 Supreme Court decision, *KSR v. Teleflex*, which eliminated a relatively inventor-friendly test for determining obviousness.

54.7.4 Adequately Described

You must disclose your invention in sufficient detail that one ordinarily skilled in the art can understand it. For a medical invention this would mean say, another OB/GYN, not just your 10 closest academic competitors in the world.

You must also disclose the best way you know of to carry out the invention at the time you file the patent application – the "best mode". You don't have to file updates if you subsequently learn even better ways of carrying out the invention.

You do not even have to actually carry out all of the invention and prove that it works. You can file a predictive patent application, politely called a "constructive reduction to practice". For example, the University of Rochester obtained a patent (US Patent 6,048,850 "Method of inhibiting prostaglandin synthesis in a human host") claiming all uses of drugs which selectively inhibited cyclooxygenase 2, but not cylcooxygenase 1. At the time the patent was filed, the university only had possession of two cell lines, one of which stably expressed Cox 1 and the other of which stably expressed Cox 2. The rest of the patent is devoted to predicting how one would use these two cell lines to identify compounds which inhibit Cox 2, but not Cox 1. Rochester subsequently sued Pfizer claiming infringement of the patent by Celebrex [8] and after an enormous (and enormously expensive) legal fight, the patent was found invalid for lack of enablement (and then Cox 2 inhibitors were found to have severe side effects and were withdrawn from the market!).

54.7.5 Patent Systems

There are two patent systems in the world:

- First-to-invent
- First-to-file

The US is now alone in operating on a "First-to-invent" system. In this system, if two inventors can show that they are entitled to be awarded the same patent, then the patent will be awarded to the inventor who can show they were the first to make the invention. The process by which this determination is made, if there are two competing inventors, is called an "interference". It is an adversarial process conducted not in court, but before a special board of the Patent Office – the Board of Patent Appeals and Interferences. Their decision is appealable to the US Federal District Court and from there to the US Court of Appeals of the Federal Circuit, the national court of appeals for patent cases. An interference is an expensive process and can take a long time to complete – the battle between Shmuel Cabilly of City of Hope Hospital in Los Angeles and Michael Boss of Celltech in the UK over coexpression of both chains of a monoclonal antibody in a single cell – an enormously valuable patent, that is required in the production of any recombinant antibody – took 18 years from application to a final (negotiated) settlement after appeal to Federal District Court. (The patent has since been invalidated on re-examination by the US PTO, a decision itself being appealed to the Board of Patent Appeals and Interferences! [9], so the fight still isn't over!).

The rest of the world operates on a first to file system. In this system, if two inventors can show that they are entitled to be awarded the same patent, then the patent will be awarded to the inventor who first filed their application somewhere in the world.

There are other differences between the two patent systems. Most notably, as noted earlier, outside the US "absolute novelty" applies – a patent application must be filed before the invention is published anywhere in the world. In the US and Canada, the inventor has 12 months from when they publish enabling details of the invention to file a patent application. In Japan, under some circumstances, the inventor has 6 months from publication to file a patent application.

What this means is that even the US applications should be filed before details of the invention are published, or else worldwide rights will be lost. In the past, this presented academics with a dilemma – should they risk losing scientific credit for being first to publish while they took one to two months to file a patent application, or should they publish first, take advantage of the one year "grace period" and file after publication and be content with the US rights only? Happily, since 1995, as discussed in the next section, a new form of patent application has been available that can be filed much more quickly and now it is possible to "have your academic cake and eat it too."

Another important difference between the US and European systems is that patents cannot be obtained for methods of treating people (e.g., a new use for an existing drug). Patent attorneys can formulate alternative ways to claim the invention to overcome this limitation.

54.8 Types of Patent Application

You will encounter a number of different types of patent applications.

54.8.1 Provisional Patent Application

Provisional patent applications have only been available in the US since 1995 when the GATT treaty came into effect [10]. A provisional patent application may be filed by an inventor by him or herself or their technology transfer office for a filing fee of $100 plus an Express Mail fee. A provisional application doesn't have to include any claims or even name any inventors. It must merely enable at least as broad a scope as the inventors ultimately wish to claim. A provisional patent application merely plants a stake in the ground and gives the inventor a year to convert the provisional application to a full utility application or PCT application and gain the benefit of the earlier filing date. If the inventor does nothing, then the provisional application dies and is never seen. A significant benefit of a provisional application is that the one-year duration does not count toward the maximum 20 year lifetime of a utility application from initial filing. While nothing happens during that year toward examination and issuance of a patent, this de facto extension of the term of the patent is very valuable with life sciences invention, which will have to go through a protracted period of development before they can be commercialized. Pharmaceutical companies frequently prepare full utility applications on their inventions, but file them as provisional applications and then merely refile them as utility applications at their one-year anniversary.

54.8.2 Utility Application

A utility patent application is the main sort of US patent application and is intended to lead to issuance of the most important category of US patent, the utility patent (the others, which are encountered much less frequently are design patents and plant patents – only asexually reproduced plants such as potatoes).

Under the American Inventors Protection Act of 1999, US applications have been published since March 15, 2001. Previously, US patent applications were confidential until the patent was issued. You can also read the discussion between the inventor and his or her attorney and the patent examiner as prosecution proceeds.

54.8.3 PCT Application

The Paris Convention of 1883 allowed inventors a year to file corresponding foreign applications after the initial filing in one of the signatory countries. Today 169 countries are signatures to the Paris Convention.

PCT is an abbreviation for the Patent Cooperation Treaty and is the primary form of international patent application. The Patent Cooperative Treaty came into effect in 1978 and allows for a single worldwide filing to fulfill the Paris Convention requirements. There are currently around 133 signatories and they include all major economies except Taiwan, Malaysia, Thailand, Uruguay, and Venezuela. PCT applications are typically filed a year after the initial ("priority") application.

A PCT application can be filed in any language though effectively the choice is limited to Arabic, Chinese, English, French, German, Japanese, Russian or Spanish, and Dutch, Korean and certain Nordic languages. The overwhelming majority are filed in English.

A PCT application can undergo a preliminary examination at the international level, which can be helpful. A PCT application is published 18 months after its priority date, or six months after the PCT filing date.

After a further 12 months (i.e., 30 months from the priority date), the PCT application expires and applications must be filed in individual countries.

54.8.4 National Phase Patent Applications

These are applications in individual country patent offices or regional patent offices such as the European Patent Office. Academic institutions will generally not file outside the US unless they have a licensee to reimburse the costs.

Most licensees other than the very largest pharmaceutical companies will only file patent applications in developed countries. A typical group of foreign counterparts might include:

- European Patent Office ("EPO")
- Japan
- Australia
- New Zealand
- Canada

The next tier of countries might include China, India and South Africa.

54.8.5 European Patent Office

The European Patent Office is based in Munich, Germany and examines patents on behalf of 34 (as of January 1, 2008) European countries. All western European countries currently belong, and the countries formed by the breakup of the former Yugoslavia recognize EPO patents.

All examination and approval of patents, including the opportunity for companies to object to the issuance of a patent that has been approved for granting, occurs at the EPO level. The EPO doesn't issue patents – this is still done at the individual country level, and translation costs were substantial. In October 2000, the London Agreement substantially reduced the number of translations required. The London Agreement came into effect on May 1, 2008.

54.9 Prosecuting a Patent Application

When the patent attorney has finished working with you to prepare the patent, he or she mails it to the patent office using Express Mail. At the patent office, it is assigned to a patent examiner, who probably has a backlog of 120 or so cases. Examiners have to work through their backlog and dispose of eight cases per two week period.

Eventually, your invention will reach the top of the examiner's pile and the examiner reads it for the first time. The examiner's normal first reaction to a patent application is to decide that there are actually two or more separate inventions contained in the application and to split it up into two or more separate applications. Since the patent lies in the claims, the examiner may say something like: "The first invention is claims 1–4 and 6–10; the second invention is claims 5, and 11–15, and the third invention is claims 16–26." This is called a restriction requirement. The inventor now has to pick the application he/she wants to prosecute first. The inventor will normally pick either:

(a) The invention they think they have the best chance of getting issued; or
(b) The invention that they want the patent issued first for commercial reasons.

The inventions that the inventor doesn't pick sit at the patent office, and the inventor can come back and start prosecuting them when the one they prosecute first is allowed. The so sidelined inventions are called "Divisional applications."

After the inventor, through their attorney, picks which set of claims to prosecute, the substantive prosecution will commence in earnest. The next communication from the Examiner is likely to be a rejection of all claims, for a combination of prior art, obviousness lack of enablement or lack of specificity, and citing references. The attorney will have views on some of the Examiner's arguments and will write to the inventor laying out the Examiner's concerns, his proposed responses and asking for the inventors' views. It is critical that the inventor be engaged in the process, read these somewhat dry pieces of correspondence (the communications from the Examiner tend to be particularly dry), read the references and help the attorney mount the strongest possible response.

The prosecution will go back and forth in this way, with the attorney and the inventor hopefully whittling away at the Examiners' objections. An inventor has a right to talk to the Examiner, either by phone or in person at the Patent Office in Washington. This is often an effective way to overcome objections and get an allowance – it makes a very strong statement to the Examiner that the inventor truly believes they're entitled to something – and the inventor should be prepared to put in the effort to take advantage of such an opportunity if it is offered.

Hopefully, the Examiner will eventually be convinced and will mail a "Notice of Allowance" to the attorney. At that point, the attorney will pay the Issue Fee and about three months later, on a Tuesday [11], the patent will issue.

In the interim between when the fee is paid and the patent issues, it is time to go back and revisit the Divisional applications that were left on the table at the outset of the process. If the inventor wants to pursue them, the additional applications must be filed before the patent issues.

54.10 How Much Does it Cost to Get a Patent?

How long is a piece of string? As any attorney or economist likes to say: "It depends". However, in overview, healthcare inventions tend to be relatively expensive. The examples are highly technical, and the inventor will generally want to claim much more broadly than the specific examples they've carried out.

There are three elements to the cost of obtaining a patent:

- Attorney's fees
- Official fees
- Translation costs

Attorneys charge by the hour, in increments generally of 6 min (0.1 h). As of this writing in early 2008, partners at major law firms are charging $500–$750 per h; associates $250–$475 per hour, technical specialists with PhD's $125–$400 per hour, depending on experience. In New York City, rates may be even higher. Smaller firms are variable. Some may have very similar rates overall. Typically, the partners' rates will be lower, but the associate and technical specialist's rate may be essentially the same.

By retaining an attorney and asking them to do something for you, you are essentially giving them a blank check – you are saying "Take as long as you need to get this job done, multiply by your hourly rate and send me the bill and I'll pay it." To avoid unpleasant surprises, it's advisable to ask the firm to cap the fees, by asking them to commit to a "Not to exceed" figure. For repetitive matters such as writing a patent, firms have a lot of experience and will generally be ready to do this.

Official fees are reasonable in the US. The US PTO charges modest fees and gives a 50% discount to small companies (less than 500 employees), not-for-profits and individuals. Once a US patent is issued, maintenance fees are only due at 3½, 7, and 11½ years and are reasonable -- $490, $1,240 and $2,055 respectively for small entities.

Foreign patent office fees tend to be higher. PCT filing costs are $3,000–$4,000. EPO fees are substantial and there are significant maintenance fees each year.

Technical translation costs are expensive. The major cost of filing a Japanese patent application is the cost of translating the application into Japanese.

In ball park terms, it should be possible to file a provisional patent application for a healthcare invention for $2,000–$7,000, depending how much additional work is put into converting a publication into a patent application. Converting this to a utility application will cost up to $20,000. Prosecuting a typical application to issuance will typically cost a further $20,000 over its life in the U.S. Filing a US utility application as a PCT application will cost $3,000–$5,000 in filing fees. A modest suite of national phase filings – Japan, EPO, Canada and Australia – will cost $25,000–$30,000. The costs to obtain and issue a patent are relatively modest in Canada and Australia. They are substantially higher in the EPO and Japan, typically about the same as in the U.S. In addition, the official fees for maintaining both the pending patent applications and the issued patents in effect in these countries is quite expensive – typically from $500–$1,500 per year per country. Thus, a lot of thought needs to be given to foreign filings.

54.11 Licensing The Patent

Getting a patent is relatively straightforward – have an original, creative idea, pay your attorney, and you will get a patent. However, the only reason for an academic scientist or physician to get a patent is to use it to induce a company to make the necessary commitment of human and financial resources to develop the invention and bring it to the market, and this is a lot more difficult. Anecdotally, one hears it said that fewer than 5% of patents are actually practiced though the data to support this is hard to come by.

Just as with prosecuting the patent, it is critical – in fact even more critical – that the inventor be very involved in the process. In a long term study [12] of 1,140 licenses completed by six institutions – the University of Florida; Massachusetts Institute of Technology; Oak Ridge National Laboratory; Oregon Health Sciences University; Tulane University; and the University of Utah – the authors confirmed the results of a preliminary study that had been carried out at MIT that the bulk of the leads that lead to completed licenses come from faculty (Table 54.4).

This may lead the inventor to ask: "If I made the invention and I find the licensee, what do I need these guys for, and in particular, why on earth are they going to get 70% of the money the technology brings in?"

The reason why the inventor is the source for over half the leads is quite simply that the inventor lives, eats, and breaths the science underlying the technology, while the technology transfer office has to work with the technologies of every professor and physician at the university. The inventor will know which companies are publishing in that space, attending the conferences and professional association meetings in that field, hiring his graduate students and post docs and so forth.

Table 54.4 Sources of leads that lead to signed license agreements at six institutions

Source	%
Inventor	56%
Marketing efforts of OTT	19%
Company called university	10%
Research sponsor requested license	7%
Unknown	7%

What the technology transfer office brings to the table is a business perspective on how to translate the invention into products, sources of information and experience in valuing the technology and in negotiating with companies. And of course the funds to pay for the patent application process.

54.11.1 Types of Licensee

Universities classify the companies that license their inventions into three categories:

- Large companies
- Small companies
- Start-up companies

In this scheme, a start-up company is one that is formed specifically to develop the technology. Small companies are those with fewer than 500 companies, which makes them eligible for various forms of government support, such as reduced fees at the patent office, access to the facilities of the Small Business Administration and eligibility for Small Business Innovation Research (SBIR) and Small Business Technology Transfer (STTR) grants.

In general, academic technologies tend to be so early stage, uncertain and with such a low probability of leading to a successful product that large companies find it hard to make the sorts of commitments that universities require from licensees, so the majority of academic licenses are with small companies, and only a third or so are with large companies. Table 54.5 shows the data for 2006 [13]:

This distribution between the types of licensee companies has held fairly constant for approaching 20 years.

Clearly, starting a new company is an important pathway for commercializing academic technology and we will consider this in some detail later in the chapter.

54.11.2 Finding a Licensee

Universities usually use a combination of passive and active marketing to find potential licensees.

Table 54.5 Licensees of US academic inventions in 2006

Type of company	Number	%
Large companies	1,648	34.1%
Small companies	2,416	50.0%
Start-up companies	764	15.8%
Total	4,828	

54.11.2.1 Passive Marketing

Passive marketing is usually achieved through having a searchable website where a non-confidential description of the technology is posted. This website is usually reached through the technology transfer office's section of the university's website. It is still laborious for prospective licensees to search each universities website in turn, so there are a number of websites that accumulate technologies from a number of sources. Some of these are commercial – e.g., Yet2.com [14] and UTEK [15] – though this has turned out to be a difficult business model to generate a return on capital (at the height of the dot.com boom there were over 40 technology matchmaking sites). Others are not-for-profit. The pioneer was created by the Massachusetts Association of Technology Transfer Offices and the Massachusetts Technology Transfer Center and provides access to technologies from all the universities, teaching hospitals and research institutes in Massachusetts [16]. The states of Florida and Texas have implemented similar systems. The Kauffman Foundation has supported another not-for-profit, iBridge, to create another website that appears set to become the dominant standard [17].

An important component of passive marketing is a one or two page (no more) non-confidential description ("NCD") of the technology that can be freely distributed to "sell" the technology. This document should focus on the advantages of the technology and the benefits it can bring to the users of it, not on the technical features, and should summarize all the work that has been done to demonstrate that the invention works – animal data, prototypes, etc.

Another powerful passive marketing tool is the press. Issuing a press release to coincide with the publication of a key paper in a respected journal, or receipt of an important grant can generate coverage in the business press that can reach the attention of prospective licensees.

Active marketing involves directly approaching companies with interests in the area. The normal course of events would be to identify a contact, either technical or in business development and establish contact by phone or email and send them the NCD. Another highly effective active marketing approach is for the inventor to give talks at professional association meetings. There are also companies which organize small, expensive conferences on areas of science that are "hot" areas of innovation. Attendance is free for speakers.

54.11.2.2 Reeling the Prospect In

Once a company has been identified which is interested in the technology, the next step may be to send them the patent application. The next step will usually be a technical meeting conducted under a confidentiality agreement. This may lead to the company doing some work to replicate the scientific conclusions, perhaps using samples provided by the inventor under a Material Transfer Agreement. The step after that will be to send the company a term sheet, a high level, 4 or 5 page documents that summarizes the key aspects of the agreement. If the parties can reach an agreement on a term sheet, the next step will be negotiation of a license agreement and perhaps sponsored research agreement.

The entire process can take from 3 to 12 months from initial contact to signed agreement.

54.11.2.3 Deal Structure

There are three important aspects of license agreements:

- the due diligence commitments of resources and/or progress milestones that the licensee will agree to in order to successfully bring the technology to the market;
- the business arrangements by which the university will share in the financial success of the product; and
- the contractual terms that will govern the relationship and assign risk and management responsibilities.

The term sheet will handle the first two of these in some detail, but will only summarize the contractual aspects.

Due Dilligence

Due diligence commitments are both general and specific. General legal standards include:

"Best Efforts", which means that the company will work harder on this project than any other. Companies will rarely agree to this standard.

"Commercially Reasonable Efforts", which means that the company will work as hard on this project as it will on its internal projects of comparable market potential. This is the normal standard agreed to.

Specific commitments tend to fall into two categories – resource commitments or effort and achievements or outputs.

Resource commitments could include an agreement to spend specific amounts per year for a specified number of years, or to commit to devote so many FTE's to the project or to carry out specific experiments.

Achievement commitments are usually tied to preclinical and clinical development stages – prototyping of diagnostics and devices and selection and preclinical testing (tox, ADME) of lead compounds, followed by entering successive stages of clinical testing and submission for regulatory approval.

To prepare for either resource or achievement due diligence negotiations, the inventor should prepare what (s)he believes is a reasonable development plan, estimate the resources needed and the likely timeline, and be prepared to discuss these with the company. It is critically important that there be well defined milestones every six to twelve months, particularly in the first two or three years, so that if the company reduces the priority of the project in this time frame, the university will be able to detect this, terminate the license and find a new licensee.

Business Arrangements

The business arrangements will be divided into a number of places in the license agreement. Some will pertain to reimbursing expenses – patent expenses both past and future and the costs of any technical assistance the licensee will want the university to provide – some to payments to be made while the product is in development and some to payments to be made after the product has reached the market.

As a general proposition, academic inventions are generally licensed at a very early stage, when the probability of successful product introduction is relatively low. The value of the technology at that stage is therefore relatively low, but will rise as the product moves through the development process. A lot of the negotiations will be devoted to agreeing how much the value has increased by what stage and how much of that increase in value should be shared with the university.

Another critical part of the negotiations will focus on the expected commercial pathway the licensee will follow – specifically, whether the initial licensee will be the one that takes the product to market or whether they will develop the product a certain distance down the developmental pathway and then sublicense the product to a larger company which will actually take it to market. This decision has enormous commercial implications.

Specific Business Terms

Patent Expenses

The university normally will expect to see all its patent costs reimbursed at the closing of the deal and for future expenses to be reimbursed within 30 days.

Upfront Fee

The university will expect to receive an upfront fee to reflect the initial value of the technology. This will likely be between $10,000 and $1 million.

Annual Minimum Royalties

Annual Minimum Royalties (“AMR”) are royalty payments that are made whether the product is on sale and paying earned royalties or not. They generally start at a relatively modest level of $10,000 or 20,000 per year (and may not even start for 2 or 3 years after the license is signed) and then escalate over a 5 year period to around $100,000. AMR’s are generally payable on January 1 of each year and are creditable against earned royalties, milestone payments etc. due in the remainder of the year.

As well as guaranteeing a minimum level of income, AMR’s serve as a due diligence mechanism – if the company has stopped developing a technology, then the company will generally terminate the license rather than making the AMR payment.

Milestone Payments

These are payments made to reflect the achievement of points where the technology has increased in value. These are frequently the same as some or all of the due diligence milestones, but there may be additional ones such as patent issuance, achieving certain levels of sales volume etc.

Milestone payments for starting clinical testing are generally fairly modest, but product approval milestone payments should be around $1 million for a device and upward of $5 million for a drug.

Sublicense Income Sharing

If the initial licensee is a small company, then they may well not have the resources, both financial and sales and marketing, to take the product all the way to regulatory approval and into the market. The license agreement should anticipate that the company will be sublicensing rights to a larger company, and should provide for the university to receive a percentage of all payments the licensee receives from the sublicensee. This percentage should be in the range of 15–25%, with higher rates due for payments received if the sublicense is issued closer to the date of the original license, and lower rates if the licensee spends a longer period of development and more of its own funds to get the technology to the point, where a large company is ready to take it over.

One of the difficult issues is the way the university will share in the sublicensee’s sales of products. Say the license provides for the licensee to pay a 5% royalty on its own sales of the product. Will the licensee agree that the university will receive 5% of the sublicensee’s sales? The answer is probably “No” because at the time the license is signed, the licensee will have no idea of what royalty rate they will receive from their sublicensees. If the licensee can only negotiate an 8% royalty on the sublicensee’s sales and has agreed to pay the university 5% of the sublicensee’s sales, then they will only be left with 3% to compensate them for all the time and money they put into the development of the technology. Therefore, the licensee will normally agree to pay the university a percentage of the royalties they receive from the sublicensee, perhaps the same percentage as they agree to pay of lump sums they receive from the sublicensee.

We have recently observed that if the agreed royalty rate is 3% or less, then it is generally possible to get the licensee to agree to pay that royalty rate on sublicensee sales too.

On the other hand, if the licensee is a large company, the agreement will probably provide for the university to receive the same set of payments and royalties whether the licensee sublicenses the technology to another company or takes it to market itself, and for the university not to share in any payments the company receives from sublicensing.

Royalties

Royalties are the payments the university will receive on the basis of the sales of the product. In general, royalty payments will provide the greatest economic return to the university if its technology does reach the market.

Royalties should be expressed as a percentage of sales, rather than say profits since sales is a very easy number for an auditor to verify when the university subsequently audits the licensee to ensure that the university is being paid all that it is entitled to receive.

One of the fundamental concepts of licensing is that the licensor should receive 25% and the licensee 75% of the pretax profits generated by a licensed product. This principle is known as the Goldscheider Principle or the 25% Rule, after Robert Goldscheider who first enunciated it. Goldscheider recently wrote an excellent review of the history, evolution and application of the rule [18]. The rule is a guide and provides onlya starting point only and many other considerations must be taken into account in applying it, but the clear implication is that the more profitable the product, the higher the royalty rate. So, for instance, if the licensee suggests that as sales increase the royalty rate should go down (the implication being that you've made so much money already, the rate should go down), the counter would be that since products, particularly pharmaceuticals, get more profitable as sales increase, the royalty should actually be higher at higher annual sales levels, not lower.

Another issue that comes up with royalties is royalties that have to be paid to others. The licensee will generally ask to be allowed to offset some or all of royalties that have to be paid to third parties. If you are negotiating a relatively high royalty rate – say 6 to 10% – this will probably be a legitimate request. However, the licensee should only be allowed to deduct 50% of the third party royalties so that they have a strong incentive to negotiate low third party royalties. If you are negotiating a relatively low royalty rate – say below 5% and certainly below 3% – you should reject the request. The risk of a licensee having to license a third party patent that they didn't know about at the time of the negotiation has been substantially reduced since 2001 when US patent applications started being published (as noted above, previously they were confidential till issued). It is legitimate therefore to ask a licensee to show you the third party IP they think they will need to license in order to practice the IP they're licensing form you.

Auditing: The Ronald Reagan Principle

Ronald Reagan once famously said "Trust – but verify". This is very true of license agreements. The only knowledge that the licensor has of what the licensee is doing is what the licensee chooses to tell the licensor. After product sales start, the licensee sends the licensor a quarterly statement that sys "Here's what I've sold and here's what I owe you." It is essential that the licensor have the ability to verify what the licensee is telling them. This is achieved through an audit provision.

The licensor will generally have negotiated the right to send an independent CPA into the licensor's business offices once a year, with suitable notice, with the right to examine the licensee's business records for the prior three years (which is the length of time the IRS requires companies to keep records). Audit clauses in licenses generally require the licensor to pay the costs of the audit, which will generally be around $30,000–$40,000, unless the auditor discovers a shortfall in any payment of 5% or more, in which case the licensee has to pay the cost of the audit. Most red blooded auditors will be confident of their ability to find such a discrepancy, and studies have shown that audits generally do find shortfalls.

It is therefore generally a prudent policy to audit licensees every three years when annual royalties reach $1 million and annually when they reach $5 million.

54.12 Forming a Start-Up Company

Forming a start-up company is a particularly hallowed vehicle for technology transfer. As noted earlier, a dedicated start-up is the chosen commercialization pathway for about 15% of academic technology transfer transactions. It has considerable potential for creating substantial wealth for the inventor and the university. That said however, forming a start-up is not a pathway that should be pursued lightly or without a deep appreciation of the effort and commitment that will be required of the inventor.

54.12.1 Finding a Business Partner

The first requirement for a professor who wants to form a start-up (beyond an invention that is sufficiently disruptive to attract the investment needed to successfully commercialize the invention) is going to be a business partner.

How to find such a brave soul? There turn out to be a surprisingly large number of sources in the communities in which most academic medical centers are located. Some universities can supply this capability through a group whose job it is to help faculty start companies. If the university does not directly provide this assistance, the Office of Technology Transfer may know individuals who are suitably experienced and who are looking for their next "gig."

Professional advisors whom the Office of Technology Transfer uses, particularly lawyers, frequently have good contacts with the entrepreneurial community and will know suitable individuals. The alumni or development office may be able to introduce the inventor to an alumnus or alumna who is involved in the industry. The university's Business School may have professors or alumni who have suitable industrial contacts. Other sources may be people the inventor has met through prior consulting relationships – say a VP of Business Development of a biotechnology company which has licensed one of their earlier inventions and who wants to start their own company. Other sources may be people to whom the inventor is referred by colleagues who have been down this path before. Some states have biotechnology centers with an economic development mandate that can provide contacts or provide direct assistance (e.g. Ohio's Thomas Edison Program [19]; Pennsylvania's Ben Franklin Program [20]; New York's Center of Excellence Program [21].

Many states have biotechnology associations that are natural congregating points for biotechnology entrepreneurs.

It is critical that the business partner has credibility in the life sciences start-up community. Resist the temptation to team up with say a stock broker or real estate executive or business lawyer (all of whom the author has seen inventors team up with, generally with frustrating and unsatisfactory results) because they have more with familiarity business than the professor does. They will be a negative as you move down the road and will probably quickly lead you astray.

54.12.2 Working with Students

Before sitting down with a potential business partner, the inventor needs to have captured the vision he has for the company. This presents a chicken and egg situation – you need the commercial vision to engage a business partner, yet you need the business partner to develop the commercial vision. One way of cracking this egg is to see if your business school (or a nearby business school if you are at a hospital or practice that's not part of a university) has courses that require the students to write a business plan or develop a business strategy or do a market research study. The professors who run these courses always have a need for business and product ideas for the students to work on, so finding and making contact with such professors may be productive. You'll need to keep the academic calendar in mind – most likely there will only two starting opportunities available – September and January, and the professor will want to have everything lined up at least a month, probably two, before the start of the semester. That said, the quality of work you can get from a dedicated inter-disciplinary team of students working for 14 weeks is stunning.

54.12.3 Communicating the Idea

Ultimately, you will need four documents to "sell" a company concept to all the stakeholders you're going to need – employees, investors, landlord, customers, etc.

In order of difficulty, and effort to generate them, these four documents are:

An Elevator Pitch
A PowerPoint presentation
An Executive Summary
A full Business Plan.

54.12.3.1 Elevator Pitch

The elevator pitch is a two minute summary of the opportunity – what you are doing, the scale of the opportunity, what's unique about your approach to solving the problem, how you are going to change the world and how the person will profit enormously by joining you on the adventure. The term comes from the idea that you get on an elevator and suddenly realize that your fellow passenger is an ideal potential investor/employee/customer/whatever and that you have them captive for the duration of a 60 floor elevator ride.

The inventor should have an elevator pitch integrated into their psyche and be ready to launch into it at a moment's notice, tailoring it to the specific audience – potential investor/employee/board member/customer, etc. A good elevator pitch takes a lot of practice. It's very easy to go into too much technical detail or to stay stuck on the product idea and the company concept and not get to asking your captive audience for what you think they can contribute and how they'll profit from working with you.

If you can't capture the idea in two minutes, you haven't thought about it sufficiently. To be able to bring together all the resources you need, you have to be able to boil the opportunity to a simple, attractive summary that can be communicated in two minutes.

Some people advocate practicing at the mirror or giving the pitch to your dog. As the last step before going "live," you should give it to your mother and see if she "gets it".

The sole purpose of the elevator pitch is to interest the person you're giving it to so much that they want to hear more and will agree to meet with you later to learn more.

54.12.3.2 The PowerPoint Presentation

If you get that next meeting, you'll need a PowerPoint presentation, which is the heart and soul of communicating a new company concept. Like an elevator pitch, it must flow seamlessly and communicate the opportunity, the company's approach to filling the need, the status of the technology, what's unique about the company's approach, including the management team and the intellectual property position that will keep the enemy at bay, the company's financial projections, the investment the company is looking for and how the investors will make money – the "exit".

The individual slides of the presentation should be attractively designed, not cluttered with too many words and should use visuals where ever possible – a picture is worth a thousand words, and a video's worth ten thousand. A good presenter will take one and a half or 2 minutes per slide, so a presentation for a 1 hour meeting – 40 minutes plus 20 minutes Q&A – should be no more than 20 to 25 slides. Use a large "clean" sans serif font like Arial rather than say Times Roman. Always try giving the slide show using an LCD projector in a sunny room before the first meeting – slides that look great on a computer screen can have insufficient color contrast and be difficult to read under "real world" conditions. Take and use your own laptop rather than downloading via a flash drive to their computer – that way you know you'll have compatible software versions, have all the plug-ins you'll need – particularly important if you're using video. Take a laser pointer with you to emphasize the talk.

In short, look technically competent, professional, organized and in control when you give a presentation on your company.

54.12.3.3 The Executive Summary

The executive summary is a five to ten page summary of the company's business plan that summarizes the presentation. If the audience liked the PowerPoint presentation, they'll ask for an executive summary and a copy of the PowerPoint to share with people within their firm that they want to get excited about the opportunity. It is probably the longest written description of the company that people will ever read.

54.12.3.4 Business Plan

The company must always have a Business Plan, which is a complete description of where the company is, where it's going and what it needs to get there. It documents the scale of the market and the opportunity, and demonstrates the company's ability to meet the need. It analyses the planned pricing of the product. It describes and justifies the viability of the company's business model – how the company will generate revenues. It describes the management team and how that will evolve. It identifies the partnerships with other companies that the company will need to get to the market. It looks at potential competition and how the company's intellectual property position will keep competition at bay. It contains detailed financial projections – development costs, capital needs, operating costs, profitability and financial return.

A company's business plan is constantly evolving. At a minimum, it should be reviewed every three of four months in the light of changing market circumstances and the company's progress. The initiation of a round of fund raising will normally trigger a new edition of the business plan.

Few outside the company will ever read the business plan cover-to-cover. However, your ability to answer detailed questions that come up in your presentations will critically depend on the thoroughness of the thought and analysis that went into the preparation of the business plan. You write it for yourself not for others.

54.12.4 Forming the Company

You can (and should) test the waters for your company concept without actually incorporating. You can project a very professional image for the company with do-it-yourself computer graphics without actually incorporating. Nobody will check at this stage. The story of how Larry Page and Sergei Brin raised the seed round financing for Google is a Silicon Valley legend. They were introduced to Andy Bechtolstein, the Co-Founder and Chairman of SUN Microsystems and a fellow Stanford alumnus. He liked the story, went out to his Ferrari, got his checkbook and wrote a check for $100,000. Brin and Page had to quickly incorporate the company in order to be able to open a bank account to cash the check.

You should check out that the company's name has not been taken by another company in the same technical area as yourself, together with a suitable URL. It may be worth paying the modest fee to reserve the URL at this stage.

However, if you start to get the sense that the company is going to be investable and so may be viable, then you will want to move ahead and incorporate. Although there are an enormous number of web sites that will offer to incorporate a company for you for as little as $99, you should use the services of a major law firm. Particularly in the major innovation hubs, the large law firms understand that mighty oaks from tiny acorns do indeed grow and that their future major clients start out as impoverished start-ups. Many of these law firms have fee deferral programs under which, for a small retainer, they will accumulate the fees incurred by the company until some significant funding threshold is reached, at which point the accumulated fees become due.

It will ultimately be to the company's considerable advantage to be seen to be using the services of a top tier law firm. They will have expertise, experience and contacts to contribute as well, and the quality of your advisors does speak legions for you.

They will also prevent you from making the Number One mistake of start-ups, which normally occurs at this point – giving out Founders' stock to the Founders without an earn in. Since start-ups are generally planned by people who are still working for someone else, or are looking at multiple opportunities, it is quite likely that one or more members of the Founding team at the "virtual" stage will decide not to join the company, or may quickly move on. It is critical that the same amount of the company's stock not be held by people who aren't fully committed to the company as by those who have staked their future financial well being on the company's success. Therefore, it is a standard practice to make people earn-in their stock over 4 or 5 years. If they leave sooner than this, whether of their own volition of at the company's request, they forfeit the balance. This keeps them motivated, preserves fairness and prevents unnecessary dilution of the company's stock.

A good law firm start-up package will include things like employment contracts, confidentiality agreements, consulting agreements, board meeting minutes and corporate resolutions, in addition to the standard Certificate of Incorporation, By-Laws and Shareholders agreements and share certificates.

54.12.5 The Initial Funding

The Founders will normally buy their stock in the company at "Par Value", a purely nominal value that is printed on the share certificates and is typically 1¢ or oven 0.1¢ per share. So, if they decide to issue themselves 5,000,000 shares, they will contribute \$5,000 at 0.1¢/share or \$50,000 at 1¢/share, enough to pay the legal costs of incorporation, but no more.

The first "real" money that goes into the company and that will be used to start its operations can come from any one of a number of sources:

- Second mortgage/credit cards
- Bootstrapping – selling products and services
- Friends and family
- Angels or Angel Groups
- SBIR/STTR grants
- Corporate partnerships
- Venture capital

Table 54.6 Initial sources of funding for university spin-outs, FY 2004

	Number	%
Individuals		49.34%
Friends and family	94	20.52%
No external funding	57	12.45%
Individual angel(s)	49	10.70%
Angel network	26	5.68%
Institutional sources		44.54%
Venture capital	85	18.56%
State funding	36	7.86%
SBIR/STTR	32	6.99%
Corporate partner	25	5.46%
Institutional funding	26	5.68%
Other	28	6.10%
Total	458	100.00%

In 2004, the AUTM Survey asked respondents what the initial sources of funding for their spin-out companies were. The results are shown in Table 54.6.

It is clear that university spin-outs more frequently attract their initial funding from individuals than from institutional sources.

A more detailed source of these funding sources follows.

54.12.5.1 Second Mortage/Credit Cards

This is a classical method of starting a company, but probably doesn't have much relevance to a life sciences startup because of the total financing needs the company will have.

54.12.5.2 Bootstrapping

This is when a company has early sales opportunities – say selling reagents to the research market – and can use the revenues to fund developing its main products. Bootstrapping can reduce capital needs, but will rarely totally eliminate the need for investment sources.

54.12.5.3 Friends and Family

Also known as "friends, family and fools", this approach involves passing the hat round the more affluent members of the inventor's family, social and even professional circles. This can raise a significant amount of money, but comes with strings. As several inventors have observed to the author: "It does make for some tense Thanksgiving dinners" when the company hits the inevitable patch of turbulence.

If the company plans on raising later rounds of financing from institutional sources, it may find that they won't want to have a large number of small shareholders, and it may be appropriate to have them invest by buying a membership interest in an LLC company, so that there would be a single voting entity representing all the investors in that round.

54.12.5.4 Angels or Angel Groups

Angel investors are rich individuals to whom the inventor is not related and who invest some or all of their wealth in young start-ups. They are generally people who have made their money themselves entrepreneurially rather than having inherited it when it is normally tied up in trusts and protected by zealous and very conservative trust attorneys.

Some Angel groups have a pooled fund and invest out of that, while others operate as meeting conveners and bring a number of Angels to a monthly breakfast or lunch meeting at which companies make presentations, and each individual investor decides if he/she wants to invest in a particular opportunity and, if so, how much.

The more highly developed a region is as an innovation hub, the more likely it is that there will be organized Angel groups operating. For instance, there are close to 20 organized Angel groups operating in Massachusetts.

54.12.5.5 SBIR/STTR grants

The Small Business Innovative Research Program and the Small Business Technology Transfer Research Programs [22] have been mainstays of the US economy for 30 years since the SBIR program was "test marketed" by the NSF starting in 1978 and expanded to all federal agencies in 1982.

They are Federal grant programs and so are a particularly attractive way to fund a company's development since they are nondilutive – the Government asks for nothing in return other than a commitment by the company to commercialize the research.

Currently, all Federal agencies with an external research budget of $100 million or more have to dedicate 2.5% of their budget for SBIR grants and 0.3% to STTR grants, so over $2.3 billion is available for these grants, a substantial pool of nondilutive investment funds. There are three solicitations a year and proposals are solicited for specific fields that the agency has established as a priority. The grant proposals are of limited length.

The Phase I awards are for $100,000 for six months and are intended to demonstrate feasibility or proof of principle. Phase I recipients are eligible to submit Phase II proposals, which are worth $750,000 over two years and are intended to carry out the project. These funding levels have not changed in many years, and Study Sections will frequently award significantly higher amounts than these.

The PI of an SBIR must be employed at least 51% by the company at the time of the award (not the time of the submission, and the company must be able to demonstrate that it has adequate facilities to carry out the research. A collaboration with a university is not required, but upto 30% of a Phase I award and 50% of a Phase II award can be subcontracted to a university.

A STTR is by contrast at an earlier stage. It *requires* a collaboration with a university. At least 30% and as much as 60% of the work can be done at a university. The PI can be either at the university or at the small company.

54.12.5.6 Corporate Partnerships

It may be possible to fund the company's start-up and early stage development through a partnership with a larger company though it is highly likely that at the time the technology is transferred from the university, it will be at too early a stage and too low a probability of success to be attractive to a larger company and for this to be a viable approach. Corporate partnerships tend to be important later in the company's development.

54.12.5.7 Venture Capital

Venture capital funds are pools of funds invested by university endowments, very rich individuals, insurance companies, pension funds and so forth. These investors, who are known as Limited Partners, can afford to tie up their money for a long time in order to secure a superior rate of return. This is critical for venture capital funds because the fund will make investments in early stage, privately held companies and will most likely not be able to sell the investment for many years. Therefore, the Limited Partners typically are asked to invest their funds for ten years with no right to ask to be repaid.

Some companies have their own venture capital funds, but these tend to be more fickle investors. They rely on the parent company to make new funds available each year, and corporate venture funds are frequently throttled back in times of economic downturn when the parent's cash flow suffers.

The actual investments are made by General Partners. These are the people that the founders of the company will deal with. General Partners are generally people who have had a successful operating track record in large technology-based companies, or more likely in small venture-backed companies that the venture investors have made a lot of money in. A few grow from freshly minted Associates recruited fresh from their MBA's into partners, and a very few service providers such as lawyers have become successful venture capitalists.

The General Partners will normally draw 2.5% of the funds under management each year to operate the partnership – pay the rent, salaries, travel, legal expenses etc. This means that over the ten year life of the fund, 25% of the invested funds will go to operate the fund, and only 75% will actually be invested in companies. In addition, when the fund makes a profit on an investment, the limited partners will first have their investment returned to them, and the General Partners will receive 20% of the net profits from that investment.

If a venture capital fund makes ten investments, it will expect to write off four (i.e., lose its entire investment), make a two or three times return on four, and a ten times or higher return on the final two. If you run the numbers, allowing for 25% of the fund going for operating expenses, and the General Partners getting 20% of the net profits on the successes, this will result in a 25–30% annual return to the Limited Partners. This will then allow the General Partners to go back to the same Limited Partners when they are starting to raise their next fund. Venture Capital is a very Darwinian business – their first objective is to successfully reproduce themselves!

The key conclusion from this analysis is that if you want to attract venture capital investment, you must be able to show that venture capitalist that if the company is a success, they will make 10× their investment. If you think it will take an investment of $20 million to launch your products, then you must be able to show the VC's that your company will be worth $200 million.

As Table 54.6 shows, venture capital is the second largest source of funding for university spin-outs, but is the initial source of funding less than 20% of the time. Most technologies are simply too untested when they're transferred out of the university to be ready for venture capital. This is particularly true in the case of drugs. VC's are generally going to be ready to invest in a new drug company only when the company is a year away from starting human clinical trials, and very few academic drug discoveries are that far along when federal funding runs out. The entrepreneur's challenge is going to be how to fund the gap between the expiration of federal funding and when the company is ready for venture capital. VC's are more likely to fund a start-up diagnostic or medical device company.

54.12.5.8 Who Gets How Much: The Capitalization ("Cap") Table

There are normally two types of stock in a start-up company:

Common stock

Preferred Stock

Common Stock

Common stock is generally a reward for effort or the provision of services in kind – the original "sweat equity". The founders will receive common stock, as will the management team for their future services and the university (whose investment of intellectual property in the new venture represents past effort).

Preferred Stock

Preferred stock is normally reserved for investors who pay cash for it. It's full name is generally Preferred, Redeemable, Convertible Stock.

Preferred means that the stock enjoys various preferences over common stock. Redeemable means that the investors can force the company to repay their investment under certain circumstances.

Convertible means it's convertible into Common stock under certain circumstances. The first round of investment will normally be called the Series A Preferred, the second round of investment will be called the Series B Preferred, etc. Each successive round normally takes priority over the previous round if times get tough. (When times are good, everybody does well!)

Dividing Up the Founders Stock

This will undoubtedly be the subject of intense debate between the founders. One common philosophy is that the two equal components of a start-up company are the technology and the management team that's going to stake its financial security on this new venture. The technology is equally divided between the intellectual property, which the university owns, and the know-how, which is in the inventor's head, and which he can monetize by agreeing to consult exclusively for the new venture. This philosophy would result in a Founders' stock distribution of:

25% to the inventor

25% to the university

50% to the management team

Another philosophy has the university being another founder alongside the founding management team.

In yet another philosophy, the university will ask for a relatively small stake – say 5% – but that they be protected from dilution till a specified amount of investment capital has been raised by the company – say $5 million.

It is critically important that the management team's stock be earned in over typically four years. The management team share should include adequate provision for the additional employees who will need to be hired until the next financing.

The Investor's Stake

The investors will normally expect to get control of the company for their initial investment. The implication of this is that the company should not sell itself too cheaply. If you're going to have to give up half your company, then give it up for $5 million, not $1 million. Go out with an ambitious technical plan that requires $5 million to achieve. The VC's may balk at investing $5 million in an initial investment in a totally untried management team, and one way to finesse this calculation is to stage the release of the funds – say $1 million initially, to get the company to a certain technical achievement, with another $2 million released when that milestone is reached, and the final $2 million released when the company successfully achieves a second technical (or business) milestone.

The Next Round

The number of shares in the company will normally be adjusted (by splitting or reverse splitting) so that the price of the Series A stock is $1/share. If the company makes good progress, the Series B will hopefully be sold at a higher per share price – say $2/share or $3/share, perhaps even $5/share. This means that the company will give up less of itself proportionately to raise the next round of financing, and the value of the existing shareholders stake will grow, even though they won't be able to sell their stake and it will be a paper profit only.

If the company doesn't do well, then the next round may have to be sold at a lower per share price than the previous round. That's when things start to get ugly, and is beyond the scope of this chapter. Hopefully, it'll never happen to you.

What About the Seed Investors?

If the company raises a relatively small amount of money, from friends and family or Angel investors, the investment will probably be made not by a purchase of stock, but in the form of a loan secured by a note which is convertible into stock in the future. This has a number of advantages:

- The legal costs are much lower
- The value of the company can be set when a more substantial amount of money is raised from sophisticated investors a little later

The seed round investors are generally rewarded for investing early by converting their loan into stock at a lower per share price than the Series A investors – say at a 20% discount. So, if the Series A per share price is $1/share, then the seed round loan will be converted into stock at a price of $0.80/share, so they will receive 25% more shares per dollar invested than the Series A investors.

Subsequent Rounds

The prior arguments will apply to subsequent rounds of financing, which will be labeled Series B, C, D, E etc. High tech companies will generally be expected to raise only A, B and C rounds and then to have achieved self sufficiency. Life sciences companied may need additional rounds of financing. Acusphere, an MIT spin-out developing in vivo diagnostics for cardiovascular conditions, went as far as a Series J before pulling off an IPO. Each round's investors will have priority over those in the prior round.

The Exit

At this stage, the company is still privately held, and there is no market for the stock. While the value of the company may have increased substantially, this is still all on paper, and neither management nor investors can actually sell their stock and realize any part of that value.

At the end of the day, being able to realize the value that has been created is what people will care about, and that is achieved through an exit.

There are only two possible exits that will put cash in founders', managements' and investors' pockets:

- Acquisition, for cash or for stock in a publically traded company, or
- An Initial Public Offering ("IPO") through which the company's shares are listed on a stock market, generally the NASDAQ.

Another exit mechanism is acquisition by or merger with another privately held company. This may help build value, but it will still be "paper profits" until one of the prior two events happens.

The acquisition route may seem more attractive, but venture capital investment terms and conditions, specifically "liquidation preferences", may skew distribution of the proceeds toward the investors and away from founders and management.

IPO's have become considerably more expensive and difficult to pull off since the passage of the Sarbanes–Oxley Act in the wake of the Enron debacle. The benefit of an IPO is that it allows for the stock price to increase after the IPO (and equally to decrease!). The negative is that the shareholders from the company's private days will be required to sign a lock-up agreement, in which they agree not to sell their stock for six months (12 months for European stock exchange IPO's). Most new companies founded currently are founded in the expectation that the exit will be by acquisition.

54.13 Case Study

54.13.1 CALM

Institution: McGill Univ. *Location:* Québec, Canada *Field of:* Obstetrics

Emily Hamilton, M.D., a McGill University obstetrics and gynecology professor, was teaching at Montreal's Jewish General Hospital when it occurred to her that doctors and nurses could better evaluate the progress of delivery if they knew how their patients were compared with others.

"Students were asking simple questions like, 'How do you know when labor is slow?'" Hamilton says. Doctors were relying on a small study of women conducted in the 1950s for information about delivering babies, yet a number of medical developments, such as epidurals, greatly influence the average length of labor. When Hamilton looked at the big picture, she saw that the power of computing combined with large-scale studies could tell physicians and nurses what comprised a normal labor for different women.

Her revelation occurred in the early 1990s, and today the Computer-Assisted Labor Monitoring, or CALM™, system is installed in numerous North American hospitals. Hamilton's studies show that the technology can reduce Cesarean sections. Fewer Cesareans mean less pain and quicker recuperation for women and less time required by surgeons. The CALM system tells medical personnel when a labor that appears long may, in fact, be progressing normally. After inputting information about the patient, a simple-to-read graph appears on the screen. The graph shows three lines: the woman's progression of labor, and the high and low limits of statistically normal progression, based on data from other women with similar clinical characteristics. Doctors can quickly and easily update the touch-sensitive screen.

In addition to her position on the McGill faculty, Hamilton now serves as vice president for medical research and scientific advisory board chair for LMS Medical Systems Ltd., which distributes and monitors CALM in North American facilities. The company is based in Montreal, and Hamilton continues to hire engineering and computer science graduates from McGill and Université de Montréal as the company expands. Read more at http://www.lmsmedical.com

References

1. http://www.autm.net/aboutTT/aboutTT_bayhDoleAct.cfm. 2008. Accessed 27 Oct 2008
2. AUTM (2008) http://www.autm.net/about/dsp.licensing_surverys.cfm
3. Jensen J, Wyller K, ER L, et al (2007) The role of public sector research in the discovery of new drugs. In: Annual meeting of the association of university technology managers. San Francisco, CA
4. Murray F, Stern S (2007) Do formal intellecutal property rights hinder the free flow of scientific knowledge? an empirical test of the anti-commons hypothesis. J Econ Behav Org 63(4):648–87
5. Thursby J, Thursby M (2005) Pros and cons of faulty participation in licensing. In: University entrepreneurship, intellectual property, and technology transfer. JAI Press, Tucson, AZ
6. Blumenthal D, Campbell EG, Causino N, Louis KS (1996) Participation of life-science faculty in research relationships with industry. N Eng J Med 335(23):1734–9
7. Mossinghoff G (1996) Remedies under patents on medical and surgical procedures. J Pat Trademark Off Soc 78:789–801
8. Malakoff D (2000) Patent prompts Rochester to sue for slice of drug profits. Science 288(5465):410–1
9. Waltz E (2007) Insdustry waits for the fallout from cabilly. Nat Biotechnol 25(7):699–700
10. http://www.inventionconvention.com/ncio/specialreport/007.html. 2008. Accessed 27 Oct 2008
11. US Pattent and Trademark Office (2008) http://www.uspto.gov/main/glossary/index.html#i. Accessed 27 Oct 2008)
12. Jansen C, Dillon H (1999) Where do the leads come from? Source data from six institutions. Journal of the Association of University Technology Managers. XI.
13. http://www.autm.net/about/dsp.pubDetail2.cfm?pid=41. 2006. Accessed 27 Oct 2008
14. http://www.yet2.com/app/about/home. 2008. Accessed 27 Oct 2008
15. http://www.utekcorp.com/. 2008. Accessed 27 Oct 08
16. http://www.masstechportal.org/. 2008. Accessed 27 Oct 2008
17. http://www.ibridgenetwork.org/. 2008. Accessed 27 Oct 2008
18. Goldscheider R, Jarosz J, Mulhern C (2002) Use of the 25% Rule in valuing IP. Les Nouvelles:1233–1313.
19. http://www.odod.state.oh.us/OSB.htm. 2008. Accessed 27 Oct 08
20. http://www.benfranklin.org/. 2008. Accessed 27 Oct 08
21. http://www.empire.state.ny.us/High_Tech_Research_and_Development/centers_for_excellence.asp. 2008. Accessed 27 Oct 08)
22. http://www.sba.gov/SBIR/indexsbir-sttr.html. 2008. Accessed 27 Oct 2008

Chapter 55
The Environment and Reproduction: Endocrine Disruption, Reproductive Impairment, and Epigenetics

C. Matthew Peterson, Douglas T. Carrell, Michael Varner, Joseph Stanford, Mary Croughan, and Germaine Buck Louis

Abstract This chapter reviews the evidence that environmental factors have a role in the etiology of reproductive abnormalities. The actions of hormonally active agents, such as endocrine disrupting chemicals, that may alter the synthesis, secretion, transport, binding, or elimination of natural hormones are highlighted. This chapter also highlights the need for and organized collection of data to further analyze the involvemnet of environmental factors in reproductive anomalies.

Keywords Endocrine disruptor • Epigenetics • Endometriosis • Environment • Reproductive impairment • Biomarkers • Chemical substance inventory • Chemicals • Contaminants

55.1 Introduction to Endocrine Disruption

Many observations suggest that chemical exposures in the environment and/or workplace (occupational) may be associated with endocrine disruption of the synthesis, secretion, transport, binding action, or elimination of natural hormones [1]. For the purposes of this chapter, we define the environment as "nongenetic," inclusive of occupation. Through purported endocrine disruption, endocrine disrupting chemicals (EDCs) may affect the maintenance, homeostasis, reproduction, development, and/or behavioral activities of the species. Specifically, environmental exposures resulting in endocrine disruption that affect reproduction may potentially: alter individual or multiple enzyme pathways and/or gene-dependent activities; be associated with identifiable reproductive impairments; and/or result in trans-generational effects. In the long term, these direct and indirect mechanisms may cause adaptive or disruptive reproductive effects that affect the ultimate health, reproductive capacity, and survival of the species [1].

The fetal origin of disease concept, introduced by Barker, exposes the potential conflict between fetal compensatory mechanisms to direct and/or indirect endocrine disrupting insults and their heritable effects [2]. Epigenetics refers to those mechanisms that act above the expression of genes and that have particular application when considering the indirect effects of environmental chemicals. The term was first proposed by the developmental biologist, Conrad H. Waddington [3]. He noted that heat-treated Drosophila pupae developed altered wing patterns that persisted trans-generationally [4]. He referred to this phenomenon as "genetic assimilation" or "epigenetics." This recognition has expanded the previous gene-centric viewpoint to one which includes the possibility of "nongenomic inheritance," explaining the complex variations between individuals and adaptive, as well as maladaptive, alterations that result from environmental changes or exposure [5, 6]. Primary epigenetic modifiers include histone modification, DNA methylation, and non-coding RNAs. These modifications control genome stability, gene imprinting, reprogramming of nonimprinted genes, X-chromosome inactivation, and the plasticity of gene expression resulting in the permanent alteration of structure and function of multiple organs.

Multiple animal studies point to an association between environmental synthetic chemicals, or xenobiotics, and human reproduction and development. However, the direct and indirect, multiple, long-term, and recently recognized

C.M. Peterson (✉)
Utah Center for Reproductive Medicine, Department of Obstetrics and Gynecology, University of Utah School of Medicine, 30 N. Medical Drive, 2B200, Salt Lake City, UT, 84132, USA
e-mail: c.matthew.peterson@hsc.utah.edu

D.T. Carrell
Departments of Surgery (Urology), Obstetrics and Gynecology, and Physiology, University of Utah School of Medicine, Salt Lake City, UT, USA

M. Varner
Department of Obstetrics and Gynecology, University of Utah school of Medicine, Salt Lake City, UT, USA

J. Stanford
Department of Family and Preventive Medicine, University of Utah Health Sciences Center, Salt Lake City, UT, USA

M. Croughan
Departments of Obstetrics, Gynecology, Reproductive Sciences, and Epidemiology and Biostatistics, University of California, San Francisco, CA, USA

G.B. Louis
Epidemiology Branch, Division of Epidemiology, Statistics, and Prevention Research, Eunice Kennedy Shriver National Institute of Child Health and Human Development, Bethesda, MD, USA

D.T. Carrell and C.M. Peterson (eds.), *Reproductive Endocrinology and Infertility: Integrating Modern Clinical and Laboratory Practice*, 781
DOI 10.1007/978-1-4419-1436-1_55, © Springer Science+Business Media, LLC 2010

epigenetic effects of such substances – individually, cumulatively, and in high- and low-dose exposures – on humans are only understood in a cursory fashion. This chapter reviews our preliminary understanding of both the direct and indirect endocrine disrupting and potential epigenetic effects of environmental EDCs on reproduction, and the important role investigations will play in the future of reproductive endocrinology. As a platform for discussion, endometriosis is examined as a potential marker for the reproductive impact of specific endocrine disrupting chemicals. Furthermore, previously identified environmental chemicals and contaminants with reproductive effects are introduced in Table 55.1, along with a summary of their documented animal, cell line and human adverse reproductive effects. PubMed search terms used to identify adverse reproductive effects detailed in Table 55.1 include all chemicals/contaminants identified combined with the search terms: abortion, birth defect, fertility, endometriosis, menstrual irregularity, reproduction, reproductive tract, and sperm.

55.2 The Chemical Substance Inventory

There are now over 87,000 known chemical substances in commerce in the United States [7]. Unfortunately, the majority of these chemicals never have been specifically tested for reproductive and/or developmental toxicity. Studies now suggest that many of these chemicals may bioaccumulate and biomagnify within the food chain [8, 9], and even combine to deliver a total body burden within toxic exposure ranges. Contemporary human toxicity testing of synthetic chemicals has yet to: systematically characterize; assess potential additive chemical interactions; determine epigenetic effects; or define the dosing responsible for the mechanisms of action (Environmental Working Group 2003; Physicians for Social Responsibility 2003) [10].

55.3 Identified Environmental Chemicals and Contaminants

A number of unregulated chemicals and contaminants are found in toys, beauty products, pets, homes, lawns, food and beverage containers, automobiles, fabrics, carpets, furniture, building materials, electrical equipment, and agricultural products. They permeate our air, food, homes, transportation systems, schools, soil, water, and workplaces. Concern regarding the reproductive effects of these contaminants is justified in light of accumulating animal evidence. In February 2005, the Stanford University School of Medicine's Women's Health and the Collaborative on Health and the Environment convened a multidisciplinary group of experts to assess the contribution of environmental chemicals and contaminants to human infertility. A list of concerning chemicals/contaminants are found in their summary report (http://www.healthandenvironment.org/working_groups/fertility).

Subsequently, this list of environmental chemicals and contaminants was expanded to include not only male and female effects, but was divided into adult exposures and developmental exposures [11]. A majority of the environmental chemicals/contaminants identified in those documents are presented in Table 55.1. Table 55.1 utilizes the identified environmental chemicals/contaminants and the PubMed search strategy listed above to detail our current knowledge of animal/cell line and human adverse reproductive effects.

A number of the chemicals/contaminants listed in Table 55.1, as well as pharmaceutical chemicals, are excreted in the urine and enter the sewer system. Wastewater treatment plants have avoided regulating these chemicals and contaminants. Furthermore, many compounds resist filtration during municipal waste treatment processes. During testing for Organic Wastewater Contaminants, scientists found prescription and nonprescription drugs and their metabolites, fragrance compounds, flame retardants, plasticizers, and cosmetic contaminants in each sample [12]. The authors concluded that the tap water in 42 states is contaminated with more than 140 unregulated chemicals that presently lack safety standards [13].

In a recent exposure study, it was noted that all 150 environmental contaminants studied were found in some segment of the US population and that the majority of the US population is measurably exposed to tobacco smoke, lead, mercury, and phthalates [14]. Increasingly, reproductive medicine specialists will be asked to weigh in with couples regarding the risk of various environmental and occupational chemicals and contaminants. An understanding of the individual and cumulative risks of various exposures, including those associated with assisted reproductive techniques, will be important in providing an appropriate perspective, reassurance, as well as precautionary evidence-based information.

55.4 Reproductive Concerns Regarding Environmental Chemicals and Contaminants

A broad range of studies now document significant reproductive concerns with environmental chemicals/contaminants in a number of species. Biologists now report that male fish in detergent-contaminated water express female characteristics [15], turtles can be sex-reversed by polychlorinated biphenyls

Table 55.1 Reproductive health effects of environmental and occupational chemical/contaminant exposure in animal/human cell lines and relevant human studies

Substance	Animal/cell line effects	Human effects
Arsenic (As) – treated lumber and contaminated drinking water are the most common exposures	Adrenal and ovarian tumors and cardiovascular disease [87, 88]	Birth defects [89]
Bisphenol A (BPA) – critical in polycarbonate plastic and epoxy resins Found in: adhesives, baby toys, CD and DVDs, cell phones, computers, enamels, dental sealants, hard plastic water bottles, sports helmets and safety products, automobiles, protective lining of food and drink cans, microwaveable and/or reuseable food and drink containers, plastic baby bottles, pacifiers, paints, and varnishes; Canadian government recently banned their use in food and beverage containers for children	Decreased birth weight [90] Hormonal changes [90, 91] Mammary and prostate cancer [21–23] Obesity [92] Oocyte chromosome abnormalities [93] Recurrent miscarriage [94] Altered prostate development [95, 96] Altered pubertal onset [92] Deceased semen quality [91, 92, 95–98]	
Cadmium – found in industrial and consumer products including batteries, pigments, metal alloys and coatings, and plastics	DNA methylation alterations [99, 100]Reduced fertility [101] Birth defects [102] Low birth weight [103] Immune parameters changes [104] Decreased ovarian reserve in offspring [105] Reduced assisted reproduction rates [106] Impaired follicle development [107] Decreased reproductive development in male offspring [108]	Fetal loss [109–111] Reduced fertility [101, 110–115] Hormonal changes [110, 113, 114, 116, 117] Menstrual irregularities [110, 115] Altered pubertal onset [118] Abnormal sperm [113, 119, 120]
Chromium	Sperm cell development abnormalities[121, 122] Germ cell abnormalities [123]	
Cigarette smoke	DNA damage [124]	Reduced fertility [101, 104, 105, 125–130] Birth defects [131–136] Small for gestational age [137] Hormonal changes [126, 138] Early menopause [126] IUGR [139] Low birth weight [139, 140] Preterm delivery [139, 141, 142] Miscarriage [126] Decreased semen quality [126, 138, 143–145] Ovarian failure [146] Reduced assisted reproduction [147]
Coumestrol	Hypermethylation of oncogene c-H-ras [148] Hormonal changes [149] Gonad development [130, 150] Reproductive behavior [149]	Endometrial cancer [151]

(continued)

Table 55.1 (continued)

Substance	Animal/cell line effects	Human effects
Diethylstilbestrol (DES)	Testicular and uterine cancer [152–158]Altered gonad development [159, 160]	Reduced fertility [110, 117] Reproductive tract malformations [161] Miscarriage [110] Menstrual irregularities [110] Uterine fibroids [117] Sperm formation abnormalities [162] Altered sex ratio [163] Hypospadias [164]
Dioxin/furans – byproducts of manufacturing or burning of products that contain chlorine including industrial bleaching and polyvinyl chloride production; dioxin is a prototypical polyhalogenated (PHAH); estimated that 95% of exposure is through food Chlorinated hydrocarbon group	Altered estrus cycle [117] Reduced fertility [117] Malformations of reproductive tract [165–167] Decreased semen quality [167, 168] Delayed time to pregnancy [169] Altered spermatogenesis [170] Sexual precocity [171] Gene expression changes [172, 173] Altered sex ratio [174] Altered testicular development [175] Altered progesterone gene expression [176]	Endometriosis [32, 110, 177] Fetal loss [178–180] Reduced fertility [110, 179] Hormonal changes [110, 114, 179, 181–183] Malformations of reproductive tract [179] Altered menarche [118, 184–186] Menstrual irregularities [33, 110, 179, 183, 187–189] Altered pubertal onset [185, 190, 191] Decreased semen quality [178, 179, 192–195] Altered sex ratio [110, 113, 179, 196–198] Embryogenesis [199] Male reproductive axis [200]
Disinfectants – there are 600 compounds formed by the reactions of chemical disinfectants (most often chlorine containing) with organic materials; trihalomethananes and trichloroethylenes are most common	DNA hypomethylation [201] Menstrual irregularities [202]	Menstrual irregularities [196, 203–205] Problem birth [206]
(-)-Epigallocatechin-3-O-gallate (EGCG) – major catechin found in green tea (*Camellia sinensis* L. Ktze. (Theaceae)).	DNA methylation [207, 208]	
Ethylene oxide – chemical sterilizer used in medical and dental practices		Fetal loss [110, 125] Miscarriage in female partner [125, 209] Decrease semen quality [125]
Fat intake	Mammary gland tumors [210] Altered male gonad development [211]	
Glucose intake	DNA demethylation alteration [212] Decreased oocyte and embryo quality [213]	Type II diabetes and obesity [214] Male fertility [215] Reduced fertility [216]
Glycol ethers – used in paints, varnishes, thinners, printing inks, electronics, semiconductors, leather, photographic film, varnishes, enamels, cosmetics, perfumes, brake fluids, wood stains		Fetal loss [217, 218] Reduced fertility [217, 219–222] Longer menstrual cycles [223] Decreased semen quality [113, 218] Birth defects [224]

Lead – found in batteries, ammunition, metal products, X-ray shields; previously a component of gasoline, paints, ceramic items, caulking, and pipe solder; most common exposures in the United States are paint in older homes, lead-containing house dust, soil, and vinyl	Tumorigenesis [225] Brain and liver toxicity [226]	Fetal loss [109–111] Reduced fertility [110, 111, 113, 114, 227] Hormonal changes [110, 113, 114, 116, 117] Menstrual irregularities [110, 228] Altered pubertal onset [118, 229, 230] Abnormal sperm [113, 119, 120] Miscarriage [231] Preterm birth [231] Low birth weight [231]
Nickel	Carcinogenesis [220, 232]	
Manganese – found in batteries, dietary supplements, ceramics, and fertilizers; a gasoline additive	Premature puberty [233, 234] Oxidative stress indicators increased [235] Abnormal sperm [236]	Fetal loss [109–111] Reduced fertility [110, 111, 113, 114] Hormonal changes [110, 113, 114, 116, 117] Menstrual irregularities [110] Altered pubertal onset [118, 229, 230] Abnormal sperm [113] Intrauterine growth retardation [237] Behavioral disinhibition [238]
Mercury – found in thermometers, dental fillings, and batteries; air and water contamination by industry and coal and waste incineration; contaminated seafood is the most common exposure in the United States	Abnormal sperm [239]	Fetal loss [109–111]Reduced fertility [110–114, 240] Hormonal changes [110, 113, 114, 116, 117] Menstrual irregularities [110] Altered pubertal onset [118] Abnormal sperm [113] Impaired neurodevelopment [241]
Octylphenol, nonylphenol – used to make surfactants (detergents), pesticides, paints, plasticizers and UV stabilizers in plastics; main exposure through the water and runoff	Hormonal changes [91, 117, 242] Altered pubertal development [243] Decreased semen quality [91, 244] Decreased testes size [242, 244] Gene expression changes [245, 246] Testicular dysgenesis [123] Sulfotransferase inhibition [247] Anemia [248]	

(continued)

Table 55.1 (continued)

Substance	Animal/cell line effects	Human effects
Organochlorine pestcides – primarily, insecticides like DDT, chlordane, Mirex, Aldrin, and HCB; banned in the United States; bioaccumulate in the environment Chlorinated hydrocarbon group	Altered estrus cycle [117] Reduced fertility [117] Malformations of reproductive tract [165–167] Decreased semen quality [167, 168] Delayed time to pregnancy [169] Male gonadotoxicity [249, 250]	Endometriosis [32, 110, 177] Fetal loss [178–180] Reduced fertility [110, 179] Hormonal changes [110, 114, 179, 181–183] Malformations of reproductive tract [179] Altered menarche [118, 184–186] Menstrual irregularities [33, 110, 179, 183, 187–189] Altered pubertal onset [185, 190, 191] Decreased semen quality [178, 179, 192] Altered sex ratio [110, 113, 179, 196, 197, 251] Miscarriage [252] Infertility [252] Cryptorchism [253] Delayed time to pregnancy [254] Sperm chromatin integrity [255]
Pentachlorophenol – coating/preservative for telephone poles, utility poles, railroad Chlorinated hydrocarbon group	Altered estrus cycle [117] Reduced fertility [117] Malformations of reproductive tract [165–167] Decreased semen quality [167, 168] Delayed time to pregnancy [169]	Endometriosis [32, 110, 177] Fetal loss [178–180] Reduced fertility [110, 179] Hormonal changes [110, 114, 179, 181–183] Malformations of reproductive tract [179] Altered menarche [118, 184, 185, 190] Menstrual irregularities [33, 110, 179, 183, 187–189] Altered pubertal onset [185, 190, 191] Decreased semen quality [178, 179, 192] Altered sex ratio [110, 113, 179, 196, 197]
Pesticides – includes insecticides, fungicides, fumigants, herbicides, rodenticides used in or around food, home, and industrial settings; exposures occur in home, food, or drinking water exposures	Malformations of reproductive tract [256, 257] Altered pubertal onset [258–260] Male CYP enzyme inhibition [261] Reduced male androgen synthesis [262] Decreased sperm concentration [263] Transgenerational reproductive effects [264, 265] Male sexual differentiation effects [123, 200, 266]	Reduced fetal growth (IUGR) [267–269] Reduced fertility [114, 125, 252, 270–276] Hormonal changes [113, 114, 277] Menstrual irregularities [188, 278] Miscarriage in female partner [252, 274, 279–283] Malformations of reproductive tract [284, 285] Altered sex ratio [113, 286] Deceased semen quality [114, 218, 287, 288] Sperm chromosomes abnormalities [289, 290] Ovarian development [291] Implantation [291] Adverse pregnancy outcomes [292] Testicular germ cell tumors [293] Sperm damage [195, 294]

Perflourinated compounds (PFOS, PFOAs) – used in textiles and carpets for stain and water-resistance, coatings for cooking pans, floor polish, insecticides, food wrap coatings; accumulate environment and food chain	Decreased birth weight [295] Fetal loss [295, 296] Hormonal changes [297] Immune system alterations [298]	Reduced birth length and abdominal circumference [299] Reduced birth weight [300]
Polybrominated diphenol ethers (PBDEs) – used as a flame retardant in furniture foam, textiles, mattresses, computers, and electronics	Decreased semen quality [301] Alter steroidogenesis [302] Sexual development and behavior [303]	Cryptorchidism [304]
Polychlorinated biphenols (PCBs) – found in industrial insulators and lubricants; bioaccumulates and persistent; banned in United States in 1976Chlorinated hydrocarbon group	Altered estrus cycle [117] Reduced fertility [117] Malformations of reproductive tract [165–167] Decreased semen quality [167, 168] Delayed time to pregnancy [169] Altered AhR activities [305] Vitamin A and thyroid homeostasis [306]	Endometriosis [32, 110, 177] Fetal loss [178–180] Reduced fertility [110, 179] Hormonal changes [110, 114, 179, 181–183] Malformations of reproductive tract [179] Altered menarche [118, 184–186] Menstrual irregularities [33, 110, 179, 183, 187–189] Altered pubertal onset [185, 190, 191] Decreased semen quality [178, 179, 192] Altered sex ratio [110, 113, 179, 196, 197, 307]
Phthalates – plasticizers added to soften PVC; also found in cosmetics, perfumes, toys, pharmaceuticals, medical devices, lubricants and wood finishes; some banned in Europe	Fetal loss [110] Hormonal changes [308] Shortened anogenital distance [309] Malformations in reproductive tract [308] Decreased semen quality [308, 310] Decreased testicular steroidogenic activity [195, 311, 312] Antiandrogenic activity [313–315] Hypospadias [316, 317]	Endometriosis [318, 319] Reduced fertility [320] Early menarche [190] Decreased semen quality [309] Altered birth weight [321] Altered sperm concentration [322]
Solvents – benzene, toluene, xylene, styrene, 1- bromopropane, perchloroethyelene, and trichloroethylene and others; used in plastics, resins, nylon, synthetic fibers, rubbers, lubricants, dyes, detergents, drugs, pesticides, glues, paints, paint thinners, fingernail polish, lacquers, printing and leather tanning processes, insulation, fiberglass, food containers, carpet backing, cleaning products, and a component of cigarette smoke; exposures are mainly through the air; referred to as volatile and semivolatile organic chemicals (VOC and SVOCs)	Reduced fertilization [323] Decreased spermatogenesis [324–326]	Fetal loss [110, 114, 125, 327] Reduced fertility [125, 126, 328–331] Hormonal changes [177] Miscarriage in female partner [125] Menstrual irregularities [110, 114, 125] Deceased semen quality [111, 113, 125, 330, 332, 333] Luteal dysfunction [334] Reproductive tract abnormalities [335]

Fecundity is the biologic capacity for reproduction regardless of pregnancy intentions. Fertility is demonstrated fecundity as measured by live births. Reduced fertility includes sterility, infertility (infecund), and impaired fecundity. Hormonal changes involve abnormalities in the normal pattern of sex steroid or gonadotropin secretion. Malformations of reproductive tract comprise shortened anogenital distance in animals, hypospadias, cryptorchidism, hypoplastic ovaries or testes, and epididymal abnormalities, and structural abnormalities of the ovaries, fallopian tubes, uterus, cervix, or vagina. Menstrual irregularities denote amenorrhea, meno/menometrorrhagia, oligo/anovulation. Decreased sperm quality is defined as oligo/terato/astheno/spermia individually or combined and low semen volume

(PCBs) [16], male frogs exposed to a common herbicide form multiple ovaries [17], pseudohermaphroditic offspring are produced by polar bears exposed to endocrine disruptors [18], seals in contaminated water have an excess of uterine fibroids [19], and normal human development may be altered by exposure to estrogenic chemicals [20]. Developmental exposure to bisphenol A (BPA) has been associated with morphologic and functional abnormalities of the genital tract and mammary gland, infertility and breast and prostate malignancies [21, 22]. Finally, neonatal exposure to BPA at environmentally relevant levels in mice results in alteration of the prostate genome [23]. Specifically, prostate phosphodiesterase type 4 variant 4 (PDE4D4) is the target of BPA-induced epigenetic reprogramming. PDE4D4 normally undergoes age-dependent transcriptional silencing via progressive hypermethylation of its promoter. Neonatal exposure of male mice to BPA or estrogen disengages the predestined silencing and, hence, may predispose to prostatic hypertrophy or precancerous lesions [23].

55.5 Endocrine Disruption Study Design Challenges

The identification and characterization of "early exposure–late effect" patterns of insult by endocrine disruptors (direct, indirect, reproductive, and epigenetic) pose significant challenges for investigators. To address some of these challenges, there is an ongoing international effort to develop, validate, and update contemporary animal toxicological testing methodologies. The 28-day oral toxicity study (Organization for Economic Co-operation and Development (OECD) Guideline 407), and the routine subacute toxicity test applied to chemicals, has been enhanced to now detect potential endocrine disrupting actions by adding measurements that include serum hormone concentrations, estrus cycle features and weights of endocrine-related organs (ovaries, uterus, testis, prostate, and other organs [24]). The assay remains, however, inadequate in fully characterizing dose–response relationships, varying durations of exposures and developmental stages at exposure.

The two-generation reproductive toxicity study (OECD Guideline, 416) is used to evaluate alterations in endocrine homeostasis during the entire developmental and reproductive period. Because exposure to endocrine disruptors is continual across the lifespan, multigenerational studies administer the test chemical continuously to parental (P) and subsequent offspring generations (F1, F2…). This testing protocol provides more information regarding effects on male and female reproductive performance, and fertility. Furthermore, pregnancy outcomes, maternal lactation and offspring care, prenatal and postnatal health and survival, growth and development of the offspring, subsequent reproductive capacity, as well as potential epigenetic effects may also be evaluated. Presently, these multigenerational studies are the only reliable, nonhuman, experimental tools for the identification of environmental chemicals with the complex exposure patterns described, and potentially pervasive effects on all aspects of reproduction.

Contemporary epidemiologic studies seek to identify reproductive and/or developmental toxicants. Not only does such work attempt to identify critical doses, but also the additive and/or syngeristic effects of chemical mixtures in keeping with the manner in which humans are exposed. Careful attention to the epidemiologic method is required to ensure valid results. Unfortunately, credible studies using current experimental models demonstrate equivocal low-dose effects with the same chemicals (National Institute of Environmental Health Sciences 2001). Thus, while increasingly sensitive screening programs and experimental models for chemicals and pesticides with low-dose endocrine disrupting effects are under development, adequately powered epidemiologic studies with individually (or pooled) measured concentrations reflecting dose are still needed. An example of such a study is the ENDO Study funded by the Eunice Kennedy Shriver National Institute of Child Health and Development (http://www.endostudy.utah.edu). The ENDO Study's aim is to determine if environmentally relevant concentrations of persistent organochlorine compounds (e.g., PCBs, DDT) are associated with endometriosis or other gynecologic pathology. Transdisciplinary approaches are needed (e.g., epidemiology, gynecology, biostatistics, toxicology, risk assessment) for answering the many critical data gaps and in communicating findings to targeted populations.

55.6 Endometriosis: A Marker for Endocrine Disruption

In light of the available experimental and human data, concerted study of EDCs and endometriosis is needed. This is further underscored by the marked declines in human fertility as measured by the number of live births throughout the developed and, increasingly the developing, world. These trends support the interplay of both macro (e.g., environmental pollution) and micro (e.g., behavior, diet) factors affecting human fecundity and fertility. Increased prevalence of gynecologic (and urologic) diseases may be an earlier marker of diminished human fecundity, defined as the biologic capacity of men and women for reproduction irrespective of pregnancy intentions. Recognition of a purported relation between dioxin, (2,3,7,8-tetrachlorodibenzo-p-dioxin or TCDD), and endometriosis first emerged in 1993 when Rier and colleagues reported a significant dose-dependent increase in the incidence and severity of endometriosis in exposed Rhesus monkeys [25]. Subsequently, Yang et al. investigated the effects of dioxin on survival and growth of ectopic endometrium in monkeys following auto transplantation [26]. Additional evidence supporting an association between PHAHs and endometriosis arose from experimental studies involving rodents in whom human endometrial implants were surgically transplanted [27]. In addition, endometriosis has been experimentally produced in rats and mice following surgical placement of endometriosis and repeated dioxin exposure [28]. These findings support dioxin's ability to promote the growth of surgically placed endometriosis in species that normally do not develop endometriosis.

Human evidence for an association between dioxin, PHAHs and PCBs primarily comes from seven published studies, available at the time this chapter was prepared. Four research groups reported significant positive associations between dioxin [29] and PCBs [30–32] and endometriosis. Two studies noted twofold to fourfold increases in risk of endometriosis in relation to dioxin and PCB exposure, respectively, but had confidence intervals inclusive of 1 [33–35], respectively. One final study failed to find an association between PCB congeners and endometriosis [36]. A clinical study comprising women with peritoneal endometriosis or deep endometriotic nodules compared with control women seeking gynecologic consultation for unknown reasons also reported higher concentrations of total toxic equivalency quotients (TEQ) levels for PCDDs, PCDFs, and dioxin-like PCBs. However, laparoscopic confirmation of disease was not required nor did final logistic models retain potential confounders [37].

Ecologic evidence is consistent with observational research. Specifically, Belgium has some of the highest breast milk dioxin concentrations in the world, and also a high prevalence of endometriosis [38]. Significantly, higher incidence rates of endometriosis were reported among women aged 25–44 years who resided in federally or state-designated national priority and superfund sites and who were discharged from New York State hospitals in comparison to three other groups of women: (1) New York State resident women, (2) Upstate New York (exclusive of New York City) women residing in geographic areas without concern, and (3) Upstate New York residents residing in other federal or state superfund sites [39].

While the pathophysiologic mechanisms underlying exposure to dioxin and other PHAHs and the development of endometriosis are not fully documented, a number of pathways have been suggested: (1) alterations in the synthesis and metabolism of estradiol; (2) alterations in the production of proinflammatory growth factors or cytokines; and (3) misexpression of remodeling enzymes [40]. Exposure profiles of PHAHs in humans and primates have been compared. Rier and Foster compared lipid adjusted body burdens of PCDDs, PCDFs, PCBs, and total PHAHs (ppt) in human and monkey samples and reported 2–20-fold higher concentrations in humans than TCDD-exposed monkeys with endometriosis [40]. These findings suggest that current background exposures for human females may be in the range where adverse human health effects could be anticipated. The facts described above and the ubiquitous nature of endocrine-disrupting chemicals raise significant concerns and warrant further study. Some hypothesized xenobiotic mechanisms of action include: (1) altered enzyme pathways and/or gene-dependent activities; (2) reproductive impairments; and/or (3) transgenerational effects. A brief review of each follows.

55.7 Altered Enzyme Pathways and/or Gene-Dependent Activities

55.7.1 *The Arylhydrocarbon Receptor*

Dioxin is a general term that describes a group of polyhalogenated aromatic hydrocarbon (PHAHs) chemicals that are highly persistent in the environment. Tetrachlorodibenzo-p-dioxin (TCDD) is the prototypical polyhalogenated aromatic hydrocarbon (PHAH), whose chemical structure is illustrated in Fig. 55.1. Dioxin is an unintentional by-product of many industrial processes involving chlorine such as waste incineration, chemical and pesticide manufacturing, and pulp or paper bleaching. It was the primary toxic component of Agent Orange, the pollutant found at Love Canal in Niagara Falls, NY and was the basis for evacuations at Times Beach, MO and Seveso, Italy. Dioxin and related chemicals resist degradation and, therefore, bioaccumulate and biomagnify within the food chain because of their lipophilic nature. The ingestion of contaminated foods is the most common source of TCDD and PHAH exposure in humans. Industrial accidents, accidental exposures, and wartime are additional sources of acute exposure. The xenobiotics PHAH, PCDD, PCDF, PCBs possess endocrine disrupting activities, having an affinity for the arylhydrocarbon receptor (AhR).

Multiple studies suggest that the toxicity of (TCDD) and other PHAH-like chemicals is mediated via the arylhydrocarbon receptor [41–45]. The cytosolic AhR has a basic helix–loop–helix configuration, which acts as a signal transducer

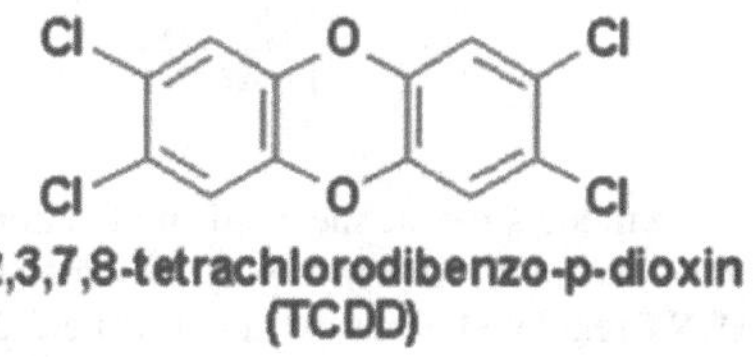

Fig. 55.1 Structure of dioxin (TCDD)

and transcription factor. With receptor activation, the receptor–ligand complex is translocated by the AhR nuclear translocator (ARNT) to the nucleus resulting in subsequent transcriptional activation. Targeted genes of this activation complex include the cytochrome P-450 complex [42] as well as genes involved in cellular growth, differentiation, immune regulation, and inflammation. A number of potential mechanisms of TCDD action have been proposed [43] (Fig. 55.2). Other xenobiotics demonstrating a high affinity for AhR with similar toxic effects include polychlorinated dibenzo-p-dioxins (PCDDs) and dibenzofurans (PCDFs) substituted in the 2,3,7,8 lateral positions. Additionally, nonortho and monoortho polychlorinated biphenyls (PCBs) are AhR agonists and participate in the toxicity of PHAHs [44–49].

55.7.1.1 Ahr Activation and Its Effect on Cytochrome P450 Aromatase

Human endometrial explants treated with TCDD demonstrate increased expression of AhR mRNA as well as the mRNA of the dioxin-responsive gene P-4501A [46, 47]. Ovarian endometriotic cells also demonstrate increased AhR mRNA and an eightfold increase in P-4501A1 mRNA compared to uterine endometrium [48, 49]. Endometriotic tissues demonstrate increased expression of P-450 aromatase, and de novo estrogen synthesis [50] and endometriotic lesions have been observed to regress following treatment with an aromatase inhibitor indicating a role for aromatase in the maintenance of the lesions [51]. Therefore, dioxins may act to promote endometriosis through aberrant activation/induction of P-450 isoenzyme expression and the resultant local increase in estrogen production and its growth-enhancing estrogenic effects on the endometriotic tissues as well as other possible agonist and antagonistic effects (Fig. 55.2). Of concern to toxicologists is the myriad of AhR-interacting xenobiotics. A number of outcomes with AhR and ARNT are possible including the direct effect of the activation of AHR-ARNT-regulated genes or an indirect effect resulting from decreased availability of either the AHR or ARNT to participate in different transactivation complexes [45–50] (Fig. 55.2).

55.7.1.2 Activation of Inflammatory Cascades

Endometriosis is associated with chronic inflammation and local expression of proinflammatory mediators and cytokines by the ectopic endometriotic cells and associated leukocytes. These inflammatory mediators affect endometrial growth, tissue remodeling and immune system function. The role of dioxin in the creation of inflammatory cytokines

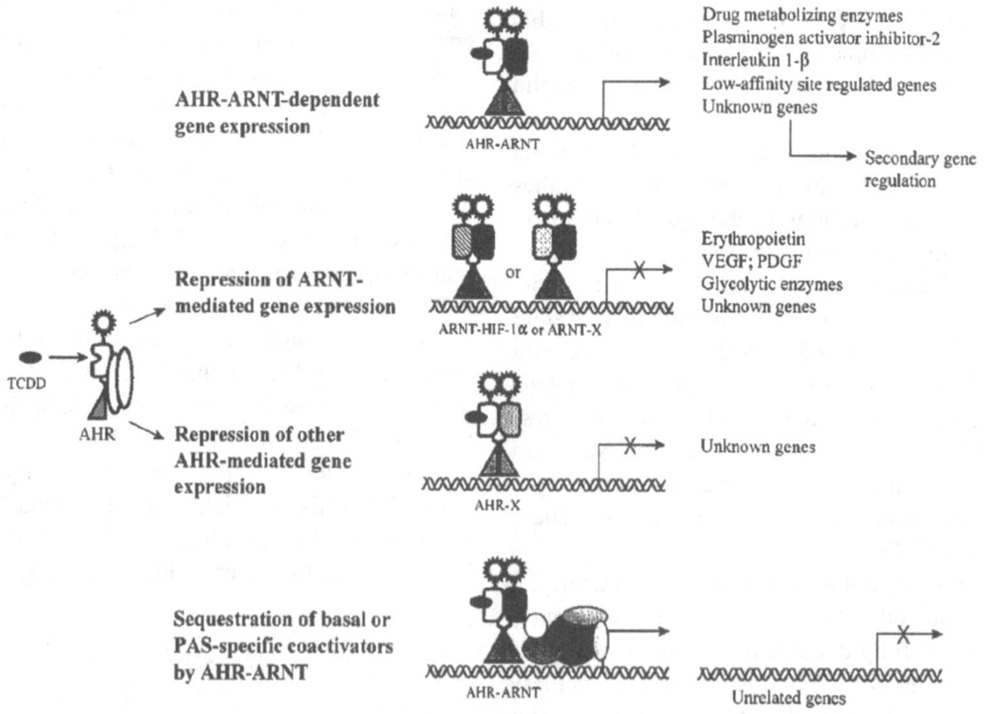

Fig. 55.2 Possible models for the mechanism of action of TCDD toxicity, which most likely results from alterations in gene expression induced by arylhydrocarbon receptor (AHR) – arylhydrocarbon receptor nuclear translocator ARNT activity. This may be either a direct effect of the activation of AHR-ARNT-regulated genes or an indirect effect resulting from a decrease in the availability of either the AHR or ARNT to participate in different transactivation complexes [45]. (Reprinted from Schmidt JV, Bradfield CA. Ah receptor signaling pathways. Annu Rev Cell Dev Biol 1996;12:55–89 with permission from Elsevier)

interleukins 1 and 6 (IL-1, Il-6), tumor necrosis factor- alpha (TNF-α), interferon gamma (IFN-gamma), transforming growth factors (TGF-α, TGF-α), and remodeling matrix metalloproteinase enzymes (MMPs) is well-documented including within endometriotic tissues [52, 53]. Furthermore, the dioxin-response element (DRE) of AhR is present in the genes of many potent inflammatory mediators including TNF-alpha, IL-1b, IL-6, and IFN-gamma [54, 55].

In particular, the cytokine TNF-α may play a significant role in TCDD-induced toxicity and promotion of endometriosis. Both TCDD and TNF-alpha administration to rodents enhanced the leukocyte inflammatory responses and cellular infiltration of macrophages and neutrophils into the peritoneal cavity following antigenic challenge that could be blocked by neutralizing the endogenous TNF-α activity [56]. Other investigators have shown that acute TCDD exposure increases both peritoneal and peripheral blood leukocyte production of TNF-α [57]. Moreover, the fact that dexamethasone or TNF antibody can reverse the morbidity or mortality associated with TCDD toxicity in the rodent serve as additional evidence implicating TNF-α [58]. Activating the inflammatory network locally results in the production of cyclooxygenase 2 (COX-2) and prostaglandin E2 (PGE2), which also induces chronic local estrogen production that may foster the development and maintenance endometriotic lesions [59, 60]. In addition to the induction of increased estradiol production, activation of the inflammatory network also suppresses progesterone action causing an increase in estradiol production [61], and causes the misexpression of the remodeling enzymes matrix metalloproteinases (MMPs) [27, 53, 62–64], which may prolong endometriotic cell survival [65, 66]. Dioxin has been shown to facilitate the survival of endometrial implants in cynmologous monkeys [26].

55.7.1.3 Local Dysregulation of Steroidogenesis

Although the total amount of estrogen produced locally by endometriotic lesions through aromatase activity is small, its local biological effect may be substantial. Aromatase activity in endometriosis has been extensively studied [60, 61, 67]. High levels of aromatase expression in the endometriotic lesions, a positive feedback loop involving PGE2, and increased aromatase mRNA in the eutopic (intrauterine) endometrial samples of women with moderate or severe endometriosis, but not in disease free (intrauterine) endometrial samples, are some of the notable findings in these studies. Recent studies confirm that local dysregulation of aromatase plays a significant role in local estrogen production [68].

The most important substrate for aromatase in endometriotic lesions is androstenedione giving rise to estrone (E1), a weak estrogen. For full activity, E1 must be converted to estradiol (E2). The 17β hydroxysteroid dehydrogenase (17β-HSD) enzyme is key in the biosynthesis of both estradiol and testosterone, with 17β-HSD type 1 catalyzing the conversion of E1 to E2 and 17β-HSD type 2 converting E2 to E1 [69, 70]. Progesterone stimulates 17β-HSD type 2 activity, however, in endometriotic lesions, 17β-HSD type 2 activity in the epithelium is deficient, giving rise to locally increased levels of estradiol [71].

Although the evidence is indirect, TCDD has been shown to selectively downregulate stromal PR-B expression and increase matrix metalloproteinases (MMP) expression in both stromal and epithelial cells suggesting that exposure to this toxin may negatively impact P-mediated cell–cell communication (and possibly 17β-HSD type 2) in the human endometrium and likely also in endometriotic lesions [72]. TCDD alters tissue remodeling processes and promotes endometriosis by disrupting progesterone regulated expression of MMPs in a nude mouse model. The MMPs are critical to endometriosis establishment. Progesterone, in the absence of TCDD, suppresses MMP production. TCDD exposure blocks the routine progesterone induced suppression of MMP [27, 53, 62–64]. These studies provide background data suggesting an association between the agents of concern and the evolution of the endometriotic lesion in animal models. Their potential role in the development of endometriosis in women remains to be proven.

55.7.2 Abberant Endometriotic Gene Expression

Giudice and colleagues have elucidated the intrinsic abnormalities in gene expression of eutopic endometrium in women with endometriosis [73]. Some of the genes and gene products aberrantly expressed in eutopic endometrium of endometriosis patients include: aromatase, endometrial bleeding factor, 17β-hydroxysteroid dehydrogenease (17β-HSD), HoxA10, HoxA11, Leukemia inhibitory factor, matrix metalloproteinase 7 and 11, and the progesterone receptors. Endometriotic tissues may show dysregulation of the following genes or gene products compared to eutopic endometrium: matrix metalloproteinase 1, 2, 3, 7, 11; cathepsin D, plasminogen activator, vascular endothelial growth factor; aromatase; 17β-HSD, progesterone receptors, haptoglobin (ENDO-1); and, tumor necrosis factor α [74]. The complex patterns demonstrated suggest potential underlying genetic predispositions to the establishment of endometrial cells refluxed to the pelvic peritoneum. These genetic predispositions may set the stage for xenobiotic induced endometriosis and at the same time obscure the effects of xenobiotics in a study of endometriosis which does not also account for such predispositions. Thus, contemporary investigations must include adjustments for the genetic diversity in the population studied.

55.7.3 Reproductive Impairment

In addition to the disrupting events on enzyme pathways and/or gene-dependent activities noted above, the potential reproductive impairment resulting from environmentally induced endometriosis include the following observations in humans. Endometriosis is a leading cause of infertility and, therefore, a major health concern to our population. Endometriosis has a prevalence of 0.5–5% in fertile and 25–40% in infertile women as reported in a recent review [75]. Clearly the choice of the study population may have important implications when assessing the role of environmental factors and endometriosis. According to the Centers for Disease Control and Prevention [14], the number of couples who report difficulty becoming pregnant or carrying a pregnancy to term has grown from 6.1 million in 1995, to 7.3 million in 2002. Using data from the US National Survey of Family Growth, there has been cross-sectional evidence that infertility rates have continually increased for women aged 20–24 years and in black women. Worldwide data confirm the decline in fertility, but do not quantify responsible factors including behavior, biology, or a combination of the two (Fig. 55.3).

Few studies have estimated the incidence of endometriosis, especially in a population-based design. One notable exception was conducted in Rochester, Minnesota, from 1970–1979. The estimated age-specific incidence of surgically reported and histologically confirmed endometriosis among white women aged 25–29 and 30–34 years was 150 and 200 cases per 100,000 person years, respectively [77, 78]. The peak incidence was observed for women aged 40–44 years (approximately 350 cases/100,000 person-years) (Fig. 55.4). The National Hospital Discharge Survey indicated that the prevalence of endometriosis requiring hospitalization peaked between the ages of 40–44 years, supporting the age-specific incidence finding [79].

Using data from the Nurses Health Study, II, the incidence rate of endometriosis among women aged 25–29 years without a prior history of infertility was 300 cases/100,000 person-years [80] (Fig. 55.5). However, incidence increased to 3,360 cases/100,000 person-years among similarly aged infertile women. Diagnostic criteria, disease recognition, healthcare-seeking behavior including the increased utilization of laparoscopy may explain, in part, the increase in incidence. However, these findings also are consistent from an ecologic perspective of an environmental etiology.

In addition to the potential increase in the incidence of infertility and endometriosis, the outcomes of pregnancies associated with endometriosis may be compromised. In a recent retrospective cohort study, the preterm birth rate increased among women with ovarian endometriosis when

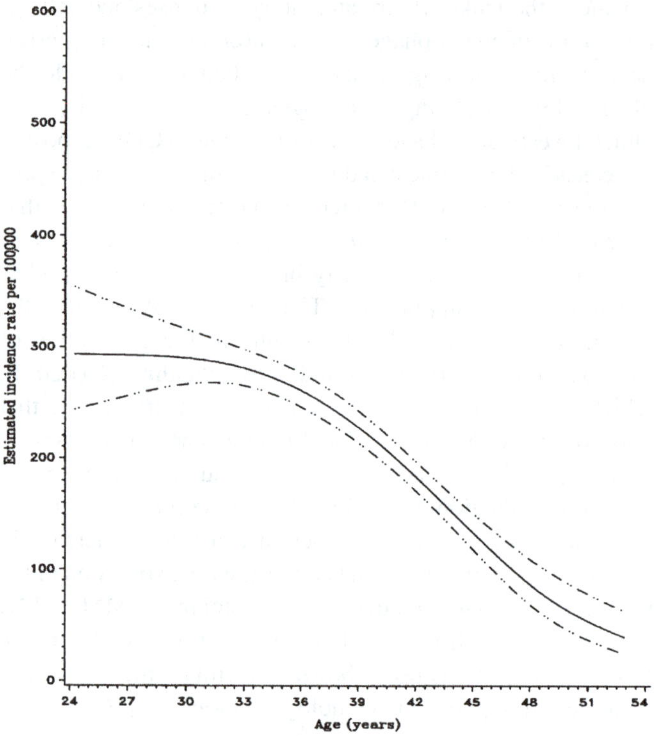

Fig. 55.4 Age-specific incidence rates of pelvic endometriosis per 100,000 person-years for white females 15–49 years of age in Rochester, MN, during 1970–1979, by types of cases included in rate numerators. *HC* histologically confirmed, *SV* surgically visualized, *CPR* clinically probable, *CPO* clinically possible [77, 78]. (Reprinted from Houston DE. Evidence for the risk of pelvic endometriosis by age, race and socioeconomic status. Epidemiol Rev 1984;6:167–191 by permission of Oxford University Press)

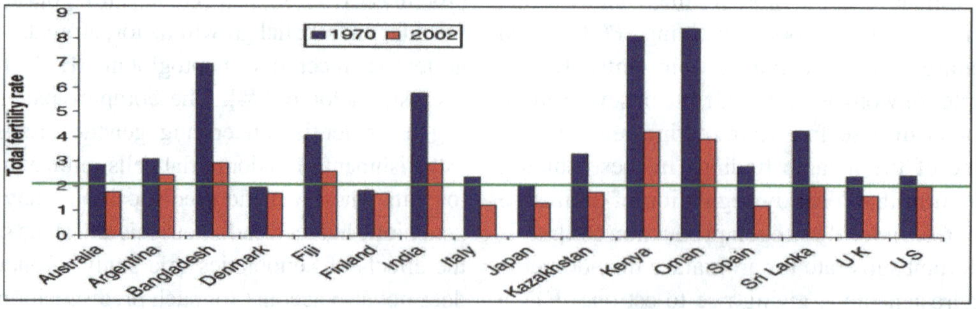

Fig. 55.3 Changes in fertility rates in developing and industrialized countries. The green line is the 2.1 fertility rate, which is necessary to sustain a population at its current level (from World Bank 2005) [76]. (Graph adapted from data provided by the World Bank)

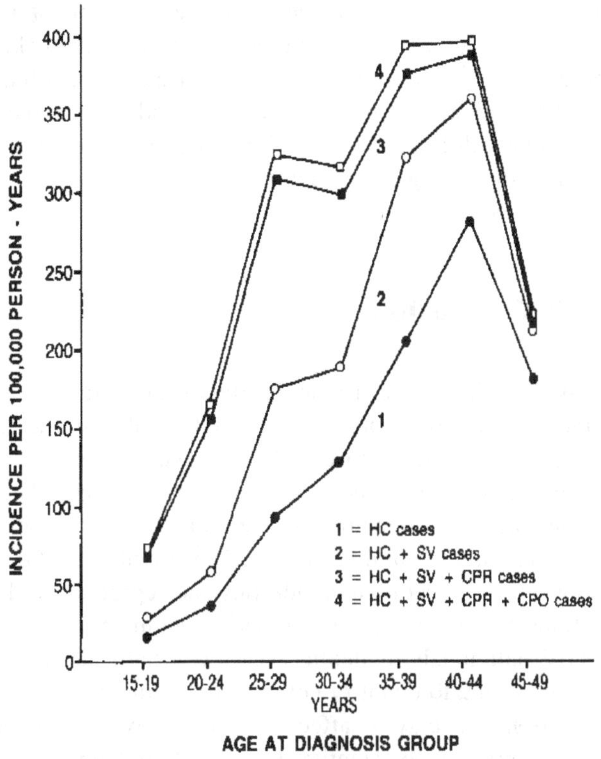

Fig. 55.5 Nonparametric regression curve of the age-specific incidence of laparoscopically confirmed endometriosis among premenopausal women with no past infertility in the Nurses' Health Study II (1989–1999) (not adjusted for covariates). *Dashed and dotted lines,* 95% confidence intervals [80]. (Reprinted from Missmer SA, Hankinson SE, Spiegelman D, Barbieri RL, Marshall LM, Hunter DJ. Incidence of laparoscopically confirmed endometriosis by demographic, anthropometric, and lifestyle factors. Am J Epidemiol 2004;160:784–796 by permission of Oxford University Press)

compared to unaffected women using community birth records ($n = 850{,}000$). Furthermore, in women with ovarian endometriomata utilizing assisted reproductive technologies, a statistically significant increase in small for gestational age (<10th percentile of weight for gestation) deliveries was found when compared to women with other forms of endometriosis [81].

55.7.4 Epigenetic Effects

While epigenetic alterations from endocrine disrupting chemicals are yet to be fully elucidated with regard to endometriosis, indirect evidence is accumulating. In a recent study, the expression of HOXA10 in the eutopic endometrium of baboons with induced endometriosis showed a notable decrease in HOXA10 mRNA which was observed after 12 and 16 months of disease. HOXA10 protein levels were decreased in both the epithelial and stromal cells of the endometrium. Furthermore, expression of beta 3 integrin (ITGB3), which is upregulated by HOXA10, was decreased, whereas EMX2, a gene that is inhibited by HOXA10, was increased. Methylation patterns of the HOXA10 gene were analyzed in both diseased and control animals. The F1 region on the promoter was found to be the most significantly methylated in the endometriosis animals, and this may account for the decrease in HOXA10 expression. These methylation patterns may set the stage for generational effects [82]. Although not yet identified in endometriosis, epigenetic effects of the PHAH endocrine disrupting chemicals has been reported by Couture and colleagues [83]. Exposure of mouse preimplantation embryos to TCDD was found to inhibit fetal growth in a response characterized by changes in the methylation status of the imprinted genes H19 and IGF [84]. Additionally, TCDD has been shown to induce histone modifications in normal human mammary epithelial cells [85].

55.8 Reproductive Health Effects of Environmental Chemical Exposure

Using endometriosis as an example for weighing evidence that environmental chemicals may affect gynecologic health, it is important to appreciate that other conditions may have a similar etiology. It remains plausible that a structural grouping or mixture of chemicals may give rise to various gynecologic disorders. Recently, some authors have suggested the need to develop a paradigm for considering the effects of EDCs on gynecologic health similar to the approach used for males. Borrowing from this collective body of work known as the testicular dysgenesis syndrome (TDS), Buck Louis and Cooney advocated for considering ovarian dysgenesis syndrome (ODS) [86]. To this end, the authors posit that in utero exposure to hormonally active agents such as EDCs may permanently reprogram the fetus and, thereby, increasing susceptibility for later onset gynecologic disorders. This hypothesis supports considering a spectrum of gynecologic disorders (e.g., endometriosis, fibroids, premature ovarian insufficiency, and polycystic ovaries) as possibly sharing similar etiologic mechanisms that arise in utero. As demonstrated using endometriosis as a marker, we have only a cursory knowledge of the potential reproductive health effects of environmental chemicals. Recently, the term Ovarian Dysgenesis Syndrome has been proposed for a number of adverse reproductive effects, including endometriosis, attributed to endocrine-disrupting chemicals as reviewed by Buck Louis and Cooney [86].

Table 55.1 summarizes select experimental and observational data including animal, human cell line and human data focusing on environmental exposures and their effect(s) on reproduction.

55.9 Actions

While the animal evidence for EDCs reproductive impairment and potential epigenetic affects has accumulated over time, epidemiologic research has lagged especially from a population perspective. In 1996, the EPA's Office of Research and Development identified endocrine disruption as one of its top six research priorities and developed a risk-based research approach to address concerns (http://www.epa.gov/ORD/WebPubs/final). Three long-term goals were identified:

First, providing a better understanding of the science underlying the effects, exposure, assessment, and risk management of endocrine disruptors. Research in this area includes determining dose–response relationships, the effects of exposure to multiple endocrine disruptors, major sources of exposure, and approaches for managing risks.

Second, determining the extent of the impact of endocrine disruptors on humans, wildlife, and the environment. Research includes determining what effects are occurring in human and wildlife populations, the chemical classes of greatest concern, the ambient levels of exposure, and how unreasonable risks can be mitigated.

Third, supporting EPA's screening and testing program. Developing needed computational tools as well as in vitro and in vivo assays in support of the implementation of a screening and testing program for endocrine disruptors, required by the 1996 Food Quality Protection Act.

The Eunice Kennedy Shriver National Institute of Child Health and Human Development is completing two population-based epidemiologic studies designed to evaluate a number of persistent environmental chemicals and their associations with couple fecundity and gynecologic disorders. (http://www.lifestudy.us and http://www.endostudy.utah.edu) Advocacy groups continue to press for additional studies, information, and regulation. Government agencies, in concert with advocacy and industry groups, hopefully will develop adequate testing paradigms, establish toxic exposure levels, clean up and eliminate documented endocrine disrupting chemicals, and recommend steps to avoid future unrecognized toxic exposures.

Scientists, health-care professionals, community activists, and politicians met in 2007 for the Summit on "Environmental Challenges to Reproductive Health and Fertility," wherein directions for the advancement of reproductive environmental health through research, health-care policy, and community action were outlined. These recommendations included: longitudinal animal and human studies including the full life cycle; leveraging existing mechanisms for data collection to include semen analyses into the CDC's NHANES study; biomarker discovery; overcoming regulatory obstacles; increased funding for research of individual and mixed chemical exposures, fetal programming and transgenerational effects, low-dose effects, nontraditional dose–response curves, cross-talk among endocrine receptors, and the identification of new emerging contaminants [11]. Future scientists in the field of reproductive endocrinology are well-advised to keep abreast of and participate in the basic, clinical and epidemiologic studies that will be required to keep our environment free of endocrine disrupting chemicals.

55.10 Conclusion

A considerable body of research offers support for an environmental etiology for adverse male and female reproductive effects gynecologic diseases. Of key concern are the hormonally active agents such as endocrine disrupting chemicals that may alter the synthesis, secretion, transport, binding, or elimination of natural hormones. The complexity of diagnosing many gynecologic conditions and reproductive dysfunctions coupled with the healthcare-seeking behaviors of affected individuals including access to healthcare make it difficult, as yet, to quantify how much and in what capacity the environment may be affecting reproductive and general health. Reproductive scientists have a role in helping to fill these and other critical data gaps. Working as a part of research teams to help recruit individuals, obtain biologic specimens for quantifying exposure or assessing biomarkers or disease susceptibility, as well as participating in interdisciplinary teams to develop strategies for communicating risk and uncertainty will be critical roles for reproductive specialists in the future.

References

1. Colborn T, vom Saal FS, Soto AM (1993) Developmental effects of endocrine-disrupting chemicals in wildlife and humans. Environ Health Perspect 101:378–384
2. Barker DJ (1994) Programming the baby. In: Mothers, babies and disease in later in life. BMJ Publishing Group, London, p 14–36
3. Van Speybroeck L (2002) From epigenesis to epigenetics: the case of C. H. Waddington. Ann N Y Acad Sci 981:61–81
4. Waddington CH (1957) The strategy of the genes: a discussion of some aspects of theoretical biology. Allen and Unwin, London
5. Godfrey KM, Lillycrop KA, Burdge GC, Gluckman PD, Hanson MA (2007) Epigenetic mechanisms and the mismatch concept of the developmental origins of health and disease. Pediatr Res 61:5R–10R
6. Jaenisch R, Bird A (2003) Epigenetic regulation of gene expression: how the genome integrates intrinsic and environmental signals. Nat Genet 33(Suppl):245–254
7. United States Environmental Protection Agency (2006) what is the chemical substance inventory? United States Environmental Protection Agency, Washington, DC
8. Kelly BC, Ikonomou MG, Blair JD, Morin AE, Gobas FA (2007) Food web-specific biomagnification of persistent organic pollutants. Science 317:236–239

9. Mackay D, Fraser A (2000) Kenneth Mellanby Review Award. Bioaccumulation of persistent organic chemicals: mechanisms and models. Environ Pollut 110:375–391
10. Myers J (2004) Gene expression and environmental exposures: new opportunities for disease prevention. San Franc Med 77:29–31
11. Woodruff TJ, Carlson A, Schwartz JM, Giudice LC (2008) Proceedings of the summit on environmental challenges to reproductive health and fertility: executive summary. Fertil Steril 89:281–300
12. Stackelberg PE, Furlong ET, Meyer MT, Zaugg SD, Henderson AK, Reissman DB (2004) Persistence of pharmaceutical compounds and other organic wastewater contaminants in a conventional drinking-water-treatment plant. Sci Total Environ 329:99–113
13. Environmental Working Group (2005) A national assessment of tap water quality. Environmental Working Group, Washington, DC
14. CDC (2005) Third national report on human exposure to environmental chemicals. Centers for Disease Control and Prevention, Atlanta, GA
15. Miles-Richardson SR, Pierens SL, Nichols KM et al (1999) Effects of waterborne exposure to 4-nonylphenol and nonylphenol ethoxylate on secondary sex characteristics and gonads of fathead minnows (*Pimephales promelas*). Environ Res 80:S122–S137
16. Willingham E, Crews D (1999) Sex reversal effects of environmentally relevant xenobiotic concentrations on the red-eared slider turtle, a species with temperature-dependent sex determination. Gen Comp Endocrinol 113:429–435
17. Hecker M, Giesy JP, Jones PD et al (2004) Plasma sex steroid concentrations and gonadal aromatase activities in African clawed frogs (*Xenopus laevis*) from South Africa. Environ Toxicol Chem 23:1996–2007
18. Wiig O, Derocher AE, Cronin MM, Skaare JU (1998) Female pseudohermaphrodite polar bears at Svalbard. J Wildl Dis 34:792–796
19. Backlin BM, Eriksson L, Olovsson M (2003) Histology of uterine leiomyoma and occurrence in relation to reproductive activity in the Baltic gray seal (*Halichoerus grypus*). Vet Pathol 40:175–180
20. Foster WG (1998) Endocrine disruptors and development of the reproductive system in the fetus and children: is there cause for concern? Can J Public Health 89(Suppl 1):S37–S41, S52, S41–S6
21. Maffini MV, Rubin BS, Sonnenschein C, Soto AM (2006) Endocrine disruptors and reproductive health: the case of bisphenol-A. Mol Cell Endocrinol 254–255:179–186
22. Welshons WV, Nagel SC, vom Saal FS (2006) Large effects from small exposures. III. Endocrine mechanisms mediating effects of bisphenol A at levels of human exposure. Endocrinology 147:S56–S69
23. Ho SM, Tang WY, Belmonte de Frausto J, Prins GS (2006) Developmental exposure to estradiol and bisphenol A increases susceptibility to prostate carcinogenesis and epigenetically regulates phosphodiesterase type 4 variant 4. Cancer Res 66:5624–5632
24. Kunimatsu T, Yamada T, Miyata K et al (2004) Evaluation for reliability and feasibility of the draft protocol for the enhanced rat 28-day subacute study (OECD Guideline 407) using androgen antagonist flutamide. Toxicology 200:77–89
25. Rier SE, Martin DC, Bowman RE, Dmowski WP, Becker JL (1993) Endometriosis in rhesus monkeys (*Macaca mulatta*) following chronic exposure to 2, 3, 7, 8-tetrachlorodibenzo-p-dioxin. Fundam Appl Toxicol 21:433–441
26. Yang JZ, Agarwal SK, Foster WG (2000) Subchronic exposure to 2, 3, 7, 8-tetrachlorodibenzo-p-dioxin modulates the pathophysiology of endometriosis in the cynomolgus monkey. Toxicol Sci 56:374–381
27. Bruner KL, Matrisian LM, Rodgers WH, Gorstein F, Osteen KG (1997) Suppression of matrix metalloproteinases inhibits establishment of ectopic lesions by human endometrium in nude mice. J Clin Invest 99:2851–2857
28. Cummings AM, Metcalf JL, Birnbaum L (1996) Promotion of endometriosis by 2,3,7,8-tetrachlorodibenzo-p-dioxin in rats and mice: time-dose dependence and spices comparison. Toxicology and applied pharmacology 138:131–9
29. Mayani A, Barel S, Soback S, Almagor M (1997) Dioxin concentrations in women with endometriosis. Hum Reprod 12:373–375
30. Louis GM, Whitcomb BW, Sperrazza R, Schisterman EF, Lobdell DT et al (2005) Environmental polychlorinated biphenylexposure and risk of endometriosis. Obstet Gynecol Surv 60:243–244
31. Gerhard I, Runnebaum B (1992) The limits of hormone substitution in pollutant exposure and fertility disorders. Zentralbl Gynakol 114:593–602
32. Porpora MG, Ingelido AM, di Domenico A et al (2006) Increased levels of polychlorobiphenyls in Italian women with endometriosis. Chemosphere 63:1361–1367
33. Eskenazi B, Mocarelli P, Warner M et al (2002) Serum dioxin concentrations and endometriosis: a cohort study in Seveso, Italy. Environ Health Perspect 110:629–634
34. Eskenazi B, Warner M, Mocarelli P et al (2002) Serum dioxin concentrations and menstrual cycle characteristics. Am J Epidemiol 156:383–392
35. Pauwels A, Schepens PJ, D'Hooghe T et al (2001) The risk of endometriosis and exposure to dioxins and polychlorinated biphenyls: a case-control study of infertile women. Hum Reprod 16: 2050–2055
36. Lebel G, Dodin S, Ayotte P, Marcoux S, Ferron LA, Dewailly E (1998) Organochlorine exposure and the risk of endometriosis. Fertil Steril 69:221–228
37. Heilier JF, Ha AT, Lison D, Donnez J, Tonglet R, Nackers F (2004) Increased serum polychlorobiphenyl levels in Belgian women with adenomyotic nodules of the rectovaginal septum. Fertil Steril 81:456–458
38. Koninckx PR, Braet P, Kennedy SH, Barlow DH (1994) Dioxin pollution and endometriosis in Belgium. Hum Reprod 9:1001–1002
39. Carpenter DO, Shen Y, Nguyen T, Le L, Lininger LL (2001) Incidence of endocrine disease among residents of New York areas of concern. Environ Health Perspect 109(Suppl 6):845–851
40. Rier S, Foster WG (2002) Environmental dioxins and endometriosis. Toxicol Sci 70:161–170
41. Safe SH (1995) Environmental and dietary estrogens and human health: is there a problem? Environ Health Perspect 103:346–351
42. Fujii-Kuriyama Y, Mimura J (2005) Molecular mechanisms of AhR functions in the regulation of cytochrome P450 genes. Biochem Biophys Res Commun 338:311–317
43. Peters JM, Narotsky MG, Elizondo G, Fernandez-Salguero PM, Gonzalez FJ, Abbott BD (1999) Amelioration of TCDD-induced teratogenesis in aryl hydrocarbon receptor (AhR)-null mice. Toxicol Sci 47:86–92
44. Whitlock JP Jr (1990) Genetic and molecular aspects of 2, 3, 7, 8-tetrachlorodibenzo-p-dioxin action. Annu Rev Pharmacol Toxicol 30:251–277
45. Schmidt JV, Bradfield CA (1996) Ah receptor signaling pathways. Annu Rev Cell Dev Biol 12:55–89
46. Bofinger DP, Feng L, Chi LH et al (2001) Effect of TCDD exposure on CYP1A1 and CYP1B1 expression in explant cultures of human endometrium. Toxicol Sci 62:299–314
47. Pitt JA, Feng L, Abbott BD et al (2001) Expression of AhR and ARNT mRNA in cultured human endometrial explants exposed to TCDD. Toxicol Sci 62:289–298
48. Khorram O, Garthwaite M, Golos T (2002) Uterine and ovarian aryl hydrocarbon receptor (AHR) and aryl hydrocarbon receptor nuclear translocator (ARNT) mRNA expression in benign and malignant gynaecological conditions. Mol Hum Reprod 8:75–80

49. Bulun SE, Zeitoun KM, Kilic G (2000) Expression of dioxin-related transactivating factors and target genes in human eutopic endometrial and endometriotic tissues. Am J Obstet Gynecol 182:767–775
50. Noble LS, Simpson ER, Johns A, Bulun SE (1996) Aromatase expression in endometriosis. J Clin Endocrinol Metab 81:174–179
51. Takayama K, Zeitoun K, Gunby RT, Sasano H, Carr BR, Bulun SE (1998) Treatment of severe postmenopausal endometriosis with an aromatase inhibitor. Fertil Steril 69:709–713
52. Rier SE, Yeaman GR (1997) Immune aspects of endometriosis: relevance of the uterine mucosal immune system. Semin Reprod Endocrinol 15:209–220
53. Osteen KG, Bruner KL, Sharpe-Timms KL (1996) Steroid and growth factor regulation of matrix metalloproteinase expression and endometriosis. Semin Reprod Endocrinol 14:247–255
54. Lai ZW, Hundeiker C, Gleichmann E, Esser C (1997) Cytokine gene expression during ontogeny in murine thymus on activation of the aryl hydrocarbon receptor by 2, 3, 7, 8-tetrachlorodibenzo-p-dioxin. Mol Pharmacol 52:30–37
55. Lai ZW, Pineau T, Esser C (1996) Identification of dioxin-responsive elements (DREs) in the 5′ regions of putative dioxin-inducible genes. Chem Biol Interact 100:97–112
56. Kerkvliet NI, Oughton JA (1993) Acute inflammatory response to sheep red blood cell challenge in mice treated with 2, 3, 7, 8-tetrachlorodibenzo-p-dioxin (TCDD): phenotypic and functional analysis of peritoneal exudate cells. Toxicology Appl Pharmacol 119:248–257
57. Clark GC, Taylor MJ, Tritscher AM, Lucier GW (1991) Tumor necrosis factor involvement in 2, 3, 7, 8-tetrachlorodibenzo-p-dioxin-mediated endotoxin hypersensitivity in C57BL/6J mice congenic at the Ah locus. Toxicol Appl Pharmacol 111:422–431
58. Taylor MJ, Lucier GW, Mahler JF, Thompson M, Lockhart AC, Clark GC (1992) Inhibition of acute TCDD toxicity by treatment with anti-tumor necrosis factor antibody or dexamethasone. Toxicol Appl Pharmacol 117:126–132
59. Huang JC, Liu DY, Yadollahi S, Wu KK, Dawood MY (1998) Interleukin-1 beta induces cyclooxygenase-2 gene expression in cultured endometrial stromal cells. J Clin Endocrinol Metab 83:538–541
60. Noble LS, Takayama K, Zeitoun KM et al (1997) Prostaglandin E2 stimulates aromatase expression in endometriosis-derived stromal cells. J Clin Endocrinol Metab 82:600–606
61. Zeitoun K, Takayama K, Sasano H et al (1998) Deficient 17beta-hydroxysteroid dehydrogenase type 2 expression in endometriosis: failure to metabolize 17beta-estradiol. J Clin Endocrinol Metab 83:4474–4480
62. Bruner KL, Rodgers WH, Gold LI et al (1995) Transforming growth factor beta mediates the progesterone suppression of an epithelial metalloproteinase by adjacent stroma in the human endometrium. Proc Natl Acad Sci USA 92:7362–7366
63. Bruner-Tran KL, Rier SE, Eisenberg E, Osteen KG (1999) The potential role of environmental toxins in the pathophysiology of endometriosis. Gynecol Obstet Invest 48(Suppl 1):45–56
64. Osteen KG, Keller NR, Feltus FA, Melner MH (1999) Paracrine regulation of matrix metalloproteinase expression in the normal human endometrium. Gynecol Obstet Invest 48(Suppl 1):2–13
65. Watson AJ (1998) Chemopreventive effects of NSAIDs against colorectal cancer: regulation of apoptosis and mitosis by COX-1 and COX-2. Histol Histopathol 13:591–597
66. Yeh WC, Hakem R, Woo M, Mak TW (1999) Gene targeting in the analysis of mammalian apoptosis and TNF receptor superfamily signaling. Immunol Rev 169:283–302
67. Kitawaki J, Noguchi T, Amatsu T et al (1997) Expression of aromatase cytochrome P450 protein and messenger ribonucleic acid in human endometriotic and adenomyotic tissues but not in normal endometrium. Biol Reprod 57:514–519
68. Hudelist G, Czerwenka K, Keckstein J et al (2007) Expression of aromatase and estrogen sulfotransferase in eutopic and ectopic endometrium: evidence for unbalanced estradiol production in endometriosis. Reprod Sci 14:798–805
69. Andersson S, Moghrabi N (1997) Physiology and molecular genetics of 17 beta-hydroxysteroid dehydrogenases. Steroids 62:143–147
70. Labrie F, Luu-The V, Labrie C et al (1989) Characterization of two mRNA species encoding human estradiol 17 beta-dehydrogenase and assignment of the gene to chromosome 17. J Steroid Biochem 34:189–197
71. Zeitoun KM, Bulun SE (1999) Aromatase: a key molecule in the pathophysiology of endometriosis and a therapeutic target. Fertil Steril 72:961–969
72. Igarashi TM, Bruner-Tran KL, Yeaman GR et al (2005) Reduced expression of progesterone receptor-B in the endometrium of women with endometriosis and in cocultures of endometrial cells exposed to 2, 3, 7, 8-tetrachlorodibenzo-p-dioxin. Fertil Steril 84:67–74
73. Giudice LC (2003) Genomics' role in understanding the pathogenesis of endometriosis. Semin Reprod Med 21:119–124
74. Giudice LC, Telles TL, Lobo S, Kao L (2002) The molecular basis for implantation failure in endometriosis: on the road to discovery. Ann N Y Acad Sci 955:252–264; discussion 93–95, 396–406
75. Ozkan S, Murk W, Arici A (2008) Endometriosis and infertility: epidemiology and evidence-based treatments. Ann N Y Acad Sci 1127:92–100
76. Skakkebaek NE, Jorgensen N, Main KM et al (2006) Is human fecundity declining? Int J Androl 29:2–11
77. Houston DE (1984) Evidence for the risk of pelvic endometriosis by age, race and socioeconomic status. Epidemiol Rev 6:167–191
78. Houston DE, Noller KL, Melton LJ 3rd, Selwyn BJ, Hardy RJ (1987) Incidence of pelvic endometriosis in Rochester, Minnesota, 1970–1979. Am J Epidemiol 125:959–969
79. Velebil P, Wingo PA, Xia Z, Wilcox LS, Peterson HB (1995) Rate of hospitalization for gynecologic disorders among reproductive-age women in the United States. Obstet Gynecol 86:764–769
80. Missmer SA, Hankinson SE, Spiegelman D, Barbieri RL, Marshall LM, Hunter DJ (2004) Incidence of laparoscopically confirmed endometriosis by demographic, anthropometric, and lifestyle factors. Am J Epidemiol 160:784–796
81. Fernando S, Breheny S, Jaques AM, Halliday JL, Baker G, Healy D (2008) Preterm birth, ovarian endometriomata, and assisted reproduction technologies. Fertil Steril 91:325–330
82. Kim JJ, Taylor HS, Lu Z et al (2007) Altered expression of HOXA10 in endometriosis: potential role in decidualization. Mol Hum Reprod 13:323–332
83. Couture LA, Abbott BD, Birnbaum LS (1990) A critical review of the developmental toxicity and teratogenicity of 2, 3, 7, 8-tetrachlorodibenzo-p-dioxin: recent advances toward understanding the mechanism. Teratology 42:619–627
84. Wu Q, Ohsako S, Ishimura R, Suzuki JS, Tohyama C (2004) Exposure of mouse preimplantation embryos to 2, 3, 7, 8-tetrachlorodibenzo-p-dioxin (TCDD) alters the methylation status of imprinted genes H19 and Igf2. Biol Reprod 70:1790–1797
85. Bradley C, van der Meer R, Roodi N et al (2007) Carcinogen-induced histone alteration in normal human mammary epithelial cells. Carcinogenesis 28:2184–2192
86. Buck Louis GM, Cooney MA (2007) Effects of environmental contaminants on ovarian function and fertility. In: Gonzalez-Bulnes A (ed) Novel concepts in ovarian endocrinology. Transworld Research Network, Kerala, India, pp 249–268
87. Waalkes MP, Liu J, Ward JM, Diwan BA (2004) Mechanisms underlying arsenic carcinogenesis: hypersensitivity of mice exposed to inorganic arsenic during gestation. Toxicology 198:31–38
88. Waalkes MP, Ward JM, Diwan BA (2004) Induction of tumors of the liver, lung, ovary and adrenal in adult mice after brief maternal gestational exposure to inorganic arsenic: promotional effects of postnatal phorbol ester exposure on hepatic and pulmonary, but not dermal cancers. Carcinogenesis 25:133–141

89. Kwok RK, Kaufmann RB, Jakariya M (2006) Arsenic in drinking-water and reproductive health outcomes: a study of participants in the Bangladesh Integrated Nutrition Programme. J Health Popul Nutr 24:190–205
90. Savabieasfahani M, Kannan K, Astapova O, Evans NP, Padmanabhan V (2006) Developmental programming: differential effects of prenatal exposure to bisphenol-A or methoxychlor on reproductive function. Endocrinology 147:5956–5966
91. Herath CB, Jin W, Watanabe G, Arai K, Suzuki AK, Taya K (2004) Adverse effects of environmental toxicants, octylphenol and bisphenol A, on male reproductive functions in pubertal rats. Endocrine 25:163–172
92. Howdeshell KL, Hotchkiss AK, Thayer KA, Vandenbergh JG, vom Saal FS (1999) Exposure to bisphenol A advances puberty. Nature 401:763–764
93. Hunt PA, Koehler KE, Susiarjo M et al (2003) Bisphenol A exposure causes meiotic aneuploidy in the female mouse. Curr Biol 13:546–553
94. Sugiura-Ogasawara M, Ozaki Y, Sonta S, Makino T, Suzumori K (2005) Exposure to bisphenol A is associated with recurrent miscarriage. Hum Reprod 20:2325–2329
95. Gupta C (2000) Reproductive malformation of the male offspring following maternal exposure to estrogenic chemicals. In: Proceedings of the society for experimental biology and medicine society for experimental biology and medicine, vol 224. New York, pp 61–68
96. Timms BG, Howdeshell KL, Barton L, Bradley S, Richter CA, vom Saal FS (2005) Estrogenic chemicals in plastic and oral contraceptives disrupt development of the fetal mouse prostate and urethra. Proc Natl Acad Sci USA 102:7014–7019
97. Al-Hiyasat AS, Darmani H, Elbetieha AM (2002) Effects of bisphenol A on adult male mouse fertility. Eur J Oral Sci 110:163–167
98. Sakaue M, Ohsako S, Ishimura R et al (2001) Bisphenol-A affects spermatogenesis in the adult rat even at a low dose. J Occup Health 43:185–190
99. Poirier LA, Vlasova TI (2002) The prospective role of abnormal methyl metabolism in cadmium toxicity. Environ Health Perspect 110(Suppl 5):793–795
100. Takiguchi M, Achanzar WE, Qu W, Li G, Waalkes MP (2003) Effects of cadmium on DNA-(Cytosine-5) methyltransferase activity and DNA methylation status during cadmium-induced cellular transformation. Exp Cell Res 286:355–365
101. Talbot P (2008) In vitro assessment of reproductive toxicity of tobacco smoke and its constituents. Birth Defects Res C Embryo Today 84:61–72
102. Thompson J, Bannigan J (2008) Cadmium: toxic effects on the reproductive system and the embryo. Reprod Toxicol 25: 304–315
103. Esposito ER, Horn KH, Greene RM, Pisano MM (2008) An animal model of cigarette smoke-induced in utero growth retardation. Toxicology 246:193–202
104. Ng SP, Zelikoff JT (2008) The effects of prenatal exposure of mice to cigarette smoke on offspring immune parameters. J Toxicol Environ Health A 71:445–453
105. Zilaitiene B, Dirzauskas M, Preiksa RT, Matulevicius V (2007) Cigarette smoking and waiting time to pregnancy: results of a pilot study. Medicina (Kaunas) 43:959–963
106. Hassa H, Gurer F, Tanir HM et al (2007) Effect of cigarette smoke and alpha-tocopherol (vitamin E) on fertilization, cleavage, and embryo development rates in mice: an experimental in vitro fertilization mice model study. Eur J Obstet Gynecol Reprod Biol 135:177–182
107. Neal MS, Zhu J, Holloway AC, Foster WG (2007) Follicle growth is inhibited by benzo-[a]-pyrene, at concentrations representative of human exposure, in an isolated rat follicle culture assay. Hum Reprod 22:961–967
108. Fowler PA, Cassie S, Rhind SM et al (2008) Maternal smoking during pregnancy specifically reduces human fetal desert hedgehog gene expression during testis development. J Clin Endocrinol Metab 93:619–626
109. Klaassen CD (2001) Casarett and Doull's toxicology: the basic scince of poisons, 6th edn. McGraw Hill, New York
110. Sharara FI, Seifer DB, Flaws JA (1998) Environmental toxicants and female reproduction. Fertil Steril 70:613–622
111. Winker R, Rudiger HW (2006) Reproductive toxicology in occupational settings: an update. Int Arch Occup Environ Health 79:1–10
112. Choy CM, Lam CW, Cheung LT, Briton-Jones CM, Cheung LP, Haines CJ (2002) Infertility, blood mercury concentrations and dietary seafood consumption: a case-control study. BJOG 109:1121–1125
113. Figa-Talamanca I, Traina ME, Urbani E (2001) Occupational exposures to metals, solvents and pesticides: recent evidence on male reproductive effects and biological markers. Occup Med 51:174–188
114. Protecting Your Health.org (2003) Infertility and related reproductive disorders http://www.protectingyourhealth.org/newscience/infertility/2003-04peerreviewinfertility.htm, http://www.protectingourhealth.org/
115. Wu SY, Tian J, Wang MZ, et al. (2004) [The effect of cadmium pollution on reproductive health in females]. Zhonghua Liu Xing Bing Xue Za Zhi 25:852–855
116. Jurasovic J, Cvitkovic P, Pizent A, Colak B, Telisman S (2004) Semen quality and reproductive endocrine function with regard to blood cadmium in Croatian male subjects. Biometals 17:735–743
117. Miller KP, Borgeest C, Greenfeld C, Tomic D, Flaws JA (2004) In utero effects of chemicals on reproductive tissues in females. Toxicol Appl Pharmacol 198:111–131
118. Denham M, Schell LM, Deane G, Gallo MV, Ravenscroft J, DeCaprio AP (2005) Relationship of lead, mercury, mirex, dichlorodiphenyldichloroethylene, hexachlorobenzene, and polychlorinated biphenyls to timing of menarche among Akwesasne Mohawk girls. Pediatrics 115:e127–e134
119. Benoff S, Jacob A, Hurley IR (2000) Male infertility and environmental exposure to lead and cadmium. Hum Reprod Update 6:107–121
120. Bonde JP, Joffe M, Apostoli P et al (2002) Sperm count and chromatin structure in men exposed to inorganic lead: lowest adverse effect levels. Occup Environ Med 59:234–242
121. Cheng RY, Hockman T, Crawford E, Anderson LM, Shiao YH (2004) Epigenetic and gene expression changes related to transgenerational carcinogenesis. Mol Carcinog 40:1–11
122. Shiao YH, Crawford EB, Anderson LM, Patel P, Ko K (2005) Allele-specific germ cell epimutation in the spacer promoter of the 45S ribosomal RNA gene after Cr(III) exposure. Toxicol Appl Pharmacol 205:290–296
123. Veeramachaneni DN (2008) Impact of environmental pollutants on the male: effects on germ cell differentiation. Anim Reprod Sci 105:144–157
124. Lima PH, Damasceno DC, Sinzato YK et al (2008) Levels of DNA damage in blood leukocyte samples from non-diabetic and diabetic female rats and their fetuses exposed to air or cigarette smoke. Mutat Res 653:44–49
125. Hruska KS, Furth PA, Seifer DB, Sharara FI, Flaws JA (2000) Environmental factors in infertility. Clin Obstet Gynecol 43:821–829
126. Younglai EV, Holloway AC, Foster WG (2005) Environmental and occupational factors affecting fertility and IVF success. Hum Reprod Update 11:43–57
127. Soares SR, Melo MA (2008) Cigarette smoking and reproductive function. Curr Opin Obstet Gynecol 20:281–291
128. Younglai EV, Wu YJ, Foster WG (2007) Reproductive toxicology of environmental toxicants: emerging issues and concerns. Curr Pharm Des 13:3005–3019

129. Jauniaux E, Burton GJ (2007) Morphological and biological effects of maternal exposure to tobacco smoke on the feto-placental unit. Early Hum Dev 83:699–706
130. Serrano H, Perez-Rivero JJ, Aguilar-Setien A, De-Paz O, Villa-Godoy A (2007) Vampire bat reproductive control by a naturally occurring phytooestrogen. Reprod Fertil Dev 19:470–472
131. Suarez L, Felkner M, Brender JD, Canfield M, Hendricks K (2008) Maternal exposures to cigarette smoke, alcohol, and street drugs and neural tube defect occurrence in offspring. Matern Child Health J 12:394–401
132. Richthoff J, Elzanaty S, Rylander L, Hagmar L, Giwercman A (2008) Association between tobacco exposure and reproductive parameters in adolescent males. Int J Androl 31:31–39
133. Faure AK, Aknin-Seifer I, Frerot G et al (2007) Predictive factors for an increased risk of sperm aneuploidies in oligo-astheno-teratozoospermic males. Int J Androl 30:153–162
134. Mostafa T, Tawadrous G, Roaia MM, Amer MK, Kader RA, Aziz A (2006) Effect of smoking on seminal plasma ascorbic acid in infertile and fertile males. Andrologia 38:221–224
135. Lie RT, Wilcox AJ, Taylor J et al (2008) Maternal smoking and oral clefts: the role of detoxification pathway genes. Epidemiology 19:606–615
136. Rogers JM (2008) Tobacco and pregnancy: overview of exposures and effects. Birth Defects Res C Embryo Today 84:1–15
137. Ness RB, Zhang J, Bass D, Klebanoff MA (2008) Interactions between smoking and weight in pregnancies complicated by preeclampsia and small-for-gestational-age birth. Am J Epidemiol 168:427–433
138. Vine MF (1996) Smoking and male reproduction: a review. Int J Androl 19:323–337
139. US Department of Health and Human Services (2001) Women and smoking: a report of the surgeon general. US Department of Health and Human Services (PHS), Washington, DC
140. Vahdaninia M, Tavafian SS, Montazeri A (2008) Correlates of low birth weight in term pregnancies: a retrospective study from Iran. BMC Pregnancy Childbirth 8:12
141. Tsai HJ, Liu X, Mestan K et al (2008) Maternal cigarette smoking, metabolic gene polymorphisms, and preterm delivery: new insights on GxE interactions and pathogenic pathways. Hum Genet 123:359–369
142. Haskins A, Mukhopadhyay S, Pekow P et al (2008) Smoking and risk of preterm birth among predominantly Puerto Rican women. Ann Epidemiol 18:440–446
143. Jensen TK, Jorgensen N, Punab M et al (2004) Association of in utero exposure to maternal smoking with reduced semen quality and testis size in adulthood: a cross-sectional study of 1, 770 young men from the general population in five European countries. Am J Epidemiol 159:49–58
144. Coutts SM, Fulton N, Anderson RA (2007) Environmental toxicant-induced germ cell apoptosis in the human fetal testis. Hum Reprod 22:2912–2918
145. Pasqualotto FF, Umezu FM, Salvador M, Borges E Jr, Sobreiro BP, Pasqualotto EB (2008) Effect of cigarette smoking on antioxidant levels and presence of leukocytospermia in infertile men: a prospective study. Fertil Steril 90:278–283
146. Chang SH, Kim CS, Lee KS et al (2007) Premenopausal factors influencing premature ovarian failure and early menopause. Maturitas 58:19–30
147. Waylen AL, Metwally M, Jones GL, Wilkinson AJ, Ledger WL (2009) Effects of cigarette smoking upon clinical outcomes of assisted reproduction: a meta-analysis. Hum Reprod Update 15:31–44
148. Lyn-Cook BD, Blann E, Payne PW, Bo J, Sheehan D, Medlock K (1995) Methylation profile and amplification of proto-oncogenes in rat pancreas induced with phytoestrogens. In: Proceedings of the society for experimental biology and medicine society for experimental biology and medicine, vol 208. New York, pp 116–119
149. Kouki T, Okamoto M, Wada S, Kishitake M, Yamanouchi K (2005) Suppressive effect of neonatal treatment with a phytoestrogen, coumestrol, on lordosis and estrous cycle in female rats. Brain Res Bull 64:449–454
150. Tarrago-Castellanos CR, Garcia-Lorenzana CM, Diaz-Sanchez V, Velazquez-Moctezuma J (2006) Gonadotrophin levels and morphological testicular features in rats after different doses of the phytoestrogen coumestrol. Neuro Endocrinol Lett 27:487–492
151. Al-Zoughool M, Dossus L, Kaaks R et al (2007) Risk of endometrial cancer in relationship to cigarette smoking: results from the EPIC study. Int J Cancer 121:2741–2747
152. Alworth LC, Howdeshell KL, Ruhlen RL et al (2002) Uterine responsiveness to estradiol and DNA methylation are altered by fetal exposure to diethylstilbestrol and methoxychlor in CD-1 mice: effects of low versus high doses. Toxicol Appl Pharmacol 183:10–22
153. Li S, Hansman R, Newbold R, Davis B, McLachlan JA, Barrett JC (2003) Neonatal diethylstilbestrol exposure induces persistent elevation of c-fos expression and hypomethylation in its exon-4 in mouse uterus. Mol Carcinog 38:78–84
154. Li S, Washburn KA, Moore R et al (1997) Developmental exposure to diethylstilbestrol elicits demethylation of estrogen-responsive lactoferrin gene in mouse uterus. Cancer Res 57:4356–4359
155. Newbold RR, Padilla-Banks E, Jefferson WN (2006) Adverse effects of the model environmental estrogen diethylstilbestrol are transmitted to subsequent generations. Endocrinology 147:S11–S17
156. Ruden DM, Xiao L, Garfinkel MD, Lu X (2005) Hsp90 and environmental impacts on epigenetic states: a model for the trans-generational effects of diethylstibesterol on uterine development and cancer. Hum Mol Genet 14(Spec No 1):R149–R155
157. Sato K, Fukata H, Kogo Y, Ohgane J, Shiota K, Mori C (2006) Neonatal exposure to diethylstilbestrol alters the expression of DNA methyltransferases and methylation of genomic DNA in the epididymis of mice. Endocr J 53:331–337
158. Tang W, Barker J, Jewfferson WN, Newbold RR, Ho S (2007) Early exposure to diethylstilbestrol or genistein and uterine cancer risk: investigating nucleosomal binding protein 1 (Nsbp1) as a gene susceptible to estrogen reprogramming in the mouse uterus. In: Endocrine society's 89th annual meeting proceeding, p 95
159. Ikeda Y, Tanaka H, Esaki M (2008) Effects of gestational diethylstilbestrol treatment on male and female gonads during early embryonic development. Endocrinology 149:3970–3979
160. Li HC, Chen Q, Wang ZM et al (2008) Effects of prepubertal exposure to diethylstilbestrol on testicular development and function of SD rats. Zhonghua Nan Ke Xue 14:142–148
161. Storgaard L, Bonde JP, Ernst E et al (2003) Does smoking during pregnancy affect sons' sperm counts? Epidemiology 14:278–286
162. Bennetts LE, De Iuliis GN, Nixon B et al (2008) Impact of estrogenic compounds on DNA integrity in human spermatozoa: evidence for cross-linking and redox cycling activities. Mutat Res 641:1–11
163. Wise LA, Palmer JR, Hatch EE et al (2007) Secondary sex ratio among women exposed to diethylstilbestrol in utero. Environ Health Perspect 115:1314–1319
164. Brouwers MM, Feitz WF, Roelofs LA, Kiemeney LA, de Gier RP, Roeleveld N (2007) Risk factors for hypospadias. Eur J Pediatr 166:671–678
165. Hamm JT, Chen CY, Birnbaum LS (2003) A mixture of dioxins, furans, and non-ortho PCBs based upon consensus toxic equivalency factors produces dioxin-like reproductive effects. Toxicol Sci 74:182–191
166. Hosie S, Loff S, Witt K, Niessen K, Waag KL (2000) Is there a correlation between organochlorine compounds and undescended testes? Eur J Pediatr Surg 10:304–309
167. Wolf CJ, Ostby JS, Gray LE Jr (1999) Gestational exposure to 2, 3, 7, 8-tetrachlorodibenzo-p-dioxin (TCDD) severely alters

reproductive function of female hamster offspring. Toxicol Sci 51:259–264
168. Guo YL, Hsu PC, Hsu CC, Lambert GH (2000) Semen quality after prenatal exposure to polychlorinated biphenyls and dibenzofurans. Lancet 356:1240–1241
169. Cohn BA, Cirillo PM, Wolff MS et al (2003) DDT and DDE exposure in mothers and time to pregnancy in daughters. Lancet 361:2205–2206
170. Choi JS, Kim IW, Hwang SY, Shin BJ, Kim SK (2008) Effect of 2, 3, 7, 8-tetrachlorodibenzo-p-dioxin on testicular spermatogenesis-related panels and serum sex hormone levels in rats. BJU Int 101:250–255
171. Rasier G, Parent AS, Gerard A, Lebrethon MC, Bourguignon JP (2007) Early maturation of gonadotropin-releasing hormone secretion and sexual precocity after exposure of infant female rats to estradiol or dichlorodiphenyltrichloroethane. Biol Reprod 77:734–742
172. Tanaka J, Yonemoto J, Zaha H, Kiyama R, Sone H (2007) Estrogen-responsive genes newly found to be modified by TCDD exposure in human cell lines and mouse systems. Mol Cell Endocr 272:38–49
173. Hsu PC, Pan MH, Li LA, Chen CJ, Tsai SS, Guo YL (2007) Exposure in utero to 2, 2′, 3, 3′, 4, 6′-hexachlorobiphenyl (PCB 132) impairs sperm function and alters testicular apoptosis-related gene expression in rat offspring. Toxicol Appl Pharmacol 221:68–75
174. Ishihara K, Warita K, Tanida T, Sugawara T, Kitagawa H, Hoshi N (2007) Does paternal exposure to 2, 3, 7, 8-tetrachlorodibenzo-p-dioxin (TCDD) affect the sex ratio of offspring? J Vet Med Sci 69:347–352
175. Taketoh J, Mutoh J, Takeda T et al (2007) Suppression of fetal testicular cytochrome P450 17 by maternal exposure to 2, 3, 7, 8-tetrachlorodibenzo-p-dioxin: a mechanism involving an initial effect on gonadotropin synthesis in the pituitary. Life Sci 80:1259–1267
176. Nayyar T, Bruner-Tran KL, Piestrzeniewicz-Ulanska D, Osteen KG (2007) Developmental exposure of mice to TCDD elicits a similar uterine phenotype in adult animals as observed in women with endometriosis. Reprod Toxicol 23:326–336
177. Louis GMB, Cooney MA, Lynch CD, Handal A (2008) Periconception window: advising the pregnancy-planning couple. Fertil Steril 89:e119–e121
178. Rogan WJ, Chen A (2005) Health risks and benefits of bis(4-chlorophenyl)-1, 1, 1-trichloroethane (DDT). Lancet 366:763–773
179. Toft G, Hagmar L, Giwercman A, Bonde JP (2004) Epidemiological evidence on reproductive effects of persistent organochlorines in humans. Reprod Toxicol 19:5–26
180. Venners SA, Korrick S, Xu X et al (2005) Preconception serum DDT and pregnancy loss: a prospective study using a biomarker of pregnancy. Am J Epidemiol 162:709–716
181. Gerhard I, Frick A, Monga B, Runnebaum B (1999) Pentachlorophenol exposure in women with gynecological and endocrine dysfunction. Environ Res 80:383–388
182. Perry MJ, Ouyang F, Korrick SA et al (2006) A prospective study of serum DDT and progesterone and estrogen levels across the menstrual cycle in nulliparous women of reproductive age. Am J Epidemiol 164:1056–1064
183. Windham GC, Lee D, Mitchell P, Anderson M, Petreas M, Lasley B (2005) Exposure to organochlorine compounds and effects on ovarian function. Epidemiology 16:182–190
184. Axmon A (2006) Menarche in women with high exposure to persistent organochlorine pollutants in utero and during childhood. Environ Res 102:77–82
185. Den Hond E, Roels HA, Hoppenbrouwers K et al (2002) Sexual maturation in relation to polychlorinated aromatic hydrocarbons: Sharpe and Skakkebaek's hypothesis revisited. Environ Health Perspect 110:771–776
186. Ouyang F, Perry MJ, Venners SA et al (2005) Serum DDT, age at menarche, and abnormal menstrual cycle length. Occup Environ Med 62:878–884
187. Cooper GS, Klebanoff MA, Promislow J, Brock JW, Longnecker MP (2005) Polychlorinated biphenyls and menstrual cycle characteristics. Epidemiology 16:191–200
188. Farr SL, Cai J, Savitz DA, Sandler DP, Hoppin JA, Cooper GS (2006) Pesticide exposure and timing of menopause: the Agricultural Health Study. Am J Epidemiol 163:731–742
189. Yu ML, Guo YL, Hsu CC, Rogan WJ (2000) Menstruation and reproduction in women with polychlorinated biphenyl (PCB) poisoning: long-term follow-up interviews of the women from the Taiwan Yucheng cohort. Int J Epidemiol 29:672–677
190. Colon I, Caro D, Bourdony CJ, Rosario O (2000) Identification of phthalate esters in the serum of young Puerto Rican girls with premature breast development. Environ Health Perspect 108:895–900
191. Krstevska-Konstantinova M, Charlier C, Craen M et al (2001) Sexual precocity after immigration from developing countries to Belgium: evidence of previous exposure to organochlorine pesticides. Hum Reprod 16:1020–1026
192. Hauser R, Chen Z, Pothier L, Ryan L, Altshul L (2003) The relationship between human semen parameters and environmental exposure to polychlorinated biphenyls and p, p'-DDE. Environ Health Perspect 111:1505–1511
193. Long M, Stronati A, Bizzaro D et al (2007) Relation between serum xenobiotic-induced receptor activities and sperm DNA damage and sperm apoptotic markers in European and Inuit populations. Reproduction 133:517–530
194. Mocarelli P, Gerthoux PM, Patterson DG Jr et al (2008) Dioxin exposure, from infancy through puberty, produces endocrine disruption and affects human semen quality. Environ Health Perspect 116:70–77
195. Phillips KP, Tanphaichitr N (2008) Human exposure to endocrine disrupters and semen quality. J Toxicol Environ Health B Crit Rev 11:188–220
196. del Rio Gomez I, Marshall T, Tsai P, Shao YS, Guo YL (2002) Number of boys born to men exposed to polychlorinated byphenyls. Lancet 360:143–144
197. Ryan JJ, Amirova Z, Carrier G (2002) Sex ratios of children of Russian pesticide producers exposed to dioxin. Environ Health Perspect 110:A699–A701
198. Tiido T, Rignell-Hydbom A, Jonsson BA, Rylander L, Giwercman A, Giwercman YL (2007) Modifying effect of the AR gene trinucleotide repeats and SNPs in the AHR and AHRR genes on the association between persistent organohalogen pollutant exposure and human sperm Y:X ratio. Mol Hum Reprod 13:223–229
199. Hutt KJ, Shi Z, Albertini DF, Petroff BK (2008) The environmental toxicant 2, 3, 7, 8-tetrachlorodibenzo-p-dioxin disrupts morphogenesis of the rat pre-implantation embryo. BMC Dev Biol 8:1
200. Sikka SC, Wang R (2008) Endocrine disruptors and estrogenic effects on male reproductive axis. Asian J Androl 10:134–145
201. Tao L, Wang W, Li L, Kramer PK, Pereira MA (2005) DNA hypomethylation induced by drinking water disinfection by-products in mouse and rat kidney. Toxicol Sci 87:344–352
202. Windham GC, Waller K, Anderson M, Fenster L, Mendola P, Swan S (2003) Chlorination by-products in drinking water and menstrual cycle function. Environ Health Perspect 111:935–941; discussion A409
203. Bove F, Shim Y, Zeitz P (2002) Drinking water contaminants and adverse pregnancy outcomes: a review. Environ Health Perspect 110(Suppl 1):61–74
204. Nieuwenhuijsen MJ, Toledano MB, Eaton NE, Fawell J, Elliott P (2000) Chlorination disinfection byproducts in water and their association with adverse reproductive outcomes: a review. Occup Environ Med 57:73–85
205. Tardiff RG, Carson ML, Ginevan ME (2006) Updated weight of evidence for an association between adverse reproductive and

developmental effects and exposure to disinfection by-products. Regul Toxicol Pharmacol 45:185–205

206. Joyce SJ, Cook A, Newnham J, Brenters M, Ferguson C, Weinstein P (2008) Water disinfection by-products and pre-labor rupture of membranes. Am J Epidemiol 168:514–521
207. Fang MZ, Wang Y, Ai N et al (2003) Tea polyphenol (-)-epigallocatechin-3-gallate inhibits DNA methyltransferase and reactivates methylation-silenced genes in cancer cell lines. Cancer Res 63:7563–7570
208. Lee WJ, Shim JY, Zhu BT (2005) Mechanisms for the inhibition of DNA methyltransferases by tea catechins and bioflavonoids. Mol Pharmacol 68:1018–1030
209. Gresie-Brusin DF, Kielkowski D, Baker A, Channa K, Rees D (2007) Occupational exposure to ethylene oxide during pregnancy and association with adverse reproductive outcomes. Int Arch Occup Environ Health 80:559–565
210. Yenbutr P, Hilakivi-Clarke L, Passaniti A (1998) Hypomethylation of an exon I estrogen receptor CpG island in spontaneous and carcinogen-induced mammary tumorigenesis in the rat. Mech Ageing Dev 106:93–102
211. Barth AD, Brito LF, Kastelic JP (2008) The effect of nutrition on sexual development of bulls. Theriogenology 70:485–494
212. Yokomori N, Tawata M, Onaya T (1999) DNA demethylation during the differentiation of 3T3–L1 cells affects the expression of the mouse GLUT4 gene. Diabetes 48:685–690
213. Robker RL (2008) Evidence that obesity alters the quality of oocytes and embryos. Pathophysiology 15:115–121
214. Dabelea D, Hanson RL, Lindsay RS et al (2000) Intrauterine exposure to diabetes conveys risks for type 2 diabetes and obesity: a study of discordant sibships. Diabetes 49:2208–2211
215. Hammoud AO, Gibson M, Peterson CM, Meikle AW, Carrell DT (2008) Impact of male obesity on infertility: a critical review of the current literature. Fertil Steril 90:897–904
216. Jokela M, Elovainio M, Kivimaki M (2008) Lower fertility associated with obesity and underweight: the US National Longitudinal Survey of Youth. Am J Clin Nutr 88:886–893
217. Correa A, Gray RH, Cohen R et al (1996) Ethylene glycol ethers and risks of spontaneous abortion and subfertility. Am J Epidemiol 143:707–717
218. LaDou J (2004) Occupational and environmental medicine, 3rd edn. Lange Medical/McGraw Hill, Stamford, CT
219. Eskenazi B, Gold EB, Samuels SJ et al (1995) Prospective assessment of fecundability of female semiconductor workers. Am J Ind Med 28:817–831
220. Chen H, Ke Q, Kluz T, Yan Y, Costa M (2006) Nickel ions increase histone H3 lysine 9 dimethylation and induce transgene silencing. Mol Cell Biol 26:3728–3737
221. Cicolella A (2006) Glycol ethers reproductive risks. Gynecol Obstet Fertil 34:955–963
222. Timour Q, Biggi-Bernard U, Descotes J (2007) Hormone replacement therapy: toxicity of glycol ethers. J Gynecol Obstet Biol Reprod (Paris) 36:62–67
223. Hsieh GY, Wang JD, Cheng TJ, Chen PC (2005) Prolonged menstrual cycles in female workers exposed to ethylene glycol ethers in the semiconductor manufacturing industry. Occup Environ Med 62:510–516
224. Chevrier C, Dananche B, Bahuau M et al (2006) Occupational exposure to organic solvent mixtures during pregnancy and the risk of non-syndromic oral clefts. Occup Environ Med 63:617–623
225. Silbergeld EK, Waalkes M, Rice JM (2000) Lead as a carcinogen: experimental evidence and mechanisms of action. Am J Ind Med 38:316–323
226. Uzbekov MG, Bubnova NI, Kulikova GV (2007) Effect of prenatal lead exposure on superoxide dismutase activity in the brain and liver of rat fetuses. Bull Exp Biol Med 144:783–785
227. Sallmen M, Anttila A, Lindbohm ML, Kyyronen P, Taskinen H, Hemminki K (1995) Time to pregnancy among women occupationally exposed to lead. J Occup Environ Med 37:931–934
228. Tang N, Zhu ZQ (2003) Adverse reproductive effects in female workers of lead battery plants. Int J Occup Med Environ Health 16:359–361
229. Selevan SG, Rice DC, Hogan KA, Euling SY, Pfahles-Hutchens A, Bethel J (2003) Blood lead concentration and delayed puberty in girls. N Engl J Med 348:1527–1536
230. Wu T, Buck GM, Mendola P (2003) Blood lead levels and sexual maturation in U.S. girls: the Third National Health and Nutrition Examination Survey, 1988-1994. Environ Health Perspect 111:737–741
231. Cleveland LM, Minter ML, Cobb KA, Scott AA, German VF (2008) Lead hazards for pregnant women and children: part 2: more can still be done to reduce the chance of exposure to lead in at-risk populations. Am J Nurs 108:40–47; quiz 7–8
232. Salnikow K, Costa M (2000) Epigenetic mechanisms of nickel carcinogenesis. J Environ Pathol Toxicol Oncol 19:307–318
233. Lee B, Hiney JK, Pine MD, Srivastava VK, Dees WL (2007) Manganese stimulates luteinizing hormone releasing hormone secretion in prepubertal female rats: hypothalamic site and mechanism of action. J Physiol 578:765–772
234. Lee B, Pine M, Johnson L, Rettori V, Hiney JK, Dees WL (2006) Manganese acts centrally to activate reproductive hormone secretion and pubertal development in male rats. Reprod Toxicol 22:580–585
235. Erikson KM, Dorman DC, Fitsanakis V, Lash LH, Aschner M (2006) Alterations of oxidative stress biomarkers due to in utero and neonatal exposures of airborne manganese. Biol Trace Elem Res 111:199–215
236. Kaur P, Kalia S, Bansal MP (2006) Effect of diethyl maleate induced oxidative stress on male reproductive activity in mice: redox active enzymes and transcription factors expression. Mol Cell Biochem 291:55–61
237. Vigeh M, Yokoyama K, Ramezanzadeh F et al (2008) Blood manganese concentrations and intrauterine growth restriction. Reprod Toxicol 25:219–223
238. Ericson JE, Crinella FM, Clarke-Stewart KA, Allhusen VD, Chan T, Robertson RT (2007) Prenatal manganese levels linked to childhood behavioral disinhibition. Neurotoxicol Teratol 29:181–187
239. Rao MV, Gangadharan B (2008) Antioxidative potential of melatonin against mercury induced intoxication in spermatozoa in vitro. Toxicol In Vitro 22:935–942
240. Al-Saleh I, Coskun S, Mashhour A et al (2008) Exposure to heavy metals (lead, cadmium and mercury) and its effect on the outcome of in-vitro fertilization treatment. Int J Hyg Environ Health 211:560–579
241. Park S, Johnson MA (2006) Awareness of fish advisories and mercury exposure in women of childbearing age. Nutr Rev 64:250–256
242. Sweeney T, Nicol L, Roche JF, Brooks AN (2000) Maternal exposure to octylphenol suppresses ovine fetal follicle-stimulating hormone secretion, testis size, and sertoli cell number. Endocrinology 141:2667–2673
243. Sharpe RM, Fisher JS, Millar MM, Jobling S, Sumpter JP (1995) Gestational and lactational exposure of rats to xenoestrogens results in reduced testicular size and sperm production. Environ Health Perspect 103:1136–1143
244. Bogh IB, Christensen P, Dantzer V et al (2001) Endocrine disrupting compounds: effect of octylphenol on reproduction over three generations. Theriogenology 55:131–150
245. Lee MJ, Lin H, Liu CW et al (2008) Octylphenol stimulates resistin gene expression in 3T3–L1 adipocytes via the estrogen receptor and extracellular signal-regulated kinase pathways. Am J Physiol Cell Physiol 294:C1542–C1551

246. Turan N, Cartwright LS, Waring RH, Ramsden DB (2008) Wide-ranging genomic effects of plasticisers and related compounds. Curr Drug Metab 9:285–303
247. Waring RH, Ayers S, Gescher AJ et al (2008) Phytoestrogens and xenoestrogens: the contribution of diet and environment to endocrine disruption. J Steroid Biochem Mol Biol 108: 213–220
248. Barlas N, Aydogan M (2009) Histopathologic effects of maternal 4-tert-octylphenol exposure on liver, kidney and spleen of rats at adulthood. Arch Toxicol 83:341–349
249. Rosenberg BG, Chen H, Folmer J, Liu J, Papadopoulos V, Zirkin BR (2008) Gestational exposure to atrazine: effects on the postnatal development of male offspring. J Androl 29:304–311
250. Sitarek K, Stetkiewicz J (2008) Assessment of reproductive toxicity and gonadotoxic potential of N-methyl-2-pyrrolidone in male rats. Int J Occup Med Environ Health 21:73–80
251. Tiido T, Rignell-Hydbom A, Jonsson B et al (2005) Exposure to persistent organochlorine pollutants associates with human sperm Y:X chromosome ratio. Hum Reprod 20:1903–1909
252. Bloom MS, Buck-Louis GM, Schisterman EF, Kostyniak PJ, Vena JE (2008) Changes in maternal serum chlorinated pesticide concentrations across critical windows of human reproduction and development. Environ Res 109:93–100
253. Damgaard IN, Skakkebaek NE, Toppari J et al (2006) Persistent pesticides in human breast milk and cryptorchidism. Environ Health Perspect 114:1133–1138
254. Axmon A, Thulstrup AM, Rignell-Hydbom A et al (2006) Time to pregnancy as a function of male and female serum concentrations of 2, 2'4, 4'5, 5'-hexachlorobiphenyl (CB-153) and 1, 1-dichloro-2, 2-bis (p-chlorophenyl)-ethylene (p, p'-DDE). Hum Reprod 21:657–665
255. Spano M, Toft G, Hagmar L et al (2005) Exposure to PCB and p, p'-DDE in European and Inuit populations: impact on human sperm chromatin integrity. Hum Reprod 20:3488–3499
256. Gray LE, Ostby J, Furr J et al (2001) Effects of environmental antiandrogens on reproductive development in experimental animals. Hum Reprod Update 7:248–264
257. Fernandez MF, Olmos B, Granada A et al (2007) Human exposure to endocrine-disrupting chemicals and prenatal risk factors for cryptorchidism and hypospadias: a nested case-control study. Environ Health Perspect 115(Suppl 1):8–14
258. Laws SC, Ferrell JM, Stoker TE, Schmid J, Cooper RL (2000) The effects of atrazine on female wistar rats: an evaluation of the protocol for assessing pubertal development and thyroid function. Toxicol Sci 58:366–376
259. Monosson E, Kelce WR, Lambright C, Ostby J, Gray LE Jr (1999) Peripubertal exposure to the antiandrogenic fungicide, vinclozolin, delays puberty, inhibits the development of androgen-dependent tissues, and alters androgen receptor function in the male rat. Toxicol Ind Health 15:65–79
260. Stoker TE, Guidici DL, Laws SC, Cooper RL (2002) The effects of atrazine metabolites on puberty and thyroid function in the male Wistar rat. Toxicol Sci 67:198–206
261. Moustafa GG, Ibrahim ZS, Ahmed MM et al (2008) Downregulation of male-specific cytochrome P450 by profenofos. Jpn J Vet Res 56:109–118
262. Multigner L, Kadhel P, Pascal M et al (2008) Parallel assessment of male reproductive function in workers and wild rats exposed to pesticides in banana plantations in Guadeloupe. Environ Health 7:40
263. Ngoula F, Watcho P, Bouseko TS, Kenfack A, Tchoumboue J, Kamtchouing P (2007) Effects of propoxur on the reproductive system of male rats. Afr J Reprod Health 11:125–132
264. Anway MD, Rekow SS, Skinner MK (2008) Transgenerational epigenetic programming of the embryonic testis transcriptome. Genomics 91:30–40
265. Nilsson EE, Anway MD, Stanfield J, Skinner MK (2008) Transgenerational epigenetic effects of the endocrine disruptor vinclozolin on pregnancies and female adult onset disease. Reproduction 135:713–721
266. Hass U, Scholze M, Christiansen S et al (2007) Combined exposure to anti-androgens exacerbates disruption of sexual differentiation in the rat. Environ Health Perspect 115(Suppl 1):122–128
267. Levario-Carrillo M, Amato D, Ostrosky-Wegman P, Gonzalez-Horta C, Corona Y, Sanin LH (2004) Relation between pesticide exposure and intrauterine growth retardation. Chemosphere 55:1421–1427
268. Perera FP, Rauh V, Tsai WY et al (2003) Effects of transplacental exposure to environmental pollutants on birth outcomes in a multiethnic population. Environ Health Perspect 111:201–205
269. Whyatt RM, Rauh V, Barr DB et al (2004) Prenatal insecticide exposures and birth weight and length among an urban minority cohort. Environ Health Perspect 112:1125–1132
270. Abell A, Juul S, Bonde JP (2000) Time to pregnancy among female greenhouse workers. Scand J Work Environ Health 26:131–136
271. Anway MD, Cupp AS, Uzumcu M, Skinner MK (2005) Epigenetic transgenerational actions of endocrine disruptors and male fertility. Science 308:1466–1469
272. Fuortes L, Clark MK, Kirchner HL, Smith EM (1997) Association between female infertility and agricultural work history. Am J Ind Med 31:445–451
273. Greenlee AR, Arbuckle TE, Chyou PH (2003) Risk factors for female infertility in an agricultural region. Epidemiology 14: 429–436
274. Bretveld RW, Hooiveld M, Zielhuis GA, Pellegrino A, van Rooij IA, Roeleveld N (2008) Reproductive disorders among male and female greenhouse workers. Reprod Toxicol 25:107–114
275. Mendola P, Messer LC, Rappazzo K (2008) Science linking environmental contaminant exposures with fertility and reproductive health impacts in the adult female. Fertil Steril 89:e81–e94
276. Peiris-John RJ, Wickremasinghe R (2008) Impact of low-level exposure to organophosphates on human reproduction and survival. Trans R Soc Trop Med Hyg 102:239–245
277. Garry VF, Holland SE, Erickson LL, Burroughs BL (2003) Male reproductive hormones and thyroid function in pesticide applicators in the Red River Valley of Minnesota. J Toxicol Environ Health A 66:965–986
278. Farr SL, Cooper GS, Cai J, Savitz DA, Sandler DP (2004) Pesticide use and menstrual cycle characteristics among premenopausal women in the Agricultural Health Study. Am J Epidemiol 160:1194–1204
279. Arbuckle TE, Savitz DA, Mery LS, Curtis KM (1999) Exposure to phenoxy herbicides and the risk of spontaneous abortion. Epidemiology 10:752–760
280. Crisostomo L, Molina VV (2002) Pregnancy outcomes among farming households of Nueva Ecija with conventional pesticide use versus integrated pest management. Int J Occup Environ Health 8:232–242
281. Goldsmith JR (1997) Dibromochloropropane: epidemiological findings and current questions. Ann N Y Acad Sci 837:300–306
282. Savitz DA, Arbuckle T, Kaczor D, Curtis KM (1997) Male pesticide exposure and pregnancy outcome. Am J Epidemiol 146:1025–1036
283. Settimi L, Spinelli A, Lauria L et al (2008) Spontaneous abortion and maternal work in greenhouses. Am J Ind Med 51:290–295
284. Fisher JS (2004) Environmental anti-androgens and male reproductive health: focus on phthalates and testicular dysgenesis syndrome. Reproduction 127:305–315
285. Kristensen P, Irgens LM, Andersen A, Bye AS, Sundheim L (1997) Birth defects among offspring of Norwegian farmers, 1967–1991. Epidemiology 8:537–544
286. Garry VF, Schreinemachers D, Harkins ME, Griffith J (1996) Pesticide appliers, biocides, and birth defects in rural Minnesota. Environ Health Perspect 104:394–399

287. Oliva A, Spira A, Multigner L (2001) Contribution of environmental factors to the risk of male infertility. Hum Reprod 16:1768–1776
288. Swan SH, Kruse RL, Liu F et al (2003) Semen quality in relation to biomarkers of pesticide exposure. Environ Health Perspect 111:1478–1484
289. Recio R, Robbins WA, Borja-Aburto V et al (2001) Organophosphorous pesticide exposure increases the frequency of sperm sex null aneuploidy. Environ Health Perspect 109: 1237–1240
290. Sanchez-Pena LC, Reyes BE, Lopez-Carrillo L et al (2004) Organophosphorous pesticide exposure alters sperm chromatin structure in Mexican agricultural workers. Toxicol Appl Pharmacol 196:108–113
291. Tiemann U (2008) In vivo and in vitro effects of the organochlorine pesticides DDT, TCPM, methoxychlor, and lindane on the female reproductive tract of mammals: a review. Reprod Toxicol 25:316–326
292. Windham G, Fenster L (2008) Environmental contaminants and pregnancy outcomes. Fertil Steril 89:e111–e116; discussion e7
293. McGlynn KA, Quraishi SM, Graubard BI, Weber JP, Rubertone MV, Erickson RL (2008) Persistent organochlorine pesticides and risk of testicular germ cell tumors. J Natl Cancer Inst 100:663–671
294. Meeker JD, Barr DB, Hauser R (2008) Human semen quality and sperm DNA damage in relation to urinary metabolites of pyrethroid insecticides. Hum Reprod 23:1932–1940
295. Butenhoff JL, Kennedy GL Jr, Frame SR, O'Connor JC, York RG (2004) The reproductive toxicology of ammonium perfluorooctanoate (APFO) in the rat. Toxicology 196:95–116
296. Luebker DJ, Case MT, York RG, Moore JA, Hansen KJ, Butenhoff JL (2005) Two-generation reproduction and cross-foster studies of perfluorooctanesulfonate (PFOS) in rats. Toxicology 215:126–148
297. Lau C, Butenhoff JL, Rogers JM (2004) The developmental toxicity of perfluoroalkyl acids and their derivatives. Toxicol Appl Pharmacol 198:231–241
298. Keil DE, Mehlmann T, Butterworth L, Peden-Adams MM (2008) Gestational exposure to perfluorooctane sulfonate suppresses immune function in B6C3F1 mice. Toxicol Sci 103:77–85
299. Fei C, McLaughlin JK, Tarone RE, Olsen J (2008) Fetal growth indicators and perfluorinated chemicals: a study in the Danish National Birth Cohort. Am J Epidemiol 168:66–72
300. Fei C, McLaughlin JK, Tarone RE, Olsen J (2007) Perfluorinated chemicals and fetal growth: a study within the Danish National Birth Cohort. Environ Health Perspect 115:1677–1682
301. Kuriyama SN, Talsness CE, Grote K, Chahoud I (2005) Developmental exposure to low dose PBDE 99: effects on male fertility and neurobehavior in rat offspring. Environ Health Perspect 113:149–154
302. He Y, Murphy MB, Yu RM et al (2008) Effects of 20 PBDE metabolites on steroidogenesis in the H295R cell line. Toxicol Lett 176:230–238
303. Lilienthal H, Hack A, Roth-Harer A, Grande SW, Talsness CE (2006) Effects of developmental exposure to 2, 2, 4, 4, 5-pentabromodiphenyl ether (PBDE-99) on sex steroids, sexual development, and sexually dimorphic behavior in rats. Environ Health Perspect 114:194–201
304. Main KM, Kiviranta H, Virtanen HE et al (2007) Flame retardants in placenta and breast milk and cryptorchidism in newborn boys. Environ Health Perspect 115:1519–1526
305. Hombach-Klonisch S, Pocar P, Kietz S, Klonisch T (2005) Molecular actions of polyhalogenated arylhydrocarbons (PAHs) in female reproduction. Curr Med Chem 12:599–616
306. Ellis-Hutchings RG, Cherr GN, Hanna LA, Keen CL (2006) Polybrominated diphenyl ether (PBDE)-induced alterations in vitamin A and thyroid hormone concentrations in the rat during lactation and early postnatal development. Toxicol Appl Pharmacol 215:135–145
307. Hertz-Picciotto I, Jusko TA, Willman EJ et al (2008) A cohort study of in utero polychlorinated biphenyl (PCB) exposures in relation to secondary sex ratio. Environ Health 7:37
308. Gray LE Jr, Ostby J, Furr J, Price M, Veeramachaneni DN, Parks L (2000) Perinatal exposure to the phthalates DEHP, BBP, and DINP, but not DEP, DMP, or DOTP, alters sexual differentiation of the male rat. Toxicol Sci 58:350–365
309. Duty SM, Silva MJ, Barr DB et al (2003) Phthalate exposure and human semen parameters. Epidemiology 14:269–277
310. Zhang YH, Lin L, Liu ZW, Jiang XZ, Chen BH (2008) Disruption effects of monophthalate exposures on inter-Sertoli tight junction in a two-compartment culture model. Environ Toxicol 23:302–308
311. Howdeshell KL, Wilson VS, Furr J et al (2008) A mixture of five phthalate esters inhibits fetal testicular testosterone production in the sprague-dawley rat in a cumulative, dose-additive manner. Toxicol Sci 105:153–165
312. Lin H, Ge RS, Chen GR et al (2008) Involvement of testicular growth factors in fetal Leydig cell aggregation after exposure to phthalate in utero. Proc Natl Acad Sci USA 105:7218–7222
313. Gunnarsson D, Leffler P, Ekwurtzel E, Martinsson G, Liu K, Selstam G (2008) Mono-(2-ethylhexyl) phthalate stimulates basal steroidogenesis by a cAMP-independent mechanism in mouse gonadal cells of both sexes. Reproduction 135:693–703
314. Howdeshell KL, Furr J, Lambright CR, Rider CV, Wilson VS, Gray LE Jr (2007) Cumulative effects of dibutyl phthalate and diethylhexyl phthalate on male rat reproductive tract development: altered fetal steroid hormones and genes. Toxicol Sci 99:190–202
315. Lague E, Tremblay JJ (2008) Antagonistic effects of testosterone and the endocrine disruptor mono-(2-ethylhexyl) phthalate on INSL3 transcription in Leydig cells. Endocrinology 149:4688–4694
316. Ge RS, Chen GR, Tanrikut C, Hardy MP (2007) Phthalate ester toxicity in Leydig cells: developmental timing and dosage considerations. Reprod Toxicol 23:366–373
317. Liu X, He DW, Zhang DY, Lin T, Wei GH (2008) Di(2-ethylhexyl) phthalate (DEHP) increases transforming growth factor-beta1 expression in fetal mouse genital tubercles. J Toxicol Environ Health A 71:1289–1294
318. Cobellis L, Latini G, De Felice C et al (2003) High plasma concentrations of di-(2-ethylhexyl)-phthalate in women with endometriosis. Hum Reprod 18:1512–1515
319. Reddy BS, Rozati R, Reddy BV, Raman NV (2006) Association of phthalate esters with endometriosis in Indian women. BJOG 113:515–520
320. Lovekamp-Swan T, Davis BJ (2003) Mechanisms of phthalate ester toxicity in the female reproductive system. Environ Health Perspect 111:139–145
321. Wolff MS, Engel SM, Berkowitz GS et al (2008) Prenatal phenol and phthalate exposures and birth outcomes. Environ Health Perspect 116:1092–1097
322. Wirth JJ, Rossano MG, Potter R et al (2008) A pilot study associating urinary concentrations of phthalate metabolites and semen quality. Syst Biol Reprod Med 54:143–154
323. Wu KL, Berger T (2008) Reduction in rat oocyte fertilizability mediated by S-(1, 2-dichlorovinyl)-L-cysteine: a trichloroethylene metabolite produced by the glutathione conjugation pathway. Bull Environ Contam Toxicol 81:490–493
324. Banu S, Ichihara S, Huang F et al (2007) Reversibility of the adverse effects of 1-bromopropane exposure in rats. Toxicol Sci 100:504–512
325. Chamkhia N, Sakly M, Rhouma KB (2006) Male reproductive impacts of styrene in rat. Toxicol Ind Health 22:349–355
326. Garner CE, Sloan C, Sumner SC et al (2007) CYP2E1-catalyzed oxidation contributes to the sperm toxicity of 1-bromopropane in mice. Biol Reprod 76:496–505
327. Kyyronen P, Taskinen H, Lindbohm ML, Hemminki K, Heinonen OP (1989) Spontaneous abortions and congenital malformations

among women exposed to tetrachloroethylene in dry cleaning. J Epidemiol Community Health 43:346–351
328. Beliles RP (2002) Concordance across species in the reproductive and developmental toxicity of tetrachloroethylene. Toxicol Ind Health 18:91–106
329. Eskenazi B, Wyrobek AJ, Fenster L et al (1991) A study of the effect of perchloroethylene exposure on semen quality in dry cleaning workers. Am J Ind Med 20:575–591
330. Ichihara G (2005) Neuro-reproductive toxicities of 1-bromopropane and 2-bromopropane. Int Arch Occup Environ Health 78:79–96
331. Sallmen M, Lindbohm ML, Kyyronen P et al (1995) Reduced fertility among women exposed to organic solvents. Am J Ind Med 27:699–713
332. Mendiola J, Torres-Cantero AM, Moreno-Grau JM et al (2008) Exposure to environmental toxins in males seeking infertility treatment: a case-controlled study. Reprod Biomed Online 16:842–850
333. Tan LF, Wang SL, Sun XZ et al (2002) Effects of fenvalerate exposure on the semen quality of occupational workers. Zhonghua Nan Ke Xue 8:273–276
334. Chen H, Song L, Wang X, Wang S (2000) Effect of exposure to low concentration of benzene and its analogues on luteal function of female workers. Wei Sheng Yan Jiu 29:351–353
335. Ohyama K, Satoh K, Sakamoto Y, Ogata A, Nagai F (2007) Effects of prenatal exposure to styrene trimers on genital organs and hormones in male rats. Exp Biol Med (Maywood) 232:301–308

Index

D

F

R